Clinical Tuberculosis

Sixth Edition

Clinical Tuberculosis

Sixth Edition

Edited by

Lloyd N. Friedman, MD
Clinical Professor of Medicine
Section of Pulmonary, Critical Care, and Sleep Medicine
Director of Inpatient Quality and Safety
Department of Internal Medicine
Yale School of Medicine
New Haven, Connecticut

Martin Dedicoat, PhD, FRCP, BSc, DTM&H
Consultant Physician in Infectious Diseases
University Hospitals Birmingham
Birmingham, United Kingdom
and
University of Warwick
Coventry, United Kingdom

Peter D. O. Davies, MA, DM, FRCP
Professor and Consultant Physician (retired)
Liverpool University
Liverpool, United Kingdom

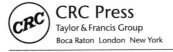

CRC Press
Taylor & Francis Group
Boca Raton London New York

CRC Press is an imprint of the
Taylor & Francis Group, an **informa** business

Sixth edition published 2020
by CRC Press
6000 Broken Sound Parkway NW, Suite 300, Boca Raton, FL 33487-2742

and by CRC Press
2 Park Square, Milton Park, Abingdon, Oxon, OX14 4RN

First issued in paperback 2022

Fourth Edition published by Hodder Arnold 2008
Fifth Edition published by CRC Press 2014

Visit the Taylor & Francis Web site at
http://www.taylorandfrancis.com

and the CRC Press Web site at
http://www.crcpress.com

Library of Congress Cataloging-in-Publication Data

Names: Friedman, Lloyd N., editor. | Dedicoat, Martin, editor. | Davies, P. D. O., editor.
Title: Clinical tuberculosis / edited by Lloyd N. Friedman, Martin Dedicoat, Peter D.O. Davies.
Description: Sixth edition. | Boca Raton, FL : CRC Press/Taylor & Francis Group, 2020. | Includes bibliographical references and index. | Summary: "Entirely updated and revised, the 6th edition of Clinical Tuberculosis continues to provide the TB physician with a definitive and erudite account of the latest techniques in diagnosis, treatment and control of TB, including an overview of the latest guidelines from the CDC and WHO"-- Provided by publisher.
Identifiers: LCCN 2020013349 (print) | LCCN 2020013350 (ebook) | ISBN 9780815370239 (hardback) | ISBN 9781351249980 (ebook)
Subjects: MESH: Tuberculosis
Classification: LCC RC311 (print) | LCC RC311 (ebook) | NLM WF 200 | DDC 616.99/5--dc23
LC record available at https://lccn.loc.gov/2020013349
LC ebook record available at https://lccn.loc.gov/2020013350

ISBN: 978-0-367-52996-3 (pbk)
ISBN: 978-0-8153-7023-9 (hbk)
ISBN: 978-1-351-24998-0 (ebk)

DOI: 10.1201/9781351249980

Typeset in Minion Pro
by Nova Techset Private Limited, Bengaluru & Chennai, India

Printed in the UK by Severn, Gloucester on responsibly sourced paper

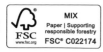

We would like to dedicate this book to all people in the world who are suffering from tuberculosis. Also to our wives and children who have supported us in our work.

Contents

Foreword

INTRO

This is the story of one overprotective mother and one lazy teenager. That "overprotective" mother turned out to be right and that "lazy teenager" went on to study English Literature and Language at Oxford University. Both lived with undiagnosed TB for over 18 years.

1997

In 1997, I (Kate) was 5 years old and had always been a happy and healthy child. My mum (Lorraine) was diagnosed with celiac disease when she was 20 years old but this was now 17 years on and it was very much under control. My grandparents, on my father's side, owned dairy farms in Ireland and it was on a visit to County Kerry in the summer of 1997 that our lives changed. We were given a jug of warm, creamy milk to put on our cornflakes. Looking back now, it seems so obvious but back then it was nothing out of the ordinary.

LORRAINE

Less than two weeks after returning from this trip to Ireland, I started to rapidly lose weight. Within a week I had lost over half a stone. At this point I had no other symptom. The following week I developed night sweats and vividly remember lying in bed, watching beads of sweat spring from nowhere and roll down my legs. By now, I also had a persistent dry, non-productive cough, accompanied by an overwhelming feeling of weakness. During this period I had seen my GP three times but there was nothing remarkable to guide him to a diagnosis. Later that week, I was admitted to the hospital, having lost over a stone of weight in less than two weeks and was subsequently diagnosed with "pneumonia." I was told that the "pneumonia" hadn't presented itself in the usual way—no temperature, no chesty cough, no chest pain or breathing difficulties, and only a faint mark on the chest x-ray. The consultants asked whether I had been outside of Europe but no one asked about Ireland. After a week of IVs I was discharged. However, on returning home I was still too weak to walk and would have to crawl on my hands and knees to make it up the stairs. The weakness remained overwhelming and even trying to lift the kettle to make a drink caused me to retch. A physio was sent to the house to try to help me to get back on my feet. It took weeks for me to master even climbing up the stairs which eventually led the medics to believe this weakness must be in some way psychosomatic. Three months later I still had no appetite and had not put on any weight.

I was later given a pneumonia vaccine but within just a few weeks, I was told the pneumonia had returned. This characterized the next few years: recurrent chest infections, antibiotics, and IVs.

I underwent extensive tests, but no one could identify the cause. In the end I was told that it must be because I was a celiac; I "obviously had a weak immune system."

KATE

Aged 10, I came home from school and collapsed in the hallway with what I can only describe as extreme weakness, a feeling I came to recognize as the years progressed. Prior to this, I had been an active and energetic child. That evening, the shivers began and then the sickness. At this point, I had no cough and no temperature. Yet, my "overprotective" mother recognized the sensation of being too exhausted and feeling too weak to even speak. "I think my daughter has pneumonia," she said to the local GP's surgery, to which they told her to calm down, "Stop overreacting, Mrs. Tuohy." Later that day, I was admitted to the hospital and diagnosed with pneumonia.

The following year my appendix burst. Meanwhile, I continued to have recurrent chest infections which were treated with oral antibiotics. A chest infection meant losing weight, extreme weakness, feeling too unwell to speak or move, no appetite, and feeling sick. Our infections were 100% debilitating.

I was aged 14 when the situation worsened. I lost a stone in a month, next my appetite went (and never returned), then the sweats and shivers began, and only when I began to feel really ill did the dry cough emerge. This was a pattern which repeated itself over the next 8 years; that dry cough used to send us into panic mode. I was constantly being diagnosed with "pneumonia" and the endless tests began. I was referred to numerous hospitals but every test came back negative. Then my tummy began to grow, a bit of bloating to start with; "Stop fussing and do some exercise," I was told again and again. The reality, without laxatives I never went to the toilet and, by the time I was 16, I was regularly being asked by doctors whether I was, in fact, pregnant.

My body was slim but my tummy was rock solid and distended. They ruled out celiac disease with a biopsy and then I underwent x-rays, ultrasounds, barium meals, and MRIs. The consultants eventually concluded that they had never seen anything like it and the only option was a laparoscopy.

In the middle of the laparoscopy, the surgeon came out to my parents and informed them that he was going to have to resect part of my terminal ileum which, for no apparent reason, was non-functioning and blocked with undigested food. The surrounding intestine also didn't look normal. The surgeon had never come across this before. Over four hours later, I emerged from the operation. For a few weeks, my gastro symptoms improved, but slowly my lower abdomen began to grow and was doughy in texture, I was back to taking laxatives, on painkillers for spasms, and occasionally admitted with violent sickness and given IV pain relief. This was my GCSE year and, by this point, there had been large gaps in my education. My school advised that I shouldn't bother taking my GCSEs and instead focus on getting better.

However, at the start of this horrible journey of ill health, one day in the Easter holidays aged 10, when I was recovering from my burst appendix, my parents had taken me for a day out in Oxford. After stumbling across a sign outside Balliol College inviting the public to look around, I made up my mind that I was going to Oxford University. In the years which followed, my academics got me through. When everything else was so beyond my control, studying became my unwavering focus. I taught myself from the hospital and home and while, over time, other aspects of my life became more limited, studying was the one thing I could do "from the sofa." Oxford University constantly remained the goal. You can, therefore, imagine the frustration and upset when doctors would suggest I was a "lazy teenager," who needed to "get off the sofa" and "do some exercise," and that I must stop labelling myself as "ill." This couldn't have been further from the truth. All I wanted was to be "normal."

LORRAINE

Over the years, a distinct pattern emerged; exertion equalled pneumonia. Now by this, I do not mean going to the gym or going on a run, but rather walking to the shop at the end of the road, climbing a flight of stairs or, in later years, having a shower. This was a pattern which emerged again and again. Kate was getting worse; how could I help her if I was too ill myself? By this stage I had given up my career, hardly went out and the saving grace turned out to be living in a bungalow. While I was far from well, losing weight every year (at my worst a BMI of 16), having a persistent dry cough throughout the day and night, having recurrent chest infections and depleted energy levels, I found that by moving as little as possible, I could prevent myself from becoming seriously ill. I resigned myself to this but Kate was a teenager and was desperately trying to live a "normal" life, which meant she became seriously ill more frequently. The crazy thing was we knew the recipe; we could force ourselves to move in the moment but we knew the end result would be the same—more weight loss, sweats, shivers, exhaustion, days of lying down, eventually sickness and a dry cough, and ultimately, more antibiotics or IVS.

Initially, the reason each of Kate's admissions proved so scary and each appointment proved so frustrating was that we were constantly battling to be believed. I was very much labelled the "overprotective mother" and fought for years to be listened to. The more we told doctors about this overwhelming weakness, the fact that we couldn't stand up for long periods and spent most of our lives lying down, the more we were labelled. In between these infections, Kate was always smiling, always positive, was achieving brilliant grades on her exams and most significantly, never showed the usual signs, leading to the consensus that she "couldn't be that ill." The only time anyone really saw how bad things could get was in A&E and even then it was a fight, a fight to convince the doctors to give her the IVs. She would be drenched in sweat and uncontrollably shaking but her temperature never reached higher than 36.8. The only person who really understood was our GP. He had been Kate's GP since birth and had seen this entire journey unravel. He became adept at spotting the signs and realized that for Kate, 36.8 was a

very high temperature. He would make phone call after phone call trying to warn and convince A&E and hospital departments to listen to us. He'd seen what happened if they waited too long; it seemed from nowhere Kate's body realized it was ill and started showing every sign—violent tremors, pain, cough, sickness, diarrhea, sweats, and shivers but still no temperature.

By now all different parts of Kate's body were being affected:

Gastroenterology

- Bloating
- No appetite
- Laxatives
- Pain
- Vomiting

Respiratory

- Recurrent infections
- Persistent cough
- Pain in right lung
- Sinusitis

Dermatology

- Skin infections
- Crumbling nails

Rheumatology

- Erythromelalgia

Endocrinology

- FSH/LH levels
- Period lasting for months
- Then periods stopped for years

Blood Pressure

- Postural orthostatic tachycardia syndrome (POTS)
- Severely low blood pressure

Sleep

- Heart palpitations
- Night sweats
- Awake all night

The list was endless and each department was treating the symptoms but not the cause.

The diagnosis ranged from polycystic ovaries, to hypermobility, to blood cancer, a sodium channelopathy, IBS, cystic fibrosis; the list goes on but we knew none of these fit the whole picture. Occasionally, I'd bring myself in, trying to illustrate that we shared many of the same symptoms, hoping it might help them with their investigations. The doctors treated me as the overbearing mother: "This appointment is for Kate, Mrs. Tuohy."

KATE

By this stage I hardly went to school, but somehow I managed to achieve my grades and was offered a place to study English Literature and Language at Jesus College, Oxford University.

The next problem: how was I going to obtain a degree at the top university in the world when my life was becoming increasingly restricted to lying on the sofa? Well, I was given a ground floor room (stairs meant pneumonia), the dining hall was just a few steps away, and a member of staff delivered my books to my door. However, as I said previously, my worst fear was being labelled and I so desperately wanted to take part in all that Oxford had to offer. It was a constant toss-up—Is this night out worth being ill for? Is this party worth ending up in the hospital for?

Prophylactic antibiotics were now a way of life but even these weren't preventing the recurrent infections. It was in my second year of uni that things hit rock bottom. I was admitted to the hospital with yet another bout of pneumonia and given 2 weeks of IV meropenem. The problem was, the antibiotics weren't as effective as they once were and this infection returned within a few days. This meant a further week of IVs and 6 weeks (out of an 8-week term) off uni. I'd surpassed the 6-week residency rule at Oxford University and was told I needed to take a year off to focus on getting better. I knew I wasn't getting better, only worse; what difference would a year make? My GP had referred me to the Mayo Clinic and it was around this time that I was supposed to be going. This was our final resort but I was turned down, deemed too ill to travel. The doctors in the UK told me every test had been done. They had stopped looking for the cause; it was now a case of palliative care. Whatever it was, was going to kill me.

Lorraine

It was our bodies, not our minds which were affected. I spent years researching on the Internet. I knew this was a physical illness which in some way responded to antibiotics, in particular clarithromycin. By now we had worked out the pattern: exertion led to pneumonia which would only be dampened down by oral clarithromycin or IVS.

It was in Kate's second year of university, after weeks of meropenem, that I insisted the doctors did more tests. After Kate was discharged from this particular admission, the consultant called me at home. She had requested a QuantiFERON Gold blood test and she was calling to say it had come back positive. This was the first test in 12 years which had given a positive result. The more I read, the more I realized we had every symptom of TB.

Sadly, the next part of our journey was far from straightforward. In between this phone call and Kate's subsequent appointment, I made it my mission to learn everything I could about TB. At the appointment, the consultant began drawing up the prescription for 3 months of latent TB drugs. To me, this made no sense. Kate had every symptom of active TB—night sweats, weight loss, no appetite, recurrent pneumonias, extreme weakness, all exacerbated by even the mildest exertion. I'd even read that the terminal ileum was often affected. By this stage, we had reflected on the unpasteurized milk we had drunk in 1997 and the picture was coming together. It was in this appointment that I questioned whether QuantiFERON Gold tested for bovine TB. When the consultant said it did not test for that strain, I knew I couldn't let Kate take the latent drugs. I was certain I had read online that it did.

That evening I emailed the scientists in America who produced the test. By the next morning my email had been forwarded to Professor Peter Davies in Liverpool. I received a response saying QuantiFERON did test positive for bovine TB and under no circumstance must my daughter take those latent drugs.

Kate

Professor Davies was one of the first doctors, other than our GP, who seemed to listen. He took on board every symptom and the entire history.

During one of my previous laparoscopies, the surgeon had taken images which we were meant to give to the Mayo Clinic. He had noticed some strange white spots on my intestine. Professor Davies noticed them immediately and felt they could well be tubercles. While he was prepared to treat me for active TB, he knew I would need to be carefully monitored and that really, I needed to be under the care of my local hospital.

The hospital who had carried out the initial QuantiFERON test still wanted to treat me for latent TB. Professor Davies then referred me to another hospital who said I was "British, white, middle class," and it did not make sense that I had TB at all and discharged me.

In the end, under the care of my local GP (the only doctor willing to work with Professor Davies), I started a course of 9 months of isoniazid, rifampicin, and pyrazinamide. Unfortunately, within two weeks, three hard lumps appeared on my neck and my body went into anaphylactic shock. After being rushed to A&E in an ambulance, it was concluded that I could never take those drugs again. This was one of our lowest points. What we never expected was that, once I'd recovered from the shock, in 12 years I had never appeared healthier; my symptoms depleted, my energy levels improved, and most significantly, I didn't develop a chest infection for 5 months, which was unheard of. Something in the treatment had worked.

Professor Davies observed this and eventually decided on a combination of moxifloxacin and ethambutol for 18 months.

This treatment transformed my life.

Lorraine

The treatment had worked for Kate and although I never had a positive test, I was prescribed the same combination of drugs.

I'd coughed every day and night for 18 years but within a few weeks of the treatment commencing, my cough had completely disappeared. I started to put on weight and I was more active than I could ever remember.

Summary

In total we went to 15 hospitals and were seen by over 30 consultants.

We describe this illness as a "cruel" one, for our journey was not just a case of being ill, the way the TB manifested itself meant it was a battle; a battle to be listened to, a battle to be believed and eventually a battle to be treated.

The picture is now very different, we have our lives back. I (Kate) obtained my Oxford degree (albeit in 4, rather than 3 years) and have set up my own business. I (Lorraine) have returned to work and have an active social life. We eat, we exercise and, most importantly, we no longer spend our lives on the sofa.

Kate and Lorraine Tuhoy, 2018

AFTERWORD

Though I have never quite encountered this combination of history, symptoms, and signs, after over a year of consultations with Kate, I came to the conclusion that she was suffering from some form of occult or cryptic disseminated bovine tuberculosis. I decided to treat her empirically for this disease. First-line treatment proved almost fatal to Kate because of an anaphylactic reaction. Rethinking the drug regimen, I treated her as though she had a resistant form of TB, giving moxifloxacin and ethambutol for 18 months. This seemed to provide cure.

When then consulted by Lorraine, who I had seen on every visit with Kate and who had very similar symptoms dating from the same event, empirical treatment again seemed appropriate. Lorraine refused the shorter first-choice regimen on the grounds that Kate had such a bad reaction so again we chose moxifloxacin and ethambutol for 18 months. Again cure seemed to be achieved.

Even in developed countries with all laboratory tests available, almost 50% of patients with non-respiratory tuberculosis are treated empirically. Here, in all probability, are two more such cases.

Peter D. O. Davies

Preface

If you were to ask anyone outside the small circle of enthusiasts in the fight against communicable diseases to place the following burdens of death by the disease they relate to, I am sure the answers you would receive would be mostly incorrect: 1.8 million, 1.4 million and 0.5 million: HIV/AIDS, TB, malaria.

When individuals are asked, no one scores more than 1/3 of answers correctly. The perception is that HIV and malaria are the big killers while TB comes a distant third. In fact, the correct disease mortalities are 1.8 million for TB, 1.4 million for HIV, 400,000 of whom also die from TB, and under 500,000 for malaria.

An article in *The Economist* published in October 2017 devoted four pages to the diseases of poverty and how they are being defeated. The majority concerned AIDS and malaria, and a bit about the rarer tropical diseases, but not a mention of TB.

When the millennium goals to defeat HIV, TB, and malaria were set up almost 20 years ago, HIV was perceived as the biggest threat. Perhaps rightly, from that time, malaria has received twice as much money as TB, and HIV twice as much as malaria, leaving TB with 1/7 of the total. It is perhaps no surprise that after so much money and publicity over HIV and malaria, the battle against these killers is doing well while the battle against TB is hardly succeeding at all.

As a consequence, TB has been left behind in terms of resources to combat the disease. It is not surprising therefore that deaths from this communicable disease now nearly exceed those from HIV/AIDS and malaria combined.

The publication of the sixth edition of *Clinical Tuberculosis* therefore is timely. The intent is to supply those joining us in the war with the essential knowledge, both academic and practical, to help conquer this disease. The book is aimed at all those working in tuberculosis, whether in public health, clinical, or laboratory-based work. As more resources become available, even in the poorest settings, it is hoped the book will be of practical value in the first and third worlds.

Diligent readers of prefaces might wonder why I (PD) am continuing to edit a textbook on tuberculosis. Reading the preface of the fifth edition it seemed as though I was retiring from the fray. I wrote in 2014 "Should there be a call for subsequent editions…I can pass the baton on to [a younger generation] knowing that it is in safe hands." As so often happens I am here again out of simple serendipity. At every American Thoracic Society meeting I attend I find myself in close company with Lloyd Friedman. Our common interest in tuberculosis would always throw us together. Lloyd had edited two editions of his textbook, which was similar to my own: a single-volume synopsis of practical and theoretical aspects of the disease. By a series of sales of titles between publishers, my title had come to rest on the desk of Taylor & Francis Group, who had been the publishers of Lloyd's book.

It therefore made sense to me that when Lloyd suggested that we combine a joint editorship for a third and sixth joint edition, respectively, that we join forces to do so. Because I have now retired from the National Health Service and no longer manage patients directly I have asked Martin Dedicoat from Birmingham, UK to join the team and he has graciously agreed.

By mutual agreement we have used the opportunity of a joint venture between the USA and the UK to seek authorship for most chapters from both sides of the pond. We can then combine the science and experience of much wider sources than if we were to "go it alone." As rates of tuberculosis have declined in both the USA and UK over the past decade, expertise in tuberculosis is more and more associated with joint work in developing countries, particularly on the continent of Africa and countries of South and Southeast Asia. Most of our authors therefore have extensive experience from these areas. As one of the editors-in-chief of the *International Journal of Tuberculosis and Lung Disease* I see many papers submitted from developing countries with joint authorship from the USA and/or a Western European country.

I am most grateful to my two co-editors for their hard work and dedication in drawing this edition together. The task of trans-Atlantic co-ordination has often not been easy. I am also very grateful to all the authors who have put in so much time and hard work to what I believe is a world-class and groundbreaking textbook on tuberculosis. Having authored many chapters in my 40 years of tuberculosis work, I know how back-breaking the task can be, but also how enjoyable it can be as the current scientific knowledge and experience on an aspect of tuberculosis is brought together into a readable synopsis.

My thanks go especially to two patients, Kate and Lorraine Tuohy, who have recorded their experience as tuberculosis sufferers in the Foreword. Not since the second edition have we had a patient contribution to the book and it is high time we did. Their experience of being misdiagnosed and fobbed off by a host of medical professionals with a supposed expertise in tuberculosis is salutary. All workers in the field would do well to read their stories.

The outline and contents of the sixth edition follow the patterns of previous editions with sections on background, diagnosis, drugs, clinical aspects, prevention and control, HIV, and drug resistance. In addition, we have included a section on transmission. The chapter on BCG (Bacille Calmette–Guérin) also references diseases caused by BCG, particularly in the treatment of bladder cancer. We have continued with a chapter on TB in animals as it remains a topic of considerable interest, especially in the UK.

We no longer have a chapter on the so-called non-tuberculous mycobacteria as this has become such a large topic that a separate book on the subject is proceeding through a long gestation process.

Lastly, we are gratified that the TB community is focusing on preventing latent tuberculosis from developing into active disease. As many as 80% of new cases each year are derived from the infected pool. Short-course treatment of latent tuberculosis infection (LTBI) has been a welcome addition, and a new vaccine in trial phase that prevents the development of active tuberculosis in individuals with latent tuberculosis is a promising addition to the armamentarium. A good vaccine will obviate the issues with treatment compliance and the worry about drug-resistant infection. We are looking forward to further development in this area.

Lloyd Friedman, Martin Dedicoat and Peter Davies
New Haven, CT, Birmingham, UK, and Liverpool, UK
January 2020

Editors

Lloyd N. Friedman, MD is a clinical professor of Pulmonary, Critical Care and Sleep Medicine at the Yale School of Medicine, New Haven, CT. He is director of Inpatient Quality and Safety for the Department of Internal Medicine.

Dr. Friedman graduated in 1975 from Columbia University, New York with a BA in biochemistry and obtained his MD in 1979 from Yale University. He completed an internship in Internal Medicine at Beth Israel Medical Center in 1980, and residency training at Oregon Health Sciences University in 1983. He completed his fellowship training in Pulmonary and Critical Care Medicine at Yale School of Medicine in 1988.

Dr. Friedman began his work with tuberculosis in 1984 when he evaluated welfare applicants who used drugs or alcohol in New York City at the beginning of the AIDS crisis. He has had numerous grants, scientific publications, chapters, and speaking engagements, and has participated in the development of regional and national guidelines. He has published two editions of his book, *Tuberculosis: Current Concepts and Treatment*. He is a recipient of the David Russell Lyman Award for Meritorious Achievement in Tuberculosis.

Dr. Friedman is a member of the American Thoracic Society, a member of the Society of Critical Care Medicine, a fellow of the American College of Chest Physicians, and a member of the International Union Against Tuberculosis and Lung Disease. He is Chairman of the Connecticut Tuberculosis Elimination Advisory Committee.

Martin Dedicoat, PhD, FRCP, BSc, DTM&H is a consultant physician in infectious diseases at the University Hospitals Birmingham.

Dr. Dedicoat qualified in medicine from University College London in 1992. He trained in internal medicine, infectious diseases, and tropical medicine in Birmingham and South Africa.

He is currently clinical lead for tuberculosis for Birmingham and Solihull, UK. His main research interests center around tuberculosis transmission in urban settings.

Dr. Dedicoat is a member of the British Thoracic Society drug-resistant tuberculosis management group advising on management of complex tuberculosis patients across the UK. He also sits on the National Tuberculosis board for England.

Peter D. O. Davies graduated in 1966 from Marlborough College, Wiltshire, UK and obtained his BM, BCh, and MA from University College, Oxford, UK in 1971 and St. Thomas's Hospital in London in 1973. He gained a DM from Oxford in 1984. He was a consultant general and respiratory physician at Aintree University Hospital from 1988 to 2011 and at Liverpool Heart and Chest Hospital from 1988 to 2015.

Dr. Davies has published over 100 peer-reviewed papers and has given over 600 invited lectures. He is or has been a member of the British Medical Association, the British Thoracic Society, the European Respiratory Society, the Royal College of Physicians of London (Fellow), the Royal Society of Medicine, the American Thoracic Society, the North Western Society of Respiratory Physicians where he served as president in 2007, the International Union Against Tuberculosis and Lung Disease where he was chair of the Tuberculosis Section, president of the European Section, and editor in chief of the *International Journal of Tuberculosis and Lung Disease*, and a member of NICE where he was chair of the Tuberculosis Section. He co-founded the UK-based TB charity in 1998.

Dr. Davies is an expert in tuberculosis, edited the inaugural edition of the textbook *Clinical Tuberculosis* in 1994, and has continued as editor for the subsequent five editions.

Contributors

Laura F. Anderson
Global Tuberculosis Programme
World Health Organization
Geneva, Switzerland

Mercedes C. Becerra
Harvard Medical School
and
Brigham and Women's Hospital
and
Partners In Health
Boston, Massachusetts

and

Advance Access & Delivery
Durham, North Carolina

Graham Bothamley
Homerton University Hospital
NHS Foundation Trust
London, United Kingdom

Jane E. Buikstra
School of Human Evolution and Social Change
Arizona State University
Tempe, Arizona

Lindsay H. Cameron
Baylor College of Medicine
Texas Children's Hospital
Houston, Texas

Ted Cohen
Epidemiology of Microbial Diseases
Yale School of Public Health
New Haven, Connecticut

Anne McB. Curtis
Department of Radiology and Biomedical Imaging
Yale School of Medicine
New Haven, Connecticut

Charles L. Daley
Department of Medicine
National Jewish Health
Denver, Colorado

and

Department of Medicine
University of Colorado Aurora, Colorado

Gerry Davies
Institutes of Infection and Global Health & Translational
Medicine
University of Liverpool
Liverpool, United Kingdom

J. Lucian Davis
Epidemiology of Microbial Diseases
Yale School of Public Health
and
Section of Pulmonary, Critical Care, and Sleep
Medicine
Department of Internal Medicine
Yale School of Medicine
New Haven, Connecticut

Martin Dedicoat
University Hospitals Birmingham
Birmingham, United Kingdom

and

University of Warwick
Coventry, United Kingdom

Charles S. Dela Cruz
Section of Pulmonary, Critical Care, and Sleep
Medicine
Department of Internal Medicine
Yale School of Medicine
New Haven, Connecticut

Keertan Dheda
Centre for Lung Infection and Immunity
Division of Pulmonology
Department of Medicine
and
UCT Lung Institute & South African MRC/UCT
Centre for the Study of Antimicrobial Resistance
University of Cape Town
Cape Town, South Africa

and

Faculty of Infectious and Tropical Diseases
Department of Immunology and Infection
London School of Hygiene and Tropical Medicine
London, United Kingdom

Anzaan Dippenaar
Centre of Excellence for Biomedical Tuberculosis Research
Division of Molecular Biology and Human Genetics
Stellenbosch University
Tygerberg, South Africa

Lucica Ditiu
Stop TB Partnership
Geneva, Switzerland

Christopher Dye
Department of Zoology
University of Oxford
Oxford, United Kingdom

Jerrold J. Ellner
Division of Infectious Disease
Department of Internal Medicine
Rutgers New Jersey Medical School
Newark, New Jersey

Aliasgar Esmail
Centre for Lung Infection and Immunity
Division of Pulmonology
Department of Medicine
and
UCT Lung Institute & South African MRC/UCT
Centre for the Study of Antimicrobial Resistance
University of Cape Town
Cape Town, South Africa

Paul E. Farmer
Harvard Medical School
and
Brigham and Women's Hospital
and
Partners In Health
Boston, Massachusetts

Clementine Fraser
Respiratory Infections Section
Imperial College London and Imperial College Healthcare
NHS Trust
London, United Kingdom

Gerald Friedland
Epidemiology and Public Health
Yale School of Public Health
Section of Infectious Diseases
Department of Internal Medicine
Yale School of Medicine
New Haven, Connecticut

Lloyd N. Friedman
Section of Pulmonary, Critical Care, and Sleep Medicine
Department of Internal Medicine
Yale School of Medicine
New Haven, Connecticut

Jennifer Furin
T.H. Chan School of Public Health
Harvard Medical School
Boston, Massachusetts

William R. Jacobs, Jr.
Department of Microbiology and Immunology
and
Department of Molecular Genetics
Albert Einstein College of Medicine
Bronx, New York

Salmaan Keshavjee
Harvard Medical School
and
Brigham and Women's Hospital
and
Partners In Health
Boston, Massachusetts

and

Advance Access & Delivery
Durham, North Carolina

Aamir J. Khan
Interactive Research and Development
Singapore

Ajit Lalvani
Respiratory Infections Section
Imperial College London
and
Imperial College Healthcare NHS Trust
London, United Kingdom

Christoph Lange
Clinical Infectious Diseases Research Center
and
German Center for Infection Research (DZIF)
Clinical Tuberculosis Unit
Borstel, Germany

and

International Health/Infectious Diseases
University of Lübeck
Lübeck, Germany

and

Department of Medicine
Karolinska Institute
Stockholm, Sweden

Charisse Mandimika
Section of Infectious Diseases
Department of Internal Medicine
Yale University School of Medicine
New Haven, Connecticut

Helen McShane
The Jenner Institute
and
Nuffield Department of Medicine
University of Oxford
Oxford, United Kingdom

James Millard
Institute of Infection and Global Health
University of Liverpool
Liverpool, United Kingdom

and

Africa Health Research Institute
Durban, KwaZulu-Natal, South Africa

Edward A. Nardell
Harvard Medical School
Boston, Massachusetts

Tom Nicholson
Advance Access & Delivery
Durham, North Carolina

Camus Nimmo
Division of Infection and Immunity
University College London
London, United Kingdom

and

Africa Health Research Institute
Durban, KwaZulu-Natal, South Africa

Manish Pareek
Department of Infection, Immunity and Inflammation
University of Leicester
Leicester, United Kingdom

Charles Peloquin
Department of Pharmacotherapy and Translational Research
College of Pharmacy
University of Florida
Gainesville, Florida

Alexander S. Pym
Africa Health Research Institute
Durban, KwaZulu-Natal South Africa

Divya B. Reddy
Division of Pulmonary Medicine
Department of Medicine
Albert Einstein Medical College/Montefiore Medical Center
Bronx, New York

Charlotte A. Roberts
Department of Archaeology
Durham University
Durham, United Kingdom

Barbara Seaworth
University of Texas Health Science Center
Tyler, Texas

Benjamin J. Silk
Division of Tuberculosis Elimination
U.S. Centers for Disease Control and Prevention
Atlanta, Georgia

Lynn E. Sosa
Connecticut Department of Public Health
Hartford, Connecticut

Jeffrey R. Starke
Baylor College of Medicine
Texas Children's Hospital
Houston, Texas

Richard S. Steyn
University Hospitals Birmingham Foundation Trust
Birmingham Heartlands Hospital
Bordesley Green East
Birmingham, United Kingdom

Sarah Talarico
Division of Tuberculosis Elimination
U.S. Centers for Disease Control and Prevention
Atlanta, Georgia

Rachel Tanner
The Jenner Institute
Nuffield Department of Medicine
University of Oxford
Oxford, United Kingdom

Grant Theron
DST/NRF Centre of Excellence for Biomedical Tuberculosis Research
SA MRC Centre for Tuberculosis Research
Division of Molecular Biology and Human Genetics
Faculty of Medicine and Health Sciences
Stellenbosch University
Tygerberg, South Africa

Robin Warren
South African Medical Research Council Centre for Tuberculosis Research
Department of Science and Technology/National Research Foundation Centre of Excellence for Biomedical Tuberculosis Research
Division of Molecular Biology and Human Genetics
Stellenbosch University
Tygerberg, South Africa

Catherine Wilson
Wellcome Trust Clinical PhD Fellow
Faculty of Health Sciences
University of Liverpool
Liverpool, United Kingdom

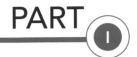

BACKGROUND

The History of Tuberculosis from Earliest Times to the Development of Drugs

CHARLOTTE A. ROBERTS AND JANE E. BUIKSTRA

INTRODUCTION

> Tuberculosis is now a conquered disease in the British Isles and the rest of the industrialised world.[1]

How wrong can one be? In the late 1980s, we thought that tuberculosis (TB) was an infection that had been controlled and almost eradicated from the developed world. However, emergence and re-emergence of infectious diseases plague the developed and the developing world today, and the medical profession struggles to cope.[2] In 2016, there were 10.4 million people who fell ill with TB, with 1.7 million dying from the disease; 40% of HIV deaths were due to TB. TB is the ninth leading cause of death worldwide and the leading cause from a single infectious agent.[3] However, TB has the potential to "develop frequency rates with the status of the 'big killer' again" as we live through the twenty-first century.[4]

TB was as important in our ancestors' world as it is today; of course, the difference between past and present is that, in theory, we now have drugs to successfully treat the disease, health education programs to prevent TB from occurring, and mechanisms and infrastructure to ensure that poverty is not a precursor to the development of the infection. However, having coping mechanisms does not mean that TB will be controlled. In some respects, they can complicate the situation; one could argue that because one of the major predisposing factors for TB is poverty, if poverty could be alleviated then TB would decline, as would many other diseases.[5]

Our ancestors perhaps may have been in a better position to combat TB, assuming they recognized that poverty led to infection. They certainly did not have to deal with one of the key predisposing factors today—human immunodeficiency virus (HIV),[6] or so we assume. Today, the combination of poverty, HIV, and drug resistance makes for a challenging and terrifying situation for many people. The cause of TB, its associated stigma, and the different political regimes and cultures around the world can vary considerably, which then affects the treatments provided, the opportunity for access to and uptake of those treatments and their effectiveness, alongside implementation of preventive measures.[7,8] We also have to consider the possibility that treatment outcomes for men, women, and children with TB (or any health problem) may be different.[9]

Here, we focus on the long history of TB as seen mainly in skeletal remains from archeological sites. First, we will consider the primary evidence for TB in the past—in the remains of people themselves—chart the distribution of the infection through time from a global perspective, and consider historical data for the presence of the disease in the distant past. We will also examine remarkable new developments from biomolecular analyses of the tubercle bacillus in human remains that are currently illuminating aspects of the history of TB. Finally, we argue that looking at TB from a deep-time perspective can aid in understanding the problem today.

EVIDENCE FOR THE PRESENCE OF TB IN THE PAST

Scholars studying TB in our ancestors draw on a number of sources. The primary evidence derives from people themselves (Figure 1.1) who were buried in cemeteries throughout the world that have been excavated over the years and that contribute to the understanding of humankind's long history. Bioarcheologists study human remains, with paleopathology specifically focused on the study of ancient disease. Secondary sources of evidence "flesh out" the skeletal remains that we study. For example, we might consider historical sources that document TB frequency at particular points in time in specific parts of the world—something we cannot glean from the skeletal remains. Written accounts will also tell us something about whether attempts were made to treat TB and how. Illustrations in texts may indicate that the infection was present in the population and also show the deformity and/or disability that accompanied it. The following sections consider this evidence in more detail, highlighting the strengths and limitations of our data.

DIAGNOSIS OF TB IN SKELETAL AND MUMMIFIED REMAINS

Being able to securely identify TB in human remains excavated from an archeological site proves the presence of the disease in a population. This compares with a written description of the infection whose signs and symptoms may be confused with other respiratory diseases.[10] Although historical sources may provide us with more realistic estimates of TB frequency in the past, we have to be sure that the diagnosis was precise. We would argue that this is not always possible.

It has been suggested that in the 1940s and 1950s, the skeletal structure was affected in approximately 3%–5% of people with pulmonary TB (PTB), but this rose to around 30% for extra-pulmonary TB.[11] In a recent study it was found that today more skeletal TB is being seen. This is because people are living longer due to long-term antibiotic use. This gives more time for lesions to develop.[12] The spine is most affected, with the hip and knee

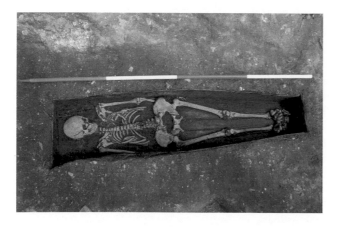

Figure 1.1 Skeleton in the ground before excavation.

being common joints that are involved. Skeletal damage is the end result of post-primary TB spreading hematogenously or via the lymphatic system to the bones. Without biomolecular analysis, we cannot identify TB in the skeletons of those people who suffered primary TB. Initial introduction of TB into a population will also lead to high and rapid mortality because of the lack of previous exposure; no bone damage would be expected. As time goes by and generations have been exposed to TB, we might expect to see it in their skeletons. In humans, TB caused by *Mycobacterium tuberculosis* and *Mycobacterium bovis* can cause skeletal damage, but there are suggestions that the latter is much more likely to do this.[13] Skeletal evidence indicates a chronic long-term process that people could have endured for many years, also suggesting that they had a relatively robust immune system.[14] However, diagnosis of TB in skeletal remains can be challenging. Unambiguous pathological lesions have to be distinguished from normal skeletal variants and changes due to post-mortem damage. Some circumstances, such as very dry, waterlogged, and frozen environments, may preserve whole bodies very well.[15] If soft tissues are preserved (e.g. in mummies), the potential amount of retrievable data can be impressive, and diagnosis of disease can be easier. Nevertheless, most archeological evidence for TB is gathered from skeletons rather than from preserved bodies.

Disease can affect the skeleton only in two ways, through bone formation and in bone destruction, although both can be found together. In studies of paleopathology, such changes are recorded for each bone of the skeleton, their distribution pattern noted and differential diagnoses provided. Because the skeleton can react only in limited ways to disease, the same changes can occur with different diseases. This is why providing a detailed description of the lesions and a list of possible differential diagnoses, based on the presence and distribution of the lesions (and clinical information), is essential if diagnoses are to be verified and/or re-evaluated in the future. This point is emphasized repeatedly.[14,16–19] Recognition of TB relies mainly on the presence of destructive lesions in the spine, termed Pott's disease after Percivall Pott, the nineteenth-century physician who first described the changes. The bacilli focus on the red bone marrow, and there is gradual destruction of the bony tissue. Jaffe[11] indicates that 25%–50% of people with skeletal TB will develop spinal changes. Once the vertebral integrity is lost, the structure collapses and angulation (kyphosis) of the spine develops (Figure 1.2), sometimes followed by fusion of vertebrae (ankylosis).

Other parts of the skeleton may also be affected, for example, the hip and knee joints (Figure 1.3), and non-specific changes can occur that may be related to TB (e.g., new bone formation on ribs: Figure 1.4).[20–24]

Most paleopathologists will diagnose TB using spinal evidence. However, it is not possible to detect all people with TB using this approach. Over the last 25 years or so, methods developed in biomolecular science have been applied to the diagnosis of disease in skeletal and mummified remains. This approach, discussed in more detail later in this chapter, includes considering the remains of a human without any evidence of disease who may have died before bone damage, as well as remains with pathological changes. TB has been the main focus of ancient biomolecular studies, with its diagnosis based upon identifying ancient DNA (aDNA) and mycolic acids of the tubercle bacillus.[25,26] Although

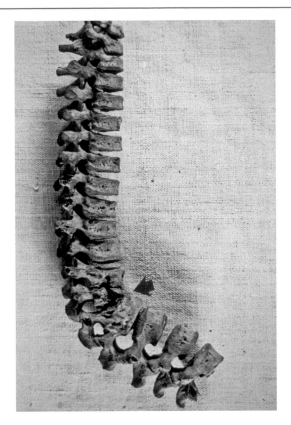

Figure 1.2 Spinal tuberculosis in a 17th century English person buried at Abingdon Abbey, Oxfordshire.

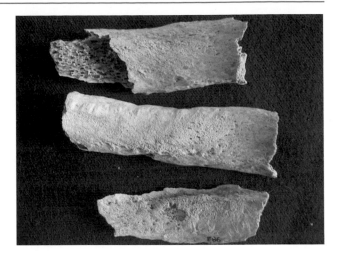

Figure 1.4 New bone formation on the visceral (internal) surface of ribs (a non-specific bone change possibly related to TB of the lungs).

there can be inevitable problems of survival and then extraction of ancient biomolecules from human remains,[27] this new line of evidence alongside modern genomic data indicating susceptibility and resistance genes has already significantly revised our models of human–pathogen (TB) co-evolution.[28,29]

HISTORICAL AND PICTORIAL DATA

We are not historians or art historians, and therefore we are not trained in the analysis and interpretation of texts and illustrations related to the history of disease and medicine.

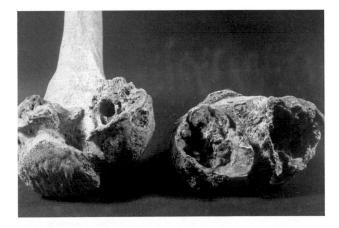

Figure 1.3 Probable joint tuberculosis (knee joint).

Even so, we recognize that historical sources can generate interpretative problems. The signs and symptoms of TB may include shortness of breath, coughing up blood, anemia and pallor, fatigue, night sweats, fever, pain in the chest, and the effects of associated skeletal changes (e.g., kyphosis of the back and paralysis of the limbs). Clearly, all these features, visible to an author or artist, could be associated with other health problems. For example, pallor may be seen in anemia, shortness of breath in chronic bronchitis, and coughing up blood in cancer of the lung. Likewise, kyphotic deformities of the back may be the result of osteoporosis of the spine or trauma. Biases abound in written sources including the interpretation of causes of death rates said to reflect TB. For example, Hardy[30] reminds us that because TB was associated with stigma in the nineteenth century, it was not always recorded as a cause of death. In addition, people could have had more than one condition contributing to their death, and we must not assume that those who diagnosed disease in the past were competent to make a correct diagnosis. Even today, some causes listed on death certificates may not be correct.[31] Despite these problems, we will consider some of this evidence following our discussion of skeletal data.

THE ANTIQUITY OF TB FROM A GLOBAL PERSPECTIVE

Before embarking on a temporal and global perspective of TB, we should emphasize that North America and parts of Europe have received much more archeological attention than many other parts of the world.[32] There are many regions into which paleo-pathologists have not yet ventured and, therefore, evidence for TB is, to date, absent from these areas. This does not mean that the disease did not exist there in the past, just that the evidence has not been sought (or excavated). This presents a challenge to scientists who wish to trace and map the origin, evolution, and transmission of TB globally. With this caveat in mind, we first consider the factors that were probably important in the development of TB in past human populations.

WHAT LED TO TB APPEARING IN HUMAN POPULATIONS?

EVIDENCE RELATING TO ANIMALS AND DOMESTICATION

If we think about farming and domestication in the Near East, domesticated sheep and goats were present by 8000 BC; by 6500 BC, this situation had occurred in Northern Europe, the Mediterranean, and India.[33]

In the New World, domestication is believed to have been established in Central Mexico by 2700 BC, in the eastern United States by 2500 BC, and in the South Central Andes in South America by 2500 BC.[34] Assuming that domesticated animals were infected by TB, and if animal to human transmission is accepted, a potential for transmission was clearly present. However, prior to domestication, hunter-gatherers could have contracted the disease through capture, butchery, and consumption of their (wild) kill. Corroborative data from Kapur et al.[35] suggest that mycobacterial species first appeared 15,000–20,000 years ago, long before domestication, and while this work has been debated as to its authenticity, Rothschild et al.[36] have revealed *M. tuberculosis* complex aDNA in the remains of an extinct, long-horned bison from North America dated to 15,870 (±230 years) BC. Brosch et al.[37] have furthermore indicated, based upon the genomic structure of tubercle bacilli, that *M. tuberculosis* did not evolve from *M. bovis*. Other researchers suggest that TB is the culmination of a global history originating in Africa, thereby affecting our hominine ancestors and extending more than 3 million years in the Old World.[38] Clearly from the genomic data it has been found that different phylogenetic lineages of *Mycobacterium tuberculosis* complex (MTBC) are associated with different geographic regions. These data will further help elucidate the long history of co-evolution of TB in humans and other animals.[39]

HUMANS, URBANIZATION, AND INDUSTRIALIZATION

Today, transmission of the human form of TB requires close contact with those infected. Because earlier peoples lived in small, mobile groups, they seldom formed settled communities.[40] With the development of agriculture, population density increased rapidly, thus enabling density-dependent diseases such as TB to flourish. Even so, it was not until the 1100s AD in North America and the late medieval period (twelfth to sixteenth centuries AD) in Europe that the disease really increased.[4]

During this period in Europe, conditions were ideal for a marked increase in TB. Poverty, the development of trade, and the migration of people from rural communities to urban centers (usually for work) enabled the transmission of TB to previously unexposed people. In addition, working with animals and their products also may have exposed populations to the infection. For example, processing animal skins in the tanning industry, working with bone and horn, and processing food products from animals all placed people at risk for the infection. Working in industries that produced particulate pollution, such as in the textile trade,

also irritated the lungs and probably predisposed people to TB. The post-medieval period and the Industrial Revolution provided potentially explosive conditions for TB. Of special interest here is the suggestion that people who have been urbanized for a long time become resistant to TB through natural selection.[41] This may explain part of the decline of TB starting in the late nineteenth and early twentieth centuries.[42]

We might also ask what people consumed in the past and whether their diet was balanced and nutritious. Quality of diet affects immune systems and how strong their resistance is to infection. If people become malnourished, they are more susceptible to TB; for example, iron and protein are important for immune function and infection outcome in TB, and diet may influence the potential for TB to disseminate from the lungs to the skeleton.[43] Skeletal and dental evidence suggests that health tends to deteriorate with increasing social complexity and the development of agriculture,[44–46] when diets were less varied. People ate less protein, which is needed to produce antibodies to fight infection, and wheat lacks certain amino acids.

As is the case today, many risk factors would have influenced the prevalence of TB in the past, especially population density and poverty. Animals—initially thought to have been central to the development and maintenance of TB in humans—probably became a key factor more recently, rather than at the time of domestication (see Chapter 22).

SKELETAL REMAINS FROM THE OLD WORLD

It can be argued that archeological human remains are the primary evidence for estimating the timing of TB's first appearance, but it is emphasized that biomolecular models predict co-evolution over a much longer time period when compared with the skeletal evidence for the disease.[35,38] We can define the Old World as the world that was known before a European presence in the Americas, comprising Europe, Asia, and Africa.[47] Most of the evidence of TB in human remains in the Old World comes from Europe, reflecting the intensity of study by paleopathologists compared with the rest of the Old World (Figure 1.5).[48] In some areas, this may be due to non-survival of human remains, non-excavation and/or analysis, and particular funerary rites that do not preserve remains well.[4] However, those Old World areas with no evidence may truly be areas with no TB in the past. We can divide the extant data into three broad areas in the Old World, which reflect similar climatic and environmental features: the Mediterranean, Northern Europe, and Asia and the Pacific islands.

THE MEDITERRANEAN

Italy has some of the earliest evidence of skeletal TB in the world, although earlier evidence has been recently reported for Northern Europe (see the next section). A female skeleton aged around 30 years at death is dated to 3800 (±90) BC and comes from the Neolithic cave of Arma dell'Aquila in Liguria,[49] and a child who lived 4500 years ago with probable TB has been found more recently in Pollera Cave, also in Liguria.[50] In the Near East, there are early skeletons with TB from Bab edh-Dhra in Jordan, dated 3150–2200 BC,[51] although Israel does not show evidence of the disease until AD 600, at the monastery of John the Baptist in the Judean Desert.[52]

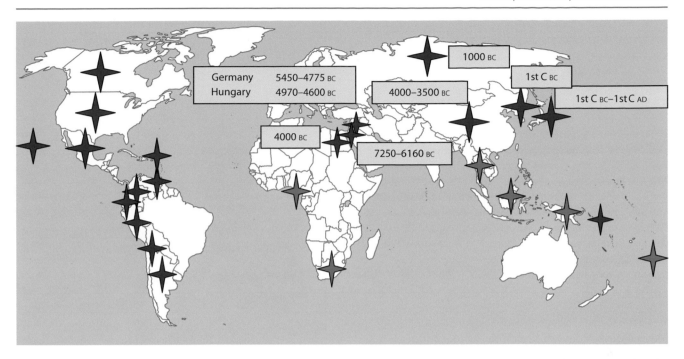

Figure 1.5 Distribution map of occurrences of skeletal tuberculosis in the world, excluding Europe (light stars = evidence that needs to be verified; dark stars = definite evidence).

Egypt reveals evidence of TB dated to 4000 BC,[53] although there is no definite evidence from sub-Saharan Africa. Data on TB in human remains have been published since early last century in this part of the world.[54] The most widely cited data are from the mummy Nesperehãn who was excavated in Thebes, where a psoas abscess and spinal changes were recorded; this established TB's presence in Egypt between 1069 and 945 BC.[53] In 1938, Derry's summary[55] indicated that the earliest occurrence dated to 3300 BC, although Morse et al.[53] record evidence from Nagada dated to as early as 4500 BC. In Egypt, there has been considerable research on soft-tissue evidence for TB. For example, Nerlich et al.[56] and Zink et al.[57] isolated and sequenced DNA from lung tissue from a male mummy found in a tomb of nobles (1550–1080 BC), providing a positive diagnosis for TB.

Spain comes next in chronological sequence with possible TB in skeletal remains dated to the Neolithic.[58] TB appears in Greece by 900 BC.[59] Since Angel's work, there have been very little skeletal data on TB from Greece, but by the fifth century BC, Hippocratic writings described the infection.[60] France, like Lithuania and Austria (Northern Europe), reveals TB around the fourth century AD.[61–63] Evidence has appeared in early, late, and post-medieval southeast France, but northern France has probably seen the most extensive paleopathological effort,[61] with nearly 2500 skeletons being examined from 17 sites dated to between the fourth and twelfth centuries AD. Twenty-nine skeletons with TB were identified, and most came from urban sites. Other Mediterranean countries, such as Serbia,[64] Turkey,[65] and Portugal,[66] provide the first evidence of the infection much more recently—in the medieval period (from around the twelfth century AD). At that time, there appeared to be significant numbers of groups with TB.[4] It should also be noted that controversial data from Israel dated to 7250–6160 BC have been published.[67,68]

NORTHERN EUROPE

In Northern Europe, the Neolithic site of Zlota (5000 BC) in Poland reveals some of the earliest published evidence for TB.[69] As in many other European countries, the frequency of the disease increased during the later medieval period. Data from the Bronze Age site of Manych, in southern Russia, suggest TB was present by 1000 BC,[64] but there is much more paleopathological work to be done in that huge country. More recently, data have been presented from Germany and Hungary, suggesting early evidence dated to 5450–4775 BC and 4970–4600 BC, respectively.[70–72]

In Denmark, the presence of TB begins during the Iron Age (500–1 BC) at Varpelev, Sjælland.[73] In Britain, the first evidence has been recovered from an Iron Age site at Tarrant Hinton, Dorset, dated to 400–230 BC.[74] Austria and Lithuania have skeletal evidence by the fourth century AD, and for Austria this coincides with the late Roman occupation.

The United Kingdom has had a long history of paleopathological study and, therefore, the evidence for TB is much more plentiful there than in other countries. Of particular interest in Britain is research that contradicts the idea that TB in rural human populations was most likely the result of transmission from animals. aDNA analysis of human remains at the rural medieval site of Wharram Percy suggests that TB was the result of *M. tuberculosis* and not *M. bovis*.[75]

In Lithuania, extensive work has documented the frequency of TB in skeletal remains,[76] with the record beginning at the late Roman site of Marvelé. In addition to diagnostic skeletal lesions, remains from Marvelé also produced positive aDNA results for the *M. tuberculosis* complex.[77] Over time, TB frequencies increased, along with population density and intensification of agriculture. Jankauskas[78] suggests that cattle probably transmitted the infection to humans, and in the early medieval period he found that people appeared to be surviving the acute stages of the infection.

By the seventh century AD, Norway and Switzerland feature in the history of TB,[79] followed by Hungary, and then by Sweden and the Netherlands during the eleventh to thirteenth centuries AD, respectively. There also has been extensive published work in Hungary documenting the frequency of TB over time.[80–82] Clearly, TB was fairly common in the seventh to eighth centuries and also in the fourteenth to seventeenth centuries; an obvious gap in the evidence in the tenth century may be due to the Hungarian population's semi-nomadic way of life at that time (burial sites not identified). Skeletal and mummified remains from Hungary that display TB have also been subject to extensive biomolecular research, which has allowed the confirmation of possible tuberculous skeletons.[81,82] In Sweden, an extensive study of more than 3000 skeletons from Lund dated between AD 990 and 1536 showed TB of the spine in one individual (AD 1050–1100), although more than 40 had possible TB in one or more joints.[83] The Czech Republic also provides its first evidence of TB during the later medieval period.[84]

ASIA AND THE PACIFIC ISLANDS

Asia and the Pacific islands reveal TB in skeletal remains much later than the Mediterranean and Northern European areas. China has evidence from a mummy dated between 206 BC and the seventh century AD,[85] although the first written description of TB treatment is dated to 2700 BC,[86] with the first accepted description of the disease dated to 2200 BC.[85] Japan has skeletal evidence dated from 454 BC to AD 124; Korea has evidence from the first century BC[87,88] and Thailand has evidence dated to the first two centuries AD.[89] Papua New Guinea and Hawaii[90–92] produce data much later (pre-European, i.e., pre–late-fifteenth century AD), with possible TB being recorded in human remains from Tonga and the Solomon Islands.

SUMMARY OF DATA FROM THE OLD WORLD

Although the Old World data for skeletal TB appear quite plentiful, there are many areas where there is no evidence (Figures 1.5 and 1.6).

This may be because:

- It really does not exist even though extensive skeletal analysis has been undertaken.
- Skeletal remains are not traditionally studied in a particular country.
- Management of the burial of the dead at a specific time may not preserve them well enough for the evidence to be observed (e.g., cremation in Bronze Age Britain).
- Skeletal remains do not survive burial because of the climate or environment in a specific geographic area, for example, the acidic soils of Wales or Scotland.
- For some time periods in certain countries, no skeletal remains have been excavated (e.g., the Roman period in Poland).

On the basis of the evidence published to date, TB has an early focus in the Mediterranean and Northern European areas. There are later appearances in Asia and other parts of Northern Europe and also in parts of the Mediterranean. However, it is not until the hazards of urban living and the increase in population size

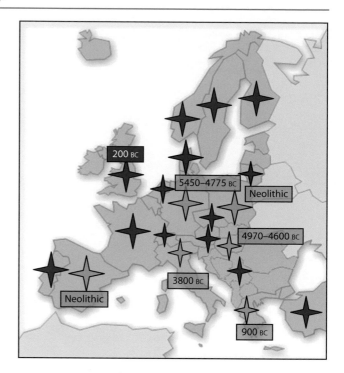

Figure 1.6 Distribution map of occurrences of skeletal tuberculosis in Europe (light stars = early evidence).

and density of the later medieval period[93,94] that we see a rise in the frequency of the disease in most places. In addition, at this time, a practice known as "Touching for the King's Evil" was developing—a monarch could apparently cure somebody with TB by touching them on the head and giving them a gold piece.[95] Whether all people "touched" were tuberculous is debatable.

SKELETAL REMAINS FROM THE NEW WORLD

In the New World, particularly in North America, skeletal remains have been studied for a considerable time. For example, the first reported human remains with TB were found in 1886,[96] although they have since been critically reviewed.[9] By the mid-twentieth century, evidence for the disease had increased considerably in Eastern North America,[97] the North American Southwest,[98] and South America.[99] Some have raised doubts concerning the presence of TB in the New World prior to the sixteenth century,[100] but current evidence, both skeletal and biomolecular, confirms that TB was present in the prehistoric Americas. A major argument for its absence in prehistoric populations was the suggestion that sufficiently large population aggregates did not exist. However, the existence of very large prehistoric communities effectively counters this argument.[4,101] For example, estimates of population size at Cahokia in the Central Mississippi Valley, circa AD 1100, have ranged from 3500[102] to 35,000,[103] with a population density of 21–27 individuals per square kilometer.[102] Although there have been doubts about the need for large populations in order for TB to flourish,[104] there were certainly wild and domesticated animals that could have provided a reservoir for the infection.

The evidence from the Americas can be divided into northern, central, and southern areas. Most of the evidence comes from North and South America.

NORTH AMERICA

There are two areas of North America where the skeletal evidence for TB derives—Eastern North America, especially the mid-continent, and the Southwest.[101] Both these areas were large population centers in late prehistory, that is, before AD 1492. However, Eastern North America provides most of the data, with four sites producing more than 10 individuals with TB: Uxbridge,[105] Norris Farms,[106] Schild,[107] and Averbuch.[108] This may reflect not only the intensity of skeletal analysis there, but also the frequency of destructive burial practices along with casual disposal of the dead in the Southwest. However, the earliest evidence of TB in North America does derive from the Southwest during the same time that there were major population concentrations in large pueblos (permanent agricultural settlements).[109] For example, the site of Pueblo Bonito had more than 800 rooms, with some of the sites having buildings up to five stories high.[110] All the evidence in North America thus post-dates AD 900 and is more recent than that in South America.

MESOAMERICA

Despite large numbers of people living in Mesoamerica before European contact, along with considerable skeletal analysis, there is a virtual absence of TB until very late prehistory.[4] This may be explained by poor preservation in some areas of Mesoamerica, but there have also been excavations and analysis of very large well-preserved cemeteries with no evidence of TB forthcoming.[111] One explanation for the absence of TB is that people were dying in Mesoamerica before bone changes occurred. However, similar stresses are also identified in North America where evidence of TB exists.[109] One could also argue that those with TB, manifested by Pott's disease of the spine, were buried away from the main cemetery or laid to rest in a different way from those without the disease. In Mesoamerica, we also know that people with "hunchbacks" (the deformity seen in spinal TB) appear to have been awarded special status, as depicted on painted ceramics,[112] and that their treatment in society may have been very different from that of the rest of the population, including their final resting place.[105]

SOUTH AMERICA

The earliest evidence for TB in the New World is seen in South America in Peru,[113] Venezuela,[114] Chile,[114] and Colombia,[115] with the oldest evidence recovered from the Caserones site in northern Chile's Atacama Desert.[116] Three individuals with TB were recorded and dated originally to around AD 290 by Allison et al.,[115] but Buikstra,[101] in considering radiocarbon dating problems in coastal environments, dates them to no earlier than AD 700. Within the larger South American sites, it is interesting to note that more males than females are affected (as is seen generally today), whereas in North American sites the sexes are equally affected.[4] Although men and women herded, caravans—groups of travelers—were composed of men; a possible reason for the South American asymmetry would be that males were placed more at risk due to their proximity to camelids while engaged in long-distance trade.[4] Stead et al.[117] also suggest that prehistoric TB in the Americas is likely due more to the *bovis* organism from infected animal products. *M. bovis*, compared with *M. tuberculosis*, is also 10 times more likely to produce skeletal damage. Thus, in North and South America, we see TB increasing after about AD 1000 and into the early historic period.[118,119]

SUMMARY OF THE DATA FROM THE NEW WORLD

The earliest evidence of skeletal TB in the New World is in South America by AD 700, with later appearances in North America. This suggests a transmission route of south to north, although Mesoamerica generally does miss the encounter until relatively late prehistory. One model suggests transmission by sea, coincident with material evidence of trade between western Mexico and Ecuador.[4] The only relatively early Mesoamerican sites with multiple skeletons with Pott's disease being found in western Mexico. However, the south to north transmission is now compatible with the molecular evidence. One of the lessons we learn from the New World data is the degree to which TB can and did move between mammalian hosts, including human.

HISTORICAL AND PICTORIAL DATA

Although we would argue that the presence of TB in past communities should rely primarily on evidence from skeletal or mummified remains, including that from biomolecular studies, there are large bodies of written and illustrative evidence that have contributed to tracing the origin, evolution, and history of this infectious disease. However, these data are less convincing than those derived from human remains. Unfortunately, the clinical expression of pulmonary TB may mimic other lung diseases such as cancer and pneumonia, and kyphotic deformities of the spine could be caused by spinal conditions other than TB. We also have to remember that authors and artists often wrote about and depicted the most disturbing diseases (especially those that were visually dramatic), and therefore they may not always include TB in their renderings. Thus, using historical sources as an indicator of the presence and frequency of TB remains challenging, and what is represented in these sources may provide a biased portrayal of what diseases were present at any point in time.

HISTORICAL DATA

In the Old World, a Chinese text (2700 BC) provides a description of possible TB in the neck's lymph nodes and in expectoration of blood,[120] while the Ebers Papyrus (1500 BC) also describes TB of the lymph glands. In India, the *Rig Veda*, of the same date, describes "phthisis," and a possible example of TB in a skeleton from Mesopotamia (675 BC) has also been described.[86] Numerous references are encountered in Classical Antiquity ranging from Homer (800 BC) through Hippocrates (460–377 BC) to Pliny (first century AD); Arabian writers during the ninth to eleventh centuries AD also suggested that animals may be affected by the disease.

The late medieval period in Europe produced considerable written evidence. For example, Fracastorius (1483–1553), in *De Contagione*, was the first to suggest that TB was due to invisible "germs" carrying the disease. From the beginning of the seventeenth century, the impression (in England at least) is that TB was becoming very common. The London Bills of Mortality report that 20% of deaths in England by the mid-1600s were due to TB.[121]

TB was also associated with romanticism and genius. By the eighteenth century, appearing pale and thin was considered attractive, especially for women, and TB led to this appearance in many.[122] For example, the heroines in some of the famous operas, such as *La Traviata* and *Mimi*, were beautiful women with TB.[122] Authors were said to have been especially inspired during fevers. During the nineteenth century, many authors and artists died of TB, thus perpetuating the myth that genius was associated with the disease. At a time when much of the population in Europe was succumbing to TB, this is hardly surprising.

When historical data are available, they can potentially provide a window on frequency rates of TB, but the numbers of those actually dying from TB may be inaccurate. This could be due to many reasons, including non-diagnosis (some due to evading a diagnosis because of the stigma attached to TB and the effect on life's prospects) and misdiagnosis. Until 1882, when the tubercle bacillus was identified, diagnosis was based on the analysis of signs and symptoms.[123] Later, sputum tests and radiography played their part, but a post-mortem examination is the only sure way of achieving a diagnosis of cause of death.

ARTISTIC REPRESENTATIONS

Artistic representations come in a variety of forms, including paintings, drawings, reliefs, and sculpture. However, we must remember that artistic conventions must be considered, that artists may be biased in what they portray, and that depiction may not be accurate and will be dependent on the artists' interpretation and skills. There appear to be two types of possible depictions of TB, the kyphotic spine and pale, thin, tired young women.[124] The former is more commonly represented than the latter. In North Africa, Morse et al. describe spinal deformities in "plastic" art dating to before 3000 BC,[53] and similar appearances are seen in Egyptian (3500 BC) and North American contexts. A figurine on a clay pot from Egypt (4000 BC) has for a long time been identified with spinal TB and emaciation, but the spinal deformity is in the cervical region (rare in TB) and we have already noted the possible differential diagnoses for such kyphotic deformities. In TB, it is important to note that angular deformities are more common than those that are more rounded.[97] In the later and post-medieval periods in Europe, more illustrations of people with deformed spines are seen, such as those by Hogarth in London. In Central America, of course, similar evidence is recorded on pottery.[112] Although potential evidence exists for TB in the past, in writings and in art, the interpretation of such data, until more recent times, is more problematic than the skeletal evidence.

BIOMOLECULAR EVIDENCE FOR TB FROM ANCIENT SKELETAL REMAINS

Humans may acquire TB from each other, and from other mammals who are infected by bacteria of the MTC or *Mycobacterium tuberculosis* complex. The MTC includes three species that are most commonly found in humans (*M. tuberculosis*, *M. africanum*, and *M. canettii*). Other forms, including *M. microti*, *M. bovis*, and *M. pinnipedi* are most commonly found in non-human mammals. Before the development of twenty-first century genomic models, researchers assumed that the more ancient forms included *M. bovis*, which is either a distinct species or polytypic form that also affects animals such as the oryx, seals, and sea lions. The pathogen, so the story went, was thought to have "jumped" species to humans as pastoralism developed in the Eastern Mediterranean.[125] TB in America remained enigmatic, perhaps derived independently from a bovine form of the Americas affecting deer or bison. Speculation also included New World domesticates such as the dog or the guinea pig. Turkeys, possible avian sources, were also kept near households in, for example, the American Greater Southwest, primarily for secondary products such as feathers rather than for meat. Biomolecular evidence for TB from human remains is a rapidly emerging analytical method for interpreting the origin, evolution, and paleoepidemiology of the disease. The study of ancient biomolecules using polymerase chain reaction (PCR) as a tool for diagnosing disease has had a short history, spanning the past 25 years or so (for a summary of the use of aDNA analysis in human remains, see Brown and Brown[126] and Stone[127]). Although there are certainly quality control issues to consider in aDNA analysis,[128–130] it has allowed theories about the origin and evolution of infectious disease, especially TB, to be explored. The most common research problems addressed have been confirmation of diagnoses,[131,132] diagnosis of individuals with no pathological changes from TB,[133] and identification of the organism that caused TB in humans.[134–136] More recently, this has been supplemented by phylogenetic research that has been able to identify different TB strains in archeological human remains, including seal/sea lion strains in South America.[137, 138]

Research diagnosing TB using aDNA analysis started in the United Kingdom and the Americas. In 1993, Spigelman and Lemma documented the amplification of *M. tuberculosis* complex DNA in British skeletal remains.[139] Around the same time, Salo et al.[25] successfully amplified *M. tuberculosis* DNA from the South American site of Chiribaya Alta; a calcified subpleural nodule was noticed during the autopsy of a woman who had died 1000 years ago. A 97 base pair segment of the insertion sequence (IS) 6110, which is considered specific to the *M. tuberculosis* complex, was identified and directly sequenced. Three other sites have yielded the same *M. tuberculosis* complex aDNA, two in Eastern North America (Uxbridge and Schild)[140] and one in South America (SR1 in northern Chile)[141]: in Uxbridge (AD 1410–1483)—a pathological vertebra from an ossuary site; in Schild (AD 1000–1200)—a pathological vertebra from a female; and in Chile (AD 800)—an affected vertebra of an 11- to 13-year-old child.

In the Old World, most biomolecular research to date has been focused on samples from skeletons and mummies from the United Kingdom, Lithuania, and Hungary. For example, Gernaey et al. confirmed a diagnosis of TB in an early medieval skeleton from Yorkshire, England with Pott's disease using aDNA and mycolic acid analyses.[26] Taylor et al. provided positive diagnoses for skeletons from the fourteenth century site of the Royal Mint in London.[131–142] Gernaey et al. established that 25% of the population buried at a post-medieval site at Newcastle in north-eastern England experienced TB, although most had no bone changes typical of the disease.[133] In Hungary, Pálfi et al. and Haas et al., using aDNA analysis, confirmed a number of TB diagnoses in human remains dating back to the seventh and eighth centuries and up to the seventeenth century,[132,143] and analysis of four eighteenth- to nineteenth-century mummies from Vac (two with TB) revealed positive diagnoses for three of them. Fletcher et al. also analyzed TB aDNA in a family group from the same site.[136] In Lithuania, Faerman et al. have also confirmed diagnoses of TB in skeletal remains, including individuals with no diagnostic osseous changes.[144]

With the genomic "revolution" of the twenty-first century, new models have identified the human predilected members of the MTC (*M. africanum*, *M. tuberculosis* and basal *M. canettii*) as being the more genetically complex and therefore the more ancient forms, when compared to *M. microti* and *M. bovis*.[37] Such models argue for a much longer co-evolution between humans and the MTC more than previously thought, beginning in Africa. Even so, the earliest skeletal evidence for human TB appears in the Eastern Mediterranean, associated with the Neolithic. This increased time depth for human–pathogen co-evolution led researchers to speculate that humans brought a form of the MTC when they migrated from East Asia to North America along the coast, or across the Bering Strait land bridge. More recently, however, it has been demonstrated that the ancient American forms of TB jumped species from pinnipeds—either seals or sea lions—who had brought the pathogen with them as they migrated from the horn of Africa.[138] Studies are currently underway to explore the path taken by the pinniped-derived human TB in the ancient and early colonial Americas.

Thus, in the last edition of this book, the use of biomolecular analyses to identify TB in human remains was beginning to answer questions impossible to contemplate prior to the early 1990s (e.g., on TB bacterial strains). However, it is clear that new methodologies and ideas have moved us forward. This and related fields hold significant future potential.[145,146] One promising line of study focuses on estimating which species of the *M. tuberculosis* complex infected humans over time in different regions of the world. A second branch of study identifies whether the strains of the organism are the same today as in the past; that is, it compares the phylogenetic relationships of organisms causing TB in the past and present and estimates how the organisms have evolved. Both these areas of research are currently receiving attention from the authors, as well as other scholars around the world.[138,147] As Guichón et al. have said, this type of research is "Moving beyond simple confirmatory analysis of diseased bone, researchers are now asking nuanced research questions capable of confronting the debate regarding TB's origins and evolution."[148]

OVERVIEW OF DATA FROM ANCIENT HUMAN REMAINS

Clearly, there is much evidence from human remains for TB from around the world, with most data derived from North America and Europe. An early focus for the infection appears in Germany, Hungary, Italy, Poland, and Spain in the Neolithic and in Egypt from 4000 BC, but TB does not increase with any real frequency until the later and post-medieval periods in the Old World. This latter observation is corroborated by historical sources. There is very little evidence, if at all, in Asia, most likely reflecting the lack of intense skeletal analysis in those parts of the world. In the New World, TB appears for the first time in South America by AD 700 and is not seen until around AD 1000 in North America, largely bypassing Mesoamerica. The current biomolecular evidence suggests that *M. tuberculosis* did not evolve from *M. bovis*. In the prehistoric Americas, population size and aggregation contributed to the flourishing of TB via droplet infection. However, in Europe and the Americas, wild and domesticated animals may also have been a reservoir of infection.

TB IN THE NINETEENTH AND TWENTIETH CENTURIES

We have thus far considered the evidence for TB in populations from very far distant eras. To bring us to the introduction of antibiotics in the mid-twentieth century, we must now turn to records of TB in the late nineteenth and early twentieth centuries. In the eighteenth century, John Bunyan referred to TB as the "captain of all these men of death."[149] By the beginning of the nineteenth century, TB was the leading cause of death in most European countries, reaching up to 500–800 cases per 100,000 population.[150] During the Victorian period in Britain, it was one of the main causes of death.[151] In the late 1800s, the start of the Industrial Revolution in Britain and rapid urbanization, including rural to urban migration, favored the spread of TB. By the mid-nineteenth century, the concept of the sanatorium had been established. Fresh air, a good healthy diet, rest, and graded exercise was the regime offered to people with TB, with surgery—such as lung collapse and rib resection—being undertaken for some. Patients were isolated from their families in an attempt to control the spread of the infection. The first sanatorium was opened in Germany in 1859, with many more founded over the next 100 years, even ones for children.[152]

In 1882, Robert Koch first described the tubercle bacillus, and in 1895, Conrad Roentgen discovered the x-ray, which provided a new method for diagnosing TB. By 1897, the theory of transmission of TB via droplet infection was established,[153] and by the early twentieth century, it was known that animals could contract the infection. By the second half of the nineteenth century and into the twentieth, there was an obvious decline in TB.[154] This is largely attributed to improvements in living conditions and diet, although Davies et al. have shown that none of the other poverty-related diseases showed such a decline, thus making interpretations difficult[42] (but see Barnes et al.[41]). An anti-tuberculosis campaign, which included controls on the quality of meat and milk, started soon after Koch discovered the bacillus.[123] In 1889, the Tuberculosis Association was established in the United States; in the 1890s, the League Against Tuberculosis was founded in France to encourage the control of TB in Europe. In 1898, the National Association for the Prevention of Tuberculosis and other Forms of Consumption (NAPT) was established in Britain as part of an international movement. The International Union against

TB was founded in 1902 to encourage a system of control; this included the notification of all cases, contact tracing, and the provision of dispensaries and sanatoria. Mass radiography during the two world wars allowed higher detection rates, while rehabilitation schemes, the Bacillus Calmette Guerin (BCG) vaccination in the 1950s (in Britain), health education, and pasteurization of milk were all seriously considered.[123] This trend towards tackling TB continued with the introduction of antibiotics in the midtwentieth century. Although TB has been with us for thousands of years and despite once being thought of as a conquered infection, it still remains a plague on a global scale.

CONCLUSION

The history of TB has been traced through the analysis and interpretation of evidence from human remains derived from archeological sites around the world. Although there may be biases in these data with respect to tracing the origin, epidemiology, and long history of TB, these are the most reliable sources we have at our disposal. The origin in Northern Europe of Old World TB nearly 8000 years ago and its appearance in the Americas by AD 700 truly illustrate TB's antiquity. We have seen that in both contexts, TB increased with human population size, which allowed transmission of the infection through exhaled and inhaled bacteria-laden droplets. Infection of humans by wild and domesticated animals was also a risk. TB continued to increase over time, with high frequencies in Europe during the Industrial Revolution of the 1800s. In the late nineteenth and early twentieth centuries, a decline preceded the introduction of antibiotics in Europe and North America. The reasons for this pattern remain speculative. Improvements in living conditions and diet (and its quality), better diagnosis, health education, vaccination and immunization, pasteurization of milk, and isolation of people with TB from the uninfected may all have helped to lower the rate of TB.

We have seen that skeletal evidence can provide us with a global picture of this ancient malady from its very earliest times. It can also direct us to the areas of the world that have revealed the earliest evidence, and we can thus begin to explore the epidemiological factors that allowed the infection to flourish. We can see that the factors that influenced TB frequencies appear very similar to those today (poverty, high population density, urban living, poor access to health care, infected animals, migrating populations, and certain occupations). How much trade and contact, and travel and migration, contributed to the tuberculous load in past populations is yet to be established with certainty, but stable isotope analysis is showing that people were very mobile in the past. Of course, HIV, acquired immune deficiency syndrome (AIDS), and antibiotic resistance were not issues with which our ancestors had to contend. Biomolecular studies of TB in the past will continue to contribute to our understanding of the paleoepidemiology of this infection, by identifying the causative organisms and their similarities and differences from the strains of TB today. We anticipate that paleopathological research in TB will also help our understanding of TB today and hopefully contribute to its decline.[155]

ACKNOWLEDGMENTS

Our thanks go to the many researchers listed in Roberts and Buikstra[4] who gave freely of their time and data during the writing of this book.

REFERENCES

1. Smith ER. *The Retreat of Tuberculosis 1850–1950*. London: Croom Helm, 1988.
2. Harper K, and Armelagos GJ. The changing disease-scape in the third epidemiological transition. *Int J Environ Res Public Health*. 2010;7:675–97.
3. WHO (World Health Organization). *Global Tuberculosis Control*. Geneva: WHO, 2011.
4. Roberts CA, and Buikstra JE. *Bioarchaeology of Tuberculosis: Global Perspectives on a Re-emerging Disease*. Gainesville: University Press of Florida, 2003.
5. Wilkinson R, and Pickett K. *The Spirit Level. Why Equality is Better for Everyone*. London: Penguin Books, 2009.
6. Pawlowski A et al. Tuberculosis and HIV co-infection. *PLoS Pathog*. 2012;8:e1002464.
7. Mason PH, Roy A, Spilllane J, and Singh P. Social, historical and cultural dimensions of tuberculosis. *J Biosco Sci* 2016; 48:206–32.
8. Walt G. The politics of tuberculosis: The role of power and process. In: Porter JDH, and Grange JM (eds.). *Tuberculosis: An Interdisciplinary Perspective*. London: Imperial College Press, 1999, 67–98.
9. Mukherjee A, Saha I, Sarkar A, and Chowdhury R. Gender differences in notification rates, clinical forms and treatment outcome of tuberculosis patients under the RNTCP. *Lung India* 2012;29:120–2.
10. Mitchell PD. Retrospective diagnosis and the use of historical texts for investigating disease in the past. *Int J Paleopath* 2011;1:81–8.
11. Jaffe HL. *Metabolic, Degenerative and Inflammatory Diseases of Bones and Joints*. Philadelphia: Lea and Febiger, 1972.
12. Steyn M, Scholtz Y, Botha D, and Pretorius S. The changing face of tuberculosis: Trends in tuberculosis-associated skeletal changes. *Tuberculosis* 2013; 93:467–74.
13. Stead WW. What's in a name? Confusion of *Mycobacterium tuberculosis* and *Mycobacterium bovis* in ancient DNA analysis. *Paleopathol Assoc Newslett* 2000;110:13–6.
14. Wood JW, Milner GR, Harpending HC, and Weiss KM. The osteological paradox: Problems of inferring prehistoric health from skeletal samples. *Curr Anthropol*. 1992;33:343–70.
15. Aufderheide AC. *The Scientific Study of Mummies*. Cambridge: Cambridge University Press, 2003.
16. Roberts CA, and Manchester K. *The Archaeology of Disease*, 3rd ed. Stroud: Sutton Publishing, 2005.
17. Buikstra JE, and Ubelaker D (eds.). *Standards for Data Collection from Human Skeletal Remains*. Arkansas: Archaeological Research Seminar Series, 1994, 44.
18. Ortner DJ. Theoretical and methodological issues in palaeopathology. In: Ortner DJ, and Aufderheide AC (eds.). *Human Paleopathology. Current Syntheses and Future Options*. Washington, DC: Smithsonian Institution Press, 1991, 5–11.
19. Ortner DJ. *Identification of Pathological Conditions in Human Skeletal Remains*, 2nd ed. London: Academic Press, 2003.
20. Schultz M. The role of tuberculosis in infancy and childhood in prehistoric and historic populations. In: Pálfi G, Dutour O, Deák J, and Hutás I (eds.). *Tuberculosis: Past and Present*. Szeged: Golden Book Publishers, 1999, 503–7.

21. Lewis ME. Endocranial lesions in non-adult skeletons: Understanding their aetiology. *Int J Osteoarchaeol.* 2004;14:82–97.

22. Kelley MA, and Micozzi M. Rib lesions in chronic pulmonary tuberculosis. *Am J Phys Anthrop* 1984;65:381–6.

23. Roberts CA, Lucy D, and Manchester K. Inflammatory lesions of ribs: An analysis of the Terry Collection. *Am J Phys Anthropol.* 1994;85:169–82.

24. Santos AL, and Roberts CA. Anatomy of a serial killer: Differential diagnosis of tuberculosis based on rib lesions of adult individuals from the Coimbra Identified Skeletal Collection, Portugal. *Am J Phys Anthropol.* 2006;130:38–49.

25. Salo WL, Aufderheide AC, Buikstra JE, and Holcomb TA. Identification of *Mycobacterium tuberculosis* DNA in a pre-Columbia mummy. *Proc Natl Acad Sci USA.* 1994;91:2091–4.

26. Gernaey A et al. Mycolic acids and ancient DNA confirm an osteological diagnosis of tuberculosis. *Tuberculosis* 2001;81:259–65.

27. Müller R, Roberts CA, and Brown TA. Complications in the study of ancient tuberculosis: Non-specificity of IS6110 PCRs. *Sci Technol Archaeol Res.* 2015; 1(1):112054892314Y.0000000002.

28. Galagan JE. Genomic insights into tuberculosis. *Nat Rev Genet.* 2014; 15: doi: 10.1038/nrg3664.

29. van Tong H, Velavan TP, Thye T, and Meyer CG. Human genetic factors in tuberculosis: An update. *Trop Med Int Health.* 2017; 22:1063–71.

30. Hardy A. Death is the cure of all diseases. Using the General Register Office cause of death statistics for 1837–1920. *Soc Hist Med.* 1994;7:472–92.

31. Payne D. Death keeps Irish doctors guessing. *Br Med J* 2000;321:468.

32. Buikstra JE, and Roberts CA (eds.). *The Global History of Palaeopathology. Pioneers and Prospects.* Oxford: Oxford University Press, 2012.

33. Renfrew C, and Bahn P. *Archaeology. Theories, Methods and Practice.* London: Thames and Hudson, 2012.

34. Smith BD. *The Emergence of Agriculture.* New York: Scientific American Library, 1995.

35. Kapur V, Whittam TS, and Musser JM. Is *Mycobacterium tuberculosis* 15,000 years old? *J Infect Dis.* 1994;170:1348–9.

36. Rothschild BM et al. *Mycobacterium tuberculosis* complex DNA from an extinct bison dated 17,000 years before present. *Clin Infect Dis.* 2001;33:305–11.

37. Brosch R et al. A new evolutionary sequence for the *Mycobacterium tuberculosis* complex. *Proc Natl Acad Sci USA.* 2002;99:3684–9.

38. Gutierrez MC et al. Ancient origin and gene mosaicism of the progenitor of *Mycobacterium tuberculosis.* *PLoS Pathol* 2005;1:e5.

39. Brites D, and Gagneux S. Co-evolution of *Mycobacterium tuberculosis* and *Homo sapiens.* *Immunol Rev.* 2015; 264:6–24.

40. Lee RB, and De Vore I (eds.). *Man the Hunter.* Chicago: Aldine, 1968.

41. Barnes I, Duda A, Pybus O, and Thomas MG. Ancient urbanization predicts genetic resistance to tuberculosis evolution. *Evolution.* 2011;65:842–8.

42. Davies RPO et al. Historical declines in tuberculosis in England and Wales: Improving social conditions or natural selection? *Int J Tuberc Lung Dis.* 1999;3:1051–4.

43. Wilbur AK, Farnbach AW, Knudson KJ, and Buikstra JE. Diet, tuberculosis and the paleopathological record. *Curr Anthropol.* 2008;49:963–91.

44. Cohen MN. *Health and the Rise of Civilisation.* New York: Yale University Press, 1989.

45. Steckel R, and Rose JC (eds.). *The Backbone of History. Health and Nutrition in the Western Hemisphere.* Cambridge: Cambridge University Press, 2002.

46. Roberts CA, and Cox M. *Health and Disease in Britain. Prehistory to the Present Day.* Stroud: Sutton Publishing, 2003.

47. Hanks P. *Collins Dictionary of the English Language.* London: Collins, 1979.

48. Roberts CA. Old World tuberculosis: Evidence from human remains with a review of current research and future prospects. *Tuberculosis* 2015;95:S117–21.

49. Canci A, Minozzi S, and Borgognini Tarli S. New evidence of tuberculous spondylitis from Neolithic Liguria (Italy). *Int J Osteoarchaeol.* 1996;6:497–501.

50. Sparacello VS, Roberts CA, Kerudin A, and Müller R. A 6500-year-old Middle Neolithic child from Pollera Cave (Liguria, Italy) with probable multifocal osteoarticular tuberculosis. *Int J Paleopathol.* 2017;17:67–74.

51. Ortner DJ. Disease and mortality in the Early Bronze Age people of Bab edh-Dhra, Jordan. *Am J Phys Anthropol.* 1979;51:589–98.

52. Zias J. Leprosy and tuberculosis in the Byzantine monasteries of the Judaean Desert. In: Ortner DJ, and Aufderheide AC (eds.). *Human Palaeopathology. Current Syntheses and Future Options.* Washington, DC: Smithsonian Institution Press, 1991, 197–9.

53. Morse D, Brothwell DR, and Ucko PJ. Tuberculosis in ancient Egypt. *Am Rev Respir Dis* 1964;90:526–41.

54. Elliot-Smith G, and Ruffer MA. Pottsche Krakheit an einer ägyptischen Mumie aus der Zeit der 21 dynastie (um 1000 v. Chr.). In: *Zur Historichen Biologie der Kranzheit Serreger.* Leipzig, 1910, 9–16.

55. Derry DE. Pott's disease in ancient Egypt. *Med Press Circ* 1938;197:196–9.

56. Nerlich AG et al. Molecular evidence for tuberculosis in an ancient Egyptian mummy. *Lancet.* 1997;35:1404.

57. Zink A et al. Morphological and molecular evidence for pulmonary and osseous tuberculosis in a male Egyptian mummy. In: Pálfi G, Dutour O, Deák J, and Hutás I (eds.). *Tuberculosis: Past and Present.* Szeged: Golden Book Publishers, 1999, 371–91.

58. Santoja M. Estudio antropológico. In: Canellada AZ (ed.). *Excavaciones de la Cueva de la Vaquera, Torreiglesias.* Segovia: Edad del Bronce, 1975, 74–87.

59. Angel JL. Health as a crucial factor in the changes from hunting to developed farming in the Eastern Mediterranean. In: Cohen MN, and Armelagos GJ (eds.). *Paleopathology at the Origins of Agriculture.* London: Academic Press, 1984, 51–74.

60. Grmek M. *Diseases in the Ancient Greek World.* London: Johns Hopkins University Press, 1989.

61. Moyart V, and Pavaut M. La tuberculose dans le nord de la France du IVe à la 62IIe siecle. *Thèse pour le Diploma d'état de Docteur en Médecine.* Lille 2, U du Droit et de la Santé, Faculté de Médecine Henri Warembourg, 1998.

62. Molnar E et al. Skeletal tuberculosis in Hungarian and French Medieval anthropological material. In: Guerci A (ed.). *La cura della mallattie. Itinerari storici.* Genoa: Erga Edizione, 1998, 87–99.

63. Blondiaux J et al. Epidemiology of tuberculosis: A 4th to 12th century AD picture in a 2498-skeleton series from Northern France. In: Pálfi G, Dutour O, Deák J, and Hutás I (eds.). *Tuberculosis: Past and Present.* Szeged: Golden Book Publishers, 1999, 521–30.

64. Djuric-Srejic M, and Roberts CA. Palaeopathological evidence of infectious disease in later medieval skeletal populations from Serbia. *Int J Osteoarchaeol.* 2001;11:311–20.

65. Brothwell D. The human bones. In: Harrison RM (ed.). *Excavations at Saraçhane in Istanbul. Volume 1: The Excavations, Structures, Architectural Decoration, Small Finds, Coins, Bones and Molluscs.* Princeton: Princeton University Press, 1986, 374–98.

66. Cunha E. Paleobiologia des populacoes Medievals Portuguesas-os-casos de Fão e. S. oãoda Almedina. FCT, University of Coimbra, *Portugal,* unpublished PhD thesis, 1994.

67. Hershkovitz I et al. Detection and molecular characterization of 9000-year-old *Mycobacterium tuberculosis* from a Neolithic settlement in the Eastern Mediterranean. *PLOS ONE* 2008;3:e3426.

68. Wilbur AK et al. Deficiencies and challenges in the study of ancient tuberculosis DNA. *J Archaeol Sci.* 2009;36:1990–7.

69. Gladykowska-Rzeczycka JJ. Tuberculosis in the past and present in Poland. In: Pálfi G, Dutour O, Deák J, and Hutás I (eds.). *Tuberculosis: Past and Present.* Szeged: Golden Book Publishers, 1999, 561–73.

70. Rokhlin DG. *Diseases of Ancient Men. Bones of the Men of Various Epochs – Normal and Pathologic Changes.* Moscow: Nauka, 1965. [in Russian].

71. Nicklisch N, Maixner F, Ganslmeier R, Friederich S, Dresely V, Meller H, Zink A, and Alt KW. Rib lesions in skeletons from early neolithic sites in Central Germany: On the trail of tuberculosis at the onset of agriculture. *Am J Phys Anthropol.* 2012; 149:391–404.

72. Masson M, Bereczk Z, Molnár E, Donoghue HD, Minnikin DE, Lee OYC, Wu HH, Besra GS, Bull ID, and Pálfi G. Osteological and biomolecular evidence of a 7000-year-old case of hypertrophic pulmonary osteopathy secondary to tuberculosis from Neolithic Hungary. *PLOS ONE* 2013;8(10):e78252.

73. Bennike P. Facts or myths? A re-evaluation of cases of diagnosed tuberculosis in Denmark. In: Pálfi G, Dutour O, Deák J, and Hutás I (eds.). *Tuberculosis: Past and Present.* Szeged: Golden Book Publishers, 1999, 511–18.

74. Mays S, and Taylor GM. A first prehistoric case of tuberculosis from Britain. *Int J Osteoarchaeol.* 2003;13:189–96.

75. Mays S et al. Paleopathological and biomolecular study of tuberculosis in a medieval skeletal collection from England. *Am J Phys Anthropol.* 2001;114:298–311.

76. Jankauskas R. History of human tuberculosis in Lithuania: Possibilities and limitations of paleoosteological evidences. *Bull Mém Soc Anthropol Paris. New Ser* 1998;10:357–74.

77. Faerman M, and Jankauskas R. Osteological and molecular evidence of human tuberculosis in Lithuania during the last two millennia. *Sci Israel Technol Adv.* 1999;1:75–8.

78. Jankauskas R. Tuberculosis in Lithuania: Palaeopathological and historical correlations. In: Pálfi G, Dutour O, Deák J, and Hutás I (eds.). *Tuberculosis: Past and Present.* Szeged: Golden Book Publishers, 1999, 551–8.

79. Morel MMP, Demetz J-L, and Sauetr M-R. Un mal de Pott du cimitère burgonde de Saint-Prex, canton de Vaud (Suisse) (5me, 6me, 7me siècles). *Lyon Med.* 1961;40:643–59.

80. Pálfi G, and Marcsik A. Paleoepidemiological data of tuberculosis in Hungary. In: Pálfi G, Dutour O, Deák J, and Hutás I (eds.). *Tuberculosis: Past and Present.* Szeged: Golden Book Publishers, 1999, 533–9.

81. Haas CJ, Zink A, and Molnár E. Molecular evidence for tuberculosis in Hungarian skeletal samples. In: Pálfi G, Dutour O, Deák J, and Hutás I (eds.). *Tuberculosis: Past and Present.* Szeged: Golden Book Publishers, 1999, 385–91.

82. Pap I et al. 18th–19th century tuberculosis in naturally mummified individuals (Vác, Hungary). In: Pálfi G, Dutour O, Deák J, and Hutás I (eds.). *Tuberculosis: Past and Present.* Szeged: Golden Book Publishers, 1999, 421–42.

83. Arcini C. *Health and Disease in Early Lund. Osteo-Pathologic Studies of 3,305 Individuals Buried in the First Cemetery Area of Lund 990–1536.* Lund: Department of Community Health Sciences, University of Lund, 1999.

84. Horácková L, Vargová L, Horváth R, and Bartoš M. Morphological, roentgenological and molecular analyses in bone specimens attributed to tuberculosis, Moravia (Czech Republic). In: Pálfi G, Dutour O, Deák J et al. (eds.). *Tuberculosis: Past and Present.* Szeged: Golden Book Publishers, 1999, 413–17.

85. Kiple K (ed.). *The Cambridge World History of Human Disease.* Cambridge: Cambridge University Press, 1993.

86. Morse D. Tuberculosis. In: Brothwell D, and Sandison AT (eds.). *Diseases in Antiquity.* Springfield: Charles C Thomas, 1967, 249–71.

87. Suzuki T, and Inoue T. Earliest evidence of spinal tuberculosis from the Neolithic Yaoi period in Japan. *Int J Osteoarchaeol.* 2007;17:392–402.

88. Suzuki T, Fujita H, and Choi JG. Brief communication: New evidence of tuberculosis from prehistoric Korea—Population movement and early evidence of tuberculosis in Far East Asia. *Am J Phys Anthropol.* 2008;136:357–60.

89. Tayles N, and Buckley HR. Leprosy and tuberculosis in Iron Age Southeast Asia? *Am J Phys Anthropol.* 2004;125:239–56.

90. Pietruwesky M, and Douglas MT. An osteological assessment of health and disease in precontact and historic (1778) Hawai'i. In: Larsen CS, and Milner GR (eds.). *In the Wake of Contact. Biological Responses to Conquest.* New York: Wiley-Liss, 1994, 179–96.

91. Pietrusewsky M, Douglas MT, Kalima PA, and Ikehara R. *Human skeletal and dental remains from Honokahua burial site, Hawai'i.* Paul H Rosendahl Inc. Archaeological, Historical and Cultural Resource Management Studies and Services. Report 246-041091, 1991.

92. Trembly D. A germ's journey to isolated islands. *Int J Osteoarchaeol.* 1997;7:621–4.

93. Platt C. *Medieval England. A Social History and Archaeology from the Conquest to 1600 AD.* London: Routledge, 1997.

94. Dyer C. *Standards of Living in the Later Middle Ages. Social Change c.1200–1520,* Rev ed. Cambridge: Cambridge University Press, 1989.

95. Crawfurd R. *The King's Evil.* Oxford: Oxford University Press, 1911.

96. Whitney WF. Notes on the anomalies, injuries and diseases of the bones of the native races of North America. *Annu Rep Trustees Peabody Museum Am Archeol Ethnol* 1886;3:433–48.

97. Lichtor J, and Lichtor A. Paleopathological evidence suggesting pre-Columbian tuberculosis of the spine. *J Bone Joint Surg* 1952;39A:1398–9.

98. Judd NM. *The Material Culture of Pueblo Bonito.* Washington, DC: Smithsonian Institution Miscellaneous Collections, Vol. 124, 1954.

99. García-Frías JE. La tuberculosis en los antiguos Peruanos. *Actualidad Médica Peruana* 1940;5:274–91.

100. Morse D. Prehistoric tuberculosis in America. *Am Rev Respir Dis* 1961;85:489–504.

101. Buikstra JE. Paleoepidemiology of tuberculosis in the Americas. In: Pálfi G, Dutour O, Deák J et al. (eds.). *Tuberculosis: Past and Present.* Szeged: Golden Book Publishers, 1999, 479–94.

102. Milner GR. *The Cahokia Chiefdom: The Archeology of a Mississippian Society.* Washington, DC: Smithsonian Institution Press, 1998.

103. Gregg ML. A population estimate for Cahokia. *Perspectives in Cahokia Archeology.* Bulletin 10. Urbana: Illinois Archaeological Survey, 1975, 126–36.

104. Black FL. Infectious disease in primitive societies. *Science.* 1975;187:515–18.

105. Pfeiffer S. Rib lesions and New World tuberculosis. *Int J Osteoarchaeol.* 1991;1:191–8.

106. Milner GR, and Smith VG. Oneota human skeletal remains. In: Santure SK, Harn AD, and Esarey D (eds.). *Archeological Investigations at the Morton Village and Norris Farms 36 Cemetery.* Reports of Investigations 45. Springfield: Illinois State Museum, 1990, 111–48.

107. Buikstra JE. Differential diagnosis: An epidemiological model. *Yearb Phys Anthropol.* 1977;20:316–28.

108. Eisenberg LE. Adaptation in a 'marginal' Mississippian population from Middle Tennessee. Biocultural insights from palaeopathology. New York University, unpublished PhD thesis, 1986.

109. Dean JS, Doelle WH, and Orcutt JD. Adaptive stress, environment and demography. In: Gumerman GJ (ed.). *Themes in Southwest Prehistory*. Santa Fe: School of American Research Press, 1994, 53–86.

110. Cordell LS. *Archaeology of the Southwest*, 2nd ed. San Diego: Academic Press, 1997.

111. Storey R. *Life and Death in the Ancient City of Teotihuacan*. Tuscaloosa: University of Alabama Press, 1992.

112. Kerr J. *The Maya Vase Book. A Corpus of Rollout Photographs of Maya Vases*. New York: Kerr Associates, 1989.

113. Buikstra JE, and Williams S. Tuberculosis in the Americas: Current perspectives. In: Ortner D, and Aufderheide AC (eds.). *Human Paleopathology. Current Syntheses and Future Options*. Washington, DC: Smithsonian Institution Press, 1991, 161–72.

114. Requena A. Evidencia de tuberculosis en la América pre-Columbia. *Acta Venezolana* 1945;1:1–20.

115. Allison MJ et al. Tuberculosis in pre-Columbian Andean populations. In: Buikstra JE (ed.). *Prehistoric Tuberculosis in the Americas*. Evanston: Northwestern University, 1981, 49–51.

116. Romero Arateco WM. *Estudio bioanthropologico de las momias de la Casa del Marque de San Jorge de Fondo de Promocion de la Cultura, Banco Popular, Bogota*. Carrera de Antropologia, Universidad Nacional de Colombia, 1998.

117. Stead WW et al. When did M. tuberculosis infection first occur in the New World? An important question for public health implications. *Am J Resp Crit Care Med* 2000;151:1267–8.

118. Clabeaux MS. Health and disease in the population of an Iroquois ossuary. *Yearb Phys Anthropol*. 1977;20:359–70.

119. Pfeiffer S, and Fairgrieve S. Evidence from ossuaries: The effect of contact on the health of Iroquians. In: Larsen CS, and Milner GR (eds.). *In the Wake of Contact. Biological Responses to Conquest*. New York: Wiley-Liss, 1994, 47–61.

120. Keers RY. Laënnec: A medical history. *Thorax*. 1981;36:91–4.

121. Lutwick LI. Introduction. In: Lutwick LI (ed.). *Tuberculosis*. London: Chapman and Hall Medical, 1995, 1–4.

122. Sontag S. *Illness as Metaphor. AIDS and Its Metaphors*. London: Penguin, 1991.

123. Bryder L. 'A health resort for consumptives'. Tuberculosis and immigration to New Zealand 1880–1914. *Med Hist*. 1996;40: 453–71.

124. Clarke HD. The impact of tuberculosis on history, literature and art. *Med Hist*. 1962;6:301–18.

125. Cockburn A. *The Evolution and Eradication of Infectious Disease*. Baltimore: Johns Hopkins University Press, 1963.

126. Brown T, and Brown K. *Biomolecular Archaeology. An Introduction*. New York: Wiley-Liss, 2011.

127. Stone AC. DNA analysis of archaeological remains. In: Katzenberg MA, and Saunders SR (eds.). *Biological Anthropology of the Human Skeleton*. New York: Wiley-Liss, 2008, 461–83.

128. Cooper A, and Poinar HN. Ancient DNA: Do it right or not at all. *Science*. 2000;289:1139–41.

129. Wilbur AK et al. Deficiencies and challenges in the study of ancient tuberculosis DNA. *J Archaeol Sci*. 2009;36:1990–7.

130. Roberts CA, and Ingham S. Using ancient DNA analysis in palaeopathology: A critical analysis of published papers and recommendations for future work. *Int J Osteoarchaeol*. 2008;18:600–13.

131. Taylor MM, Crossley M, Saldanha J, and Waldron T. DNA from M. tuberculosis identified in Medieval human skeletal remains using PCR. *J Archaeol Sci*. 1996;23:789–98.

132. Haas CJ et al. Molecular evidence for different stages of tuberculosis in ancient bone samples from Hungary. *Am J Phys Anthrop* 2000;113:293–304.

133. Gernaey A et al. Correlation of the occurrence of mycolic acids with tuberculosis in an archaeological population. In: Pálfi G, Dutour O,

Deák J, and Hutás I (eds.). *Tuberculosis: Past and Present*. Szeged: Golden Book Publishers, 1999, 275–82.

134. Taylor GM et al. First report of *Mycobacterium bovis* DNA human remains from the Iron Age. *Microbiology* 2007;153:1243–9.

135. Zink AR et al. Molecular history of tuberculosis from ancient mummies and skeletons. *Int J Osteoarchaeol*. 2007;17:380–91.

136. Fletcher HA et al. Molecular analysis of *Mycobacterium tuberculosis* DNA from a family of 18th century Hungarians. *Microbiology* 2003;149:143–51.

137. Müller R, Roberts CA, and Brown TA. Genotyping of ancient *Mycobacterium tuberculosis* strains reveals historic genetic diversity. *Proc Roy Soc. B* 2014; 281(1781): 20133236.

138. Bos K et al. pre-Columbian mycobacterial genomes reveal seals as a source of New World human tuberculosis. *Nature*, 2014;514(7523): 494–7.

139. Spigelman M, and Lemma E. The use of polymerase chain reaction (PCR) to detect *Mycobacterium tuberculosis* in ancient skeletons. *Int J Osteoarchaeol*. 1993;3:137–43.

140. Braun M, Cook D, and Pfeiffer S. DNA from *Mycobacterium tuberculosis* complex identified in North American pre-Columbian human skeletal remains. *J Archaeol Sci*. 1998;25:271–7.

141. Arriaza B, Salo W, Aufderheide AC, and Holcomb TA. Pre-Columbian tuberculosis in Northern Chile: Molecular and skeletal evidence. *Am J Phys Anthrop* 1995;98:37–45.

142. Taylor GM et al. Genotypic analysis of *Mycobacterium tuberculosis* from medieval human remains. *Microbiology* 1999;145:899–904.

143. Pálfi G et al. Coexistence of tuberculosis and ankylosing spondylitis in a 7th–8th century specimen evidenced by molecular biology. In: Pálfi G, Dutour O, Deák J, and Hutás I (eds.). *Tuberculosis: Past and Present*. Szeged: Golden Book Publishers, 1999, 403–9.

144. Faerman M et al. Prevalence of human tuberculosis in a Medieval population of Lithuania studied by ancient DNA analysis. *Anc Biomol* 1997;1:205–14.

145. Mehaafy MC, Kruh-Garcia NA, and Dobos KM. Prospective on *Mycobacterium tuberculosis* proteomics. *J Proteom Res* 2012;11: 17–25.

146. Boros-Major A et al. New perspectives in biomolecular palaeopathology of ancient tuberculosis: A proteomic approach. *J Archaeol Sci*. 2011;38:197–201.

147. Bouwman AS, Bunning SL, Müller R, Holst M, Caffell AC, Roberts CA, and Brown TA. The genotype of a historic strain of *Mycobacterium tuberculosis*. *Proceedings of the National Academy of Science* 2012;109:18511–6.

148. Guichón RA, Buikstra JE, Stone AC, Harkins KM, Suby JA, Massone M, Wilbur A, Constantinescu F, and Martín CR. Pre-Columbian tuberculosis in Tierra del Fuego? Discussion of the paleopathological and molecular evidence. *Int J Paleopathol*. 2015; 11:92–101.

149. Guthrie D. *A History of Medicine*. London: Thomas Nelson, 1945.

150. Pesanti EL. A short history of tuberculosis. In: Lutwick LI (ed.). *Tuberculosis*. London: Chapman and Hall Medical, 1995, 5–19.

151. Howe GM. *People, Environment, Disease and Death. A Medical Geography of Britain through the Ages*. Cardiff: University of Wales Press, 1997.

152. Roberts CA, and Bernard MC. Tuberculosis: A biosocial study of admissions to a children's sanatorium (1936–1954) in Stannington, Northumberland, England. *Tuberculosis* 2015; 95:S105–8.

153. Meachen NG. *A Short History of Tuberculosis*. London: Staples Press, 1936.

154. Bryder L. *Below the Magic Mountain. A Social History of Tuberculosis in 20th Century Britain*. Oxford: Clarendon Press, 1988.

155. Glaziou P et al. Lives saved by tuberculosis control and prospects for achieving the 2015 global target for reducing tuberculosis mortality. *Bull World Health Organ*. 2011;89:573–82.

Epidemiology

GRANT THERON, TED COHEN, AND CHRISTOPHER DYE

THE LENGTH AND BREADTH OF TUBERCULOSIS EPIDEMIOLOGY

Why did tuberculosis (TB) decline in Europe and North America for much of the nineteenth and twentieth centuries but not elsewhere? What is the current direction of the global TB epidemic? How can we improve control of TB epidemics in line with ambitious global policy goals to end TB by 2035[1]? This overview of TB epidemiology is structured around ten such questions about the distribution and control of the disease in human populations (Table 2.1).

The chapter has two more general themes. The first is that we cannot fully address the questions in Table 2.1 without considering the disease agent (*M. tuberculosis*), the host (humans), and the environment (e.g., migration, living conditions) as dynamic, interacting entities. Conventional tools of epidemiology such as cross-sectional, case–control, cohort studies and experimental trials,[2] which often employ molecular methods to analyze and trace strains (i.e., molecular epidemiology), allow us to assess risk factors for infection, disease, and treatment outcomes, but these studies do not usually inform long-term projection of disease trends or population-wide impact of interventions. For instance, a new vaccine found to have a protective efficacy of 70% against pulmonary TB in adults would be a breakthrough for TB control, but by knowing only the protective efficacy, we could not predict the community-wide impact of a vaccination program over 10 years. That understanding requires a knowledge of events that happen through interactions among individuals and across bacterial and human generations—of processes that can be understood and measured in terms of case reproduction numbers, heterogeneity in transmission, herd immunity, feedback loops, equilibrium, and evolutionary selective pressure.[3]

The second theme is that ending TB will require epidemiologists to take an imaginative and unrestricted view of the opportunities for intervention. Over the past 25 years, the chemotherapy of active TB, delivered initially under the rubric of the WHO directly observed therapy strategy (DOTS) (first extended as the stop TB strategy[4] and now succeeded by the end TB strategy[1]), has come to be accepted as the cornerstone of good TB management. As a model of delivery, standardization, and evaluation, DOTS represented a major advance in the attack, not just on TB, but also on the principal endemic diseases of the developing world.[3–5] However, DOTS did not sufficiently explain how TB programs could improve case detection and cure, especially by addressing broader social (e.g., financial support), behavioral (e.g., tobacco smoking), environmental (e.g., air pollution), and clinical (e.g., HIV) risks. The elimination of TB will depend on this, rather than just improving detection and care for individuals with active disease.

The Global Plan to End TB Strategy (2016–2020), framed by the objective of achieving Universal Health Coverage and nested

Table 2.1 Ten leading questions about TB epidemiology

1. What is the burden of TB worldwide, and which countries are most affected?
2. Why does *M. tuberculosis* cause epidemics of a low-incidence disease that run over centuries?
3. Why do some people get TB and not others?
4. Why did TB decline in Europe and North America for most of the twentieth century?
5. What factors explain resurgences of TB, like those seen in Africa and the former Soviet countries since 1990?
6. Do differences in *M. tuberculosis* strains modify the natural history, epidemiology, and control of TB epidemics?
7. How does TB interact with other diseases?
8. How can current tools, including broader interventions that address risk factors for poor health and strengthen health systems, be used to better control TB epidemics?
9. Will TB become resistant to all antibiotics?
10. How can the use of novel tools and pharmacological interventions (e.g., diagnostics, drugs, and vaccines) be informed by lessons learned from the recent implementation of advances (e.g., Xpert MTB/RIF)?

within the Sustainable Development Goals, represents a new plan by which the global community hopes to end TB by 2035.[173] The End TB Strategy requires treating 29 million people with TB, preventing 45 million people from getting TB, and averting the catastrophic costs that patients and their families face due to TB. The objective of Universal Health Coverage will address some of DOTS' prior limitations and ultimately enhance the End TB Strategy not only by drawing attention to cross-cutting risk factors that impact TB (e.g., alcohol) and were previously siloed by most national TB programs, but by incorporating these factors into the global TB reporting infrastructure, highlighting opportunities for targeted interventions. If widely implemented, the plan could result in a reduction in TB deaths by 90% and reduce the incidence rate (defined as the number of new cases per 100,000 population per year) by 80% (<20/100,000) compared to 2015.[1,5] As we argue in this chapter, new perspectives, tools, and approaches are needed to accomplish these lofty goals. This requires, but by no means is limited to, drastically accelerating the hitherto slow decline in the epidemic, reducing the incidence of multidrug-resistant (MDR) TB, increasing the targeting of vulnerable populations in a cost-effective manner using new tools, and, importantly, empowering national TB programs to better use local epidemiological data for decision making. Ultimately, all of this is underscored by a need to massively increase funding for TB, to support both research and programmatic implementation.[6]

WHAT IS THE BURDEN OF TB WORLDWIDE, AND WHICH COUNTRIES ARE MOST AFFECTED?

Based on notification reports and surveys, there were an estimated 10.4 million new TB cases in 2016. Assuming lifelong infection, about a quarter of humanity is infected with *M. tuberculosis*.[7] Most of the estimated cases in 2016 occurred in the WHO Southeast Asian Region (45%) followed by the WHO African Region (25%), where the burden of HIV-associated TB is highest and exceeds 50% in southern Africa. Despite having a lower incidence, extremely populous countries like India nevertheless account for a large proportion of the new cases (∼1 in 5) and TB deaths (∼1 in 4) worldwide.[8]

Although the overall burden of disease is still large, there has been substantial progress in worldwide TB control. In a reversal of patterns in the 1990s, the global incidence rate of TB has been declining since 2002 and the absolute number of new cases per year has been decreasing since 2006.[5] While this represents an achievement, the overall rate of decline in per capita is slow (2% per year), and needs to accelerate (4%–5% per year) to reach the 2020 milestones of the End TB Strategy (Figure 2.1).[5,8] Furthermore, some countries and regions (e.g., China, India) are still experiencing an increase in TB incidence and MDR TB.

Over the past two decades, while Asian countries had the most cases, countries in Africa and Eastern Europe have reflected global trends in incidence (Figure 2.1). Countries within sub-Saharan Africa and the former Soviet Union showed the greatest increases in case load during the 1990s and, despite falling case numbers in other parts of the world (principally West and Central Europe, the Americas, and the Eastern Mediterranean regions), were responsible for the overall rise in TB incidence per capita during the late 1990s and early 2000s. However, since 2013, most of the global increase in notifications is driven by India, with an estimated 37% increase from 2013 to 2016.[8]

TB prevalence (the estimated number of extant TB cases at a specific time) is falling more quickly than incidence (Figure 2.2). At the present rate, the global TB incidence will decrease from ∼125/100,000 to ∼100/100,000 by 2035 yet, under the Global Plan accelerated investment scenario, it is expected to reach ∼100/100,000 before 2020, before finally reaching elimination levels by 2035 (≤10/100,000).

There were approximately 1.7 million deaths from TB in 2016, of which one in five were in HIV co-infected individuals. TB is the world's leading killer among infectious agents,[3] with an overall estimated case fatality of 16% (deaths among all TB cases/total number of incident TB cases). Mortality is substantially higher among individuals with untreated HIV-co-infection and for individuals with drug-resistant TB. While these statistics are grim, both regional and global mortality estimates are declining. From 1990 to 2010, global TB mortality had declined by more than one-third in HIV-uninfected patients while the incidence in HIV-infected patients slowly declined (Figure 2.2).[8] The Stop TB Partnership goal of halving overall TB mortality rates compared with a 1990 baseline was met by 2015, but not in all regions (most notably Africa).

Although TB is among the top ten overall causes of illness and disability,[11] estimation of burden remains imprecise, especially in high-burden countries where precision is most needed.[12,13] Since 2002, national surveys of the prevalence of TB disease, which are done in a random cross-section of the population, have been undertaken in well over 20 countries and more are scheduled within the next few years. These surveys provide vital data in high-burden settings, but the world as a whole cannot be feasibly surveyed. Investment in high-quality routine surveillance

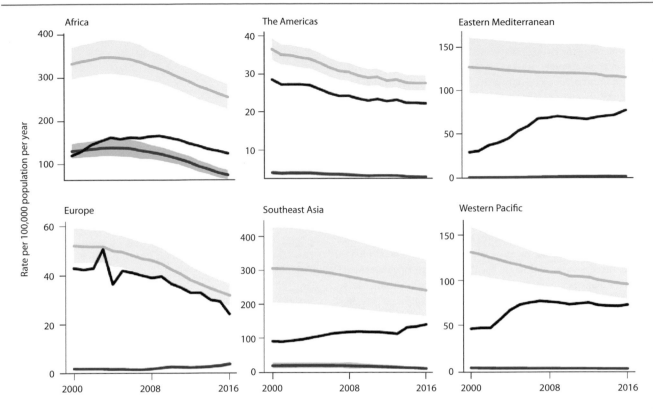

Figure 2.1 Regional trends in estimated TB incidence rates by WHO region, 2000–2016. Total TB incidence rates are shown in green and incidence rates of HIV-positive TB are shown in red. Shaded areas represent uncertainty intervals. The black lines show notifications of new and relapse cases for comparison with estimates of the total incidence rate. (Taken from the WHO.[8])

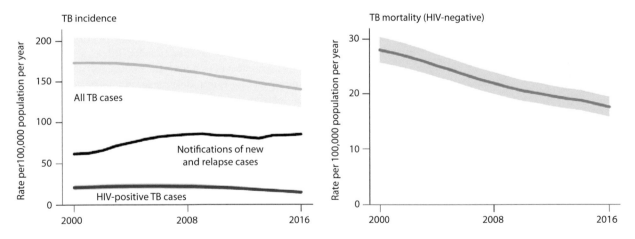

Figure 2.2 Global trends in estimated TB incidence and mortality rates, 2000–2016. Shaded areas represent uncertainty intervals. (Taken from the WHO.[8])

and innovative targeted sampling methods that build on systems already in place are needed to produce robust data for assessment and future planning.[13,14]

WHY DOES *M. TUBERCULOSIS* CAUSE EPIDEMICS OF A LOW-INCIDENCE DISEASE THAT RUN OVER CENTURIES?

Remarkably, the interaction between *M. tuberculosis* and humans is relatively low compared to the enormous burden of suffering

in at least three respects. First, as a rule of thumb, untreated sputum smear-positive cases infect 5–10 other individuals each year.[15-17] For a prevalence of smear-positive disease of 0.1% (i.e., 100/100,000, a little less than the estimated global average of 122/100,000) an average contact rate of 10 per year would generate an annual risk of infection of 1%. Second, only about 5%–10% of infected individuals (in the absence of other predisposing conditions) develop "progressive primary" disease following infection and this proportion is lower in children and higher in adults.[18-20] Third, the progression from infection to disease is slow, averaging 2–4 years.[21,22] After 5 years, there is a low annual risk of developing TB by "reactivation" of infection that is then said to be "latent."

Augmenting the strong innate resistance to developing disease, infection is associated with an acquired immune response. This acquired immunity can be only partially protective against active disease,[18–20,23] however, infected persons living in an endemic area remain at high risk of TB because of the continuing threat of reinfection.[19,24–28]

The low probability of progression to symptomatic disease explains why population-level incidence of active TB is low. Thus, tuberculosis's importance among infectious diseases is largely attributable to the high case fatality rate among untreated or improperly treated cases (e.g., only half of MDR cases are diagnosed worldwide). About two-thirds of untreated smear-positive cases die within 5–8 years, the majority within the first 2 years.[15,29] The case fatality rate for untreated smear-negative cases, who generally have less advanced disease and fewer bacilli in sputum (making them harder to diagnose by microscopy and even new PCR tests[30]), is lower but still 10%–15%.[31,32] Even among smear-positive patients receiving treatment, case fatality can exceed 10% if adherence is low, or if rates of HIV infection and drug resistance are high.[5]

The longer-term consequences of this host–pathogen relationship can be explored by a simple mathematical model (Figure 2.3).[33] Individuals in a population are assigned to mutually exclusive states of infection and disease, and the natural history described previously specifies the rates of flow between states. TB models generate slow epidemics that peak after several

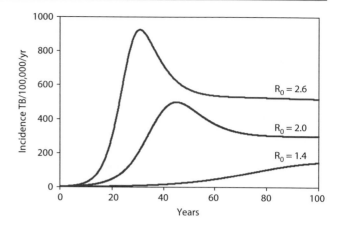

Figure 2.4 Model TB epidemics generated for three different basic case reproduction numbers (R_0). The mathematical model is described in Dye and Williams.[279]

decades, typically at an incidence rate below 1% (Figure 2.4).[24,34–36] More complex models with additional compartments that reflect, for example, heterogeneity in disease and transmission are often required, and the parameters depend on the question for which the model is designed. The accuracy and usefulness of models is, of course, dependent on how well described these parameters are for different settings, making those that are poorly characterized yet influential for model behavior important focus areas for clinical research.[37] Even though models are often based on assumptions, they are useful where there is limited data and policy makers or health programs need to make urgent decisions and focus limited resources on key areas.

One composite epidemic parameter of critical importance is the basic case reproduction number (R_0), which is defined as the average number of secondary infectious cases generated when one infectious case is introduced into an uninfected population. For an infection to spread, R_0 must exceed 1. Because active TB can arise via three different routes, and typically with a considerable time delay after infection, it is not straightforward to calculate an exact R_0.[38] However, rough estimates of R_0 for TB are relatively low among infectious diseases, on the order of 2 in untreated populations.[39] For $R_0 = 2$, the expected doubling time of a TB epidemic in its early stages is 4–5 years, meaning that epidemics of a single strain can extend for many decades (Figure 2.4).[35] Although large human populations uninfected with TB no longer exist, the concept of R_0 remains useful because it guides thinking about a wide range of epidemiological processes. This could, for example, include the transition from predominantly acquired drug-resistant TB in the past to an epidemic that is now dominated by primary transmission,[40] requiring a new look at the projected efficacy of different control methods on epidemics' trajectories.

WHY DID TB DECLINE IN EUROPE AND NORTH AMERICA FOR MOST OF THE TWENTIETH CENTURY?

The model described earlier can be used to produce projections of the trajectory of epidemics. Figure 2.4 shows the incidence of

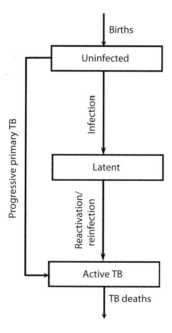

Figure 2.3 A simple compartmental model of TB epidemiology. Individuals within a population are assigned to the mutually exclusive states uninfected, latent, and with active TB (boxes), and the arrows represent possible transitions between states. Active TB (progressive primary disease, usually taken to be within 5 years) can develop soon after infection, or after a period of latency by reactivation or reinfection. Most mathematical models are more complex than the scheme represented here, distinguishing, for example, infectious from non-infectious disease, or allowing for different rates of progression among HIV-infected and uninfected individuals.

TB eventually reaching a steady state. Case reports suggest that TB incidence has been nearly steady for at least two decades in some Southeast Asian countries (Figure 2.1), but equilibrium was never reached in Western Europe or the Americas. TB has been in decline since per capita incidence rates peaked in industrialized countries, probably sometime during the early nineteenth century and certainly before chemotherapy began in the 1950s (Figure 2.5).[41] Some of this decline could be due to the natural waning of the epidemic (Figure 2.4),[35] but the trend was too prolonged for this to provide the whole explanation. In this respect, then, this very basic model appears to be wrong.

The reasons for the sustained 150-year decline have been the subject of perennial debate,[42] with three broad proposed explanations: (1) reduced opportunities for transmission per case, (2) reduced susceptibility of contacts, and (3) reduced virulence of the pathogen. Fewer transmissions per infectious case may have occurred because of lower living density or better ventilation within homes or because of patient isolation within sanatoria. As the disease declined, an upward shift in the average age of cases may have resulted in less opportunity for spread in the population if elderly cases had fewer contacts.[43] Assuming that no other concomitant change in risk of disease occurred, one analysis suggested that the number of effective contacts per infectious case fell from 22 in England and Wales in 1900 to about 10 by 1950.[44]

Yet, there also may have been other factors affecting susceptibility of contacts that contributed to this decline. Nutrition improved,[45] and is linked to susceptibility[46] and can reduce incidence in children (but not transmission).[47] Susceptibility is also under genetic control and, with 15%–30% of deaths in cities of the USA attributable to TB during the early nineteenth century,[48] most of them among young adults of reproductive age, there must have been some selective pressure. However, at least one analysis suggests that natural selection by pulmonary TB is unlikely to have played a major role in the decline of TB prior to the availability of anti-TB drugs.[49]

The third explanation is that *M. tuberculosis* has generally become less pathogenic. Intriguingly, irreversible genetic deletions may have produced phenotypes of *M. tuberculosis* less likely to cause cavitary pulmonary disease,[50,51] but it remains to be proven that these types of deletion events occurred more rapidly than the sporadic appearance of novel, virulent variants. Indeed, some apparently virulent strains are associated with novel genetic deletions[52] and more generally, some emergent strains of *M. tuberculosis*, including some in the Beijing group, are relatively virulent and harbor significant levels of drug resistance with a propensity toward developing compensatory mutations.[53,54]

It is not possible to disentangle the factors contributing to TB decline before the widespread introduction of chemotherapy. For example, the city of Cape Town, which had a similar incidence as New York City and London at the start of the twentieth century, introduced contemporaneous measures of TB control prior to chemotherapy (e.g., tuberculin testing, pneumothorax, milk pasteurization), yet while incidence and mortality fell in New York City and London, they diverged dramatically in Cape Town.[41] Whatever the exact causes of this decline in the West are, however, these processes together caused a fall in the TB death rate per capita in Western Europe of only 5% per year in the era before chemotherapy. Environmental and nutritional improvements will have benefits beyond those related to a specific disease, but it is doubtful that they can be employed as powerful instruments for TB control, especially in the short term. However, this requires investigation (e.g., observational data on TB incidence as cities embark on initiatives to reduce air pollution, community cluster randomized-controlled trials of a school feeding program in impoverished areas).

WHY DO SOME PEOPLE GET TB AND NOT OTHERS?

The simple model described earlier captures some of the typical behavior of TB epidemics, but there are important variations on this basic theme. Some variations have been discovered through investigations of epidemiological "risk factors" that influence the probability of infection, disease, or outcome and operate on many scales (e.g., physiological, genetic, and behavioral). The goal of risk factor analysis is to try to identify the principal causal and modifiable factors affecting TB epidemiology.

A small selection of known host-related risk factors is given in Table 2.2, classified in terms of the *M. tuberculosis* life cycle rather than an epidemiologic scale.[32] HIV co-infection dramatically increases the risk of TB disease following primary infection, and promotes the reactivation of latent infection. In HIV-co-infected versus uninfected individuals, the average relative risk of developing TB was found in one study to be 28 over 25 months.[55] This risk increases as host immunity is progressively impaired.[56–61]

Although HIV is much more detrimental than other documented risk factors such as diabetes,[62,63] alcohol,[64] silicosis,[65] malnutrition,[46,66–68] and indoor air pollution,[40] the cumulative impact of a risk factor at population level depends on the number of people exposed as well as the risk to each person exposed. Consequently, some factors that only minimally elevate risks among individuals can be responsible for a large proportion of disease in a population if those factors are very common. As determinants of the total

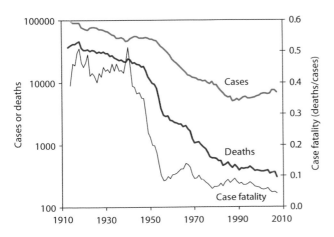

Figure 2.5 Decline in TB cases and deaths in England and Wales from 1912. Case fatality remained at 40%–50% until TB drugs became available during the 1940s, fell sharply into the 1950s and more slowly thereafter. (Data from UK Health Protection Agency.)

Table 2.2 Selected host-related risk factors for infection, progression to active TB, and adverse outcomes of disease. Factors can elevate risk across multiple phases of TB disease

Risk factor	Type of study	Source
Infection		
Increased risk of TB among healthcare workers	Retrospective ecologic	[70]
TB among the homeless associated with recent transmission	Retrospective analysis of strain clusters	[71]
HIV-positive TB patients less likely to infect contacts than HIV-negatives	Cohort	[72]
Childhood infection linked to consumption of unpasteurized milk or cheese	Case—control	[73]
Household contacts of infectious TB case at increased risk of infection	Case—control	[74]
Cigarette smokers at increased risk of infection	Meta-analysis of cohort and case—control studies	[75,76]
Progression to disease		
HIV increases the risk of recurrent TB via reinfection	Cohort	[77]
TB associated with cigarette smoking	Meta-analysis of cohort and case—control studies	[75,76]
TB associated with diabetes mellitus	Meta-analysis of cohort and case—control studies	[63]
TB associated with exposure to smoke from biomass stoves	Case—control	[78]
TB associated with intake of dietary iron from traditional beer	Case—control	[79]
Vitamin D deficiency associated with active TB, facilitated by polymorphism in the vitamin D receptor gene	Case—control	[80,81]
NRAMP1 polymorphisms associated with smear-positive pulmonary TB	Case—control	[82]
Adverse outcome of disease		
Malnutrition associated with early mortality in a cohort of patients with high HIV infection	Cohort	[83]
Women at higher risk of carrying MDR-TB	Retrospective analysis of strain clusters	[84]
Previously treated TB patients less likely to adhere to therapy	Cohort	[85]
Severity of pulmonary disease associated with death among hospitalized patients	Cross-sectional	[86]
Non-adherence to treatment linked to alcoholism, injection drug use, homelessness, less morbidity, psychological distress, and poorer health literacy	Cohort	[87,88]
Mortality is higher for cigarette smokers	Meta-analysis of cohort and case—control studies	[75,76]
Diabetes mellitus is associated with increased rates of mortality and relapse	Meta-analysis of cohort and case—control studies	[89]
Cavitation on initial chest radiograph or 2-month positive culture associated with relapse	Retrospective cohort study	[90]

number of TB cases, tobacco smoking in Asia and malnutrition in Africa could rival the importance of HIV.[8,69]

Besides environmental factors and concomitant illness, infection and the progression to active TB are also under human genetic control. That TB runs in families is well known but this observation confounds genes and possible transmission due to close contact. Among the genes associated with susceptibility to TB (e.g., twin studies, case—control studies) are those encoding the vitamin D receptor, natural resistance associated macrophage protein (NRAMP1), HLA, mannose binding lectin (MBL), ASAP1 actin and membrane remodeling protein, and the Toll-like receptors.[91–100] Associations between human genetic polymorphisms and disease risk, clinical presentation, or outcome are typically determined by the interactions between genes and their environment.[101,102] Investigations of genetic determinants have thus not yielded consistent results, as illustrated by studies of vitamin D receptor polymorphisms[97,103] and clinical trials evaluating vitamin D supplementation describing an overall lack of impact on TB treatment outcomes.[104]

In sum, the standard picture of *M. tuberculosis* as the agent of slow epidemics is a useful frame of reference, but certain co-factors can profoundly alter TB epidemiology. Above all, we still have no more than a superficial understanding of why only a small fraction of infections ultimately result in clinical disease. Unlocking this is a major research priority, and could reveal targets for TB control (e.g., vaccine development to prevent progression to active disease), diagnostics (e.g., to identify and triage patients who will imminently progress), and permit more accurate modeling (and thus targeting of interventions to high-risk groups).

WHAT FACTORS CAN EXPLAIN RESURGENCES OF TB, LIKE THOSE SEEN IN AFRICA AND THE FORMER SOVIET COUNTRIES SINCE 1990?

Preventing and controlling epidemics of TB requires measuring and understanding the factors that drive increases in incidence. In Africa, spatial and temporal variation in TB incidence is correlated strongly with HIV prevalence.[105] The WHO Africa region contributes 34% of the HIV-positive TB caseload. In 2016,

82% of TB patients in Africa had a documented HIV test result, however, Africa had the lowest rate of antiretroviral treatment (ART) initiation in HIV-positive TB cases.[8] Globally, an estimated 13% of all new adult TB cases were HIV-co-infected in 2016 and the percentage of incident TB cases with HIV varied greatly (as low as 2% in the Western Pacific Region). The extent to which HIV is fueling TB transmission (in addition to provoking reactivation) remains poorly understood: one analysis suggested that 1%–2% of all transmission events were from HIV-infected, smear-positive TB cases in 2000[106] and another showed that HIV-infected patients are more likely to be reactivated TB cases rather than primary TB cases.[107] The fraction of the overall force of TB infection attributable to HIV-infected cases depends on the prevalence of HIV as well as the relative infectiousness of HIV-associated TB compared with TB cases not affected by HIV. The relative infectiousness of HIV-associated TB is affected by both host and microbiological factors (e.g., the probability of sputum smear-positive pulmonary disease) and environmental factors that determine the expected duration of infectiousness (e.g., how rapidly cases can access diagnosis and effective treatment). The duration of HIV-associated TB infectiousness appears to vary, being shorter than for HIV-negative TB[108] or about the same[109] depending on the setting; reductions in the per-day infectiousness may be the case where there is a diagnostic delay for HIV-infected patients.[110]

The rise in TB incidence attributable to HIV has evidently peaked in most countries, following the peak in HIV incidence.[111] However, the number of notified HIV-positive TB cases was, in 2016, only 46% of the estimated incidence of TB among people living with HIV[8] suggesting massive under-detection of TB in this vulnerable population. More aggressive implementation of ART,[111,112] combined with other interventions targeted at TB (such as isoniazid preventive therapy [IPT][113] or systematic testing of HIV-positive patients[114]) will help further to reduce the burden of HIV-associated TB.

In Russia and other former-Soviet countries, TB incidence and death increased sharply between 1990 and 2000, but stabilized and now are falling.[8] Understanding precisely why this increase happened is as difficult as understanding the preceding decline. It is clear that there was a marked deterioration in case finding and cure rates in Russia, but this cannot explain all of the rise.[115] Other factors that may have shaped the post-1990 epidemic in Russia include enhanced transmission due to mixing of prison and civilian populations, an increase in susceptibility to disease following infection (possibly linked to stress, malnutrition, and alcoholism), poor service delivery, the spread of drug resistance, and, latterly, HIV infection.[116–119]

Immigration from high-incidence countries is part of the reason why the decline of TB in Western Europe, North America, and the Gulf States has stalled. Many immigrants are infected in their countries of origin and they cause, in varying degrees, further transmission and outbreaks after arrival.[120–125] Furthermore, from 2008 to 2018, the proportion of TB cases in the Western Europe region with an HIV test result that was HIV-positive increased from 3% to 15%.[8]

TB incidence is no longer falling in some East Asian settings, notably Singapore.[8,111] Part of the explanation could be that more cases are arising by reactivation from an aging TB epidemic in an aging human population.[126,127] TB deaths are not frequent enough to cause significant demographic change, but demographic changes can markedly affect TB epidemiology.

DOES VARIATION BETWEEN *M. TUBERCULOSIS* STRAINS MODIFY THE NATURAL HISTORY, EPIDEMIOLOGY, AND CONTROL OF TB EPIDEMICS?

While early targeted genetic analyses (e.g., multilocus sequence typing) suggested minimal within-species diversity of *M. tuberculosis*,[128,129] recent advances using whole genome sequencing and ultra-deep sequencing to uncover minority sub-populations, combined with large public collections of sequencing data from clinical isolates, are allowing new insights into the molecular epidemiology of *M. tuberculosis*.[130,131] These include substantial within-host genetic diversity (especially in immunocompromised patients) that can also be associated with different phenotypes (e.g., drug susceptibility by anatomical site),[132,133] and a new understanding of the global population structure of *M. tuberculosis* lineages (including drug-resistant varieties) and how they have spread around the world[54,130,134–136] (Figure 2.6).

This appreciation of diversity within *M. tuberculosis* has been accompanied by investigations that aim to discover whether differences between (or within[137]) lineages modify the ability of the pathogen to infect hosts or are associated with differences in the natural history of disease.[138] Accumulating evidence suggests that strain lineages vary in strength and mechanism of host-immune stimulation after infection,[53] within-host competitive ability,[139] and in the rates of acquiring mutations[140] and in the specific mutations they preferentially acquire.[141] Each of these dimensions may affect the within-host course of infection, disease, response to therapy, drug susceptibility, and transmission fitness. Early mathematical modeling efforts suggested potential effects of strain diversity on the emergence of drug resistance[142] and the effects of potential interventions.[143,144] Recently, molecular epidemiology studies suggest that, contrary to early work in the 1950s,[145] certain *M. tuberculosis* lineages (e.g., the Beijing family under lineage two) have inherent capacity for rapid evolution of drug resistance and compensatory mutations, which afford the organism more opportunities to develop resistance-causing and/or fitness-promoting mutations, and increased virulence and transmission.[130,146–148] Improving our understanding of the genetic variation in *M. tuberculosis* strains will doubtless improve our ability to predict and intervene in emergent epidemics. This will require additional data on strain molecular epidemiology. Importantly, the routine use of sequencing technologies for drug resistance in the medium term[149,150] may serve as a readily available source of such data. Critically, the value of molecular epidemiology data is enhanced dramatically when paired with patient and other microbiological metadata.[27] On a larger scale, *M. tuberculosis* molecular data can be combined with data on human genetic diversity and movement and, when paired with knowledge of migration explain the dissemination of strains.[148,151,152]

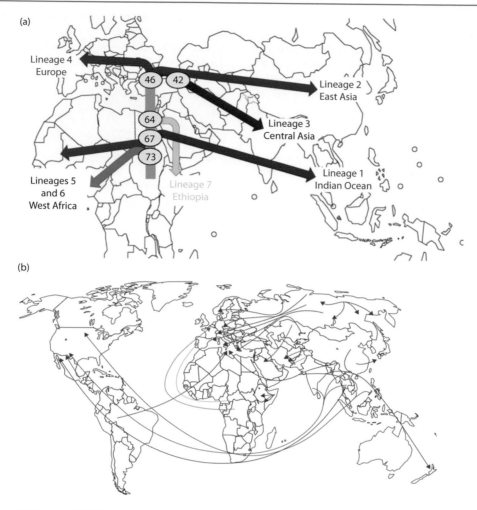

Figure 2.6 The genetic history of MTB corresponds with human migration and movement. (a) Out-of-Africa and Neolithic expansion of MTB reconstructed from phylogeographic and dating analyses that shows a correlation with human migration events, starting ~67 000 years ago with a split in Lineage 1. Major splits are annotated with the median value (in thousands of years) of the dating of the relevant node. Lineage 7 diverged subsequent to the proposed Out-of-Africa migration of MTB complex; it may have arisen among a human population that remained in Africa or a population that returned to Africa. (b) Worldwide spread of drug-resistant strains of MTB. Red = Beijing strain. Green = LAM9 strain. Light blue = Haarlem1 strain. Purple = T1 strain. Dark blue = untyped strains. ([a] From Comas I et al.[152]; [b] From Dheda K et al.[240])

DOES TB INFLUENCE THE EPIDEMIOLOGY OF OTHER DISEASES (OR VICE VERSA)?

Mammalian adaptive immune responses fall into two antagonistic subclasses—Th1 and Th2—each with its own set of cytokine mediators. Microbial infections have the potential to influence the balance between Th1 and Th2 responses by altering cytokine profiles, with positive or negative consequences for health. By influencing Th1/Th2 balance, bacterial infections can play a role in atopy, an allergic state producing mucosal inflammation characteristic of asthma that is characterized by over-reactive Th2 responses.

Because mycobacteria elicit strong Th1 responses, shifting the Th1/Th2 balance away from Th2, *M. tuberculosis* infection may protect against asthma. One study of Japanese children found that strong tuberculin responses, probably attributable to *M.*

tuberculosis exposure, were associated with less asthma, rhinoconjunctivitis, and eczema in later childhood.[153] A study of South African children found an inverse association between *M. tuberculosis* infection and atopic rhinitis.[154] Comparisons among countries have found that asthma tends to be more common where TB is not.[155,156] The implication of the majority of these results of association is that TB may inhibit the spread of atopic disorders in some settings, though there are notable exceptions.[157]

Besides the link between TB and asthma, interactions between other infections have come under investigation. Vigorous Th2 responses are seen in protective immune reactions to helminth infections, and helminths could modulate atopic disease while compromising the immune response to bacille Calmette-Guerin (BCG) and *M. tuberculosis*.[158–160] Another common organism *Helicobacter pylori*, estimated to infect over 4 billion people, may play a role in TB: *H. pylori*-infected macaques challenged with low doses of *M. tuberculosis* are less likely to progress to active TB compared to *H. pylori*-uninfected macaques and, in humans, latently infected household contacts who did not develop active TB within two years were more likely to be infected with *H. pylori* than contacts that go on to develop active disease.[161] Conversely, mice with *Helicobacter hepaticus* (a human pathogen) gut infection have subclinical inflammation, and drastic impairment of immune control of the growth of subsequently administered *M. tuberculosis*, which results in severe lung tissue pathology.[162]

Inversely, a mycobacterial vaccine might be constructed to prevent atopy and asthma. BCG could already serve that purpose, and although the evidence is ambiguous,[158] it may improve non-specific mortality.[163,164] *M. tuberculosis* infection may protect against leprosy, as does BCG,[165] and natural TB transmission could have contributed to the decline of leprosy in Europe.[166] While the synergistic and antagonistic interactions between bacterial, viral, and parasitic infections are complex and unresolved, these examples raise the possibility that mycobacteria influence, and are influenced by, the presence of other infections.

Recently, rapidly rising living standards in settings with a high TB burden (e.g., India) and the increased likelihood of new types of co-epidemics have received attention.[167] For example, obesity will increase and, concomitantly, type II diabetes. Diabetes increases risk of TB 2–3 fold, tuberculosis worsens glycemic control, and drug–drug interactions add complexity to patient management.[168] The number of people with diabetes is expected to grow from 387 million in 2014 to 592 million by 2030, with three-fourths of diabetics living in countries presently classified as low or middle income.[169,170] While the underlying immunological interactions between TB and diabetes are studied,[171] this interaction (as well as that of TB with other non-communicable diseases [NCDs]) requires an integration of health screening and delivery services and has implications for the future reporting of case notifications and monitoring disease. However, it also presents new opportunities for diagnosing and treating both TB and diabetes.[170,172]

HOW CAN CURRENT STRATEGIES BE ENHANCED TO IMPROVE CONTROL OF TB EPIDEMICS?

With this epidemiological background, we can now explore the impact of past control methods of TB. The cornerstone of TB control traditionally focused on the prompt treatment of symptomatic cases with combination chemotherapy, administered through the End TB Strategy's predecessor—the Stop Strategy. Well-implemented standard short-course regimens can cure over 90% of new, drug-susceptible TB cases and these provide a foundation for more complex strategies for control where, for example, rates of drug resistance or HIV infection are high.

Many national TB control programs show that they can achieve high cure rates: the average treatment success rate in 2016 among the 6.3 million new cases was 83%, however, it was worse for drug-resistant TB (54% for MDR/rifampicin-resistant TB and 30% for XDR TB, both 2014 data).[8] The most substantial deviations below the average for drug-susceptible TB treatment were in the WHO European Region (due to high rates of treatment failure and death) and the Region of the Americas (high loss to follow-up and missing

data). From a higher-level perspective, reasons for suboptimal treatment completion include deficiencies inherent in DOTS or its implementation that need strengthening (e.g., improved funding, increased patient autonomy and alignment with patients' needs, and reduced patient financial costs).[174,175] The global TB community recently has aspired to meet the 90–90–90 targets, where 90% of patients started on treatment successfully complete it; however, in 2016, just seven of the designated 30 high burden countries met this criterion. Critically, the quality of data used to measure progress toward these goals requires improvement (useful tools and guidance to accomplish these exist,[176–178] however, investment and incentives are required so that programs meet reporting standards).

High case detection and cure rates are essential if incidence, prevalence, and death rates are to be reduced.[179] Mathematical modeling suggests that the incidence of endemic TB will decline at 5%–10% per year with ≥70% passive case detection and ≥85% cure.[20,181] In principle, TB incidence could be reduced more rapidly, by as much as 30% per year, if new cases could be found soon enough to eliminate transmission,[182] but given the slow onset of symptoms in many cases and the suboptimal limits of detection of current TB diagnostic tests, this has been hard to achieve. It is possible, however, that new ultra-sensitive nucleic acid amplification tests (e.g., Xpert MTB/RIF Ultra) may offer improved sensitivity in paucibacillary patients with early-stage disease.[183] Furthermore, promising tests based on correlates of risk signatures, which aim to rule out the likely development of active TB within months of infection and, when positive, can be used to monitor patients or give them confirmatory testing, may serve as powerful ways of identifying patients at high risk.[184,185] However, in general, the decline driven by such interventions will be faster when a larger fraction of cases (primary progressive or exogenous disease) arises from recent infection, i.e., in areas where transmission rates are high. As TB transmission and incidence decrease, a higher proportion of cases may arise from the reactivation of latent infection, and the rate of decline in incidence may slow (Figure 2.7).

In the control of endemic TB largely by chemotherapy, the best results have been achieved in communities of Alaskan, Canadian, and Greenland Inuit, where the incidence was reduced by 13%–18%

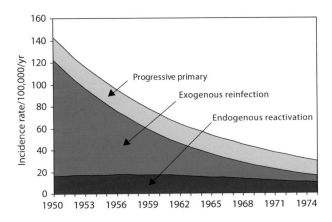

Figure 2.7 The changing etiology of TB in decline, modeled on 45–49 year-olds in the Netherlands. (From Dye C.[182]; Adapted from Styblo K.[15])

per year from the early 1950s onward[15] (Figure 2.8). Over a much wider area in Western Europe, TB declined at 7%–10% per year after drugs became available during the 1950s, though incidence was already falling at 4%–5% per year before chemotherapy.[15]

Case notification series from some countries show that incidence is not falling in the manner anticipated by modeling studies, even though national TB control programs have apparently achieved high rates of case detection and cure. Vietnam is a case in point. WHO targets for case detection and cure had, on the available evidence, been met by 1997, and yet the numbers of notified TB cases have remained more or less stable. Closer inspection of the data reveals that falling case rates among adults 35–64 years old (especially women) have been offset by a rise in the age group 15–34 years old (especially men).[186,187]

Although the long-term aim of TB control is to prevent new cases, the immediate goals are to reduce prevalence and deaths. About 90% of the burden of TB, as measured in terms of years of healthy life lost (or disability-adjusted life years, DALYs) is due to premature death, and prevalence and deaths can be reduced faster than incidence by community-wide chemotherapy. Thus, the TB

death rate among Alaskan Inuit dropped at an average of 30% per year in the interval 1950–1970, and at 12% per year throughout the Netherlands from 1950 to 1990 (faster at first, slower later).[15,188] Indirect assessments of DOTS' impact suggest that 70% of TB deaths were averted in Peru between 1991 and 2000, and more than half the expected TB deaths have been prevented each year in in provinces in China that implemented DOTS.[189,190] Nationwide surveys carried out in China showed a reduction in the prevalence of smear-positive disease from 169/100,000 in 2000 to 66/100,000 in 2010, a reduction of 61%. This rate of decline is almost as fast as previously recorded in the Republic of Korea (Figure 2.8).[5]

Recently, in line with the Universal Health Care umbrella of the Sustainable Development Goals (specifically Goal 3, Good Health and Well-being for People, which aims to ensure healthy lives and promote the well-being for all at all ages), the emphasis on prompt treatment initiation has expanded to incorporate aspects of universal health care focusing on the broader social and economic risk factors (and repercussions) of TB.[1,8] Monitoring frameworks that include key indicators of progress toward universal health coverage are now incorporated into reporting indicators (e.g., malnourishment). This

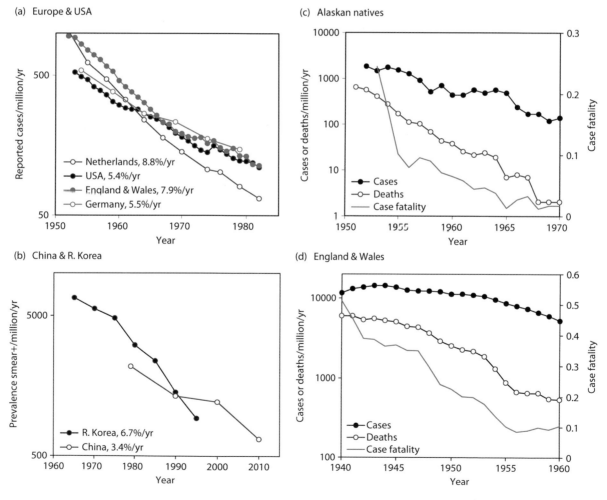

Figure 2.8 Examples of the decline in TB incidence, prevalence, and mortality nationally and sub-nationally, under the influence of large-scale programs of drug treatment. (a) Case notifications from three European countries plus the USA.[15,280–282] (b) National population-based prevalence surveys in the Republic of Korea (1965–1995) and China (1979–2010).[210,283,284] (c) TB cases and deaths recorded from an intensively studied population of Alaskan natives (1952–1970). Case fatality is estimated as the ratio of deaths/cases.[188] (d) National case and death notifications from England and Wales, 1940–1960, with case fatality estimated as in (c).[281]

broadening of what is now considered to fall under the remit of TB control programs is an advance that ultimately will likely reduce the TB epidemic; however, important research and data on the type of interventions or improvements that target these indicators in a manner most impactful for TB are needed.

USING TB DRUGS MORE EFFECTIVELY: ACTIVE CASE FINDING AND TREATMENT

DOTS embraced passive case detection for three reasons: most smear-positive disease develops more quickly than any reasonable frequency of mass screening of symptoms or by radiography; the majority of patients severely ill with a life-threatening disease are likely to seek help quickly[191]; and countries that have not yet implemented effective systems for passive case detection will have difficulty pursuing cases more actively.

But the drawback of passive case finding is that it is often very passive indeed. Population surveys of disease commonly find large numbers of TB patients that have not sought treatment of any kind, or have sought treatment but were not diagnosed. Symptom screening, which is often done sub-optimally,[192] still misses one-fifth of cases when done well[193] and near-future technologies might later become suitable for mass screening in people without or with minimal symptoms (and are thus a major research and development priority[194]). Furthermore, while drug treatment after a long illness can prevent death, it may not impact transmission as most transmission occurs prior to presentation.[195] Strategies for increasing screening among sub-populations in which TB is concentrated such as refugees,[196] those sleeping in shelters for the homeless,[197] contacts of active cases,[198,199] health workers,[70] drug users and prisoners,[200] people in very high incidence areas,[201,202] HIV-positive people,[203] and people with a history of TB[204] can be feasible and cost-effective.

Because active case finding cuts delay to treatment, the benefits for individual patients are clear, but the benefits for whole populations through reduced transmission are harder to detect. One cluster randomized trial has demonstrated that some forms of active case finding can reduce the prevalence of TB in high HIV incidence communities.[202] However, studies of the epidemiological impact of active case finding have not found significant effects on reducing community TB incidence,[205] including the large community-randomized ZAMSTAR study that covered nearly one million individuals in South Africa and Zambia.[206] This large and expensive study is unlikely to be repeated and not only highlights the difficulties in attempting to empirically research key TB epidemiology questions, but also the limitations of our understanding of the effect of active case finding.[207]

Nevertheless, mathematical models (as well as intuition) suggest that, even in the midst of a major HIV epidemic, early detection and cure of TB are effective ways to cut TB burden.[208] New models to understand how best to implement active case finding policies are being developed[209] and, by combining the assault on active TB with other methods, such as the prevention and treatment of HIV infection, the treatment of latent TB infection,[208,211] and infection control in key settings it should be possible to achieve a synergistic effect, thereby making TB control still more effective.[212] But these beneficial effects remain to be demonstrated in practice and there continues to be a need to design and rigorously evaluate interventions to halt transmission, and then prioritize those interventions most likely to achieve population-level impact for implementation.[213] Indeed, recent work (Figure 2.9) comparing the long-term impact of interventions using independent models, shows that scale-up of current tools is probably insufficient to meet the End TB goals in India and China, but may succeed in South Africa,[212] and the further context-specific interventions are likely required (e.g., tackling undernutrition in India or the latent infection reservoir in elderly Chinese).

The TB patient care cascade, which quantifies the number of patients with a favorable outcome at each step of the care continuum, has recently emerged as a useful tool to identify diagnostic (and many other) gaps where patients are "lost" by the system.[192,214] On a local level, such a tool can be used to identify types of people who are under-represented and do disproportionally worse at each step of the cascade.[215]

USING TB DRUGS MORE EFFECTIVELY: TREATMENT OF LATENT TB INFECTION

Persons at high risk of TB can be given a test for latent TB infection and those found to be positive can be offered treatment for latent infection, most commonly IPT. Studies among contacts of active cases have demonstrated that 12 months of daily isoniazid gives 30%–100% protection against active TB,[216] and yet IPT is not widely used. The main challenges are (1) active disease must be excluded (e.g., by radiography) or culture before isoniazid is taken alone, (2) compliance to six or more months of daily treatment tends to be poor among healthy people, and (3) side effects including a hepatitis risk of 1% per year. Even with the resources available in the USA, the implementation of contact tracing and IPT has fallen short of recommendations.[217]

Current WHO guidelines recommend that HIV-infected individuals free of symptoms suggestive of TB receive treatment with IPT for at least 6 months.[218] In 2016, 920,269 HIV-positive individuals received IPT, a number that has grown substantially since 2009.[8] The high risk of TB among persons co-infected with *M. tuberculosis* and HIV motivates those individuals, encouraging wider use of preventive therapy, especially in Africa,[219] but questions have been raised about the methods of screening to ensure that those most likely to benefit receive this treatment[220,221] and that those with subclinical TB are not inadvertently treated with monotherapy.[166–168] Although trials of IPT in skin-test-positive adults infected with HIV have averaged about 60% protection, the effects have been lost soon after the IPT treatment has ended and there has been little or no impact on mortality.[222–228] Studies have suggested that the benefits of IPT appear to be limited to those with positive TST and IPT does not appear to reduce adult mortality,[229] however, in HIV-positive patients receiving ART there is evidence from a high burden setting showing that IPT's effect is not restricted to patients who are TST-positive.[230] Furthermore, the benefits of IPT do not outlast treatment in high-incidence settings where reinfection can occur[231] and there is not yet evidence that widely offering IPT alone within high incidence settings improves TB control.[211] By contrast, IPT has been shown to reduce both TB incidence and mortality among HIV-infected

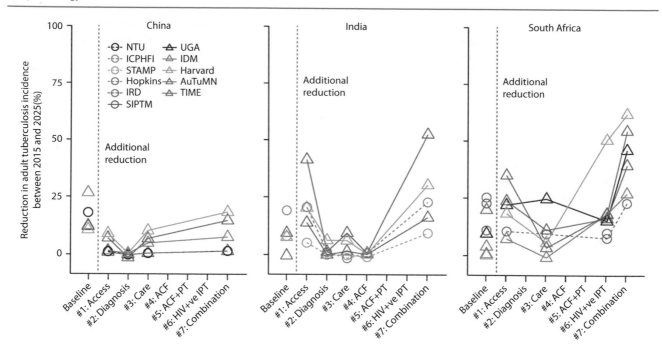

Figure 2.9 An example showing the projected impact of different interventions on the incidence of TB. Models had to reflect activities planned by national TB programs to address specific targets in the TB care cascade (e.g., a reduction in the proportion of patients not accessing TB care). The figure shows the variable project impact of baseline (left of dotted line) and incremental (excluding baseline, right of dotted line) impact of individual intervention scenarios (triangles and circles) from independent models (shapes). Lines between models are for illustration of within-model impact of interventions. Critically, this shows that setting-specific interventions based on currently available tools can, in South Africa, help reach the End TB goals but in China and India they will likely be insufficient. Interventions: Access (increase access to high quality care), Diagnosis (diagnosis of disease and MDR), Care (improve post-diagnosis care), ACF (active case finding in general population), ACF+PT (active case finding followed by preventive therapy of latent TB), HIV+ive IPT (continuous IPT for ART-receiving population), Combination (scale up all interventions simultaneously). Study countries: NTU (China), ICPHFI (India), STAMP (India), Hopkins (South Africa), IRD (South Africa), SIPTM (South Africa), UGA (South Africa), IDM (South Africa, China), Harvard (South Africa, India, China), AutuMN (South Africa, India, China), TIME (South Africa, India, China). (From Houben et al.[212])

children.[232] Recently, there is some population-level evidence of efficacy in medium incidence settings, but it is hard to estimate the independent effect of IPT.[233] In a community-randomized trial in Brazil that included treatment of infection (alongside active case finding), incidence decreased by 15% compared to standard procedure.[234] In another cluster-randomized trial in Brazil in HIV-infected people, strengthening active TB screening, tuberculin testing, and IPT provision reduced the adjusted hazard of TB incidence and death by 25%–30%.[235]

There remain significant logistic hurdles to providing IPT for people who are co-infected,[236] especially if IPT must be administered for many years to have a durable effect. A key challenge in providing IPT is identifying the subset of people who will benefit from treatment. Studies are underway on the efficacy of preventive treatment in patients with so-called incipient TB (i.e., patients identified through correlate of risk signatures, rather than TST, as having high probability of soon progressing to culture-positive TB),[237,238] which may make widespread IPT more feasible to programs.

WILL TB BECOME RESISTANT TO ALL ANTIBIOTICS?

Efforts to systematically document the global burden of drug-resistant forms of TB date back to the mid-1990s. At that time,

the prevalence of MDR TB was highest in countries of the former Soviet Union and the spread of resistance there was linked to the resurgence of TB after dissolution of the Union in 1991. Surveys and surveillance indicate that the severity of the MDR crisis in the former Soviet and Eastern European region remains high; data collected between 2007 and 2010 indicate that the proportion of new cases with MDR was greater than 20% in Belarus, the Republic of Moldova, and six oblasts of the Russian Federation. Among previously treated cases, MDR prevalence was at least 50% in Belarus, Lithuania, the Republic of Moldova, and five oblasts of the Russian Federation.[239]

Although the proportion of cases with MDR is highest in the countries of the former Soviet Union and Eastern Europe, the greatest numbers of MDR cases are in India and China due to their large populations. Drug-resistant TB remains underdiagnosed and under-treated: of the 600,000 estimated incident MDR cases in 2016, only 129,689 were started on second-line treatment (India and China alone accounted for 39% of this incidence-notification gap).[8] This is despite recent advances in the detection of MDR TB.[240] In 2011, the WHO endorsed Xpert MTB/RIF (a frontline PCR test for TB that also detects rifampicin resistance).[241,242] It has become a standard-of-care in many high burden countries (at the end of 2016, nearly 30,000 machine modules had been installed and over 23 million cartridges procured by the public sector).[8] In sub-Saharan African countries, the precise effects of HIV on the burden of drug-resistant TB is not clear[243–245] but, in 2006, reports of the spread and high case fatality associated with XDR TB among HIV-co-infected patients in KwaZulu-Natal, South Africa captured global attention,[246] and subsequent studies have documented very high rates of resistance to available drugs in XDR patients, raising the specter of essentially untreatable epidemics of TB.[247-250] Alarmingly, this has been followed with reports of patients with persistently culture-positive highly drug-resistant forms of TB being discharged back into communities resulting in primary transmission.[247,248]

The extent to which drug resistance threatens global control of TB depends on the absolute and relative genetic fitness of susceptible and resistant strains. As detailed earlier, there now is a substantial body of evidence that most drug resistance is caused by primary transmission.[40,54,130] More highly drug-resistant strains appear to be transmitted less, however, the proportion of cases attributed to transmission appears to increase year on year as strains have more opportunities to mitigate fitness costs through compensatory mutation.[251,252] Importantly, while transmitted drug-resistant cases outnumber those caused by acquired resistance by orders of magnitude, the prevalence of drug resistance in previously treated cases remains higher (19% vs. 4%).[8] While it is true that transmission is driving drug-resistant TB globally, there is heterogeneity on a local level and efforts to infer relative case reproduction numbers from molecular epidemiological studies (e.g., clusters of genotypically similar strains) have produced variable results.[253-256] Encouragingly, when some countries (e.g., Latvia and Estonia) with a high fraction of MDR TB (likely due to transmission) implemented aggressive new TB programs that included treatment of MDR TB, overall incidence decreased.

While individualized regimens are efficacious in the treatment of highly drug-resistant forms of disease[257-259] and the new shortened MDR regimen treatment holds promise,[260] there is substantial progress to be made to ensure that all TB cases receive appropriate therapy, regardless of resistance. This is complicated by a lack of rapid diagnostics for susceptibility to several drugs (e.g., pyrazinamide, ethambutol) within the new second-line regimen and high levels of background resistance to these drugs in MDR strains (40%–50% in some settings). This threatens the emergence of resistance to critical drugs like the fluoroquinolones and could comprise the new MDR regimen.[261-263]

HOW CAN NOVEL TOOLS AND PHARMACOLOGICAL INTERVENTIONS CONTRIBUTE TO ENDING TB EPIDEMICS?

Recent years have seen unprecedented innovation pertaining to new diagnostic tests and drugs for TB. These have served to galvanize research, policy, and healthcare provider communities after long periods of slow progress, and also stimulated commercial research and development where there was previously little.[150] Here, we summarize what is known about the epidemiological impact of these recent tools, lessons learned from their implementation, and the potential epidemiological effect of future interventions.

REDUCING THE RISK OF TB BEFORE INFECTION

The current vaccine, BCG, has low efficacy in preventing infectious TB in countries with a high disease burden.[264] Thus, even with the very high coverage now achieved, BCG is unlikely to have any substantial impact on transmission, and hence incidence, because its main effect is to prevent serious (but non-infectious) disease in children. The manufacture of a new, high-efficacy vaccine would change the focus of TB control from treatment to prevention. In some models, a "pre-exposure" vaccine that prevents infection may have a greater impact than a "post-exposure" vaccine that stops progression to disease among those already infected (Figure 2.10).[180] However, it is difficult to predict the impact of different vaccines until we know more about their mode of action and their efficacy in clinical trials. Furthermore, although the effect of different theoretical vaccines with pre-specified characteristics can be comparatively modeled, it should be noted there is a lack of consensus on the potential epidemiological effect of pre- versus post-exposure vaccines.[265] There are approximately 20 vaccine candidates at different stages of clinical trial pipeline.[266]

REDUCING THE RISK OF TB AFTER INFECTION

Vaccines or drugs delivered to individuals with latent infection can improve TB control; the development of new diagnostic tools that target these individuals most at risk of progression is needed. Neither tuberculin skin tests nor novel commercially available diagnostics for latent infection such as interferon-gamma release assays appear to be particularly good predictors of the

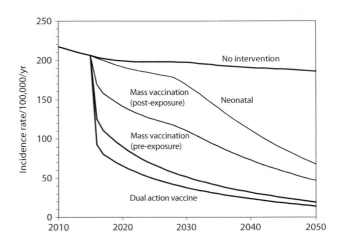

Figure 2.10 Hypothetical impact of four vaccination strategies on TB incidence rate. Calculations have been carried out with an age-structured mathematical model[20] set up to investigate the effect of vaccination on a TB epidemic like that in South Asia with an annual incidence set at about 200 per 100,000 population in 2015. Mass vaccination of uninfected populations (pre-exposure) would reduce the annual incidence to 20 per 100,000 in 2050. In a country the size of India, this would correspond to prevention of 50 million cases. A dual-action vaccine active both pre- and post-exposure would prevent a further 5 million cases, reducing the incidence to 14 per 100,000. (From Young DB, and Dye C.[180])

risk of developing active TB (sensitivity and specificity of ~80%). However, the aforementioned correlates of risk-based tests represent recent significant advances that likely outperform interferon-gamma release assays, which do not meet minimum diagnostic test characteristic criteria for active TB, are undergoing evaluation in clinical trials.[184,267,268]

While averting progression to disease from latency is beneficial for individuals affected, the projected epidemiological impact of such an intervention is dependent on the proportion of total TB incidence that is due to reactivation from latency as compared to recent infection and rapid progression or reinfection. This proportion differs between settings and depends on local forces of infection; where the prevalence of disease is high and the risk of infection (and reinfection) is substantial, preventing cases of reactivation disease may not have as marked an impact on TB control as other interventions. However, synergistic effects can be realized when efforts to reduce reactivation are combined with other control efforts that reduce transmission.

REDUCING THE SPREAD OF INFECTION: WHY HAVE RECENT SIGNIFICANT ADVANCES IN DIAGNOSTICS STRUGGLED TO SHOW IMPACT?

The End TB Strategy, like its predecessors the DOTS and Stop TB strategies, emphasizes the detection and rapid initiation of effective treatment for individuals with infectious TB. Xpert MTB/RIF, in terms of sensitivity (60%–80% for smear-negative TB), degree of automation (reduced reliance on scarce skilled personnel), and the simultaneous detection of resistance, has doubtless been a major advance. However, in contrast to what had been projected, multiple randomized-clinical trials showed no impact of Xpert MTB/RIF on long-term patient health (morbidity, mortality), despite significant improvements in rates of bacteriological diagnosis, treatment initiation, and time-to-treatment initiation.[269–272] In addition to Xpert MTB/RIF not being a true point of care test (it does not meet the target product profile criteria[194]), there are additional overarching reasons for this apparent lack of impact that we only partly understand. In many high burden settings, rapid empiric treatment was (and still continues to be) frequent (due to deficiencies in previous microscopy-based diagnostic algorithms) and Xpert MTB/RIF's main effect appeared to be the displacement of true-positive empiric treatment decision making.[273] Furthermore, poor linkage to care, which resulted in diagnostic capacity outstripping capacity for effective treatment initiation (including for MDR) undermined Xpert MTB/RIF's impact.[274] In a routine health systems context, national programs also faced challenges with implementation (e.g., training, quality assurance, technical support) and did not have data systems in place to easily assess Xpert MTB/RIF's effect in this context. This latter aspect represents a major missed opportunity: early adopters of Xpert MTB/RIF like South Africa could be useful—to researchers, other national programs, and policy makers—as massive natural experiments in TB control interventions. However, the type, quality, and accessibility of data is restricted.

Xpert MTB/RIF has recently been succeeded by Xpert MTB/RIF Ultra, which offers an important incremental (but likely not transformative) improvement.[275] The obvious importance of the context in which the test is placed adds considerable complexity to the projection and evaluation of the impact of new tests and underscores how linkage to care must be emphasized. This difficulty in detecting long-term impact has, given patients' complex and highly varied pathways to care, led to calls that the importance of long-term surrogate endpoints in diagnostic studies is overstated.[276]

NEW DRUG REGIMENS

Epidemiologically, not only are drugs important for reducing morbidity, but they are likely the most rapid way to render a patient non-infectious and thereby directly curtail transmission (provided the strain is susceptible to the regimen). Optimized regimens will also reduce non-adherence driven by side effects, however, regimen efficacy is likely the single most important characteristic of long-term impact on incidence and mortality (e.g., more so than regimen duration).[277] Recent drug development and evaluation activity has focused on shorter regimens for both drug-susceptible and drug-resistant TB. For drug-susceptible TB, shorter fluoroquinolone-containing regimens have generated mixed evidence but overall failed to show superiority to the standard six-month regimen. For drug-resistant TB, regimens to improve poor cure rates lead to serious side effect profiles stemming from use of the second-line injectables. The new shortened regimen for drug-resistant TB should help close the MDR diagnosis-treatment gap and high burden countries need to focus on improving access to effective drugs.

CONCLUSIONS

Overall, our assessment of the current scale and direction of the TB epidemic is a mixed report. The positive news is that the global TB epidemic is declining, but progress has been slow and not shared equally across the world. Incidence and death rates grew during the 1990s, due mainly to the spread of HIV in Africa and to social and economic decline in former Soviet countries, but reached a maximum before 2005.

While the sustained decline in incidence and mortality rates of TB overall is encouraging, these declines must be greatly accelerated to reach the End TB goals.[278] Given that such a rapid rate of decline has never been achieved, new perspectives, tools and strategies will be needed to meet this goal, while re-doubling our focus on traditional key priorities for TB control (i.e., early diagnosis and effective treatment). Key to accelerating TB's decline is embracing the principles of universal health coverage in the context of the Sustainable Development Goals. This requires accepting that modifiable poverty and social economic factors are critical drivers of the TB epidemic that need to be integrated into TB reporting, research, and local context-aware interventions. Broader initiatives that modify population-level risk factors (e.g., nutrition) will also doubtless improve TB control and should be encouraged. Gaps in the TB care cascade—and the requisite health systems strengthening—remain key priorities and are most acute for drug-resistant TB where the MDR epidemic is unlikely to abate unless many more cases can be correctly diagnosed and effectively treated each year.

Innovative technologies, especially within the diagnostics sphere, continue to arrive and the TB community must be poised to rapidly evaluate these tools and determine the places and strategies in which such technologies can deliver sufficient health benefits to balance costs. The comparative lack of activity in the TB drug pipeline and the absence of a promising late-phase vaccine candidate stand out as major deficiencies (the latter especially as most models suggest that global control targets are unlikely to be met without an improved vaccine). Nevertheless, far better control of the epidemic can be achieved with existing and near-future technologies, including addressing the underlying causes of TB. Epidemiologists must provide the evidence to promote uptake of these tools and strategies and motivate further for the resources needed to help End TB.

REFERENCES

1. Stop TB Partnership, *The paradigm shift 2016–2020, Global Plan to End TB.* United Nations Office for Project Services, UNOPS, Geneva Switzerland, 2015.
2. Streiner DL, Norman GR, and Blum HM. *PDQ Epidemiology.* Toronto: B.C. Decker Inc, 1989.
3. Keeling MJ, and Rohani P. *Modeling Infectious Diseases in Humans and Animals.* Princeton: Princeton University Press, 2007.
4. Raviglione MC, and Uplekar MW. WHO's new Stop TB Strategy. *Lancet.* 2006;367:952–955.
5. World Health Organization. *Global Tuberculosis Control: Who Report 2011.* Geneva: World Health Organization, 2011.
6. Frick M. *2016 report on tuberculosis research funding trends, 2005–2015: no time to lose.* Treatment Action Group, 2016.
7. Houben RM, and Dodd PJ. The global burden of latent tuberculosis infection: A re-estimation using mathematical modelling. *PLoS Med.* 2016;13(10):e1002152.
8. World Health Organization. *Global Tuberculosis Report:* Geneva, Switzerland, 2017.
9. Straetemans M et al. Assessing tuberculosis case fatality ratio: A meta-analysis. *PLOS ONE.* 2011;6(6):e20755.
10. Houben R, Odone A, and Grant A. TB Case Fatality Ratio by patient stratum for Spectrum TB. 2013.
11. Lopez A et al., eds. *Global Burden of Disease and Risk Factors.* New York: The World Bank and Oxford University Press, 2006.
12. Dye C et al. Global burden of tuberculosis. Estimated incidence, prevalence, and mortality by country. *JAMA.* 1999;282(7):677–686.
13. Dye C et al. Measuring tuberculosis burden, trends and the impact of control programmes. *Lancet Infect Dis.* 2008;8:233–243.
14. Robertson SE, and Valadez JJ. Global review of health care surveys using lot quality assurance sampling (LQAS), 1984–2004. *Soc Sci Med.* 2006;63(6):1648–1660.
15. Styblo K. *Epidemiology of Tuberculosis.* 2nd ed. The Hague: KNCV Tuberculosis Foundation. 136, 1991.
16. Bourdin Trunz B, Fine P, and Dye C. Effect of BCG vaccination on childhood tuberculous meningitis and miliary tuberculosis worldwide: A meta-analysis and assessment of cost-effectiveness. *Lancet.* 2006;367:1173–1180.
17. van Leth F, Van der Werf MJ, and Borgdorff MW. Prevalence of tuberculous infection and incidence of tuberculosis: A re-assessment of the Styblo rule. *Bull WHO.* 2008;86:20–26.
18. Sutherland I, Svandova E, and Radhakrishna S. The development of clinical tuberculosis following infection with tubercle bacilli. 1. A theoretical model for the development of clinical tuberculosis following infection, linking from data on the risk of tuberculous infection and the incidence of clinical tuberculosis in the Netherlands. *Tubercle.* 1982;63:255–268.
19. Vynnycky E, and Fine PEM. The natural history of tuberculosis: The implications of age-dependent risks of disease and the role of reinfection. *Epidemiol Infect.* 1997;119:183–201.
20. Dye C et al. Prospects for worldwide tuberculosis control under the WHO DOTS strategy. Directly observed short-course therapy. *Lancet.* 1998;352:1886–1891.
21. Sutherland I. *The ten-year incidence of clinical tuberculosis following "conversion" in 2,550 individuals aged 14 to 19 years.* Tuberculosis Surveillance and Research Unit Progress Report, KNCV, The Hague. 1968.
22. Borgdorff MW et al. The incubation period distribution of tuberculosis estimated with a molecular epidemiological approach. *Int J Epidemiol.* 2011;40:964–970.
23. Andrews JR et al. Risk of progression to active tuberculosis following reinfection with *Mycobacterium tuberculosis. Clin Infect Dis.* 2012;54:784–791.
24. Dye C et al. Prospects for worldwide tuberculosis control under the WHO DOTS strategy. *Lancet.* 1998;352:1886–1891.
25. de Viedma DG, Marin M, Hernangomez S, Diaz M, Serrano MJR, Alcala L, and Bouza E. Reinfection plays a role in a population whose clinical/epidemiological characteristics do not favor reinfection. *Arch Intern Med.* 2002;162:1873–1879.
26. Richardson M et al. Multiple *Mycobacterium tuberculosis* strains in early cultures from patients in a high-incidence community setting. *J Clin Microbiol.* 2002;40:2750–2754.
27. Mathema B et al. Molecular epidemiology of tuberculosis: Current insights. *Clin Microbiol Rev.* 2006;19(4):658–685.
28. Chiang CY, and Riley LW. Exogenous reinfection in tuberculosis. *Lancet Infect Dis.* 2005;5:629–636.
29. Tiemersma EW et al. Natural history of tuberculosis: Duration and fatality of untreated pulmonary tuberculosis in HIV negative patients: A systematic review. *PLOS ONE.* 2011;6:e17601.
30. Dorman SE et al. Xpert MTB/RIF Ultra for detection of *Mycobacterium tuberculosis* and rifampicin resistance: A prospective multicentre diagnostic accuracy study. *Lancet Infect Dis.* 2017.
31. Krebs W. Die Fälle von Lungentuberkulose in der aargauischen Heilstätte Barmelweid aus den Jahren 1912–1927. *Beiträge zur Klinik der Tuberkulose.* 1930;74:345–379.
32. Rieder HL. *Epidemiologic Basis of Tuberculosis Control.* 1st ed. Paris: International Union Against Tuberculosis and Lung Disease, 1999, 1–162.
33. Dye C. *The Population Biology of Tuberculosis.* Princeton University Press, 2015.
34. Grigg ERN. The arcana of tuberculosis. With a brief epidemiologic history of the disease in the U.S.A. *Am Rev Tuberc.* 1958;78:151–172.
35. Blower SM et al. The intrinsic transmission dynamics of tuberculosis epidemics. *Nat Med.* 1995;1:815–821.
36. Murray CJL, and Salomon JA. Modeling the impact of global tuberculosis control strategies. *Proc Natl Acad Sci USA.* 1998;95:13881–13886.
37. Dowdy DW, Dye C, and Cohen T. Data needs for evidence-based decisions: A tuberculosis modeler's 'wish list'. *Int J Tuberc Lung Dis.* 2013;17(7):866–877.
38. Vynnycky E, and Fine PEM. The long-term dynamics of tuberculosis and other diseases with long serial intervals: Implications of and for changing reproduction numbers. *Epidemiol Infect.* 1998;121:309–324.

39. Dye C, and Espinal MA. Will tuberculosis become resistant to all antibiotics? *Proceedings of the Royal Society of London Series B, Biological Sciences.* 2001;268:45–52.

40. Kendall EA, Fofana MO, and Dowdy DW. Burden of transmitted multidrug resistance in epidemics of tuberculosis: A transmission modelling analysis. *Lancet Respir Med.* 2015;3(12):963–972.

41. Hermans S, Horsburgh Jr CR, and Wood R. A century of tuberculosis epidemiology in the Northern and Southern Hemisphere: The differential impact of control interventions. *PLOS ONE.* 2015;10(8):e0135179.

42. Davies RPO et al. Historical declines in tuberculosis in England and Wales: Improving social conditions or natural selection? *Int J Tuberc Lung Dis.* 1999;3:1051–1054.

43. McFarlane N. Hospitals, housing and tuberculosis in Glasgow. *Soc Hist Med.* 1989;2(59–85):59–85.

44. Vynnycky E, and Fine PEM. Interpreting the decline in tuberculosis: The role of secular trends in effective contact. *Int J Epidemiol.* 1999;28:327–334.

45. McKeown T, and Record RG. Reasons for the decline in mortality in England and Wales in the nineteenth century. *Popul Stud.* 1962;16:94–122.

46. Edwards LB et al. Height, weight, tuberculous infection, and tuberculous disease. *Arch Environ Health.* 1971;22:106–112.

47. Bhargava A et al. Can social interventions prevent tuberculosis? The Papworth experiment (1918–1943) revisited. *Am J Respir Crit Care Med.* 2012;186(5):442–449.

48. Lowell AM, Edwards LB, and Palmer CE. *Tuberculosis. Vital and Health Statistics Monographs, American Public Health Association.* Cambridge: Harvard University Press, 1969.

49. Lipsitch M, and Sousa AO. Historical intensity of natural selection for resistance to tuberculosis. *Genetics.* 2002;161:1599–1607.

50. Kato-Maeda M et al. Comparing genomes within the species *Mycobacterium tuberculosis. Genome Res.* 2001;11:547–554.

51. Mostowy S et al. Genomic deletions suggest a phylogeny for the *Mycobacterium tuberculosis* complex. *J Infect Dis.* 2002;186(1):74–80.

52. Newton SM et al. A deletion defining a common Asian lineage of *Mycobacterium tuberculosis* associates with immune subversion. *Proc Natl Acad Sci USA.* 2006;103:15594–15598.

53. Lopez B et al. A marked difference in pathogenesis and immune response induced by different *Mycobacterium tuberculosis* genotypes. *Clin Exp Immunol.* 2003;133:30–37.

54. Merker M et al. Evolutionary history and global spread of the *Mycobacterium tuberculosis* Beijing lineage. *Nat Genet.* 2015.

55. Shafer RW, and Edlin BR. Tuberculosis in patients infected with human immunodeficiency virus: Perspective on the past decade. *Clin Infect Dis.* 1996;22:683–704.

56. Freedberg KA, Losina E, Weinstein MC, Paltiel AD, Cohen CJ, Seage GR, Craven DE, Zhang H, Kimmel AD, and Goldie SJ. The cost effectiveness of combination antiretroviral therapy for HIV disease. *N Engl J Med.* 2001;344:824–831.

57. Badri M, Wilson D, and Wood R. Effect of highly active antiretroviral therapy on incidence of tuberculosis in South Africa: A cohort study. *Lancet.* 2002;359:2059–2064.

58. Antonucci G et al. Risk factors for tuberculosis in HIV-infected persons. A prospective cohort study. The Gruppo Italiano di Studio Tubercolosi e AIDS (GISTA). *JAMA.* 1995;274:143–148.

59. Selwyn PA et al. A prospective study of the risk of tuberculosis among intravenous drug users with human immunodeficiency virus infection. *N Engl J Med.* 1989;320:545–550.

60. Williams BG, and Dye C. Antiretroviral drugs for tuberculosis control in the era of HIV/AIDS. *Science.* 2003;301:1535–1537.

61. Yazdanpanah Y et al. Incidence of primary opportunistic infections in two human immunodeficiency virus-infected French clinical cohorts. *Int J Epidemiol.* 2001;30:864–871.

62. Stevenson CR et al. Diabetes and the risk of tuberculosis: A neglected threat to public health? *Chronic Illn,* in press.

63. Jeon CY, and Murray MB. Diabetes mellitus increases the risk of active tuberculosis: A systematic review of 13 observational studies. *PLoS Med.* 2008;5:e152.

64. Imtiaz S et al. Alcohol consumption as a risk factor for tuberculosis: Meta-analyses and burden of disease. *Eur Respir J.* 2017;50(1):1700216.

65. Corbett EL et al. Risk factors for pulmonary mycobacterial disease in South African gold miners. A case-control study. *Am J Respir Crit Care Med.* 1999;159(1):94–99.

66. van Lettow M, Fawzi WW, and Semba RD. Triple trouble: The role of malnutrition in tuberculosis and human immunodeficiency virus co-infection. *Nutr Rev.* 2003;61:81–90.

67. Cegielski JP, and McMurray DN. The relationship between malnutrition and tuberculosis: Evidence from studies in humans and experimental animals. *Int J Tuberc Lung Dis.* 2004;8:286–298.

68. Comstock GW, and Palmer CE. Long-term results of BCG vaccination in the southern United States. *Am Rev Resp Dis.* 1966;93:171–183.

69. Lönnroth K et al. Tuberculosis control and elimination 2010–50: Cure, care, and social development. *Lancet.* 2010;375:1814–1829.

70. Cuhadaroglu C et al. Increased risk of tuberculosis in health care workers: A retrospective survey at a teaching hospital in Istanbul, Turkey. *BioMed Central Infect Dis.* 2002;2:14.

71. Geng E et al. Changes in the transmission of tuberculosis in New York City from 1990 to 1999. *N Engl J Med.* 2002;346:1453–1458.

72. Carvalho AC et al. Transmission of *Mycobacterium tuberculosis* to contacts of HIV-infected tuberculosis patients. *Am J Respir Crit Care Med.* 2001;164:2166–2171.

73. Besser RE et al. Risk factors for positive mantoux tuberculin skin tests in children in San Diego, California: Evidence for boosting and possible foodborne transmission. *Pediatrics.* 2001;108(2):305–10.

74. van Geuns HA, Meijer J, and Styblo K. Results of contact examination in Rotterdam, 1967–1969. *Tuberculosis Surveillance Research Unit Report No. 3.* 1975;50:107–121.

75. Lin HH, Ezzati M, and Murray M. Tobacco smoke, indoor air pollution and tuberculosis: A systematic review and meta-analysis. *PLoS Med.* 2007;4–e20:173–189.

76. Slama K et al. Tobacco and tuberculosis: A qualitative systematic review and meta-analysis. *Int J Tuberc Lung Dis.* 2007;10:1049–1061.

77. Sonnenberg P et al. HIV-1 and recurrence, relapse, and reinfection of tuberculosis after cure: A cohort study in South African mineworkers. *Lancet.* 2001;358(9294):1687–93.

78. Perez-Padilla R et al. Cooking with biomass stoves and tuberculosis: A case control study. *Int J Tuberc Lung Dis.* 2001;5:441–447.

79. Gangaidzo IT et al. Association of pulmonary tuberculosis with increased dietary iron. *J Infect Dis.* 2001;184:936–939.

80. Wilkinson RJ et al. Influence of vitamin D deficiency and vitamin D receptor polymorphisms on tuberculosis among Gujarati Asians in west London: A case-control study. *Lancet.* 2000;355:618–621.

81. Nnoaham KE, and Clarke A. Low serum vitamin D levels and tuberculosis: A systematic review and meta-analysis. *Int J Epidemiol.* 2008;37:113–119.

82. Bellamy R et al. Variations in the NRAMP1 gene and susceptibility to tuberculosis in West Africans. *N Engl J Med.* 1998;338:640–644.

83. Zachariah R et al. Moderate to severe malnutrition in patients with tuberculosis is a risk factor associated with early death. *Trans R Soc Trop Med Hyg.* 2002;96:291–294.

84. Toungoussova OS et al. Drug resistance of *Mycobacterium tuberculosis* strains isolated from patients with pulmonary tuberculosis in Archangels, Russia. *Int J Tuberc Lung Dis.* 2002;6:406–414.

85. Sevim T et al. Treatment adherence of 717 patients with tuberculosis in a social security system hospital in Istanbul, Turkey. *Int J Tuberc Lung Dis.* 2002;6:25–31.

86. Abos-Hernandez R, and Olle-Goig JE. Patients hospitalised in Bolivia with pulmonary tuberculosis: Risk factors for dying. *Int J Tuberc Lung Dis.* 2002;6(6):470–4.

87. Pablos-Méndez A et al. Nonadherence in tuberculosis treatment: Predictors and consequences in New York City. *Am J Med* 1997;102: 164–170.

88. Theron G et al. Psychological distress and its relationship with nonadherence to TB treatment: A multicentre study. *BMC Infect Dis.* 2015;15(1):253.

89. Baker MA et al. The impact of diabetes on tuberculosis treatment outcomes: A systematic review. *BMC Med.* 2011;9:81.

90. Jo K-W et al. Risk factors for 1-year relapse of pulmonary tuberculosis treated with a 6-month daily regimen. *Respir Med.* 2014;108(4):654–659.

91. Abel L et al. Genetics of human susceptibility to active and latent tuberculosis: Present knowledge and future perspectives. *Lancet Infect Dis.* 2017.

92. Grange JM et al. Historical declines in tuberculosis: Nature, nurture and the biosocial model. *Int J Tuberc Lung Dis.* 2001;5:208–212.

93. Goldfeld AE et al. Association of an HLA-DQ allele with clinical tuberculosis. *JAMA.* 1998;279:226–228.

94. Hill AV. Aspects of genetic susceptibility to human infectious diseases. *Annu Rev Genet.* 2006;40:469–486.

95. Fernando SL, and Britton WJ. Genetic susceptibility to mycobacterial disease in humans. *Immunol Cell Biol.* 2006;84:125–137.

96. Liu PT et al. Toll-like receptor triggering of a vitamin D-mediated human antimicrobial response. *Science.* 2006;311:1770–1773.

97. Gao L et al. Vitamin D receptor genetic polymorphisms and tuberculosis: Updated systematic review and meta-analysis. *Int J Tuberc Lung Dis.* 2010;14:15–23.

98. Greenwood CM, Fujiwara TM, and Boothroyd LJ. Linkage of tuberculosis to chromosome 2q35 loci, including NRAMP1, in a large aboriginal Canadian family. *Am J Hum Genet.* 2000; 67:405–416.

99. Curtis J et al. Susceptibility to tuberculosis is associated with variants in the ASAP1 gene encoding a regulator of dendritic cell migration. *Nat Genet.* 2015;47(5):523.

100. Salie M et al. Association of toll-like receptors with susceptibility to tuberculosis suggests sex-specific effects of TLR8 polymorphisms. *Infect Genet Evol.* 2015;34:221–229.

101. Alm JS et al. Atopy in children in relation to BCG vaccination and genetic polymorphisms at SLC11A1 (formerly NRAMP1) and D2S1471. *Genes Immun.* 2002;3:71–77.

102. Schurr E. Is susceptibility to tuberculosis acquired or inherited? *J Intern Med.* 2007;261(2):106–111.

103. Lewis SJ, Baker I, and Davey Smith G. Meta-analysis of vitamin D receptor polymorphisms and pulmonary tuberculosis risk. *Int J Tuberc Lung Dis.* 2005;9:1174–1177.

104. Martineau AR et al. High-dose vitamin D3 during intensive-phase antimicrobial treatment of pulmonary tuberculosis: A double-blind randomised controlled trial. *Lancet.* 2011;377(9761):242–250.

105. Corbett EL et al. HIV-1/AIDS and the control of other infectious diseases in Africa. *Lancet.* 2002;359:2177–2187.

106. Corbett EL et al. The growing burden of tuberculosis: Global trends and interactions with the HIV epidemic. *Arch Intern Med.* 2003;163:1009–1021.

107. Middelkoop K et al. Transmission of tuberculosis in a South African community with a high prevalence of HIV infection. *J Infect Dis.* 2014;211(1):53–61.

108. Corbett EL et al. Human immunodeficiency virus and the prevalence of undiagnosed tuberculosis in African gold miners. *Am J Respir Crit Care Med.* 2004;170:673–679.

109. Wood R et al. Undiagnosed tuberculosis in a community with high HIV prevalence: Implications for tuberculosis control. *Am J Respir Crit Care Med.* 2007;175:87–93.

110. Getahun H et al. Diagnosis of smear-negative pulmonary tuberculosis in people with HIV infection or AIDS in resource-constrained settings: Informing urgent policy changes. *Lancet.* 2007;369:2042–2049.

111. Williams BG et al. Antiretroviral therapy for tuberculosis control in nine African countries. *Proc Natl Acad Sci USA.* 2010;107:19485–19489.

112. Suthar AB et al. Antiretroviral therapy for prevention of HIV-associated tuberculosis in developing countries: A systematic review and meta-analysis. *PLoS Med.* 2012;9:e1001270.

113. Akolo C et al. Treatment of latent tuberculosis infection in HIV infected persons. *Cochrane Database Syst Rev.* 2010;(1):CD000171.

114. Lawn SD et al. Screening for HIV-associated tuberculosis and rifampicin resistance before antiretroviral therapy using the Xpert MTB/RIF assay: A prospective study. *PLoS Med.* 2011;8(7):e1001067.

115. Shilova MV, and Dye C. The resurgence of tuberculosis in Russia. *Philos Trans Roy Soc London. Ser B, Biol Sci.* 2001;356:1069–1075.

116. Toungoussova OS, Bjune G, and Caugant DA. Epidemic of tuberculosis in the former Soviet Union: Social and biological reasons. *Tuberculosis (Edinb).* 2006;86:1–10.

117. Atun RA et al. Barriers to sustainable tuberculosis control in the Russian Federation health system. *Bull WHO.* 2005;83:217–223.

118. Stone R. Social science. Stress: The invisible hand in Eastern Europe's death rates. *Science.* 2000;288:1732–1733.

119. Leon DA et al. Hazardous alcohol drinking and premature mortality in Russia: A population based case-control study. *Lancet.* 2007;369(9578):2001–2009.

120. Borgdorff MW et al. Analysis of tuberculosis transmission between nationalities in the Netherlands in the period 1993–1995 using DNA fingerprinting. *Am J Epidemiol.* 1998;147(2):187–195.

121. Murray MB. Molecular epidemiology and the dynamics of tuberculosis transmission among foreign-born people. *CMAJ.* 2002;167(4):355–356.

122. Lillebaek T et al. Persistent high incidence of tuberculosis in immigrants in a low-incidence country. *Emerg Infect Dis.* 2002;8:679–684.

123. Verver S et al. Tuberculosis infection in children who are contacts of immigrant tuberculosis patients. *Eur Respir J.* 2005;26:126–132.

124. Borgdorff MW et al. Transmission of *Mycobacterium tuberculosis* depending on the age and sex of source cases. *Am J Epidemiol.* 2001;154:934–943.

125. Pareek M et al. Screening of immigrants in the UK for imported latent tuberculosis: A multicentre cohort study and cost-effectiveness analysis. *Lancet Infect Dis.* 2011;11:435–444.

126. Vynnycky E et al. Limited impact of tuberculosis control in Hong Kong: Attributable to high risks of reactivation disease. *Epidemiol Infect.* 2008;136:943–952.

127. Wu P et al. The transmission dynamics of tuberculosis in a recently developed Chinese city. *PLOS ONE.* 2010;5:e10468.

128. Sreevatsan S et al. Restricted structural gene polymorphism in the *Mycobacterium tuberculosis* complex indicates evolutionarily recent global dissemination. *Proc Natl Acad Sci USA.* 1997;94:9869–9874.

129. Musser JM, Amin A, and Ramaswamy S. Negligible genetic diversity of *Mycobacterium tuberculosis* host immune system protein targets: Evidence of limited selective pressure. *Genetics*. 2000;155:7–16.

130. Gagneux S. Ecology and evolution of *Mycobacterium tuberculosis*. *Nat Rev Microbiol*. 2018; 16(4):202–13.

131. Metcalfe JZ et al. Cryptic microheteroresistance explains mycobacterium tuberculosis phenotypic resistance. *Am J Respir Crit Care Med*. 2017 November 1;196(9):1191–201.

132. Lieberman TD et al. Genomic diversity in autopsy samples reveals within-host dissemination of HIV-associated *Mycobacterium tuberculosis*. *Nat Med*. 2016;22(12):1470.

133. Prideaux B et al. The association between sterilizing activity and drug distribution into tuberculosis lesions. *Nat Med*. 2015;21(10):1223.

134. Gutacker MM et al. Single-nucleotide polymorphism-based population genetic analysis of *Mycobacterium tuberculosis* strains from 4 geographic sites. *J Infect Dis*. 2006;193:121–128.

135. Filliol I et al. Global phylogeny of *Mycobacterium tuberculosis* based on single nucleotide polymorphism (SNP) analysis: Insights into tuberculosis evolution, phylogenetic accuracy of other DNA fingerprinting systems, and recommendations for a minimal standard SNP set. *J Bacteriol*. 2006;188:759–772.

136. Hershberg R et al. High functional diversity in *Mycobacterium tuberculosis* driven by genetic drift and human demography. *PLoS Biol*. 2008;6:e311.

137. Mathema B et al. Epidemiologic consequences of microvariation in *Mycobacterium tuberculosis*. *J Infect Dis*. 2012;205:964–974.

138. Nicol MP and Wilkinson RJ. The clinical consequences of strain diversity in *Mycobacterium tuberculosis*. *Trans R Soc Trop Med Hyg*. 2008;102:955–965.

139. Barczak AK et al. In vivo phenotypic dominance in mouse mixed infections with *Mycobacterium tuberculosis* clinical isolates. *J Infect Dis*. 2005;192:600–606.

140. De Steenwinkel JEM et al. Drug susceptibility of *Mycobacterium tuberculosis* Beijing genotype, association with MDR TB. *Emerg Infect Dis*. 2012;18:660–663.

141. Fenner L et al. Effect of mutation and genetic background on drug resistance in *Mycobacterium tuberculosis*. *Antimicrob Agents Chemother*. 2012;56:3047–3053.

142. Basu S, Orenstein E, and Galvani AP. The theoretical influence of immunity between strain groups on the progression of drug-resistant tuberculosis epidemics. *J Infect Dis*. 2008;198:1502–1513.

143. Cohen T, Colijn C, and Murray M. Modeling the effects of strain diversity and mechanisms of strain competition on the potential performance of new tuberculosis vaccines. *Proc Natl Acad Sci USA*. 2008;105:16302–16307.

144. Colijn C, Cohen T, and Murray M. Latent coinfection and the maintenance of strain diversity. *Bull Math Biol*. 2009;71:247–263.

145. Middlebrook G and Cohn ML. Some observations on the pathogenicity of isoniazid-resistant variants of tubercle bacilli. *Science*. 1953;118(3063):297–299.

146. Gagneux S et al. The competitive cost of antibiotic resistance in *Mycobacterium tuberculosis*. *Science*. 2006;312(5782):1944–1946.

147. Ford CB et al. *Mycobacterium tuberculosis* mutation rate estimates from different lineages predict substantial differences in the emergence of drug-resistant tuberculosis. *Nat Genet*. 2013;45(7):784.

148. Eldholm V et al. Armed conflict and population displacement as drivers of the evolution and dispersal of *Mycobacterium tuberculosis*. *Proc Natl Acad Sci USA*. 2016;113(48):13881–13886.

149. Köser CU et al. Routine use of microbial whole genome sequencing in diagnostic and public health microbiology. *PLoS Pathog*. 2012;8(8):e1002824.

150. UNITAID. *Tuberculosis Diagnostic Technology Landscape*. Geneva, Switzerland: World Health Organization, 2017 [cited 2017 October 25]; Available from: https://unitaid.eu/assets/2017-Unitaid-TB-Diagnostics-Technology-Landscape.pdf.

151. Cain KP et al. The movement of multidrug-resistant tuberculosis across borders in East Africa needs a regional and global solution. *PLoS Med*. 2015;12(2):e1001791.

152. Comas I et al. Out-of-Africa migration and Neolithic coexpansion of *Mycobacterium tuberculosis* with modern humans. *Nat Genet*. 2013;45(10):1176.

153. Shirakawa T et al. The inverse association between tuberculin responses and atopic disorder. *Science*. 1997;275(5296):77–9.

154. Obihara CC et al. Inverse association between *Mycobacterium tuberculosis* infection and atopic rhinitis in children. *Allergy*. 2005;60:1121–1125.

155. von Mutius E et al. International patterns of tuberculosis and the prevalence of symptoms of asthma, rhinitis, and eczema. *Thorax*. 2000;55:449–453.

156. Shirtcliffe P, Weatherall M, Beasley R. An inverse correlation between estimated tuberculosis notification rates and asthma symptoms. *Respirology*. 2002;7:153–155.

157. Baccioglu Kavut A et al. Association between tuberculosis and atopy: Role of the CD14-159C/T polymorphism. *J Investig Allergol Clin Immunol*. 2012;22:201–207.

158. Hopkin JM. Atopy, asthma, and the mycobacteria. *Thorax*. 2000;55:443–445.

159. Obihara CC et al. Respiratory atopic disease, Ascaris-immunoglobulin E and tuberculin testing in urban South African children. *Clin Exp Allergy*. 2006;36:640–648.

160. Ferreira AP et al. Can the efficacy of bacille Calmette-Guerin tuberculosis vaccine be affected by intestinal parasitic infections? *J Infect Dis*. 2002;186(3):441–442.

161. Perry S et al. Infection with *Helicobacter pylori* is associated with protection against tuberculosis. *PLOS ONE*. 2010;5(1):e8804.

162. Majlessi L et al. Colonization with *Helicobacter* is concomitant with modified gut microbiota and drastic failure of the immune control of *Mycobacterium tuberculosis*. *Mucosal Immunology*. 2017.

163. Aaby P et al. Randomized trial of BCG vaccination at birth to low-birth-weight children: Beneficial nonspecific effects in the neonatal period? *J Infect Dis*. 2011;204(2):245–252.

164. Storgaard L et al. Development of BCG scar and subsequent morbidity and mortality in rural Guinea-Bissau. *Clin Infect Dis*. 2015;61(6):950–959.

165. Group KPT. Randomised controlled trial of single BCG, repeated BCG, or combined BCG and killed *Mycobacterium leprae* vaccine for prevention of leprosy and tuberculosis in Malawi. *Lancet*. 1996;348:17–24.

166. Lietman T, Porco T, and Blower S. Leprosy and tuberculosis: The epidemiological consequences of cross-immunity. *Am J Public Health*. 1997;87:1923–1927.

167. NCD Alliance, 2018 is the year to stand together against NCDs and TB [cited 2018 March 28]; Available from: https://ncdalliance.org/news-events/blog/2018-is-the-year-to-stand-together-against-ncds-and-tb.

168. The Lancet Diabetes Endocrinology, Diabetes and tuberculosis —a wake-up call. *Lancet Diabetes Endocrinol*. 2014;2(9):677.

169. Whiting DR et al. IDF diabetes atlas: Global estimates of the prevalence of diabetes for 2011 and 2030. *Diabetes Res Clin Pract*. 2011;94(3):311–321.

170. Creswell J et al. Tuberculosis and noncommunicable diseases: Neglected links and missed opportunities. *Eur Respiratory Soc*. 2011.

171. Martinez N, and Kornfeld H. Diabetes and immunity to tuberculosis. *Eur J Immunol*. 2014;44(3):617–626.

172. Riza AL et al. Clinical management of concurrent diabetes and tuberculosis and the implications for patient services. *Lancet Diabetes Endocrinol.* 2014;2(9):740–753.

173. Uplekar M et al. WHO's new End TB Strategy. *Lancet.* 2015;385 (9979):1799–1801.

174. Munro SA et al. Patient adherence to tuberculosis treatment: A systematic review of qualitative research. *PLoS Med.* 2007;4(7):e238.

175. Garner P et al. Promoting adherence to tuberculosis treatment. *Bull WHO.* 2007;85(5):404–406.

176. World Health Organization, Manual on use of routine data quality assessment (RDQA) tool for TB monitoring. 2011.

177. World Health Organization, Standards and benchmarks for tuberculosis surveillance and vital registration systems: Checklist and User Guide. *WHO/JTM/TB/2014.02.* 2014: Geneva, Switzerland.

178. World Health Organization, *Understanding and Using Tuberculosis Data.* 2014: World Health Organization.

179. Dye C et al. Targets for global tuberculosis control. *Int J Tuberc Lung Dis.* 2006;10:460–462.

180. Young DB, and Dye C. The development and impact of tuberculosis vaccines. *Cell.* 2006;124:683–687.

181. Dowdy DW, and Chaisson RE. The persistence of tuberculosis in the age of DOTS: Reassessing the effect of case detection. *Bull WHO.* 2009;87:296–304.

182. Dye C. Tuberculosis 2000–2010: Control, but not elimination. *Int J Tuberc Lung Dis.* 2000;4:S146–152.

183. Chakravorty S et al. The new Xpert MTB/RIF Ultra: Improving detection of *Mycobacterium tuberculosis* and resistance to rifampin in an assay suitable for point-of-care testing. *mBio.* 2017;8(4): e00812–17.

184. Petruccioli E et al. Correlates of tuberculosis risk: Predictive biomarkers for progression to active tuberculosis. *Eur Respir J.* 2016:ERJ-01012-2016.

185. Zak DE et al. A blood RNA signature for tuberculosis disease risk: A prospective cohort study. *Lancet.* 2016;387(10035):2312–2322.

186. Vree M et al. Tuberculosis trends, Vietnam. *Emerg Infect Dis.* 2007;13:332–333.

187. Buu TN et al. Decrease in risk of tuberculosis infection despite increase in tuberculosis among young adults in urban Vietnam. *Int J Tuberc Lung Dis.* 2010;14:289–295.

188. Grzybowski S, Styblo K, and Dorken E. Tuberculosis in Eskimos. *Tubercle.* 1976;57(supplement):S1–S58.

189. Dye C et al. Evaluating the impact of tuberculosis control: Number of deaths prevented by short-course chemotherapy in China. *Int J Epidemiol.* 2000;29:558–564.

190. Suarez PG et al. The dynamics of tuberculosis in response to 10 years of intensive control effort in Peru. *J Infect Dis.* 2001;184:473–478.

191. Toman K. *Tuberculosis Case-Finding and Chemotherapy. Questions and Answers.* 1st ed. Geneva: World Health Organization, 1979, 1–239.

192. Naidoo P et al. The South African tuberculosis care cascade: Estimated losses and methodological challenges. *J Infect Dis.* 2017;216(suppl_7):S702–S713.

193. Getahun H et al. Development of a standardized screening rule for tuberculosis in people living with HIV in resource-constrained settings: Individual participant data meta-analysis of observational studies. *PLoS Med.* 2011;18;8(1):e1000391.

194. World Health Organization, High-priority target product profiles for new tuberculosis diagnostics: Report of a consensus meeting. Geneva, Switzerland, 2014.

195. Kasaie P et al. Timing of tuberculosis transmission and the impact of household contact tracing. An agent-based simulation model. *Am J Respir Crit Care Med.* 2014;189(7):845–852.

196. Marks GB et al. Effectiveness of postmigration screening in controlling tuberculosis among refugees: A historical cohort study, 1984–1998. *Am J Public Health.* 2001;91:1797–1799.

197. Solsona J et al. Screening for tuberculosis upon admission to shelters and free-meal services. *Eur J Epidemiol.* 2001;17:123–128.

198. Noertjojo K et al. Contact examination for tuberculosis in Hong Kong is useful. *Int J Tuberc Lung Dis.* 2002;6:19–24.

199. Claessens NJM et al. High frequency of tuberculosis in households of index TB patients. *Int J Tuberc Lung Dis.* 2002;6:266–269.

200. Nyangulu DS et al. Tuberculosis in a prison population in Malawi. *Lancet.* 1997;350:1284–1287.

201. Calligaro GL et al. Effect of new tuberculosis diagnostic technologies on community-based intensified case finding: A multicentre randomised controlled trial. *Lancet Infect Dis.* 2017; 17(4):441–450.

202. Corbett EL et al. Comparison of two active case-finding strategies for community-based diagnosis of symptomatic smear-positive TB and control of infectious TB in Harare, Zimbabwe (DETECTB): A cluster-randomised trial. *Lancet.* 2010;376:1244–1253.

203. Golub JE et al. Active case finding of tuberculosis: Historical perspective and future prospects. *Int J Tuberc Lung Dis.* 2005; 9:1183–1203.

204. Marx FM et al. Tuberculosis control interventions targeted to previously treated people in a high-incidence setting: A modelling study. *Lancet Glob Health.* 2018;6(4):e426–e435.

205. Kranzer K et al. A systematic literature review of the benefits to communities and individuals of screening for active tuberculosis disease. In preparation, 2012.

206. Ayles H et al. Effect of household and community interventions on the burden of tuberculosis in southern Africa: The ZAMSTAR community-randomised trial. *Lancet.* 2013; 382(9899):1183–1194.

207. Getahun H, and Raviglione M. Household tuberculosis interventions—How confident are we? *Lancet.* 2013;382(9899):1157–1159.

208. Currie CS et al. Tuberculosis epidemics driven by HIV: Is prevention better than cure? *AIDS.* 2003;17:2501–2508.

209. Dodd PJ, White RG, and Corbett EL. Periodic active case finding: When to look? *PLOS ONE.* 2012;6:e29130.

210. Wang L et al. Prevalence and trends in smear-positive and bacteriologically-confirmed pulmonary tuberculosis in China in 2010. Unpublished. 2012.

211. Churchyard G et al. Community-wide isoniazid preventive therapy does not improve TB control among gold miners: The Thibela TB study, South Africa. in *19th Conference on Retroviruses and Opportunistic Infections.* 2012. Seattle.

212. Houben RM et al. Feasibility of achieving the 2025 WHO global tuberculosis targets in South Africa, China, and India: A combined analysis of 11 mathematical models. *Lancet Glob Health.* 2016;4(11):e806–e815.

213. Dowdy DW et al. Designing and evaluating interventions to halt the transmission of tuberculosis. *J Infect Dis.* 2017;216(suppl_6):S654–S661.

214. Subbaraman R et al. The tuberculosis cascade of care in India's public sector: A systematic review and meta-analysis. *PLoS Med.* 2016;13(10):e1002149.

215. Cazabon D et al. Quality of tuberculosis care in high burden countries: The urgent need to address gaps in the care cascade. *Int J Infect Dis.* 2017;56:111–116.

216. Cohn DL, and El-Sadr WM. Treatment of latent tuberculosis infection. In: Reichman LB, and Hershfield E (eds.). *Tuberculosis: A comprehensive international approach.* New York: Marcel Dekker, 2000.

217. Lee LM et al. Low adherence to guidelines for preventing TB among persons with newly diagnosed HIV infection, United States. *Int J Tuberc Lung Dis.* 2006;10:209–214.

218. World Health Organization, *Guidelines for intensified tuberculosis case-finding and isoniazid preventive therapy for people living with HIV in resource-constrained settings:* Geneva: World Health Organization, 2011.

219. Stop TB Partnership and World Health Organization, The Global Plan to Stop TB, 2006–2015. 2006, Geneva: Stop TB Partnership.

220. Boyles TH, and Maartens G. Should tuberculin skin testing be a prerequisite to prolonged IPT for HIV-infected adults? *Int J Tuberc Lung Dis.* 2012;16:857–859.

221. Lawn SD, and Wood R. Short-course untargeted isoniazid preventive therapy in South Africa: Time to rethink policy? *Int J Tuberc Lung Dis.* 2012;16:995–996.

222. Wilkinson D Squire SB, and Garner P. Effect of preventive treatment for tuberculosis in adults infected with HIV: Systematic review of randomised placebo controlled trials. *Br Med J.* 1998;317:625–629.

223. Bucher HC et al. Isoniazid prophylaxis for tuberculosis in HIV infection: A meta-analysis of randomized controlled trials. *AIDS.* 1999;13:501–507.

224. Johnson JL et al. Duration of efficacy of treatment of latent tuberculosis infection in HIV-infected adults. *AIDS.* 2001;15:2137–2147.

225. Quigley MA et al. Long-term effect of preventive therapy for tuberculosis in a cohort of HIV-infected Zambian adults. *AIDS.* 2001;15(2):215–222.

226. Whalen CC et al. A trial of three regimens to prevent tuberculosis in Ugandan adults infected with the human immunodeficiency virus. Uganda-Case Western Reserve University Research Collaboration. *N Engl J Med.* 1997;337(12):801–8.

227. Mwinga A et al. Twice weekly tuberculosis preventive therapy in HIV infection in Zambia. *AIDS.* 1998;12:2447–2457.

228. Woldehanna S, and Volmink J. Treatment of latent tuberculosis infection in HIV infected persons. *Cochrane Database Syst Rev.* 2004;(1):CD000171.

229. Samandari T et al. 6-month versus 36-month isoniazid preventive treatment for tuberculosis in adults with HIV infection in Botswana: A randomised, double-blind, placebo-controlled trial. *Lancet.* 2011;377:1588–1598.

230. Rangaka MX et al. Isoniazid plus antiretroviral therapy to prevent tuberculosis: A randomised double-blind, placebo-controlled trial. *Lancet.* 2014;384(9944):682–690.

231. Samandari T et al. TB incidence increase after cessation of 36 months' isoniazid prophylaxis in HIV+ adults: Botswana. in *19th Conference on Retroviruses and Opportunistic Infections.* 2012. Seattle.

232. Zar HJ et al. Effect of isoniazid prophylaxis on mortality and incidence of tuberculosis in children with HIV: Randomised controlled trial. *BMJ.* 2006. 1–7.

233. Rangaka MX et al. Controlling the seedbeds of tuberculosis: Diagnosis and treatment of tuberculosis infection. *Lancet.* 2015;386(10010):2344–2353.

234. Durovni B et al. Effect of improved tuberculosis screening and isoniazid preventive therapy on incidence of tuberculosis and death in patients with HIV in clinics in Rio de Janeiro, Brazil: A stepped wedge, cluster-randomised trial. *Lancet Infect Dis.* 2013;13(10):852–858.

235. Golub JE et al. Long-term protection from isoniazid preventive therapy for tuberculosis in HIV-infected patients in a medium-burden tuberculosis setting: The TB/HIV in Rio (THRio) study. *Clin Infect Dis.* 2014;60(4):639–645.

236. Ayles H, and Muyoyeta M. Isoniazid to prevent first and recurrent episodes of TB. *Trop Dr.* 2006;36:83–86.

237. Penn-Nicholson A et al. A novel blood test for tuberculosis prevention and treatment. *SAMJ: South African Medical Journal.* 2017;107(1):4–5.

238. Suliman S et al. Four-gene Pan-African blood signature predicts progression to tuberculosis. *Am J Respir Crit Care Med.* 2018;197:1198–1208.

239. Zignol M et al. Surveillance of anti-tuberculosis drug resistance in the world: An updated analysis, 2007–2010. *Bull WHO.* 2012;90:111–119D.

240. Dheda K et al. The epidemiology, pathogenesis, transmission, diagnosis, and management of multidrug-resistant, extensively drug-resistant, and incurable tuberculosis. *Lancet Respir Med.* 2017;5(4):291–360.

241. World Health Organization, Automated real-time nucleic acid amplification technology for rapid and simultaneous detection of tuberculosis and rifampicin resitance: Xpert MTB/RIF SYSTEM. *Publication number WHO/HTM/TB/2011.4.* 2011: Geneva, Switzerland.

242. Boehme C et al. Rapid molecular detection of tuberculosis and rifampin resistance. *N Engl J Med.* 2010;363:1005–1015.

243. Sergeev R et al. Modeling the dynamic relationship between HIV and the risk of drug-resistant tuberculosis. *Sci Transl Med.* 2012;4:135ra67.

244. Lukoye D et al. Variation and risk factors of drug resistant tuberculosis in sub-Saharan Africa: A systematic review and meta-analysis. *BMC Public Health.* 2015;15(1):291.

245. Mesfin YM et al. Association between HIV/AIDS and multi-drug resistance tuberculosis: A systematic review and meta-analysis. *PLOS ONE.* 2014;9(1):e82235.

246. Raviglione MC, and Smith IM. XDR tuberculosis—Implications for global public health. *N Engl J Med.* 2007;356:656–659.

247. Dheda K et al. Outcomes, infectiousness, and transmission dynamics of patients with extensively drug-resistant tuberculosis and home-discharged patients with programmatically incurable tuberculosis: A prospective cohort study. *Lancet Respir Med.* 2017;5(4):269–281.

248. Pietersen E et al. Long-term outcomes of patients with extensively drug-resistant tuberculosis in South Africa: A cohort study. *The Lancet.* 2014.

249. Klopper M et al. Emergence and spread of extensively and totally drug-resistant tuberculosis, South Africa. *Emerg Infect Dis.* 2013;19(3):449.

250. Velayati AA et al. Emergence of new forms of totally drug-resistant tuberculosis bacilli: Super extensively drug-resistant tuberculosis or totally drug-resistant strains in Iran. *Chest.* 2009;136(2):420–425.

251. Streicher E et al. Genotypic and phenotypic characterization of drug-resistant *Mycobacterium tuberculosis* isolates from rural districts of the Western Cape Province of South Africa. *J Clin Microbiol.* 2004;42(2):891–894.

252. Streicher EM et al. Emergence and treatment of multidrug resistant (MDR) and extensively drug-resistant (XDR) tuberculosis in South Africa. *Infect Genet Evol.* 2012;12(4):686–694.

253. World Health Organization, *Towards universal access to diagnosis and treatment of multidrug-resistant and extensively drug-resistant tuberculosis by 2015: WHO progress report 2011.* 2011.

254. Dye C et al. Erasing the world's slow stain: Strategies to beat multidrug-resistant tuberculosis. *Science.* 2002;295:2042–2046.

255. Cohen T, Sommers B, and Murray M. The effect of drug resistance on the fitness of *Mycobacterium tuberculosis*. *Lancet Infect Dis.* 2003;3:13–21.

256. Cohen T et al. Mathematical models of the epidemiology and control of drug-resistant TB. *Expert Review of Respiratory Medicine.* 2009;3(1):67–79.

257. Mitnick C et al. Community-based therapy for multidrug-resistant tuberculosis in Lima, Peru. *N Engl J Med.* 2003;348:119–128.

258. Mitnick CS et al. Comprehensive treatment of extensively drug-resistant tuberculosis. *N Engl J Med.* 2008;359:563–574.

259. Van Deun A et al. Short, highly effective, and inexpensive standardized treatment of multidrug-resistant tuberculosis. *Am J Respir Crit Care Med.* 2010;182:684–692.

260. World Health Organization, Guidelines for the programmatic management of drug-resistant tuberculosis - 2011 update, W.H. Organization, Editor. 2011, World Health Organization: Geneva.

261. Dowdy DW et al. Of testing and treatment: Implications of implementing new regimens for multidrug-resistant tuberculosis. *Clin Infect Dis.* 2017;65(7):1206–1211.

262. Zignol M et al. Population-based resistance of *Mycobacterium tuberculosis* isolates to pyrazinamide and fluoroquinolones: Results from a multicountry surveillance project. *Lancet Infect Dis.* 2016.

263. National Institute for Communicable Diseases, *South African Tuberculosis Drug Resistance Survey 2012–14.* [accessed 18 June 2018] Available from: http://www.nicd.ac.za/assets/files/K-12750%20 NICD%20National%20Survey%20Report_Dev_V11-LR.pdf. 2016: Johannesburg, South Africa.

264. Fine PEM. BCG vaccines and vaccination, in *Tuberculosis: a Comprehensive International Approach*, L.B. Reichman, Hershfield, E.S., Editor. 2001, Marcel Dekker: New York.

265. Harris RC et al. Systematic review of mathematical models exploring the epidemiological impact of future TB vaccines. *Hum Vaccines Immunotherapeut.* 2016;12(11):2813–2832.

266. Kaufmann SH et al. Progress in tuberculosis vaccine development and host-directed therapies—A state of the art review. *Lancet Respir Med.* 2014;2(4):301–320.

267. Haas CT et al. Diagnostic 'omics' for active tuberculosis. *BMC Med.* 2016;14(1):37.

268. Denkinger CM et al. Defining the needs for next generation assays for tuberculosis. *J Infect Dis.* 2015;211(suppl_2):S29–S38.

269. Theron G et al. Feasibility, accuracy, and clinical effect of point-of-care Xpert MTB/RIF testing for tuberculosis in primary-care settings in Africa: A multicentre, randomised, controlled trial. *The Lancet.* 2013;383(9915):424–35.

270. Churchyard GJ et al. Xpert MTB/RIF versus sputum microscopy as the initial diagnostic test for tuberculosis: A cluster-randomised trial embedded in South African roll-out of Xpert MTB/RIF. *Lancet Global Health.* 2015;3(8):e450–e457.

271. Cox HS et al. Impact of Xpert MTB/RIF for TB diagnosis in a primary care clinic with high TB and HIV prevalence in South Africa: A pragmatic randomised trial. *PLoS Med.* 2014;11(11):e1001760.

272. Durovni B et al. Impact of replacing smear microscopy with Xpert MTB/RIF for diagnosing tuberculosis in Brazil: A stepped-wedge cluster-randomized trial. *PLoS Med.* 2014;11(12):e1001766.

273. Theron G et al. Do high rates of empirical treatment undermine the potential effect of new diagnostic tests for tuberculosis in high-burden settings? *Lancet Infect Dis.* 2014;14(6):527–532.

274. Albert H et al. Development, roll-out and impact of Xpert MTB/RIF for tuberculosis: What lessons have we learnt and how can we do better? *Eur Respir J.* 2016:ERJ-00543–2016.

275. García-Basteiro AL, Saavedra B, and Cobelens F. The good, the bad and the ugly of the next-generation Xpert Mtb/Rif (*) ultra test for tuberculosis diagnosis. *Arch Bronchoneumol.* 2017.

276. Pai M, Schumacher SG, and Abimbola S. Surrogate endpoints in global health research: Still searching for killer apps and silver bullets? *BMJ Specialist J.* 2018.

277. Kendall EA et al. Priority-setting for novel drug regimens to treat tuberculosis: An epidemiologic model. *PLoS Med.* 2017;14(1):e1002202.

278. Dye C et al. Prospects for tuberculosis elimination. *Annu Rev Public Health.* 2013;34.

279. Dye C, and Williams BG. Criteria for the control of drug-resistant tuberculosis. *Proc Natl Acad Sci USA.* 2000;97:8180–8185.

280. Centers for Disease Control and Prevention. *Tuberculosis (TB).* 2012 [cited 2012 April 25]; Available from: http://www.cdc.gov.

281. Health Protection Agency. Tuberculosis (TB). 2012 [cited 2012 April 25]; Available from: http://www.hpa.org.uk.

282. Styblo K, Broekmans JF, and Borgdorff MW. Expected decrease in tuberculosis incidence during the elimination phase. How to determine its trend? *Tuberculosis Surveillance Research Unit, Progress Report 1997.* 1997;1:17–78.

283. Hong YP et al. The seventh nationwide tuberculosis prevalence survey in Korea, 1995. *Int J Tuberc Lung Dis.* 1998;2:27–36.

284. China Tuberculosis Control Collaboration. The effect of tuberculosis control in China. *Lancet.* 2004;364:417–422.

PATHOLOGY AND IMMUNOLOGY

3

Mycobacterium tuberculosis
The Genetic Organism

WILLIAM R. JACOBS, JR.

INTRODUCTION: THE GLOBAL PROBLEM AND TB IN INFECTIOUS DISEASE HISTORY

Tuberculosis (TB) has been a leading cause of death throughout human history. The World Health Organization reported over 1.6 million deaths from TB and over 10 million new cases of TB in 2017, making TB the single leading cause of death from an infectious agent today.[1] The TB problem has worsened in the last 50 years, with the emergence of the HIV epidemic, which has caused increased transmission, increased incidence, and the emergence of drug resistance. *Mycobacterium tuberculosis* strains have evolved that are resistant to the two front-line TB drugs—Isoniazid (INH) and Rifampicin. These strains are called multi-drug-resistant *M. tuberculosis* (MDR).[2] Ominously, extensively drug-resistant strains (XDR) have also evolved that are resistant to as many as 10 TB drugs.[3] This emergence of resistance is surprising as TB is a disease for which control programs are employed around the world: (1) rapid diagnostic tests, (2) a vaccine, BCG (bacilli Calmette and Guerine), and (3) a sterilizing chemotherapy. If so many solutions are available, then why is TB still a major global health threat and economic burden?

The question of whether TB was caused by a transmissible agent or was merely a manifestation of an inherited disposition was a controversial subject in the nineteenth century, but the 1868 demonstration by Jean Antoine Villemin that inoculation of tuberculous materials from humans and cattle into rabbits elicited characteristic granulomatous lesions swung the argument strongly in favor of an infectious cause.[4] The matter was finally and irrefutably settled on March 24, 1882 when Robert Koch described a series of meticulous studies in which he had not only isolated the causative bacilli but also rigorously demonstrated causality by fulfilling criteria laid out in his well-known postulate.[5,6] In that 1882 paper, Robert Koch wrote: "To prove that tuberculosis was caused by the invasion and multiplication of bacilli, it was necessary to: (1) isolate the bacilli; (2) grow them in pure culture, and (3) administer them to an animal to produce the same moribund condition."[3,4]

While others had hypothesized that many diseases were caused by microbes, the inability to grow these microbes in pure cultures prevented stringent testing of this hypothesis. Robert Koch, like Louis Pasteur, developed methods to grow pure cultures of microbes, providing a new tool to visualize and characterize these organisms. Jean Antoine Villemin performed the first TB animal experiment when he showed the transfer of tubercles from patients with TB caused the disease in rabbits.[4,7] As a surgeon, Villemin could see the differences between the tubercles in TB patients compared to the tumors he observed in patients with lung cancers. Brilliantly, he demonstrated the transfer of cancerous lesions to rabbits caused no disease whereas transfer of tubercle lesions always caused TB. Villemin concluded TB was not a cancer, but rather was caused by an infectious agent.[7] Robert Koch actually first fulfilled the conditions of the Henle–Koch theory with the anthrax bacillus and published this work in 1876.[8] By obtaining fluid from a cow's eye, he had a sterile fluid he could inoculate with anthrax bacillus *in vitro* to obtain pure cultures of the pathogen. He went on to show that these pure cultures reproducibly caused disease in rabbits and mice, thus fulfilling the three conditions of Koch's postulate to prove that the anthrax bacillus was the etiologic agent of the disease. The same approach enabled Robert Koch to demonstrate that TB was caused by a bacillus. For growing the tubercle bacilli, Koch needed larger amounts of growth media and so he decided to use sera from cows.[8] After drawing blood and allowing the red cells to settle, he sterilized the sera by repeated cycles of heating to 65°C and cooling. At the end of the seventh cycle, he would allow the serum to solidify in a slanted tube. A gelatinous surface would form, which upon inoculation, enabled the growth of tubercle bacilli. Koch used these pure cultures of tubercle bacilli to infect rabbits, mice, guinea pigs, cows, and cats; all developed TB-like disease. For the first time in history, we knew TB was caused by an infectious agent. For his foundational work, Robert Koch received the Nobel Prize in 1905.

GENE TRANSFER IN *M. TUBERCULOSIS*

Gregor Mendel published his work in 1866 establishing the concept of discreet units of hereditary (genes) caused by characteristics (phenotypes in plants).[9] Interestingly, the molecular basis for a gene was not determined until 80 years later and this was achieved by an experiment selecting for a virulent bacterium in a mouse.[10]

Phenotypes are characteristics of an organism that result from a genotype and its environment. For bacteria, common phenotypes refer to characteristics such as virulence, drug-resistance, and dye-staining properties or colony morphologies. Molecular Koch's postulate was a concept first proposed by Stanley Falkow for establishing causality of a phenotype.[11] A paraphrased version of Koch's postulate would be: To prove that a phenotype such as drug resistance of an organism is caused by a specific genotype, it was necessary to: (1) isolate a mutant exhibiting drug resistance, (2) clone the genotype from the drug-resistant mutant, and (3) transfer the cloned genotype to a parental strain and demonstrate the acquisition of drug resistance. This is the essence of genetics.

Sixty years after Koch discovered the tubercle bacillus and before DNA was known to encode genetic material, molecular genetics began with Beadle and Tatum in 1941[12] where mutants of *Neurospora crassa* were generated by irradiation and plated on complex media. These mutants, referred to as auxotrophic mutants, required single nutrients such as pyridoxine, thiamine, or para-amino benzoic acid and later amino acids. In completing the requirement of gene transfer, Beadle and Tatum fulfilled the third condition of Molecular Koch's postulate and discovered, for the first time, that one gene encoded one enzyme. In fact, the discovery of the molecular nature transforming principle (an isolated fraction of a virulent cell extract of *Streptococcus pneumoniae*) allowed Avery, MacLeod, and McCarty to discover in 1941 that DNA was the genetic material.[13]

In contrast to *Neurospora*, which was a diploid organism that underwent meiosis, transfer of DNA directly into *Streptococcus* was called transformation. The question as to whether bacteria had genes was answered convincingly when Salvador Luria and Max Delbruck used phages (bacterial viruses) as selecting agents, providing evidence that Charles Darwin's survival of the fittest premise existed even for bacteria.[14] Gene transfer studies exploded when Joshua Lederberg and Edward Tatum demonstrated in 1946 that *Escherichia coli* could transfer genes from cell to cell (conjugation) using double auxotrophic mutants.[15] *E. coli* would become the model organism for molecular genetics for the next 30 years. The lingering debate as to whether DNA, not protein, was the genetic material was convincingly proved by Hershey and Chase's experiment with phages, bacteria, and radiolabeled DNA

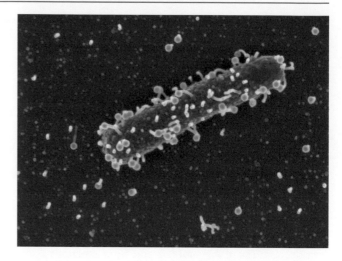

Figure 3.1 Scanning electron micrograph of TM4-based shuttle phasmids attached to *M. tuberculosis*. The TM4-based shuttle phasmids provided a facile system for delivering foreign DNA into *M. tuberculosis*. These phages have been used to: (1) systematically develop transformation for mycobacteria, (2) deliver transposons for transposon mutant libraries, (3) move mutated alleles into *M. tuberculosis* strains (specialized transduction), and (4) deliver reporter genes such as firefly luciferase to rapidly assess drug susceptibilities.

or protein.[16] Notably, Norton Zinder, while trying to repeat the Lederberg experiment for *Salmonella*, discovered phages could transfer genes to other bacterial cells—a process he named transduction.[17] Thus transformation, conjugation, and transduction became the key tools for the successful fulfillment of the third condition of Molecular Koch's postulate. The slow growth and virulence precluded successful gene transfer in *M. tuberculosis* until 1987.[18] Using the first chimeric mycobacteriophage–*E. coli* shuttle vector, termed a shuttle phasmid—it became possible to transfer genes in *M. tuberculosis* (Figure 3.1). Nearly 100 years later, plasmid transformation, efficient transposon mutagenesis systems, specialized transduction, and reporter mycobacteriophages have enabled the acquisition of many phenotypes of *M. tuberculosis*, opening the doors for new therapeutic approaches (see reviews[19–21]).

THE GENOME OF *M. TUBERCULOSIS*

A landmark in TB research occurred with the publication of the genome sequence of *M. tuberculosis* in 1998[22] on a widely used reference strain, H37Rv. No extrachromosomal genetic elements were detected. The genome of *M. bovis* has also been sequenced and shows more than 99.95% similarity with that of *M. tuberculosis* although it is very slightly smaller, with 4,345,492 base pairs.[23] In contrast, the genome of *M. leprae*,[24] with 3.27 million base pairs, is considerably smaller than that of *M. tuberculosis*, and it differs from the latter in that many of its genes, around a half, are defective and non-functional, explaining why this organism has never been cultivated *in vitro* and is an obligate intracellular pathogen.

The chemical structure of the genome of *M. tuberculosis* is remarkably uniform with a high guanine + cytosine content

(65.6%) throughout, indicating that it has evolved with minimal incorporation of DNA from extraneous sources. Other notable differences between this genome and those of other bacteria have been determined. In particular, *M. tuberculosis* has a very large number of genes coding for enzymes involved in lipid metabolism, around 250 compared to only 50 in *E. coli*. All known lipid biosynthesis pathways encountered elsewhere in nature, as well as several unique ones, are detectable in the mycobacteria. Most of these enzymes are involved in the synthesis of the extremely complex lipid-rich mycobacterial cell walls.

The mycobacterial genome is also unique in containing a large number of genes, up to 10% of the total coding potential, that code for two unrelated families, Pro-Glu and Pro-Pro-Glu, of acidic, glycine-rich proteins that contribute to the diversity in antigenic structure and virulence. Because they undergo frequent genetic remodeling by various mechanisms, they may have contributed substantially to the evolution of the *M. tuberculosis* complex and adaptation of its various members to different hosts.[25] Despite much research in the decade since their discovery, the function of the PE/PPE group of proteins remains poorly understood, although they induce or modulate a range of innate and acquired immune reactions.[26]

Four main types of genomic differences among strains within the *M. tuberculosis* complex have been described: those involving single-nucleotide variations (single-nucleotide polymorphisms, or SNPs),[27] those involving several sequential nucleotides (long-sequence polymorphisms, or LSPs), minisatellites, and microsatellites. Although there are 1075 SNP differences between *M. tuberculosis* H37Rv and a recent clinical isolate, and 2437 between H37Rv and the sequenced strain of *M. bovis*, these differences are small in relation to the four million or more nucleotide pairs in the genomes of these strains. The LSPs are much fewer in number than the SNPs in the *M. tuberculosis* complex and include 20 well-defined regions of difference (RD) that are described here.

The function of bacterial minisatellites is unknown, but their analogues in eukaryotic genomes contribute to genetic diversity by mediating chromosome recombination during meiosis.[28] In the mycobacteria, they often occur as tandem repeats in the regions between functional genes and some are designated mycobacterial interspersed repetitive units (MIRUs). Minisatellites are utilized in a typing system known as variable number tandem repeat (VNTR) analysis, as described in Chapter 5. By insertion or deletion, microsatellites, also known as single sequence repeats, cause reversible frame-shift mutations at a relatively high rate and impart a genetic "plasticity" to the genomes of pathogens, enabling them to adapt readily to different hosts.[29,30]

The genome of *M. tuberculosis* contains mobile units of DNA, informally known as "jumping genes" that contribute to genetic variation and evolution. These mobile elements include a class termed insertion sequences (ISs) of which 56 different types, grouped in several families, are present in the genome of strain H37Rv. Most, but not all, strains of *M. tuberculosis* contain copies, usually numbering from 4 to 14, of the insertion sequence IS6110.[31] With some exceptions, strains of *M. bovis* contain fewer copies of IS6110 than *M. tuberculosis*, with, as described earlier, daughter strains of BCG containing either one or two copies. The considerable variation in the numbers and position of copies of IS6110 between strains forms the basis of the restriction fragment-length polymorphism (RFLP) typing system used in epidemiological purposes.

The genome of members of *M. tuberculosis* contains a complex termed the direct repeat (DR) locus consisting of repetitive 36 base-pair units of DNA separated by non-repetitive 34–41 base-pair spacer oligonucleotides. The DR region of *M. tuberculosis* is an example of a region present in all bacterial genomes and is termed clustered regularly interspaced short palindromic repeats (CRISPR). The function of this region is unknown, but it may be the bacterial analogue of the centromere found in eukaryote chromosomes. There are numerous possible combinations of spacer oligonucleotides, and these are very stable, providing a highly discriminative typing scheme known as spacer oligonucleotide typing, or "spoligotyping",[32] as described in Chapter 5. There is evidence that variation in the DR locus is due to mutational events in the spacer oligonucleotides, including their disruption by translocations of the ISs.[33] Such mutational events occur at a very slow rate and serve as an evolutionary "clock."

Since the year 2000, there has been intense interest in a class of small, non-coding, RNA molecules (microRNAs) that regulate cellular metabolism by binding to messenger RNA, thereby blocking transcription in the ribosome and "silencing" gene expression. Interest has principally focused on microRNAs in eukaryotic, including human, cells as possible therapeutic agents, but analogous molecules, sRNAs, are present in bacteria. Many sRNAs have been detected in *M. tuberculosis*, and their expression varies considerably according to growth conditions, particularly between bacilli in exponential growth and stationary phases of cultivation and between those extracted from infected lungs and those grown *in vitro*.[34] Therefore, sRNAs may play a key role in the adaptation of *M. tuberculosis* to a wide range of *in vivo* and *in vitro* environments.

The nomenclature of the causative organisms of human and mammalian TB is not entirely logical. As described here, analysis of their genomes has shown that these bacilli, grouped in the *M. tuberculosis* complex, are very closely related, with less than 0.1% genomic difference between them; thus, they clearly belong to what should be regarded as a single species.

The great majority of strains of *M. tuberculosis* produce rough colonies on solid media (Figure 3.1), but one rare variant, termed the Canetti type and also but unofficially *M. canetti*, produces smooth colonies due to large amounts of lipopolysaccharides on their cell surfaces.[35,36] This variant, almost all strains of which have been isolated in the Horn of Africa, appears to be a primitive "living fossil" form of *M. tuberculosis* (see the following section). Human-to-human transmission has not been confirmed, and epidemiological findings suggest that human infection is acquired from animate or non-animate non-human sources.[37]

Strains of *M. bovis* differ from *M. tuberculosis* in several respects including resistance to the anti-TB agent pyrazinamide. However, isolates susceptible to this agent, though in most other respects similar to *M. bovis*, have been isolated from animals, principally goats, in Spain and Germany. Because there are genomic differences between these strains and *M. bovis*, they have been allocated to the separate species *M. caprae*.[38] Occasional strains of otherwise typical *M. bovis* are also susceptible to pyrazinamide.[39]

TB caused by *M. caprae* has also been reported in humans, notably in Germany where one-third of 166 strains of human origin initially identified as *M. bovis*, isolated between 1999 and 2001 from patients principally living in south Germany, were found to be *M. caprae*.[40] The patients were in the same elderly age range as those infected with *M. bovis*, suggesting that disease due to both types represents reactivation of old infections.

An important "man-made" variant of *M. bovis* is the BCG vaccine that was derived, by 230 sub-cultivations on a potato-bile medium between the years 1908 and 1921, from a strain ("Lait Nocard") isolated from a case of bovine mastitis. Some currently available daughter strains of BCG, including the Brazilian, Japanese, Romanian, Russian, and Swedish strains, were issued by the Institut Pasteur before 1932. These differ from those daughter strains issued after this date in their cell wall structure, their active secretion of an antigenic protein, MPB70, and having two copies, rather than one, of the insertion sequence IS6110 (see the following section).[41]

A group of tubercle bacilli principally isolated from humans in equatorial Africa and in migrants from that region have properties intermediate between *M. tuberculosis* and *M. bovis* and have been given the separate species name *M. africanum*. Originally, two geographical variants of this species were described: Type I strains, principally from West Africa, resembling *M. bovis*, and Type II, mainly found in East Africa, resembling *M. tuberculosis*.[42] More recently, it has been suggested that Type I strains should be subdivided into West African Types 1 and 2 of *M. africanum* and Type II strains reclassified as the Uganda genotype of *M. tuberculosis*.[43] Around half the cases of human TB in West Africa are caused by *M. africanum,* and there is a tendency for patients to be older, more frequently infected with HIV, and more malnourished than those with disease caused by classical *M. tuberculosis*, indicating that the former is of lower virulence.[42]

In addition to *M. bovis*, there are strains that clearly belong to the *M. tuberculosis* complex with unique distinguishing properties that cause disease in various animals, with humans as rare secondary hosts. The first to be described was *M. microti*, so-named because it was first isolated from the vole, *Microtus agrestis*, and originally termed the vole tubercle bacillus. It was regarded as being attenuated in humans, having the same order of virulence as BCG vaccine, and was evaluated as a vaccine for human use in comparison with BCG in clinical trials,[44] but there have been several reports of human TB due to *M. microti* in immunocompetent and immunocompromised patients in recent years.[45] A very similar organism has been isolated from the dassie, or rock hyrax, and the llama.

Strains with sufficient genomic differences to justify the separate species name *M. pinnepedii* have been isolated from tuberculous lesions in free and captive seals and sea lions in Australia, New Zealand, South America, and the Netherlands, and transmission to animal keepers has been confirmed by tuberculin skin testing and interferon-gamma release assays.[46,47] A further cluster termed *M. mungi* has been isolated from the banded mongoose (*Mungos mungo*) in Botswana.[48] Strains with distinct features have been isolated from tuberculous lesions in other animals including oryx, water buffaloes, and cats but have not been given separate species names.

KNOWLEDGE OF *M. TUBERCULOSIS* PHENOTYPES, GENOTYPES, AND CLINICAL IMPLICATIONS

Before the development of gene transfer we did not know: (1) acid-fastness is regulated by a signal transduction pathway; (2) the primary attenuation of BCG is a loss of a Type VII secretion system; (3) *M. tuberculosis* lives an autarkic lifestyle; (4) the targets of isoniazid, its mechanisms of action, and its mechanism of resistance; (5) the targets for other TB-specific drugs; and (6) persistence is mediated by a unique expression profile and can be reversed by stimulating respiration. These unknown facts seemed surprising for the pathogen that Koch demonstrated to be the cause of an infectious disease. A brief summary follows of how genetics provides the critical mutants for elucidating the facts.

ACID-FAST STAINING IS REGULATED BY A SIGNAL TRANSDUCTION PATHWAY

Microscopic analysis of clinical samples remains one of the fastest way to diagnose infections. The Gram stain, developed by Christian Gram, remains a standard test for distinguishing Gram-positive organisms (such as *Staphylococci* or *Streptococci*) from Gram-negative organisms (such *E. coli* or *Pseudomonas*). *M. tuberculosis* and the leprosy bacillus stain acid-fast positive. Dyes can be removed from the cell walls of Gram-negative bacteria when treated with alcohol, whereas Gram-positive organisms retain the dye. During the process of investigating the role of specific genes of mycolic acid biosynthesis, it was discovered that a mutant of *M. tuberculosis* that had the *kasB* gene deleted no longer stained acid fast. The *kasB* gene encodes a keto–acyl synthase enzyme that mediates the addition of the last six carbons on the mycolic acid chain increasing the length from 76 carbons to 82 carbons. Surprisingly, the elimination of this enzyme makes the *M. tuberculosis* cells lose their acid-fast staining property.[49] Importantly, a year after Koch discovered the tubercle bacillus, another group found *M. tuberculosis* strains that did not stain acid-fast positive still caused TB. This was called Koch's paradox.[50] Interestingly, this kasB deletion has been shown to infect and kill mice lacking T and B cells (SCID mice), but is unable to kill immunocompetent isogenic parents. Surprisingly, the enzyme activity of the KasB keto–acyl synthase is turned off when two of the threonines located within the amino acid sequence of the protein are phosphorylated, demonstrating that this enzyme activity is regulated by a signal transduction pathway of a serine/threonine kinase.[51] Unlike most bacteria, *M. tuberculosis* possess 11 of these serine/threonine kinases that are well-known to regulate different pathways in eukaryotic cells. This enzyme regulation activity provides an explanation for Koch's paradox as it demonstrates there exist strains of *M. tuberculosis* that can infect, multiply in hosts, and are not virulent unless the patient's immune system is compromised. Moreover, the acid-fast negative bacteria represent a variation of *M. tuberculosis* that can persist in the host. Finally, since acid-fast staining represents the method by which *M. tuberculosis* cells are detected, subpopulations of acid-fast *M. tuberculosis* cells may represent an unidentified and unappreciated set of

M. tuberculosis cells representing a significant, unidentified set of organisms in TB patients. The development of a reagent such as a monoclonal antibody that selectively identifies these acid-fast-negative organisms might be a useful tool for characterizing these persistent forms of the organism.

THE PRIMARY ATTENUATION OF BCG IS A LOSS OF A TYPE VII SECRETION SYSTEM

BCG (bacilli Calmette and Guerine) is a TB vaccine still given to children at birth or within the first two weeks of birth in most developing countries. While it has not eliminated TB, numerous studies demonstrate BCG reduces severe forms of TB in children and hence WHO recommends its administration in countries where TB is highly present.[52] The strain was originally isolated from a bovine tubercle bacillus in 1904 and demonstrated by Drs. Calmette and Guerin to be highly attenuated in animals. In 1921, Dr. Calmette administered the strain orally to a child whose mother had died of TB.[53] The child never developed TB and by 1928, the League of Nations had recommended it be given to all children at birth. The efficacy results with BCG have proven to be variable with over 70% protection in some trials and no protection in others. These differences have been postulated to be due to: (1) genetic differences in BCG isolates, (2) human population differences, and/or (3) differences in exposure to environmental mycobacteria.[54]

Before genome sequences and gene transfer, there was no way to know the molecular genetic basis for the attenuation of BCG. The lab of Ken Stover was the first to discover genome differences between BCG and *M. tuberculosis* using genomic subtractive hybridization methodology.[55] This elegant study clearly showed many genomic deletions amongst various BCG strains but also reported one deletion, the RD1 deletion, was common to all BCG strains. The availability of microarrays from the original *M. tuberculosis* genome sequence demonstrated significant accumulations of various deletions of BCG strains that had been passaged in independent labs over the years.[56] It is noteworthy to point out that this group was unable to restore full virulence to BCG by transferring in the deleted genes. In fact, virulence in SCID mice was restored when a cosmid spanning RD1 was introduced into BCG.[57] Precise deletions of only the RD1 region in virulent *M. tuberculosis* and *M. bovis* showed that this deletion was sufficient for a high degree of attenuation.[58] The RD1 region has been extensively studied and found to be involved in generating connections between the phagolysosomal vacuole in which *M. tuberculosis* resides and the cytoplasm of the infected cell.[59,60] The clinical implications are numerous. First, the deletion of the genes encoding ESAT-6 and CFP-10 explains why the QuantiFERON test can distinguish BCG vaccination from *M. tuberculosis* infection. Second, the attenuation of BCG is related to its ability to cause lysis of lung pneumocytes or its connection of phagosomal vacuole to the cytoplasm of *M. tuberculosis* cells providing tools for probing the cell biology of macrophages and dendritic cells. Lastly, the precise deletion of RD1 from *M. tuberculosis* or *M. bovis* failed to improve, or only slightly improved, vaccine derivative efficacy. Therefore, the hypothesis became that even if the original BCG was found, its protectiveness was not going to be improved in the current human population. The world needs a better TB vaccine that elicits a different protective immune response than BCG.

THE AUTARKIC LIFESTYLE OF *M. TUBERCULOSIS*

By studying the biology of the auxotrophic mutants of *M. tuberculosis*, it is clear that the tubercle bacillus, unlike many other intracellular pathogens, has evolved to have an autarkic or self-sufficient lifestyle. Other intracellular pathogens, such as *Francisella* or *Legionella*, are naturally occurring amino acid auxotrophs. Whereas, *M. tuberculosis* and *M. leprae* sequences reveal intact genes to synthesize all 20 amino acids,[22,24] *M. tuberculosis* fails to be able to multiply in mice if it is unable to make leucine,[10] methionine,[61] or arginine.[62] Plants, fungi, and most bacteria have the ability to make all 20 amino acids. *Legionella* cannot make arginine, methionine, cysteine, leucine, valine, isoleucine, phenylalanine, and tyrosine. Interestingly, leucine starvation for *M. tuberculosis* is bacteriostatic whereas starvation for methionine or arginine is rapidly bactericidal thereby suggesting the enzymes to make these amino acids might be excellent drug targets.

THE TARGET OF ISONIAZID

Isoniazid was discovered in 1952[63,64] as an analogue of nicotinamide, which was serendipitously discovered to kill *M. tuberculosis* while it was used as a remedy to treat the ill effects of cancer therapies.[65] During the synthesis of one of these synthetic molecules, namely γ-pyridyaldehyde thiosemicarbazone, an intermediate was discovered to have surprisingly strong activity against TB. This intermediate was called isonicotinic acid hydrazide or INH.[63,64] The combination of Streptomycin, *p*-amino salicylic, and Isoniazid was the first combination therapy that led to sterilizing chemotherapy.

Although researchers had found this wunderkind of a drug, a major hurdle still remained: how exactly did it work? The answer to this question lingered over TB research for the next 50 years.

For five decades following the discovery of INH, many researchers attempted to determine its mechanism of action. The specificity to act only on mycobacteria and the lack of gene transfer in mycobacteria made it impossible to discover the target of INH and thereby elucidate its precise mechanism of action. A drug target is a component of a cell (usually an enzyme or a protein component of a complex cellular machine) to which a drug binds and inhibits, and this inhibition leads to the death of the cell. The mapping and sequencing of genes conferring drug resistance allows for the elucidation of the mechanism of drug action and drug resistance.

For example, streptomycin—the first drug discovered to have bactericidal activity against *M. tuberculosis*—was also found to be active against *E. coli*. By isolating mutants and mapping the locations of their resistance alleles, researchers concluded that resistance was due to a ribosomal protein (S12) of the small subunit designated rpsL.[66] Consistent with this conclusion, the recent elucidation of the three-dimensional structure of the ribosome with streptomycin shows the binding to streptomycin to the S12 protein.[67]

Without gene transfer, early published reports on INH mechanisms of action were associated with inhibition of DNA biosynthesis, inhibition of NAD glycosylase, and disruption of cell walls (reviewed in Vilcheze and Jacobs Jr.[2]). Frank Winder was the first to find evidence that INH inhibited mycolic acid biosynthesis.[68] Importantly, Kuni Takayama, showed that the death of *M. tuberculosis* cells correlated with the inhibition of mycolic acid biosynthesis.[69] Moreover, Takayama demonstrated that the inhibition of mycolic acid biosynthesis resulted in an accumulation of a monounsaturated fatty acid allowing him to conclude that the specific target had to be: (1) a desaturase, (2) a cyclopropane, or (3) an enzyme component of the fatty acid elongation pathway.[70] The question of the target was further complicated by the fact that most of INH-resistant mutants that had been isolated were found to correlate with a loss of a catalase peroxidase activity.[71] A resolution of the mechanism of action of INH would not be resolved until gene transfers could be performed in mycobacteria.

To prove that a phenotype (INH-resistance) was mediated by a specific genotype (a specific DNA sequenced allele), it was necessary to: (1) isolate a mutant that was INH-resistant; (2) clone the mutant allele; and (3) transfer the allele and demonstrate it conferred INH-resistance to the parental strain. While this set of three conditions seemed simple enough, performing allelic exchanges in *M. tuberculosis* chromosome had never been demonstrated. The easiest way to clone a gene was to clone it on a plasmid, but plasmid transformation would have to wait until a plasmid transformable *M. smegmatis* mutant mc²155 was

developed.[72,73] Using mc²155, INH-resistant mutants were isolated that either had a loss of function (a loss of the INH activator activity[74]) or a gain of INH-resistance in a gene named *inhA*.[75] The loss of function did indeed correlate with a loss of a *katG*-catalase-peroxidase activity, which suggested that the catalase peroxidase was an activator that activated INH. The InhA encodes a NADH-dependent enoyl-reductase (Figure 3.2), which is involved in elongating the mycolic acid chain from C18 to a C50 or C56 (reviewed in Vilcheze and Jacobs Jr.[2]). Surprisingly, X-ray crystallographic analyses revealed the actual inhibitor of InhA to be an INH-NAD adduct.[76] Importantly, the genetic data found in *M. smegmatis* was confirmed with *M. tuberculosis*.[77–79]

Thus, we know that that INH, when activated by the *katG*-encoded catalase peroxidase, forms an adduct with NAD that inhibits the enoyl reductase of mycolic acid synthase. As predicted for a drug target, a mutation within the structural gene that confers resistance would display reduced binding of the drug. This was observed for the INH-NAD adduct.[79] In addition to structural mutations, target proteins can also confer resistance by target overexpression thereby titrating the inhibitor.[51]

PERSISTENCE: THE SINGLE GREATEST IMPEDIMENT TO TB CONTROL

Persistence was defined by Walsh McDermott as the capacity of the tubercle bacillus to survive sterilization in mouse tissues.[80] Numerous clinical trials had demonstrated that curing

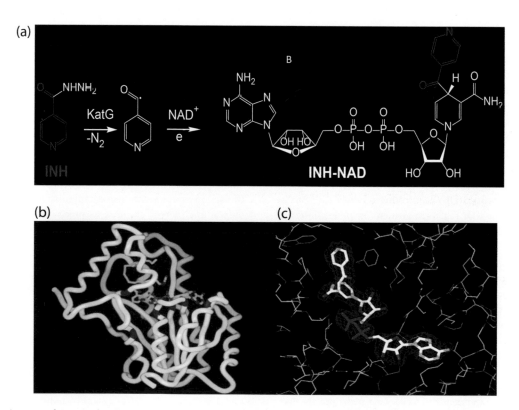

Figure 3.2 Mechanism of isoniazid action. (a) Isoniazid is a pro-drug that is activated by the *katG*-encoded catalase peroxidase to form a radical that binds to NAD resulting in an INH-NAD adduct. (b) The *inhA*-encoded NAD-specific enoyl reductase (three-dimensional structure) is part of mycolic acid biosynthesis. (c) Binding of the INH-NAD adduct to the InhA protein inhibits the enoyl reductase activity resulting in inhibition of mycolic acid biosynthesis and the death of *M. tuberculosis* cells. (Courtesy of Catherine Vilcheze Jim Sacchettini.)

TB required long therapies as too short a therapy would lead to reactivated TB with *M. tuberculosis* strains that are fully drug sensitive. These studies demonstrated that TB has the ability to persist during treatment.[81] In order to better understand this phenomenon of persistence, a highly reproducible *in vitro* model was developed for *M. tuberculosis* and INH.[2,82,83] For this model, if 10^6 exponentially growing *M. tuberculosis* cells are freshly inoculated into media with or without INH and samples are taken daily for the next 28 days, 99%–99.9% of the INH-treated cells are killed in the first 3 days, but the remaining cells are not sterilized (Figure 3.3). The 0.1%–1% survivors are INH-sensitive when regrown. These represent a subpopulation of *M. tuberculosis* cells that are expressing phenotypic resistance. By analyzing the mRNA

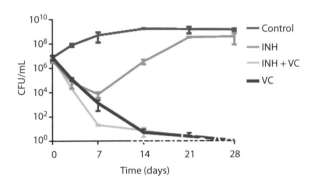

Figure 3.3 *In vitro* model revealing Isoniazid persisters and their sterilization when INH is combined with vitamin C. Exponentially growing *M. tuberculosis* cells are mixed with or without INH and viable colony forming units are quantitated at various days post-addition as can be seen by day 3, 99%–99.9% of the cells are killed but 0.1%–1% of cells express phenotypic INH resistance and eventually lead to the emergence of genetically resistant INH cells. The addition of vitamin C with INH leads to the rapid sterilization of the *M. tuberculosis* culture.

expression pattern microarrays, we discovered that these INH-persister cells had down-regulated many of the normal growth genes involved in cell division or respiration but were upregulated for stress responses.[84] These INH-tolerant cells can be visualized using a dual reporter mycobacteriophage (Figure 3.4), which expresses an RFP fused to a highly upregulated *dnaK* promoter but will not express a GFP that is fused to a strong phage promoter.[84] Importantly, we have discovered that in the setting of INH administration, the addition of vitamin C or *N*-acetyl cysteine results in sterilization of the cultures and this correlates with increased respiration.[82]

CONCLUDING REMARKS

Although TB was one of the first diseases proven to be caused by an infectious agent over 135 years ago, it remains the single leading infectious cause of death in the world today. Success in controlling many other infectious diseases has come about with rapid sterilizing chemotherapies and/or effective vaccines. Moreover, the ability to observe gene transfer by conjugation, transformation, or transduction has allowed for the discovery of drug-resistance genes, virulence genes, and many genes involved in evading host defenses. This knowledge has led to improved therapies for many other pathogens.

The characteristic slow growth of *M. tuberculosis* and its virulence have slowed down its research. However, the ability to perform gene transfer in *M. tuberculosis* and other mycobacteria has provided many new ways to understand the tubercle bacillus and its biology. Moreover, the availability of thousands of genomic sequences of *M. tuberculosis* and efficient means for generating transposon mutagenesis and targeted gene disruptions will most

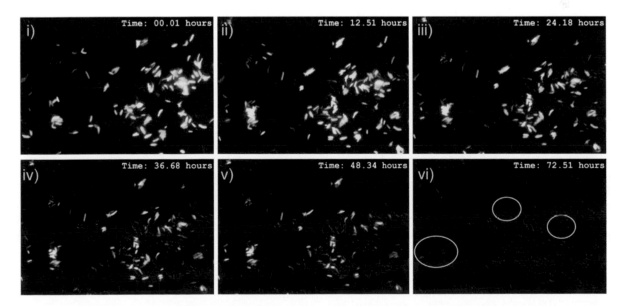

Figure 3.4 Time lapsed images of *M. tuberculosis* infected with a dual reporter mycobacteriophage and treated with INH. Initially *M. tuberculosis*, the dual reporter mycobacteriophage, and INH were mixed together on a microfluidic chip and images were taken every 12 hours for 3 days. As can be seen, initially most of the cells fluoresced green and yellow because of GFP and RFP co-expression. By day 3, all of the yellow cells had died leaving only red cells fluorescing. The GFP had been fused to a highly efficient phage promoter and is expressed in actively growing cells, whereas the RFP is only expressed in non-dividing, INH-persistent cells.

certainly lead to many new chemotherapeutic and immunotherapeutic interventions.

It is likely that the single greatest impediment to TB control is the ability of *M. tuberculosis* to persist when assaulted by bactericidal drugs or immune effectors. The phenomenon of persistence is particularly relevant for this slowly replicating organism and has been difficult to study. There are now ways to study *M. tuberculosis* persistence with precisely defined genomes and reproducible methodologies. The slow growth of the tubercle bacillus still makes the analysis of this phenomenon challenging. Resistance is not mediated by specific singular genes, as can be observed for drug-resistant mutants but rather, a complex genetic array of expression patterns that confer phenotypic resistance. By understanding the mechanisms that *M. tuberculosis* uses to enter into this persistence state, novel strategies can be developed to treat this deadly disease.

REFERENCES

1. WHO. WHO endorses new rapid tuberculosis test. 2010 [cited 2019 April 26]; Available from: https://www.who.int/mediacentre/news/releases/2010/tb_test_20101208/en/.
2. Vilcheze C, and Jacobs WR, Jr. The isoniazid paradigm of killing, resistance, and persistence in *Mycobacterium tuberculosis*. *J Mol Biol*. 2019.
3. WHO. Drug-resistant TB: XDR-TB FAQ. 2019 [cited 2019 8/5/2019]; Available from: https://www.who.int/tb/areas-of-work/drug-resistant-tb/xdr-tb-faq/en/.
4. Villemin JA. Cause et nature de la tuberculose. *Bull Acad Méd*. 1865;31:211–6.
5. Koch R. Die Atiologie der Tuberkulose. *Berliner Klinischen Wochenschrift*. 1882;15:221–30. English translation; Available from: http://www.asm.org/ccLibraryFiles/FILENAME/0000000228/1882p109.pdf.
6. Pinner M. The aetiology of tuberculosis. *Am Rev Tuberc*. 1932:48.
7. Villemin JA. *Études sur la tuberculose : preuves rationnelles et expérimentales de sa spécificité et de son inoculabilité*. 1868, Paris: J.- B. Baillière et fils.
8. Koch R. Die A ̈tiologie der Milzbrandkrankheit, begru ̈ndet auf dieEntwicklungsgeschichte des *Bacillus Anthracis*. *Beitra ̈ge zur Biologie der Pflanzen*. 1876;2:277–310.
9. Mendel G. Versuche über Plflanzenhybriden, in Verhandlungen des naturforschenden Vereines in Brünn, Bd. IV für das Jahr. 1865.
10. McAdam RA et al. In vivo growth characteristics of leucine and methionine auxotrophic mutants of *Mycobacterium bovis* BCG generated by transposon mutagenesis. *Infect Immun*. 1995;63(3):1004–12.
11. Falkow S. Molecular Koch's postulates applied to microbial pathogenicity. *Rev Infect Dis*. 1988;10(Suppl 2):S274–6.
12. Beadle GW, and Tatum EL. Genetic control of biochemical reactions in *Neurospora*. *Proc Natl Acad Sci USA*. 1941;27(11):499–506.
13. Avery OT, Macleod CM, and McCarty M. Studies on the chemical nature of the substance inducing transformation of pneumococcal types: Induction of transformation by a desoxyribonucleic acid fraction isolated from *Pneumococcus* Type III. *J Exp Med*. 1944;79(2):137–58.
14. Luria SE, and Delbruck M. Mutations of bacteria from virus sensitivity to virus resistance. *Genetics*. 1943;28(6):491–511.
15. Lederberg J, and Tatum EL. Gene recombination in *Escherichia coli*. *Nature*. 1946;158(4016):558.
16. Hershey AD, and Chase M. Independent functions of viral protein and nucleic acid in growth of bacteriophage. *J Gen Physiol*. 1952;36(1):39–56.
17. Zinder ND. Bacterial transduction. *J Cell Physiol Suppl*. 1955;45(Suppl. 2):23–49.
18. Jacobs WR, Jr, Tuckman M, and Bloom BR. Introduction of foreign DNA into mycobacteria using a shuttle phasmid. *Nature*. 1987;327(6122):532–5.
19. Glickman MS, and Jacobs WR, Jr. Microbial pathogenesis of *Mycobacterium tuberculosis*: Dawn of a discipline. *Cell*. 2001;104(4):477–85.
20. Jacobs WR, Jr. Gene transfer in *Mycobacterium tuberculosis*: Shuttle phasmids to enlightenment. *Microb Spectr*. 2014;2(2).
21. Jacobs WR, Jr et al. Development of genetic systems for the mycobacteria. *Acta Leprol*. 1989;7(Suppl 1):203–7.
22. Cole ST et al. Deciphering the biology of *Mycobacterium tuberculosis* from the complete genome sequence. *Nature*. 1998;393(6685):537–44.
23. Garnier T et al. The complete genome sequence of *Mycobacterium bovis*. *Proc Natl Acad Sci USA*. 2003;100(13):7877–82.
24. Cole ST et al. Massive gene decay in the leprosy bacillus. *Nature*. 2001;409(6823):1007–11.
25. Brennan MJ, and Delogu G. The PE multigene family: A 'molecular mantra' for mycobacteria. *Trends Microbiol*. 2002;10(5):246–9.
26. Sampson SL. Mycobacterial PE/PPE proteins at the host-pathogen interface. *Clin Dev Immunol*. 2011;2011:497203.
27. Filliol I et al. Global phylogeny of *Mycobacterium tuberculosis* based on single nucleotide polymorphism (SNP) analysis: Insights into tuberculosis evolution, phylogenetic accuracy of other DNA fingerprinting systems, and recommendations for a minimal standard SNP set. *J Bacteriol*. 2006;188(2):759–72.
28. Supply P et al. Variable human minisatellite-like regions in the *Mycobacterium tuberculosis* genome. *Mol Microbiol*. 2000;36(3):762–71.
29. Sreenu VB et al. Microsatellite polymorphism across the *M. tuberculosis* and *M. bovis* genomes: Implications on genome evolution and plasticity. *BMC Genomics*. 2006;7:78.
30. Qin L et al. Perspective on sequence evolution of microsatellite locus (CCG)n in Rv0050 gene from *Mycobacterium tuberculosis*. *BMC Evol Biol*. 2011;11:247.
31. Cave MD et al. Stability of DNA fingerprint pattern produced with IS6110 in strains of *Mycobacterium tuberculosis*. *J Clin Microbiol*. 1994;32(1):262–6.
32. Groenen PM et al. Nature of DNA polymorphism in the direct repeat cluster of *Mycobacterium tuberculosis*; application for strain differentiation by a novel typing method. *Mol Microbiol*. 1993;10(5):1057–65.
33. Legrand E et al. Use of spoligotyping to study the evolution of the direct repeat locus y IS6110 transposition in *Mycobacterium tuberculosis*. *J Clin Microbiol*. 2001;39:1595–9.
34. Arnvig KB et al. Sequence-based analysis uncovers an abundance of non-coding RNA in the total transcriptome of *Mycobacterium tuberculosis*. *PLoS Pathog*. 2011;7(11):e1002342.
35. Pfyffer GE et al. *Mycobacterium canettii*, the smooth variant of *M. tuberculosis*, isolated from a Swiss patient exposed in Africa. *Emerg Infect Dis*. 1998;4(4):631–4.
36. Fabre M et al. Molecular characteristics of "*Mycobacterium canettii*" the smooth *Mycobacterium tuberculosis* bacilli. *Infect Genet Evol*. 2010;10(8):1165–73.
37. Koeck JL et al. Clinical characteristics of the smooth tubercle bacilli '*Mycobacterium canettii*' infection suggest the existence of an environmental reservoir. *Clin Microbiol Infect*. 2011;17(7):1013–9.

38. Aranaz A et al. Elevation of *Mycobacterium tuberculosis* subsp. *caprae* Aranaz et al. 1999 to species rank as *Mycobacterium caprae* comb. nov., sp. nov. *Int J Syst Evol Microbiol.* 2003;53(Pt 6):1785–9.

39. Niemann S, Richter E, and Rusch-Gerdes S. Differentiation among members of the *Mycobacterium tuberculosis* complex by molecular and biochemical features: Evidence for two pyrazinamide-susceptible subtypes of *M. bovis. J Clin Microbiol.* 2000;38(1):152–7.

40. Kubica T, Rusch-Gerdes S, and Niemann S. *Mycobacterium bovis* subsp. *caprae* caused one-third of human *M. bovis*-associated tuberculosis cases reported in Germany between 1999 and 2001. *J Clin Microbiol.* 2003;41(7):3070–7.

41. Fomukong NG et al. Use of gene probes based on the insertion sequence IS986 to differentiate between BCG vaccine strains. *J Appl Bacteriol.* 1992;72:126–33.

42. Grange JM, Yates MD, and de Kantor IN. *Guidelines for Speciation within the Mycobacterium tuberculosis Complex.* 2nd ed. 1996: Geneva: World Health Organization.

43. de Jong BC, Antonio M, and Gagneux S. *Mycobacterium africanum*—Review of an important cause of human tuberculosis in West Africa. *PLoS Negl Trop Dis.* 2010;4(9):e744.

44. Hart PD, and Sutherland I. BCG and vole bacillus vaccines in the prevention of tuberculosis in adolescence and early adult life. *Br Med J.* 1977;2(6082):293–5.

45. Panteix G et al. Pulmonary tuberculosis due to *Mycobacterium microti*: A study of six recent cases in France. *J Med Microbiol.* 2010;59(Pt 8):984–9.

46. Cousins DV et al. Tuberculosis in seals caused by a novel member of the *Mycobacterium tuberculosis* complex: *Mycobacterium pinnipedii* sp. nov. *Int J Syst Evol Microbiol.* 2003;53(Pt 5):1305–14.

47. Kiers A et al. Transmission of *Mycobacterium pinnipedii* to humans in a zoo with marine mammals. *Int J Tuberc Lung Dis.* 2008;12(12):1469–73.

48. Alexander KA et al. Novel *Mycobacterium tuberculosis* complex pathogen, *M. mungi. Emerg Infect Dis.* 2010;16(8):1296–9.

49. Bhatt A et al. Deletion of kasB in *Mycobacterium tuberculosis* causes loss of acid-fastness and subclinical latent tuberculosis in immunocompetent mice. *Proc Natl Acad Sci USA.* 2007;104(12):5157–62.

50. Vilcheze C, and Kremer L., Acid-fast positive and acid-fast negative *Mycobacterium tuberculosis*: The Koch paradox. *Microbiol Spectr.* 2017;5(2).

51. Vilcheze C et al. Phosphorylation of KasB regulates virulence and acid-fastness in *Mycobacterium tuberculosis. PLoS Pathog.* 2014;10(5):e1004115.

52. WHO. BCG (Tuberculosis). 2018 07/05/2018; Available from: https://www.who.int/biologicals/areas/vaccines/bcg/Tuberculosis/en/.

53. Calmette A. Preventive vaccination against tuberculosis with BCG. *Proc R Soc Med.* 1931;24(11):1481–90.

54. Bloom B et al. Tuberculosis: Old lessons unlearnt? *Lancet.* 1997;350(9071):149.

55. Mahairas GG et al. Molecular analysis of genetic differences between *Mycobacterium bovis* BCG and virulent *M. bovis. J Bacteriol.* 1996;178(5):1274–82.

56. Behr MA et al. Comparative genomics of BCG vaccines by whole-genome DNA microarray. *Science.* 1999;284(5419):1520–3.

57. Pym AS et al. Loss of RD1 contributed to the attenuation of the live tuberculosis vaccines *Mycobacterium bovis* BCG and *Mycobacterium microti. Mol Microbiol.* 2002;46(3):709–17.

58. Hsu T et al. The primary mechanism of attenuation of bacillus Calmette-Guerin is a loss of secreted lytic function required for invasion of lung interstitial tissue. *Proc Natl Acad Sci USA.* 2003;100(21):12420–5.

59. Brosch R et al. A new evolutionary scenario for the *Mycobacterium tuberculosis* complex. *Proc Natl Acad Sci USA.* 2002;99(6):3684–9.

60. Tiwari S et al. Infect and inject: How *Mycobacterium tuberculosis* exploits its major virulence-associated type VII Secretion System, ESX-1. *Microbiol Spectr.* 2019;7(3).

61. Berney M et al. Essential roles of methionine and S-adenosylmethionine in the autarkic lifestyle of *Mycobacterium tuberculosis. Proc Natl Acad Sci USA.* 2015;112(32):10008–13.

62. Tiwari S et al. Arginine-deprivation-induced oxidative damage sterilizes *Mycobacterium tuberculosis. Proc Natl Acad Sci USA.* 2018;115(39):9779–84.

63. Fox HH. The chemical approach to the control of tuberculosis. *Science.* 1952;116(3006):129–34.

64. Bernstein J et al. Chemotherapy of experimental tuberculosis. V. Isonicotinic acid hydrazide (nydrazid) and related compounds. *Am Rev Tuberc.* 1952;65(4):357–64.

65. Chorine V. Action of nicotinamide on bacilli of the species *Mycobacterium. C. R. Acad. Sci.* 1945;220:150–1.

66. Davies JE. Studies on the ribosomes of streptomycin-sensitive and resistant strains of *Escherichia coli. Proc Natl Acad Sci USA.* 1964;51:659–64.

67. Carter AP et al. Functional insights from the structure of the 30S ribosomal subunit and its interactions with antibiotics. *Nature.* 2000;407(6802):340–8.

68. Winder FG, Collins P, and Rooney SA. Effects of isoniazid on mycolic acid synthesis in *Mycobacterium tuberculosis* and on its cell envelope. *Biochem J.* 1970;117(2):27P.

69. Takayama K, Keith AD, and Snipes W. Effect of isoniazid on the protoplasmic viscosity in *Mycobacterium tuberculosis. Antimicrob Agents Chemother.* 1975;7(1):22–4.

70. Takayama K et al. Site of inhibitory action of isoniazid in the synthesis of mycolic acids in *Mycobacterium tuberculosis. J Lipid Res.* 1975;16(4):308–17.

71. Middlebrook G, and Cohn ML. Some observations on the pathogenicity of isoniazid-resistant variants of tubercle bacilli. *Science.* 1953;118(3063):297–9.

72. Snapper SB et al. Lysogeny and transformation in mycobacteria: Stable expression of foreign genes. *Proc Natl Acad Sci USA.* 1988;85(18):6987–91.

73. Snapper SB et al. Isolation and characterization of efficient plasmid transformation mutants of *Mycobacterium smegmatis. Mol Microbiol.* 1990;4(11):1911–9.

74. Zhang Y et al. The catalase-peroxidase gene and isoniazid resistance of *Mycobacterium tuberculosis. Nature.* 1992;358(6387):591–3.

75. Banerjee A et al. inhA, a gene encoding a target for isoniazid and ethionamide in *Mycobacterium tuberculosis. Science.* 1994;263(5144):227–30.

76. Rozwarski DA et al. Modification of the NADH of the isoniazid target (InhA) from *Mycobacterium tuberculosis. Science.* 1998;279(5347):98–102.

77. Zhang Y, Garbe T, and Young D., Transformation with katG restores isoniazid-sensitivity in *Mycobacterium tuberculosis* isolates resistant to a range of drug concentrations. *Mol Microbiol.* 1993;8(3):521–4.

78. Larsen MH et al. Overexpression of inhA, but not kasA, confers resistance to isoniazid and ethionamide in *Mycobacterium smegmatis, M. bovis* BCG and *M. tuberculosis. Mol Microbiol.* 2002;46(2):453–66.

79. Vilcheze C et al. Transfer of a point mutation in *Mycobacterium tuberculosis* inhA resolves the target of isoniazid. *Nat Med.* 2006;12(9):1027–9.

80. McCune RM et al. Microbial persistence. I. The capacity of tubercle bacilli to survive sterilization in mouse tissues. *J Exp Med.* 1966;123(3):445–68.

81. Kerantzas CA, and Jacobs WR, Jr., Origins of combination therapy for tuberculosis: Lessons for future antimicrobial development and application. *MBio.* 2017;8(2).

82. Vilcheze C et al. *Mycobacterium tuberculosis* is extraordinarily sensitive to killing by a vitamin C-induced Fenton reaction. *Nat Commun.* 2013;4:1881.

83. Vilcheze C et al. Enhanced respiration prevents drug tolerance and drug resistance in *Mycobacterium tuberculosis. Proc Natl Acad Sci USA.* 2017;114(17):4495–500.

84. Jain P et al. Dual-reporter mycobacteriophages (Phi2DRMs) reveal preexisting *Mycobacterium tuberculosis* persistent cells in human sputum. *MBio.* 2016;7(5).

4

Pathogenesis of Tuberculosis

DIVYA B. REDDY AND JERROLD J. ELLNER

OVERVIEW

Tuberculosis (TB) outranks infection with human immunodeficiency virus (HIV) and all other infectious diseases as a leading cause of mortality worldwide and is one of the top 10 causes of death.[1] Current understanding of the pathogenesis of TB derives from experimental observations in infected animals and clinical observations in humans; pathologic and immunologic studies of the blood and tissues of infected animals and humans with TB; and microbiologic, biochemical, and genetic studies of *Mycobacterium tuberculosis* (MTB) and its molecular constituents. There are corresponding levels of complexity to the understanding of TB. No single approach to the elucidation of the pathogenesis of TB encompasses its entirety. Recent progress in the understanding of TB and MTB allows a more complete view of how this pathogen interacts with the host.

This chapter begins with a brief review of the natural history of TB and virulence factors, and then focuses on the major new developments in the pathogenesis of TB. Acquired immunity to MTB infection will be discussed from the standpoint of animal studies; from *in vitro* studies of phagocytosis and T-cell-independent growth inhibition of MTB by mononuclear phagocytes; and from host-genetic influences on acquiring MTB infection and development of TB. Adaptive immunity to MTB will include discussions of the role of CD4 and CD8 T cells, TH-1 and TH-2 type responses and γδ and natural killer (NK) T-cells in the control of MTB infection in addition to emerging concepts on the role of humoral immunity in TB-directed host immunity. The role of cytokines in macrophage activation and deactivation in the modulation of T-cell responses and in tissue damage and granuloma formation will be considered. Class I- and class II-restricted cytotoxicity and their role in protection and immunopathology will be considered. Immune responses in human TB will be reviewed in the blood, pleural, and lung compartments separately. Finally, the impact of HIV-1 on the development of TB and the effect of TB on HIV disease will be considered.

NATURAL HISTORY AND IMMUNOPATHOLOGY

Exposure to an individual with active pulmonary TB carries a substantial risk of acquiring infection. In household contacts of TB cases, this risk is approximately 50%–80%; it is higher if exposure is more prolonged in sustained close quarters and highest in those sharing a bed or sleeping in the same room as a TB case. Inhalation of microdroplets (droplet nuclei) containing MTB may result in infection. Although large droplets are deposited in the upper airways (trachea and bronchi) and removed by mucociliary clearance mechanisms, smaller droplets (approximately 1–5 μm) that contain three or fewer bacilli may reach the alveoli.[2–6] Thus, the first line of defense against MTB consists of the innate cells including the alveolar macrophages that line the alveoli. MTB organisms that are able to survive intracellular killing may grow to a limited extent within alveolar macrophages. During the time required to develop adaptive immunity to contain bacterial growth, MTB infection can spread by lymphohematogenous dissemination to other sites, including the upper lung fields. With the development of immunity (4–6 weeks), small granulomas form at the sites of initial MTB inoculation and dissemination, and the tuberculin skin test (TST) and interferon gamma release assays (IGRA) convert to positive. Alternatively, and especially if protective immunity does not intercede in a timely manner, the bacilli may continue to replicate and manifest as progressive primary TB. This is the most common scenario in high-prevalence countries.

In the majority of infected individuals, the development of adaptive immunity leads either to local destruction of MTB or persistence of the organisms in a latent phase within tissue macrophages and perhaps elsewhere, for a lifetime. Foci with latent MTB organisms are the sites of the original dissemination and include the apices of the lungs, the cortices of the kidneys, and the growth plates of long bones. A characteristic common to these tissues is a high local concentration of oxygen. *In vitro* studies confirm that higher levels of ambient oxygen increase intracellular MTB growth within human macrophages.[7] Conversely, as oxygen is gradually depleted from MTB cultures, the bacilli become tolerant to anaerobic conditions and enter a phase of non-replicating persistence.[8] The mechanism of this shift in MTB metabolism leading to MTB dormancy, and the factors that permit or interfere with latent MTB infection, are not known. However, in approximately 5%–10% of cases, due to the failure of immunologic surveillance against MTB infection, bacillary multiplication resumes and manifests as clinical TB. The pathologic hallmark of TB is granuloma formation in various tissues.[9] Tuberculous granulomas are characterized by accumulations of blood-derived macrophages, epithelioid cells (i.e., differentiated macrophages), multinucleated giant cells (i.e., fused macrophages with nuclei around the periphery of the giant cell [Langhans' type of giant cells]), and T lymphocytes around the periphery of the granuloma. Thus, mononuclear phagocytes are the main cellular constituents of tuberculoid granulomas. Whether the epithelioid cells and multinucleated giant cells are adapted for mycobacterial killing is not known, although activated macrophages may be more microbicidal than blood monocytes.[10] In tuberculous granulomas, acid fast bacilli (AFB) are found almost exclusively within the macrophages.[9]

Latent foci of MTB infection retain the ability to undergo reactivation, most commonly in the lung. This is the predominant pathogenic mechanism in low- and middle-prevalence countries. Pulmonary TB is the most common manifestation of TB in adults. Although MTB infection provides protection against exogenous reinfection in young and healthy individuals, reinfection TB is common in high-prevalence settings. Pulmonary TB, generally, is localized to the apical and posterior segments of the upper lobes or the superior segment of the lower lobes.[11] Caseous necrosis of granulomas is the pathologic hallmark of both primary progressive and reactivation TB. In some granulomas, liquefaction of the caseous material occurs and it is believed that MTB replicates better in this liquefied material than in caseous material. Caseous necrosis and cavity formation likely result from immune and inflammatory responses to MTB constituents. It is of interest, therefore, that cavity formation is prevented in rabbits by desensitizing the animals with a tuberculin-active peptide before infecting them.[12] Healing occurs by fibrosis and contraction of the affected structures. A characteristic feature of active TB is the concurrent findings of caseation, liquefaction, cavity formation, and fibrosis in lungs and other organs of affected individuals. It is assumed that destructive enzymes such as matrix metalloproteinases and oxygen radicals produced by macrophages and neutrophils mediate much of the tissue damage with resulting liquefaction of granulomas and cavity formation.[9] In addition, cytokines (see subsection "Mononuclear Phagocytes") produced by mononuclear cells at sites of active MTB infection most likely contribute to the pathology as do neutrophils. However, the cellular and molecular basis for the immunopathology of TB is not fully understood. It is becoming clear, as well, that lung damage and chronic obstructive pulmonary disease may be a sequelae of TB.

VIRULENCE FACTORS

MTB virulence factors have been the subject of intense research. Previously, three major virulence factors from the outer layer of the complex mycobacterial cell wall have been characterized molecularly: mycobacterial glycolipids (cord factor), mycobacterial sulfolipids (SL), and mycosides. Cord factor(s) are trehalose-6,6'-dimycolates,[13] that exist in either a non-toxic and protective micellar conformation or a toxic and immunogenic monolayer conformation. The latter is capable of killing macrophages in minutes, exacerbates acute and chronic TB in mice, and interferes with the ability of isoniazid to kill MTB.[14] The toxic effects of cord factor have been attributed to an interaction with mitochondrial membranes resulting in reduction of the activity of nicotinamide adenine dinucleotide-dependent microsomal enzymes in various tissues (lung, liver, and spleen).[15,16] As the most abundant lipid produced by virulent MTB, it is directly responsible for MTB multiplication in lung cavities with consequent expulsion into the environment and person-to-person spread.[17]

SLs are trehalose-2'-sulfates acylated with pthioceranic, hydroxypthioceranic, or saturated straight-chain fatty acids resulting in highly hydrophobic compounds.[18,19] SLs kill mice when injected intraperitoneally and enhance the toxicity of the cord factor.[20,21] The production of SLs by MTB correlates with their virulence; avirulent strains are deficient and virulent strains produce SL abundantly.[22] Importantly, SLs inhibit the fusion of MTB phagosomes with lysosomes, thus allowing MTB to evade host microbicidal molecules,[23] although inhibition of phagosome–lysosome fusion may also be mediated by other molecules, such as ammonia produced by MTB.[18]

Mycosides are species-specific glycolipids and peptidoglycolipids of mycobacteria.[19] The complex chemical structure of many of these compounds has been elucidated by Brennan et al.[24] The surface glycolipids of MTB consist of trehalose-containing lipooligosaccharides. Biochemical differences between the surface mycosides of virulent MTB and nonpathogenic strains of MTB have[18] been described.[24,25] Also, certain mycosides of mycobacteria induce the formation of an electron transparent zone in bacilli phagocytized by macrophages.[26] The role of the electron-transparent zone in protecting MTB against intracellular killing has not been determined.

More recently, an abundant lipoglycan of the mycobacterial cell wall, lipoarabinomannan (LAM), has been ascribed to virulence function(s).[24] LAM, being a key immunomodulator, counteracts interferon (IFN)-γ-induced macrophage activation, arrests phagosomal maturation in infected macrophages, reduces phagocytosis, and blocks induction of cellular genes. By modulating the cytokine milieu toward one of deactivations, LAM may allow the persistence of MTB within tissues.[22,27] Gaur et al. showed that LprG, a cell envelope lipoprotein, is essential for normal surface expression of LAM and its functions.[28]

Other virulence factors relate to MTB genes that allow the organism to survive during the stationary phase.[29] For example, sigma factors, which are small transcription factors, regulate the transcriptional activity of MTB during its adaptive states, and may be indispensable for its virulence.[30] Of note is the description of a small (16 kDa) heat shock protein, α-crystallin (Acr), by Barry et al.,[31] that has a chaperoning function. Acr-knockout MTB mutants are able to grow normally, but are unable to persist *in vivo*, and therefore may not establish latent foci.

There has been a paradigm shift in the understanding of MTB virulence factors that depends on single-nucleotide polymorphism (SNP) analysis of the genome. For example,[32] a study of an outbreak strain in Denmark showed SNPs in 23 genes associated with virulence compared to a reference strain including genes associated with hypervirulence. For example, the *MazE2* gene, a toxin–antitoxin gene that induces dormancy and persistence, and the *pks 1/15* gene which suppresses the human immune response.

CONTROL OF MTB INFECTION: INNATE MECHANISMS

With regard to understanding the innate responses of the host against MTB, animal models and, more recently, *in vitro* studies of human mononuclear cells have been most informative.

ANIMAL MODELS

In classic studies, Lurie et al. followed the course of mycobacteria in the lung and in other tissues after inhalation of bacilli by inbred-resistant versus inbred-susceptible rabbits.[5,6] In resistant rabbits, alveolar macrophages contained more mycobacteria than susceptible rabbits initially, and the drainage of bacilli to tracheobronchial nodes also was higher. However, 7 days after inhalation of bacilli (Bacilli Calmette–Guérin [BCG]), susceptible rabbits had 20- to 30-fold higher levels of bacilli in the lung compared to resistant rabbits,[33] and died sooner. Other histopathologic characteristics of resistant rabbits were increased differentiation of macrophages, enhanced interstitial inflammation, and faster progression through the caseous process. By contrast, the susceptible phenotype was associated with higher pneumonic inflammation, and increased number and size of tubercles in the lung. In this model, the native resistance of alveolar macrophages, conceivably through increased uptake and killing of mycobacteria by macrophages, was believed to underlie the differences between the two phenotypes. After this first stage of mycobacterial infection, both resistant and susceptible rabbits develop a state of symbiosis with the organism during which mycobacteria grow logarithmically within cells, but the cells are not lysed.[6,33] It appears that recently recruited monocyte-derived macrophages[11] of early granulomata contain more bacilli than differentiated tissue macrophages. This finding has been attributed to the efficiency of phagocytosis, to undeveloped microbicidal mechanisms, and to less MTB-induced cytotoxicity of immature macrophages.[6,31] Similar rates of logarithmic growth, in this stage and when MTB growth reaches a plateau with the development of adaptive immunity (after 3 weeks), was observed in both groups of animals. Interestingly, as compared to susceptible rabbits, the resistant animals developed a more robust acquired immunity to MTB after BCG vaccination.[5] Thus, it appears that innate resistance may be important to the development of antimycobacterial immunity. Studies of murine TB have shown the relative resistance of this animal model to MTB. However, much important information regarding the development of the adaptive response, and the role of T cells has been derived from this animal model.[34] Other studies have shown the importance of the route of infection in mice, i.e., mice infected with MTB by aerosolization were predisposed to chronic MTB infection of the lung.[35] In fact, after the initial period of containment of MTB growth subsequent to aerosol infection, a chronic granulomatous inflammation developed, followed by resumption of MTB growth, and subsequently, death.

In a guinea pig model developed by Smith et al., 3 weeks after infection by the aerosol route, bacilli had disseminated hematogenously back to the lung in large numbers.[36] However, both in the lung and at distant sites, adaptive immunity finally controlled bacillary growth. In fact, of all animal models of MTB infection, the guinea pig model most closely resembles human infection. Aiyaz et al., using microarray-based whole-genomic analysis, showed that guinea pigs infected with a low dose aerosol of Atypical Beijing Western Cape TT372 strain of MTB and previously vaccinated with BCG showed lower levels of genes involving lung healing, response to oxidative stress, and cell trafficking compared to infected and unvaccinated guinea pigs.[37]

In vitro human studies have shown the ease with which mononuclear phagocytes can get parasitized with MTB, i.e., the capacity to develop bacteriostasis but not to kill MTB, and the relative superiority of alveolar macrophages compared to monocytes in MTB growth containment. The contribution of cytokines and various pathways to MTB infection and growth containment is described below.

MACROPHAGES

MTB, phagocytosed by macrophages, can evade intracellular bactericidal mechanisms and replicate within the cell. It is agreed generally that the degree of virulence of MTB depends on its relative capacity to multiply within host macrophages. There are three ways that the growth of MTB may be inhibited; each involves mononuclear phagocytes and two require both lymphocytes and mononuclear phagocytes. First, mononuclear phagocytes have a natural armamentarium against the bacillus known as natural resistance (see later in this section). Second, mononuclear phagocytes can be activated to kill MTB through cytokines or other mediators, and when such activation is conferred by sensitized T lymphocytes, acquired resistance has evolved, i.e., cell-mediated immunity (CMI) in its strictest sense. Third, mononuclear phagocytes containing bacilli may be lysed by cytotoxic T cells, but the *in vivo* significance for the containment of MTB by this mechanism is still not clear; presumably, bacilli that are released when macrophages are lysed may be taken up by more activated macrophages which are better able to control their growth (these latter two mechanisms will be discussed in following sections).

Macrophages are functionally heterogeneous. The classically activated or M1 macrophage is intrinsically pro-inflammatory, whereas the alternatively activated M2 macrophage is immuno-regulatory. After priming by IFN-γ and then stimulated with a second signal such as tumor necrosis factor-alpha (TNF-α) the M1 macrophage demonstrates more efficient antigen (Ag) presentation and phagocytosis and release of inflammatory mediators. M2 macrophages are generated by interleukin (IL)-4 and IL-13 produce immunosuppressive cytokines IL-10 and transforming growth factor-beta (TGF-β) are anti-inflammatory and less efficient at intracellular killing and Ag presentation. They appear to play a role in resolution of inflammation and healing.

Alveolar macrophage function is tightly regulated as they are the primary defense against invading pathogens but also limit inflammation and the subsequent lung damage. Pattern recognition receptors (PRRs) such as toll-like receptors (TLRs) recognize pathogen-associated molecular patterns initiate an inflammation which is perpetuated through their receptors for TNF-α, IL-1 β, and IFN-γ. In balance signaling through non-TLR PRRs such as the mannose receptor and signaling through IL-10 and TGF-β limit inflammation. Macrophages are important sources of Type 1 IFNs. These limit anti-TB effector mechanisms by inhibiting the production of IL-12p40, IL-1α, and IL-1-β while inducing immunosuppressive mediators such as IL-10 and IL-1-R antagonists.

TLRs are generally considered to be pro-inflammatory as their ligation leads to nuclear factor (NF)-κb activation. However, TLRs also activate signaling molecules TRIF and IRF increasing expression of IFN-β and an anti-inflammatory response. Relative to monocytes, alveolar macrophages express lower levels of TL-R2, increased TLR-9, and comparable TLR-4. Mycobacterial Ags and even DNA differentially activate TLRs leading to a complex and nuanced response.[310]

PHAGOCYTOSIS AND MTB GROWTH CONTAINMENT

Swartz et al. have observed that different species of mycobacteria vary in their extent of ingestion by blood monocytes.[38] *Mycobacterium avium* complex was taken up by many monocytes, whereas MTB, *Mycobacterium kansasii*, and other mycobacteria were taken up by fewer monocytes. Serum was found to be important for the uptake of *M. avium* complex and to a lesser extent for MTB. Complement played a major role in this effect of serum.[38] Complement receptor 1 (CR1) and CR3 mediate phagocytosis of virulent MTB by blood monocytes, and the C3 component of complement is the bacterial-bound ligand.[39] More recently, Schlesinger et al. have shown that avirulent and virulent MTB are comparable in adherence and phagocytosis by macrophages, and thus phagocytosis alone is not a determinant of virulence.[40] Other host molecules shown to have roles in phagocytosis of MTB are the mannose receptor and cell surface fibronectin (reviewed in ref.[41]); the MTB ligands for these molecules are LAM and the cell wall 30 kDa Ag, respectively.

Hirsch et al.[42] assessed the phagocytosis and growth inhibition of MTB by human alveolar macrophages in comparison with blood monocytes. Alveolar macrophages from healthy subjects phagocytosed and inhibited the growth of this strain of MTB significantly

better than blood monocytes. Phagocytosis by alveolar macrophages was mediated through CR4 to a greater extent compared to CR1 or CR3. In addition, pulmonary surfactant protein A mediated enhanced phagocytosis of MTB, possibly through mannose receptors.[43] In a study by Hirsch et al., the basis for improved growth inhibition of MTB by alveolar macrophages was attributed, in part, to an increased expression of TNF-α by alveolar macrophages after phagocytosis of the organisms.[42] Previous studies have shown that BCG and purified protein derivative[24] (PPD) stimulate the production of the macrophage-activating molecule, TNF-α, by human alveolar macrophages,[44] and that the capacity to produce TNF-α and its regulator p38 mitogen-activated protein (MAP) kinase by alveolar macrophages exceeds that of blood monocytes.[45,46] Because healthy subjects were the source of alveolar macrophages in these studies, the growth inhibition by these cells is a reflection of the natural resistance of these cells. However, in addition to production of macrophage-activating cytokines, MTB and its PPD and secreted components induce the production of macrophage-deactivating cytokines such as TGF-β and IL-10.[47]

LYSOSOMAL ENZYMES

The fusion of the MTB phagosomes with the lysosomes that contain lysosomal enzymes (including proteases, lysozyme, acid hydrolases, and cationic proteins) is critical to the containment of the intracellular growth of bacilli. The capacity of virulent strains of MTB to disrupt the phagosomal membrane and multiply freely in the cytoplasm of rabbit alveolar macrophages,[48] has also been shown in a mouse model,[49] indicating that MTB may evade the lysosomal contents totally. Lurie and Dannenberg's histologic studies in rabbits showed an increase in lysosomal enzymes in activated macrophages that appeared to be killing tubercle bacilli; the macrophages in granulomas with fewer AFB contained high numbers of lysosomal granules.[6,33] Moreover, lysosomes from activated cells contained higher levels of lysosomal contents, such as cathepsins. In another study, Armstrong and d'Arcy Hart have shown that only after the phagocytosis of nonviable MTB, but not intact MTB, will mouse peritoneal macrophage phagosomes fuse with lysosomes.[50] Therefore, it appears that the digestion of MTB by the lysosomal enzymes of activated macrophages is important in the control of bacillary growth.

Autophagy is a homeostasis pathway wherein discrete portions of the cytoplasm are sequestered into an "autophagosome," and delivered to lysosomes for degradation. Gutierrez and Singh have demonstrated that induction of autophagic pathways by drugs such as rapamycin can enhance host resistance to MTB by promoting phagosome maturation. In fact, IFN-γ-induced activation of p47 GTPases such as LRG-47 in MTB-infected macrophages leads to formation of large organelles with autophagolysosomal properties and in part, explains the reactive nitrogen- and oxygen-independent pathways of IFN-γ antimicrobial action.[51] Similarly, Yuk et al. have shown that vitamin D3 exhibits antimycobacterial properties, by inducing autophagy in human monocytes via cathelicidin driven transcription of the autophagy-related genes *Beclin-1* and *Atg5*.[52] The role of autophagy in controlling bacterial burden and limiting tissue damaging inflammation is now becoming apparent and it is potentially a pathway for pharmacological manipulation.[53]

OXYGEN RADICALS

Mitchison et al. have found that resistance of MTB to hydrogen peroxide is associated with virulence.[54] Other studies have shown, in contrast, that although resistance to peroxide is necessary, it is not sufficient for virulence, and differences in susceptibility to peroxidative killing do not correlate with MTB virulence.[55,56] Furthermore, Douvas et al. have shown that the increased growth inhibition of MTB by monocyte-derived macrophages as compared to monocytes was not associated with increased release of reactive oxygen species.[56] Although mycobacteria are sensitive to oxygen radicals, scavengers of toxic oxygen metabolites failed to influence the capacity of IFN-γ-activated mouse bone marrow macrophages to inhibit the growth of *Mycobacterium bovis*.[51] A number of MTB products, such as LAM and phenolic glyco-lipids, interfere with the production of oxygen radicals; however, presently, the relevance of reactive oxygen intermediaries (ROIs) to MTB growth containment by phagocytes is not clear.

REACTIVE NITROGEN INTERMEDIARIES (RNIS)

The L-arginine-dependent pathway to produce nitric oxide (NO) and other nitrogen intermediaries is important in the control of intracellular microbes, including MTB. Compelling evidence for the role of RNIs as mediators of microbicidal activity first was shown in the mouse model.[57] Recently, it has been shown that in NO synthase (NOS) knockout mice, MTB replication is dramatically increased. Also, the inhibitors of inducible NOS (iNOS) increased the growth of MTB in wild-type mice.[58] MTB induces the production of NO in human alveolar macrophages (but not monocytes). The levels of NO produced by alveolar macrophages from different donors varied, and correlated inversely with intracellular MTB growth.[311]

NEUTROPHILS

Injection of mycobacteria or their products into tissues or the pleural space of animals produces an inflammatory response, initially dominated by neutrophils that can persist for up to 48 hours.[59] Although neutrophils are the first cells to arrive at the site of tuberculous infection, they are the less studied components of host immune response. It is now becoming apparent that in early stages of TB infection and disease (<1 week), neutrophils are largely protective, however, in established disease, they are associated with poorer prognosis and more tissue destruction and are representative of a malfunctioning immune system. For example, lipopolysaccharide-induced recruitment of neutrophils to the lungs of rats infected with MTB, lead to a decrease in the number of CFUs recovered from the lung during the course of the disease.[60] Correspondingly, depleting granulocytes in mice prior to intratracheal infection with MTB lead to an increase in CFUs recovered subsequently from lung and spleen.[61] In chronic infection, however, the opposite response was observed by Zhang et al.; depletion of neutrophils with the monoclonal antibody NIMP-R14 showed a decrease in CFU rather than an increase.[62] Additionally, the discovery of a neutrophil-driven IFN-inducible whole blood transcriptomic signature that correlates with TB disease severity highlights the potential role of neutrophils in exacerbating TB pathology.[63]

Recruitment of neutrophils to the site of infection is followed by internalization of MTB. Brown et al. have demonstrated first that neutrophils from healthy humans are capable of killing MTB *in vitro*.[64] The mechanism of killing of MTB by neutrophils, however, is not clear. May et al. have found that MTB induces a respiratory burst in neutrophils.[65] However, neutrophils from patients with chronic granulomatous disease killed MTB as well as neutrophils from healthy subjects, suggesting nonoxidative mechanisms are involved in the mycobactericidal process.[64] Furthermore, inhibitors of oxygen radical formation do not neutralize the killing of MTB by human neutrophils.[66] These data suggest that oxygen radicals are unlikely to be important in the killing of MTB by neutrophils. The role of human neutrophil peptides (HNPs), members of the α-defensin family stored in azurophilic granules in the neutrophils, in controlling MTB by disrupting plasma membranes and damaging DNA is being increasingly recognized. HNP concentrations are high in the areas of TB infection and they likely play an integral role in chemotaxis of mononuclear phagocytes and T cells, T cell/B cell interactions, antibody-mediated killing and cytokine production.[67] Cathelicidin, a 19 kDa protein stored in neutrophilic granules, is a potent macrophage chemotactic agent and likely aids in MTB killing by enhancing autophagy.[52]

In summary, the exact role neutrophils play in MTB-induced host immunity depends upon the stage of infection. The extent to which neutrophils contribute to intracellular/extracellular killing of MTB is unclear. They however, through release of chemokines/cytokines and granular products in response to mycobacteria, participate in the initial influx of monocytes from the blood to the infected region (usually the lung).

NATURAL KILLER CELLS

A role for NK cells in MTB containment by mononuclear phagocytes has been suggested both in the mouse model and in human *in vitro* systems. NK cells mediate their effect by production of IFN-γ and thereby activation of MTB-parasitized phagocytes, or by direct cytotoxicity against infected cells. Yoneda et al. have shown comparable activity of NK cells and CD4 cells in the containment of MTB growth in infected monocytes.[68]

NK cells are traditionally consider as innate cells but recent studies suggest that NK cells can distinguish Ags, and that memory NK cells expand and protect against viral pathogens and have an important role in mycobacterial infections.[69] In fact, a subpopulation of memory-like NK cells (CD3-NKp46+CD27+KLRG1+) expand in BCG-vaccinated mice and LTBI+ individuals to provide protection against MTB infection.[70]

Band T cells

T cells bearing γ or δ T-cell receptors (TCR), which comprise up to 5% of circulating T cells, also are able to produce IFN-γ and mediate cytolysis of MTB-infected targets. δ cells do not require major histocompatibility (MHC) Ags for activation and effector function. Both murine and human *in vitro* studies indicate a possible role for γδ T cells in natural resistance to MTB infection. Because γδ T cells often are found in the lung and epithelia, it has been suggested that they may act as a first line of defense against foreign Ags. γδ T cells have been shown to be expanded in the lymph nodes and the lung following exposure to mycobacterial Ags.[71,72] Havlir et al. have found that live MTB, but not heat-killed organisms, ingested by monocytes, selectively induce the expansion of human peripheral blood γδ T cells.[73] The ability of other infectious pathogens such as *Salmonella*, *Listeria monocytogenes*, and *Staphylococcus aureus* to induce γδ T cells further suggests that this subpopulation has a general role in the primary immune response to infectious agents.[74] Whether γδ T cells ultimately will prove to be of major importance in protection against MTB remains to be determined.

MAIT CELLS

Mucosal-associated invariant T (MAIT) cells are an innate-like T cell subset prevalent in humans and distributed throughout the blood and mucosal sites. MR1-restricted MAIT cells have been shown to facilitate the control of *M. bovis* BCG.[75,76] In subjects with TB, MR1Ts are often depleted in the peripheral circulation,[77–79] and return following therapy.[80]

IMMUNOGENETICS OF TB

Recently, a significant number of findings have accrued to define the role of host-genetic make-up in the susceptibility to MTB infection. Overall, immunogenetics may affect three separate phenomena during MTB infection. Despite the obvious interdependence of these phenomena, they may be viewed as affecting MTB infection independently. The host-genetic make-up may affect: (1) the susceptibility to MTB infection, (2) the susceptibility to develop TB, or (3) the clinical expression of TB.

About 20% of individuals with long standing exposure to MTB fail to mount an immune response to the TST suggesting an intrinsic resistance to MTB infection. Cobat et al. conducted a genome wide linkage scan for loci associated with TST reactivity (positive vs. negative [TST1] and extent of TST [TST2]) in a hyperendemic region in South Africa. A significant linkage signal for TST1 was found on the chromosomal region 11p14 (lod score = 3.81, $p = 1.4 \times 10^{-5}$) and for TST2 on chromosome 5p15 (lod score = 4.00, $p = 9 \times 10^{-6}$).[81] Subsequently they also mapped a locus controlling production of TNF, a major immune mediator and macrophage activator in TB, by blood cells stimulated by BCG and BCG plus IFN-γ in the region of TST1.[82] This genetic connection offers a potential mycobacteria-driven TNF-mediated resistance to MTB infection.

In the murine model of BCG infection, resistance has been attributed to the natural resistance-associated macrophage protein (Nramp1) gene.[83] Mice with a functional deletion of this gene are susceptible to other intracellular pathogens, such as salmonella and leishmania. Nramp1 is a membrane component of macrophage cytoplasmic vesicles, which translocates to the phagosome subsequent to phagocytosis.[84] Nramp1 also was believed to confer susceptibility to MTB infection in mice.[83] In recent studies, however, North et al. have shown unequivocally that Nramp1 plays no role in the determination of resistance against MTB infection in mice.[85] In humans, the homolog for Nramp1 is on chromosome 2q35, and polymorphisms have been shown to be associated with susceptibility to leprosy.[86] A small effect of Nramp1 has been observed in resistance to TB.[87] In another recent study looking at polymorphisms of Nramp1 in a Brazilian population,[88] an effect of this gene on susceptibility to TB was not observed. However, as the genetic approach and the Nramp1 loci studied were different in these two reports, it is hard to compare these findings.

In humans, evidence for a genetic predisposition to develop fatal mycobacterial infections has been established recently. Patients with severe recurrent atypical mycobacterial or salmonella infections have been shown to have mutations in their IFN-γ or IL-12 receptor genes.[89–91] Earlier studies have shown that blacks are more likely than whites to convert their TST to positive after exposure to a case of TB in an institutional setting.[92] Also, identical twins and blood relatives in a household with a case of TB are more likely to be concordant for disease than nonidentical twins and nonblood relatives.[93] Also, TB siblings in India demonstrate excess haplotype sharing.[94]

Several efforts have been made to show an association between human leukocyte antigen (HLA) phenotype and TB; the results have been widely divergent. For example, expression of some HLA-B and HLA-DR2 Ags in various populations is associated with the development of TB. These Ags include B8, Bw15, Bw35, B27, and DR2.[95–100] The association of other Class I and Class II MHC phenotypes with TB have been reported in other populations.[100–104] Each of these studies was performed on unrelated subjects. Because there was no *a priori* hypothesis that a specific HLA type was associated with TB, the statistical analysis is questionable as it did not correct for the multiple alleles under study. The fact that different phenotypes identified in disparate populations are associated with TB is not discouraging in itself, because the HLA genes may be in linkage disequilibrium with one or a few genes that determines susceptibility to TB. Linkage studies of HLA phenotypes among multiple family members with or without TB or tuberculous infection are required to confirm further the genetic predisposition for resistance or susceptibility to MTB in humans.

Cox et al. have assessed HLA-DR in a group of Mexican Americans with TB.[105] There was no association of a class II MHC locus with disease or TST reactivity. Of interest, however, was a relationship between HLA-DR and *in vitro* lymphocyte responses to PPD. In fact, the haplotype HLA-B14-DR1 was associated with low blastogenic responses. This is of considerable interest because this haplotype is associated with nonclassical adrenal 21-hydroxylase deficiency[106]; the gene for this abnormality maps to chromosome 6, within the class II MHC, and is a trait that is associated with altered expression of HLA-DR1 such that there is failure to activate alloreactive or class II-restricted T-cell clones.

Pathologic studies show that TB is a more aggressive disease in blacks. TB also reportedly is more difficult to treat in black than in white people.[107–110] The incidence is higher among people of Asian origin than white people in the UK.[111] The basis for the epidemiologic and clinical observations of differences in susceptibility to TB among races of people, however, is far from understood. Crowle and Elkins addressed this issue by studying the growth of MTB in monocytes and monocyte-derived macrophages from black and white people.[112] Both monocytes and monocyte-derived macrophages from black people killed MTB better after phagocytosis, but significantly less well during culture thereafter, especially in the presence of black donor serum. Furthermore, the macrophage-activating factor 1,25-(OH)-vitamin D3 provided less protection against the growth of tubercle bacilli in macrophages from black compared to white donors. Although these data implicate a genetic predisposition to the development of TB observed among black people, larger studies will be required to confirm this observation and to understand more fully the basis for the susceptibility.

An interesting link between genetic and environmental factors in the racial predisposition to TB was noted by Davies in an effort to explain the increased incidence of TB among Asians compared to white people in the UK.[111] Metabolites of vitamin D activate macrophages to kill MTB, but food in the UK is not supplemented with this vitamin. Thus, a dietary deficiency in vitamin D may predispose to the development of TB. Recently, polymorphisms in the vitamin D receptor gene were found to contribute to the susceptibility to TB in this population, particularly in combination with dietary deficiencies (Wilkinson RJ, personal communication). This study, underscores the importance of the cumulative effect of genetic and environmental factors in the predisposition to TB.

In a study of Indians in the UK, polymorphisms in the IL1 receptor antagonist (IL-1Ra) were associated with the clinical expression of TB; IL-1Ra allele (A) A2 positive patients had a lower incidence of pleural and peritoneal TB, and reduced PPD skin test reactivity. This polymorphism, however, was similar in TB patients and their healthy household contacts, indicating that it did not have an effect on the development of TB.[113] However, Zhang et al. identified a polymorphism in the promoter gene of IL-1β (high-IL-1β-producing rs1143627T allele) that correlated with the development of TB disease and severity in a Chinese population. IL-1β-driven IFN-γ/IL-17 dependent neutrophilic inflammation in the lungs likely explains severe pathology before TB treatment and permanent lung damage and functional decline after treatment.[114] Thus, a genetic basis for the development of clinical forms of TB exists.

There is now evidence for a significant role for host-genetic factors in progression from MTB infection to disease.[115,116] Early studies of twins demonstrated TB to be highly heritable, with some estimates of heritability (h2) approaching 70%. Mendelian disorders of immune function also result in an immune-compromised state that increases susceptibility to mycobacteria disease.[117] These disorders are characterized by rare, protein-damaging variation and have linked dysregulation of genes and transcription factors within the IL-12/IFN-γ immune cascade with the development of active disease. In addition, a number of TB susceptibility loci—class II HLA, 11p13, 18q11, ASP1, and PTX3121 have been identified from genome wide association studies (GWAS).[118] The implicated genes and loci also converged upon IFN-γ as a major immunological pathway in the susceptibility of disease.

A recent GWAS focusing on TB infection-resistant individuals from Tanzania and Uganda identified a locus on chromosome 5q33.3—100 kb downstream of the putative TB candidate gene IL12B and overlapping a putative transcription enhancer—that conferred a 70% protection from TB infection (OR: 0.23).[119] This finding mirrors a recently described recessive Mendelian disorder caused by rare, protein-damaging variants in IL-12B that increases susceptibility to MTB.[120]

ACQUIRED RESISTANCE TO MTB

ADAPTIVE IMMUNITY

Adaptive immunity is a consequence of the activation of macrophages by products of sensitized T lymphocytes such as IFN-γ. In general, cellular immune responses are initiated by exposure to a foreign Ag. The Ag is taken up, processed, and presented on the surface of Ag-presenting cells (accessory cells), such as macrophage and dendritic cells, to T lymphocytes.

Subsequently, T-cell activation and proliferation in response to the presented Ag occurs if such presentation is accompanied by HLA molecules on the surface of Ag-presenting cells as well as by amplifying cytokines such as IL-1 and IL-6. CD4 helper T cells react with class II HLA molecules, whereas CD8 cytotoxic/suppressor T cells react with class I HLA molecules. The interaction of Ag, T cells, and Ag-presenting cells results not only in the immediate proliferation of T cells and cytokine release but also in the development of sensitized or memory T cells that will respond to the Ag within 1 or 2 days of subsequent exposure. Cytotoxic effector cells are a second effector arm and may lyse overburdened macrophages.

Evidence for a definitive role for CMI in acquired resistance to MTB infection initially came from animal studies; specific antisera did not confer passive protection to mycobacterial Ags whereas protection was conferred by the transfer of T cells.[121–124] Over the last two decades, the occurrence of TB in HIV-infected subjects has underscored the importance of CMI in resistance to MTB.

Koch reported in 1891 that guinea pigs infected for 4–6 weeks with MTB and then challenged intracutaneously with a small number of virulent bacilli developed a localized area of induration and necrosis at the dermal inoculation site within 48 hours.[125] The Koch phenomenon is the classical tuberculin delayed-type hypersensitivity (DTH) reaction. A half-century later, Chase demonstrated that tuberculin DTH was transferred by lymphocytes.[126] Animal studies have indicated that CMI (protective immunity) and DTH are mediated by different T-cell subsets, although they occur concurrently.[127] The argument that DTH and protective immunity are dissociable stems from studies demonstrating that animals can be desensitized without loss of protection; they can be rendered hypersensitive without causing an increase in protection; and certain fractions of tubercle bacilli incur resistance without producing cutaneous hypersensitivity.[128] Furthermore, Orme and Collins have demonstrated that DTH and protective antituberculous immunity are mediated by separate subpopulations of T lymphocytes in mice (Ly-1 for DTH and Ly-2 for protection).[127] In humans, protection and DTH are linked epidemiologically in that TST-positive subjects are relatively resistant to exogenous reinfection.[129]

Perhaps Rook summarized this issue of the relationship between protective immunity and DTH best by acknowledging their complexity.[130] Thus, it appears that DTH and CMI are dissociable yet overlapping and complex events, and are linked by mononuclear cells to the expression of an intricate network of suppressive and injurious vs. beneficial cytokines, with cross-modulatory capacity. This scenario is complicated further by the accumulating evidence that CMI is differentially expressed in various tissues. The following sections seek to summarize the knowledge to date about the functions of each of the major cellular players in response to MTB or its products *in vitro* and in patients with TB.

PROTECTIVE IMMUNITY AND T-LYMPHOCYTE-DEPENDENT MACROPHAGE ACTIVATION

ANIMAL STUDIES

Immunization of mice with BCG results in the acquisition of the ability of splenic lymphocytes to transfer protective immunity adoptively after an aerogenic challenge with virulent MTB. Furthermore, immunization with live- but not heat-killed organisms generates protective immunity in mice.[131] Heat-killed organisms transfer nonspecific resistance and DTH. These data suggest that products of metabolically active mycobacteria may be particularly important in the protective response against MTB. Cooper et al. have shown that the memory immune response to MTB develops slowly in the lung following an aerosol challenge, but despite its strength, does not protect against the reestablishment of infection.[132]

CD4 AND CD8 SUBSETS

During the course of intravenous infection with MTB, protective CD4 lymphocytes appear early in the spleen, produce large quantities of IFN-γ, and are associated temporally with the onset of bacterial elimination; cytolytic T cells appear later and are less clearly associated with a role in protective immunity.[133] Depletion experiments using monoclonal antibodies against CD4 and CD8 cells in mice indicate that protection against mycobacteria can be conferred by both CD4[133-135] and by CD8[135] T lymphocytes. In mice, however, there is evidence of a functional separation of CD4 lymphocytes into IFN-γ secreting type 1 (TH-1) and IL-4 (and IL-5, IL-10, and IL-13) secreting type 2 cells.[136] TH-1 and TH-2 cytokines also are cross-modulatory. In mice, TH-1 CD4 cells confer protection against intracellular pathogens, including MTB.

Although the mechanism by which CD4 and CD8T cells protect mice against subsequent challenge with MTB still is not totally clear, studies indicate that there are two potential mechanisms for protection. Secretion of macrophage-activating cytokines such as IFN-γ, and possibly other molecules such as granulocyte—macrophage colony stimulating factor, induces MTB growth inhibition within macrophages. Studies using mice with genetic disruption of IFN-γ have shown the absolute necessity for this TH-1 cytokine in the control of MTB infection.[137,138] The other mechanism by which T cells may be protective is by cytotoxicity for mycobacterial-laden macrophages. Thus, class I MHC dysfunctional mice were more susceptible to MTB infection.[139] However, mice with genetic disruption of perforin, a molecule involved in CD8 cytotoxicity, did not demonstrate enhanced susceptibility to MTB infection.[140] Current thinking is that the IFN-γ/IL-12 axis is critical to protection. IL-12 is produced early in infection by Ag-presenting cells, and promotes the differentiation of T-helper cells and production of IFN-γ. IFN-γ further activates macrophages to produce TNF-α and other protective cytokines that promote intracellular killing of MTB.

Infection with MTB results in the differentiation of naïve T cells into effector T cells that expand to great numbers in the host. CD4T cells differentiate into Th1 and Th2 cells, whereas CD8T cells differentiate into cytotoxic T cells. Together, the effector CD4 and CD8T cell compartments of the adaptive immune response put forth a coordinated effort to clear the infection. As infection clears, the effector T cells (TE) undergo extensive apoptosis and T cell numbers return to homeostasis in the host. Importantly, during this time period, a small number of Ag-specific T cells survives either as short-lived T effector memory (TEM) or as long-lived central memory T cells (TCM).[141]

There is ample evidence that TE, TEM, and TCM can be distinguished from each other biochemically, phenotypically, and functionally. For example, effector and memory T cells generated in response to *Listeria* infection can be distinguished by the reciprocal expression of the transcription factors T-bet and eomesodermin, respectively.[142] Although the underlying mechanisms are not well understood, T effector cells undergo increased apoptosis compared to memory cells. A key difference between TEM and TCM is that TEM migrate to inflamed tissue and have immediate effector function, whereas TCM home to secondary lymphoid organs and have little effector function initially, but rapidly proliferate to become effector cells during a recall response. CD4 TEMs retain their Th1 and Th2 phenotype and rapidly secrete their signature cytokines under appropriate stimulating conditions and CD8 TEMs can be distinguished by their high expression of perforin. Contrarily, TCM, like naïve T cells, requires the appropriate biasing conditions to acquire a Th1 or Th2 phenotype.[143] Consistent with this notion, analysis of histone acetylation at promoters of cytokine genes shows that the pattern and level of chromatin remodeling is similar between TEMs and TEs, whereas TCM are more similar to naïve T cells (reviewed in ref.[119]). Additionally, TCMs are less dependent on co-stimulation for full activation as compared to TEMs. Human TCMs are CD45RO$^+$ and constitutively express CCR7 and CD62L. In contrast, TEMs have lost constitutive expression of CCR7 and express differing levels of CD62L. CD8 effector T cells can be distinguished from T cells by their high expression of CD38, HLA DR, CD27, and Ki-67, and low level expression of BCl-2 and CCR7. Additional memory populations have been defined as stem cell memory, transitional memory, and T-effectory memory reexpressing cells. Memory subsets can be characterized by differential surface expression of CD45RA and CD45RO isotypes, CCR7, CD27, and CD95.[144-146]

HUMAN STUDIES

T-cell responses of healthy subjects

MTB-infected persons are identified on the basis of a positive tuberculin PPD skin test. As noted, such infected individuals are relatively immune to exogenous reinfection and therefore protective T cells are likely to be present in their blood as well as in other compartments. Because the blood is the most accessible source in humans, the reactivity of blood T cells to mycobacterial Ags has been assessed most readily. Overall, these studies have shown the prominence of T cells in the production of cytokines, in particular IFN-γ, and cytotoxicity to MTB-infected mononuclear phagocytes.[147] However, as the antigenic repertoire of MTB is shared to a large extent with other mycobacteria, including environmental mycobacteria and BCG, these immunologic responses have to be understood in the context of the mycobacterial sensitization of the subjects recruited to these *in vitro* studies. In this regard, *in vitro* studies of household members of cases of TB may be most informative. In particular, studies of these households may allow analysis of responses over the spectrum of MTB infection, based on epidemiologic characterization. One such study demonstrated a correlation of PPD skin testing with heightened responses to T-cell IFN-γ release assay responses (spectrum of MTB-related Ags (ESAT-6, CFP-10, 16 kDa, 19 kDa, MPT64, Ag 85B, 38 kDa, hsp65, PPD, and BCG).[148] However, to date, T-cell responses of PPD skin test-reactive household contacts to only a few MTB Ags have been used to understand the responses of TB patients (see subsection "Antigenic targets of the T-cell response to MTB").

Bronchoalveolar lavage has allowed access to the immune cells that protect the alveoli. Studies of lung cells from healthy household members of TB cases may finally allow identification of important MTB protective mechanisms and Ags. Recently, Tan et al. have demonstrated that bronchoalveolar lymphocytes were prominent in the cytolytic lysis of MTB-infected alveolar macrophages.[149]

Pleural TB

Pleural TB generally is a self-limited process, suggesting that immune responses in this form of paucibacillary disease are highly protective.[150] However, 60% of patients with pleural TB present later with reactivation TB, indicating that the protection is compartmentalized to the pleural space alone. Pleural fluid from patients with pleural TB contains increased numbers of MTB-reactive CD4T lymphocytes compared to blood,[150,151] and these cells are predominantly of the CD4+CDw29+ T-cell phenotype, which are thought to represent memory T cells.[152] Fujiwara et al. have shown that the frequency of Ag-reactive blood lymphocytes in patients with tuberculous pleurisy is normal, whereas the frequency is increased in pleural fluid.[153] Therefore, the increase in pleural fluid Ag-reactive CD4T cells may be the result of *in situ* expansion rather than sequestration of such cells from the circulating pool. Despite adequate numbers of Ag-reactive T cells, however, the response of blood mononuclear cells to PPD in a third of patients is depressed relative to healthy tuberculin reactors and relative to the pleural fluid responses in the same patients.[154] This finding is due to the presence of suppressive monocytes (see subsection "Suppression by Monocytes and Regulatory T-cells") in the blood but not the pleural fluid. Pleural fluid also contains several fold increased levels of IFN-γ, TNF-α, and 1,25-dihydroxycholecalciferol (vitamin D) relative to serum,[155] consistent with the vigorous and effective local immune response.

Because local protective mechanisms are effective at containing the pleural infection despite the inadequacy of the systemic response, Wallis et al. sought to identify potential protective Ags using cells from the pleural fluid.[156] Upon transformation with Epstein Barr virus, pleural fluid B lymphocytes from two subjects with pleural TB spontaneously elaborated immunoglobulins (Igs). The frequency of MTB-reactive clones was 54% and 9% in these two subjects. Most (83%) of the clones secreted IgM, and the remainder IgG, antibodies. Western blot analysis using these antibodies identified predominantly a 31.5 kDa band reactive to MTB culture filtrate. The 30 kDa

α-Ag (antigen 6) is a secreted mycobacterial protein, which has been shown to be protective (see subsection "Regulation by Monocyte-Stimulatory Antigens").

The "Catch 22" of protective immunity is an immune mechanism that can only be established as protective in the context of a TB vaccine that demonstrates efficacy. The paradox is that to develop effective vaccines one needs immune correlates of protection as endpoints in early efficacy trials. There are two promising results in recent trials. Revaccination with BCG prevented stable IGRA conversion,[157] and a subunit vaccine M72 in adjuvant provided 53% protection against progression from LTBI to TB disease.[158]

ANTIGENIC TARGETS OF THE T-CELL RESPONSE TO MTB

A number of mycobacterial Ags have been characterized molecularly that stimulate T cells in tuberculin reactors. Due to the complexity of MTB infection, and the enormous heterogeneity of the human immune response, Ags that are targets of protective immunity still are not fully identified. Host responses at different stages of MTB infection are likely to be directed at particular MTB Ags, which in turn may induce various degrees of anti-MTB immunity.[159] It is also possible that the heterogeneity in Ags recognized by T cells at least partly reflects the diversity of T-cell subpopulations and functions.

Initial studies identified human responses to highly conserved bacterial and eukaryotic heat shock proteins, such as the 65 and 71 kDa proteins of MTB. Blastogenic responses of human blood T cells to these Ags have been reported in some, but not all studies.[160,161] Animal studies confirm that these Ags do not appear to be major targets of protective T-cell responses.[156] They are somatic Ags; murine T cells that confer protective immunity against TB do not recognize these molecules. However, the heat shock proteins may be involved in autoimmune processes targeted to peptides shared by mycobacteria and humans, and thereby in MTB-associated immunopathology. The 65 kDa heat shock protein of BCG is a target molecule for CD4 cytotoxic T cells that in turn lyse human monocytes pulsed with this protein.[160] However, only 20% of BCG vaccinees respond to this 65 kDa protein.

Another approach to define targets of the T-cell response to MTB has been to separate lysates and filtrates of MTB by physicochemical techniques and assess the relative reactivity of T cells to the separated fractions. The most consistent finding has been heterogeneity of the targets of the human T-cell response. For example, we found that T cells from tuberculin-positive healthy donors showed peaks of reactivity to fractions of culture filtrate of MTB H37Rv of 30, 37, 44, 57, 71, and 88 kDa.[162] Western immunoblotting indicated that three of these fractions contained previously defined Ags (30, 64, and 71 kDa). This technique does not allow determination of whether these previously identified proteins account for the activity found in the respective fractions. Schoel et al. have found numerous and diverse responses to 400 fractions prepared by 2D gel electrophoresis of lysates of MTB, underscoring the extensive heterogeneity of the mycobacterial Ag targets of human T cells.[163]

As protective immunity is conferred by living MTB only, the search for a protective Ag has focused primarily on secreted, not somatic, MTB Ags. Of the wide variety of secreted mycobacterial proteins identified,[164] the 85th complex of MTB is the subject of intense interest. The 85th complex is a group of three major extracellular Ags of MTB encoded by separate genes and secreted by actively proliferating MTB cultures.[165–169] Two of these Ags, 85A and 85B, bind to fibronectin and are of molecular weights 30–32 kDa. Ag 85B is identical to a previously recognized MTB Ag termed Ag 6, or the α-Ag,[170] the gene of which has been cloned by Matsuo et al.[171] This protein, which will be designated 30 kDa here, contains specific and cross-reactive determinants, stimulates blastogenesis and IFN-γ production by T cells from healthy donors, and elicits DTH in sensitized guinea pigs. Immunization with 85th complex proteins confers protection against respiratory challenge with MTB in guinea pigs.[172] Also T-cell responses to the 30 and 32 kDa Ags are preserved in tuberculin reactors, but not in patients with active TB.[173] It is possible that the 30 kDa Ag is involved in virulence[174] and/or immunosuppressive circuits.[47] The 30 kDa α-Ag recently has been identified as MTB mycolyl transferase.[175]

CYTOKINES IN RESISTANCE TO MTB AND IMMUNOPATHOLOGY OF TB

MTB and its components are potent inducers of cytokine production by monocytes/macrophages. Initial studies have shown that PPD directly stimulates monocytes to produce IL-1,[176] TNF-α,[44] IL-2R,[177] and TGF-β.[178] Also, purified proteins of MTB culture filtrate, such as the 58 kDa Ag (identified as MTB glutamine synthetase[179,180]), are potent inducers of TNF-α. Binding of fibronectin by the 30 kDa Ag enhances cytokine production by monocytes[174] and, therefore, the interaction of MTB and the host may lead to further in situ amplification of cytokines. Furthermore, the 30 kDa Ag induces both IL-10[47] and TGF-β.[46] MTB and its cell wall component, LAM, also induce TGF-β.[27] Therefore, it appears that the cytokine milieu of the tuberculous lesion, containing mycobacteria and its constituents, may be particularly biased to excess expression of TGF-β. In fact, immunoreactive TGF-β was present both in Langhans' giant cells and epithelioid cells of tuberculous granulomas of patients with untreated TB.[181]

TNF AND TGF IN RESISTANCE TO MTB, GRANULOMA FORMATION, AND TISSUE DAMAGE

Rook first suggested in 1983 that the secretory products of mononuclear phagocytes may induce the characteristic symptoms (fever and weight loss) and tissue necrosis of TB.[182] Although TNF-α is the most likely candidate, other cytokines such as TGF-β have also been associated with cachexia.[183] Although both TGF-β and TNF-α may be involved in tissue damage, the stimulation of collagenase production by fibroblasts, activation of endothelial cells by TNF-α, and inhibition of endothelial growth by TGF-β have been reported. Additionally, TGF-β promotes fibrosis,[184] and excess TGF-β has been implicated in the pathogenesis of a number of diseases associated with fibrosis.[185]

TNF-α may have beneficial as well as detrimental effects. TNF-α leads to the inhibition of growth of M. avium in human monocytes and monocyte-derived macrophages. TNF-α activates macrophages through the enhancement of both ROI and RNI.[186] Bermudez et al. have demonstrated that injection of TNF-α with or without IL-2 inhibits the growth of M. avium complex in vivo.[187]

The role of TNF-α, however, in the intracellular growth containment of MTB by mononuclear phagocytes is not totally clear. The combination of IFN-γ, calcitriol, and TNF-α, however, decreased the growth of MTB in blood monocytes.[188] TNF-α is an important mediator of growth inhibition of MTB by human alveolar macrophages.[42] Together with the heightened production of TNF-α,[45] and the limitation of production of the macrophage-deactivating cytokine, TGF-β,[189] alveolar macrophages may be poised to inhibit initial MTB growth. Because IFN-γ enhances the production and effects of TNF-α, the MTB growth inhibitory effect of TNF-α may be even greater after the development of CMI. By contrast, pretreatment of human blood monocytes with TGF-β increases intracellular mycobacterial growth. As noted, MTB induces TGF-β, and through autoinduction, TGF-β may amplify its own production at the sites of MTB infection.[46]

In addition, the local synthesis of TNF-α correlates with granuloma formation in mice infected with BCG, and injection of the anti-TNF-α antibody has been shown to decrease the number and size of granulomas and the development of epithelioid cells, allowing for massive replication of BCG.[190] Granuloma formation is critical to the containment of mycobacteria. The effect of TGF-β on the formation of granulomas presently is not known. However, because TGF-β inhibits the production of a number of chemokines, its effect may be one of altering the cellularity of granulomas. Overall, the balance of production of deactivating and activating cytokines as well as other products of the cellular constituents of granulomas likely contributes to the fate of infecting mycobacteria within them and ultimately to the expression of disease.

MACROPHAGE ACTIVATION BY IFN-Γ AT SITES OF MTB INFECTION

Murine peritoneal macrophages respond to IFN-γ by increasing their control of the replication of MTB.[191,192] Murine bone marrow macrophages also are activated by IFN-γ for increased containment of MTB, but the response to IFN-γ is specific to the strain of MTB used; some are more affected than others. In contrast to these animal studies, Douvas et al. have reported that IFN-γ does not activate growth containment of MTB in human blood monocyte-derived macrophages and, in fact, enhances MTB growth.[193] Rook et al., however, have found that although IFN-γ has little effect on MTB growth inhibition in human blood monocytes, it enhances MTB growth inhibition by monocyte-derived macrophages.[194] We found a modest effect of IFN-γ on MTB growth inhibition by human monocytes.[195] The mechanism by which IFN-γ exerts its macrophage activation is partly through the induction of the enzymes necessary for conversion of 25-hydroxyvitamin D3 to the active metabolite of vitamin D, i.e., 1,25-dihydroxyvitamin D3.[188] This metabolite in turn induces the differentiation of monocytes into macrophages with increased capacity to contain MTB growth. In addition, IFN-γ induces the production of RNIs which have been found to be bactericidal against MTB.[57] Bermudez has shown that TGF-β produced by monocytes upon ingestion of M. avium blocks the activity of IFN-γ.[196] This effect of TGF-β may in part be secondary to inhibition of the expression of IFN-γ receptors or the IFN-γ response. In MTB-infected human monocytes, the modest growth inhibition by TNF-α and

IFN-γ were mitigated by TGF-β.[195] In addition, neutralization of TGF-β activity enhanced MTB growth containment.[197] Inhibition of iNOS and, thereby, reduced production of NO, may in part be the basis for macrophage deactivation by TGF-β.[198] In addition, TGF-β inhibits the production of IFN-γ by T cells in response to MTB and other stimuli.[199] This effect occurs in part by counteracting the TH-1 promoting cytokine, IL-12, which is necessary for induction of IFN-γ expression.

Infection of macrophages by MTB leads to either apoptosis (decreased viability and enhanced immunity) or necrotic cell death (spread of infection) which in turn determines the outcome of infection. The type of cell death is regulated by eicosanoid lipid mediators, prostaglandin E2 (PGE2, proapoptotic) and lipoxin A4 (LXA4, pronecrotic); the latter being induced by the more virulent mycobacterial strains.[200] Arachidonic acid derivatives leukotrienes, PGE2, and lipoxin A4 (LXA4) have opposing roles in mycobacterial immunity. PGE2 induces macrophage apoptosis and restricts MTB growth in macrophages whereas LXA4 ablates the protective effect of PGE2 in the macrophage leading to necrosis. Mayer-Barber et al. recently outlined the role of IL-1-induced eicosanoids in the counter regulation of type 1 IFNs in mice. Inability to produce IL-1 and/or excess production of type 1 IFNs has been attributed to an eicosanoid imbalance (decreased prostaglandins and increase leukotrienes) that correlates with severe pathology and tissue necrosis.[201] PGE2 expression is enhanced by IL-1β but reduced by type 1 IFN, a potent inhibitor of IL-1β. In addition, IL-10 also leads to reduced PGE2 as IL-10 promotes type 1 IFN production. Thus, in the presence of IL-10 and type 1 IFN, IL-1β expression is abrogated and consequently PGE2 levels decrease. This results in macrophage necrosis and increased growth of MTB. Together these findings demonstrate that the balance of cytokines mediating macrophage resistance against MTB can be modulated by the levels of type 1 IFNs.

Studies assessing host-directed therapies targeting eicosanoids to enhance host immunity and limit long term sequelae of TB disease are therefore warranted.

CLASS II-RESTRICTED CYTOTOXICITY—ROLE IN PROTECTION AND IMMUNOPATHOLOGY

As noted, cytolytic T lymphocytes (CTL) appear during the course of experimental MTB infections.[135] Most of the support for CTL as an effector mechanism in MTB is based on *in vitro* studies. Blood T lymphocytes from MTB or *Mycobacterium leprae*-infected individuals are cytotoxic for monocytes pulsed with mycobacterial Ags. The cytotoxicity was found to be a property of CD4T cells. Recently, Boom et al. demonstrated that CD4 T-cell clones from PPD-reactive individuals were cytotoxic to mycobacterial Ag-pulsed or MTB-infected monocytes.[202] The cytotoxicity was independent of the profile of cytokines released by these clones (IL-2 vs. IL-4) and was a common property of these T-cell clones.

CD4 blood lymphocytes and clones from BCG-vaccinated subjects have been shown to be cytotoxic to mycobacterial-Ag-pulsed monocytes.[203] Interestingly, the cytotoxic CD4 clones also suppressed proliferation of BCG-specific T-cell clones in response to BCG. Whether the suppression of T-cell responses was a consequence of cytotoxicity for Ag-presenting cells or direct

suppression of T-cell responses was not resolved by this study. Macrophages that have ingested MTB or have been pulsed with soluble products such as PPD are targets of the CTL response.[160,203] Recent studies have indicated that human alveolar lymphocytes that were expanded *in vitro* by IL-2 and PPD performed well both in class I- and class II-mediated cytotoxicity against MTB-pulsed target cells.

Most investigators have speculated that the cytotoxicity mediated by CD4 cells may be a default mechanism by which MTB is released from overburdened and, therefore, dysfunctional effector cells. Presumably, once the organisms are released, they will be ingested and killed by fresh monocytes drawn to the fray. Alternatively, CTL, by lysing host cells, must be considered a factor in immunopathology. Clearly, additional *in vivo* studies in experimental animals will be necessary to resolve the relative importance of these two diverse sequelae of CTL.

ROLE OF HUMORAL IMMUNITY AGAINST MTB

Although animal and human studies continue to define the role of CMI in TB,[204] emerging evidence also suggests a significant role of B-cell and humoral immunity in host response to MTB.[205] Seibert and colleagues were the first to study antibody responses to MTB proteins and polysaccharides (LAM) following BCG vaccination in rabbits. They showed that antibody responses to MTB polysaccharides in addition to MTB proteins conferred more protection against TB disease as compared to rabbits who developed antibodies to MTB proteins alone. Likewise, inability to mount an antibody response following immunization to MTB polysaccharides was also associated with more extensive disease and higher mortality in rabbits.[206] Inadequate B-cell function and humoral host immune responses have been similarly associated with increased susceptibility to TB by multiple studies in humans, including children and HIV-infected individuals.[207] Demonstration of the benefits in survival, CFU reduction, Ag clearance, and mycobacterial dissemination in mice after administration of monoclonal antibodies against mycobacterial polysaccharides such as arabinomannan and LAM and mycobacterial proteins such as 16 kDa α-Acr, MPB83, and heparin binding hemagglutinin further solidifies the notion that humoral immunity has an important role in protection against MTB.[205,206]

Antibody-mediated protection against MTB occurs through several mechanisms. Intracellular killing after antibody mediated opsonization due to phagolysosomal fusion, increased macrophage Ca+ signaling, and enhanced oxidative burst has been demonstrated.[205,207] Additionally through TH1 activation, cytokine-driven immunomodulation, complement activation, and direct antimycobacterial activity, it is very likely that humoral immunity hugely contributes to MTB host responses.[207,208]

Mouse,[209] non-human primate (NHP), and human studies[210–212] show that B cells and Ab regulate anti-TB immunity. Notably, serum IgG from subjects with latent TB (LTBI) is superior to that from those with active disease in mediating macrophage anti-TB functions *in vitro*.[211] Monoclonal and serum-purified IgA derived from LTBI subjects inhibit MTB infection in epithelial cells, whereas monoclonal IgG from patients with active TB promotes infection of these cells.[212] Sera from healthcare workers that remain uninfected despite prolonged TB exposure protect against MTB in an Ab-dependent manner, suggesting innate resistance mediated via natural Ab may play a role in TB control,[210] a notion supported by our finding that blood and/or bronchoalveolar lavage fluid (BALF) of uninfected mice, NHP, and humans harbor Ig (IgM/IgG), that recognize MTB Ags including carbohydrates. These data implicate IgM, IgG, IgA, and natural Ab in regulating immune responses to MTB to modulate protection and/or influence disease and infection outcomes. B cells and Ig are required for (i) optimal granulomatous response and protection against MTB,[209] modulating lung neutrophil infiltration, IL-10 production, and immunopathology; (ii) activating Fcγ receptor (FcγR)-deficient mice are more susceptible to MTB, and those lacking the inhibitory FcγRIIB, more resistant,[209] suggesting that Ig can regulate anti-TB immunity by engaging FcγR on Ag-presenting cells with Ag–Ab complexes; (iii) B cells are required for optimal BCG-elicited Th1 response,[209] which, together with ability of B cells to modulate T-cell memory,[209] suggest a role for B cells in vaccine-engendered protection against MTB.

Although the extent of protection provided by B-cells and humoral immunity against MTB is yet to be ascertained, it is becoming increasingly clear that TB vaccines that can additionally induce antibody-mediated host response will likely be more effective.

THE MICROBIOME

There is growing appreciation that the gut microbiota can extend its influence to distal sites. A direct link to the microbiota was established when introduction of a species of gut-residing filamentous bacteria resulted in the generation of Th17 cells and rapid induction of autoimmune arthritis.[213] Gut dysbiosis has been shown to enhance systemic release of PGE2 and subsequent development and accumulation of M2 Macs in the lung. The beneficial effects of undigested dietary fiber and its fermentation products, especially short chain fatty acids (SCFAs) are now well documented.[214] SCFAs, notably acetate, propionate, and butyrate regulate cellular B cell antibody responses and T-cell effector functions.[214] Indole-3-propionic acid, a metabolite produced by *Clostridium sporogenes* and other gut commensals, has recently been shown to exhibit anti-mycobacterial activity.[215] However, another study found that anaerobic specifically SCFAs potentially increased TB susceptibility by blocking IFN-γ and IL-17A production via induction of regulatory T cell (Treg) expansion.[216] These studies underscore the power of the gut microbiota-released metabolites in influencing disease outcome at distal sites.

IMMUNE RESPONSES IN HUMAN TB

ANERGY

From 17% to 25% of patients with active TB are unresponsive to PPD skin tests.[217–219] In a more recent population study in which TB was newly introduced into the community, the prevalence of TB morbidity and mortality were high, and tuberculin anergy was present in as much as 50% of patients.[220] These data indicate that the expression of anergy in a population may depend upon the length of time that they are exposed to TB. In patients with pulmonary TB, tuberculin anergy correlates with the activity of TB; patients with far-advanced disease have a higher frequency of tuberculin anergy. Tuberculin anergy correlates with measurements of *in vitro* T-cell responses (see "T-cell Responses").

T-CELL RESPONSES

In vitro blastogenic responses of blood T cells to PPD are absent in approximately 40% of patients with active TB, including most skin test-nonreactors and some reactors.[221–225] Hyporesponsiveness to mycobacterial Ags has been described in various geographic areas and, therefore, seems to be relatively constant regardless of prior immunization with BCG. Several studies have indicated that the responses to nonmycobacterial Ags and mitogens are intact, so that depression of tuberculin reactivity is relatively specific.[221–224,226,236,312] The basis for the lower mononuclear cell responsiveness during TB is due to functional suppression of T-cell production of the TH-1 cytokine, IL-2, and the expression of IL-2 receptors.[225,228] However, the relative number of the main T-cell subpopulations, namely CD4 and CD8 cells, are unaltered.[222,228] Moreover, the frequency of PPD-reactive T cells is not significantly lower than that of healthy skin test-reactive subjects.[229] In a recent study, both blastogenesis and IFN-γ production by blood mononuclear cells were decreased, but improved during treatment.[230] Importantly, suppression of MTB-induced IFN-γ production also appears to correlate with the extent of pulmonary TB.[231] Rakotosamimanana et al. recently showed that "modern" mycobacterial strains such as Beijing and Central Asia strains tend to induce lower levels of IFN-γ production from peripheral blood mononuclear cells (PBMCs) compared to the "ancient" strains such as East African-Indian strains in index TB cases and their household contacts.[232] Similarly, multidrug-resistant TB patients show significantly less IFN-γ production and dysregulated IL-10, IL-8, and IL-12 levels compared to drug sensitive TB strains.[233] These concerning findings are likely suggestive of adaptation and evolution in the more pathological strains.

Frequencies of MTB-specific IFN-γ+CD4+ T cells that expressed immune activation markers CD38 and HLA-DR as well as intracellular proliferation marker Ki-67 were substantially higher in subjects with active TB (ATB) compared to those with LTBI.[234] Further, there are higher frequencies of MTB-specific caspase-3+IFN-γ+CD4+ T cells in ATB compared to LTBI.[235] Caspase-3 is expressed by CD4 T-cells downstream of anti-CD3 mediated TCR activation and modulates apoptosis during bacterial infection. Caspase-3+IFN-γ+CD4+ T cells were also more activated compared to their caspase-3-negative counterparts.[187] Furthermore, the frequencies of caspase-3+IFN-γ+CD4+ T cells decreased in response to anti-TB treatment.

A lack of correction of low T-cell responses by IL-2, which has been observed in two of three studies,[225,231,236] may reflect low lymphocyte IL-2R expression.[225] However, the possibility of interference with the interaction of IL-2 and IL-2R by another mediator has been sought (see subsection "Suppression by Monocytes and Regulatory T-cells"). In parallel to the dysregulation of IL-2 and its receptor, other studies have shown that patients with TB have a defect in the production of IFN-γ to different Ags of MTB.[231–235,237–239] Overall, the results of these *in vitro* experiments indicate that CD4T cells from patients with TB are limited in their expression of the TH-1 cytokines, IL-2, and IFN-γ, in response to MTB Ags.

Evidence for involvement of TH-2 cytokines derives from studies of protozoal infections and leprosy.[240,241] The TH-2 cytokines, IL-4 and IL-10, are cross-modulatory in that they limit TH-1 responses and increase antibody production.[242] Both of these cytokines have been shown to have macrophage-deactivating effects.[243,244] An increase in the frequency of IL-4 producing T cells in TB has been shown.[245] However, no correlation to low blastogenesis or IFN-γ production in response to mycobacterial Ags was found. Hirsch et al. also showed that stimulation of PBMCs with PPD or 30 kDa α-Ag induced higher secretion of TGF-β but not TNF-α or IL-10 in TB patients compared to PPD reactive household contacts.

SUPPRESSION BY MONOCYTES AND REGULATORY T-CELLS

A predominant role for blood monocytes in the suppression of T-cell responses has been indicated by several studies examining immune responses of patients with TB. Depletion of adherent monocytes from PBMCs of patients caused enhanced T-cell blastogenesis,[221] and production of IL-2[225] and IFN-γ.[246] Conversely, small numbers of monocytes (2% of T cells) added back to T-cell cultures have been shown to suppress T-cell production of IL-2.[224] Blood monocytosis is a well-documented feature of active TB. DNA-labeling studies indicate that monocytes from patients appear to be less mature than those of healthy subjects.[247] Furthermore, monocytes from tuberculous subjects display stigmata of *in vivo* activation as they spontaneously express IL-2R mRNA, display surface IL-2R, and release IL-2R upon *in vitro* culture.[176] We have shown that in freshly obtained mononuclear cells from patients with active TB, NF-κB) is already activated.[248] The cytokine profile of monocytes from patients with TB is also consistent with the notion that these cells are activated *in vivo*. When compared to monocytes of healthy subjects, production of the proinflammatory cytokines, TNF-α,[91] IL-1,[34] and IL-6[60] are enhanced by tuberculous monocytes upon *in vitro* stimulation with PPD or lipopolysaccharide. As noted, expression of IL-2R is similarly increased.[176] The presence of NF-κB-binding motifs in the promoters of these molecules links their transcriptional upregulation with the activation of NF-κB.

The mechanisms by which monocytes suppress T-cell responses in TB have been partially clarified. As noted, monocytes from TB patients express low numbers of IL-2R and shed IL-2R upon *in vitro* culture. When cultured with exogenous IL-2, monocytes from patients remove IL-2 from supernatants.[176] However, consumption of IL-2 by monocytes is not sufficient to explain lowered T-cell responses.[225] Other studies have indicated that upon isolation, monocytes from TB patients with active pulmonary TB contain immunoreactive TGF-β, and that the concentration of TGF-β in cultures of unstimulated and MTB-stimulated monocytes from TB patients is higher than that in PPD skin test-reactive healthy subjects.[181] Importantly, neutralization of TGF-β enhanced both

T-cell blastogenesis and production of IFN-γ in response to PPD in mononuclear cells of TB patients. Overall, excess production of TGF-β by monocytes may be central to low *in vitro* T-cell responses during TB. However, cytotoxic CD4 lymphocytes[160] and Fcγ-receptor-positive T cells[222] may also contribute to the suppression of T-cell responses during TB.

A critical and as yet unanswered question is the significance of the suppression of T-cell responses to mycobacterial Ags in patients with TB. Depressed T-cell responses may be a factor in the pathogenesis of reactivation TB. Alternatively, depressed T-cell responses may be an associated feature of active TB. Also, the relationship between suppressed responses in the blood and regulation of the immune response locally at the site of infection must be addressed.

Maintaining an efficacious anti-TB Th1 T effector (Teff) response is dependent on counter-regulation by an additional subset of CD4+ T cells, termed natural regulatory T cells (Tregs). Treg cells are commonly identified by constitutive expression of CD25 (IL-2 receptor), FoxP3 (transcription factor), and reduced expression of CD127 (IL-7 receptor) and are responsible for suppressing Teff cell proliferation and cytokine expression.[226] The main suppressive mediators expressed by Tregs are IL-10 and TGF-β. Tregs are recognized as important in regulating inflammation. Treg have been reported to be increased in number and suppressive of MTB-stimulated production of IFN-γ[227] but this has not been a consistent finding. Blocking studies that a subpopulation expanded in TB, HLA-DR+ Teff are compromised to Treg-mediated suppression mediated through the β-chemokine receptor CCR5 as well as through the negative regulatory molecule, PD-L1.[249] Both CCR5 and PD-L1 are reported to promote Treg suppression. HLA-DR+ Teff express higher levels of Th1/Th17 cytokines (IFN-γ, IL-17, and IL-22) that negatively regulate Tregs.

REGULATION BY MONOCYTE-STIMULATORY AGS

The basis for the Ag specificity of suppression in TB has been studied intensively. As noted, PPD is a direct stimulus for monocytes to produce IL-1,[171] TNF-α,[44] IL-2R,[177] and TGF-β.[175] As noted, both the polysaccharide, LAM, and protein mycobacterial products also have the capacity to stimulate the production of TGF-β by monocytes.[46] The 30 kDa α-Ag of MTB also has the capacity to stimulate the expression of TNF-α, TGF-β, and IL-10 by monocytes. Thus, the intense interaction of MTB with mononuclear phagocytes may create a cytokine milieu that is conducive to immunoprotection during latent MTB infection, and one of the immunosuppressions during active TB. The direct stimulatory properties of MTB components with the host mononuclear phagocytes most likely underlie the extensive tissue damage in TB.

IMMUNOPATHOGENESIS OF TB: BRONCHOALVEOLAR LAVAGE CELLS

Studies indicate that alveolar cells and their functions reflect the pattern of activity found in the interstitium. A fundamental observation is that the cells from the lung do not represent the cells from the blood either phenotypically or functionally. Initially, Lenzini et al. analyzed the cellular pattern in the BALF of several patients with various lung diseases.[250] One patient with acute TB had 53% lymphocytes and 45% alveolar macrophages (normal 6% to 10% lymphocytes, 90% to 95% macrophages). In another patient with chronic TB, there were 20% lymphocytes and 80% macrophages. Recent studies also have demonstrated a lymphocytic alveolitis.[251–256] Schwander et al. have demonstrated an alveolitis in TB-involved BAC, characterized by an abundance of immature macrophages (20%–25%) and alveolar lymphocytes. However, the presence of memory (CD45RO⁺) alveolar lymphocytes and their state of activation were similar.[256]

Schwander et al. have found that BAC from TB patients have enhanced blastogenic responses to PPD, the 30 kDa Ag, and LAM, and an increased PPD-induced frequency of IFN-γ producing cells.[257] The frequency of IL-4- and IL-10-producing cells were not expanded. Others have reported an enhanced production of IFN-γ and IL-12 by BAC of TB patients.[258]

There has been an explosion of new information derived from studies of the transcriptome.[259,260] TNF-α, IFN-γ, and the Th1 axis appear to be important in protective immunity in mice and humans. During active TB, the dominant signature is that of IFN-inducible genes, complement-related genes, myeloid function, and inflammation. By contrast, B and T-cell signals are decreased.[261] The neutrophils and monocytes are the principal sources of type 1 IFNs. Furthermore, in TB, overexpression of IFN response genes, including STAT1, IFITs, GBPs, MX1, OAS1, IRF1, and other genes, were also detected early in TB contacts who progressed to active disease. *In vitro* studies have shown that distinct mycobacterial molecules and signaling pathways are involved in the induction of this family of type 1 IFNs during MTB infections. High levels of type 1 IFN are preferentially induced by virulent strains because of the mycobacterial virulence factor ESX-1 protein secretion system. Several mechanisms underlying the pathogenic role of type 1 IFN in TB have been described, including induction of IL-10 and negative regulation of the IL-12/IFN-γ and IL-1β/PGE2 host-protective responses. However, there is also evidence that type 1 IFN may play a protective role in certain contexts. Although high levels of type 1 IFN have negative effects during the course of MTB infection, tonic I IFN signaling or low levels of type 1 IFN in the context of low mycobacterial loads may in turn have positive effects by priming host-protective responses.

HIV AND PATHOGENESIS OF TB

TB IN HIV INFECTION

HIV is the greatest known risk both for reactivation of latent MTB infection[262,263] and for the development of primary TB upon exposure to infectious persons.[263] However, the main impact of HIV on TB has occurred in developing countries where the prevalence of both MTB and HIV infection is high. The range of the median CD4 count at the time of diagnosis of TB varies widely,[264] and includes both normal and low CD4 counts. In the US, TB occurs relatively early in HIV infection; in 50%–67% of cases, it occurs at a mean of 6–9 months before another acquired immunodeficiency

syndrome (AIDS)-defining condition.[265] The early onset of TB in HIV-infected individuals underscores the virulence of MTB, and suggests a strict requirement for a fully competent cell-mediated immune response for protection against MTB. HIV infection increases the likelihood of a negative TST in MTB-infected people,[266] which correlates with the number of CD4 cells.

Although anergy is common in HIV infection, HIV-infected patients with TB often have a positive cutaneous DTH response to PPD. Over two-thirds of HIV-infected patients with active TB who do not have other AIDS-defining conditions are tuberculin reactive, whereas only one-third is tuberculin reactive once another AIDS-defining condition has developed.[267] MTB-induced T-cell proliferation and cytokine production (IFN-γ and TNF-α) have been shown to be increased in symptomatic and asymptomatic TST-positive HIV-infected TB women who were studied as part of a mother–infant cohort.[268] These data support the concept that T-cell responses to MTB are boosted by active TB even in the presence of HIV-related immunosuppression. However, more subtle defects in CMI may be sufficient to increase susceptibility to TB. Also, defects in native resistance may account for some of the increase in predisposition to TB. The known abnormalities in T cell and mononuclear phagocyte function in HIV infection may provide clues.

Immunosuppression makes the diagnosis of TB in persons living with HIV challenging. Several biosignatures that can accurately detect active TB from other lung diseases in HIV-infected individuals have now been identified.[269–273] Differential gene expression of activating Fcγ receptor (FcGR1A) is of particular interest as it has been shown to successfully distinguish active TB from latent TB regardless of HIV status or genetic background.[274] Gene expression of BATF2 has also been shown to have a high-negative predictive value in diagnosing active TB-coinfected individuals.[275] In fact, recently Verma et al. have shown that gene expression of FcGR1A and BATF2 in addition to plasma protein levels of IFN-γ and CXCL10 have the potential to identify active TB even in advanced HIV patients with a CD4 count of <100 cells/μL).[276]

TB-associated immune reconstitution syndrome (TB-IRIS) in HIV patients initiated on anti-retroviral therapy (ART) can occur due to paradoxical worsening of TB features or due to unmasking of TB infection and is characterized by an exaggerated inflammatory response. Low baseline CD4 counts (50–100 cells/μL), short interval between initiation of ART and TB treatment, and disseminated TB are considered as major risk factors for TB-IRIS.[277] The immunopathogenesis of TB-IRIS, however, is poorly understood. The role of mycobacteria PPD—specifically, IFN-γ-producing Th1 cells in TB-IRIS,[278] enhanced NK cell activation[279] and, increased neutrophils and its mediators such as S100A8/S100A9[280] have been recognized. Tran et al. interestingly also showed that HIV-TB-coinfected patients who developed TB-IRIS showed dysregulation of the complement system and imbalance between the effector C1Q and the inhibitor C1-INH prior to the initiation of ART.[281] They also observed differences in monocyte gene expression at baseline prior to initiation of ART among TB-HIV-coinfected patients who developed TB-IRIS suggesting a possible role.[282] Narendran et al. in a prospective cohort study showed that elevated baseline levels of IL-6 and C-reactive protein in HIV-TB-coinfected patients may have a predictive role in TB-IRIS as well.[283] Corticosteroids are the mainstay of TB-IRIS treatment and have been shown to rapidly improve symptoms and decrease need for hospitalizations.[284] A double-blind randomized, placebo-controlled study proved that initiating prednisone with ART in TB-HIV-coinfected patients with CD4 counts of <100 cells/L (after exclusion of rifampin-resistant TB, hepatitis B, and Kaposi's sarcoma) reduces the risk of TB-IRIS by 30% and can be used as a preventive strategy.[285] TB-IRIS causes significant morbidity and possibly mortality in resource poor countries and there is a need for better diagnostic tests, prognostic biomarkers, and novel therapeutic interventions.

T LYMPHOCYTES

During infection with HIV, CD4T helper cells are progressively depleted and profoundly impaired with respect to proliferation and production of TH-1 cytokines.[286] HIV and MTB-induced synergistic immune activation leading to apoptosis of HIV-infected CD4+ lymphocytes and bystander uninfected CD4+ and CD8+ lymphocytes partly explains the cell loss.[287] In contrast, B-lymphocyte activity increases during HIV infection resulting in a polyclonal hypergammaglobulinemia. The mechanisms of progressive T-cell dysfunction include selective loss and functional impairment of memory T cells, immunoregulatory dysfunction of mononuclear phagocytes, active immunosuppression by products of HIV such as gp120 and tat, and excessive production of immunosuppressive cytokines.[288] Each of these mechanisms also may impact on susceptibility to TB in HIV infection. The production of immunoregulatory cytokines in HIV infection may be especially important with regard to TB. In a cohort of over 100 HIV-positive individuals, a selective loss of IL-2 and IFN-γ production in response to recall Ags correlated with an increase in phytohemagglutinin-stimulated IL-4 and IL-10 production,[263] indicating that a decline in TH-1 function and an increase in TH-2 function occur concurrently during HIV infection. However, Zhang et al. have shown that despite low TH-1 responses, IL-4 and IL-10 were comparable in HIV-infected and -uninfected TB patients.[289] Thus, the switch in the balance toward TH-2 function in HIV infection does not entirely explain the increased susceptibility to TB in HIV-infected persons.

MONONUCLEAR PHAGOCYTES

Mononuclear phagocytes, including blood monocytes and tissue macrophages, may be infected with HIV in vitro and in vivo.[290] Because MTB is an intracellular pathogen, mononuclear phagocytes may be affected particularly by dual infection with HIV and MTB. Cumulatively, studies indicate that the number of monocytes; expression of cytokines including IL-1 and TNF-α; production of oxygen radical production; expression of phenotypic markers such as class II MHC, CR1, and CR3; and microbicidal activity against several pathogens are preserved.[290,291] Ag presentation by monocytes, however, is decreased, whereas accessory cell function for T-cell responses to mitogens is normal.[292] Microbicidal activity of alveolar macrophages from subjects with AIDS is normal for *Toxoplasma gondii* and *Chlamydia psittaci* and killing is upregulated by IFN-γ.[293] However, these latter responses for MTB have not been studied fully.

Several immunologic and effector functions of alveolar macrophages from HIV-infected subjects are up-regulated, including the expression of markers of activation[294] and the expression of cytokines such as IL-1,[295] IL-6,[296] and TNF-α.[297] Whether these findings relate to the immunopathogenesis of TB in coinfected subjects is not clear. Furthermore, there is an expansion of CD8 lymphocytes in the lungs of patients with HIV infection. As noted, CD8T cells lyse Ag-pulsed alveolar macrophages in a class I-restricted manner.[298] Whether CD8 cytotoxicity against MTB-infected alveolar macrophages is blunted in coinfected patients and/or contributes to pathology is unknown.

IMPACT OF TB ON HIV INFECTION

The impact of TB on the progression of HIV infection has been recognized widely. However, to date, this effect is most notable in Africa where 12 of the 15 million coinfected patients have originated.[299] Because the response of HIV-infected TB patients to antituberculous drugs is similar to HIV-uninfected TB patients, the increased morbidity[300] and mortality[300,301] in coinfected patients is attributable to worsening of HIV disease. For example, in Uganda, the mortality of TB in HIV-infected patients is 30%; this finding has been found to be due primarily to progressive HIV disease, and not to the TB disease.[302] Serum levels of $\beta2$ microglobulin, a marker of HIV disease progression, were twofold higher in HIV-infected Ugandan patients with pulmonary TB than in HIV-infected nontuberculous subjects and HIV-seronegative patients with TB.[268] Data from the US have shown that HIV-infected patients with TB have reduced survival, more opportunistic infections, and a greater decrease in CD4 counts relative to CD4-matched controls.[300] In fact, the development of TB and associated immune activation leads to induction of HIV viral replication and an increase in plasma HIV RNA.[303] This increase is particularly significant in HIV-infected TB patients with higher CD4 counts and at the site of TB infection.[304]

Replication of HIV in vitro and presumably in vivo in both lymphocytes and monocytes requires activation by various stimuli such as Ags, mitogens, growth factors, and cytokines including TNF-α, IL-1, and IL-6. These stimuli initiate viral replication in part through activation of NF-κB that, in turn, binds to the long-terminal repeat in the promoter region of HIV, thereby stimulating viral transcription. Recent research has suggested that the activation of MAP kinase pathways, especially p38 MAP kinase pathway, is also critical in HIV-1 replication.[304] Blood monocytes from patients with TB release increased amounts of TNF-α, IL-1, and IL-6 upon stimulation,[46] and display spontaneous NF-κB and p38 MAP kinase activation.[248] Furthermore, mycobacteria, and protein and polysaccharide constituents of mycobacteria, enhance HIV replication in latently infected cell lines[305] and in HIV-infected monocytes.[304] Finally, MTB and PPD induce HIV replication in alveolar macrophages from HIV-infected patients.[306] Monocytes from patients with pulmonary TB have been found to be more susceptible to infection with HIV in vitro than monocytes from healthy subjects.[307] The increased susceptibility was not attributable to increased viral entry, reverse transcription, or the number of infected cells, suggesting that either integration or viral transcription was upregulated in these cells. The role of monocyte-derived cytokines in the enhanced replication of HIV in patients with TB is being examined. Other studies have indicated that TB generates a cytokine microenvironment (TNF-α, IL-6, and IL-2) enhancing the infection of lymphocytes by HIV.[308] Cumulatively, these data indicate that the cytokines that may be relevant to protection against MTB may be deleterious for persons with HIV infection, and that anticytokine therapy may be effective at limiting HIV replication during the treatment of active TB in HIV-positive subjects.

Recently, we have shown that TB occurring prior to initiation of ARTs is associated with diminished latent reservoirs of virus.[309] The underlying mechanism is not yet known. This may, however, be proof of principle for purging latent reservoirs by immune activation.

REFERENCES

1. World Health Organization (WHO). Global Tuberculosis Report 2018. Geneva: WHO; 2018. https://www.who.int/tb/publications/global_report/tb18_ExecSum_web_4Oct18.pdf?ua=1.

2. Wells WF, Wells MW, and Wilder TS. The environmental control of epidemic contagion: I. An epidemiologic study of radiant disinfection of air in day schools. *Am J Hyg.* 1942;35:97.

3. Riley RL, Mills CC, O'Grady F, Sultan LU, Wittstadt F, and Shivpuri DN. Infectiousness of air from a tuberculosis ward. Ultraviolet irradiation of infectiousness of different patients. *Am Rev Respir Dis.* 1962;85:511.

4. Smith DW, McMurray DN, Wiegeshaus EH, Grover AA, and Harding GE. Host–parasite relationships in experimental airborne tuberculosis. IV. Early events in the course of infection in vaccinated and nonvaccinated guinea pigs. *Am Rev Respir Dis.* 1970;102:937.

5. Lurie MB, *Resistance to Tuberculosis: Experimental Studies in Native and Acquired Defensive Mechanisms.* Cambridge, MA: Harvard University Press, 1964.

6. Lurie MB and Dannenberg AM, Jr. Macrophage function in infectious disease with inbred rabbits. *Bacteriol Rev.* 1965;29(466).

7. Meylan PR, Richman DD, and Kornbluth RS. Reduced intracellular growth of mycobacteria human macrophages cultivated at physiologic oxygen pressure. *Am Rev Respir Dis.* 1992;145:947.

8. Wayne LG and Hayes LG. An *in vitro* model for sequential study of shiftdown of *Mycobacterium tuberculosis* through two stages of nonreplicating persistence. *Infect Immun.* 1996;64:2062.

9. Dannenberg AM. Immune mechanisms in the pathogenesis of pulmonary tuberculosis. *Rev Infect Dis.* 1989;52:369.

10. North RJ. T-cell dependence of macrophage activation and mobilization during infection with *Mycobacterium tuberculosis. Infect Immun.* 1974;10:66.

11. Medlar EM. The behavior of pulmonary tuberculous lesions: A pathological study. *Am Rev Tuberc.* 1955;71:1.

12. Yamamura Y, Ogawa Y, Maeda H, and Yamamura Y. Prevention of tuberculous cavity formation by desensitization with tuberculin-active peptide. *Am Rev Respir Dis.* 1974;109:594.

13. Noll H. The chemistry of cord factor, a toxic glycolipid of *M. tuberculosis. Adv Tuberc Res.* 1956;7:149.

14. Hunter RL, Olsen MR, Jagannath C, and Actor JK. Multiple roles of cord factor in the pathogenesis of primary, secondary, and cavitary tuberculosis, including a revised description of the pathology of secondary disease. *Ann Clin Lab Sci.* 2006;36(4).

15. Artman M, Bekierkunst A, and Goldenberg I. Tissue metabolism in infection: Biochemical changes in mice treated with cord factor. *Arch Biochem Biophys.* 1964;105:80.

16. Kato M. Site II-specific inhibition of mitochondrial oxidative phosphorylation by trehalose-6,6′-dimycolate (cord factor) of *Mycobacterium tuberculosis. Arch Biochem Biophys.* 1970;140:379.

17. Hunter RL, Venkataprasad N, and Olsen MR. The role of trehalose dimycolate (cord factor) on morphology of virulent *M. tuberculosis in vitro. Tuberculosis (Edinburgh).* 2006;86:349–56.

18. Gordon AH, D'Arcy Hart P, and Young MR. Ammonia inhibits phagosome–lysosome fusion in macrophages. *Nature (London).* 1980;286:79.

19. Smith DW, Randall HM, Gaastambide-Odier MD, and Koevoet AL. Mycosides: A new class of type-specific glycolipids of mycobacteria. *Ann NY Acad Sci.* 1960;69:145.

20. Goren MB. Sulfolipid I of *Mycobacterium tuberculosis* strain H37Rv. II. Structural studies. *Biochem Biophys Acta.* 1970;210:127.

21. Kato M and Goren MB. Synergistic action of cord factor and mycobacterial sulfatides on mitochondria. *Infect Immun.* 1974;10:733.

22. Mishra AK, Driessen NN, Appelmelk BJ, and Besra GS. Lipoarabinomannan and related glycoconjugates: Structure, biogenesis and role in *Mycobacterium tuberculosis* physiology and host–pathogen interaction. *FEMS Microbiol Rev,* 1 November 2011;35(6):1126–57, https://doi.org/10.1111/j.1574–6976.2011.00276.x

23. Goren MB, D'Arcy Hart P, Young WR, and Armstrong JA. Prevention of phagosome-lysosome fusion in cultured macrophages by sulfatides of *Mycobacterium tuberculosis. Proc Nat Acad Sci USA.* 1976;73:2510.

24. Brennan PJ, Hunter SW, McNeil M, Chatterjee D, and Daffe M. Reappraisal of the chemistry of mycobacterial cell walls, with a view to understanding the roles of individual entities in disease processes. In: Ayoub EM, Cassell GH, Branch WC, Jr., and Henry TJ, (eds). *Microbial Determinants of Virulence and Host Response.* Washington, D.C.: American Society for Microbiology, 1990.

25. Daffe M, Lacave C, Lanelle M-A, Gillois M, and Lanelle G. Polyphthinenacyl trehalose, glycolipids specific for virulent strains of the tubercle bacillus. *Eur J Biochem.* 1988;112:579.

26. Rastogi N. Recent observations concerning structure and function relationships in the mycobacterial cell envelope: Elaboration of a model in terms of mycobacterial pathogenicity, virulence and drug resistance, *Res Microbiol.* 1991;142:464.

27. Chan J, Fan XD, Hunter SW, Brennan PJ, and Bloom R. Lipoarabinomannan, a possible virulence factor involved in persistence of *Mycobacterium tuberculosis* within macrophages. *Infect Immun.* May 1991;59(5):1755–61.

28. Gaur RL et al. LprG-mediated surface expression of lipo-arabinomannan is essential for virulence of *Mycobacterium tuberculosis*. *PLoS Pathog.* 2014;10(9):e1004376. https://doi.org/10.1371/journal.ppat.1004376

29. Parrish N and Bishai WR. Mechanisms of latency in *Mycobacterium tuberculosis*. *Trends Microbiol.* 1998;6:107.

30. Gomez JE, Chen, J-M., and Bishai WR. Sigma factors of *Mycobacterium tuberculosis*. *Tuberc Lung Dis.* 1997;78:175.

31. Yuan Y, Crane DD, Simpson RM, Zhu YQ, Hickey MJ, Sherman DR, and Barry CE III. The 16-kDa alpha-crystallin (Acr) protein of *Mycobacterium tuberculosis* is required for growth in macrophages. *Proc Natl Acad Sci.* 1998;95:9578.

32. Folkvardsen DB, Norman A, Andersen AB, Rasmussen EM, Lillebaek T, and Jelsbak L. A major *Mycobacterium tuberculosis* outbreak caused by one specific genotype in a low prevalence country: Exploring gene profile virulence explanations. *Sci Rep.* 2018;8:118669.

33. Dannenberg AM, Jr. Delayed-type hypersensitivity and cell mediated immunity in the pathogenesis of tuberculosis. *Immunol Today.* 1991;12:228.

34. Orme I and Collins FM. Mouse model of tuberculosis. In: Bloom B (ed). *Tuberculosis, Pathogenesis, Protection, and Control*. Materials Park, OH: ASM Press 1994.

35. Rhoades ER, Frank AA, and Orme IM. Progression of chronic pulmonary tuberculosis in miceaerogenically infected with virulent *Mycobacterium tuberculosis*. *Tuberc Lung Dis.* 1997;78:57.

36. Smith DW, McMurray DN, Wiegeshaus EH, Grover AA, and Harding GE. Host–parasite relationships in experimental airborne tuberculosis. IV. Early events in the course of infection in vaccinated and nonvaccinated guinea pigs. *Am Rev Resp Dis.* 1970;102:937.

37. Aiyaza, M, Bipina C, and Pantulwara V. Whole genome response in guinea pigs infected with the high virulence strain *Mycobacterium tuberculosis* TT372. *Tuberculosis (Edinburgh).* 2014 December;94(6):606–15.

38. Swartz RP, Naal D, Vogel, C-W, and Yeager H, Jr. Differences in uptake of mycobacteria by human monocytes: A role for complement. *Infect Immun.* 1988;56:2223.

39. Schlessinger L, Bellinger-Kawahara CG, Payne NR, and Horwitz MA. Phagocytosis of *Mycobacterium tuberculosis* is mediated by human monocyte complement receptors and complement component C3. *J Immunol.* 1990;144:2771.

40. Schlesinger LS, Kaufman TM, Iyer S, Hull SR, and Marchiando LK. Differences in mannose receptor-mediated uptake of lipoarabinomannan from virulent and attenuated strains of *Mycobacterium tuberculosis* by human macrophages. *J Immunol.* 1996;157:4568.

41. Schlesinger LS. Entry of *Mycobacterium tuberculosis* into mononuclear phagocytes. *Curr Top Microbiol Immunol.* 1996;215:71.

42. Hirsch CS, Ellner JJ, Russell DG, and Rich EA. Complement receptor mediated uptake and tumor necrosis-α-mediated growth inhibition of *Mycobacterium tuberculosis* by human alveolar macrophages. *J Immunol.* 1994;152:743.

43. Gaynor CD, McCormack FX, Voelker DR, McGowan SE, and Schlesinger LS. Pulmonary surfactant protein A mediates enhanced phagocytosis of *Mycobacterium tuberculosis* by a direct interaction with human macrophages. *J Immunol.* 1995;55:5343.

44. Valone SE, Rich EA, Wallis RR, and Ellner JJ. Expression of tumor necrosis factor *in vitro* by human mononuclear phagocytes stimulated with BCF and mycobacterial antigens. *Infect Immun.* 1988;56:3313.

45. Rich EA, Panuska JR, Wallis RS, Wolf CB, and Ellner JJ. Dyscoordinate expression of tumor necrosis factor-alpha by human blood monocytes and alveolar macrophages. *Am Rev Respir Dis.* 1989;139:1010.

46. Surewicz K, Aung H, Kanost RA, Jones L, Hejal R, and Toossi Z. The differential interaction of p38 MAP kinase and tumor necrosis factor-α in human alveolar macrophages and monocytes induced by *Mycobacterium tuberculosis*. *Cell Immunol.* 2004;228:34–41.

47. Torres M, Herrera T, Villareal H, Rich EA, and Sada E. Cytokine profiles for peripheral blood lymphocytes from patients with active pulmonary tuberculosis and healthy household contacts in response to the 30-kilodalton antigen of *Mycobacterium tuberculosis*. *Infect Immun.* 1998;66:176.

48. Myrvik QN, Leake EE, and Wright MJ. Disruption of phagosomal membranes of normal alveolar macrophages by the H37Rv strain of *Mycobacterium tuberculosis*: A correlate of virulence. *Am Rev Respir Dis.* 1984;129:322.

49. McDonough KA, Kress Y, and Bloom BR. Interaction of *Mycobacterium tuberculosis* with macrophages. *Infect Immun.* 1993;61:2763.

50. Armstrong JA and d'Arcy Hart P. Phagosome-lysosome interactions in cultured macrophages infected with virulent tubercle bacilli. Reversal of the usual nonfusion pattern and observations on bacterial survival. *J Exp Med.* 1975;142:1.

51. Gutierrez, MG et al. Autophagy is a defense mechanism inhibiting BCG and *Mycobacterium tuberculosis* survival in infected macrophages. *Cell.* 2004;119(6), 753–66

52. Yuk JM, Shin DM, Lee HM, Yang CS, Jin HS, Kim KK, Lee ZW, Lee SH, Kim JM, and Jo EK. Vitamin D3 induces autophagy in human monocytes/macrophages via cathelicidin. *Cell Host Microbe.* 2009;6: 231–43.

53. Castillo EF et al. Autophagy protects against active tuberculosis by suppressing bacterial burden and inflammation. *Proc Natl Acad Sci U S A.* 2012 Nov 13;109(46):E3168–76. doi: 10.1073/pnas.1210500109. Epub 2012 Oct 23.

54. Mitchison DA, Selkon JB, and Lloyd J. Virulence in the guinea-pig, susceptibility to hydrogen peroxide, and catalase activity of isoniazid-sensitive tubercle bacilli from South Indian and British patients. *J Pathol Bacteriol.* 1963;86:377.

55. Jackett PS, Aber VR, and Lowrie DB. Virulence of *Mycobacterium tuberculosis* and susceptibility of peroxidative killing systems. *J Gen Microbiol.* 1978;106:273.

56. Douvas GS, Berger EM, Repine JE, and Crowle AJ. Natural mycobacteriostatic activity inhuman monocyte-derived adherent cells. *Am Rev Respir Dis.* 1986;134:44.

57. Chan J, Tanaka D, Caroll D, Flynn KJ, and Bloom BR. Effects of nitric oxide synthase inhibitors on murine infection with *Mycobacterium tuberculosis*. *Infect Immun*. 1995;63:736.

58. Macmicking AD, North RJ, La Course R, Mudgett JS, Shah SK, and Nathan CF. Identification of nitric oxide synthase as a protective locus against tuberculous. *Proc Natl Acad Sci*. 1997;94:5243.

59. Martin SP, Pierce CH, Middlebrook G, and Dubos RJ. The effect of tubercle bacilli on the polymorphonuclear leukocytes of normal animals. *J Exp Med*. 1950;91:381.

60. Sugawara I et al. Rat neutrophils prevent the development of tuberculosis. *Infect Immun*. 2004;72:1804–6.

61. Barrios-Payan J et al. Neutrophil participation in early control and immune activation during experimental pulmonary tuberculosis. *Gac Med Mex*. 2006;142:273–81.

62. Zhang X et al. Coactivation of Syk kinase and MyD88 adaptor protein pathways by bacteria promotes regulatory properties of neutrophils. *Immunity*. 2009;31:761–71.

63. Brown AE, Holzer TJ, and Andersen BR. Capacity of human neutrophils to kill *Mycobacterium tuberculosis*. *J Infect Dis*. 1987;156:985.

64. Berry MP et al. An interferon-inducible neutrophil-driven blood transcriptional signature in human tuberculosis. *Nature*. 2010;466:973–7.

65. May ME and Spagnuolo PJ. Evidence for activation of a respiratory burst in the interaction of human neutrophils with *Mycobacterium tuberculosis*. *Infect Immun*. 1987;55:2304.

66. Jones GS, Amirault HJ, and Andersen BR. Killing of *Mycobacterium tuberculosis* by neutrophils: A nonoxidative process. *J Infect Dis*. 1990;162:700.

67. Fu LM. The potential of human neutrophil peptides in tuberculosis therapy. *Int J Tuberc Lung Dis*. 2003;7:1027–32.

68. Yoneda T and Ellner JJ. CD4(+) T cell and natural killer cell-dependent killing of *Mycobacterium tuberculosis* by human monocytes, *Am J Respir Crit Care Med*. 1998;158:395.

69. Cheekatla SS et al. NK-CD11c+ cell crosstalk in diabetes enhances IL-6-mediated inflammation during *Mycobacterium tuberculosis* infection. *PLoS Pathog*. 2016;21:e1005972.

70. Venkatasubramanian S, Cheekatla S, Paidipally P, Tripathi D, Welch E, Tvinnereim AR, Nurieva R, and Vankayalapati R. IL-21-dependent expansion of memory-like NK cells enhances protective immune responses against *Mycobacterium tuberculosis*. *Mucosal Immunol*. 2017;10:1031.

71. Janis EM, Kaufmann SHE, Schwartz RH, and Pardoll DM. Activation of γδ T-cells in the primary immune response to *Mycobacterium tuberculosis*. *Science* 1989;244:2754.

72. Augustin A, Kubo RT, and Sim G. Resident pulmonary lymphocytes expressing the γδ T-cell receptor. *Nature* 1989;340:239.

73. Havlir DV, Ellner JJ, Chervenak KA, and Boom WH. Selective expansion of human γδ T-cells by monocytes infected by live *Mycobacterium tuberculosis*. *J Clin Invest*. 1991;87:729.

74. Munk ME, Gatrill AJ, and Kaufman SHE. Target cell lysis and IL-2 secretion by γδ T-lymphocytes after activation with bacteria. *J Immunol*. 1990;145:2434.

75. Chua WJ, Truscott SM, Eickhoff CS, Blazevic A, Hoft DF, and Hansen TH. Polyclonal mucosa-associated invariant T cells have unique innate functions in bacterial infection. *Infect Immun*. 2012;80:3256.

76. Sakala IG et al. Functional heterogeneity and antimycobacterial effects of mouse mucosal-associated invariant T cells specific for riboflavin metabolites. *J Immunol*. 2015;195:587.

77. Gold MC et al. Human mucosal associated invariant T cells detect bacterially infected cells. *PLoS Biol*. 2010;8:e1000407.

78. Le Bourhis L et al. Antimicrobial activity of mucosal-associated invariant T cells. *Nat Immunol*. 2010;11:701.

79. Kwon YS et al. Mucosal-associated invariant T cells are numerically and functionally deficient in patients with mycobacterial infection and reflect disease activity. *Tuberculosis (Edinburgh)*. 2015;95:267

80. Wong EB et al. Low levels of peripheral CD161++CD8+ mucosal associated invariant T (MAIT) cells are found in HIV and HIV/TB co-infection. *PLOS ONE*. 2013;8:e83474.

81. Cobat A et al. Two loci control tuberculin skin test reactivity in an area hyperendemic for tuberculosis. *J Exp Med*. 2009;206:2583–91. doi:10.1084/jem.20090892

82. Cobat A et al. Identification of a major locus, *TNF1*, that controls BCG-triggered tumor necrosis factor production by leukocytes in an area hyperendemic for tuberculosis. *Clin Infect Dis*. 2013;57:963–70.

83. Skamene E. Genetic control of susceptibility to mycobacterial infections. *Rev Infect Dis*. 1989;2(Suppl. 1):S394.

84. Vidal SM, Pinner E, Lepage P, Gauthier S, and Gros P. Natural resistance to intracellular infections: Nramp1 encodes a membrane phosphoglycoprotein absent in macrophages from susceptible mice. *J Immunol*. 1996;157:3559.

85. North RJ and Medina E. How important is Nramp1 in tuberculosis? *Trends Microbiol*. 1998;6:441.

86. Abel L, Sanchez FO, Oberti J, Thuc NV, Hoa LV, Lap VD, Skamene E, Lagrange PH, and Schurr E. Susceptibility to leprosy is linked to the human Nramp1 gene. *J Infect Dis*. 1998;177:133.

87. Bellamy R, Ruwende C, Corrah T, McAdam KP, Whittle HC, and Hill AV. Variations in the NRAMP1 gene and susceptibility to tuberculosis in West Africans. *N Engl J Med*. 1998;338:640.

88. Shaw MA et al. Evidence that genetic susceptibility to *Mycobacterium tuberculosis* in a Brazilian population is under oligogenic control: Linkage study of the candidate genes NRAMP1 and TNFA. *Tuberc Lung Dis*. 1997;78:35.

89. Newport MJ, Huxley CM, Huston S, Hawrylowicz CM, Oostra BA, Williamson R, and Levin M. A mutation in the interferon-γ receptor gene and susceptibility to mycobacterial infection. *N Engl J Med*. 1996;335:1941.

90. Jong R et al. Severe mycobacterial and salmonella infections in interleukin-12 receptor-deficient patients. *Science*. 1998;280:1435.

91. Altare F et al. Impairment of mycobacterial immunity in human interleukin-12 receptor deficiency. *Science*. 1998;280:1432.

92. Stead WW. Racial differences in susceptibility to infection by *Mycobacterial tuberculosis*. *N Engl J Med*. 1990;322:422.

93. Comstock GW. Tuberculosis in twins: A re-analysis of the prophit survey. *Am Rev Respir Dis.* 1978;117:621.

94. Singh SPN, Mehra NK, Dingley HB, Pande JN, and Vaidya MC. HLA haplotype segregation study in multiple case families of pulmonary tuberculosis. *Tissue Antigens* 1984;23:84.

95. Selby R, Barnard JM, Buehler SK, Crumley J, Larsen B, and Marshall WH. Tuberculosis associated with HLA-B8, BfS in a Newfoundland community study. *Tissue Antigens* 1978;11:403.

96. Al-Arif LI, Goldstein RA, Affronti LF, and Janicki JW. HLA Bw15 and tuberculosis in a North American black population. *Am Rev Respir Dis.* 1979;120:1275.

97. Jian ZF, An JB, Sun YP, Mittal KK, and Lee TD. Association of HLA-BW35 with tuberculosis in the Chinese. *Tissue Antigens.* 1983;22:86.

98. Khomenko AG, Litvinov VI, Chukanova VP, and Pospelov LE. Tuberculosis in patients with various HLA phenotypes. *Tubercle.* 1990;71:187.

99. Bothamley GH, Beck JS, Schreuder GMTh, D'Amaro J, deVries RRP, Kardjito T, and Ivanyi J. Association of tuberculosis and MTB-specific antibody levels with HLA. *J Infect Dis.* 1989;159:549.

100. Hwange CH, Khan S, Ende N, Mangura BT, Reichman LB, and Chou J. The HLA-A, -B, and -DR phenotypes and tuberculosis, *Am Rev Respir Dis.* 1985;132:382.

101. Hafez M, El-Salab SH, El-Shennawy F, and Bassiony MR. HLA-antigens and tuberculosis in the Egyptian population. *Tubercle.* 1985;66:35.

102. Zervas J, Castantopoulos C, Toubis M, Anagnostopoulos D, and Cotsovoulou V. HLA-A and B antigens and pulmonary tuberculosis in Greeks. *Br J Dis Chest.* 1987;81:147.

103. Cox RA, Arnold DR, Cook D, and Lundberg DI. HLA phenotypes in Mexican Americans with tuberculosis. *Am Rev Respir Dis.* 1982;126:653.

104. Singh SPN, Mehra NK, Dingley HB, Pande JN, and Vaidya MC. HLA-A, -B, -C, and -DR antigen profile in pulmonary tuberculosis in North India. *Tissue Antigens.* 1983;21:380.

105. Cox RA, Downs M, Neimes RE, Ognibene AJ, Yamashita TS, and Ellner JJ. Immunogenetic analysis of human tuberculosis. *J Infect Dis.* 1988;158:1302.

106. Davis JE, Rich RR, Van M, Le MV, Pollach MS, and Cook RG. Defective antigen presentation and novel structural properties of DR1 from an HLA haplotype associated with 21 hydroxylase deficiency. *J Clin Invest.* 1987;80:898.

107. Centers for Disease Control. A strategic plan for the elimination of tuberculosis in the United States. *J Am Med Assoc.* 1989;261:2929.

108. Rook GAW. The role of vitamin D in tuberculosis. *Am Rev Respir Dis.* 1988;138:768.

109. Snider DE. Reorientation of tuberculosis control programs in the USA. *Bull Int Union Tuberc.* 1989;64:25.

110. Snider DE and Hutton MD. Tuberculosis in correctional institutions. *J Am Med Assoc.* 1989;261:436.

111. Davies PDO. A possible link between vitamin D deficiency and impaired host defence to *Mycobacterium tuberculosis.* *Tubercle.* 1985;66:301.

112. Crowle A and Elkines N. Relative permissiveness of macrophages from black and white people for virulent tubercle bacilli. *Infect Immun.* 1990;58:632.

113. Wilkinson R, Patel P, Llewlyn M, Hirsh CS, Passoval G, Snounou G, Davidson RN, and Toossi Z. Influence of polymorphism in the genes for Interleukin (IL)-1 beta and IL-1 receptor antagonist on tuberculosis. *J Exp Med.* 1999;189:1863.

114. Zhang G et al. Allele-specific induction of IL-1β expression by C/EBPβ and PU.1 contributes to increased tuberculosis susceptibility. *PLoS Pathog.* 2014;10(10):e1004426. https://doi.org/10.1371/journal.ppat.1004426

115. Raghavan S, Alagarasu K, and Selvaraj P. Immunogenetics of HIV and HIV-associated tuberculosis. *Tuberculosis (Edinburgh).* 2012;92:18.

116. Kinnear C, Hoal EG, Schurz H, van Helden PD, and Moller M. The role of human host genetics in tuberculosis resistance. *Expert Rev Respir Med.* 2017;11:72.

117. Cottle LE. Mendelian susceptibility to mycobacterial disease. *Clin Genet.* 2011;79:17.

118. Olesen RM et al. DC-SIGN (CD209), pentraxin 3 and vitamin D receptor gene variants associate with pulmonary tuberculosis risk in West Africans. *Genes Immun.* 2007;8:456.

119. Sobota RS et al. A locus at 5q33.3 confers resistance to tuberculosis in highly susceptible individuals. *Am J Hum Genet.* 2016;98(3):514–24.

120. Remus N, El Baghdadi J, Fieschi C, Feinberg J, Quintin T, Chentoufi M, Schurr E, Benslimane A, Casanova JL, and Abel L. Association of IL12RB1 polymorphisms with pulmonary tuberculosis in adults in Morocco. *J Infect Dis.* 2004 Aug 1;190(3):580–7. Epub 2004 Jul 6.

121. North RJ. Importance of thymus-derived lymphocytes in cell-mediated immunity to infection. *Cell Immunol.* 1973;7:166.

122. Lefford MJ. Transfer of adoptive immunity to tuberculosis in mice. *Infect Immun.* 1975;11:1174.

123. Orme IM and Collins FM. Passive transfer of tuberculin sensitivity from anergic mice. *Infect Immun.* 1984;46:850.

124. Orme IM and Collins FM. Protection against *Mycobacterium tuberculosis* infection by adoptive immunotherapy. *J Exp Med.* 1983;158:74.

125. Koch R. Weitere mitteilungen uber ein heilmittel gegen tuberculose. *Dtsch Med Wschr.* 1891;17:101.

126. Chase MW. The cellular transfer of cutaneous hypersensitivity to tuberculin. *Proc Soc Exp Biol Med.* 1945;59:134.

127. Orme IM and Collins FM. Adoptive protection of the *Mycobacterium tuberculosis*-infected lung; dissociation between cells that passively transfer protective immunity and those that transfer delayed type hypersensitivity to tuberculin. *Cell Immunol.* 1984;84:113.

128. Boom WH, Wallis RS, and Chervenak KA. Human MTB-reactive CD4+ T-cell clones: Heterogeneity in antigen recognition, cytokine production, and cytotoxicity for mononuclear phagocytes. *Infect Immun.* 1991;59:2737.

129. Lanier LL, Ruitenberg JJ, and Phillips JH. Human CD3+ T-lymphocytes that express neither CD4+ nor CD8+ antigens. *J Exp Med.* 1986;164:339.

130. Rook GAW. Immunity and hypersensitivity. *Practitioner.* 1983;227:iv.

131. Orme IM. Induction of nonspecific acquired resistance and delayed type hypersensitivity, but not specific acquired resistance, in mice inoculated with killed mycobacterial vaccines. *Infect Immun.* 1988;56:3310.

132. Cooper AM, Callahan JE, Keen M, Belisle JT, and Orme IM. Expression of memory immunity in the lung following re-exposure to *Mycobacterium tuberculosis. Tuberc Lung Dis.* 1997;78:67.

133. Orme IM, Miller ES, Roberts AD, Furney SK, Griffin JP, Dobos EM, Chi D, Rivoire B, and Brennan PJ. T-lymphocytes mediating protection and cellular cytolysis during the course of *Mycobacterium tuberculosis. J Immunol.* 1992;148:189.

134. Orme IM. Characteristics and specificity of acquired immunologic memory to MTB infection. *J Immunol.* 1988;140:3589.

135. Muller I, Cobbold S, Waldmann H, and Kaufmann SME. Impaired resistance to MTB after selective *in vivo* depletion of L3T4+ and Lyt -2+ T-cells. *Infect Immun.* 1987;55:2037.

136. Fiorentino DF, Bond MW, and Mosmann TR. Two types of mouse T helper cell IV. TH-2 clones secrete a factor that inhibits cytokine production by TH-1 clones. *J Exp Med.* 1989;170:2081.

137. Cooper MA, Dalton DK, Stewart TA, Griffin JP, Russell DG, and Orme IM. Disseminated tuberculosis in interferon-γ gene-disrupted mice. *J Exp Med.* 1993;178:2243.

138. Flynn JL, Chan J, Triebold KJ, Dalton DK, Stewart TA, and Bloom BR. An essential role for interferon-γ in resistance to *Mycobacterium tuberculosis. J Exp Med.* 1993;178:2249.

139. Flynn JL, Goldstein MM, Triebold KJ, Koller B, and Bloom BR. Major histocompatibility complex class I-restricted T cells are required for resistance to *Mycobacterium tuberculosis* infection. *Proc Natl Acad Sci USA.* 1992;89:12013.

140. Cooper AM, D'Souza C, Frank AA, and Orme IM. The course of *Mycobacterium tuberculosis* infection in the lungs of mice lacking expression of either perforin- or granzyme-mediated cytolytic mechanisms. *Infect Immun.* 1997;65:1317.

141. Kaech SM, and Wherry EJ. Heterogeneity and cell-fate decisions in effector and memory CD8+ T cell differentiation during viral infection. *Immunity* 2007;27:39.

142. Takemoto N, Intlekofer AM, Northrup JT, Wherry EJ, and Reiner SL. Cutting edge: IL-12 inversely regulates T-bet and eomesodermin expression during pathogen-induced CD8+ T cell differentiation. *J Immunol.* 2006;177:755.

143. Sallusto F, Geginat J, and Lanzavecchia A. Central memory and effector memory T cell subsets: Function, generation, and maintenance. *Annu Rev Immunol.* 2004;22:745.

144. Sallusto F, Lenig D, Forster R, Lipp M, and Lanzavecchia A. Two subsets of memory T lymphocytes with distinct homing potentials and effector functions Nature. 1999;401:708–12.

145. Fritsch RD, Shen X, Sims GP, Hathcock KS, Hodes RJ, and Lipsky PE. Stepwise differentiation of CD4 memory T cells defined by expression of CCR7 and CD27. *J Immunol.* 2005;175:6489.

146. Gattinoni L et al. A human memory T cell subset with stem cell-like properties. *Nat Med.* 2011 Sep 18;17(10):1290–7. doi: 10.1038/nm.2446.

147. Boom WH, Wallis RS, and Chervenak KA. Human MTB-reactive CD4+ T-cell clones: Heterogeneity in antigen recognition, cytokine production, and cytotoxicity for mononuclear phagocytes. *Infect Immun.* 1991;59:2737.

148. Vilaplana C, Ruiz-Manzano J, Gil O, Cuchillo F, Montané E, Singh M, Spallek R, Ausina V, and Cardona PJ. The tuberculin skin test increases the responses measured by T cell interferon-gamma release assays. *Scand J Immunol.* 2008;67:610–7.

149. Tan JS, Canaday DH, Boom WH, Balaji KN, Schwander SK, and Rich EA. Human alveolar T lymphocyte responses to *Mycobacterium tuberculosis* antigens. *J Immunol.* 1997;159:290.

150. Berger HW and Mejia E. Tuberculous pleurisy. *Chest.* 1973;63:88.

151. Fujiwara H, Okuda Y, Fukukawa T, and Tsuyuguchi I. *In vitro* tuberculin reactivity of lymphocytes from patients with tuberculous pleurisy, *Infect Immun.* 1982;35:402.

152. Barnes PF, Mistry SD, Cooper CL, Pirmez C, Rea TH, and Modlin RL. Compartmentalization of a CD4+ T-lymphocyte subpopulation in tuberculous pleuritis. *J Immunol.* 1989;142:1114.

153. Fujiwara H and Tsuyuguchi I. Frequency of tuberculin-reactive T-lymphocytes in pleural fluid and blood from patients with tuberculous pleurisy. *Chest* 1984;89:530.

154. Ellner JJ. Pleural fluid and peripheral blood lymphocyte function in tuberculosis, *Ann Int Med.* 1978;89:932.

155. Barnes PF, Fong SJ, Brennan PJ, Twomey PE, Mazumder A, and Modlin RL. Local production of tumor necrosis factor and interferon-g in tuberculous pleuritis. *J Immunol.* 1990;145:149.

156. Wallis RS, Alde SL, Havlir DV, Amir-Tahmasseb H, Daniel TM, and Ellner JJ. Identification of antigens of *Mycobacterium tuberculosis* using human monoclonal antibodies. *J Clin Invest.* 1989;84:214.

157. Nemes E et al. C-040-404 Study Team. Prevention of *M. tuberculosis* infection with H4:IC31 vaccine or BCG revaccination. *N Engl J Med.* 2018;379:138.

158. Van Der Meeren O et al. Phase 2b controlled trial of M72/AS01$_E$ vaccine to prevent tuberculosis. *N Engl J Med.* 2018.

159. Anderseen P. Host responses and antigens involved in protective immunity to *Mycobacterium tuberculosis. Scand J Immunol.* 1997;45:115.

160. Ottenhoff THM, Kale B, van Embden JDA, Thole JER, and Kiessling R. The recombinant 65 kD heat shock protein of *Mycobacterium bovis* Bacillus Calmette-Guérin/MTB is a target molecule for CD4+ cytotoxic T-lymphocytes that lyse human monocytes. *J Exp Med.* 1988;168:1947.

161. Munk ME, Schoel B, and Kaufmann SHE. T cell responses of normal individuals towards recombinant protein antigens of MTB. *Eur J Immunol.* 1988;18:1835.

162. Havlir DV, Wallis RS, Boom WH, Daniel TM, Chervenak K, and Ellner JJ. Human immune response to MTB antigens. *Infect Immun.* 1991;59:665.

163. Schoel B, Gulle M, and Kaufmann SHE. Heterogeneity of the repertoire of T cells of tuberculosis patients and healthy contacts to MTB antigens separated by high resolution techniques. *Infect Immun.* 1992;60:1717.

164. Young DB, Kaufmann SHE, Hermans PWM, and Thole JER. Mycobacterial proteins, a compilation. *Mol Microbiol.* 1992;6:133.

165. Wiker HG, Sletten K, Nagai S, and Harboe M. Evidence for three separate genes encoding the proteins of the mycobacterial antigen 85 complex. *Infect Immun.* 1990;58:272.

166. Rambukkhan A, Das PK, Chand A, Baas JG, Grothuis DG, and Kold AHJ. Subcellular distribution of monoclonal antibody-defined epitopes on immunuo dominant 33-kilodalton proteins of MTB: Identification and localization of 29/33 kilodalton doublet proteins in mycobacterial cell walls. *Scand J Immunol.* 1991;33:763.

167. Abou-Zeid C, Ratliff TL, Wiker HG, Harboe M, Bennedsen J, and Rook GAW. Characterization of fibronectin-binding antigens released by MTB and *M. bovis* BCG. *Infect Immun.* 1988;56:3046.

168. Abou-Zeid C, Smith I, Grange JM, Ratliff TL, Steele J, and Rook GAW. The secreted antigens of MTB and their relationship to those recognized by the available antibodies. *J Gen Microbiol.* 1988;134:531.

169. Wiker HG, Harboe M, and Lea TE. Purification and characterization of two protein antigens from the heterogeneous BCG 85 complex in *M. bovis* BCG. *Int Arch Allerg Appl Immunol.* 1986;81:298.

170. Salata RA, Sanson AJ, Malhotra IJ, Wiker HG, Harboe HG, Phillips NB, and Daniel TM. Purification and characterization of the 30,000 dalton native antigen of *Mycobacterium tuberculosis* and characterization of six monoclonal antibodies reactive with a major epitope of this antigen. *J Lab Clin Med.* 1991;118:589.

171. Matsuo K, Yamaguchi R, Yamakazi A, Tasaka H, and Yamada T. Cloning and expression of the *M. bovis* BCG gene for extracellular alpha antigen. *J Bacteriol.* 1988;160:3847.

172. Pal PG and Horowitz MA. Immunization with extracellular proteins of *M. tuberculosis* induces cell-mediated immune responses with substantial protective immunity in a guinea pig model of pulmonary tuberculosis. *Infect Immun.* 1992;60:4782.

173. Huygen K, van Vooren JP, Turneer M, Bosmans R, Dierckx P, and De Bruyn J. Specific lymphoproliferation, gamma interferon production, and serum immunoglobulin G directed against a purified 32 kDA mycobacterial protein antigen (P32) in patients with active tuberculosis. *Scand J Immunol.* 1988;27:187.

174. Abou-Zeid C, Ratliff TL, Wiker HG, Harboe M, Bennedsen J, and Rook GAW. Characterization of fibronectin-binding antigens released by MTB and *M. bovis* BCG. *Infect Immun.* 1988;56:3046.

175. Yuan Y, Lee RE, Besra GS, Belisle JT, and Barry CE, III. Identification of a gene involved in the biosynthesis of cyclopropanated mycolic acids in *Mycobacterium tuberculosis*. *Proc Natl Acad Sci USA.* 1995;92:6630.

176. Wallis RS, Fujiwara H, and Ellner JJ. Direct stimulation of monocyte release of interleukin-1 by mycobacterial protein antigens. *J Immunol.* 1986;36:193.

177. Toossi Z, Lapurga JP, Ondash R, Sedor JR, and Ellner JJ. Expression of functional interleukin-2 receptors by peripheral blood monocytes from patients with active pulmonary tuberculosis. *J Clin Invest.* 1990;85:1777.

178. Toossi Z, Young TG, Averill LE, Hamilton BD, Shiratsuchi H, and Ellner JJ. Induction of transforming growth factor-β (TGF-β) by purified protein derivative (PPD) of *Mycobacterium tuberculosis*. *Infect Immun.* 1995;63:224.

179. Harth G, Clemens DL, and Horwitz MA. Glutamine synthetase of *Mycobacterium tuberculosis*: Extracellular release and characterization of its enzymatic activity. *Proc Natl Acad Sci USA.* 1994;91:9342.

180. Wallis RS, Raranjape R, and Phillips M. Identification of 2-D gel electrophoresis of a 58 kD TNF-α-reducing protein of MTB. *J Immun.* 1993;61:627.

181. Toossi Z, Gogate P, Shiratsuchi H, Young T, and Ellner JJ. Enhanced production of TGF-β by blood monocytes from patients with active tuberculosis and presence of TGF-β in tuberculosis granulomatous lung lesions. *J Immunol.* 1995;154:465.

182. Rook GAW. Importance of recent advances in our understanding of antimicrobial cell-mediated immunity to the International Union for the Prevention of Tuberculosis. *Bull Int Union Tuberc.* 1983;58:60.

183. Zugmaier G et al. Transforming growth factor β1 induces cachexia and systemic fibrosis without an antitumor effect in nude mice. *Cancer Res.* 1991;51:3590.

184. Broekelmann TJ, Limper AH, Colby TV, and McDonald JA. Transforming growth factor β is present at sites of extracellular matrix gene expression in human pulmonary fibrosis. *Proc Natl Acad Sci USA.* 1991;88:6642.

185. Border WA and Noble NA. Transforming growth factor β in tissue fibrosis. *N Engl J Med.* 1994;331:1286.

186. Denis M. Tumor necrosis factor and granulocyte macrophage-colony stimulating factor stimulates human macrophages to restrict growth of virulent *Mycobacterium avium* and to kill avirulent *M. avium*. Killing effector mechanism depends on the generation of reactive nitrogen intermediates. *J Leuk Biol.* 1991;49:380.

187. Bermudez LE M. and Young LS. Tumor necrosis factor alone or in combination with IL-2 but not IFN-gamma, is associated with macrophage killing of *Mycobacterium avium* complex. *J Immunol.* 1988;140:3006.

188. Rook GAW, Steele J, Fraber L, Barker S, Karmali R, O'Riordan J, and Standford J. Vitamin D3, gamma interferon and control of proliferation of *Mycobacterium tuberculosis* by human monocytes. *Immunology* 1986;56:159.

189. Toossi Z, Hirsch CS, Hamilton BD, Kunuth CK, Friedlander MA, and Rich EA. Decreased production of transforming growth factor β1 (TGF-β1) in human alveolar macrophages. *J Immunol.* 1996;156:3461.

190. Kindler V, Sappino AP, Grau GE, Piquet PI, and Vassali P. The reducing role of tumor necrosis factor in the development of bactericidal granulomas during BCG infection. *Cell* 1989;56:731.

191. Flesch I and Kaufmann SH E. Mycobacterial growth inhibition by interferon-gamma activated bone marrow macrophages and differential susceptibility among strains of MTB. *J Immunol.* 1987;138:4408.

192. Flesch IE and Kaufmann SH E. Mechanisms involved in mycobacterial growth inhibition by gamma interferon-activated bone marrow macrophages: Role of reactive nitrogen intermediates. *Infect Immun.* 1991;59:3213.

193. Douvas GS, Looker DL, Vatter AE, and Crowle AJ. Gamma interferon activates human macrophages to become tumoricidal and leishmanicidal but enhances replication of macrophage associated mycobacteria. *Infect Immun.* 1985;50:1.

194. Rook GAW, Steele J, Fraher L, Barker S, Karmali R, O'Riordan J, and Stanfor J. Vitamin D3, gamma interferon, and control of proliferation of *Mycobacterium tuberculosis* by human monocytes. *Immunology* 1986;57:159.

195. Hirsch CS, Yoneda T, Ellner JJ, Averill LE, and Toossi Z. Enhancement of intracellular growth of *M. tuberculosis* in human monocytes by transforming growth factor beta. *J Infect Dis.* 1994;170:1229.

196. Bermudez LE. Production of transforming growth factor-β by *Mycobacterium avium*-infected human macrophages is associated with unresponsiveness to IFN-γ. *J Immunol.* 1993;150:1838.

197. Hirsch CS, Jerrold JE, Blinkhorn R, and Toossi Z. *In vitro* restoration of T-cell responses in tuberculosis and augmentation of monocyte effector function against *Mycobacterium tuberculosis* by natural inhibitors of transforming growth factor-β. *Proc. Natl. Acad. Sci. USA* 1997;94:3926.

198. Ding A, Nathan C, and Srimal S. Macrophage deactivating factor and TGF-β inhibit of macrophage nitrogen oxide synthesis by IFN-γ. *J Immunol.* 1990;145:940.

199. Toossi Z, Mincek M, Seeholtzer E, Fulton SA, Hamilton BD, and Hirsch CS. Modulation of IL-12 by transforming growth factor-β (TGF-β) in *Mycobacterium tuberculosis*-infected mononuclear phagocytes and in patients with active tuberculosis. *J Clin Lab Immunol.* 1997;49:59.

200. O'Garra A, Redford PS, McNab FW, Bloom CI, Wilkinson RJ, and Berry MPR. The immune response in tuberculosis. *Annu Rev Immunol.* 2013;31(1):475–527

201. Mayer-Barber KD et al. Host-directed therapy of tuberculosis based on interleukin-1 and type I interferon crosstalk. *Nature* 03 July 2014;**511**:99–103, doi:10.1038/nature13489

202. Boom WH, Wallis RS, and Chervenak KA. Human MTB-reactive CD4+ T-cell clones: Heterogeneity in antigen recognition, cytokine production, and cytotoxicity for mononuclear phagocytes. *Infect Immun.* 1991;59:2737.

203. Mustafa AS and Godal T. BCG-induced CD4+ cytotoxic T cells from BCG vaccinated healthy subjects: Relation between cytotoxicity and suppression *in vitro*. *Clin Exp Immunol.* 1987;69:255.

204. Orme I, Andersen P, and Boom WH. T-cell responses to *Mycobacterium tuberculosis. J Infect Dis.* 1993;167:1481.

205. Chan J, Mehta S, Bharrhan S, Chen Y, Achkar JM, Casadevall A, and Flynn J. The role of B cells and humoral immunity in *Mycobacterium tuberculosis* infection. *Semin Immunol.* 2014;26(6):588–600. http://doi.org/10.1016/j.smim.2014.10.005

206. Glatman-Freedman A. The role of antibody-mediated immunity in defense against *Mycobacterium tuberculosis*: Advances toward a novel vaccine strategy. *Tuberculosis (Edinburgh)* 2006;86:191–7. [PubMed: 16584923]

207. Achkar JM, Chan J, and Casadevall A. Role of B cells and antibodies in acquired immunity against *Mycobacterium tuberculosis. Cold Spring Harb Perspect Med.* 2015;5(3):a018432. http://doi.org/10.1101/cshperspect.a018432

208. Maglione PJ, and Chan J. How B cells shape the immune response against *Mycobacterium tuberculosis. Eur J Immunol.* 2009;39:676–86.

209. Chan J, Mehta S, Bharrhan S, Chen Y, Achkar JM, Casadevall A, and Flynn J. The role of B cells and humoral immunity in *Mycobacterium tuberculosis* infection. *Semin Immunol.* 2014;26:588.

210. Li H, Wang XX, Wang B, Fu L, Liu G, Lu Y, Cao M, Huang H, and Javid B. Latently and uninfected healthcare workers exposed to TB make protective antibodies against *Mycobacterium tuberculosis. Proc Natl Acad Sci U S A.* 2017;114:5023.

211. Lu LL et al. A functional role for antibodies in tuberculosis. *Cell* 2016;167:433.

212. Zimmermann N et al. Human isotype-dependent inhibitory antibody responses against *Mycobacterium tuberculosis. EMBO Mol Med.* 2016;8:1325.

213. Wu HJ, Ivanov II, Darce J, Hattori K, Shima T, Umesaki Y, Littman DR, Benoist C, and Mathis D. Gut-residing segmented filamentous bacteria drive autoimmune arthritis via T helper 17 cells. *Immunity* 2010;32:817.

214. Trompette A, Gollwitzer ES, Pattaroni C, Lopez-Mejia IC, Riva E, Pernot J, Ubags N, Fajas L, Nicod LP, and Marsland BJ, Dietary fiber confers protection against flu by shaping Ly6c− patrolling monocyte hematopoiesis and CD8+ T cell metabolism. *J Immunity.* 2018;4:992.

215. Negatu DA, Liu JJJ, Zimmerman M, Kaya F, Dartois V, Aldrich CC, Gengenbacher M, and Dick T. Whole-cell screen of fragment library identifies gut microbiota metabolite indole propionic acid as antitubercular. *Antimicrob Agents Chemother.* 2018;62:31.

216. Segal LN et al. Anaerobic bacterial fermentation products increase tuberculosis risk in antiretroviral-drug-treated HIV patients. *Cell Host Microbe.* 2017;21:530.

217. Daniel TM, Oxtoby MJ, Pinto E, and Moreno E. The immune spectrum in patients with pulmonary tuberculosis. *Am Rev Respir Dis.* 1981;123:556.

218. Nash DR and Douglass JE. Anergy in pulmonary tuberculosis: Comparison between positive and negative reactors and an evaluation of 5TU and 250 TU skin test doses, *Chest,* 1980;77:32.

219. Rooney JJ, Crocco JA, Kramer S, and Lyons HA. Further observations on tuberculin reactions in tuberculosis. *Am J Med.* 1976;60:517.

220. Sousa AO, Salem JI, Lee FK, Vercosa MC, Cruad P, Bloom BR, Lagrange PH, and David HL. An epidemic of tuberculosis with a high rate of tuberculin anergy among a population previously unexposed to tuberculosis, the Yanomami Indians of the Brazilian Amazon. *Proc Natl Acad Sci USA.* 1997;94:13227.

221. Ellner JJ. Suppressor adherent cells in human tuberculosis. *J Immunol.* 1978;121:2573.

222. Kleinhenz ME and Ellner JJ. Antigen responsiveness during tuberculosis: Regulatory interaction of T-cell subpopulations and adherent cells. *J Lab Clin Med.* 1987;110:31.

223. Kleinhenz ME and Ellner JJ. Immunoregulatory adherent cells in human tuberculosis: Radiation sensitive antigen-specific suppression by monocytes. *J Infect Dis.* 1985;152:171.

224. Toossi Z, Edmonds KL, Tomford WJ, and Ellner JJ. Suppression of PPD-induced interleukin2 production by interaction of Leu-22 (CD16) lymphocytes and adherent mononuclear cells in tuberculosis. *J Infect Dis.* 1989;159:352.

225. Toossi Z, Kleinhenz ME, and Ellner JJ. Defective interleukin-2 production and responsiveness in human pulmonary tuberculosis. *J Exp Med.* 1986;163:1162.

226. Josefowicz SZ, Lu LF, and Rudensky AY. Regulatory T cells: Mechanisms of differentiation and function. *Annu Rev Immunol.* 2012;30:531–64. https://doi.org/10.1146/annurev.immunol.25.022106.141623

227. Ribeiro-Rodrigues R, Resende Co T, Rojas R, Toossi Z, Dietze R, Boom WH, Maciel E, and Hirsch CS. A role for CD4+CD25+ T cells in regulation of the immune response during human tuberculosis. *Clin Exp Immunol.* 2006 Apr;144(1):25–34.

228. Vanham G et al. Generalized immune activation in pulmonary tuberculosis: Co-activation with HIV infection. *Clin Exp Immunol.* 1996;103:30.

229. Fujiwara H and Tsuyuguchi I. Frequency of tuberculin-reactive T-lymphocytes in pleural fluid and blood from patients with tuberculous pleuritis. *Chest* 1984;89:530.

230. Carlucci S, Beschin A, Tuosto L, Ameglio F, Gandolfo G, Cocito C, Fiorucci F, Saltini C, and Piccolella E. Mycobacterial antigen complex A60-specific T-cell repertoire during the course of pulmonary tuberculosis, *Infect Immun.* 1993;61:439.

231. Hirsch CS, Hussain R, Toossi Z, Dawood G, Shahid F, and Ellner JJ. Cross modulation by transforming growth factor β in human tuberculosis: Suppression of antigen-driven blastogenesis and interferon γ production. *Proc Natl Acad Sci (USA).* 1995;93:3193.

232. Rakotosamimanana N et al. Variation in gamma interferon responses to different infecting strains of *Mycobacterium tuberculosis* in acid-fast bacillus smear-positive patients and household contacts in Antananarivo, Madagascar. *Clin Vaccine Immunol.* 2010;**17**:1094–103.

233. Lee J-S et al. Profiles of IFN-γ and its regulatory cytokines (IL-12, IL-18 and IL-10) in peripheral blood mononuclear cells from patients with multidrug-resistant tuberculosis. *Clin Exp Immunol.* 2002;128(3):516–24.

234. Adekambi T, Ibegbu CC, Cagle S, Kalokhe, AS, Wang YF, Hu Y, Day CL, Ray SM, and Rengarajan J. Biomarkers on patient T cells diagnose active tuberculosis and monitor treatment response. *J Clin Invest.* 2015;125:1827.

235. Adekambi T, Ibegbu CC, Cagle S, Ray SM, and Rengarajan J. High Frequencies of caspase-3 expressing *Mycobacterium tuberculosis*-specific cD4+ T cells are associated with active tuberculosis. *Front Immunol.* 2018;25:1481.

236. Andrade-Arzabe R, Machado IV, Fernandez B, Blanca I, Ramirez R, and Bianco NE. Cellular immunity in current active pulmonary tuberculosis. *Am Rev Respir Dis.* 1991;143:496.

237. Shiratsuchi H, Okuda Y, and Tsuyuguchi I. Recombinant human interleukin-2 reverses *in vitro* deficient cell-mediated immune responses to tuberculin purified protein derivative by lymphocytes of tuberculous patients. *Infect Immun.* 1987;55:2126.

238. Huygen K, van Vooren JP, Turneer M, Bosmans R, Dierckx P, and De Bruyn J. Specific lymphoproliferation, gamma interferon production, and serum immunoglobulin G directed against a purified 32 kDA mycobacterial protein antigen (P32) in patients with active tuberculosis. *Scand J Immunol.* 1988;27:187.

239. Vilcek J, Klion A, Henriksen-DeStefano D, Zemtsov A, Davidson DM, Davidson M, and Friedman-Kien A. Defective gamma-interferon production in peripheral blood leukocytes of patients with acute tuberculosis. *J Clin Immunol.* 1986;6:146.

240. Gazzinelli RT, Hieny S, Wynn TA, Wolf S, and Sher A. Interleukin 12 is required for the T-lymphocyte-independent induction of interferon γ by an intracellular parasite and induces resistance in T-cell-deficient hosts. *Proc Natl Acad Sci.* 1993;90:6115.

241. Sieling PA, Abrams JS, Yamamura M, Salgame P, Bloom BR, Rea TH, and Modlin RL. Immunosuppressive roles for IL-10 and IL-4 in human infection. *J Immunol.* 1993;150:5501.

242. Street NE and Mossman TR. Functional diversity of T lymphocytes due to secretion of different cytokine patterns, *FASB J.* 1991;5:171.

243. Bogdan C, Vodovotz Y, and Nathan C. Macrophage deactivation by interleukin 10. *J Exp Med.* 1991;174:1549.

244. Lehn MW, Weisner WY, Engelhorn S, Gillis S, and Remold HG. IL-4 inhibits H_2O_2 production and antileishmanial capacity of human cultured monocytes mediated by IFN gamma. *J Immunol.* 1989;143:3020.

245. Sucrel HM, Tory-Blomberg M, Paulie S, Anderson G, Moreno C, Pasvol G, and Ivanyi J. TH-1/TH-2 profiles in tuberculosis, based on the proliferation and cytokine response of blood lymphocytes to mycobacterial antigens. *Immunology* 1994;81:171.

246. Hirsch CS, Toossi Z, Hussain R, and Ellner JJ. Suppression of T-cell responses by TGF-β in tuberculosis. *J Invest Med.* 1995;43:365A.

247. Schmitt E, Meuret G, and Stix L. Monocyte recruitment in tuberculosis and sarcoidosis. *Brit J Hematol.* 1977;35:11.

248. Toossi Z, Hamilton BD, Phillips MH, Averill LE, Ellner JJ, and Salvekar A. Regulation of nuclear factor-kB and its inhibitor IkB-a/ MAD-3 in monocytes by *Mycobacterium tuberculosis* and during human tuberculosis. *J Immunol.* 1997;159:4109.

249. Ahmed A, Adiga V, Nayak S, Uday Kumar JAJ, Dhar C, Sahoo PN, Sundararaj BN, Souza GD, and Vyakarnam A. Circulating HLA-DR+CD4+ effector memory T cells resistant to CCR5 and PD-L1 mediated suppression compromise regulatory T cell function in tuberculosis. *PLoS Pathog.* 2018;14(9):e1007289. https://doi.org/10.1371/journal.ppat.1007289

250. Lenzini L, Heather CJ, Rottoli L, and Rottoli P. Studies on bronchoalveolar cells in humans. I. Preliminary morphological studies in various respiratory diseases. *Respiration* 1978;36:145.

251. Venet A, Niaudet P, Bach JF, and Even P. Study of alveolar lymphocytes obtained by bronchoalveolar lavage. *Ann Anesthesiol Fr.* 1980;6:634.

252. Sharma SK, Pande JN, and Verma K. Bronchoalveolar lavage (BAL) in miliary tuberculosis. *Tubercle* 1988;69:175.

253. Dhank R, De A, Ganguly NK, Gupta N, Jaswal S, Malik SK, and Kohli KK. Factors influencing the cellular response in bronchoalveolar lavage and peripheral blood of patients with pulmonary tuberculosis. *Tubercle* 1988;69:161.

254. Baughman RP, Dohn MN, Loudon RG, and Trame PT. Bronchoscopy with bronchoalveolar lavage in tuberculosis and fungal infections. *Chest* 1991;99:92.

255. Ozaki T, Nakahira S, Tani K, Ogushi F, Yasuoka S, and Ogura T. Differential cell analysis in bronchoalveolar lavage fluid from pulmonary lesions of patients with tuberculosis. *Chest* 1992;102:54.

256. Schwander SK, Sada E, Torres M, Escobedo D, Sierra JG, Alt S, and Rich EA. T lymphocytic and immature macrophage alveolitis in active pulmonary tuberculosis. *J Infect Dis.* 1996;176:1267.

257. Schwander SK, Torres M, Sada E, Carranza C, Ramos E, Tary-Lehmann M, Wallis RS, Sierra J, and Rich EA. Enhanced responses to *Mycobacterium tuberculosis* antigens by human alveolar lymphocytes during active pulmonary tuberculosis. *J Infect Dis.* 1998;178:1434.

258. Taha RA, Kotsimbos TC, Song, Y-L., Menzies D, and Hamid Q. IFN-γ and IL-12 are increased in active compared with inactive tuberculosis. *Am J Respir Crit Care Med.* 1997;155:1135.

259. Berry MPR et al. An interferon-inducible, neutrophil-driven, blood transcriptional signature in tuberculosis. *Nature.* 2010;466:973.

260. Cliff JM, Kaufmann SHE, McShane H, and van Helden P. The human immune response to tuberculosis and its treatment; a view from the blood. *Immunol Rev.* 2015;264:88.

261. Moreira-Teixeira T, Mayer-Barber K, Sher A, and O'Garra A. Type 1 interferons in tuberculosis: Foe and occasionally friend. *J Exp Med.* 2018.

262. Reider HL, Cauthen GM, Bloch AB, Cole CH, Holtzman D, Snider DE, Bigler WJ, and Witte JJ. Tuberculosis and AIDS: Florida. *Arch Intern Med.* 1989;149:1268.

263. Daley CL, Small GF, Schecter GK, Schoolnik GK, McAdam RA, Jacobs WR, and Hopewell PC. An outbreak of tuberculosis with accelerated progression among persons infected with HIV. *N Engl J Med.* 1992;326:2131.

264. Lucas S and Nelson AM. Pathogenesis of tuberculosis in human immunodeficiency virus-infected people. In: Bloom B. (ed.). *Tuberculosis Pathogenesis, Protection, and Control.* ASM Press: Materials Park, OH, 1994.

265. Ellner JJ. [Editorial] Tuberculosis in the time of AIDS: The facts and the message. *Chest* 1990;98:1051.

266. Okwera A, Eriki PP, Guay LA, Ball P, and Daniel TM. Tuberculin reactions in HIV-seropositive and HIV-seronegative healthy women in Uganda. *MMWR.* 1990;39:638.

267. Johnson JL et al. Impact of human immunodeficiency virus type 1 infection on the initial bacteriologic and radiographic manifestations of pulmonary tuberculosis in Uganda (Makerere University-Case Western Reserve Research Collaboration). *Int J Tuberc Lung Dis.* 1998;2:397.

268. Wallis RS, Vjecha M, Amir-Tahmasseb M, Okwera A, Byekwaso F, Nyole J, Kabengera J, Mugerwa RD, and Ellner JJ. Influence of tuberculosis on HIV: Enhanced cytokine expression and elevated B2 microglobulin in HIV-1 associated tuberculosis. *J Infect Dis.* 1992;167:43.

269. Kaforou M et al. Detection of tuberculosis in HIV-infected and -uninfected African adults using whole blood RNA expression signatures: A case-control study. *PLoS Med.* 2013;10(10):e1001538.

270. Dawany N, Showe LC, Kossenkov AV, Chang C, Ive P, Conradie F, Stevens W, Sanne I, Azzoni L, and Montaner LJ. Identification of a 251 gene expression signature that can accurately detect *M. tuberculosis* in patients with and without HIV co-infection. *PLOS ONE* 2014;9(2):e89925.

271. Maertzdorf J, McEwen G, Weiner J 3rd, Tian S, Lader E, Schriek U, Mayanja-Kizza H, Ota M, Kenneth J, and Kaufmann SH. Concise gene signature for point-of-care classification of tuberculosis. *EMBO Mol Med.* 2016;8(2):86–95.

272. Laux da Costa L, Delcroix M, Dalla Costa ER, Prestes IV, Milano M, Francis SS, Unis G, Silva DR, Riley LW, and Rossetti ML. A real-time PCR signature to discriminate between tuberculosis and other pulmonary diseases. *Tuberculosis (Edinburgh)* 2015;95(4):421–5.

273. Sweeney TE, Braviak L, Tato CM, and Khatri P. Genome-wide expression for diagnosis of pulmonary tuberculosis: A multicohort analysis. *Lancet Respir Med.* 2016;4(3):213–24.

274. Sutherland JS et al. Differential gene expression of activating Fcgamma receptor classifies active tuberculosis regardless of human immunodeficiency virus status or ethnicity. *Clin Microbiol Infect.* 2014;20(4):O230–8.

275. Roe JK et al. Blood transcriptomic diagnosis of pulmonary and extrapulmonary tuberculosis. *JCI Insight* 2016;1(16):e87238.

276. Verma S et al. Tuberculosis in advanced HIV infection is associated with increased expression of IFNγ and its downstream targets. *BMC Infect Dis.* 2018;18(1):220. Published 2018 May 15. doi:10.1186/s12879-018-3127-4

277. Lai RP, Nakiwala JK, Meintjes G, and Wilkinson RJ. The immunopathogenesis of the HIV tuberculosis immune reconstitution inflammatory syndrome. *Eur J Immunol* 2013;43:1995–2002.

278. Meintjes G et al. Type 1 helper T cells and FoxP3-positive T cells in HIV–tuberculosis-associated immune reconstitution inflammatory syndrome. *Am J Respir Crit Care Med.* 2008;178(10):1083–9.

279. Conradie F et al. Natural killer cell activation distinguishes *Mycobacterium tuberculosis*-mediated immune reconstitution syndrome from chronic HIV and HIV/MTB coinfection. *J Acquired Immune Defic Syndr.* 2011;58(3):309–18.

280. Jinmin Ma J et al. Zinc finger and interferon-stimulated genes play a vital role in TB-IRIS following HAART in AIDS. *Per Med.* 2018;15(4):251–69.

281. Tran HTT et al. Geert for the TB-IRIS study group. Modulation of the complement system in monocytes

contributes to tuberculosis-associated immune reconstitution inflammatory syndrome. *AIDS* July 17th, 2013; 27(11):1725–34.

282. Tran HTT, Van der Bergh R, Vu TN, Laukens K, Worodria W, Loembe MM, Colebunders R, Kestens L, De Baetselier P, Raes G for the TB-IRIS Study Group. The role of monocytes in the development of tuberculosis-associated immune reconstitution inflammatory syndrome. *Immunobiology* January 2014;219(1):37–44.

283. Narendran G et al. Paradoxical tuberculosis immune reconstitution inflammatory syndrome (TB-IRIS) in HIV patients with culture confirmed pulmonary tuberculosis in India and the potential role of IL-6 in prediction. *PLOS ONE* 2013;8(5):e63541. https://doi.org/10.1371/journal.pone.0063541

284. Meintjes G et al. Randomized placebo-controlled trial of prednisone for paradoxical tuberculosis-associated immune reconstitution inflammatory syndrome. *AIDS* 2010;24(15):2381–90.

285. Meintjes G et al. PredART Trial Team. Prednisone for the prevention of paradoxical tuberculosis-associated IRIS. *N Engl J Med.* 2018 Nov 15;379(20):1915–25. doi: 10.1056/NEJMoa1800762.

286. Cohen OJ, Kinter A, and Fauci AS. Host factors in the pathogenesis of HIV disease, *Immunol Rev.* 1997;159:31.

287. Lawn SD, Butera ST, and Shinnick TM. Tuberculosis unleashed: The impact of human immunodeficiency virus infection on the host granulomatous response to *Mycobacterium tuberculosis. Microbes Infect* 2002;4:635e46.

288. Clerici M, and Shearer GM. A TH-1/TH-2 switch is a critical step in the etiology of HIV infection. *Immunol Today* 1993;14:107.

289. Zhang M, Gong J, Iyer D, Jones BE, Modlin RL, and Barnes PF. T-cell cytokine responses in persons with tuberculosis and human immunodeficiency virus infection. *J Clin Invest.* 1994;94:2435.

290. Orenstein JM, Fox C, and Wahl MS. Macrophages as a source of HIV during opportunistic infections, *Science* 1997;276:1857.

291. Meltzer MS, Skillman DR, Gomatos PJ, Kalter DC, and Gendelman HE. Role of mononuclear phagocytes in the pathogenesis of human immunodeficiency virus infection. *Ann Rev Immunol.* 1990;8:169.

292. Twigg HL, Lipscomb MF, Yoffe B, Barbaro DJ, and Weissler JC. Enhanced accessory cell function by alveolar macrophages from patients infected with the human immunodeficiency virus: Potential role for depletion of CD4+ cells in the lung. *Am J Respir Cell Mol Biol.* 1989;1:391.

293. Murray HW, Gellene RA, Libby DM, Roth E, Armmel CD, and Rubin BY. Activation of tissue macrophages from AIDS patients: *in vitro* responses of AIDS alveolar macrophages to lymphokines and interferon-γ. *J Immunol.* 1985; 135:2374.

294. Buhl R, Jaffe HA, Holroyd KJ, Borok Z, Roum JH, Mastrangeli A, Wells FB, Kirby M, Saltini C, and Crystal RG. Activation of alveolar macrophages in asymptomatic HIV-infected individuals. *J Immunol.* 1993;150:1019.

295. Twigg HL, Iwamoto GK, and Soliman DM. Role of cytokines in alveolar macrophage accessory cell function in HIV-infected individuals. *J Immunol.* 1992;149:1462.

296. Trentin L, Barbisa S, Zambello R, Agostini C, Caenazzo C, di Francesco C, Cipriani A, Francavalla E, and Semenzato G. Spontaneous production of IL-6 by alveolar macrophages form human immunodeficiency virus type 1-infected patients. *J Infect Dis.* 1992;166:731.

297. Agostini C et al. Alveolar macrophages from patients with AIDS and AIDS-related complex constitutively synthesize and release tumor necrosis factor alpha. *Am Rev Respir Dis.* 1991;144:195.

298. Plata F, Autran B, Pedroza Martins L, Wain-Hobson S, Raphael M, Mayaud C, Denis M, Guillon JM, and Debre P. AIDS virus-specific cytotoxic T-lymphocytes in lung disorders. *Nature (London)* 1987;328:348.

299. De Cock KM, Soro B, Coulibaly IM, and Lucas SB. Tuberculosis and HIV infection in sub-Saharan Africa. *JAMA* 1992;268:1581.

300. Whalen C, Horsburgh CR, Hom D, Lahart C, Simberkoff M, and Ellner JJ. Accelerated course of human immunodeficiency virus infection after tuberculosis. *Am J Respir Crit Care Med.* 1995;151:129.

301. Braun MM, Nsanga B, and Ryder RW. A retrospective cohort study of the risks of tuberculosis among women of childbearing age with HIV infection in Zaire. *Am Rev Respir Dis.* 1991;143:501.

302. Vjecha M et al. Predictors of mortality and drug toxicity in HIV-infected patients from Uganda treated for pulmonary tuberculosis, *8th International Conference on AIDS/3rd STD World Congress*, Amsterdam, Netherlands, July 1992.

303. Goletti D, Weissman D, Jackson RW, Graham NM, Vlahov D, Klein RS, Munsiff SS, Ortona L, Cauda R, and Fauci AS. Effect of *Mycobacterium tuberculosis* on HIV replication: Role of immune activation. *J Immunol.* 1996;157:1271.

304. Toossi Z. Virological and immunological impact of tuberculosis on human immunodeficiency virus type 1 disease. *J Infect Dis.* 15 October 2003;188(8):1146–55, https://doi.org/10.1086/378676

305. Lederman MM, Georges DL, Kusner DJ, Mudido P, Giam, C-Z, and Toossi Z. *Mycobacterium tuberculosis* and its purified protein derivative activate expression of the human immunodeficiency virus. *J Acquired Immune Defic Syndr.* 1994;7:727.

306. Toossi Z, Nicolacakis K, Xia L, Ferrari NA, and Rich EA. Activation of latent HIV-1 by *Mycobacterium tuberculosis* and its purified protein derivative in alveolar macrophages from HIV infected individuals *in vitro. J Acquired Immune Defic Syndr Hum Retrovirol.* 1997;15:325.

307. Toossi Z, Sierra-Madero JG, Blinkhorn RA, Mettler MA, and Rich EA. Enhanced susceptibility of blood monocytes from patients with pulmonary tuberculosis to productive infection with human immunodeficiency virus-1 (HIV-1). *J Exp Med.* 1993;177:1511.

308. Garrait CJ, Esvant H, Henry I, Morinet P, Mayaud C, and Israel-Biet D. Tuberculosis generates a microenvironment enhancing the productive infection of local lymphocytes by HIV. *J Immunol.* 1997;159:2824.

309. Olson A, Ragan EJ, Nakiyingi L, Lin N, Jacobson KR, Ellner JJ, Manabe YC, and Sagar M. Pulmonary tuberculosis is associated with persistent systemic inflammation and decreased HIV-1 reservoir markers in co-infected Ugandans. *J Acquired Immune Defic Syndr.* 2018 Jul 26. doi: 10.1097/QAI.0000000000001823. [Epub ahead of print]

310. Murugesan VS, Bin N, Dodd CE, and Schesinger LS. Macrophage immunoregulatory pathways in tuberculosis. *Semin Immunol.* 2014;26:471.

311. Rich EA, Torres M, Sada E, Finegan CK, Hamilton BD, and Toossi Z. Mycobacterium tuberculosis (MTB)-stimulated production of nitric oxide by human alveolar macrophages and relationship of nitric oxide production to growth inhibition of MTB. *Tuberc Lung Dis* 1997;78:247.

312. Hussain R, Dawood G, Obaid M, Toossi Z, Wallis RS, Minai A, Dojki M, Sturm AW, and Ellner JJ. Depressed cellular and augmented humoral responses in patients with active tuberculosis from Pakistan. *Clin Diag Lab Immunol.* 1995;2:726.

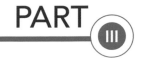
TRANSMISSION

5

Using Genotyping and Molecular Surveillance to Investigate Tuberculosis Transmission

SARAH TALARICO, LAURA F. ANDERSON, AND BENJAMIN J. SILK

INTRODUCTION

Tuberculosis (TB) control programs prevent transmission of *Mycobacterium tuberculosis* by identifying and treating active cases of TB disease and ensuring that contacts of infectious cases are also identified, screened, and treated for active disease or latent infection. Genotyping and molecular surveillance methods can identify clusters of cases that share genetically similar *M. tuberculosis* strains, which may be related by recent transmission. Public health tools to investigate TB transmission have advanced by combining technologies for DNA sequencing and phylogenetic analysis with clinical and epidemiological information. Outbreak investigations are a priority because they can establish epidemiological links among patients and direct prevention measures toward populations and settings with ongoing transmission. The chapter reviews the use of genotyping to investigate transmission as well as how genotyping methods have been applied to study transmission dynamics, lineage, recurrent TB disease, mixed infections, and laboratory contamination.

GENOTYPING METHODS

Genotyping methods for *M. tuberculosis* can be divided into two main categories: (1) conventional genotyping methods that examine variation affecting a small portion of the *M. tuberculosis* genome and (2) whole-genome sequencing (WGS), which examines most of the *M. tuberculosis* genome at the nucleotide level. The three most commonly used conventional genotyping methods are restriction fragment length polymorphism (RFLP), spacer oligonucleotide typing (spoligotyping), and mycobacterial interspersed repetitive units-variable number tandem repeats (MIRU-VNTR). These methods are all based on repetitive DNA sequences found either interspersed throughout the bacterial

genome (insertion sequences) or at specific loci. Changes in these repetitive DNA sequences serve as a proxy for genetic diversification that is occurring throughout the entire genome. However, as DNA sequencing technologies have advanced, WGS is replacing the use of conventional genotyping methods for public health purposes to provide direct analysis of phylogenetic relationships at the nucleotide level.

CONVENTIONAL METHODS BASED ON REPETITIVE SEQUENCES

RFLP typing for *M. tuberculosis* is based on the 1.3 kilobase repetitive insertion sequence IS*6110*, which is unique to *M. tuberculosis* complex (MTBC).[1] IS*6110* varies in the number of copies from 0 to 25 per strain and also by insertion site in the genome.[2] These variations produce highly diverse hybridization patterns that are used to discriminate between strains (Figure 5.1). In the 1990s, IS*6110* was the gold standard for genotyping *M. tuberculosis* due to the high discriminatory power and the stability of the biomarker, which has a half-life of approximately 3.2 years (i.e., the time it takes for a hybridization pattern to change).[3] Disadvantages of IS*6110*-RFLP are that the technique itself is time-consuming, technically demanding, lacks inter-laboratory reproducibility, and requires specialized software for the analysis of results, which are difficult to compare between different laboratories and over time. Furthermore, the discriminatory power is poor for strains without a copy of IS*6110* and for strains with a low (<6) copy number, such as *M. bovis*.

Spoligotyping is based on the presence or absence of 43 unique DNA "spacer" sequences that are interspersed between 36 base pair sequences.[4,5] The results consist of binary data and the number and position of absent spacer sequences can be compared between strains (Figure 5.2). Results are reproducible, easy to interpret,

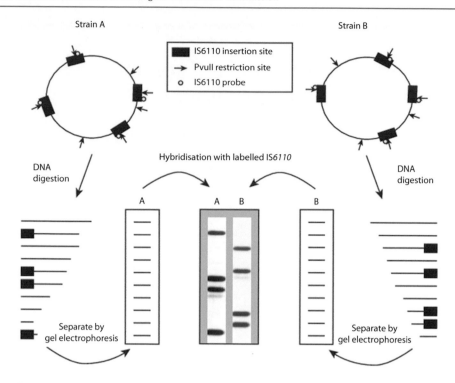

Figure 5.1 IS*6110*-based RFLP analysis. The DNA from two strains of *M. tuberculosis* are depicted schematically. After the DNA has been extracted from the mycobacteria (this step is not illustrated), the DNA is cleaved using *Pvu*II, a specific restriction endonuclease (arrows). In reality, thousands of fragments of DNA are created and then separated according to molecular weight by gel electrophoresis. At this stage, thousands of bands produce a nearly confluent image that is difficult to interpret. By hybridization with an IS*6110* probe (circle), only those fragments containing IS*6110* will be visible on the gel. In this example, the two strains each have four copies of IS*6110*, but they differ in location on the gel.

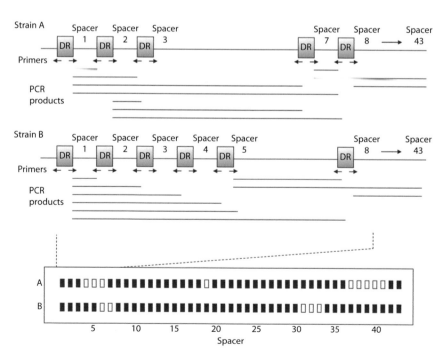

Figure 5.2 Spoligotyping. In the upper part of the figure, the direct repeat (DR) region is illustrated for two strains of *M. tuberculosis*. In this example, only spacers 1–8 are illustrated in detail. Strain A is missing spacers 4–6 and strain B is missing spacers 6–7 (additional spacers are missing but not highlighted in the figure). Polymerase chain reaction (PCR) amplification of the conserved DR locus is performed using two sets of primers depicted with the arrows. The resulting PCR products are hybridized to a membrane containing covalently bound oligonucleotides corresponding to each of the 43 spacers. Each strain of *M. tuberculosis* produces a positive (black) or negative (white) signal at each spacer location. In this example, strain A is missing eight spacers and strain B is missing five. The resulting genotype pattern can be converted into a binary code for easy data sharing.

and can be recorded in binary or octal format to facilitate intra-laboratory comparisons. The procedure is rapid and requires small amounts of DNA, which means it can be carried out on non-viable organisms. A disadvantage of spoligotyping is the lower discriminatory power,[6,7] which occurs partly because spoligotyping focuses on the direct repeat region only. Spoligotyping can be used to detect lineages that are characterized by spacer deletions, such as Beijing strains that have lost 34 spacer sequences.[8] In combination with other genotyping methods, spoligotyping can provide a highly accurate discriminatory system.[6,9]

MIRU-VNTR typing detects the number of tandem repeats at multiple loci in the genome (Figure 5.3). The discriminatory power of MIRU-VNTR increases in proportion to the number of loci that are included.[10–12] It is rapid, can be carried out on very early cultures, shows excellent reproducibility between laboratories,[13,14] and is cheaper than other typing methods. The results are produced as a numerical string, so they can easily be compared on a national and international level, when loci are reported in the same order. The proposed international standard is 24 locus MIRU-VNTR,[10] and has been implemented prospectively for public health use in the United States,[9,15] the Netherlands, and the United Kingdom.[16] Studies have shown that the discriminatory power of MIRU-VNTR typing is slightly lower than IS6110-RFLP for identifying molecular clusters[10,17] but is more discriminatory for low IS6110 copy strains.[18–20] The discriminatory power is higher than spoligotyping[9,21–23] and, if used in combination, is comparable to IS6110-RFLP for detecting clusters in both low[9,21,22,24] and high[11,25] TB incidence settings.

WHOLE-GENOME SEQUENCING

The *M. tuberculosis* genome was first sequenced in 1998 using the dideoxy-chain-termination method;[26] however, time and cost considerations precluded large-scale WGS of *M. tuberculosis* isolates for molecular surveillance purposes. Next-generation sequencing technologies have allowed WGS of *M. tuberculosis* isolates to become more rapid and affordable. Unlike genotyping methods that examine only a small portion (~1%) of the *M. tuberculosis* genome, WGS analysis examines ~90% of the genome. Approximately 10% of the remaining *M. tuberculosis* genome is comprised of PE and PPE genes; homology among members of this large gene family make these genes difficult to analyze accurately. By expanding the genomic coverage and examining variation at the nucleotide level, WGS analysis captures much more of the genetic diversity among *M. tuberculosis* isolates and allows for greater resolution to distinguish differences among strains.

WGS data can be used to perform single nucleotide polymorphism (SNP) analyses. Using SNP data, a phylogenetic tree can then be generated showing the evolutionary relationships among the isolates in the analysis (i.e., the direction of genetic change) in relation to a most recent common ancestor (MRCA). The MRCA is a hypothetical genome type from which all isolates on the tree are descended and serves as a reference point for examining the direction of SNP accumulation (Figure 5.4). For reference, Walker et al. estimated the rate of change in *M. tuberculosis* DNA sequences is approximately 0.5 SNPs per genome per year (95% CI 0.3–0.7), and the rate of change was rarely more than five SNPs

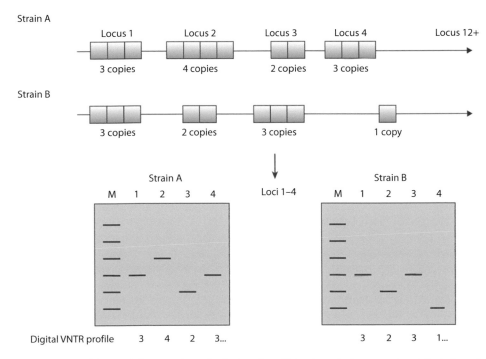

Figure 5.3 MIRU-VNTR. Portions of the DNA from two hypothetical strains of *M. tuberculosis* are depicted. Only four of the standard 24 loci are illustrated. In this example, strains A and B have three copies of the repeat at locus 1, whereas strain A has four copies at locus 2 and strain B has only two copies. In the lower half of the figure, the loci are depicted along the top of the gels. There is a molecular weight standard (M) on the left side of each gel. The loci move down the gel, based on molecular weight, so those at the top of the gels are larger pieces of DNA that contain more copies of the repeat than those at the bottom of the gel. This information can be digitized to provide an easy way to share information between laboratories. For example, strain A would be given the identifier 3423 and strain B would be given the identifier 3231.

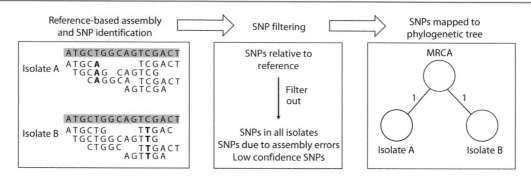

Figure 5.4 Whole-genome single nucleotide polymorphism (wgSNP) analysis. The first step of the analysis is reference-based assembly and SNP identification (left of figure). Isolate sequence reads are first aligned to a reference genome (shown in gray) and SNPs relative to the reference genome are identified (bold). Isolate A has a T → A SNP and isolate B has a C → T SNP. SNPs are then filtered to produce a list of informative, high-quality SNPs (middle of figure). High-quality SNPs can then be mapped to a phylogenetic tree to diagram the direction of genetic change in relation to a MRCA. The MRCA is a hypothetical genome type from which all isolates on the tree are descended. Isolates A and B differ by two SNPs and each has diverged one SNP from the MRCA (right of the figure).

in a three-year period.[27] Other studies have produced remarkably similar estimates of the "molecular clock" (e.g., 0.3 or 0.4 SNPs per genome per year).[28–30] Thus, investigators can assess whether it is likely that recent transmission has occurred by examining the number of SNP differences between isolates from individuals in a cluster. However, since there is no standard method for SNP analysis, SNP thresholds for assessing recent transmission will vary (e.g., ≤5 or ≤12 SNPs), making them difficult to compare across studies. Furthermore, because the mutation rate may be lower during latent infection,[31] closely related isolates could also result from reactivation cases from a transmission event in the remote past. Based on U.S. experiences, relatively large SNP differences can rule out isolates from apparent clusters as very unlikely to be related by recent transmission. In contrast, isolates that are closely related may be related by recent transmission, but these isolates cannot be distinguished from isolates from cases due to reactivation based on WGS data alone. In addition, phylogenetic trees can provide some insights into plausible chains of transmission, but they are not the same as transmission diagrams. This limitation is due to many factors, including intra-host genetic diversity, asynchrony of transmission and sample collection, and because some cases that are involved in transmission will not have an isolate included in the phylogenetic analysis. For these reasons, phylogenetic trees are best understood when augmented with epidemiological and clinical data when making inferences about directionality of transmission.

The United Kingdom and United States both have recently implemented prospective WGS for all *M. tuberculosis* isolates for molecular surveillance purposes, which should allow for further insights via population-based surveillance studies. In addition, multilocus sequence typing (MLST) based on sequencing of the whole genome offers an opportunity to standardize a classification scheme. In one example, Kohl et al. used this gene-by-gene allele numbering approach to develop a core genome MLST (cgMLST) scheme that discriminated between isolates with a comparable resolution to that of whole-genome SNP analysis.[32] Aside from use in epidemiological investigation, WGS has the additional advantage of providing species identification and detection of mutations that confer drug resistance. Although WGS of *M. tuberculosis* currently requires culturing, methods for sequencing directly from

patient samples are being developed that will greatly reduce the time from sample collection to molecular epidemiology and antibiotic susceptibility results for a patient.[33,34]

RECENT TRANSMISSION

For decades, genotyping has enabled epidemiologists to estimate the amount of TB arising in communities due to recent transmission and identify associated risk factors. Most studies measured the proportion of clustered cases in a population. Many of these studies have been conducted in low-incidence, high-income countries where it is possible to genotype the majority of TB isolates from culture-confirmed cases. By detecting and monitoring transmission, TB control programs can assess the effectiveness of interventions that target groups at higher risk. A common outbreak investigation goal is to combine genotyping data with different sources of clinical, epidemiological, and programmatic data through partnerships that lead investigators to the best conclusions and public health action for control of recent transmission.

CLUSTERING AND RISK FACTORS FOR RECENT TRANSMISSION

As a proxy for recent transmission, studies have examined the proportions of clustered cases in a population within a specific period. A cluster includes two or more patients with the same genotype; the remaining cases with unmatched genotypes are considered unique. Key assumptions are made that clustered cases are in the same chain of transmission, and that unique cases arise because of reactivation of infection acquired in the remote past.[35,36] The proportion of clustering can be estimated either by the "*n* method," which calculates the proportion of cases that are clustered out of all culture-confirmed cases with a genotype. Alternatively, the "*n*−1 method" assumes that the index case has arisen as a result of reactivation; therefore, one case is subtracted from each cluster. Model predictions of transmission suggest that the proportion of clustering using the *n*−1 method underestimates recent transmission in high-incidence countries where the annual risk of infection remains stable over time.[37] This is because most cases will have arisen due to recent infection rather than the assumption that the first case results from a reactivation.

Many past studies conducted in Europe, North America, and South Africa have used conventional genotyping methods to show that the proportions of clustered TB cases vary substantially (11%–72%).[35,38–50] A meta-analysis by Fok et al.[51] found similar variability in the proportions of clustered cases (7%–72%). Irrespective of incidence rates, demographic and clinical risk factors for clustering were being native born, experiencing homelessness, and having pulmonary, sputum smear-positive disease. Male sex, younger age, and social risk factors, such as alcohol and substance use, were also frequently associated with clustering.[36,41,42,45,47,51–54] Associations between younger age and clustering may be due to increased interactions within social networks of similar age, the higher likelihood of reactivation in older patients who are more likely to have a unique genotype, or both. An association between clustering of multidrug-resistant TB (MDR TB) and bacteriologic factors also has been suggested.[55]

Molecular surveillance studies have allowed investigators to characterize patient factors associated with cluster size and growth. A surveillance period of >2 years is generally required for accurate estimates to avoid time censoring and because the periods from infection until progression to disease vary.[56,57] For example, a cluster analysis by De Vries et al.[58] found that 52% of patients in Rotterdam who were linked to an index case developed TB within one year, 19% in the second year, and 29% in two to five years subsequently. A study period of one year would have missed almost half of the secondary cases. In another Dutch study, Kik et al.[46] found that 9% of all clustered cases were part of a large cluster and the remaining 91% were part of small clusters in a two-year period. The authors compared the characteristics of the first two patients in small and large clusters and found that independent predictors for being in a large cluster were younger age, if both patients lived in an urban area or were born in sub-Saharan Africa, and if the time between diagnosis of the first and second case was less than three months. Similarly, reporting of the first two cases within three months of each other was associated with large cluster size in London.[44,59] In British Columbia, large clusters occurred more frequently among Canadian-born patients, residents of rural areas, persons reporting drug use, and the Euro-American lineage of *M. tuberculosis*.[60] In France and the United States, patients experiencing homelessness were often part of larger clusters and outbreaks.[42,61] Because these studies demonstrate how to identify specific populations at risk for cluster growth and outbreaks, TB control programs can prioritize certain clusters for further investigation and public health interventions.

Yet, TB transmission occurs when populations occupy settings and communities that facilitate transmission.[62] Studies have used geospatial software (e.g., geographic information systems, or GIS) to determine if cases cluster by residence, and, if so, where transmission is occurring. Investigators identified hotspots of TB transmission in China[63] and Brazil[64] as well as MDR TB hotspots in Moldova[65] and Peru.[66] To estimate the impact of addressing community transmission, a study in Rio de Janeiro used a steady-state compartmental transmission model.[67] They found that when 6% of residents lived in a hotspot, with the assumption that each active TB case in the hotspot caused 0.5 secondary cases in the community, then targeting individuals in the hotspot with TB control interventions had the same impact on reducing TB incidence as targeting the whole community. This suggests that interventions that target specific transmission settings may be more efficient and cost effective at reducing transmission than an approach that aims to target the entire population. Although spatial analyses of TB case distributions are common, they are heterogeneous in their methods and findings.[68]

The central problem with using genotype clustering to estimate recent transmission has been that clustered cases are not necessarily part of the same chain of transmission. When an endemic strain is circulating in the population (i.e., a common genotype), cases may have the same genotype without actually being epidemiologically linked by transmission. In low-incidence countries, individuals migrating from the same country or region where predominant strains circulate may lead to the importation of common strains; this migration pattern results in molecular clustering that may actually reflect transmission abroad, coincidental reactivations with the same genotype, or both. To help detect possible outbreaks within endemic U.S. clusters, Althomsons et al. developed a statistical method to identify unexpected growth.[69] Defining clusters based not only on matching genotypes, but also on geographic proximity, can often serve as a better proxy for recent transmission. A progression of U.S. studies of recent transmission is illustrative. In the United States, Moonan et al.[70] found that clustering based on geospatial concentrations not subject to artificial political boundaries gave the most conservative estimate (25%) of recent transmission. France et al. developed a plausible-source case method,[71] which further refined estimates of recent transmission using clinical and demographic criteria in addition to genotype-matched clustering of cases that are proximal in time and space. Applying this method, Yuen et al. estimated that 14% of U.S. cases were attributed to recent transmission.[72] Similar to past studies of clustering, transmission was associated with native birth, homelessness, and belonging to a minority race. Because molecular clustering is a function of the discriminatory power of the genotyping method, another strategy is to improve the method itself. In fact, the progression of studies coincides with a transition from using 12 to 24 loci MIRU-VNTR for genotyping in combination with spoligotyping.[73] The U.S. transition to prospective WGS for molecular surveillance is therefore expected to further lower recent transmission estimates based on the enhanced discriminatory power of WGS.

Another important issue is that only cases that are culture positive will have an *M. tuberculosis* isolate available for genotyping. Even in countries with robust surveillance systems, a significant proportion of cases will not be culture confirmed (e.g., 22% in the United States in 2017).[74] Exclusion of clinically diagnosed cases can lead to underestimates of recent transmission and may prevent timely identification of transmission chains. Estimates may be particularly affected where there are pediatric or extrapulmonary cases in clusters because these cases are more often culture negative.[75] De Vries et al.[40] showed that culture negative cases in the Netherlands frequently had a contact to a pulmonary case, which suggests that they are likely part of a recent chain of transmission.

CLUSTER AND OUTBREAK INVESTIGATION

National and regional TB control programs can design molecular surveillance systems to detect clusters of TB cases prospectively, as early indicators of transmission and possible outbreaks that might otherwise be undetected. However, these systems have several necessary requirements to function effectively as a public health intervention, which means that all aspects of a system need to be planned. These requirements include a public health laboratory service to genotype an isolate from each culture-confirmed case, timely isolate submission and linkage of genotyping results with case report data (i.e., surveillance data with basic clinical, demographic, and risk factor information), some precision locating cases geographically, and commitment to an information system for efficient dissemination and investigation of cluster-related data. For purposes of cluster detection, alerting, and investigation, programs can use a surveillance database to apply standardized classification schemes that designate new strains based on unique results of conventional genotyping or MLST, and identify matches to existing results. For example, the U.S. Centers for Disease Control and Prevention (CDC) sponsors the TB Genotyping Information Management System (TB GIMS), which detects genotype-matched clusters that are geospatially concentrated.[76] Weekly alerts are automatically sent to state and local TB program staff for cluster prioritization and possible public health action.[77] Similarly, MIRU-VNTR strain typing data are integrated within a web-based national TB surveillance system in the United Kingdom, allowing for cluster detection and investigation.[78] Although universal genotyping services and information systems require major investments, low-incidence countries could consider establishing them to help progress toward TB elimination. As an alternative, programs can selectively apply retrospective genotyping to help determine if cases in an apparent cluster are likely to be part of the same chain of transmission if cultures are routinely performed and isolates can be obtained. Retrospective genotyping results may still allow programs to make informed decisions as to whether further public health action is required, but delays obtaining this information can lead to unnecessary expenditures (e.g., extended contact tracing and screening).

When review of molecular surveillance data suggests that a cluster should be prioritized for further action, an epidemiological investigation can help determine if transmission among reported cases occurred recently and locally.[79] Early twenty-first century examples illustrated the particular challenge of determining whether transmission events were missed by an investigation or whether genotyping imprecision had falsely detected clustering that did not represent actual transmission. Using IS6110-RFLP, for example, investigations found epidemiological links in less than half of clustered cases in Germany and the Netherlands.[48,80] Studies in Canada and the U.K. demonstrated that isolates with matching MIRU-VNTR genotyping patterns were further discriminated using WGS, which indicates that recent transmission has also been overestimated by MIRU-VNTR.[27,81] A study in Switzerland used WGS to show that clustering based on MIRU-VNTR differentially misestimated recent transmission depending on nativity. WGS confirmed three quarters of clusters involving Swiss-born patients, but only one quarter of clusters involving non-native patients.[82] On the other hand, Walker et al. found that some cases with isolates that differed by one MIRU-VNTR locus were epidemiologically linked and considered to be in the same chain of transmission by WGS, meaning that clustering based on MIRU-VNTR typing where all 24 loci match can also underestimate recent transmission. However, cases with 24 loci MIRU-VNTR profiles with more than one locus mismatch mostly were not closely genetically related or epidemiologically linked (Figure 5.5).[27]

Several published investigations have also evaluated the use of WGS for investigating clustering and transmission of specific lineages. Jamieson et al. reported that WGS provided greater resolution for distinguishing isolates in the Manila sublineage, for which conventional genotyping methods had resulted in large clusters that were not epidemiologically meaningful.[83] A genomic epidemiology study of TB cluster investigations in Hawaii, where Beijing and Manila lineages are predominant, concluded that WGS is necessary because of the relatively low specificity of MIRU-VNTR for cluster identification.[84] Gurjav et al. reached a similar conclusion with SNP analyses of East-African and Beijing lineage isolates in Australia that falsely clustered by 24 loci MIRU-VNTR.[85] In Greenland, a population-based comparison of genotyping showed that SNP analyses discriminated 182 isolates of Euro-American lineage from five MIRU-VNTR clonal complexes ($\leq$2 loci differences) to four genomic clusters with further diversity described by phylogenetic branching and sub-lineage assignments.[86]

The added discriminatory resolution of WGS analyses now offers a far more powerful public health tool for investigating outbreaks of recent transmission. A 2018 Bayesian phylodynamics analysis conducted in Kinshasa, Democratic Republic of Congo quantitatively estimated how different genotyping methods performed for isolates collected from TB treatment clinics.[87] WGS allowed for discerning recent transmission within a 10-year time period (e.g., with a five SNP threshold), while time spans for clustering based on 24 loci MIRU-VNTR (several decades) and spoligotyping (hundreds of years) were far greater. Although isolates that are closely related by WGS may help provide valuable evidence of recent transmission, other types of data are usually required to distinguish these isolates from isolates due to reactivation. Furthermore, phylogenetic trees representing directionality in SNP accumulation are not equivalent to network visualizations that depict directionality of transmission, for reasons described previously (see *Whole-genome sequencing*). In a large outbreak investigation of isoniazid (INH)-resistant TB in London, for example, Casali et al. showed that nearly all of the 344 isolates from cases identified over a 14-year period were closely related or indistinguishable ($\leq$5 SNPs).[88] The investigators noted the occurrence of multiple transmission events without SNP accumulation and an inability to infer transmission directionality for most cases. Such limitations may be particularly challenging in closed populations and settings where transmission is ongoing,[89] such as isolated communities and congregate facilities (e.g., homeless shelters and prisons). Newer mathematical methods show promise for resolving some of the limitations of reliance on non-standardized SNP data and thresholds, such as incorporating detailed clinical and time data,[90,91] but have not yet been widely adopted into practice.

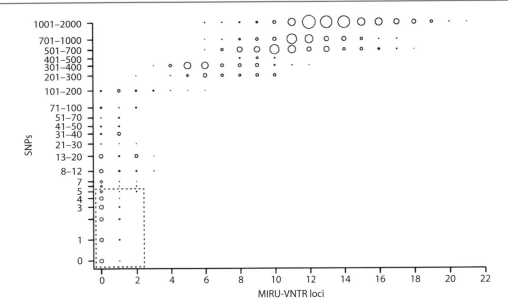

Figure 5.5 All isolates with complete 24-locus MIRU-VNTR profiles were compared. As each isolate was compared to every other isolate, the number of SNPs and MIRU-VNTR loci at which they diverge was recorded. The results are plotted on a log scale. Circle sizes are proportionate to the number of pairs diverging by a specific number of loci and SNPs. The dashed box includes isolates that differ by five or fewer SNPs. SNP = single-nucleotide polymorphism; MIRU-VNTR = mycobacterial interspersed repetitive unit-variable number tandem repeat. (Adapted from Walker TM et al. *Lancet Infect Dis.* 2013;13(7):137–46.)

Integrating WGS data with different sources of clinical, programmatic, and epidemiological data is a standard of public health practice for outbreak investigations. By interpreting WGS data in the context of these other data, TB control programs can make inferences that are not possible with any single data source. Basic clinical data on timing and degree of infectiousness for pulmonary cases (e.g., sputum smear positivity and grade, cavitation on chest radiograph), or lack of infectiousness for exclusively extrapulmonary and pediatric cases, are informative. Latent TB infection screening results from contact investigations can help determine if recent transmission has occurred (e.g., conversion rates for tuberculin skin testing or interferon-gamma release assays). This strategy is advantageous because many local TB control programs in high-income countries routinely ensure identification, screening,

and treatment of contacts of infectious cases for active disease and latent infection. Graphical representations of clustered cases can be useful to visualize epidemiological links, results of WGS analysis, common risk factors, and settings that are relevant for characterizing transmission (Figure 5.6). Yet, WGS analysis results should be reviewed as soon as available to rule out genetically distant isolates and exclude clustered cases that are unlikely to be related by recent transmission. An apparent cluster can often be redefined as one or more sub-clusters (Figure 5.7), which may narrow or refine the scope, focus, and goals of the investigation. This strategy can save considerable time and resources in subsequently pursuing epidemiological links. Estimates of efficiency gains from a Dutch study of 535 isolates genotyped by MIRU-VNTR and WGS are compelling.[92] WGS analyses reduced clustering by 50% and doubled the

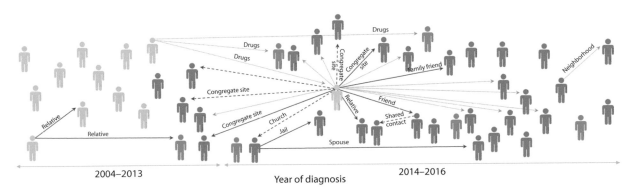

Figure 5.6 Plausible transmission network showing integrated wgSNP, clinical, and epidemiological data for a large cluster of patients with genotype-matched isolates. Patients in the pre-outbreak period (2004–2013) are shown in gray. Patients in the outbreak investigation period (2014–2016) are color coded, as orange (closely related by wgSNP analysis), blue (distant by wgSNP analysis), and yellow (highly infectious, presumed source case for most secondary cases). Solid lines denote definite epidemiological links; dashed and dotted lines denote probable and possible links, respectively. Social relationships and shared risk factors and presumed transmission settings are overlaid.

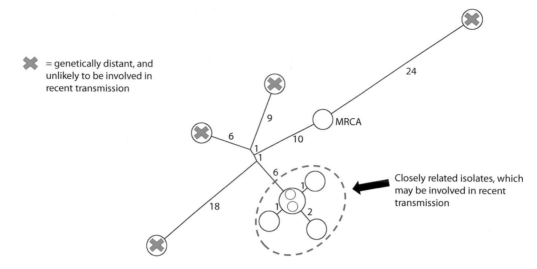

Figure 5.7 Phylogenetic tree showing wgSNP analysis results for a hypothetical cluster of genotype-matched isolates. SNPs are mapped to diagram the direction of genetic change in relation to a MRCA. In this example, a sub-cluster of five isolates that are closely related (0–2 SNPs) may be involved in recent transmission. The remaining four genetically distant isolates are unlikely to be involved in recent transmission (i.e., they can be ruled out).

proportion of epidemiological links subsequently identified. In Oxfordshire, United Kingdom, Walker et al. showed that investigators' understanding of transmission improved from 42% to 69% of 26 "transmission events" within clusters defined by WGS.[93]

Using epidemiological links to investigate transmission can be problematic because they are not necessarily equivalent to transmission events.[94,95] In Norway, an investigation of a community outbreak of 14 TB cases found that the patients all had social contact with each other and had a common link through a church, but six different genotypes were identified.[96] In fact, several studies have shown that contacts with TB disease do not necessarily have the same genotype as the index case, even if they live in the same household.[97-99] This appears to be more common in high-incidence settings where the risk of infection is higher. In Cape Town, South Africa, less than half of secondary cases were found to have the same genotype as other TB cases in the household.[99] Using WGS, Glynn et al. showed that less than 10% of TB cases in rural Malawi could be attributed to close contacts.[100] Another issue is that, even with rigorous investigation, epidemiological links can be elusive in communities where TB is stigmatized or patients are otherwise unwilling to name contacts or provide information on their social activities and relationships. Information may not be divulged by a patient because of many factors, such as the way that the questions are asked, the questions themselves, insufficient training in interviewing techniques, language barriers, and lack of trust. Nevertheless, identification of higher risk groups, social networks, and community settings can help target public health actions to prevent transmission, so various strategies that use genotyping data have been developed. Sintchenko et al. found that a second interview for patients with indistinguishable genotypes was more effective than other methods in detecting recent secondary cases.[101] Jackson et al. effectively used a combination of genotyping results and a social networking questionnaire that consisted of open-ended questions and themes relating to causes of TB and understanding transmission.[102] Gardy et al. used WGS

results and social networking questionnaires with open-ended questions, which was also very successful in identifying settings where confirmed transmission had occurred.[81]

In conclusion, genotyping results should be used in tandem with clinical, programmatic, and epidemiological data to detect and investigate TB transmission. WGS can reduce estimates of molecular clustering that do not actually represent transmission, and help avoid identification of epidemiological links that are spurious. However, WGS data also have key limitations, including an inability to characterize the relatedness of cases that are not culture-confirmed. Therefore, the most sensible strategy is to detect outbreaks early using available genotyping data and work iteratively to combine other data sources that help ensure that epidemiological information is sufficiently collected to identify transmission risk factors and settings.

CLINICAL AND PUBLIC HEALTH APPLICATIONS

TB LINEAGE, SEVERITY OF DISEASE, AND TRANSMISSION

In 2002, Fleischmann et al. reported the first whole-genome sequence comparison of two *M. tuberculosis* isolates, which identified genetic variation in the form of long sequence polymorphisms (LSPs) and SNPs.[103] In 2006, Gagneux et al. used LSPs to classify *M. tuberculosis* into six main lineages and 15 sublineages, and a significant association between lineage and world region was identified.[104] Furthermore, the study found that lineage was associated with place of birth and ethnicity in a random sample of TB cases in San Francisco. For example, East Asian lineage, which is most common in East Asia, was found in patients born in China, the Philippines, and Vietnam as well as in American-born citizens of Chinese or Filipino descent. The geographical distribution of lineages defined by Gagneux and colleagues is supported by other studies,[105–113] and there is generally good concordance for lineage assignation between SNP analysis and MIRU-VNTR,[114] spoligotyping,[115,116] and IS6110-RFLP.[117] Free web-based bioinformatics tools that facilitate assignation of TB strains to lineages based on spoligotype or MIRU-VNTR are available. These include MIRU-VNTR-*plus*[118] (http://www.miru-vntrplus.org), SpolDB4[116] (http://www.pasteur-guadeloupe.fr), and TB-Insight[119] (http://tbinsight.cs.rpi.edu/run_tb_lineage.html).

The identification of an *M. tuberculosis* phylogenetic framework has allowed for study of the effects of lineage on transmission and severity of TB disease. Several studies have demonstrated that Beijing/East Asian strains (also known as lineage 2) are more transmissible and may be more virulent compared to strains of other lineages. Beijing/East Asian strains comprise 13% of all global TB isolates and are the most widely disseminated across the world.[116] A study of 4,987 Beijing/East Asian lineage isolates from 99 countries that used MIRU-VNTR typing combined with WGS showed that this lineage originated in the Far East and had multiple expansions into other regions of the world.[120] The Beijing/East Asian lineage has been associated with pulmonary disease and sputum smear positivity as well as increased rates of molecular clustering when compared to other lineages.[121–124] The virulence of Beijing/East Asian strains has been attributed to production of a phenolic glycolipid (PGL) that is able to modulate the host immune response.[125] Beijing/East Asian strains are able to produce PGL because they have an intact polyketide synthase gene (*pks1–15*), but this gene is disrupted in other lineages. However, expression of PGL varies among Beijing/East Asian strains and effect of PGL on host immune response seems to depend on the genomic context of the strain.[126]

Strains of the Beijing/East Asian lineage can also be further divided into sublineages based on presence or absence of genomic regions of difference (RD) or SNP analysis. In epidemiological studies, modern Beijing sublineages have increased molecular clustering and ability to cause disease compared to ancestral Beijing sublineages.[127,128] This difference is apparent in animal models as well, with modern sublineages of Beijing/East Asian strains inducing a lower proinflammatory response and resulting in increased mortality in mice compared to ancestral Beijing sublineages.[129–131]

Conversely, there is also evidence to suggest that non-East Asian lineages are associated with extrapulmonary disease, lower transmissibility, or both. For example, the East African-Indian lineage, which is the predominant lineage in the Indian subcontinent, has been shown to have lower rates of transmission and cause less severe forms of TB compared with other lineages.[132,133] Indo-Oceanic and East African-Indian lineages were found to be associated with exclusively extrapulmonary disease, even when controlling for host factors.[122] Guerra-Assuncao et al. used WGS to conduct a population-based analysis of clustering and transmissibility in Malawi and found that Indo-Oceanic strains had the lowest measures of transmissibility.[134] Furthermore, Euro-American sublineages were found to vary in transmissibility, with the RD145 sublineage having the highest frequency of new infections and sublineage RD219 having the lowest.[135] On the other hand, Lee and colleagues concluded that successful transmission of Euro-American lineage *M. tuberculosis* in Nunavik, Québec was likely driven by environmental and social factors (i.e., not strain characteristics).[136]

Given the established association between lineage and geographical region, changing trends in the lineage distribution in a population are likely to be driven either by shifting demographic or migration patterns or by the introduction of foreign strains into the population that replace less transmissible native strains.[41] Therefore, the prevalence of these strains in the population should be monitored because this could have important implications for TB control strategies. For example, an increase in the frequency of Beijing strains could hypothetically lead to a higher number of rapidly growing outbreaks; active case finding to ensure early diagnosis and treatment of secondary cases and contacts may be important to control transmission and prevent additional cases. Conversely, if circulating strains are more likely to cause extrapulmonary disease, then it may be more important to raise healthcare providers' awareness of atypical disease presentations to ensure timely diagnosis.

TRANSMISSION OF DRUG-RESISTANT TB

The number of drug-resistant cases of TB continues to increase globally.[137] To predict future trends, it is important to understand the transmission dynamics of drug-resistant TB. The spread of drug-resistant strains will depend on their relative fitness compared to drug-susceptible strains, measured by their ability to reproduce and be transmitted. Mutations that confer resistance to antibiotics usually occur in genes that are essential for bacterial growth and thus could result in a "fitness cost" to the bacteria, causing them to have a lower transmission rate or reproductive rate (R_0).[138] In order to compensate for such mutations, bacterial populations can acquire secondary mutations to restore the original level of fitness.[139] If drug-resistant strains are less transmissible, then the majority of drug-resistant TB cases would be expected to result from acquired resistance.[140] However, studies using molecular and epidemiological data and modelling have indicated that primary transmission of drug-resistant strains is the main driver of increasing rates of multidrug-resistant (MDR) TB worldwide.[141,142]

There is some experimental evidence to suggest that drug-resistant strains have reduced fitness compared to sensitive strains, but conflicting results have been found in epidemiological studies. Using animal models, experiments in the 1950s showed that INH-resistant strains were less virulent than susceptible strains.[143,144] However, more recent studies found that the most common mutation in the *katG* gene, S315T, which confers INH resistance, does not affect bacterial fitness.[145,146] This finding is supported by several epidemiological studies. A large study in the Netherlands showed there was no difference between the proportion of clustering of INH-resistant strains compared to sensitive strains, and increased clustering was observed for isolates with the S315T mutation compared to INH-resistant strains with other mutations.[147] In rural China, INH-resistant strains with the S315T mutation also showed a higher proportion of clustering compared to sensitive strains.[148] In San Francisco, patients infected with INH-resistant TB only transmitted to secondary cases if isolates had this particular mutation.[149] Similarly, the S531L mutation in the *rpoB* gene, which is the most common rifampin resistance-conferring mutation in clinical isolates, had the lowest fitness cost of any of the experimentally derived *rpoB* mutations tested in a competitive fitness assay. Furthermore, clinical isolates with this mutation showed no measurable fitness cost when compared to rifampin-susceptible ancestor isolates from the same patient.[150]

Primary transmission of MDR TB has been documented in both high and low incidence countries.[121,151-154] Studies to estimate the relative contributions of primary transmission vs. acquired resistance to the overall burden of MDR and extensively drug-resistant (XDR) TB can be difficult because resistance can arise independently multiple times in the same strain, so estimates will depend on the discriminatory power of the genotyping method that is used.[155] Also, ruling out patients as having primary transmission based on past history of treatment may overestimate the contribution of acquired resistance. A study of previously treated patients in Shanghai, China found that 59% of patients with increasing drug resistance resulted from exogenous reinfection.[156] Many epidemiological studies of MDR and XDR TB transmission have been conducted in South Africa, where the burden is one of the highest globally. In KwaZulu-Natal province, where co-infection of TB and HIV is high, the majority of XDR TB cases were likely due to transmission.[157] Epidemiological links for these cases indicated that local hospitals, which typically have poor infection control measures, are an important transmission setting. This demonstrates that MDR and XDR TB are able to spread easily in settings that facilitate transmission, particularly in populations with a high prevalence of HIV and other risk factors for the development of active TB disease.

An association between MDR TB and the Beijing lineage has been consistently found globally.[106,107,158-162] It has been hypothesized that this association could be due to a biological mechanism and that Beijing strains may have a higher mutation rate compared to those of other lineages, but an *in vitro* study that compared mutation rates between lineages found that there were no differences.[163] It has also been suggested that the association between MDR TB and Beijing lineage is coincidental because Beijing strains are more common in areas of the world where the emergence of MDR TB has occurred due to poor TB treatment and control programs. Furthermore, if Beijing strains transmit more readily than other lineages, then it will appear that they have acquired mutations more easily in areas of a high incidence of MDR TB.[127] Indeed, epidemiological studies have provided some evidence that Beijing MDR TB strains are more transmissible than non-Beijing MDR TB strains.[124,162] If the combination of MDR TB and Beijing strain does lead to higher rates of transmission, the emergence of Beijing strains in South Africa[164] and the recently identified association with XDR TB is worrisome.[152]

Current evidence suggests that the fitness of drug-resistant strains may be dependent on particular mutations or lineage. However, factors associated with geographical region, host factors, and the transmission setting also appear to play an important role in predicting the likelihood of transmission and outbreaks of drug-resistant strains. Large epidemiological studies combining clinical, social risk factor, and demographic data with molecular information and contact tracing and screening results are required to further investigate the transmissibility of drug-resistant strains.

REACTIVATION VS. REINFECTION

Recurrent episodes of active TB disease in the same patient can occur because of reactivation of the previous episode of TB disease following incomplete treatment or relapse, or by exogenous reinfection during a new transmission event.[165] This distinction is programmatically important for TB control in a population because different interventions are required. Cases of recurrent TB due to relapse imply that enhanced efforts are needed to ensure treatment efficacy, possibly through greater attention to adherence, longer duration of therapy, or attention to drug choice and dosing. Recurrent TB due to reinfections indicates ongoing transmission. To help identify recurrences, some programs may add a time component to account for the period when completion of therapy or cure (e.g., sputum culture conversion to negative) is expected for the earlier episode. For example, the U.S. National TB Surveillance System (NTSS) counts in national incidence reporting a case of recurrent TB disease only $\geq$12 months after the last clinical visit for TB treatment.[166] Because most relapses occur within a year following treatment completion,[167] NTSS recurrences are sometimes described as "late recurrences."[168] NTSS also collects information on cases with recurrence within 12 months; however, these cases are not counted in national surveillance for incidence.

TB control programs can use conventional genotyping and WGS data to help differentiate between reactivation and reinfection if historical isolates are available from previous TB episodes. Genotyping results should be indistinguishable or very similar for cases of recurrent TB due to reactivation, and are expected to differ for cases of reinfection. Using conventional genotyping, numerous studies have found that reinfection is common in countries with a high incidence of TB,[169-172] presumably because the likelihood of contact with an infectious individual is high. Furthermore, HIV co-infection is associated with increased susceptibility to recurrent disease following reinfection (i.e., immunodeficiency due to untreated, advanced HIV). More recently, studies using clinical trial data from Malaysia, South Africa, and Thailand have demonstrated that SNP analyses of WGS data are superior to MIRU-VNTR for differentiation.[173,174] Population-based studies using WGS will allow for refined estimates of the proportions of TB cases arising from reinfections. In rural Karonga in Malawi, for example, 20 (27%) of 75 recurrences with paired WGS or IS6110-RFLP data were due to reinfections.[175] Reinfections were associated with HIV co-infection; the study also suggested Beijing lineages were overrepresented in cases of reinfection. Conversely, only two instances of reinfection were identified by a MIRU-VNTR and WGS study of the Nunavut, Canada outbreak where *M. tuberculosis* strains are closely related.[89] In low-incidence countries such as Australia, Finland, and the United States, several studies using MIRU-VNTR and WGS have shown that significant proportions (13%–15%) of TB cases arise from reinfection.[165,176,177] Using a network model, Cohen et al. found that transmission among individuals who are part of close social networks (i.e., non-random mixing) can result in certain individuals becoming infected multiple times even in low incidence settings.[176] This finding is consistent with findings by Interrante et al., showing that a majority of recurrent TB cases among recent U.S. immigrants from Africa (50%) and Mexico (60%) were due to reinfections.[165]

However, historical isolates may be unavailable for genotyping. Moreover, even when complete genotyping data are available, distinguishing exogenous reinfections from reactivations depends on an assumption that reinfections are more likely due to transmission of a new *M. tuberculosis* strain (i.e., a genotype that is different from the previous episode). In geographical areas or transmission settings where a single strain predominates, it is possible for an individual to be repeatedly reinfected with the same strain. These recurrent cases may be misclassified as due to reactivation, which could lead to underestimates of recent transmission. Thus, other data sources are important for characterizing recurrent disease. Based on clinical trial data, predictors of treatment failure or relapse include cavitary disease and smear positivity at completion of 2 months of treatment.[178,179] U.S. surveillance data suggest that risk factors for late recurrences differed for non-U.S.-born (HIV infection and smear positivity) and U.S.-born patients (aged 25–44 years, substance use, and treatment supervised by health departments).[168] These risk factors may also contribute to the higher mortality observed during recurrent episodes.[166] It is important to note that regardless of whether an infectious TB case is believed to have arisen due to primary infection, reactivation, or exogenous reinfection, vigorous contact tracing procedures should be initiated.

WITHIN-HOST GENETIC DIVERSITY

Most studies on TB transmission have been based on the assumption that individuals are infected with one strain of *M. tuberculosis*. However, *M. tuberculosis* genetic diversity within a single host can result from simultaneous infection with two different strains (the so-called mixed infections) or microevolution of a single strain.

Conventional genotyping methods are able to detect simultaneous infection with two different strains within the same TB episode. MIRU-VNTR typing was shown to be more sensitive at detecting mixed infections compared with RFLP or spoligotyping.[180] Different genotypes have been isolated from different sites within the body[181] and the lungs.[182] In high-incidence settings, the proportion of TB cases with mixed infections has been shown to vary between 1% and 19%.[183–191] Studies carried out in Shanghai[185] and Cape Town,[190] which are urban areas of high TB incidence, found that mixed infections were more common in retreatment cases compared to new cases. This finding highlights the importance of exogenous reinfection in recurrent episodes of TB. Conversely, Huyen et al.[180] reported that in rural South Vietnam, which has a lower TB incidence, 4.8% of TB cases had mixed infections, and these were associated with cases that were not previously treated.

Within-host genetic diversity can also result from microevolution of a single strain. Although the conventional genotyping methods IS*6110* RFLP and MIRU-VNTR have been used to detect microevolution,[3,192] these methods greatly underestimate the extent of genetic diversity because they only examine a small portion of the genome. In contrast, WGS has greatly enhanced the ability to detect *M. tuberculosis* genetic diversity within a single host. Microevolution of *M. tuberculosis* has been documented when examining a single specimen, specimens from different sites of disease within the same patient, and specimens collected over time from the same patient. Comparison of WGS data for single colonies from *M. tuberculosis* isolates revealed that subpopulations of bacteria with unique SNPs are present within an *M. tuberculosis* isolate.[155] A study by Liu et al. of a patient with MDR TB showed the patient had six anatomically distinct lesions in the lung that responded to treatment differently.[156] WGS of serial isolates found three dominant subpopulations of *M. tuberculosis* that differed by 10–14 SNPs, including mutations that are known to confer antibiotic resistance. Walker et al. performed WGS analysis on pulmonary and extrapulmonary isolates from the same patients.[27] Of 48 patients, 37 had isolates from the pulmonary and extrapulmonary sites that were identical by WGS analysis and 11 had isolates that differed by one to 11 SNPs, indicating that genetic diversity within a single infecting strain existed in these patients. The same study also examined longitudinal isolates collected from the same patients at intervals ranging from 6 to 102 months; 17 of 28 patients had isolates that differed by one to 10 SNPs.

Intra-host genetic diversity involving mutations that confer antibiotic resistance could have serious implications for patient treatment. If an individual is infected with subpopulations of *M. tuberculosis* that have different drug-resistance patterns, resistance may not be detected at diagnosis,[193] especially if the majority of the bacterial population is fully sensitive. The subsequent emergence of drug-resistant strains within an individual can then lead to treatment failure in the absence of repeated drug-sensitivity testing and also transmission of drug-resistant strains to others.[183,194,195] WGS could be used to identify individuals with a mixture of drug-resistant and drug-susceptible *M. tuberculosis* at the start of treatment who may be at higher risk of treatment failure. These individuals would then be monitored more closely throughout treatment and have their regimens modified in response to drug sensitivity results to improve their chances of treatment success.

FALSE-POSITIVE CULTURES AND CROSS-CONTAMINATION

Culture confirmation of *M. tuberculosis* is the gold standard for diagnosing active TB disease. Multiple European and U.S. studies conducted using conventional genotyping during the 1990s and 2000s have shown that false-positivity rates can be as high as 4%.[196–202] False-positive results are important to identify and prevent misdiagnoses, which can lead to unnecessary patient isolation, treatment, hospitalization, stigma, and costs as well as false clustering and misguided public health actions.[202–205] If patients are admitted to the same hospital ward, failure to detect false-positive results can also lead to erroneous inferences that nosocomial transmission has occurred. Causes of false-positive results may include clerical errors (e.g., mislabeling), contamination of medical devices and equipment (e.g., bronchoscopes), and cross-contamination of laboratory samples when *M. tuberculosis* is inadvertently inoculated into a specimen not containing the bacilli.[204] Contamination is more likely to occur during sample processing when samples are batch processed on the same day.[206]

Identifying how laboratory cross-contamination occurred can be further complicated by the need to refer specimens and isolates from clinical settings to commercial and reference laboratories for additional testing.

Laboratorians and TB control program staff can use genotyping data to monitor for and detect potential false-positive culture results. In countries with universal genotyping services, prospective strain typing of *M. tuberculosis* isolates can facilitate detection. If available, an isolate from a specimen collected on a different date can be submitted for repeat genotyping when contamination is suspected to determine if the patient's first and second genotyping results differ from one another. Unusual genotyping results, such as matches to reference strains used for proficiency testing or quality control that are not transmitted in the community (e.g., H37Rv), may indicate that a result is either falsely positive or has resulted from an occupational laboratory exposure. Genotyping results should also be reviewed if there is no alternative explanation for an unusual increase in isolates with the same drug-resistance pattern or an unexpected increase in the percentage of culture-positive results.

False-positive investigations are a multidisciplinary endeavor that should involve laboratorians, clinicians, and other TB program staff. Clinical indicators of false positivity include a single positive culture from multiple specimens collected for a new patient, prolonged incubation time with late appearing growth (liquid media) or scanty growth (solid media), the absence of clinical or radiographic findings consistent with TB, and another confirmed diagnosis that is consistent with the patient's clinical presentation. Indistinguishable genotyping results provide evidence for false positivity if isolates from different patients or reference strains were recently processed in the same laboratory or different patients' specimens were collected recently in the same facility. Reference laboratories can routinely monitor for clustering of isolates from source laboratories. Many laboratories have also developed policies and procedures to minimize and detect *M. tuberculosis* cross-contamination.

REFERENCES

1. Thierry D, Matsiota-Bernard P, Pitsouni E, Costopoulos C, and Guesdon JL. Use of the insertion element IS6110 for DNA fingerprinting of *Mycobacterium tuberculosis* isolates presenting various profiles of drug susceptibility. *FEMS Immunol Med Microbiol.* 1993;6(4):287–97.

2. Schurch AC, and van Soolingen D. DNA fingerprinting of *Mycobacterium tuberculosis*: From phage typing to whole-genome sequencing. *Infect Genet Evol.* 2012;12(4):602–9.

3. de Boer AS, Borgdorff MW, de Haas PE, Nagelkerke NJ, van Embden JD, and van Soolingen D. Analysis of rate of change of IS6110 RFLP patterns of *Mycobacterium tuberculosis* based on serial patient isolates. *J Infect Dis.* 1999;180(4):1238–44.

4. Groenen PM, Bunschoten AE, van Soolingen D, and van Embden JD. Nature of DNA polymorphism in the direct repeat cluster of *Mycobacterium tuberculosis*; application for strain differentiation by a novel typing method. *Mol Microbiol.* 1993;10(5):1057–65.

5. Kamerbeek J et al. Simultaneous detection and strain differentiation of *Mycobacterium tuberculosis* for diagnosis and epidemiology. *J Clin Microbiol.* 1997;35(4):907–14.

6. Kremer K et al. Comparison of methods based on different molecular epidemiological markers for typing of *Mycobacterium tuberculosis* complex strains: Interlaboratory study of discriminatory power and reproducibility. *J Clin Microbiol.* 1999;37(8):2607–18.

7. Goyal M, Saunders NA, van Embden JD, Young DB, and Shaw RJ. Differentiation of *Mycobacterium tuberculosis* isolates by spoligotyping and IS6110 restriction fragment length polymorphism. *J Clin Microbiol.* 1997;35(3):647–51.

8. Tsolaki AG et al. Genomic deletions classify the Beijing/W strains as a distinct genetic lineage of *Mycobacterium tuberculosis*. *J Clin Microbiol.* 2005;43(7):3185–91.

9. Cowan LS et al. Evaluation of a two-step approach for large-scale, prospective genotyping of *Mycobacterium tuberculosis* isolates in the United States. *J Clin Microbiol.* 2005;43(2):688–95.

10. Supply P et al. Proposal for standardization of optimized mycobacterial interspersed repetitive unit-variable-number tandem repeat typing of *Mycobacterium tuberculosis*. *J Clin Microbiol.* 2006;44(12):4498–510.

11. Maes M, Kremer K, van Soolingen D, Takiff H, and de Waard JH. 24-locus MIRU-VNTR genotyping is a useful tool to study the molecular epidemiology of tuberculosis among Warao Amerindians in Venezuela. *Tuberculosis.* 2008;88(5):490–4.

12. Christianson S et al. Evaluation of 24 locus MIRU-VNTR genotyping of *Mycobacterium tuberculosis* isolates in Canada. *Tuberculosis.* 2010;90(1):31–8.

13. de Beer JL, Kremer K, Kodmon C, Supply P, van Soolingen D, and Global Network for the Molecular Surveillance of T. First worldwide proficiency study on variable-number tandem-repeat typing of *Mycobacterium tuberculosis* complex strains. *J Clin Microbiol.* 2012;50(3):662–9.

14. Cowan LS et al. Evaluation of mycobacterial interspersed repetitive-unit-variable-number tandem-repeat genotyping as performed in laboratories in Canada, France, and the United States. *J Clin Microbiol.* 2012;50(5):1830–1.

15. National TB Controllers Association/CDC Advisory Group on Tuberculosis Genotyping. *Guide to the Application of Genotyping to Tuberculosis Prevention and Control.* Atlanta, GA: US Department of Health and Human Services, CDC; June 2004. Available at: https://www.cdc.gov/tb/programs/genotyping/manual.htm.

16. Anderson L et al. The national strain typing service. *Tuberculosis in the UK: annual report on tuberculosis surveillance in the UK 2010.* 2010:28–30.

17. Gopaul KK, Brown TJ, Gibson AL, Yates MD, and Drobniewski FA. Progression toward an improved DNA amplification-based typing technique in the study of *Mycobacterium tuberculosis* epidemiology. *J Clin Microbiol.* 2006;44(7):2492–8.

18. Cowan LS, Mosher L, Diem L, Massey JP, and Crawford JT. Variable-number tandem repeat typing of *Mycobacterium tuberculosis* isolates with low copy numbers of IS6110 by using mycobacterial interspersed repetitive units. *J Clin Microbiol.* 2002;40(5):1592–602.

19. Valcheva V, Mokrousov I, Narvskaya O, Rastogi N, and Markova N. Utility of new 24-locus variable-number tandem-repeat typing for discriminating *Mycobacterium tuberculosis* clinical isolates collected in Bulgaria. *J Clin Microbiol.* 2008;46(9):3005–11.

20. Barlow RE, Gascoyne-Binzi DM, Gillespie SH, Dickens A, Qamer S, and Hawkey PM. Comparison of variable number tandem repeat and IS6110-restriction fragment length polymorphism analyses for discrimination of high- and low-copy-number IS6110 *Mycobacterium tuberculosis* isolates. *J Clin Microbiol.* 2001;39(7):2453–7.

21. Allix-Beguec C, Fauville-Dufaux M, and Supply P. Three-year population-based evaluation of standardized mycobacterial interspersed repetitive-unit-variable-number tandem-repeat typing of *Mycobacterium tuberculosis*. *J Clin Microbiol.* 2008;46(4):1398–406.

22. Bidovec-Stojkovic U, Zolnir-Dovc M, and Supply P. One year nationwide evaluation of 24-locus MIRU-VNTR genotyping on Slovenian *Mycobacterium tuberculosis* isolates. *Respir Med.* 2011;105 Suppl 1:S67–73.

23. Sola C et al. Genotyping of the *Mycobacterium tuberculosis* complex using MIRUs: Association with VNTR and spoligotyping for molecular epidemiology and evolutionary genetics. *Infect Genet Evol.* 2003;3(2):125–33.

24. Oelemann MC et al. Assessment of an optimized mycobacterial interspersed repetitive-unit-variable-number tandem-repeat typing system combined with spoligotyping for population-based molecular epidemiology studies of tuberculosis. *J Clin Microbiol.* 2007;45(3):691–7.

25. Vadwai V, Shetty A, Supply P, and Rodrigues C. Evaluation of 24-locus MIRU-VNTR in extrapulmonary specimens: Study from a tertiary centre in Mumbai. *Tuberculosis.* 2012;92(3):264–72.

26. Cole ST, and Barrell BG. Analysis of the genome of *Mycobacterium tuberculosis* H37Rv. *Novartis Found Symp.* 1998;217:160–72; discussion 72-7.

27. Walker TM et al. Whole-genome sequencing to delineate *Mycobacterium tuberculosis* outbreaks: A retrospective observational study. *Lancet Infect Dis.* 2013;13(2):137–46.

28. Bryant JM et al. Inferring patient to patient transmission of *Mycobacterium tuberculosis* from whole genome sequencing data. *BMC Infect Dis.* 2013;13:110.

29. Ford CB et al. Use of whole genome sequencing to estimate the mutation rate of *Mycobacterium tuberculosis* during latent infection. *Nat Genet.* 2011;43(5):482–6.

30. Roetzer A et al. Whole genome sequencing versus traditional genotyping for investigation of a *Mycobacterium tuberculosis* outbreak: A longitudinal molecular epidemiological study. *PLoS Med.* 2013;10(2):e1001387.

31. Colangeli R et al. Whole genome sequencing of *Mycobacterium tuberculosis* reveals slow growth and low mutation rates during latent infections in humans. *PLOS ONE.* 2014;9(3):e91024.

32. Kohl TA et al. Whole-genome-based *Mycobacterium tuberculosis* surveillance: A standardized, portable, and expandable approach. *J Clin Microbiol.* 2014;52(7):2479–86.

33. Brown AC et al. Rapid whole-genome sequencing of *Mycobacterium tuberculosis* isolates directly from clinical samples. *J Clin Microbiol.* 2015;53(7):2230–7.

34. Votintseva AA et al. Same-day diagnostic and surveillance data for tuberculosis via whole-genome sequencing of direct respiratory samples. *J Clin Microbiol.* 2017;55(5):1285–98.

35. Alland D et al. Transmission of tuberculosis in New York City. An analysis by DNA fingerprinting and conventional epidemiologic methods. *N Engl J Med.* 1994;330(24):1710–6.

36. Small PM et al. The epidemiology of tuberculosis in San Francisco. A population-based study using conventional and molecular methods. *N Engl J Med.* 1994;330(24):1703–9.

37. Vynnycky E, Borgdorff MW, van Soolingen D, and Fine PE. Annual *Mycobacterium tuberculosis* infection risk and interpretation of clustering statistics. *Emerg Infect Dis.* 2003;9(2):176–83.

38. Dahle UR, Sandven P, Heldal E, and Caugant DA. Molecular epidemiology of *Mycobacterium tuberculosis* in Norway. *J Clin Microbiol.* 2001;39(5):1802–7.

39. Dahle UR, Sandven P, Heldal E, and Caugant DA. Continued low rates of transmission of *Mycobacterium tuberculosis* in Norway. *J Clin Microbiol.* 2003;41(7):2968–73.

40. de Vries G, Baars HW, Sebek MM, van Hest NA, and Richardus JH. Transmission classification model to determine place and time of infection of tuberculosis cases in an urban area. *J Clin Microbiol.* 2008;46(12):3924–30.

41. Fenner L et al. *Mycobacterium tuberculosis* transmission in a country with low tuberculosis incidence: Role of immigration and HIV infection. *J Clin Microbiol.* 2012;50(2):388–95.

42. Gutierrez MC et al. Molecular fingerprinting of *Mycobacterium tuberculosis* and risk factors for tuberculosis transmission in Paris, France, and surrounding area. *J Clin Microbiol.* 1998;36(2):486–92.

43. Heldal E, Docker H, Caugant DA, and Tverdal A. Pulmonary tuberculosis in Norwegian patients. The role of reactivation, reinfection and primary infection assessed by previous mass screening data and restriction fragment length polymorphism analysis. *Int J Tuberc Lung Dis.* 2000;4(4):300–7.

44. Hernandez-Garduno E et al. Predictors of clustering of tuberculosis in Greater Vancouver: A molecular epidemiologic study. *CMAJ.* 2002;167(4):349–52.

45. Kamper-Jorgensen Z et al. Clustered tuberculosis in a low-burden country: Nationwide genotyping through 15 years. *J Clin Microbiol.* 2012;50(8):2660–7.

46. Kik SV et al. Tuberculosis outbreaks predicted by characteristics of first patients in a DNA fingerprint cluster. *Am J Respir Crit Care Med.* 2008;178(1):96–104.

47. van Deutekom H, Gerritsen JJ, van Soolingen D, van Ameijden EJ, van Embden JD, and Coutinho RA. A molecular epidemiological approach to studying the transmission of tuberculosis in Amsterdam. *Clin Infect Dis.* 1997;25(5):1071–7.

48. van Deutekom H et al. Clustered tuberculosis cases: Do they represent recent transmission and can they be detected earlier? *Am J Respir Crit Care Med.* 2004;169(7):806–10.

49. Vanhomwegen J et al. Impact of immigration on the molecular epidemiology of tuberculosis in Rhode Island. *J Clin Microbiol.* 2011;49(3):834–44.

50. Verver S et al. Transmission of tuberculosis in a high incidence urban community in South Africa. *Int J Epidemiol.* 2004;33(2):351–7.

51. Fok A, Numata Y, Schulzer M, and FitzGerald MJ. Risk factors for clustering of tuberculosis cases: A systematic review of population-based molecular epidemiology studies. *Int J Tuberc Lung Dis.* 2008;12(5):480–92.

52. Borgdorff MW, Nagelkerke NJ, van Soolingen D, and Broekmans JF. Transmission of tuberculosis between people of different ages in The Netherlands: An analysis using DNA fingerprinting. *Int J Tuberc Lung Dis.* 1999;3(3):202–6.

53. Heldal E et al. Risk factors for recent transmission of *Mycobacterium tuberculosis*. *Eur Respir J.* 2003;22(4):637–42.

54. Maguire H et al. Molecular epidemiology of tuberculosis in London 1995–7 showing low rate of active transmission. *Thorax.* 2002;57(7):617–22.

55. Feng JY et al. Clinical and bacteriological characteristics associated with clustering of multidrug-resistant tuberculosis. *Int J Tuberc Lung Dis.* 2017;21(7):766–73.

56. Glynn JR, Vynnycky E, and Fine PE. Influence of sampling on estimates of clustering and recent transmission of *Mycobacterium tuberculosis* derived from DNA fingerprinting techniques. *Am J Epidemiol.* 1999;149(4):366–71.

57. Vynnycky E, Nagelkerke N, Borgdorff MW, van Soolingen D, van Embden JD, and Fine PE. The effect of age and study duration on the relationship between 'clustering' of DNA fingerprint patterns and the proportion of tuberculosis disease attributable to recent transmission. *Epidemiol Infect.* 2001;126(1):43–62.

58. de Vries G, van Hest NA, Burdo CC, van Soolingen D, and Richardus JH. A *Mycobacterium tuberculosis* cluster demonstrating the use of genotyping in urban tuberculosis control. *BMC Infect Dis.* 2009;9(151).

59. Hamblion EL et al. Recent TB transmission, clustering and predictors of large clusters in London, 2010–2012: Results from first 3 years of universal MIRU-VNTR strain typing. *Thorax*. 2016;71(8):749–56.

60. Guthrie JL et al. Molecular epidemiology of tuberculosis in British Columbia, Canada: A 10-year retrospective study. *Clin Infect Dis*. 2018;66(6):849–56.

61. Powell KM et al. Outbreak of drug-resistant *Mycobacterium tuberculosis* among homeless people in Atlanta, Georgia, 2008–2015. *Public Health Rep*. 2017;132(2):231–40.

62. Noppert GA, Yang Z, Clarke P, Ye W, Davidson P, and Wilson ML. Individual- and neighborhood-level contextual factors are associated with *Mycobacterium tuberculosis* transmission: Genotypic clustering of cases in Michigan, 2004–2012. *Ann Epidemiol*. 2017;27(6):371–6 e5.

63. Wang T, Xue F, Chen Y, Ma Y, and Liu Y. The spatial epidemiology of tuberculosis in Linyi City, China, 2005–2010. *BMC Public Health*. 2012;12:885.

64. Ribeiro FK et al. Genotypic and spatial analysis of *Mycobacterium tuberculosis* transmission in a high-incidence urban setting. *Clin Infect Dis*. 2015;61(5):758–66.

65. Jenkins HE et al. Assessing spatial heterogeneity of multidrug-resistant tuberculosis in a high-burden country. *Eur Respir J*. 2013;42(5):1291–301.

66. Lin HH, Shin SS, Contreras C, Asencios L, Paciorek CJ, and Cohen T. Use of spatial information to predict multidrug resistance in tuberculosis patients, Peru. *Emerg Infect Dis*. 2012;18(5):811–13.

67. Dowdy DW, Golub JE, Chaisson RE, and Saraceni V. Heterogeneity in tuberculosis transmission and the role of geographic hotspots in propagating epidemics. *Proc Natl Acad Sci USA*. 2012;109(24):9557–62.

68. Shaweno D et al. Methods used in the spatial analysis of tuberculosis epidemiology: A systematic review. *BMC Med*. 2018;16(1):193.

69. Althomsons SP et al. Statistical method to detect tuberculosis outbreaks among endemic clusters in a low-incidence setting. *Emerg Infect Dis*. 2018;24(3):573–5.

70. Moonan PK, Ghosh S, Oeltmann JE, Kammerer JS, Cowan LS, and Navin TR. Using genotyping and geospatial scanning to estimate recent *Mycobacterium tuberculosis* transmission, United States. *Emerg Infect Dis*. 2012;18(3):458–65.

71. France AM, Grant J, Kammerer JS, and Navin TR. A field-validated approach using surveillance and genotyping data to estimate tuberculosis attributable to recent transmission in the United States. *Am J Epidemiol*. 2015;182(9):799–807.

72. Yuen CM, Kammerer JS, Marks K, Navin TR, and France AM. Recent transmission of tuberculosis—United States, 2011–2014. *PLOS ONE*. 2016;11(4):e0153728.

73. Teeter LD et al. Evaluation of 24-locus MIRU-VNTR genotyping in *Mycobacterium tuberculosis* cluster investigations in four jurisdictions in the United States, 2006–2010. *Tuberculosis*. 2017;106:9–15.

74. Centers for Disease Control and Prevention. *Reported Tuberculosis in the United States, 2017*. Available at: https://www.cdc.gov/tb/statistics/reports/2017/2017_Surveillance_FullReport.pdf.

75. Bothamley GH. Strain typing and contact tracing—A clinician's viewpoint. *Tuberculosis*. 2007;87(3):173–5.

76. Ghosh S, Moonan PK, Cowan L, Grant J, Kammerer S, and Navin TR. Tuberculosis genotyping information management system: Enhancing tuberculosis surveillance in the United States. *Infect Genet Evol*. 2012;12(4):782–8.

77. Centers for Disease Control and Prevention. Prioritizing tuberculosis genotype clusters for further investigation and public health action [updated 2017]. Available at: https://www.cdc.gov/tb/programs/genotyping/Prioritizing_Tuberculosis_Genotype_Clusters_August2017.pdf.

78. Davidson JA, Anderson LF, Adebisi V, de Jongh L, Burkitt A, and Lalor MK. Creating a web-based electronic tool to aid tuberculosis (TB) cluster investigation: Data integration in TB surveillance activities in the United Kingdom, 2013 to 2016. *Euro Surveill*. 2018;23(44).

79. Hamblion EL et al. Public health outcome of Tuberculosis Cluster Investigations, England 2010–2013. *J Infect*. 2019;78(4):269–74.

80. Diel R, Rusch-Gerdes S, and Niemann S. Molecular epidemiology of tuberculosis among immigrants in Hamburg, Germany. *J Clin Microbiol*. 2004;42(7):2952–60.

81. Gardy JL et al. Whole-genome sequencing and social-network analysis of a tuberculosis outbreak. *N Engl J Med*. 2011;364(8):730–9.

82. Stucki D et al. Standard genotyping overestimates transmission of *Mycobacterium tuberculosis* among immigrants in a low-incidence country. *J Clin Microbiol*. 2016;54(7):1862–70.

83. Jamieson FB, Teatero S, Guthrie JL, Neemuchwala A, Fittipaldi N, and Mehaffy C. Whole-genome sequencing of the *Mycobacterium tuberculosis* Manila sublineage results in less clustering and better resolution than mycobacterial interspersed repetitive-unit-variable-number tandem-repeat (MIRU-VNTR) typing and spoligotyping. *J Clin Microbiol*. 2014;52(10):3795–8.

84. Koster KJ et al. Genomic sequencing is required for identification of tuberculosis transmission in Hawaii. *BMC Infect Dis*. 2018;18(1):608.

85. Gurjav U et al. Whole genome sequencing demonstrates limited transmission within identified *Mycobacterium tuberculosis* clusters in New South Wales, Australia. *PLOS ONE*. 2016;11(10):e0163612.

86. Bjorn-Mortensen K et al. Tracing *Mycobacterium tuberculosis* transmission by whole genome sequencing in a high incidence setting: A retrospective population-based study in East Greenland. *Sci Rep*. 2016;6:33180.

87. Meehan CJ et al. The relationship between transmission time and clustering methods in *Mycobacterium tuberculosis* epidemiology. *EBioMedicine*. 2018;37:410–6.

88. Casali N, Broda A, Harris SR, Parkhill J, Brown T, and Drobniewski F. Whole genome sequence analysis of a large isoniazid-resistant tuberculosis outbreak in London: A Retrospective Observational Study. *PLoS Med*. 2016;13(10):e1002137.

89. Tyler AD et al. Application of whole genome sequence analysis to the study of *Mycobacterium tuberculosis* in Nunavut, Canada. *PLOS ONE*. 2017;12(10):e0185656.

90. Didelot X, Gardy J, and Colijn C. Bayesian inference of infectious disease transmission from whole-genome sequence data. *Mol Biol Evol*. 2014;31(7):1869–79.

91. Stimson J, Gardy J, Mathema B, Crudu V, Cohen T, and Colijn C. Beyond the SNP threshold: Identifying outbreak clusters using inferred transmissions. *Mol Biol Evol*. 2019;36(3):587–603.

92. Jajou R et al. Epidemiological links between tuberculosis cases identified twice as efficiently by whole genome sequencing than conventional molecular typing: A population-based study. *PLOS ONE*. 2018;13(4):e0195413.

93. Walker TM et al. Assessment of *Mycobacterium tuberculosis* transmission in Oxfordshire, UK, 2007–12, with whole pathogen genome sequences: An observational study. *Lancet Respir Med*. 2014;2(4):285–92.

94. Lalor MK et al. The use of whole-genome sequencing in cluster investigation of a multidrug-resistant tuberculosis outbreak. *Eur Respir J*. 2018;51(6).

95. Teeter LD et al. Validation of genotype cluster investigations for *Mycobacterium tuberculosis*: Application results for 44 clusters from four heterogeneous United States jurisdictions. *BMC Infect Dis*. 2016;16(1):594.

96. Dahle UR et al. Tuberculosis in contacts need not indicate disease transmission. *Thorax*. 2005;60(2):136–7.

97. Bennett DE et al. DNA fingerprinting of *Mycobacterium tuberculosis* isolates from epidemiologically linked case pairs. *Emerg Infect Dis.* 2002;8(11):1224–9.

98. Borrell S et al. Factors associated with differences between conventional contact tracing and molecular epidemiology in study of tuberculosis transmission and analysis in the city of Barcelona, Spain. *J Clin Microbiol.* 2009;47(1):198–204.

99. Verver S et al. Proportion of tuberculosis transmission that takes place in households in a high-incidence area. *Lancet.* 2004;363(9404):212–4.

100. Glynn JR et al. Whole genome sequencing shows a low proportion of tuberculosis disease is attributable to known close contacts in rural Malawi. *PLOS ONE.* 2015;10(7):e0132840.

101. Sintchenko V, and Gilbert GL. Utility of genotyping of *Mycobacterium tuberculosis* in the contact investigation: A decision analysis. *Tuberculosis.* 2007;87(3):176–84.

102. Jackson AD et al. Characterising transmission of a tuberculosis genotype in Scotland: A qualitative approach to social network enquiry. *Int J Tuberc Lung Dis.* 2009;13(4):486–93.

103. Fleischmann RD et al. Whole-genome comparison of *Mycobacterium tuberculosis* clinical and laboratory strains. *J Bacteriol.* 2002;184(19):5479–90.

104. Gagneux S et al. Variable host-pathogen compatibility in *Mycobacterium tuberculosis*. *Proc Natl Acad Sci USA.* 2006;103(8):2869–73.

105. Kato-Maeda M et al. Strain classification of *Mycobacterium tuberculosis*: Congruence between large sequence polymorphisms and spoligotypes. *Int J Tuberc Lung Dis.* 2011;15(1):131–3.

106. Brown T, Nikolayevskyy V, Velji P, and Drobniewski F. Associations between *Mycobacterium tuberculosis* strains and phenotypes. *Emerg Infect Dis.* 2010;16(2):272–80.

107. Ghebremichael S et al. Drug resistant *Mycobacterium tuberculosis* of the Beijing genotype does not spread in Sweden. *PLOS ONE.* 2010;5(5):e10893.

108. Phyu S, Stavrum R, Lwin T, Svendsen OS, Ti T, and Grewal HM. Predominance of *Mycobacterium tuberculosis* EAI and Beijing lineages in Yangon, Myanmar. *J Clin Microbiol.* 2009;47(2):335–44.

109. Coscolla M, and Gagneux S. Does *M. tuberculosis* genomic diversity explain disease diversity? *Drug Discov Today Dis Mech.* 2010;7(1):e43–59.

110. Hershberg R et al. High functional diversity in *Mycobacterium tuberculosis* driven by genetic drift and human demography. *PLoS Biol.* 2008;6(12):e311.

111. Huang SF et al. Association of *Mycobacterium tuberculosis* genotypes and clinical and epidemiological features—A multi-center study in Taiwan. *Infect Genet Evol.* 2012;12(1):28–37.

112. Arora J et al. Characterization of predominant *Mycobacterium tuberculosis* strains from different subpopulations of India. *Infect Genet Evol.* 2009;9(5):832–9.

113. Lahlou O et al. The genotypic population structure of *Mycobacterium tuberculosis* complex from Moroccan patients reveals a predominance of Euro-American lineages. *PLOS ONE.* 2012;7(10):e47113.

114. Gibson A, Brown T, Baker L, and Drobniewski F. Can 15-locus mycobacterial interspersed repetitive unit-variable-number tandem repeat analysis provide insight into the evolution of *Mycobacterium tuberculosis*? *Appl Environ Microbiol.* 2005;71(12):8207–13.

115. Filliol I et al. Global distribution of *Mycobacterium tuberculosis* spoligotypes. *Emerg Infect Dis.* 2002;8(11):1347–9.

116. Brudey K et al. *Mycobacterium tuberculosis* complex genetic diversity: Mining the fourth international spoligotyping database (SpolDB4) for classification, population genetics and epidemiology. *BMC Microbiol.* 2006;6:23.

117. Gutacker MM et al. Single-nucleotide polymorphism-based population genetic analysis of *Mycobacterium tuberculosis* strains from 4 geographic sites. *J Infect Dis.* 2006;193(1):121–8.

118. Weniger T, Krawczyk J, Supply P, Niemann S, and Harmsen D. MIRU-VNTRplus: A web tool for polyphasic genotyping of *Mycobacterium tuberculosis* complex bacteria. *Nucleic Acids Res.* 2010;38:W326–31.

119. Shabbeer A et al. TB-Lineage: An online tool for classification and analysis of strains of *Mycobacterium tuberculosis* complex. *Infect Genet Evol.* 2012;12(4):789–97.

120. Merker M et al. Evolutionary history and global spread of the *Mycobacterium tuberculosis* Beijing lineage. *Nat Genet.* 2015;47(3):242–9.

121. Metcalfe JZ et al. Determinants of multidrug-resistant tuberculosis clusters, California, USA, 2004–2007. *Emerg Infect Dis.* 2010;16(9):1403–9.

122. Click ES, Moonan PK, Winston CA, Cowan LS, and Oeltmann JE. Relationship between *Mycobacterium tuberculosis* phylogenetic lineage and clinical site of tuberculosis. *Clin Infect Dis.* 2012;54(2):211–9.

123. Pareek M et al. Ethnicity and mycobacterial lineage as determinants of tuberculosis disease phenotype. *Thorax.* 2013;68(3):221–9.

124. van der Spuy GD et al. Changing *Mycobacterium tuberculosis* population highlights clade-specific pathogenic characteristics. *Tuberculosis.* 2009;89(2):120–5.

125. Reed MB et al. A glycolipid of hypervirulent tuberculosis strains that inhibits the innate immune response. *Nature.* 2004;431(7004):84–7.

126. Sinsimer D et al. The phenolic glycolipid of *Mycobacterium tuberculosis* differentially modulates the early host cytokine response but does not in itself confer hypervirulence. *Infect Immun.* 2008;76(7):3027–36.

127. Hanekom M, Gey van Pittius NC, McEvoy C, Victor TC, Van Helden PD, and Warren RM. *Mycobacterium tuberculosis* Beijing genotype: A template for success. *Tuberculosis.* 2011;91(6):510–23.

128. Yang C et al. *Mycobacterium tuberculosis* Beijing strains favor transmission but not drug resistance in China. *Clin Infect Dis.* 2012;55(9):1179–87.

129. Ribeiro SC et al. *Mycobacterium tuberculosis* strains of the modern sublineage of the Beijing family are more likely to display increased virulence than strains of the ancient sublineage. *J Clin Microbiol.* 2014;52(7):2615–24.

130. van Laarhoven A et al. Low induction of proinflammatory cytokines parallels evolutionary success of modern strains within the *Mycobacterium tuberculosis* Beijing genotype. *Infect Immun.* 2013;81(10):3750–6.

131. Chen YY et al. The pattern of cytokine production *in vitro* induced by ancient and modern Beijing *Mycobacterium tuberculosis* strains. *PLOS ONE.* 2014;9(4):e94296.

132. Albanna AS et al. Reduced transmissibility of East African Indian strains of *Mycobacterium tuberculosis*. *PLOS ONE.* 2011;6(9):e25075.

133. Nebenzahl-Guimaraes H, Verhagen LM, Borgdorff MW, and van Soolingen D. Transmission and progression to disease of *Mycobacterium tuberculosis* phylogenetic lineages in the Netherlands. *J Clin Microbiol.* 2015;53(10):3264–71.

134. Guerra-Assuncao JA et al. Large-scale whole genome sequencing of *M. tuberculosis* provides insights into transmission in a high prevalence area. *Elife.* 2015;4.

135. Feng JY et al. Impact of Euro-American sublineages of *Mycobacterium tuberculosis* on new infections among named contacts. *Int J Tuberc Lung Dis.* 2017;21(5):509–16.

136. Lee RS et al. Population genomics of *Mycobacterium tuberculosis* in the Inuit. *Proc Natl Acad Sci USA.* 2015;112(44):13609–14.

137. World Health Organization. *Global tuberculosis report 2017*, 2017. Available at: http://www.whoint/tb/publications/global_report/en/.

138. Dye C, Williams BG, Espinal MA, and Raviglione MC. Erasing the world's slow stain: Strategies to beat multidrug-resistant tuberculosis. *Science*. 2002;295(5562):2042–6.

139. Borrell S, and Gagneux S. Infectiousness, reproductive fitness and evolution of drug-resistant *Mycobacterium tuberculosis*. *Int J Tuberc Lung Dis*. 2009;13(12):1456–66.

140. Cohen T, Sommers B, and Murray M. The effect of drug resistance on the fitness of *Mycobacterium tuberculosis*. *Lancet Infect Dis*. 2003;3(1):13–21.

141. Fox GJ, Schaaf HS, Mandalakas A, Chiappini E, Zumla A, and Marais BJ. Preventing the spread of multidrug-resistant tuberculosis and protecting contacts of infectious cases. *Clin Microbiol Infect*. 2017;23(3):147–53.

142. Kendall EA, Fofana MO, and Dowdy DW. Burden of transmitted multidrug resistance in epidemics of tuberculosis: A transmission modelling analysis. *Lancet Respir Med*. 2015;3(12):963–72.

143. Middlebrook G, and Cohn ML. Some observations on the pathogenicity of isoniazid-resistant variants of tubercle bacilli. *Science*. 1953;118(3063):297–9.

144. Mitchison DA. Tubercle bacilli resistant to isoniazid; virulence and response to treatment with isoniazid in guinea-pigs. *Br Med J*. 1954;1(4854):128–30.

145. Pym AS, Saint-Joanis B, and Cole ST. Effect of katG mutations on the virulence of *Mycobacterium tuberculosis* and the implication for transmission in humans. *Infect Immun*. 2002;70(4):4955–60.

146. Ordway DJ, Sonnenberg MG, Donahue SA, Belisle JT, and Orme IM. Drug-resistant strains of *Mycobacterium tuberculosis* exhibit a range of virulence for mice. *Infect Immun*. 1995;63(2):741–3.

147. van Soolingen D, de Haas PE, van Doorn HR, Kuijper E, Rinder H, and Borgdorff MW. Mutations at amino acid position 315 of the katG gene are associated with high-level resistance to isoniazid, other drug resistance, and successful transmission of *Mycobacterium tuberculosis* in the Netherlands. *J Infect Dis*. 2000;182(6):1788–90.

148. Hu Y, Mathema B, Jiang W, Kreiswirth B, Wang W, and Xu B. Transmission pattern of drug-resistant tuberculosis and its implication for tuberculosis control in eastern rural China. *PLOS ONE*. 2011;6(5):e19548.

149. Gagneux S et al. Impact of bacterial genetics on the transmission of isoniazid-resistant *Mycobacterium tuberculosis*. *PLoS Pathog*. 2006;2(6):e61.

150. Gagneux S, Long CD, Small PM, Van T, Schoolnik GK, and Bohannan BJ. The competitive cost of antibiotic resistance in *Mycobacterium tuberculosis*. *Science*. 2006;312(5782):1944–6.

151. Gilpin CM et al. Evidence of primary transmission of multidrug-resistant tuberculosis in the Western Province of Papua New Guinea. *Med J Aust*. 2008;188(3):148–52.

152. Streicher EM et al. Emergence and treatment of multidrug resistant (MDR) and extensively drug-resistant (XDR) tuberculosis in South Africa. *Infect Genet Evol*. 2012;12(4):686–94.

153. Leung EC et al. Transmission of multidrug-resistant and extensively drug-resistant tuberculosis in a metropolitan city. *Eur Respir J*. 2013;41(4):901–8.

154. Senghore M et al. Whole-genome sequencing illuminates the evolution and spread of multidrug-resistant tuberculosis in Southwest Nigeria. *PLOS ONE*. 2017;12(9):e0184510.

155. Black PA et al. Whole genome sequencing reveals genomic heterogeneity and antibiotic purification in *Mycobacterium tuberculosis* isolates. *BMC Genomics*. 2015;16:857.

156. Nsofor CA et al. Transmission is a noticeable cause of resistance among treated tuberculosis patients in Shanghai, China. *Sci Rep*. 2017;7(1):7691.

157. Shah NS et al. Transmission of extensively drug-resistant tuberculosis in South Africa. *N Engl J Med*. 2017;376(3):243–53.

158. Drobniewski F et al. Rifampin- and multidrug-resistant tuberculosis in Russian civilians and prison inmates: Dominance of the Beijing strain family. *Emerg Infect Dis*. 2002;8(11):1320–6.

159. Tanveer M et al. Genotyping and drug resistance patterns of *M. tuberculosis* strains in Pakistan. *BMC Infect Dis*. 2008;8:171.

160. Niemann S, Diel R, Khechinashvili G, Gegia M, Mdivani N, and Tang YW. *Mycobacterium tuberculosis* Beijing lineage favors the spread of multidrug-resistant tuberculosis in the Republic of Georgia. *J Clin Microbiol*. 2010;48(10):3544–50.

161. Kubica T et al. The Beijing genotype is a major cause of drug-resistant tuberculosis in Kazakhstan. *Int J Tuberc Lung Dis*. 2005;9(6):646–53.

162. Sun YJ et al. Genotype and phenotype relationships and transmission analysis of drug-resistant tuberculosis in Singapore. *Int J Tuberc Lung Dis*. 2007;11(4):436–42.

163. Werngren J, and Hoffner SE. Drug-susceptible *Mycobacterium tuberculosis* Beijing genotype does not develop mutation-conferred resistance to rifampin at an elevated rate. *J Clin Microbiol*. 2003;41(4):1520–4.

164. Cowley D et al. Recent and rapid emergence of W-Beijing strains of *Mycobacterium tuberculosis* in Cape Town, South Africa. *Clin Infect Dis*. 2008;47(10):1252–9.

165. Interrante JD, Haddad MB, Kim L, and Gandhi NR. Exogenous reinfection as a cause of late recurrent tuberculosis in the United States. *Ann Am Thorac Soc*. 2015;12(11):1619–26.

166. Kim L, Moonan PK, Yelk Woodruff RS, Kammerer JS, and Haddad MB. Epidemiology of recurrent tuberculosis in the United States, 1993–2010. *Int J Tuberc Lung Dis*. 2013;17(3):357–60.

167. Nunn AJ, Phillips PP, and Mitchison DA. Timing of relapse in short-course chemotherapy trials for tuberculosis. *Int J Tuberc Lung Dis*. 2010;14(2):241–2.

168. Kim L, Moonan PK, Heilig CM, Yelk Woodruff RS, Kammerer JS, and Haddad MB. Factors associated with recurrent tuberculosis more than 12 months after treatment completion. *Int J Tuberc Lung Dis*. 2016;20(1):49–56.

169. Cohen T et al. Multiple introductions of multidrug-resistant tuberculosis into households, Lima, Peru. *Emerg Infect Dis*. 2011;17(6):969–75.

170. Sonnenberg P, Murray J, Glynn JR, Shearer S, Kambashi B, and Godfrey-Faussett P. HIV-1 and recurrence, relapse, and reinfection of tuberculosis after cure: A cohort study in South African mineworkers. *Lancet*. 2001;358(9294):1687–93.

171. van Rie A et al. Exogenous reinfection as a cause of recurrent tuberculosis after curative treatment. *N Engl J Med*. 1999;341(16):1174–9.

172. Verver S et al. Rate of reinfection tuberculosis after successful treatment is higher than rate of new tuberculosis. *Am J Respir Crit Care Med*. 2005;171(12):1430–5.

173. Bryant JM et al. Whole-genome sequencing to establish relapse or re-infection with *Mycobacterium tuberculosis*: A retrospective observational study. *Lancet Respir Med*. 2013;1(10):786–92.

174. Witney AA et al. Use of whole-genome sequencing to distinguish relapse from reinfection in a completed tuberculosis clinical trial. *BMC Med*. 2017;15(1):71.

175. Guerra-Assuncao JA et al. Recurrence due to relapse or reinfection with *Mycobacterium tuberculosis*: A whole-genome sequencing approach in a large, population-based cohort with a high HIV infection prevalence and active follow-up. *J Infect Dis*. 2015;211(7):1154–63.

176. Korhonen V, Soini H, Vasankari T, Ollgren J, Smit PW, and Ruutu P. Recurrent tuberculosis in Finland 1995–2013: A clinical and epidemiological cohort study. *BMC Infect Dis*. 2017;17(1):721.

177. Parvaresh L, Crighton T, Martinez E, Bustamante A, Chen S, and Sintchenko V. Recurrence of tuberculosis in a low-incidence setting: A retrospective cross-sectional study augmented by whole genome sequencing. *BMC Infect Dis*. 2018;18(1):265.

178. Benator D et al. Rifapentine and isoniazid once a week versus rifampicin and isoniazid twice a week for treatment of drug-susceptible pulmonary tuberculosis in HIV-negative patients: A randomised clinical trial. *Lancet*. 2002;360(9332):528–34.

179. Romanowski K et al. Predicting tuberculosis relapse in patients treated with the standard 6-month regimen: An individual patient data meta-analysis. *Thorax*. 2019;74(3):291–7.

180. Huyen MN et al. Mixed tuberculosis infections in rural South Vietnam. *J Clin Microbiol*. 2012;50(5):1586–92.

181. Garcia de Viedma D, Marin M, Ruiz Serrano MJ, Alcala L, and Bouza E. Polyclonal and compartmentalized infection by *Mycobacterium tuberculosis* in patients with both respiratory and extrarespiratory involvement. *J Infect Dis*. 2003;187(4):695–9.

182. Kaplan G et al. *Mycobacterium tuberculosis* growth at the cavity surface: A microenvironment with failed immunity. *Infect Immun*. 2003;71(12):7099–108.

183. Baldeviano-Vidalon GC, Quispe-Torres N, Bonilla-Asalde C, Gastiaburu-Rodriguez D, Pro-Cuba JE, and Llanos-Zavalaga F. Multiple infection with resistant and sensitive *M. tuberculosis* strains during treatment of pulmonary tuberculosis patients. *Int J Tuberc Lung Dis*. 2005;9(10):1155–60.

184. Das S et al. Simultaneous infection with multiple strains of *Mycobacterium tuberculosis* identified by restriction fragment length polymorphism analysis. *Int J Tuberc Lung Dis*. 2004;8(2):267–70.

185. Fang R et al. Mixed infections of *Mycobacterium tuberculosis* in tuberculosis patients in Shanghai, China. *Tuberculosis*. 2008;88(5):469–73.

186. Lazzarini LC et al. Discovery of a novel *Mycobacterium tuberculosis* lineage that is a major cause of tuberculosis in Rio de Janeiro, Brazil. *J Clin Microbiol*. 2007;45(12):3891–902.

187. Richardson M et al. Multiple *Mycobacterium tuberculosis* strains in early cultures from patients in a high-incidence community setting. *J Clin Microbiol*. 2002;40(8):2750–4.

188. Shamputa IC et al. Genotypic and phenotypic heterogeneity among *Mycobacterium tuberculosis* isolates from pulmonary tuberculosis patients. *J Clin Microbiol*. 2004;42(12):5528–36.

189. Stavrum R et al. High diversity of *Mycobacterium tuberculosis* genotypes in South Africa and preponderance of mixed infections among ST53 isolates. *J Clin Microbiol*. 2009;47(6):1848–56.

190. Warren RM et al. Patients with active tuberculosis often have different strains in the same sputum specimen. *Am J Respir Crit Care Med*. 2004;169(5):610–4.

191. Yeh RW, Hopewell PC, and Daley CL. Simultaneous infection with two strains of *Mycobacterium tuberculosis* identified by restriction fragment length polymorphism analysis. *Int J Tuberc Lung Dis*. 1999;3(6):537–9.

192. Cohen T et al. Within-host heterogeneity of *Mycobacterium tuberculosis* infection is associated with poor early treatment response: A prospective Cohort Study. *J Infect Dis*. 2016;213(11):1796–9.

193. van Rie A et al. Reinfection and mixed infection cause changing *Mycobacterium tuberculosis* drug-resistance patterns. *Am J Respir Crit Care Med*. 2005;172(5):636–42.

194. Theisen A et al. Mixed-strain infection with a drug-sensitive and multidrug-resistant strain of *Mycobacterium tuberculosis*. *Lancet*. 1995;345(8963):1512.

195. Niemann S, Richter E, Rusch-Gerdes S, Schlaak M, and Greinert U. Double infection with a resistant and a multidrug-resistant strain of *Mycobacterium tuberculosis*. *Emerg Infect Dis*. 2000;6(5):548–51.

196. Bauer J, Thomsen VO, Poulsen S, and Andersen AB. False-positive results from cultures of *Mycobacterium tuberculosis* due to laboratory cross-contamination confirmed by restriction fragment length polymorphism. *J Clin Microbiol*. 1997;35(4):988–91.

197. Bhattacharya M et al. Cross-contamination of specimens with *Mycobacterium tuberculosis*: Clinical significance, causes, and prevention. *Am J Clin Pathol*. 1998;109(3):324–30.

198. Braden CR, Templeton GL, Stead WW, Bates JH, Cave MD, and Valway SE. Retrospective detection of laboratory cross-contamination of *Mycobacterium tuberculosis* cultures with use of DNA fingerprint analysis. *Clin Infect Dis*. 1997;24(1):35–40.

199. Frieden TR, Woodley CL, Crawford JT, Lew D, and Dooley SM. The molecular epidemiology of tuberculosis in New York City: The importance of nosocomial transmission and laboratory error. *Tuber Lung Dis*. 1996;77(5):407–13.

200. Jasmer RM et al. A prospective, multicenter study of laboratory cross-contamination of *Mycobacterium tuberculosis* cultures. *Emerg Infect Dis*. 2002;8(11):1260–3.

201. Small PM, McClenny NB, Singh SP, Schoolnik GK, Tompkins LS, and Mickelsen PA. Molecular strain typing of *Mycobacterium tuberculosis* to confirm cross-contamination in the mycobacteriology laboratory and modification of procedures to minimize occurrence of false-positive cultures. *J Clin Microbiol*. 1993;31(7):1677–82.

202. Ruddy M et al. Estimation of the rate of unrecognized cross-contamination with *Mycobacterium tuberculosis* in London microbiology laboratories. *J Clin Microbiol*. 2002;40(11):4100–4.

203. Lai CC et al. Molecular evidence of false-positive cultures for *Mycobacterium tuberculosis* in a Taiwanese hospital with a high incidence of TB. *Chest*. 2010;137(5):1065–70.

204. Burman WJ, and Reves RR. Review of false-positive cultures for *Mycobacterium tuberculosis* and recommendations for avoiding unnecessary treatment. *Clin Infect Dis*. 2000;31(6):1390–5.

205. Northrup JM et al. Estimated costs of false laboratory diagnoses of tuberculosis in three patients. *Emerg Infect Dis*. 2002;8(11):1264–70.

206. Lee MR et al. Epidemiologic surveillance to detect false-positive *Mycobacterium tuberculosis* cultures. *Diagn Microbiol Infect Dis*. 2012;73(4):343–9.

6

Tuberculosis Transmission Control

EDWARD A. NARDELL

INTRODUCTION

Globally, in high burden settings, *recent* transmission, including *reinfection*, accounts for most incident TB clinical cases, compared to reactivation of remote latent infection.[1] Ongoing transmission, therefore, especially in congregate settings, is driving the TB epidemic.[2] In low-burden settings, however, where transmission is infrequent, reactivation of latent infection is relatively more important, and treatment of latent infection has been a strategy for TB elimination.[3] Even under low-burden settings, it is argued, most disease results within a year or so of transmission, and the risk from old infection may be overestimated.[1]

IMPORTANCE OF THE UNDIAGNOSED CASE OR UNDIAGNOSED DRUG RESISTANCE

This chapter will review current understanding on *Mycobacterium tuberculosis* (*Mtb*) transmission and its control, with emphasis on the importance of transmission from persons with *unsuspected* TB, or *unsuspected* drug resistance, not on effective therapy.[5] Although effective therapy has long been known to rapidly stop transmission, conventional TB infection control efforts tend to focus on known TB patients, most of whom are on effective therapy and not likely to be sources of transmission.[6,7] Guidelines and practice need to shift from a focus on known cases started on effective therapy to finding unsuspected cases in congregate settings through screening, followed by rapid molecular diagnosis and drug susceptibility testing, leading to prompt, effective treatment.[8] This re-focused, intensified administrative approach to TB transmission control has been packaged as an easy-to-remember

acronym, "F-A-S-T," Find cases Actively, Separate temporarily, and Treat effectively, based on molecular drug susceptibility testing.[8] The acronym emphasizes the need to reduce time from symptom reporting to effective treatment. In crowded congregate settings, however, such as registration areas and ambulatory clinics, effective screening for unsuspected TB may not be feasible. There, administrative measures (triage, appointments) to reduce crowding, and air disinfection through natural ventilation and upper room germicidal lamps are important interventions.[9,10] Likewise, respiratory protection for healthcare workers is less important for encounters with known TB patients on effective treatment—where they are most commonly used—and more likely to be effective for encounters with patients at high risk for undiagnosed TB or undiagnosed drug resistance.[11] Good examples are caring for patients with undiagnosed respiratory infection in the emergency room, or patients undergoing bronchoscopy for lung infiltrates where TB is prevalent.

AIRBORNE SPREAD

TB pathogenesis begins through person-to-person transmission, almost exclusively by the *airborne* route, a relatively unusual transmission route among human pathogens, shared primarily with some respiratory viruses.[12] Airborne *Mtb* infection requires host susceptibility to the extremely small dose of *Mtb*, carried as *droplet nuclei* (the 1–5 μm dried residua of larger droplets) able to traverse the structural barriers of the upper respiratory track to reach the peripheral lung where pulmonary alveolar macrophages (PAMs) reside.[13] PAMs are both a first line of innate immunity and, paradoxically, the target cell for initial *Mtb* replication. To accomplish this, *Mtb* has evolved specific mechanisms for blocking PAM intracellular killing. Airborne transport is probably facilitated by *Mtb's* uniquely thick, hydrophobic cell wall, able to protect this preferentially intracellular pathogen from the stresses of aerosolization, dehydration in room air, transport, and rehydration in the humid respiratory track of a new host.[14] Barer has described a "fat and lazy" spore-like phenotype that may be preparatory to aerosolization.[15] Exactly what microbial gene-expression signatures are necessary to facilitate airborne transport remain largely unknown, but may be important to elucidate. For example, the rapid impact of effective treatment on transmission, discussed later in this chapter, well before sputum smear and culture conversion, might be due to pharmacologic interference with specific microbial adaptive mechanisms.[16]

Particles small enough to be inhaled deep into the lung settle very slowly in still air and can remain suspended indefinitely in occupied rooms where air is rarely stagnant due to body heat, air infiltration, and other factors.[17] The 1–5 μm size of infectious droplet nuclei is defined not by organism size (0.5×1.0 μm), per se, but by the size of the entire particle containing one, or at most several (estimated 2–3) *Mtb* organisms, but also dried solute, mucous, and cellular debris found in respiratory lining liquid.[18] High airflow in the relatively narrow upper airways and trachea, generated by cough and other forced respiratory maneuvers, shears off relatively large droplets that evaporate rapidly into *droplet nuclei* once expelled, depending on fluid viscoelasticity and ambient humidity.[17] Thinner lung lining fluid may be easier to aerosolize than viscous sputum. Quiet breathing can also generate droplet nuclei as alveoli pop open with inhalation, but the contribution of this mechanism to TB transmission is unknown.[19] A hallmark of chronic TB disease is *lung cavitation*, the result of caseation necrosis of a granuloma and erosion into an airway. With cavities containing an estimated 10^8 *Mtb* organisms, expectorated sputum may contain tens of thousands of detectable *Mtb* organisms per cubic millilitre in various states of viability and infectiousness. Aerosolization by cough and other respiratory maneuvers into room air results in a variety of respiratory droplets and droplet nuclei—the majority of which, it is believed, contain damaged, dead, or dying organisms, including microbial fragments of DNA from *Mtb*, other microorganisms, and respiratory lining cells. Molecular testing of ambient air samples in an unventilated small chamber occupied by an infectious TB patient reveal orders of magnitude more *Mtb* DNA copies than the estimated numbers of viable, infectious droplet nuclei that actually reach the alveolus and result in sustained infection.[20,21] Thus, there is a steep cascade from large numbers of particles generated, many of which are dead or dying, to fewer and fewer particles that reach the distal lung and remain both viable and infectious—and succeed in causing a sustained infection.[20]

Unable to define the exact number of infectious droplet nuclei that must be inhaled to result in infection in a host, Wells applied the word *"quanta,"* a general term referring to the smallest amount of almost anything—in this case, the smallest infectious dose. For an individual infection, the lowest *infectious dose* (or quanta) of *Mtb*, cannot be less than one intact, viable, infectious *Mtb* organism, but nor can it be more than can be associated with a single airborne infectious droplet nucleus. Unlike multifocal point-source histoplasmosis infection, for example, initial (primary)

TB infection in humans (and *naturally* infected experimental animals) is rarely more than a single lung focus—usually in better ventilated dependent (lower) regions of lungs. This strongly implies a single infectious droplet nucleus. By definition, the clinical foci of infection recognized by x-ray or at autopsy likely represent only the *successful host–pathogen interactions* from the pathogen perspective, leading to persistent infection manifest by detectable adaptive inflammatory responses. Unknown are the number of host–pathogen interactions that occurred where the host (i.e., macrophage) wins the initial encounter, resulting in complete microbial clearance, leaving little or no measurable evidence (by current methods) of infection or an innate immune response, much less any evidence of any aborted adaptive immune responses.[22,23]

Understanding that inhaling particles is probabilistic, Wells introduced *Poisson's law of small chances* and defined a *"quanta"* of TB infection on a population basis—the average dose necessary to infect 63% of a population—the remaining exposed susceptible hosts escaping infection by chance. The estimated source strength from human outbreaks and human-to-guinea-pig experiments (see subsection "Source factors" and Figure 6.8), ranges from 1.25 infectious quanta per hour (qph), to 13 qph for an infectious office worker, to 60 qph for a case of laryngeal TB, and approximately 250 qph for a bronchoscopy-related TB case.[24–26]

Room air concentrations of infectious quanta vary with dilution of in-room volume, and from ventilation and die-off over time, but estimates from Riley's classic 2-year human-to-guinea-pig transmission study are as low as 1 infectious quanta in 11,000 ft³ (311 m³) of air.[27,28] These low levels of contagion, however, were sufficient to explain the rate at which student nurses became infected on hospital TB wards in the pre-chemotherapy era.[29] The more infectious a particular airborne pathogen for a particular host, the less role chance plays, for example, initial measles exposure almost always results in human infection.

MEASURING INFECTIOUSNESS

TB is routinely diagnosed in sputum by smear microscopy, culture, and by molecular detection of *Mtb*. Smear microscopy will detect about half of the organisms that will grow in sputum culture—and the newest molecular methods detect about the same as does liquid culture. However, it has not been possible to grow *Mtb* sampled from ambient room air on selective media due to overwhelming numbers of fast-growing competing environmental organisms. As noted previously, while molecular methods can detect nucleic acids, their viability and infectivity remain unknown. Coughing into a sterilized air-sampling cylinder, directly onto agar surfaces or into liquid media (cough aerosol sampling system, CASS), incorporating the host's ability to cough and generate aerosol, has allowed source strength quantification that has been shown to correlate better with household *Mtb* spread than does sputum smear or culture alone.[30] Because it is technically challenging, CASS remains a research tool. In low burden settings, accurate estimates of infectiousness of a source case requires testing human contacts for infection by tuberculin skin testing or IGRA. Under high-burden settings, however, pre-existing tuberculin hypersensitivity from vaccination or previous mycobacterial infection limits the utility of contact tracing.

Because of far fewer variables, for research purposes, the gold standard method for measuring human infectiousness remains quantitative animal studies, where hundreds of highly vulnerable guinea pigs breath the exhaust air from an experimental TB ward and are tested monthly for new infection.[22,26,31]

Although human-to-animal transmission experiments go back to the late nineteenth century, the first quantitative human-to-guinea-pig (H-GP) transmission study, envisioned by Wells and conducted by Riley in the late 1950s and the early 1960s, proved beyond doubt that *Mtb* was routinely spread via the air, that patients varied greatly from one another in infectiousness, and that effective treatment had an immediate and profound impact on transmission.[26] More recently, Escombe conducted similar studies in Peru, focused on an HIV co-infected patient population, and proved the effectiveness of upper room germicidal UV (GUV) air disinfection (see Figure 6.1 and subsection "Upper room GUV").[32] In South Africa, Nardell, Stoltz, and colleagues have used the same model for more than 14 years (Figure 6.1)—major findings include the rapid impact of effective treatment, and new regimens, on transmission of multi-drug resistant (MDR)/extensively drug-resistant (XDR)-TB, the effectiveness of surgical masks on patients, the effectiveness of upper room GUV air disinfection (with dosing specifications), the ineffectiveness of selected room air cleaning (filtration) devices, and importantly, new insights into the early events of infection in the guinea-pig model, demonstrating frequent transient infections, with spontaneous clearance, as well as reinfection. These findings are discussed further, below.[6,22,33,34]

TB primary infection (and reinfection), as noted above, follows inhalation of viable and infectious *Mtb*-containing droplet nuclei small enough (1–5 μm) to reach and impact surfaces in the peripheral lung patrolled by alveolar macrophages.[13] Macrophage recognition and phagocytosis of *Mtb* triggers a series of host innate and metabolic defense mechanisms aimed at killing the microbe at

that *stage*, and initiating specific adaptive immunity, should it be necessary. But phagocytosis of *Mtb* also triggers a series of microbial virulence factors intended to evade host defenses (see subsections "Infection: Transient and sustained" and "Host factors") and, indeed, to allow the organisms to replicate rather than die within and, ultimately, outside of host cells.[13] Stimulation of intracellular macrophage signaling also impacts the cytokine environment thereby modifying the strength of adaptive immunity, leading to *Mtb* survival and tolerance (granuloma formation, necrosis, latency) over time. Thus, the early *innate* host responses to Mtb are essential for preventing sustained TB infection as well as for developing effective adaptive immunity should infection persist.[23,35]

Development of active (clinical) TB, therefore, represents a failure of host defenses at several levels, but critically, failure of the earliest response to prevent sustained infection from relatively rare, individual *Mtb*-containing droplet nuclei. Given the natural variability in host innate immunity and microbial virulence, a spectrum of host–pathogen outcomes is inevitable, but poorly documented for TB. Not well described in the literature, transient TB infection occurs—the best documented example of which—albeit not usually resolved at the earliest stage of infection due to an extremely large microbial dose—is *BCG* vaccination, where despite clear evidence of local response to live bacteria at the injection site, measurable systemic hypersensitivity is almost always transient (months to many years) following complete clearance of this attenuated strain.[36]

INFECTION: TRANSIENT AND SUSTAINED

Despite a clear understanding that initial TB infection entails innate immune responses to one or, at most, several viable Mtb organisms able to reach the alveoli in a single focus, most experimental laboratory aerosol challenge models employ brief (10–20 min) exposures to 10–50 CFUs of cultured organisms to assure infection

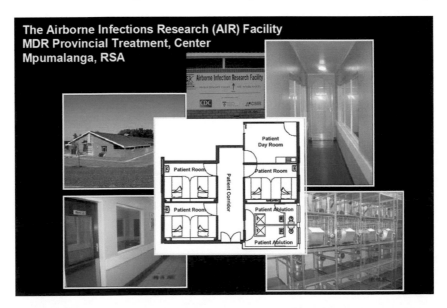

Figure 6.1 The AIR Facility, Mpumalanga, South Africa, has been a collaboration of several US and South African institutions, with funding from NIOSH, USAID, NIH, and the Bill and Melinda Gates Foundation. Clockwise from the photo of the signage, the images show the two identical guinea-pig exposure chambers, the cages in one exposure chamber, one of three patient 2-bed rooms, and the outside of the facility. In the center is a schematic of the patient suite. Air is sampled from the three patient rooms, the corridor, and the patient day room.

and disease progression. Critical early host pathogen interactions are completely obscured in these models.[37] In contrast, human-to-guinea-pig transmission studies provide a unique model that routinely shows clear evidence of the earliest, often transient, focal host–pathogen interactions produced by long-term (months) exposures of hundreds of immunologically naïve guinea pigs to the exhaust air from a TB ward in South Africa (Figure 6.1). Using this model, we routinely measure early innate immune responses that begin to trigger adaptive immunity (TST and T-cell stimulation responses), which are often aborted, and sometimes progress to sustained infection and disease progression. Evidence that these transient TST responses are due to viable, infectious, and not dead *Mtb* or environmental bacteria, is provided by the observations that they do not occur at all without exposure to exhaust air from TB patients, and are prevented if exhaust air from patients is UV irradiated.[38-40] Presumably, there are other early host–pathogen interactions that resolve with microbial death, but without stimulating measurable TST responses. This leads to the question, what exactly is infection? While not presuming to answer that question here, we suggest that if latent *Mtb*, which often persists but does not progress to disease—manifest only by adaptive immunological response—is called "latent infection," then specific immunological responses that do not persist, reflecting early innate host–pathogen interactions, also deserve to be called infection, albeit, transient infection. That this phenomenon is not better recognized than it is, although observed in the H-GP model almost 70 years ago, is attributable to the difficulty of measuring these reproducible events in exposed humans where serial TST or IGRA testing is rarely done, and to the absence of transient infection in experimental animal models employing unnaturally high doses of aerosolized laboratory strains of *Mtb* specifically intended to infect most animals and lead to disease.

REINFECTION

Smith theorized that reinfection was an integral part of TB pathogenesis under endemic conditions, allowing organisms to seed the vulnerable lung apex when systemic hematogenous seeding is blocked by adaptive immunity (Figures 6.2 and 6.3).[41] Apical lung seeding is the favored location for reactivation and lung cavitation, a critical part of airborne transmission (Figure 6.2). But beyond a secondary, airway route to the lung apex, reinfection can be considered another form of dose. Because individual airborne droplet nuclei can contain relatively few organisms and still be airborne, and because not all infections initiated in macrophages are successfully sustained, repeated inhalations and reinfection increase the probability that some "hits" progress even if many do not. In a study of household contacts of infectious cases in British Columbia, Grzybowski showed that, given infection, children in households with a sputum smear positive index case were more likely to progress to disease than children in households where the index case was culture positive, but sputum smear negative, indicating a lower bacterial burden in the source case.[42] Children in households with a sputum smear positive index case likely had many more "hits" and a greater chance that at least one would progress to disease.

DETERMINANTS OF TRANSMISSION

A convenient way to discuss the determinants of transmission and potential interventions is through the *Wells-Riley equation* (Equation 6.1), an idealized steady-state model that has been widely used to better understand the theoretical relationship among factors.[43] For this purpose, it is less important as an equation for accurately predicting risk of infection than as a single place to consider the relative importance of the major *Mtb* transmission factors.

Number of Infected Persons = Number of Susceptible Hosts
× Chance of Not Becoming Infected

$$C = S(1 - e^{-Iqpt/Q}) \qquad (6.1)$$

Equation 6.1 is the Wells–Riley mass balance equation for airborne equation—explained in the text.[43]

In this model, *C* represents the number of infected persons; *S* is the number of susceptible persons exposed to contaminated air generated by one or more infectious source or sources (*I*) at a certain generation rate (*q*) over a given time period (*t*). Infection rate (*C/S*) is directly related to the generally low probability of inhaling an infectious dose of *Mtb* as droplet nuclei in dilute air—hence the Poisson distribution (infrequent events) is used, represented

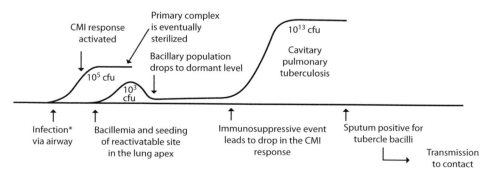

Endogenous reactivation (Endog. Path.)

CMI response activated

Primary complex is eventually sterilized

10^{13} cfu

Cavitary pulmonary tuberculosis

10^5 cfu

Bacillary population drops to dormant level

10^3 cfu

Infection* via airway

Bacillemia and seeding of reactivatable site in the lung apex

Immunosuppressive event leads to drop in the CMI response

Sputum positive for tubercle bacilli

Transmission to contact

Figure 6.2 Smith figure showing Stead unitary theory, that active disease in low burden settings where active disease almost always represents reactivation of infection early in life. (From Smith D et al. *Rev Infect Dis.* 1989;11: S385–S393.)

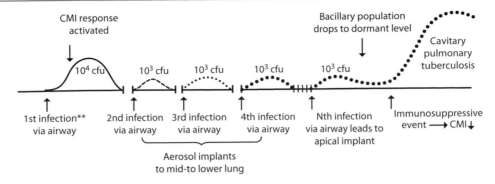

Figure 6.3 Smith concept of reinfection as an alternative pathway to cavitary disease, especially in persons with enhanced immunity from prior immunization or mycobacterial infection. (From Smith D et al. *Rev Infect Dis.* 1989; 11:S385-S393.)

by the natural logarithm (e). *C/S* is directly related to the generation rate of infectious doses ($I \times q$). *t* represents the duration of exposure. *p* represents the host pulmonary ventilation, which is a species-specific constant for the purposes of this relationship. *C/S* is *inversely related* to only one factor under steady-state conditions—building or room outdoor ventilation rate (*Q*).

Under non-steady state, non-well-mixed conditions, outside, for example, dilution is infinite and changing as infectious droplet nuclei disperse, so the equation does not apply. The relationship is simpler than the equation would suggest. For example, doubling source strength doubles infection rate and doubling ventilation rate halves it. Importantly, doubling ventilation again, reduces the risk again by half. Like all first-order kinetic processes (*target theory*), where the magnitude of the effect depends on the target concentration, it becomes increasingly difficult and expensive to decontaminate air as the concentration of contaminant (*Mtb*) falls. Put another way, a first air change removes approximately 63% of contaminated air under well-mixed conditions, and a second air change removes approximately 63% of what remains, and so on, with decreasing increments in protection from each step increase in ventilation (Figure 6.4). As discussed later, upper room air disinfection also works on first-order kinetics, allowing comparison of protection expressed as equivalent air changes (1 Eq air changes per hour (ACH) = a 63% reduction in risk) achieved by GUV with that achieved by ventilation (Figure 6.5).

From Figure 6.6 it is evident that there are other transmission factors not included in the *Wells–Riley* equation, such as those determining source strength, as detailed below. For the

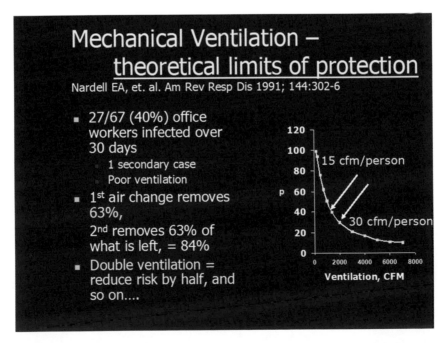

Figure 6.4 Example of using the Well–Riley equation to estimate source strength and the effect of changing room ventilation on infection rate. The graph illustrates of probability of infection as a function of ventilation, in cubic feet per minute. See ventilation discussion below. In a TB exposure in an office building, a worker exposed 67 known TST negative co-workers for 1 month, resulting in 27 documented TST conversions and one secondary case. The Well–Riley equation estimated that the source case produced approximately 13 infectious quanta (doses) per hour. It further estimated that increasing the estimated ventilation rate of 15 cfm per person to 30 cfm per person would reduce the infection rate from 40% to 20%, an example of the general rule that doubling outside ventilation reduces the transmission rate by half. (From Nardell EA et al. *Am Rev Respir Dis.* 1991;144:302–6. Reprinted with permission of the American Thoracic Society. Copyright © 2020 American Thoracic Society.)

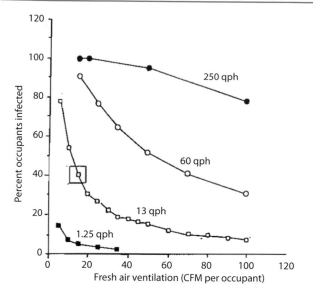

Figure 6.5 Impact of ventilation on transmission—results from a modeling exercise based on the office building exposure cited earlier. Note that while increasing ventilation always reduces transmission, protection is a function of source strength, that is, the number of quanta of infection generated per hour (qph). At very high generation rates room occupants are not protected fully even at high ventilation rates.[4]

organism, the model assumes uniform virulence and viability, and for host resistance, it assumes uniform susceptibility despite possible immunization or prior mycobacterial exposure, and it assumes no interventions, such as respiratory protection. Given several unrealistic assumptions and unknowns, the basic Wells–Riley is useful primarily for understanding general relationships among factors, but not for precise predictions, and more sophisticated mathematical enhancements are likely not warranted.[44]

SOURCE FACTORS

Human-to-human *Mtb* transmission requires the presence of an infectious source (or sources, *I*) and susceptible hosts sharing the same breathing space (shared air). Infectious droplet nuclei are generated at a certain rate (*q*) and removed from the air at a certain rate (or inhaled by susceptible hosts). Among factors known to increase source strength are: (1) the number of untreated (often unsuspected) source cases, (2) the presence of lung cavities in non-immunocompromised persons (HIV patients are less likely to cavitate but may harbor large numbers of organisms), (3) the ability to cough and generate aerosol (also related to sputum viscosity), (4) the absence of effective treatment, (5) the presence of drug resistance (often unsuspected), (6) the use of cough hygiene or surgical masks, and (7) separation or isolation of the infectious source case.

ORGANISM FACTORS

Mtb strains are well known to vary in virulence (ability to infect and cause disease) with the most dramatic examples being the vaccine strain of bovine TB, *M. bovis* and the laboratory strain, H37Ra, which have mutations leading to a loss of virulence for immunocompetent hosts, producing at most a transient infection in the case of BCG.[45] Circulating clinical strains also appear to vary in virulence with the Beijing family of strains being notoriously virulent as well. Other strains, for example CDC 1551, were suspected as being hyper-virulent because of the amount of skin test hypersensitivity produced among contacts in large outbreaks, but that appeared to represent just the opposite, a strain stimulating a greater immune response (despite the appearance of wider transmission) but perhaps, resulting in less disease as a result of a vigorous immune response.[46]

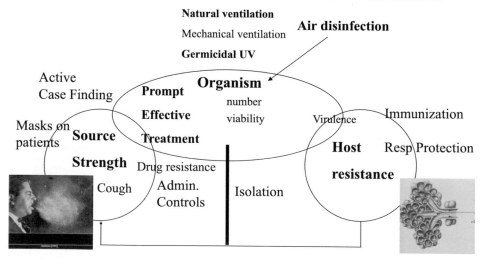

Figure 6.6 Schematic of key factors in airborne transmission and major intervention sites as discussed in the text.

ENVIRONMENTAL FACTORS

How specific environmental conditions impact *Mtb* viability is poorly understood. Person-to-person *Mtb* transmission is successful in the heat and humidity of the tropical climates as well as in dry, cold climates, although crowded, poorly ventilated indoor conditions where transmission occurs may be humid, despite dry, cold outside conditions. The primary indoor factor associated with transmission is crowding and lack of ventilation, leading to the propensity to re-breathe contaminated air. Rudnick and Milton have argued that indoor CO_2 levels may be a good surrogate for rebreathed air fraction, an important transmission risk determinant, given infectious sources in the room.[47] Ambient CO_2 is influenced by both crowding, dilution, and outdoor (non-recirculated) ventilation. High levels could result from overcrowding, underventilation, or a combination of both factors. Wood and colleagues have monitored individual ambient CO_2 levels encountered during the day to estimate where students, for example, experience the greatest rebreathed air fraction. They concluded that schools and minibuses could be important sites of TB transmission in South Africa.[32,48] We have used the same methodology to monitor the rebreathed air experience of nurses working in two somewhat differently constructed hospitals in the Cape Town, South Africa, area, finding that both were reasonably well ventilated relative to occupancy in that breezy climate, the highest CO_2 levels being experienced in the crowded tea break room where an infectious TB case is unlikely—but where influenza among staff could more easily spread from person to person.

With global warming and soaring temperatures in megacities in India and other hot climates, air conditioner use is escalating dramatically, immediately increasing the risk of airborne infection as windows are closed for efficient operation. Similar conditions have long existed in cold climates with tightly sealed windows and radiant heating, leading to high rates of transmission, especially of drug-resistant TB, compounded by prolonged hospitalization and delayed diagnosis of drug resistance. Both administrative and environmental control strategies are needed.

HOST FACTORS

Humans vary greatly in resistance to *Mtb* infection, reinfection, and disease progression, based on both inherited innate immunity, epigenetic modification, and adaptive immunity, further complicated by age, medication, and risk factors such as smoking, air pollution, diabetes and HIV co-infection. Previous exposure to mycobacteria and related organisms such as *BCG* vaccination, environmental mycobacteria, *Mtb*, and *M. leprae* are associated with greater resistance to *Mtb* infection, reinfection, and/or disease progression. Long attributed to adaptive immunity, there is growing evidence of innate *learned* immunity derived from epigenetic exposure, mediated at the level of bone marrow.[49–52] In addition, populations vary greatly in the extent to which they have co-evolved with TB infection, reflected in selective pressure for resistance in populations. For example, Stead and Bates have argued that central African populations were spared exposure to the TB epidemic raging in Western Europe and the Americas until recent centuries, resulting in less inherited resistance to infection

among black residents of Arkansas nursing homes compared to Caucasian residents. Once infected, however, the risk of progression to disease was similar, but disease clinical manifestations differed in the two populations.[53] Disease in blacks tends to be more acute whereas disease in whites more indolent and chronic. These differences they argued are not inherently racial, but strictly based on evolutionary population exposure to *Mtb*. Aboriginal populations in North America and the Pacific Islands similarly had little inherited resistance to *Mtb*, with devastating results when these naïve populations encountered European settlers.[53]

INTERVENTIONS

SOURCE STRENGTH INTERVENTIONS: THE RAPID IMPACT ON TRANSMISSION OF EFFECTIVE TREATMENT

There has long been evidence that the principle source of *Mtb* transmission in congregate settings is persons with *unsuspected* TB not on therapy, or patients with known TB, but unsuspected drug resistance, not on effective therapy. Nonetheless, most TB transmission control interventions focus almost exclusively on known or suspected cases who are likely to be on effective treatment. Hospitals focus on TB wards, on the isolation or separation of known or suspected cases. Healthcare workers focus on respiratory protection when caring for known or suspected patients even after treatment has started. Part of the problem is lack of familiarity with the evidence showing how promptly transmission stops once effective treatment starts. If asked, many healthcare workers will quote the "two-week rule"—that transmission can be assumed to cease after two weeks of effective treatment (Figure 6.5). Where does the two-week rule come from and is it valid?

Following the introduction of effective chemotherapy in the early 1950s, long-term hospitalization for TB became unnecessary, but the safety of ambulatory treatment regarding household and community transmission became an issue. The Madras study, showing the efficacy of ambulatory treatment through a controlled clinical trial (one of the first of any intervention), also demonstrated no difference in household conversion rates when patients were treated at home vs. hospital.[54] Based on several household transmission studies, Rouillion and colleagues concluded in 1976 that chemotherapy at that time (only INH, streptomycin, and PAS) was likely to render patients non-infectious quickly, probably in less than two weeks. This was more consensus than science.[7] That conclusion did not incorporate the human-to-guinea-pig studies published by Riley and colleagues over a decade earlier, below, showing that patients admitted at exactly the same time that treatment was started (not two weeks earlier) were 98% less infectious for guinea pigs (Table 6.1).[39] Guinea pigs are believed to be much more susceptible to human *Mtb* than are normal humans, so these stunning results strongly suggest that effective treatment, even treatment less effective than current regimens, rapidly shuts down human–human transmission.

As Riley stated, "The treated patients were admitted to the ward at the time treatment was initiated and were generally

Table 6.1 Outcome of human-to-guinea-pig *Mtb* transmission studies, showing the rapid impact of effective treatment on transmission among DS and DR patients

Patients with susceptible *Mtb*	Numbers of GPs infected	Relative infectiousness[a]%
Untreated	29	100
Treated	1	2
Patients with DR *Mtb*		
Untreated	14	28
Treated	6	5

Source: From Riley et al. *Am Rev Resp Dis* 1962;85:511–525. Reprinted with permission of the American Thoracic Society. Copyright © 2020 American Thoracic Society.

Note: The only available drugs at the time were isoniazid, streptomycin, and PAS, so DR patients, usually INH resistant at least, had very few treatment options.

[a] All smear positive patients, relative to the amount of time spent on the ward.

removed before the sputum became completely negative. Hence the decrease in infectiousness preceded the elimination of the organisms from the sputum, indicating that the effect was prompt as well as striking."[39] This is the clearest demonstration to date that *effective* treatment has an almost immediate effect on the ability of organisms, still viable on culture, to infect a new host. Based on our own human-to-guinea-pig studies in South Africa, we recently published evidence suggesting that even MDR-TB is rapidly rendered non-infectious for guinea pigs by effective chemotherapy, but unsuspected XDR-TB, inadvertently treated (ineffectively) as MDR-TB, continued to transmit.[6] Moreover, the addition of bedaquiline and linezolid to failed MDR treatment had not reduced transmission to guinea pigs over an 11-day period, but these drugs both require prolonged loading time to reach full therapeutic levels. However, the NIX regimen, containing the more rapidly acting pretomamid (a delamamid-like drug), promptly stopped XDR transmission (Prof. Anton Stoltz, 2018, personal communication).

FAST: FIND CASES ACTIVELY, SEPARATE, AND TREAT EFFECTIVELY BASED ON RAPID MOLECULAR DIAGNOSTIC TESTING

Renewed awareness of the rapid impact of effective treatment on transmission, combined with the broad implementation of rapid molecular diagnostic testing for TB, has led to a refocused administrative control strategy that we call "F-A-S-T."[8] The active case finding component (*A*) acknowledges the long-held belief that transmission most often occurs from persons with unsuspected TB or unsuspected drug resistance. How common is that? There are few studies. Willingham and colleagues screened 250 patients for TB admitted to a large female medical ward in a busy general hospital in Lima, Peru over a period of one year.[5] They found 40 patients who were sputum *Mtb* culture positive, including 26 (65%) smear positive and 13 (33%) unsuspected TB patients. Of the 40 culture-positive cases, 8 had MDR-TB (6 unsuspected, including 3 smear-positive cases). Without prompt identification of *Mtb* and drug resistance, followed by effective treatment, transmission

from such patients continues. Other screening efforts, in Zambia for example, have had similar results.[11] Such surveys are important as they would suggest futility of the FAST approach in low-burden settings like the US. There, depending on the population served, most cough and upper lobe chest x-ray findings would not likely be TB-related.

The FAST strategy is an attempt to prioritize TB surveillance and effective treatment as the single most important way to reduce institutional TB transmission. Thus far, FAST has been selectively implemented in Bangladesh, Vietnam, South Africa, and Russia to name a few early adopters.[55,56] Recently published results in Russia are dramatic, although limited to the profound effect of preventing delayed diagnosis of MDR-TB.[57] Before presenting those results, the unusual *Mtb* transmission situation in Eastern Europe and Central Asia deserves discussion.

HYPER-TRANSMISSION OF MDR-TB IN EASTERN EUROPE AND CENTRAL ASIA

Kendall and colleagues recently published a model to estimate the percentage of MDR-TB transmitted compared to that acquired by poor treatment globally and in selected high and low MDR-TB risk countries.[58] Overall, their model showed that WHO global estimates of 3.5% MDR-TB among new cases, and 20.5% among retreated cases translated to a median of 96% transmitted among all incident cases and 61% among retreated cases. Thus, of the countries studied, apart from low-MDR rate Bangladesh, most MDR-TB results from transmission, not poor treatment. In the 2016, WHO report, MDR-TB percentages of new cases for Belarus, Kazakhstan, Kyrgyzstan, Moldova, Russia, Tajikistan, and Ukraine, were 38, 26, 27, 26, 27, 22, and 27, respectively.[59] Clearly, these distinctly high MDR-TB rates represent hyper-transmission—resulting, we propose, from a combination of prolonged hospitalization, delayed diagnosis of DR-TB, and poor ventilation in generally cold climates in Eastern Europe and Central Asia. With the introduction of universal rapid molecular drug susceptibly testing on admission, however, can change dramatically as discussed below.[57] The following scenario from Tomsk, Siberia, provides insight into why hyper-transmission has been happening in Eastern Europe and Central Asia.

ROLE OF HOSPITALIZATION

A retrospective study of risk factors for MDR-TB in the Russian oblast of Tomsk found the unanticipated result that hospitalization among adherent patients during an initial course of treatment for drug susceptible TB was the major risk factor (OR >6) for development of MDR-TB compared to adherent patients treated in an ambulatory setting.[60] Having previously been treated, these cases would have been routinely classified as acquired drug resistance rather than primary MDR-TB, but that is clearly not the case. In many former Soviet Union (FSU) countries, patients are admitted to hospital and treated for presumed drug susceptible (DS TB) based on smear or CXR with culture pending. Not until months of clinically failing treatment are drug susceptibility tests done, and still months later when MDR-TB is diagnosed and effectively treated. In the meantime, other patients are admitted to the same poorly ventilated congregate rooms, and many of those with DS TB become re-infected with drug-resistant (DR TB). Prompt diagnosis and effective treatment based on rapid molecular testing can stop hyper-transmission and reinfection, as demonstrated, below.

SUCCESSFUL INTERVENTION

In Voronezh and Petrozavodsk, Russia, for example, investigators implemented a targeted form of F-A-S-T in two TB hospitals to reduce transmission from patients with unsuspected MDR-TB. Hospitalization was prolonged before and after implementation—an average of 20.7 weeks before, and 20.0 weeks after implementation. Universal Xpert testing was initiated on all admissions to both the 800-bed and 120-bed facilities, followed by prompt (<48 h) Xpert-directed treatment of DS and Rifampin-resistant TB. Before implementation of universal Xpert testing it took an average of 76.5 days before MDR-TB was diagnosed and patients started on effective treatment.[57] They compared the subsequent rate of MDR-TB generation associated with hospitalization to the baseline rate, pre-FAST. Of a total of 450 patients that were HR sensitive on admission before implementation, 12.2% were diagnosed with MDR-TB within 12 months of finishing treatment. Of 259 patients that were HR sensitive after implementation of universal molecular testing and prompt, effective treatment, only 3.1% were subsequently diagnosed with MDR-TB within 12 months of finishing treatment—a 78% odds reduction in MDR acquisition through the interruption of transmission by prompt, effective treatment of MDR-TB cases in hospital.[57]

ENVIRONMENTAL FACTORS

CLIMATE CHANGE

Transmission and reinfection are driving the epidemic in warm as well as cold climates. Without comparing molecular fingerprints of original and relapse isolates (infrequently available), there is no specific test for reinfection, and it is rarely discussed. As noted, reinfection is an important pathogenesis distinction because it usually implies recent transmission, whereas reactivation does not.[61,62] In rural South Africa, for example, the widely publicized report of rapidly fatal XDR-TB cases called the world's attention to the potential for rapid spread from one or more unsuspected XDR-TB cases to HIV-infected patients in multi-bed wards common throughout resource-limited regions.[63–65] Fifty-five percent of the 53 cases initially reported had not been treated previously, but two-thirds had been hospitalized, and 85% of cases had isolates with the same genotypes, strongly suggesting transmission and presumably mostly reinfection among previously infected adults. Moreover, with climate change and soaring temperatures and humidity, ductless (split system) air conditioning is being introduced widely, in India for example, resulting in windows being closed and an increased risk of transmission.[66] Although rapid diagnosis and effective treatment is essential for stopping the spread of DS and MDR-TB, stopping XDR transmission may depend more on isolation and air disinfection since evidence of a rapid effect of treatment is limited. This is also true for situations where active case finding, drug susceptibility testing, and prompt effective treatment are not yet available or feasible in the near future.

ENVIRONMENTAL CONTROL INTERVENTIONS

Even if active case finding efforts were widely implemented, some indoor situations will continue to defy prompt diagnosis and effective treatment as an administrative approach to preventing transmission. Around the world, crowded, poorly ventilated corridors continue to serve as waiting rooms in ambulatory centers (Figure 6.7). Patients and family members typically wait for hours to be seen, potentially exposing others—or being exposed—to undiagnosed infectious TB. However, the logistics of effective triage based on symptoms or screening tests, the resources and time required, and the absence of a truly simple, rapid point of care "rule in" or "rule out" test all make the "FAST" approach impractical as the main approach to transmission control in these settings. Other administrative approaches to lessen indoor crowding using outdoor waiting areas (where climate permits), creative scheduling of patients, and appointment systems, are important, but rarely implemented due to tradition, economic factors, and simple inertia.

For example, in a new MDR-TB Clinic in Karachi, Pakistan, the architect designed natural ventilation into the infrastructure in that windy location, but also planned to have patients wait outside under sun cover (see Figure 6.8, right) with small groups of patients called in according to their appointment in order to reduce indoor crowding. In this way patients are exposed to

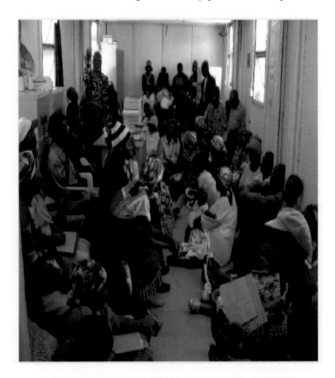

Figure 6.7 Typical corridor serving as an overcrowded waiting area. At least in the setting pictured, windows exist on both sides. Often both sides are lined by doors to clinic consultation rooms.

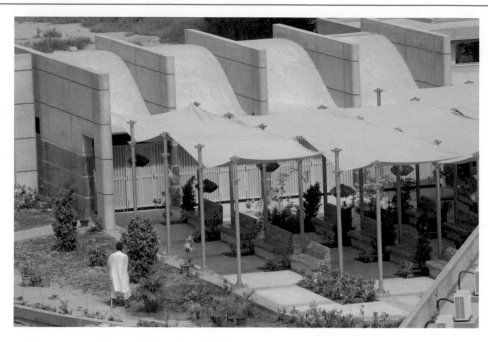

Figure 6.8 MDR-TB Clinic, Karachi, Pakistan, Tarique Alexander Qaiser, architect. Note wind scoop design in the main building and a covered outdoor waiting area to decrease crowding.

unsuspected TB cases either outside, with optimal ventilation, or inside in smaller groups to reduce transmission.

IMPORTANCE AND LIMITATIONS OF NATURAL VENTILATION

The Karachi example illustrates two of the optimal uses of natural ventilation: outdoor waiting areas and buildings designed to assure good airflow patterns. However, many buildings are not optimally designed, positioned, located, or operated for optimal natural ventilation, all day, every day, and in all seasons. Even in generally warm climates, windows are often closed at night to keep out cool air, for security or superstition, and to keep out vermin. Outdoor conditions change between day and night, by season, and wind velocity and direction can change constantly, favoring cross-contamination of rooms one second, preventing it the next. That said, in favorable climates such as Lima, Peru; Karachi, Pakistan; and Cape Town, South Africa, conditions are so consistent that generally good air disinfection can be achieved most of the time by simply keeping windows open.[9] But in high altitude Johannesburg, South Africa, for example, closed windows at night virtually assure air stagnation. In the very cold climates of Eastern Europe, Russia, and Central Asia, for example, natural ventilation is uncommonly a reliable means of air disinfection. Moreover, for heating efficiency by radiators and space heaters, windows are often made leak proof, reducing even natural infiltration of outside air.

MECHANICAL VENTILATION

Some buildings in TB high-burden settings have mechanical ventilation systems, but maintenance is an ongoing problem unless maintenance contracts are in place. Even if functioning properly, mechanical systems often mostly recirculate air with few outdoor air changes per hour (ACH). Recirculating air within a building contributes to dilution and redistribution, but not removal of infectious droplet nuclei. The risk near an infectious source may be reduced, but at the expense of a higher risk elsewhere in the building served by the heating/ventilation system for as long as droplet nuclei remain infectious.

Depending on occupancy, low outside air ventilation may be measurable as relatively high indoor CO_2 levels (above outside levels), indicating increased shared air breathing.[47] As noted above, personal monitoring of ambient CO_2 levels is being used to assess where during a typical day vulnerable persons experience the highest percentage of rebreathed air—at home, in school, on the bus, or in other congregate settings.[32, 48] As mentioned, as a research tool, we are using the same approach to assess buildings and their use from an airborne infection risk perspective. For example, do nurses working in a poorly ventilated emergency department experience a higher average rebreathed air fraction compared to nurses doing similar work in another building? Ambient CO_2 reflects building ventilation and occupancy, and personal average ambient CO_2 experience for occupants also reflects building usage by individuals or groups of individuals.

As mentioned, reducing indoor CO_2 levels by half by doubling ventilation results in half the risk of transmission. But also as noted, reducing the CO_2 levels by half again, requiring another doubling of ventilation, becomes increasingly impractical and expensive to achieve. The theoretical limits of protection by mechanical ventilation has been discussed in the literature.[4] High-level natural ventilation can overcome these limits, but as noted, is inherently inconsistent, and requires attention to building design, location, and operation. As also noted, the reduced ventilation often found in cold climates is increasingly found in hot climates where ductless cooling system are commonly being used in response to climate change. What alternative strategies are available when both natural and mechanical ventilation are not entirely reliable or protective?

UPPER ROOM GUV AIR DISINFECTION: THE ONLY PRACTICAL ALTERNATIVE TO NATURAL VENTILATION

The above claim may strike some as extreme, but consider the alternatives. Both natural and mechanical ventilation require outside air exchange for effective air disinfection, with a resulting energy cost associated with heating and cooling outdoor air for comfort. Upper room GUV air disinfection with air mixing works by inactivating airborne pathogens without energy losses due to exhausting air outside, and the need to heat, cool, and dehumidify outdoor air. With upper room GUV, outside air is required for comfort only—for odor control, for example. Here, we briefly discuss the general theory and application of upper room GUV, referring readers to published guidelines and reviews for details.[67,68]

GUV refers to short-wavelength UV (UV-C, 254–270 nm wavelength). For more than 70 years, upper room GUV lamps have been used in rooms, often with air mixing fans, to rapidly disinfect room air of airborne pathogens in the occupied space. Most commonly, GUV fixtures are mounted on walls as shown in Figure 6.9.

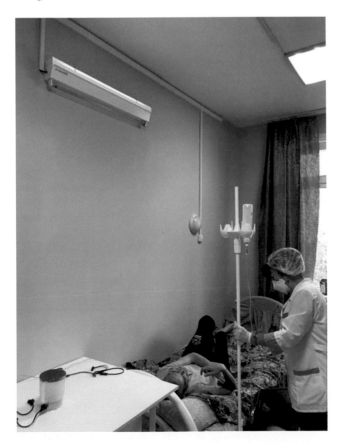

Figure 6.9 Upper room germicidal fixture in use in Russia.

Current upper room GUV utilizes mercury-based fluorescent lamps nearly identical to lamps commonly used for fluorescent room lighting. GUV differs in two ways: (1) utilize UV-transparent quartz or Vicor® glass to permit UV to escape the lamp, and (2) absent coating on the inner surface of GUV lamps that, in fluorescent lamps, produces visible light in response to UV. Good quality mercury lamps produce a narrow spike of 254 nm UV, close to the peak germicidal action spectrum of 265–270 nm, but less penetrating of skin and outer eye structures.[69–71] Newer LED GUV may be closer to 265–270 nm, more germicidal but also slightly more penetrating and potentially irritating. For safety reasons, upper room GUV fixtures are designed to confine UV irradiance to the space above peoples' heads. Although excessive direct or reflected exposure of eyes and skin to 254–270 nm UV will cause temporary irritation, properly applied germicidal UV does not cause skin cancer or cataracts because it is much less penetrating than longer wavelength UV A and B found in sunlight. A full discussion of GUV safety has been published.[72]

Despite repeated demonstrations of safety and efficacy, upper room GUV has not become a routine intervention like mechanical ventilation when air disinfection beyond natural ventilation is needed, even though it is demonstrably more effective, less expensive, and more easily adapted to existing buildings without major installation costs. Fear of UV overexposure and difficulty demonstrating efficacy are likely part of the reason for the limited adoption, as is lack of accessible expertise to plan and maintain GUV systems. Engineers trained in GUV air disinfection are available, but maintenance remains a problem for GUV and many other devices in hospitals. A maintenance manual on upper room GUV has been published by the Stop TB initiative in English, Spanish, and Russian (http://www.stoptb.org/wg/ett/assets/documents/MaintenanceManual.pdf).

The air disinfecting efficacy of upper room GUV with air mixing has been quantified three times in two very different hospital settings: an HIV ward in Peru with mostly DS TB, and an MDR-TB hospital in South Africa where the majority of patients are also HIV infected.[10,31] The most recent published study showed approximately 80% efficacy, or the equivalent of adding approximately 24 equivalent air changes to the existing 6 mechanical air changes on the ward. The effective dose was a total GUV fixture output of 17 mW/m³ of total room volume. Because air is well-mixed in the room, relevant dosing volume is the entire room, not just the irradiated volume. In that study, the average calculated UV *flux* (irradiance from multiple sources) was 6 μW/cm². A repeat study, not yet published, used less GUV flux (12 mW/m³) and also had excellent air disinfection. Based on these studies, we recommend the lower GUV dose of 12 mW/m³ total room volume.

After determining where upper room GUV is likely to be most useful, a knowledgeable GUV consultant needs to identify quality GUV fixtures, the output of which has been professionally measured by gonioradiometry or integrating sphere—two lighting laboratory methods of measuring total fixture output. It is impossible to rationally dose upper room GUV without knowing total fixture output, and ideally, total directional output, that is, gonioradiometry.[67,73] Many of the best GUV fixture manufacturers have had their fixture's output measured by established lighting laboratories. Knowing the risk areas, their room volumes and configurations, the consultant identifies locations for specific fixtures.

As important as providing sufficient upper room GUV energy (flux), adequate room air mixing is required. We recommend air turnover rates from low-velocity ceiling fans of 25 per hour. The direction of airflow, up or down, makes little difference to GUV efficacy since both directions produce airflow through the upper room. Fan speed is also not usually a critical factor. This is because more frequent, shorter transits of airborne infectious droplet nuclei through the upper room at higher fan speed, or fewer, longer exposures at low speeds result in approximately the same germicidal dose. Ideally, organisms reaching the upper, irradiated zone would be 100% inactivated on one pass, but residual exposure in the lower room still represents dramatic risk reduction for occupants.

Like new construction, before GUV systems are fully activated, they need to be commissioned, that is, tested for safety and efficacy under real-life conditions before occupants are exposed. Testing GUV systems requires a high-quality photometer sensitive at both high (upper room) and low (lower room) detection ranges. GUV systems should be re-checked every 3–6 months for lamp output and safety. The major causes of output deterioration are dust accumulation, lamp failure, or ballast failure. Although hospital staff can be trained to use a photometer properly, a better option, if available, is to hire a consultant, using frequently calibrated meters, with the correct specifications, trained to make accurate, reproducible measurements. Details on meter selection and use are available in a recently published GUV maintenance manual, referenced above.

ROOM AIR CLEANERS: PLAUSIBLE IN THEORY, BUT RARELY EFFECTIVE IN PRACTICE

Faced with unreliable natural ventilation, day and night, and season to season, and in cold climates, some facility managers purchase room air cleaners, promoted by companies as a simple, relatively inexpensive solution to air disinfection. They are generally not. As proof of efficacy, sales representatives for these devices often present data showing contaminated air entering the device, and nearly 100% decontaminated air leaving the device. What they rarely reveal is the clean air delivery rate, or CADR, essentially the flow rate of air through the machine. While it is not difficult to decontaminate air in a device using air filtration, irradiation, or even more exotic electrostatic or plasma technology, it is difficult to move enough air through the device to result in adequate numbers of equivalent air changes per hour (6–12 Eq ACH) to meet air disinfection recommendation.[74] To make matters worse, many room air cleaners by necessity have their air intake and outlet located close to one another, resulting in recapture of decontaminated air (short-circuiting), and an even lower *effective* air disinfection rate than suggested by the equivalent air changes per hour, calculated from the CADR. Disregarding the negative effects of short-circuiting of air, if a room air cleaner promoted in South Africa has a 28.3 lps CADR, and is placed in a small hospital isolation room with a 48 m³ (4×4 m, 3 m high ceilings) volume, an equivalent ACH of only 2.1 will result—less if any substantial

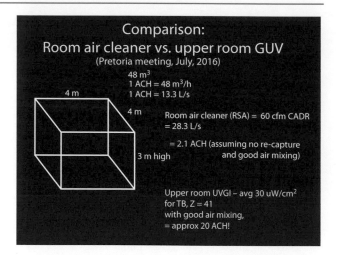

Figure 6.10 Comparision of room air cleaner vs. upper room GUV. In a hypothetical small room with a volume of 48 m³ one air cleaner with the clear air delivery rate specified would produce just 2.1 Eq ACH compared to more than 20 Eq ACH easily produced by GUV.

recapture (short-circuiting) occurs (Figure 6.10). In contrast, just one upper room GUV fixture providing 0.5 W total fixture output, with a ceiling fan, could provide approximately 20 EqACH based on the studies previously discussed. In other words, without inherent short-circuiting of air, 10 of these room air cleaners would be necessary to approach the air disinfecting effect of just one upper room GUV fixture and ceiling fan. Of course, larger room air cleaning devices are available, with much higher CADRs. Five such units, selected for optimal performance produced about 16 EqACH, and were tested twice in the South African Airborne Infection Research Facility in exactly the same way as upper room GUV had also been tested twice. The same ceiling fans were used to make conditions comparable. The results (unpublished) were surprisingly disappointing—approximately 20% protection compared to 80% with upper room GUV. The possible reasons for these poor results were thoroughly and independently investigated by the South African Council for Scientific and Industrial Research (CSIR). The CADR was re-checked and found to be correct. Some leakage around HEPA filters was found, but not enough to explain the poor results. Computerized fluid dynamic (CFD) studies failed to suggest competing interactions between the room air cleaners and the mechanical ventilation system of the AIR facility. As noted, a repeat study confirmed the poor results. Long experience with a variety of room air cleaners of many designs has convinced air disinfection experts that they are not a practical solution for most hospital and clinic applications. They may be occasionally useful in small rooms with ceilings too low (<8 m) for upper room UVGI. Where used, CADR should produce at least 6–12 Eq ACH, depending on their application.

RESPIRATORY PROTECTION, RESPIRATORS AND SURGICAL MASKS

By recent convention in the medical literature, face masks refer to surgical masks designed to protect the surgical field. Similar-looking face coverings to protect healthcare workers are called respirators. Surgical face masks stop large particles that exit the mouth or nose and can be loose fitting. For TB control they are often worn by potentially infectious patients to reduce the generation of airborne infectious droplet nuclei. This application of surgical masks is a form cough hygiene, like covering the nose or mouth with a hand or tissue. We tested the effectiveness of simple surgical masks for reducing *Mtb* transmission using the human-to-guinea-pig transmission test facility and found 56% efficacy under study conditions.[33] We did not test tighter fitting respirators for the purpose because they are too expensive for simple barrier use and are unlikely to be substantially more effective. Leakage around surgical masks with coughing is the major limitation and respirators are unlikely to resist the force of a cough. Surgical masks are also sometimes used to protect wearers from predominantly droplet spread infections, such as influenza—serving as a simple reminder not to touch your mouth with contaminated fingers, but they offer the wearer little protection from truly airborne infections such as *Mtb*.

For protecting healthcare workers from *Mtb* and other airborne infections, respirators rather than masks are used.[73-76] Respirators can be disposable, intended for limited re-use, or reusable "elastomeric" respirators with replaceable filters, primarily used in industry—although they can be economical compared to disposable masks for healthcare applications. Respirators differ from surgical masks by having a tight fit, usually designed with two elastic straps rather than one, and a design intended to create a seal to the face without gaps. Unlike surgical masks, the face-seal is critical in protecting the wearer from infection. People have a variety of face shapes that cannot be adequately fitted with any one style or size of respirator. Because face-seal leak is the major cause of respiratory protection failure, fit testing of respirators prior to selection for each wearer is required—using a distinctive volatile test substance (e.g., bitter tasting material, or banana oil) within a hood. Commercial respirator fit-testing kits are available, and a respirator fit-testing program can easily be implemented in high burden settings.[75] Given the high cost of disposable respirators and the danger of TB infection, an effective respiratory program must include fit testing and the availability of a variety of respirator models and sizes to assure adequate protection.

The major limitation of respiratory protection, apart from face-seal leak, is that they cannot be worn all day due to discomfort and may not be used when sharing air with a patient with unsuspected TB. They are essential for high-risk procedures such as bronchoscopy, autopsy, sputum induction, and other cough aerosol-generating procedures. They are far less important in caring for patients already started on effective therapy and rendered rapidly non-infectious, as noted above. Because of these limitations, respiratory protection is considered a third priority in the traditional hierarchy of airborne transmission controls—administrative, environmental (engineering), and respiratory protection. In this chapter we have prioritized FAST as a refocused, intensified approach to administrative TB transmission control, and natural ventilation as well as upper room GUV as environmental controls. There are many more comprehensive guidelines with additional details, as listed below.

MORE COMPREHENSIVE, EVIDENCE-BASED GUIDELINES

A revised WHO TB transmission control policy has recently been issued, and an accompanying implementation guide is being developed.[76] The policy document is limited by recommendations based on (scarce) hard evidence supplemented by expert opinion, whereas the implementation guide is less constrained, based on experience, with additional practical application advice.

We have presented some of experimental evidence favoring FAST and GUV, for example, but demonstrating the efficacy of most accepted interventions for preventing *Mtb* infection or disease in high burden settings has proven difficult. Sources of *Mtb* infection are common in the community; tuberculin reactivity is common among healthcare workers and in the community and confounded by BCG immunization. Newer gamma interferon release assays were designed to circumvent BCG confounding, but are expensive, complex tests, with limited routine application thus far in high burden settings.[77] *Mtb* contamination of air cannot be routinely measured, and quantifying infectiousness is even harder. Unlike drug trials, randomized-controlled clinical trials for TB prevention strategies are rare. In short, most interventions to prevent TB transmission in healthcare facilities are not supported by the highest level of data showing reduced infection or disease.

TREATMENT OF LATENT TB IN HEALTHCARE WORKERS

The treatment of latent infection is discussed elsewhere in this book. Healthcare workers are at increased risk of transmission and disease progression and should be considered for chemoprophylaxis—although this is uncommonly done in high burden settings as of this writing. It is done in low burden settings, ideally in response to true test conversions reflecting recent infection. Currently, treatment is sometimes offered in response to small changes in tuberculin skin test responses and IGRA results that may not reflect true, sustained infection.

REFERENCES

1. Behr MA, Edelstein PH, and Ramakrishnan L. Revisiting the timetable of tuberculosis. *BMJ*. 2018;362:k2738.
2. Yates TA et al. The transmission of *Mycobacterium tuberculosis* in high burden settings. *Lancet Infect Dis*. 2016;16:227–38.
3. American Thoracic Society. Targeted tuberculin testing and treatment of latent tuberculosis infection. *MMWR Recomm Rep*. 2000;49:1–51.
4. Nardell EA, Keegan J, Cheney SA, and Etkind SC. Airborne infection. Theoretical limits of protection achievable by building ventilation. *Am Rev Respir Dis*. 1991;144:302–6.
5. Willingham FF et al. Hospital control and multidrug-resistant pulmonary tuberculosis in female patients, Lima, Peru. *Emerg Infect Dis*. 2001;7:123–7.

6. Dharmadhikari AS et al. Rapid impact of effective treatment on transmission of multidrug-resistant tuberculosis. *Int J Tuberc Lung Dis.* 2014;18:1019–25.

7. Rouillion A PS, and Parrot R. Transmission of tubercle bacilli: The effects of chemotherapy. *Tubercle.* 57:275–99.

8. Barrera E, Livchits V, and Nardell E. F-A-S-T: A refocused, intensified, administrative tuberculosis transmission control strategy. *Int J Tuberc Lung Dis.* 2015;19:381–4.

9. Escombe AR et al. Natural ventilation for the prevention of airborne contagion. *PLoS Med.* 2007;4:e68.

10. Mphaphlele M et al. Institutional tuberculosis transmission. Controlled trial of upper room ultraviolet air disinfection: A basis for new dosing guidelines. *Am J Respir Crit Care Med.* 2015;192:477–84.

11. Bates M et al. Evaluation of the burden of unsuspected pulmonary tuberculosis and co-morbidity with non-communicable diseases in sputum producing adult inpatients. *PLOS ONE.* 2012;7:e40774.

12. Nardell E, and Macher J. *Respiratory Infections.* In: Macher J, (ed.) Cincinnati: ACGIH, 1999, 1–13.

13. Queval CJ, Brosch R, and Simeone R. The macrophage: A disputed fortress in the battle against *Mycobacterium tuberculosis. Front Microbiol.* 2017;8:2284.

14. Brennan PJ. Structure, function, and biogenesis of the cell wall of *Mycobacterium tuberculosis. Tuberculosis (Edinb).* 2003;83:91–7.

15. Garton NJ et al. Cytological and transcript analyses reveal fat and lazy persister-like bacilli in tuberculous sputum. *PLoS Med.* 2008;5:e75.

16. Warner DF, and Mizrahi V. Tuberculosis chemotherapy: The influence of bacillary stress and damage response pathways on drug efficacy. *Clin Microbiol Rev.* 2006;19:558–70.

17. Wells W. (ed.) *Airborne Contagion and Air Hygiene.* Cambridge: Harvard University Press, 1955.

18. Wells W, Ratcliff H, and Crumb C. On the mechanism of droplet nuclei infection II: Quantitative experimental airborne infection in rabbits. *Am J Hyg.* 1948;47:11.

19. Edwards DA et al. Inhaling to mitigate exhaled bioaerosols. *Proc Natl Acad Sci USA.* 2004;101:17383–8.

20. Nardell EA. Air sampling for tuberculosis—Homage to the lowly guinea pig. *Chest.* 1999;116:1143–5.

21. Nardell E. Wells revisited: Infectious particles vs quanta of *Mycobacterial tuberculosis* infection—Don't get them confused. *Mycobact Dis.* 2016;6.

22. Dharmadhikari AS et al. Natural infection of guinea pigs exposed to patients with highly drug-resistant tuberculosis. *Tuberculosis (Edinb).* 2011;91(4):329–38.

23. Lerner TR, Borel S, and Gutierrez MG. The innate immune response in human tuberculosis. *Cell Microbiol.* 2015;17:1277–85.

24. Sultan L, Nyka C, Mills C, O'Grady F, and Riley R. Tuberculosis disseminators—A study of variability of aerial infectivity of tuberculosis patients. *Am Rev Respir Dis.* 1960;82:358–69.

25. Catanzaro A. Nosocomial tuberculosis. *Am Rev Respir Dis.* 1982;125:559–62.

26. Riley RL MC et al. Aerial dissemination of pulmonary tuberculosis: A two-year study of contagion in a tuberculosis ward: 1959. *Am J Epidemiol.* 1995;142:3–14.

27. Riley RL. The contagiosity of tuberculosis. *Schweiz Med Wochenschr.* 1983;113:75–9.

28. Riley R, and Permutt S. Room air disinfection by ultraviolet irradiation of upper air—Air mixing and germicidal effectiveness. *Arch Environ Health.* 1971;22:208–19.

29. Riley R. Aerial dissemination of pulmonary tuberculosis—The Burns Amberson Lecture. *Am Rev Tuberc Pulmon Dis.* 1957;76:931–41.

30. Fennelly KP, Martyny JW, Fulton KE, Orme IM, Cave DM, and Heifets LB. Cough-generated aerosols of *Mycobacterium tuberculosis*: A new method to study infectiousness. *Am J Respir Crit Care Med.* 2004;169:604–9.

31. Escombe AR et al. Upper-room ultraviolet light and negative air ionization to prevent tuberculosis transmission. *PLoS Med.* 2009;6:e43.

32. Andrews JR, Morrow C, Walensky RP, and Wood R. Integrating social contact and environmental data in evaluating tuberculosis transmission in a South African township. *J Infect Dis.* 2014;210:597–603.

33. Dharmadhikari AS et al. Surgical face masks worn by patients with multidrug-resistant tuberculosis: Impact on infectivity of air on a hospital ward. *Am J Respir Crit Care Med.* 2012;185:1104–9.

34. Dharmadhikari AS, and Nardell EA. What animal models teach humans about tuberculosis. *Am J Respir Cell Mol Biol.* 2008;39:503–8.

35. Khan N, Vidyarthi A, Javed S, and Agrewala JN. Innate immunity holding the flanks until reinforced by adaptive immunity against *Mycobacterium tuberculosis* infection. *Front Microbiol.* 2016;7:328.

36. Nardell EA, and Wallis RS. Here today—Gone tomorrow: The case for transient acute tuberculosis infection. *Am J Respir Crit Care Med.* 2006;174:734–5.

37. Orme IM, and Ordway DJ. Mouse and guinea pig models of tuberculosis. *Microbiol Spectr.* 2016;4.

38. Escombe AR et al. The detection of airborne transmission of tuberculosis from HIV-infected patients, using an *in vivo* air sampling model. *Clin Infect Dis.* 2007;44:1349–57.

39. Riley RL, Mills CC, O'grady F, Sultan LU, Wittstadt F, and Shivpuri DN. Infectiousness of air from a tuberculosis ward. Ultraviolet irradiation of infected air: Comparative infectiousness of different patients. *Am Rev Respir Dis.* 1962;85:511–25.

40. Mphahlele MDA et al. Highly effective upper room ultraviolet germicidal air disinfection (UVGI) on an MDR-TB ward in Sub-Saharan Africa. 2009.

41. Smith D, and Wiengeshaus E. What animal models can teach us about the pathogenesis of tuberculosis in humans. *Rev Infect Dis.* 1989;11:S385–S93.

42. Grzybowski S, Barnett G, and Styblo K. Contacts of cases of active pulmonary tuberculosis. *Select Papers Roy Netherlands Tuber Assoc.* 1975;16:90–9.

43. Riley E, Murphy G, and Riley R. Airborne spread of measles in a suburban elementary school. *Am J Epidemiol.* 1978;107:421–32.

44. Gammaitoni L, and Nucci MC. Using a mathematical model to evaluate the efficacy of TB control measures. *Emerg Infect Dis.* 1997;3:335–42.

45. Forrellad MA et al. Virulence factors of the *Mycobacterium tuberculosis* complex. *Virulence.* 2013;4:3–66.

46. Manca C et al. *Mycobacterium tuberculosis* CDC1551 induces a more vigorous host response *in vivo* and *in vitro*, but is not more virulent than other clinical isolates. *J Immunol.* 1999;162:6740–6.

47. Rudnick SN, and Milton DK. Risk of indoor airborne infection transmission estimated from carbon dioxide concentration. *Indoor Air.* 2003;13:237–45.

48. Andrews JR, Morrow C, and Wood R. Modeling the role of public transportation in sustaining tuberculosis transmission in South Africa. *Am J Epidemiol.* 2013;177:556–61.

49. Joosten SA et al. Mycobacterial growth inhibition is associated with trained innate immunity. *J Clin Invest.* 2018;128:1837–51.

50. Kaufmann E et al. BCG educates hematopoietic stem cells to generate protective innate immunity against tuberculosis. *Cell.* 2018;172:176–90 e19.

51. Brighenti S, and Joosten SA. Friends and foes of tuberculosis: Modulation of protective immunity. *J Intern Med.* 2018. doi: 10.1111/joim.12778.

52. Arts RJW et al. Immunometabolic pathways in BCG-induced trained immunity. *Cell Rep*. 2016;17:2562–71.

53. Stead WW, Senner JW, Reddick WT, and Lofgren JP. Racial differences in susceptibility to infection by *Mycobacterium tuberculosis* [see comments]. *N Engl J Med*. 1990;322:422–7.

54. Andrews RH, Devadatta S, Fox W, Radhakrishna S, Ramakrishnan CV, and Velu S. Prevalence of tuberculosis among close family contacts of tuberculous patients in South India, and influence of segregation of the patient on early attack rate. *Bull World Health Organ*. 1960;23:463–510.

55. Le H et al. Process measure of FAST tuberculosis infection control demonstrates delay in likely effective treatment. *Int J Tuberc Lung Dis*. 2019;23:140–6.

56. Nathavitharana RR et al. FAST implementation in Bangladesh: High frequency of unsuspected tuberculosis justifies challenges of scale-up. *Int J Tuberc Lung Dis*. 2017;21:1020–5.

57. Miller AC et al. Turning off the tap: Using the FAST approach to stop the spread of drug-resistant tuberculosis in Russian Federation. *J Infect Dis*. 2018;218(4):654–58.

58. Kendall EA, Fofana MO, and Dowdy DW. Burden of transmitted multidrug resistance in epidemics of tuberculosis: A transmission modelling analysis. *Lancet Respir Med*. 2015;3:963–72.

59. WHO. Global Tuberculosis Report. In: Department ST, (ed.) Geneva: WHO, 2016.

60. Gelmanova IY et al. Non-adherence, default, and the acquisition of multidrug resistance in a tuberculosis treatment program in Tomsk, Siberia. (submitted for publication - to be resolved or listed as personal communication before publication).

61. Andrews JR et al. Exogenous reinfection as a cause of multidrug-resistant and extensively drug-resistant tuberculosis in rural South Africa. *J Infect Dis*. 2008;198:1582–9.

62. Andrews JR, Noubary F, Walensky RP, Cerda R, Losina E, and Horsburgh CR. Risk of progression to active tuberculosis following reinfection with *Mycobacterium tuberculosis*. *Clin Infect Dis*. 2012;54:784–91.

63. Moodley P et al. Spread of extensively drug-resistant tuberculosis in KwaZulu-Natal province, South Africa. *PLOS ONE*. 2011;6:e17513.

64. Lim JR et al. Incidence and geographic distribution of extensively drug-resistant tuberculosis in KwaZulu-Natal Province, South Africa. *PLOS ONE*. 2015;10:e0132076.

65. Gandhi NR et al. Extensively drug-resistant tuberculosis as a cause of death in patients co-infected with tuberculosis and HIV in a rural area of South Africa. *Lancet*. 2006;368:1575–80.

66. Davis LW, and Gertler PJ. Contribution of air conditioning adoption to future energy use under global warming. *Proc Natl Acad Sci USA*. 2015;112:5962–7.

67. Nardell E, Vincent R, and Sliney DH. Upper-room ultraviolet germicidal irradiation (UVGI) for air disinfection: A symposium in print. *Photochem Photobiol*. 2013;89:764–9.

68. Nardell EA. Environmental infection control of tuberculosis. *Semin Respir Infect*. 2003;18:307–19.

69. Brickner PW, Vincent RL, First M, Nardell E, Murray M, and Kaufman W. The application of ultraviolet germicidal irradiation to control transmission of airborne disease: Bioterrorism countermeasure. *Public Health Rep*. 2003;118:99–114.

70. First M, Nardell E, Chaission W, and Riley R. Guidelines for the application of upper-room ultraviolet germicidal irradiation for preventing transmission of airborne contagion—Part II: Design and operations guidance. *ASHRAE Trans*. 1999;105:877–87.

71. First M, Nardell E, Chaission W, and Riley R. Guidelines for the application of upper-room ultraviolet germicidal irradiation for preventing transmission of airborne contagion—Part I: Basic principles. *ASHRAE Trans*. 1999;105:869–76.

72. Nardell EA et al. Safety of upper-room ultraviolet germicidal air disinfection for room occupants: Results from the Tuberculosis Ultraviolet Shelter Study. *Public Health Rep*. 2008;123:52–60.

73. Zhang J et al. A radiometry protocol for UVGI fixtures using a moving-mirror type gonioradiometer. *J Occup Environ Hyg*. 2012;9:140–8.

74. Miller-Leiden S, Lobascio C, Nazaroff WW, and Macher JM. Effectiveness of in-room air filtration and dilution ventilation for tuberculosis infection control. *J Air Waste Manag Assoc*. 1996;46:869–82.

75. Campbell DL, Coffey CC, Jensen PA, and Zhuang Z. Reducing respirator fit test errors: A multi-donning approach. *J Occup Environ Hyg*. 2005;2:391–99.

76. *WHO Guidelines on Tuberculosis Infection Prevention and control: 2019 Update*. Geneva: 2019.

77. Pollock NR et al. Interferon gamma-release assays for diagnosis of latent tuberculosis in healthcare workers in low-incidence settings: Pros and cons. *Clin Chem*. 2014;60:714–8.

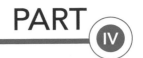

PART IV

DIAGNOSIS OF ACTIVE DISEASE AND LATENT INFECTION

7

Diagnosis of Active Pulmonary Tuberculosis

J. LUCIAN DAVIS

DIAGNOSIS OF PULMONARY TB IN A PUBLIC HEALTH CONTEXT

Globally, an estimated 10 million people developed incident tuberculosis (TB) in 2018, but nearly 30% of these individuals were never reported to public health authorities.[1] Sometimes referred to as the "missing 3 million," these individuals either never sought care because they did not have symptoms or access to diagnostic evaluation services, sought care but were not diagnosed with TB, or were diagnosed with TB but never notified to national TB authorities.[2] Undiagnosed TB is associated with substantial morbidity and mortality and with ongoing TB transmission in the community, a fact that makes improving performance and delivery of diagnostic testing services a leading priority for control and elimination of TB worldwide.[3] Nevertheless, to be effective, novel tests must facilitate early treatment initiation to minimize individual complications and prevent further TB transmission in the community. It is also important to note that TB testing itself is often time-consuming and expensive, irrespective of the diagnostic result. Thus, the major objectives of TB diagnostic evaluation should be to maximize the proportion of individuals who obtain timely and accurate diagnosis and treatment; to minimize the proportion who are harmed by missed diagnoses, delayed diagnoses, over-testing, and over-treatment; and to prevent individuals and their households from experiencing catastrophic financial costs.

The World Health Organization's annual report on the global and local epidemiology of TB provides critical context for understanding TB diagnostic practices around the world. The key indicator for evaluating diagnostic performance is known as "TB treatment coverage," and represents the ratio of annual TB case notifications to estimated annual TB incidence. The accuracy of this indicator may be limited by under-reporting of TB diagnoses, especially from the private and non-governmental sectors, and by uncertainty in TB disease estimates that are derived from country-specific mathematical models. Nonetheless, the indicator is valuable for following national trends and comparing the relative quality and effectiveness of national TB programs in detecting and initiating treatment for TB patients. The wide range in TB treatment coverage rates between countries illustrates substantial variation in the quality of TB diagnostic services between countries. In high-incidence, low-income communities that account for the majority of the world's undiagnosed TB patients, limitations in patient access to healthcare facilities and in the availability of high-quality TB diagnostic services at these facilities contributes to low TB case detection rates and high mortality from undiagnosed TB. In contrast, in low-incidence, high-income countries where clinicians encounter TB patients less frequently, missed diagnoses with resulting higher morbidity and mortality may still be common, in spite of the greater availability of high-level diagnostic capacity. Worldwide, persons living with HIV (PLWH) account for approximately 10% of all TB patients, but over a quarter of all fatalities.[4] While TB prevalence and incidence are declining among PLWH, PLWH experience unique diagnostic challenges. For example, PLWH have higher levels of poverty and stigma, which make accessing care more difficult, and also tend to have more rapidly progressive but more paucibacillary forms of TB. This combination of factors helps explain the reduced sensitivity and clinical impact of TB diagnostics among PLWH.[5] Finally, treatment coverage ratios are particularly low for individuals with drug-resistant TB: although multidrug-resistant TB affects at least a half-million new individuals each year, only about one-third receive treatment.[1] Because multiple barriers to TB diagnosis exist and vary widely between settings, the TB diagnostic process must be grounded in knowledge of local epidemics.[4]

In recent years, multiple advances in TB testing have made it more likely that widely deployable, low-cost technologies will someday close the gaps that prevent early, accurate TB case identification. This process began with new WHO diagnostic policies that reduced the number of samples required for sputum smear microscopy, simplified interpretation of microscopy results, and approved several low-cost culture methods.[6–8] In addition, the WHO issued its first-ever negative diagnostic recommendation, against the use of inaccurate commercial serodiagnostic tests for TB, a recommendation that highlighted the harms of using unvalidated commercial diagnostics.[9] Over the last decade, new WHO policies have inaugurated a new era of molecular diagnostics in low- and middle-income countries, beginning with the approval of line-probe assays for diagnosis of drug-resistant TB and semi-automated nucleic acid amplification assays for both drug-susceptible and drug-resistant TB. Whole-genome sequencing, now standard in public health laboratories in several high-income countries, promises to further revolutionize the diagnosis and management of drug-resistant TB. In 2015, the WHO approved the first non-sputum-based, point-of-care diagnostic test for TB, the urinary lipoarabinomannan (LAM) assay. This and later generation assays represent an important development as the first truly point-of-care technologies for TB diagnosis.[10]

The rapid progress in introducing new diagnostics with improved sensitivity and turn-around time has been welcome, but their impact on patient-important outcomes remains unclear. Unfortunately, regulatory bodies do not require such information for their approval processes and few studies report measures of patient impact.[11,12] Without further advances that demonstrate integrated strategies for driving down TB incidence, TB mortality, and catastrophic costs of TB, it will be difficult to advance the larger END TB Strategy goals of eliminating TB as a public health threat by 2035.[13] There is a greater need than ever for translational research in real-world settings to produce the next generation of diagnostics that can leapfrog current resource limitations and engage patients and providers.[14]

In this chapter, we focus on the principles, tools, and practices that support a high-quality evaluation for pulmonary TB. We first outline key principles of diagnostic evaluation for TB, then provide an overview of the role of the clinical history and physical examination in screening patients for active pulmonary TB. We then discuss sample collection for diagnostic testing, and conclude with a review of current and emerging diagnostic tests for TB, focusing on the principles underlying these new technologies and drawing examples from the tests most commonly implemented in routine clinical and public health practice. Table 7.1 summarizes the sensitivity and specificity of routinely available diagnostic tests for active pulmonary TB, including clinical symptoms, chest radiography, and other commonly used tests.

GUIDING PRINCIPLES OF TB DIAGNOSTIC EVALUATION

A thorough and accurate diagnostic evaluation for TB requires that clinicians integrate information from the clinical assessment with knowledge of the performance of different testing strategies using a formal or informal likelihood-based approach.[15] A fundamental aspect of diagnostic testing for TB and other diseases is that sensitivity varies widely between settings, and statistical heterogeneity is almost universally reported in systematic reviews of diagnostic test accuracy.[16] Common reasons for this variability in performance are worth noting here. First, the predictive value of diagnostic testing depends on the prior probability of disease, which is informed by knowledge of the local prevalence of the disease within the general population or within specific communities or populations to which the patient belongs. Second, the accuracy of diagnostic tests depends on the severity or spectrum of disease in the population being evaluated, as determined by the burden and distribution of *Mtb* bacilli, and/or the host response. For example, more severe illness usually increases the sensitivity of the clinical history, physical findings, and inflammatory markers for TB, often at the cost of lower specificity. In contrast, immunosuppressed patients may become ill with a lower burden of bacilli, and more commonly with extrapulmonary manifestations, reducing the sensitivity of sputum microbiologic assays for TB. Finally, performance depends on the quality with which tests are performed, so that automation, inclusion of internal controls, and external quality assurance programs are important strategies for improving accuracy and reproducibility.

The second important principle of TB diagnostics is that given the expected heterogeneity of presentation and performance, no single diagnostic test has been identified as well-suited to all settings. Moving testing closer to the point-of-care is desirable if accuracy and quality can be assured, as this is likely to make TB diagnostic evaluation more patient-centered. To do so, the ideal test would be simple, affordable, reliable, reproducible, rapid, sensitive, and specific, as well as deliverable without need for electricity, maintenance, or additional supplies or equipment.[14] It would detect both drug-susceptible and drug-resistant TB, and provide information on disease severity and prognosis. Because no single test is likely to have all desirable features, it is valuable to define different test phenotypes according to where they may fit into standard diagnostic pathways.[17] Thus, WHO has identified four high priority test types for diagnostic development and created target product profiles (TPPs) for each.[18] The first of these, a community-based triage or referral test, would improve TB screening by reducing the number of individuals who require confirmatory testing using a costly reference standard assay (i.e., nucleic acid amplification testing [NAAT] or mycobacterial culture). According to WHO, a useful triage test should provide high sensitivity ($\geq$90%) and moderate specificity ($\geq$70%) for active TB disease at low cost (<US$2) and with a short turn-around time (<30 minutes). The second test type, a rapid (<1 hour), sputum-based test for detecting TB in primary-care settings should have higher sensitivity and similar or higher specificity than smear

Table 7.1 Sensitivity and specificity of routinely available diagnostic tests for TB

Assay	Sensitivity (95% CI)	Specificity (95% CI)	Reference standard[f]	Number of studies	Number of patients	Citation
Prolonged cough[a]	35% (24–46)	95% (93–97)	Microscopy and/or culture	8	223,402	(21,24)
Any TB symptom[b]	77% (68–86)	68% (50–85)	Microscopy and/or culture	8	218,476	(21,24)
PLWH ART-naive	89% (83–94)	28% (19–40)		16	8,664	(25)
PLWH on ART	51% (28–73)	71% (48–86)		7	4,640	(25)
Chest x-ray						
Any abnormality	98% (95–100)	75% (72–79)	Microscopy, culture	3	72,065	(21,24)
TB abnormality	87% (79–95)	89% (87–92)	Microscopy, culture	5	163,646	
Microscopy						
Direct (LED FM)	73% (61–85)	97% (97–100)	Culture	23	19,797	(117)
Processed[c]	+12% (CI 1-22)	98% (92–100)[d]	Culture	4	3,609	(59)
Urinary LAM						
PLWH[e]	59% (43–77)	78% (64–88)	Culture or NAAT	6	2,402	(118)
GeneXpert						
MTB/RIF	85% (82–88)	98% (97–98)	Culture	70	37,237	(77)
Ultra	88% (85–91)	96% (94–97)	Culture	1	1,439	(103)

Abbreviations: ART, antiretroviral therapy; CI, confidence interval; NAAT, nucleic acid amplification test, PLWH, persons living with HIV; TB, tuberculosis.
[a] Prolonged cough is defined as lasting ≥2–3 weeks.
[b] Any symptom includes cough of any duration, fever, chills, night sweats, and/or weight loss
[c] Three studies of concentrated N-acetylcysteine (NALC)–sodium hydroxide (NaOH) processing method, and one of sodium hypochlorite (NaOCl) processing with polycarbonate membrane filtration.
[d] Range rather than 95% CI reported in parentheses.
[e] Median CD4 count in six studies ranged from 71 to 210.
[f] All reference standard tests performed on sputum.

microscopy at modest cost (<US$6). The third, a rapid (<1 hour), biomarker-based, non-sputum test should be as accurate as smear microscopy for pulmonary TB but should also be able to detect extrapulmonary TB and pediatric TB. A non-sputum test should also be inexpensive (<US$6) and simple enough to be offered in clinic and community settings without need for biosafety protocols that sputum tests require. Finally, in areas with a high prevalence of drug-resistance, there is a need for a rapid (<2 hours), next-generation, drug-susceptibility assay deployable in primary care settings and above. This assay would serve as an add-on test for individuals in whom a diagnosis of active TB has been confirmed via other methods.

HISTORY AND PHYSICAL EXAMINATION

The history and physical examination provide an important starting point in the diagnostic evaluation of active TB disease. A careful assessment by a competent clinician is among the most rapid and lowest cost screening tests available, and recognizing the many clinical presentations of TB is essential to obtaining additional directed diagnostic testing to confirm the diagnosis.

Furthermore, a well-done history and physical helps ground subsequent testing and interpretation of results in the patient's clinical and epidemiological circumstances.[19]

The classic symptoms of pulmonary TB can be identified by taking a careful clinical history, in which patients should be asked about the presence of cough and its duration; the presence of sputum and its physical appearance; and the presence and duration of fever, chills, night sweats, and weight loss. Among children, the failure to grow taller and gain weight appropriately should be explored as this may precede weight loss. A comprehensive history and physical should also investigate any other physical complaints or abnormalities. These may suggest extrapulmonary manifestations of TB, and may provide additional opportunities for diagnostic confirmation of TB (e.g., fine-needle aspiration of palpable lymph nodes). Thus, a comprehensive history should explore any other physical complaints or abnormalities noted by the patient. For example, the presence of headache, confusion, neck stiffness, or motor weakness could indicate TB of the central nervous system; eye pain, blurry vision, or photophobia should raise concern for uveitis; back pain could implicate spinal TB; and shortness of breath might indicate pulmonary, pericardial, or pleural TB.

Symptom screening is the most commonly used triage test for TB. The International Standards of TB Care recommend that a criterion of cough of two to three weeks' duration be used as a screening question to identify individuals who should be further evaluated for TB.[20] This range in the duration of cough that should prompt evaluation acknowledges that cough has different performance characteristics in different clinical settings and in different parts of the world. In a systematic review carried out by the WHO to inform global policy recommendations on screening for active TB, the diagnostic performance of prolonged cough was found to have 25% sensitivity and 96% specificity in low HIV-prevalence settings in Asia and 49% sensitivity and 92% specificity in high HIV-prevalence areas of sub-Saharan Africa, although wide confidence intervals surrounded these estimates.[21] In a large, community-level cluster-randomized trial in communities in Zambia and South Africa with a high prevalence of HIV, cough had a sensitivity of only 25%, while the combination of cough of any duration, fever, chills, night sweats, or weight loss was sensitive enough to detect TB in only 40% of all TB patients.[22] In the WHO-commissioned systematic review, the presence of any of these symptoms of TB was 77% sensitive and 68% specific for active TB, again with wide precision estimates. A limitation is that almost all of the contributing studies are community-based prevalence studies, and therefore likely underestimate the sensitivity and overestimate the specificity of symptoms among patients undergoing evaluation in health facilities.

One population for whom symptoms have particularly high sensitivity are PLWH. The so-called "four-symptom rule"—the reported presence of cough of any duration, fever, night sweats, or weight loss of at least three kilograms—has an extremely high sensitivity of 99% for active TB among PLWH, although the specificity of these criteria is only 30%. This combination of symptoms was identified through a systematic review of the performance and yield of many different combinations of symptoms, and in 2011 WHO recommended that these be used as the standard criteria for screening of all PLWH.[23] WHO undertook a similar evidence review process in 2011 to provide recommendations for TB screening among individuals without HIV.[24] A 2018 update of this systematic review highlights the important finding that comparing studies enrolling populations taking antiretroviral therapy to those not taking antiretroviral therapy, the four-symptom rule has a substantially lower sensitivity (51% vs. 89%) and higher specificity (71% vs. 28%).[25] The authors conclude that additional screening tests beyond symptoms should be incorporated into diagnostic testing algorithms for PLWH on antiretroviral therapy (ART).

In addition to a detailed review of the clinical history by system, a careful history should also inquire about past medical history of active TB; close contact with individuals with confirmed or possible active pulmonary TB; or prior history of TB infection (as defined by a positive tuberculin skin test or interferon gamma release assay). In the context of prior TB exposure or latent infection, risk factors for progression from latent to active TB, such as immunosuppression due to HIV or pharmacologic therapy, diabetes, and chronic kidney disease, are particularly relevant.[26]

The physical exam should usually be focused, and follow-up on the findings of the clinical history. However, if there are risk factors for extra-pulmonary TB, such as being a PLWH and/or reporting localizing symptoms outside the respiratory system, a more comprehensive physical exam is recommended. In patients for whom the history suggests TB, the physical exam should assess specific organ systems that are most commonly or most severely affected by extra-pulmonary TB: a comprehensive neurological examination to screen for meningitis, vertebral TB (Pott's disease), or TB discitis; examination for cervical, axillary, or inguinal lymphadenopathy without tenderness, cutaneous warmth or erythema; examination for abnormal breath sounds, decreased vocal fremitus and dullness to percussion suggestive of a pleural effusion; distant heart sounds and/or *pulsus alternans* suggestive of a pericardial effusion; ascites suggestive of peritoneal TB; and/or large, discrete, firm, red, raised skin nodules in a pretibial distribution consistent with *erythema nodosum*.

CHEST RADIOGRAPHY

Chest radiography is among the most widely used tests to screen for pulmonary TB. Where accessible, it is performed either as a routine part of TB diagnostic evaluation or, in more resource-constrained settings, as a follow-on test in individuals who are unable to produce sputum or test negative on rapid microbiologic examination of sputum (e.g., by smear microscopy or NAAT). Other groups in whom chest radiography is strongly recommended are persons living with HIV (PLWH), and individuals in whom chest radiography may influence additional diagnostic evaluation (e.g., physical findings suggestive of pleural effusion) or management (e.g., a patient with significant hemoptysis in whom bronchoscopy or other intervention may be indicated). During active case finding in community settings where individuals predominantly have asymptomatic and pre-clinical disease, chest radiography may dramatically increase the yield of TB diagnoses, as shown by the experience with mass radiographic screening in high-income countries at the beginning of the chemotherapy era and by more recent TB prevalence surveys in many countries.[21] This experience has promoted substantial interest in emerging, low-cost, portable digital radiography with computer-aided interpretation.

The radiographic manifestations of pulmonary TB depend on the stages of infection and disease. During primary TB, the formation of a granuloma may lead to a focal scar or persistent nodule of the parenchyma, called a Ghon lesion, and occasionally calcified lymph nodes in the hila and/or mediastinum which if seen all together are termed a Ranke complex.[27] In a significant minority of individuals, these radiographic abnormalities will persist as a scar or thickening with or without calcifications, with the clinical significance that they will be detectable on screening chest radiography or computed tomography (CT) for a lifetime. Individuals who fail to control a primary TB infection may develop a tuberculoma, or a focal or lobar infiltrate; up to 25% of individuals may have multifocal disease.[27] Among the most common and distinctive radiographic manifestations of TB are cavities, often found in the upper lung fields. Another distinctive but rare radiographic finding of TB is a diffuse and random micronodular pattern, which is highly specific for disseminated, also known as miliary, TB. It was once thought that primary disease presented with mid- and lower-lung zone infiltrates while only post-primary disease gave upper lobe infiltrates and cavities represent post-primary disease, the use of molecular epidemiology to differentiate between recently and remotely transmitted infections does not support that dogma.[28] Among individuals living with HIV, findings may often present atypically as simple pulmonary infiltrates, with manifestations more atypical among PLWH as CD4 count declines.[29,30] A substantial proportion may even have normal-appearing chest radiography, although infiltrates may blossom due to immune reconstitution after initiation of antiretroviral therapy.[31,32]

Although a subset of individuals with early-stage pulmonary TB may have negative chest radiography, the sensitivity of chest radiography is generally high; the greater limitation is poor specificity, especially among patients with advanced HIV, pre-existing chronic lung disease, and other acute pulmonary infections. In a 2013 WHO-sponsored systematic review, any abnormality on CXR had a sensitivity of 98% and a specificity of 75%. When only abnormalities deemed consistent with TB were considered, sensitivity was 87%, and specificity 89%.[21] When added to screening using the four-symptom rule among PLWH, chest radiography substantially increases the sensitivity for TB primarily among those taking ART (from 51% to 85%), albeit with a major loss of specificity (from 71% to 30%). The increment in sensitivity gained by adding chest radiography to symptom screening is much less for those not on ART (from 89% to 94%), but the loss in specificity is also diminished (from 28% to 20%).[25]

Given the wide variety of radiographic manifestations of TB and the variable performance of chest radiography, researchers have sought to develop standardized scoring systems to make interpretation simpler and more reproducible. A recent systematic review found that scoring systems provide high sensitivity (median 96%), but low specificity (median 46%).[33] An alternative approach involves the use of computer-aided detection (CAD) not only for standardization but also to reduce the workload for radiologists or technician screeners, a particular need in the use of radiography active case finding. To date, the few high-quality studies examining CAD performance show that it can provide high sensitivity and modest specificity, comparable to the results obtained for scoring systems applied by human readers.[34] This technology may help reduce the number of confirmatory tests when used in mass screening.[35]

SPECIMEN COLLECTION METHODS

SPUTUM EXPECTORATION

Examination of a sample from the lower respiratory tract—expectorated sputum, most commonly; induced sputum; or specimens obtained during bronchoscopy—is an essential initial step in testing for pulmonary TB using smear microscopy, NAAT, or mycobacterial culture. Obtaining high-quality sputum specimens is likely important but can be challenging. Expert guidance and long-standing practice recommends that the quality of a specimen be judged by an adequate volume of sputum (e.g., ≥ 0.5 mL) and gross appearance (i.e., sputum, not saliva), although there is little published evidence supporting this dogma.[36,37]

Sputum for examination may be obtained by expectoration or induction. Obtaining good quality sputum requires care in collection. Expectorated sputum should be procured by a trained and experienced health worker. WHO guidelines on sputum collection for smear microscopy recommend that a health worker follow three steps to instruct a patient how to expectorate good quality sputum, as follows. The health worker should instruct the patient to (1) take three deep breaths immediately prior to collection, (2) cough forcefully, and (3) produce sputum rather than saliva, with the appearance demonstrated to the participant using a visual aid.[38] In a study from Pakistan, instruction prior to expectoration was associated with a 63% increase in the yield of positive sputum examinations among women, although not among men.[39] A randomized-controlled trial evaluating the impact of a sputum instruction video in Tanzania was associated with a greater than two-fold increase in the proportion of men and women who tested positive, as well as increases in sputum volume and a decrease in the proportion of salivary specimens.[40] While an older practice was to reject salivary specimens for microscopic examination, current guidelines recommend that the best available specimen be examined, provided it is properly labeled with the appropriate patient identifiers and correctly packaged in a well-sealed container.[38] Specimens with a salivary appearance may still provide a positive microbiologic diagnosis with smear microscopy, and at least one large study suggests that when examined using NAATs, salivary sputum may provide higher sensitivity than other sputum types.[41] Thus, it is recommended that all respiratory specimens submitted to the laboratory be examined, especially when no other specimen can be obtained, and any concerns about the effects of the quality of the specimen on the results be explained as an annotation to the result at the time of reporting so that the clinician can adjust the interpretation.

Another important aspect of sputum examination relates to the number, time of collection, and duration of collection of specimens. Since 2007, WHO has recommended that only two sputum specimens per patient be collected for examination by smear microscopy.[6] In 2012, WHO approved a novel sputum collection approach called same-day microscopy,[42] based on high-quality data showing that examination of two samples collected one hour apart provides a similar diagnostic yield as two samples collected on different days, with reduced rates of initial losses to follow-up.[43] Early morning sputum collection has long been recommended to maximize yield of sputum smear examination, but requiring patients to return to health facilities has been associated with high rate of drop-out from the diagnostic process. Two recent high-quality studies,[44] including a systematic review of 23 studies comprising 8967 individuals undergoing evaluation for active TB,[45] found that early-morning sputum collection provided no statistically significant increase in diagnostic yield over randomly timed, "on-the-spot" sputum collection. Even pooled overnight sputum collection did not have a higher yield than spot collection directly observed by a health worker with instructions on how to produce a good quality sputum sample. There are many benefits for patients, providers, and public health in completing sputum evaluation in a single visit, including earlier diagnosis, greater convenience, and reduced costs for patients; fewer episodes of care for providers, and reduced losses to follow-up for public health.[47-49]

There are a number of operational limitations of sputum collection for TB diagnosis. Most important are infection control concerns, as expectorating sputum produces cough aerosols which may lead to nosocomial spread of TB. Thus, health workers should wear personal protective equipment such as N95 particulate respirators, and, where resources allow, sputum and respiratory samples should be collected in rooms equipped with negative-pressure ventilation and high-efficiency particulate exhaust systems; sterilization of the air with ultraviolet germicidal irradiation (UVGI) following the procedure adds an additional measure of protection.[50] If such facilities are not available, specimens should be collected away from other patients where there is adequate natural ventilation and plenty of sunlight. Second, not all patients are able to expectorate sputum, especially young children. At least 1–5 mL of good quality, non-salivary sputum, should be collected, but the best available specimen should be analyzed.[38] In individuals who cannot expectorate on an initial request and with coaching, it is worth making a second request for sputum at a later time, before moving on to sputum induction or bronchoscopy.

SPUTUM INDUCTION

In patients unable to produce sputum after coughing, a 15-minute treatment with hypertonic saline aerosolized using an ultrasonic nebulizer or pneumatic compressor and delivered via high-flow air through a mouthpiece is a well-established procedure to induce coughing and expectoration of a sample from the lower airways. Usually administered in concentrations of 3%–7% NaCl, the aerosolized saline settles in the central airways where it promotes osmotic inflow of interstitial fluid into the respiratory tract. This additional fluid appears to trigger cough via the airway receptors, leading the patient, with encouragement from the supervising health worker, to expectorate thin fluid with or without mucus that may be sent for microbiologic examination.[51] Laboratory staff should be notified via the laboratory requisition if a sample is induced to help prevent it from being inappropriately rejected as a salivary specimen. Infection control is a particular concern with sputum induction because the patient is asked to cough repeatedly over several minutes and should be carried out with careful attention to infection control measures.

BRONCHOSCOPY

Fiberoptic bronchoscopy is a semi-invasive examination that allows inspection of the central airways and collection of lower samples via bronchial wash, bronchoalveolar lavage (BAL), endobronchial brushings, endobronchial biopsy, transbronchial needle aspiration of enlarged paratracheal, mediastinal, and hilar lymph nodes in accessible locations with or without ultrasound guidance, and/or transbronchial lung biopsy. Samples may frequently be sent for cell counts, cytological staining, and/or flow cytometry, as well as microbiological examinations including AFB smear microscopy, NAAT, and mycobacterial culture. Airway inspection may rarely identify granulomatous lesions of the endobronchial mucosa, and transbronchial aspirates and biopsies may occasionally identify tissue that confirms active tuberculosis, or an alternative diagnosis such as infection due to nontuberculous mycobacteria or fungal infection, an inflammatory condition such as sarcoidosis, or malignancy. In some clinical scenarios, such as when immunocompromised patients are undergoing evaluation, bronchoscopy may be indicated to obtain samples for diagnosis of other infections. In these circumstances, the procedure is often guided by chest CT to identify radiographic patterns and locations of disease that may inform the differential diagnosis and the types of samples to be collected. In such scenarios, bronchoscopy may offer the opportunity to obtain concentrated saline washings that can reduce the time to diagnosis of TB or other infections, and lead to management changes.[52,53] In other scenarios, TB may be diagnosed unexpectedly as part of a diagnostic evaluation for another condition causing pulmonary infiltrates, cavities, or nodules, such as possible lung cancer. One particular group in whom bronchoscopy may be beneficial are patients in whom radiography shows a "miliary" pattern, characterized by diffuse 2–3 mm nodular opacities in a random distribution; these are said to resemble millet seeds and represent hematogeneously disseminated mycobacteria. Given this wide distribution of the bacilli via the vasculature, sputum samples tend to be paucibacillary and microbiologic examination is insensitive; endobronchial brushings, transbronchial biopsy, and/or bronchoalveolar lavage may confirm the diagnosis in more than half of patients with miliary TB.[54] Outside these select scenarios, studies among immunocompetent and among immunocompromised patients have found no difference in the diagnostic yield of induced sputum and BAL whether examined by either smear microscopy or mycobacterial culture.[55,56]

There are some clinical and operational considerations that influence the feasibility of bronchoscopy, most notably the respiratory status of the patients. In spontaneously breathing patients, bronchoscopy requires topical anesthetization of the upper and lower airway, and most patients also require conscious sedation with benzodiazepines and opiates for anxiolysis and control of dyspnea, discomfort, and coughing, all of which can make the procedure uncomfortable for the patient and therefore technically challenging for the proceduralist. Given the potential risks of over-sedation and respiratory failure, bronchoscopy is undertaken in a monitored setting. Patients with severe respiratory distress may require intubation and mechanical ventilation for safety, and the risk of clinical complications including pneumothorax (e.g. if transbronchial biopsy is performed) and worsening hypoxemia must be weighed against the risk of continuing care without a confirmed diagnosis.

CURRENT SPUTUM TESTS

SMEAR MICROSCOPY

Sputum smear microscopy dates back to Robert Koch's seminal discovery of *M. tuberculosis* in 1882 and remains the most common diagnostic test for TB. Usually performed on sputum, the test involves directly smearing a small sample of diagnostic material (sputum, fine-needle aspirate, or other body fluid) onto a disposable glass slide, heat-fixing the material to the glass, and applying chemical dyes that are specific for mycobacteria and a small number of other bacteria, including *Nocardia* and *Rhodococcus*. The classic carbol-fuchsin stains exploit a unique property of the mycobacterial cell wall that allows it to absorb the brilliant fuchsia-colored dye. They retain this coloring even after application of a background methylene blue counterstain and a subsequent destaining procedure with acid alcohol. Under a light microscope, deep pink bacilli may be readily viewed against the blue background and counted as semi quantitative measure of bacillary load. A limitation of the technique is that it requires the technician to view at least one 2-cm slide length under a 1000× objective over 10 minutes in order to exclude smear-positive TB.[38,57] Newer microscopes using long-lasting, low-cost LED bulbs have been adapted to visualize fluorochrome stains of the mycobacterial cytoplasm, which permit viewing at 200× and greatly reduce the time required to read a slide.[58] Nonetheless, sputum smear microscopy is limited by poor sensitivity, detecting only 50%–70% of active pulmonary TB patients. Moreover, while the technique has high specificity in settings with high TB prevalence, its specificity and positive predictive value are significantly reduced in low TB-prevalence settings, and among patients with a history of prior TB. Using mucolytic agents and centrifugation prior to processing have been shown to increase the sensitivity of smear microscopy by an average of 13%.[59] Processing methods that do not require centrifugation (e.g. bleach digestion) have also been described, but are associated with modestly reduced specificity.[60]

MYCOBACTERIAL CULTURE

Mycobacterial culture of two-to-three respiratory samples on solid or liquid media is considered the reference standard test for diagnosis of pulmonary TB. Unfortunately, mycobacterial culture requires substantial technical expertise and laboratory infrastructure, including level 3 biosafety protection, because a high concentration of bacilli in culture increases the risks of *M.tb* transmission to laboratory staff. As a result, mycobacterial culture is usually available only in centralized commercial or public health laboratories and is not routinely available in most low-income countries.

Several factors related to specimen collection and processing have a major influence on the sensitivity and specificity of mycobacterial culture. For example, because the quantity of bacilli may vary from sample to sample even within the same subject, at least three specimens should be sent for culture if resources permit. Oral commensal bacteria contaminate sputum during expectoration, and can overgrow the culture medium within days, preventing mycobacteria from growing. To limit this, laboratories decontaminate sputum using sodium hydroxide (1%–4% concentration) prior to inoculation in culture, but this may eliminate up to a third of all mycobacteria in the sample. As with microscopy, treatment with mucolytic agents such as N-acetyl-L-cysteine and concentration via centrifugation helps maximize the number of mycobacteria for inoculation.[36] In spite of these measures, around 5% of all sputa sent for mycobacterial culture will deliver an indeterminate result because of contamination. To reduce the probability of contamination, sputum sent for culture

should be stored and transported via cold chain and processed as rapidly as possible upon arrival in the laboratory. Alternatively, sputum may be treated with agents such as cetylpyridium chloride and other newer commercial agents designed to stabilize and protect mycobacterial cells from overgrowth without cold chain requirements.[61]

There are a number of different choices of media, each with advantages and disadvantages. Solid media including Lowenstein–Jensen and Ogawa media are low-cost, egg-based media that are often prepared on site in laboratories, especially in low-income countries. Newer agar-based commercial media include Middlebrook 7H10 and selective 7H11 media. Newer liquid media systems, often combined with automated, in-tube colorimetric reading, include Middlebrook 7H9 media, now commonly supplied in mycobacterial growth indicator tubes (MGIT), a colorimetric system that can be measured manually or using automated systems for early detection and reporting. In addition to using glycerol and other inorganic compounds as a primary nutrient source, liquid media are supplemented with oleic acid–albumin–dextrose–catalase (OADC) and the antibiotics polymyxin B, amphotericin B, nalidixic acid, trimethoprim, and azlocillin (PANTA) to select against more rapidly growing bacteria. Compared with solid culture, liquid culture is fosters more rapid growth of mycobacteria. Median time to positivity is 13 days, and cultures are considered negative if no bacteria are detected after 42 days of monitoring.[62] In contrast, growth on solid media is expected after a median of 26 days, and cultures are considered negative after 56 days. Liquid media provide greater sensitivity and shorter turn-around time for detection of mycobacteria, albeit at the cost of more frequent contamination by bacteria and nontuberculous mycobacteria. Solid culture is lower in cost, and the visualization of discrete mycobacterial colonies may also allow identification of multiple species or strains in the same specimen. Overall sensitivity of MGIT liquid media is 88% and specificity 99.6%, as compared with a sensitivity of 76% and specificity of 99.9% for solid media.[62]

Interestingly, there appears to be a degree of selectivity to all media, and, if resources allow, every specimen should be cultured on at least one solid and one liquid medium to minimize the consequences of selectivity and contamination.[63] Once a culture is noted to be positive, additional tests must be performed for speciation and drug susceptibility testing. Traditionally, selective culturing and biochemical assays were used to identify species of mycobacteria, but increasingly, nucleic acid amplification, MPT 64 antigen testing using lateral flow assays, and high-performance liquid chromatography are used for identification.

NUCLEIC ACID AMPLIFICATION TESTING

NAAT for TB diagnosis first became widely available in laboratories in the early 1990s, with the commercial introduction of assays targeting the IS6110 sequence.[46] Although widely endorsed by public health authorities,[64,65] first-generation assays never achieved widespread adoption[67] for a variety of clinical and operational reasons. Although there were many high-quality diagnostic accuracy studies showing NAAT to be highly sensitive and specific for TB,[66] as well as thoughtful clinical and public health guidance about how to integrate test results with clinical decision-making,[19,68] there were very few studies demonstrating an important clinical impact.[69] On the contrary, studies from both the United States[70] and the United Kingdom[71] showed that clinicians were comfortable initiating therapy for positive results, but rarely withheld therapy in the setting of negative results. Operationally, these assays were complex to perform, requiring up to 8 hours of dedicated laboratory technician time and complicated, multi-room, unidirectional work flows. The open-tube nature of these assays made them susceptible to laboratory cross-contamination, and they developed a reputation for false-positive results.[72] Given their imperfect sensitivity, there were also concerns about false-negative results, and CDC guidelines at that time recommended repeat testing if the clinical probability of active TB remained high.[68] Given low demand for first-generation NAATs from clinicians and concerns from laboratory directors that the assays were not affordable, availability of the tests decreased and turn-around time increased in high-income countries;[73] they were never routinely introduced in low-income countries because of high costs and intensive labor requirements.

In 2010, the first clinical data on next-generation NAATs was reported, launching a new era in TB diagnostics.[74–76] Unlike previous NAATs, these tests were developed specifically to address the need for rapid, low-cost assays to replace smear microscopy in low- and middle-income countries, through the novel mechanism of public–private partnerships. The first of these assays, GeneXpert MTB/RIF, applied several major technological advances to NAATs: (1) use of a novel, amplification-compatible mucolytic reagent and ultrasonic cell lysis to optimize extraction of target nucleic acids; (2) use of hemi-nested nucleic-acid amplification to improve sensitivity; (3) targeting of *rpoB*, a highly conserved 81 base-pair region of the *Mtb* genome to simultaneously provide information about TB diagnosis and about putative drug resistance to rifamycins; (4) amplification inside a closed, disposable cartridge and use of short, overlapping molecular beacon probes to improve specificity; and (5) automation of amplification using microfluidics to reduce labor requirements and turn-around time. Multiple clinical studies have shown that Xpert MTB/RIF detects virtually all sputum smear-positive TB patients and the majority of sputum smear-negative patients in most settings in both high- and low-burden countries. In 70 studies of 37,237 possible TB patients included in a Cochrane review, pooled sensitivity of Xpert MTB/RIF was 85% and pooled specificity 98%; in 48 studies enrolling 8020 participants, pooled sensitivity for rifampicin resistance was 96% and specificity 98%.[77]

Following WHO approval in 2011,[78] Xpert MTB/RIF was introduced widely in low-income countries. While it was originally targeted to persons living with HIV and those with risk factors for MDR-TB, with expansion of concessionary pricing through donor subsidies, WHO subsequently updated its policy to recommend Xpert as the first-line replacement test for smear microscopy for all forms of TB in all individuals, including children.[79] Several post-implementation studies using quasi-randomized designs have shown that Xpert can increase the proportion of individuals with microbiologically confirmed diagnoses and shorten the time-to-treatment initiation. However, studies that have examined more important patient outcomes such as morbidity and mortality,

have failed to show an important impact in routine practice.[80–82] For example, the TB-NEAT trial, a multi-country, individually randomized trial comparing nurse-performed Xpert MTB/RIF to standard sputum microscopy in several countries in southern Africa showed no change in TB-related morbidity.[82] Similarly, the XTEND study, a parallel-group, cluster-randomized trial of 4656 patients nested into the national roll-out of Xpert MTB/RIF at 20 clinics in South Africa, showed no difference in six-month mortality, with a substantial proportion (16%) of Xpert-positive TB patients never receiving their results or initiating treatment.[83] These findings were confirmed in an individual patient meta-analysis of five randomized trials, although among persons living with HIV, Xpert was shown to have a statistically significant 24% reduction in mortality. [84]

There are several potential explanations for the apparent failure of Xpert to impact clinically important outcomes in the general population of patients undergoing evaluation for active TB. Methodologists have noted that improvements in diagnostics are rarely large enough to impact downstream clinical outcomes like mortality, especially for highly curable conditions like TB.[85] Other contributing factors may include high rates of presumptive treatment of smear-negative individuals in the control arms of these trials. Observational studies have described (1) high rates of initial losses to follow-up among individuals assigned to Xpert testing as a result of difficulties that centralized laboratories experience in returning results to patients; (2) a frequent failure to refer all possible TB patients for Xpert testing and ensure that testing is completed; (3) confusion among clinicians about interpretation of Xpert results, particularly for drug resistance; and (4) technical failures of the tests and testing platforms. These failures may arise from rugged field conditions where dust, heat, power cuts, power surges, irregular supplies, and lack of regular maintenance and repair services may reduce availability of testing or increase the frequency of indeterminate results.[86,87] These observations have suggested to many that designing smaller and simpler Xpert machines and placing them at microscopy facilities could be a less costly and more effective strategy for improving diagnosis and more effectively linking these patients to care.[119] Thus, a variety of modifications to the Xpert test cartridge and platform are planned, including reducing the number of modules to one per device and integrating a solar-powered battery.

Xpert MTB/RIF has been shown to provide similar diagnostic accuracy results in low-burden settings as in an FDA-registration study that enrolled a majority of patients in the United States.[88] This study supported approval of Xpert MTB/RIF for the indications of TB diagnosis and exclusion of infectious TB.[89,90] In addition, a series of hypothetical trials that performed both conventional smear-microscopy and Xpert MTB/RIF in the United States demonstrated a substantial impact on clinical and health systems outcomes in a variety of settings. Among outpatients in an urban TB control program, these benefits included potential reductions in unnecessary empiric treatment for active TB, unnecessary contact investigations, and unnecessary evictions from congregate housing.[91] Among inpatients placed in respiratory isolation while undergoing evaluation for possible active TB, studies have projected substantial reductions in length of stay in isolation rooms and in hospital,[92–95] as well as in health-system costs.[96,97] More recently, the safety, efficiency, and cost benefits of Xpert following implementation as part of a triage algorithm for inpatients were confirmed prospectively in a large pragmatic, before-and-after study in a safety-net hospital.[98] In spite of long-standing CDC recommendations that all possible TB patients be evaluated with nucleic-acid testing, less than half of patient evaluations meet this quality metric.[65,99,100] Current guidelines state that possible TB patients may have respiratory isolation discontinued based on two negative Xpert results on expectorated or induced sputum collected at least eight hours apart.[101]

In 2017, the GeneXpert Ultra, an updated NAAT with increased sensitivity for active pulmonary TB, was approved by WHO, and is expected to gradually replace Xpert MTB/RIF in low- and middle-income countries. Xpert Ultra provides enhanced sensitivity through several technological innovations on the original Xpert assay. These include targeting the multi-copy IS6110 and IS1081 sequences of the *Mtb* genome for amplification alongside the *rpoB* targets; conversion of the *rpoB* and IS6110 assays into fully nested amplification assays; and doubling the starting volume of the processed sputum entering the amplification chamber.[102] In addition, the assay has been modified to use sloppy molecular beacon probes and melting curve analysis in order to provide more accurate rifamycin resistance results. In a multi-center diagnostic accuracy study in which all participants provided sputum for testing by both Xpert assays and serial mycobacterial culture, Xpert Ultra had 17% (95% confidence interval [CI] 10%–24%) higher sensitivity than Xpert MTB/RIF but 2.7% (95% CI 1.7%–3.9%) lower specificity; performance in detecting rifamycin resistance was similar.[103] In post-hoc analyses, two sub-groups accounted for nearly all of the false-positive results: patients with a history of prior TB and individuals with trace-positive results on Xpert Ultra testing. Repeat testing of individuals with trace-positive results eliminated the specificity differences when compared with Xpert MTB/RIF; this approach is recommended in the final WHO statement. The cartridge innovations that enabled multiplexing of targets for the Ultra assay have also facilitated development of a separate cartridge for isoniazid, fluoroquinolone, and amikacin resistance for use as a reflex text for pre-XDR/XDR TB.

An alternative next-generation molecular test for TB is the loop-mediated isothermal amplification test (TB LAMP), approved by WHO in 2016 for use as a replacement test for microscopy in peripheral centers lacking infrastructure to perform GeneXpert testing. TB LAMP is a rapid, manual, closed-tube reaction that requires only a heating block, tubes, and reagents, and can be read with the naked eye, all making it about 25% less costly than Xpert MTB/RIF. Although TB LAMP has several potential advantages over microscopy, including enhanced sensitivity, it requires a manual, multi-step process that is more labor intensive than GeneXpert and does not provide information about drug resistance. Moreover, data on its performance are based on very low-quality evidence for key populations, including PLWH.

A large number of additional NAAT assays are in development, many with multi-analyte detection capabilities for nontuberculous mycobacteria as well as *Mtb*. Many of these have acquired approvals from European and US (FDA) regulatory authorities, and a few are scheduled for WHO review. These technologies are comprehensively described in the UNITAID TB Diagnostic Landscape Report, which has been updated continually over the last few years.[104]

OTHER MOLECULAR DIAGNOSTICS FOR DRUG RESISTANCE

In addition to the GeneXpert platform, a growing number of other technologies are available or in development for molecular drug susceptibility testing (DST). Together, these technologies offer hope for being able to decrease the cost and turn-around time for diagnosis of drug-resistant TB.[104] A common challenge for these methods is limited data about the correlations among phenotypic DST, genotypic DST, and clinical outcomes. Expert guidelines therefore encourage that the reporting of molecular DST include evidence about the correlation between specific mutations and clinical outcomes to guide interpretation,[105] and WHO continues to recommend that all patients undergo culture-based phenotypic drug-susceptibility testing as the reference test.[1]

Line-probe assays (LpA) employ a generic technology for interrogating pre-amplified *Mtb* sequences using fluorescent hybridization probes on disposable test strips.[106,107] The results are easily interpretable with the naked eye. They have been harnessed for a variety of purposes, including TB diagnosis, identifying different species of mycobacteria in cultures, and targeted genotyping of drug-resistance mutations. The assays are rapid and inexpensive, but because of the limited analytic sensitivity of the hybridization probes, they must be applied to pre-amplified DNA. This requires that they be performed in advanced laboratories with infrastructure and human-resource capacity to extract and amplify DNA. These assays are performed as add-on tests after positive smear microscopy or mycobacterial culture have indicated the presence of adequate amounts of template DNA for amplification. LpA have achieved their greatest impact in screening for drug resistance to first-line agents (i.e., isoniazid and rifampin) and second-line (i.e., second-line injectable drugs and fluoroquinolones). First recommended by WHO in 2008, with updated recommendations issued in 2016,[106,107] line-probe assays are routinely available countrywide as part of the standard public health testing algorithm in South Africa.[104] They have contributed substantially to earlier and lower cost diagnosis of MDR TB, pre-XDR TB, and XDR TB in many countries with high burdens of drug resistance. The limitations of LpA are that each probe targets only a single resistance mutation and each strip can accommodate only a limited number of probes. Thus, multiple strips may be required to test for second-line drug resistance and the sensitivity of LpA may be limited for detecting resistance to drugs with multiple resistance alleles and may be unable to detect resistance for rare alleles.

Sequencing involves a diverse set of high-throughput methods with the ability to amplify DNA with higher sensitivity and specificity than other available methods. This higher resolution may facilitate identification of rare or unusual sequence variants that could be clinically important for a variety of indications including identifying rare or silent drug-resistance mutations; diagnosing mixed infections with different mycobacterial species or different Mtb strains, including strains with different resistance patterns; and revealing transmission links and their directionality. The main limitations of sequencing methods are the current high cost and complexity and lack of standardization of the process, which requires not only laboratory proficiency, but also an advanced understanding of bioinformatics to align and normalize sequences. Nonetheless, with rapidly falling costs and increasing standardization of methods, many public health programs in high-income countries now offer sequencing routinely, including the US Centers for Disease Control, many state public health laboratories, and Public Health England. At least one analysis suggests that whole genome sequencing for TB may be highly cost-effective compared with the conventional approach of mycobacterial culture, reflex species identification, and phenotypic drug-susceptibility testing.[108]

NON-SPUTUM TESTS

In spite of the many available sputum assays for TB diagnosis, there is ongoing demand for a test for TB that would not require sputum. Blood and urine are commonly considered alternatives, with a number of commercial assays with a variety of targets in development. Breath is a novel specimen type that is also being explored by a number of research groups using a variety of targets, but is at an earlier stage of development compared to blood and urine. Commercial serological tests with both antigen and antibody targets have long been widely available, especially in the private sector in Asia and Africa.[109] High-quality evidence demonstrates that these assays have poor sensitivity and specificity,[110,111] and WHO has specifically recommended that they not be used.[9] There is ongoing research by a number of groups working to develop next-generation approaches to serologic testing,[112,113] but as yet there have been no clinical studies of assays ready to be made commercially available. Interferon-gamma release assays are commercially available tests for latent TB infection. A number of studies have evaluated their performance for active pulmonary TB on peripheral blood and found them insufficiently sensitive or specific for active pulmonary TB.[114,115] Two recent studies have reported the use of gene-expression profiling based on whole-blood amplification of human RNA signatures, with most of the data coming from children.[116] The only commercially available and approved non-sputum test for TB is the urinary lipoarabinomannan (LAM) antigen test.

LIPOARABINOMANNAN ASSAYS

Antigen-based detection of LAM is a WHO-approved assay for detection of TB in patients with advanced HIV, including individuals with CD4 counts less than 100 cells/µL and individuals with severe illness regardless of CD4 count (defined by the presence of any one of the four danger signs, including respiratory rate >30/min, temperature >39°C, heart rate >120/min, or inability to walk unaided).[10] LAM is a lipopolysaccharide released from mycobacterial cell walls and found in high concentrations in urine in persons living with advanced HIV. The assay uses a lateral-flow format, with the readout interpretable using automated optical reading devices or the naked eye, with very good inter-reader and intra-reader agreement. This may be because of the higher prevalence of disseminated TB, including renal TB, in these populations,

and from higher LAM clearance rates in the renal glomeruli of individuals with severe illness. The pooled sensitivity across six studies of 2402 persons living with HIV (median CD4 71–210) undergoing evaluation for symptoms suggestive of TB was 59% (95% CrI 43–77) and the pooled specificity was 78% (95% CrI 64–88). In a subset of five studies of 859 PLWH with CD4 ≤100, pooled sensitivity was 56% (95% CrI 41–70), and pooled specificity was 90% (95% CrI 81–95). The suboptimal specificity of the assay may reflect the fact that LAM is also found in other mycobacteria, and that standards based on sputum culture and clinical assessment used in diagnostic accuracy studies may fail to capture some patients with disseminated forms of TB (e.g., miliary TB). WHO recommends against the use of LAM as a screening test, but says that it may be used for diagnosis of PLWH with CD4 ≤200 or among individuals who are seriously ill.[10] Although the diagnostic accuracy of urinary LAM is less than ideal, the approach of diagnosing TB using a urinary antigen is an important breakthrough in the field because of its simplicity and comparative biosafety. There is substantial ongoing research to enhance the capture of LAM and develop assays with improved analytic sensitivity in PLWH and others.[104] For example, a novel urinary LAM assay using monoclonal antibodies and a novel silver-based technique for visualization has recently shown enhanced sensitivity and similar specificity for TB among PLWH.[120]

CONCLUSION

Diagnosing TB remains one of the most formidable challenges in medicine, both because of the often indolent nature of the disease and because of more than a century without progress in improving testing. After over a century with very little progress in TB diagnostics, the last decade has brought enormous progress in the science, advocacy, and implementation of new tests and strategies. Much more is yet to be done to reach the more than 3 million people around the world who are still living with TB unbeknownst to themselves or public health authorities. By redoubling advocacy for increased funding and political engagement to address the disease, drawing on new scientific breakthroughs, and building on established principles of high-quality individualized assessment and patient-centered care, there is hope that we may substantially narrow and someday eliminate the diagnosis gap in TB.

REFERENCES

1. World Health Organization. *Global Tuberculosis Control: WHO Report 2019*. Geneva: World Health Organization, 2019.
2. *Implementing the WHO Stop TB Strategy: A Handbook for National Tuberculosis Control Programmes*. Geneva: World Health Organization, 2008.
3. Keeler E et al. Reducing the global burden of tuberculosis: The contribution of improved diagnostics. *Nature*. 2006;444(Suppl 1):49–57.
4. World Health Organization. *Global Tuberculosis Control: WHO Report 2017*. Geneva: World Health Organization, 2017.
5. Perkins MD, Cunningham J. Facing the crisis: Improving the diagnosis of tuberculosis in the HIV era. *J Infect Dis*. 2007;196(Suppl 1):S15–27.

6. World Health Organization. *Policy statement: Reduction of Number of Smears for Pulmonary Tuberculosis.* Geneva: World Health Organization, 2007.

7. World Health Organization. *Policy Statement: The Use of Liquid Medium for Culture and DST in Low- and Middle-Income Country Settings.* Geneva: World Health Organization, 2007.

8. World Health Organization. *Policy Statement: Noncommercial Culture and Drug-Susceptibility Testing Methods for Screening Patients at Risk for Multidrug-Resistant Tuberculosis.* Geneva: World Health Organization, 2011.

9. World Health Organization. *Commercial Serodiagnostic Tests for Diagnosis of Tuberculosis: Policy Statement.* Geneva: World Health Organization, 2011.

10. World Health Organization. *Lateral flow urine lipoarabinomannan assay (LF-LAM) for the diagnosis of active tuberculosis in people living with HIV,* 2019 Update. Geneva: World Health Organization, 2019.

11. Brunet L, Minion J, Lienhardt C, and Pai M. Mapping the landscape of tuberculosis diagnostic research. *Am J Respir Crit Care Med.* 2010;296:A2255.

12. Lessells RJ, Cooke GS, Newell M-L, and Godfrey-Faussett P. Evaluation of tuberculosis diagnostics: Establishing an evidence base around the public health impact. *J Infect Dis.* 2011; 204(suppl_4):S1187–S95.

13. World Health Organization. *The End TB Strategy.* Geneva: World Health Organization, 2015.

14. Stop TB Partnership. Pathways to better diagnostics for tuberculosis: A blueprint for the development of TB diagnostics. In: New Diagnostics Working Group, Dacombe R (ed.). Geneva: World Health Organization, 2009.

15. Pauker SG, and Kassirer JP. The threshold approach to clinical decision making. *N Engl J Med.* 1980;302(20):1109–17.

16. Leeflang MM, Deeks JJ, Gatsonis C, and Bossuyt PM. Systematic reviews of diagnostic test accuracy. *Ann Intern Med.* 2008;149(12):889–97.

17. Bossuyt PM, Irwig L, Craig J, and Glasziou P. Comparative accuracy: Assessing new tests against existing diagnostic pathways. *BMJ.* 2006;332(7549):1089–92.

18. World Health Organization. *High-Priority Target Product Profiles for New Tuberculosis Diagnostics: Report of a Consensus Meeting.* Geneva: World Health Organization, 2014.

19. Catanzaro A et al. The role of clinical suspicion in evaluating a new diagnostic test for active tuberculosis: Results of a multicenter prospective trial. *JAMA.* 2000;283(5):639–45.

20. TB CARE I. *International Standards for Tuberculosis Care.* 3rd ed. The Hague, 2014.

21. van't Hoog AH et al. *A Systematic Review of the Sensitivity and Specificity of Symptom- and Chest-Radiography Screening for Active Pulmonary Tuberculosis in HIV-Negative Persons and Persons with Unknown HIV Status.* Geneva: World Health Organization, 2013.

22. Claassens MM, van Schalkwyk C, Floyd S, Ayles H, and Beyers N. Symptom screening rules to identify active pulmonary tuberculosis: Findings from the Zambian South African Tuberculosis and HIV/AIDS Reduction (ZAMSTAR) trial prevalence surveys. *PLOS ONE.* 2017;12(3):e0172881.

23. World Health Organization. *Guidelines for Intensified Tuberculosis Case-Finding and Isoniazid Preventive Therapy for People Living with HIV in Resource-Constrained Settings.* Geneva: World Health Organization, 2011.

24. World Health Organization. Systematic screening for active tuberculosis: Principles and recommendations. In: Lonnroth K (ed.). Geneva: World Health Organization, 2013.

25. Hamada Y, Lujan J, Schenkel K, Ford N, and Getahun H. Sensitivity and specificity of WHO's recommended four-symptom screening rule for tuberculosis in people living with HIV: A systematic review and meta-analysis. *Lancet HIV.* 2018;5(9):e515–e23.

26. Lienhardt C. From exposure to disease: The role of environmental factors in susceptibility to and development of tuberculosis. *Epidemiol Rev.* 2001;23(2):288–301.

27. Skoura E, Zumla A, Bomanji J. Imaging in tuberculosis. *Int J Infect Dis.* 2015;32:87–93.

28. Geng E, Kreiswirth B, Burzynski J, Schluger NW. Clinical and radiographic correlates of primary and reactivation tuberculosis: A molecular epidemiology study. *JAMA.* 2005;293(22):2740–5.

29. Saks AM, Posner R. Tuberculosis in HIV positive patients in South Africa: A comparative radiological study with HIV negative patients. *Clin Radiol.* 1992;46(6):387–90.

30. Greenberg SD, Frager D, Suster B, Walker S, Stavropoulos C, and Rothpearl A. Active pulmonary tuberculosis in patients with AIDS: Spectrum of radiographic findings (including a normal appearance). *Radiology.* 1994;193(1):115–9.

31. Yoo SD et al. Clinical significance of normal chest radiographs among HIV-seropositive patients with suspected tuberculosis in Uganda. *Respirology.* 2011;16(5):836–41.

32. Worodria W et al. Clinical spectrum, risk factors and outcome of immune reconstitution inflammatory syndrome in patients with tuberculosis-HIV coinfection. *Antivir Ther.* 2012;17(5):841–8.

33. Pinto LM, Pai M, Dheda K, Schwartzman K, Menzies D, and Steingart KR. Scoring systems using chest radiographic features for the diagnosis of pulmonary tuberculosis in adults: A systematic review. *Eur Respir J.* 2013;42(2):480–94.

34. Pande T, Cohen C, Pai M, and Ahmad Khan F. Computer-aided detection of pulmonary tuberculosis on digital chest radiographs: A systematic review. *Int J Tuberculosis Lung Dis.* 2016;20(9):1226–30.

35. Zaidi SMA et al. Evaluation of the diagnostic accuracy of computer-aided detection of tuberculosis on chest radiography among private sector patients in Pakistan. *Sci Rep.* 2018;8(1):12339.

36. Kent PT, Kubica GP. *Public Health Mycobacteriology: A guide for the Level III Laboratory.* Atlanta: Centers for Disease Control, 1985.

37. Ho J, Marks GB, and Fox GJ. The impact of sputum quality on tuberculosis diagnosis: A systematic review. *Int J Tuberc Lung Dis.* 2015;19(5):537–44.

38. Stop TB Partnership. Laboratory diagnosis of tuberculosis by sputum microscopy. In: Global Laboratory Initiative, Lump R et al. (eds.) Adelaide, Australia: SA Pathology, 2013.

39. Khan MS, Dar O, Sismanidis C, Shah K, and Godfrey-Faussett P. Improvement of tuberculosis case detection and reduction of discrepancies between men and women by simple sputum-submission instructions: A pragmatic randomised controlled trial. *Lancet.* 2007;369(9577):1955–60.

40. Mhalu G et al. Do instructional videos on sputum submission result in increased tuberculosis case detection? A randomized controlled trial. *PLOS ONE.* 2015;10(9):e0138413.

41. Meyer AJ et al. Sputum quality and diagnostic performance of GeneXpert MTB/RIF among smear-negative adults with presumed tuberculosis in Uganda. *PLOS ONE.* 2017;12(7):e0180572.

42. World Health Organization. *Same-Day Diagnosis of Tuberculosis: Policy Statement.* Geneva: World Health Organization, 2011.

43. Davis JL, Cattamanchi A, Cuevas LE, Hopewell PC, and Steingart KR. Diagnostic accuracy of same-day microscopy versus standard microscopy for pulmonary tuberculosis: A systematic review and meta-analysis. *Lancet Infect Dis.* 2013;13(2):147–54.

44. Murphy ME et al. Spot sputum samples are at least as good as early morning samples for identifying *Mycobacterium tuberculosis*. *BMC Med*. 2017;15(1):192.

45. Datta S, Shah L, Gilman RH, and Evans CA. Comparison of sputum collection methods for tuberculosis diagnosis: A systematic review and pairwise and network meta-analysis. *Lancet Global Health*. 2017;5(8):e760–e71.

46. Eisenach KD, Sifford MD, Cave MD, Bates JH, Crawford JT. Detection of mycobacterium tuberculosis in sputum samples using a polymerase chain reaction. *Am Rev Respir Dis*. 1991;144(5):1160–3.

47. Kemp JR, Mann G, Simwaka BN, Salaniponi FM, and Squire SB. Can Malawi's poor afford free tuberculosis services? Patient and household costs associated with a tuberculosis diagnosis in Lilongwe. *Bull WHO*. 2007;85(8):580–5.

48. Davis JL, Dowdy DW, den Boon S, Walter ND, Katamba A, and Cattamanchi A. Test and treat: A new standard for smear-positive tuberculosis. *J Acquir Immune Defic Syndr*. 2012;61(1):e6–8.

49. Davis JL. Bringing patient-centered tuberculosis diagnosis into the light of day. *BMC Med*. 2017;15(1):219.

50. Jensen PA, Lambert LA, Iademarco MF, Ridzon R. Guidelines for preventing the transmission of *Mycobacterium tuberculosis* in health-care settings, 2005. *MMWR Recomm Rep*. 2005;54(RR-17):1–141.

51. Gonzalez-Angulo Y et al. Sputum induction for the diagnosis of pulmonary tuberculosis: A systematic review and meta-analysis. *Eur J Clin Microbiol Infect Dis*. 2011.

52. Dunagan D, Baker A, Hurd D, and Haponik E. Bronchoscopic evaluation of pulmonary infiltrates following bone marrow transplantation. *Chest*. 1997;111(1):135–41.

53. Rano A et al. Pulmonary infiltrates in non-HIV immunocompromised patients: A diagnostic approach using non-invasive and bronchoscopic procedures. *Thorax*. 2001;56(5):379–87.

54. Sharma SK, Mohan A, Sharma A, Mitra DK. Miliary tuberculosis: New insights into an old disease. *Lancet Infect Dis*. 2005;5(7):415–30

55. Anderson C, Inhaber N, and Menzies D. Comparison of sputum induction with fiber-optic bronchoscopy in the diagnosis of tuberculosis. *Am J Respir Crit Care Med*. 1995;152(5 Pt 1):1570–4.

56. Conde MB et al. Comparison of sputum induction with fiberoptic bronchoscopy in the diagnosis of tuberculosis: Experience at an acquired immune deficiency syndrome reference center in Rio de Janeiro, Brazil. *Am J Respir Crit Care Med*. 2000;162(6):2238–40.

57. Cambanis A, Ramsay A, Wirkom V, Tata E, and Cuevas LE. Investing time in microscopy: An opportunity to optimise smear-based case detection of tuberculosis. *Int J Tuberculosis Lung Dis*. 2007;11(1):40–5.

58. Hanscheid T. The future looks bright: Low-cost fluorescent microscopes for detection of *Mycobacterium tuberculosis* and Coccidiae. *Trans R Soc Trop Med Hyg*. 2008;102(6):520–1.

59. Steingart KR et al. Sputum processing methods to improve the sensitivity of smear microscopy for tuberculosis: A systematic review. *Lancet Infect Dis*. 2006;6(10):664–74.

60. Cattamanchi A, Davis JL, Pai M, Huang L, Hopewell PC, and Steingart KR. Does bleach processing increase the accuracy of sputum smear microscopy for diagnosing pulmonary tuberculosis? *J Clin Microbiol*. 2010;48(7):2433–9.

61. Hiza H et al. Preservation of sputum samples with cetylpyridinium chloride (CPC) for tuberculosis cultures and Xpert MTB/RIF in a low-income country. *BMC Infect Dis*. 2017;17.

62. Cruciani M, Scarparo C, Malena M, Bosco O, Serpelloni G, and Mengoli C. Meta-analysis of BACTEC MGIT 960 and BACTEC 460 TB, with or without solid media, for detection of mycobacteria. *J Clin Microbiol*. 2004;42(5):2321–5.

63. Joloba ML et al. What is the most reliable solid culture medium for tuberculosis treatment trials? *Tuberculosis (Edinb)*. 2014;94(3):311–6.

64. Nucleic acid amplification tests for tuberculosis: Guidelines from the Centers for Disease Control & Prevention. *MMWR Morb Mortal Wkly Rep* 1996;45(43):950–2.

65. Centers for Disease Control and Prevention. Updated guidelines for the use of nucleic acid amplification tests in the diagnosis of tuberculosis. *MMWR Morb Mortal Wkly Rep* 2009;58(1):7–10.

66. Greco S, Girardi E, Navarra A, Saltini C. Current evidence on diagnostic accuracy of commercially based nucleic acid amplification tests for the diagnosis of pulmonary tuberculosis. *Thorax*. 2006;61(9):783–90.

67. Dorman SE. Editorial commentary: Coming of age of nucleic acid amplification tests for the diagnosis of tuberculosis. *Clin Infect Dis* 2009;49(1):55–7.

68. Rapid Diagnostic Tests for Tuberculosis: What is the appropriate use? American Thoracic Society Workshop. *Am J Respir Crit Care Med* 1997;155(5):1804–14.

69. Taegtmeyer M et al. The clinical impact of nucleic acid amplification tests on the diagnosis and management of tuberculosis in a British hospital. *Thorax*. 2008;63(4):317–21.

70. Guerra RL et al. Use of the amplified *Mycobacterium tuberculosis* Direct test in a public health laboratory: Test performance and impact on clinical care. *Chest*. 2007;132(3):946–51.

71. Conaty SJ, Claxton AP, Enoch DA, Hayward AC, Lipman MC, and Gillespie SH. The interpretation of nucleic acid amplification tests for tuberculosis: Do rapid tests change treatment decisions? *J Infect*. 2005;50(3):187–92.

72. Thomsen VO. Diagnosis of pulmonary tuberculosis. Application of Gen-Probe amplified *Mycobacterium tuberculosis* direct test. *APMIS: Acta Pathol, Microbiol Immunol Scand*. 1998;106(7):699–703.

73. Dylewski J. Nucleic acid amplification testing for the diagnosis of tuberculosis: Not for all. *Clin Infect Dis*. 2009;49(9):1456–7.

74. Boehme CC et al. Rapid molecular detection of tuberculosis and rifampin resistance. *N Engl J Med*. 2010;363(11):1005–15.

75. Small PM, and Pai M. Tuberculosis diagnosis—Time for a game change. *N Engl J Med*. 2010;363(11):1070–1.

76. Boehme CC et al. Feasibility, diagnostic accuracy, and effectiveness of decentralised use of the Xpert MTB/RIF test for diagnosis of tuberculosis and multidrug resistance: A multicentre implementation study. *Lancet*. 2011;377(9776):1495–505.

77. Horne DJ et al. Xpert MTB/RIF and Xpert MTB/RIF Ultra for pulmonary tuberculosis and rifampicin resistance in adults. *Cochrane Database Syst Rev*. 2019;6(6):CD009593.

78. World Health Organization. *Automated Real-Time Nucleic Acid Amplification Technology for Rapid and Simultaneous Detection of Tuberculosis and Rifampicin Resistance: Xpert MTB/RIF System: Policy Statement*. Geneva: World Health Organization, 2011.

79. World Health Organization. *Automated Real-Time Nucleic Acid Amplification Technology for Rapid and Simultaneous Detection of Tuberculosis and Rifampicin Resistance: Xpert MTB/RIF System for the Diagnosis of Pulmonary and Extrapulmonary TB in Adults and Children: Updated Policy Statement*. Geneva: World Health Organization, 2013.

80. Cox HS et al. Impact of Xpert MTB/RIF for TB diagnosis in a primary care clinic with high TB and HIV prevalence in South Africa: A pragmatic randomised trial. *PLoS Med.* 2014;11(11):e1001760.

81. Lessells RJ, Cooke GS, McGrath N, Nicol MP, Newell ML, and Godfrey-Faussett P. Impact of point-of-care Xpert MTB/RIF on tuberculosis treatment initiation. A cluster-randomized trial. *Am J Respir Crit Care Med.* 2017;196(7):901–10.

82. Theron G et al. Feasibility, accuracy, and clinical effect of point-of-care Xpert MTB/RIF testing for tuberculosis in primary-care settings in Africa: a multicentre, randomised, controlled trial. *Lancet.* 2014;383(9915):424–35.

83. Churchyard GJ et al. Xpert MTB/RIF versus sputum microscopy as the initial diagnostic test for tuberculosis: A cluster-randomised trial embedded in South African roll-out of Xpert MTB/RIF. *Lancet Global Health.* 2015;3(8):e450–7.

84. Di Tanna GL et al. Effect of Xpert MTB/RIF on clinical outcomes in routine care settings: individual patient data meta-analysis. *Lancet Glob Health* 2019;7(2):e191–e9.

85. Bossuyt PM, Lijmer JG, and Mol BW. Randomised comparisons of medical tests: Sometimes invalid, not always efficient. *Lancet.* 2000;356(9244):1844–7.

86. Hanrahan CF et al. Implementation of Xpert MTB/RIF in Uganda: Missed opportunities to improve diagnosis of tuberculosis. *Open Forum Infect Dis.* 2016;3(2).

87. Creswell J et al. Results from early programmatic implementation of Xpert MTB/RIF testing in nine countries. *BMC Infect Dis.* 2014;14:2.

88. Luetkemeyer AF et al. Evaluation of Xpert MTB/RIF versus AFB smear and culture to identify pulmonary tuberculosis in patients with suspected tuberculosis from low and higher prevalence settings. *Clin Infect Dis.* 2016;62(9):1081–8.

89. U.S. Food and Drug Administration. FDA permits marketing of first U.S. test labeled for simultaneous detection of tuberculosis bacteria and resistance to the antibiotic rifampin July 25, 2013. Available from: http://www.fda.gov/NewsEvents/Newsroom/PressAnnouncements/ucm362602.htm.

90. Revised device labeling for the Cepheid Xpert MTB/RIF assay for detecting *Mycobacterium tuberculosis*. *MMWR Morb Mortal Wkly Rep.* 2015;64(7):193.

91. Davis JL et al. Impact of GeneXpert MTB/RIF on patients and tuberculosis programs in a low-burden setting. A hypothetical trial. *Am J Respir Crit Care Med.* 2014;189(12):1551–9.

92. Lippincott CK, Miller MB, Popowitch EB, Hanrahan CF, and Van Rie A. Xpert MTB/RIF assay shortens airborne isolation for hospitalized patients with presumptive tuberculosis in the United States. *Clin Infect Dis.* 2014;59(2):186–92.

93. Chaisson LH et al. Impact of GeneXpert MTB/RIF assay on triage of respiratory isolation rooms for inpatients with presumed tuberculosis: A hypothetical trial. *Clin Infect Dis.* 2014;59(10):1353–60.

94. Cowan JF et al. Clinical impact and cost-effectiveness of Xpert MTB/RIF testing in hospitalized patients with presumptive pulmonary tuberculosis in the United States. *Clin Infect Dis.* 2017;64(4):482–9.

95. Poonawala H et al. Use of a single Xpert MTB/RIF assay to determine the duration of airborne isolation in hospitalized patients with suspected pulmonary tuberculosis. *Infect Control Hosp Epidemiol.* 2018:1–6.

96. Choi HW, Miele K, Dowdy D, and Shah M. Cost-effectiveness of Xpert® MTB/RIF for diagnosing pulmonary tuberculosis in the United States. *Int J Tuberc Lung Dis.* 2013;17(10):1328–35.

97. Millman AJ et al. Rapid molecular testing for TB to guide respiratory isolation in the U.S.: A cost-benefit analysis. *PLOS ONE.* 2013;8(11):e79669.

98. Chaisson LH et al. Association of rapid molecular testing with duration of respiratory isolation for patients with possible tuberculosis in a US hospital. *JAMA Intern Med.* 2018;178(10):1380–8.

99. Institute of Medicine (U.S.). *Committee on Leading Health Indicators for Healthy People 2020. Leading health indicators for healthy people 2020: Letter report.* Washington, D.C.: National Academies Press, 2011.

100. Salfinger M. Molecular assay testing to rule out tuberculosis—be that early adopter. *JAMA Int Med.* 2018;178(10):1388–9.

101. Consensus statement on the use of Cepheid Xpert MTB/RIF® assay in making decisions to discontinue airborne infection isolation in healthcare settings. National TB Controllers Association and the Association of Public Health Laboratories, 2015.

102. Chakravorty S et al. The new Xpert MTB/RIF ultra: Improving detection of *Mycobacterium tuberculosis* and resistance to rifampin in an assay suitable for point-of-care testing. *MBio.* 2017;8(4).

103. Dorman SE et al. Xpert MTB/RIF Ultra for detection of *Mycobacterium tuberculosis* and rifampicin resistance: A prospective multicentre diagnostic accuracy study. *Lancet Infect Dis.* 2018;18(1):76–84.

104. Boyle D. UNITAID. *Tuberculosis: Diagnostics Technology Landscape.* 5th ed. Geneva: World Health Organization, 2017.

105. Dominguez J et al. Clinical implications of molecular drug resistance testing for *Mycobacterium tuberculosis*: A TBNET/RESIST-TB consensus statement. *Int J Tuberc Lung Dis.* 2016;20(1):24–42.

106. World Health Organization. *The use of molecular line probe assays for the detection of resistance to isoniazid and rifampicin.* Geneva: World Health Organization, 2016.

107. World Health Organization. The use of molecular line probe assays for the detection of resistance to second-line anti-tuberculosis drugs: Policy Guidance. *Geneva: World Health Organization*; 2016.

108. Pankhurst LJ et al. Rapid, comprehensive, and affordable mycobacterial diagnosis with whole-genome sequencing: A prospective study. *Lancet Respir Med* 2016;4(1):49–58.

109. Grenier J et al. Widespread use of serological tests for tuberculosis: Data from 22 high-burden countries. *Eur Respir J.* 2012;39(2):502–5.

110. Steingart KR et al. Performance of purified antigens for serodiagnosis of pulmonary tuberculosis: A meta-analysis. *Clin Vaccine Immunol.* 2008;16(2):260–76.

111. Dowdy DW, Steingart KR, and Pai M. Serological testing versus other strategies for diagnosis of active tuberculosis in India: A cost-effectiveness analysis. *PLoS Med.* 2011;8(8):e1001074.

112. Chegou NN et al. Diagnostic performance of a seven-marker serum protein biosignature for the diagnosis of active TB disease in African primary healthcare clinic attendees with signs and symptoms suggestive of TB. *Thorax.* 2016;71(9):785–94.

113. Shete PB et al. Evaluation of antibody responses to panels of *M. tuberculosis* antigens as a screening tool for active tuberculosis in Uganda. *PLOS ONE.* 2017;12(8):e0180122.

114. Metcalfe JZ et al. Interferon-gamma release assays for active pulmonary tuberculosis diagnosis in adults in low- and middle-income countries: Systematic review and meta-analysis. *J Infect Dis.* 2011;204(Suppl 4):S1120–9.

115. Sester M et al. Interferon-gamma release assays for the diagnosis of active tuberculosis: A systematic review and meta-analysis. *Eur Respir J.* 2011;37(1):100–11.

116. Anderson ST et al. Diagnosis of childhood tuberculosis and host RNA expression in Africa. *N Engl J Med*. 2014;370(18):1712–23.

117. Steingart KR et al. Fluorescence versus conventional sputum smear microscopy for tuberculosis: A systematic review. *Lancet Infect Dis*. 2006;6(9):570–81.

118. Shah M et al. Lateral flow urine lipoarabinomannan assay for detecting active tuberculosis in HIV-positive adults. *Cochrane Database Syst Rev*. 2016;(5).

119. Reza TF et al. Study protocol: A cluster randomized trial to evaluate the effectiveness and implementation of onsite GeneXpert testing at community health centers in Uganda (XPEL-TB). *Implement Sci*. 2020 Apr 21;15(1):24.

120. Broger T et al. Novel lipoarabinomannan point-of-care tuberculosis test for people with HIV: A diagnostic accuracy study. *Lancet Infect Dis*. 2019;19(8):852–61.

8

Radiology of Mycobacterial Disease

ANNE McB. CURTIS

PRIMARY TUBERCULOSIS

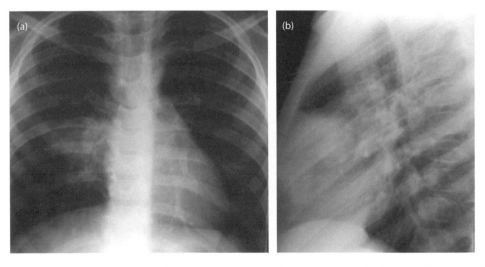

Figure 8.1 (a, b) A 12-year-old female who presented with a fever and cough. Her grandmother had active tuberculosis. The location of the lobar opacity (right middle lobe) and hilar adenopathy are typical for primary infection.

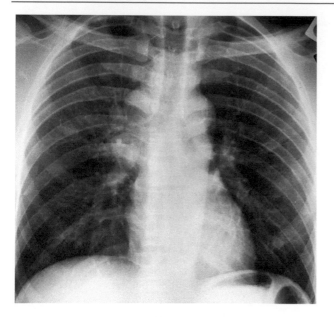

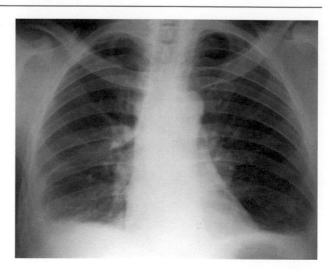

Figure 8.3 A 25-year-old male with fever and weight loss. The pleural effusion and adenopathy are characteristic of primary infection.

Figure 8.2 A 43-year-old male with carpal tunnel syndrome and right paratracheal and hilar adenopathy. The carpal tunnel syndrome was the result of caseating granulomas found at surgery. In the non-HIV-positive population, adenopathy is more common in children and non-Caucasian adults, particularly in African-Americans and persons from India. Although asymmetric adenopathy is uncommon in sarcoidosis, the patterns of tuberculous adenopathy may mimic exactly those of sarcoid and lymphoma.

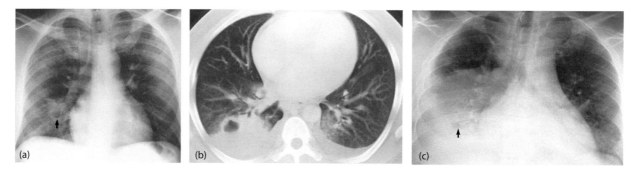

Figure 8.4 (a–c) A 40-year-old male diabetic with fever, chills, and cough of 3 weeks duration. There is an ill-defined opacity with cavitation on admission radiograph (a) (arrow), which is easily seen on computed tomography (b). A tuberculous pleural effusion developed as well (c). The patient was anergic at admission and the diagnosis was made initially by a positive smear at bronchoscopy. He then remembered that a friend had been sick with tuberculosis several months earlier (Figure 8.11 shows the contact's films).

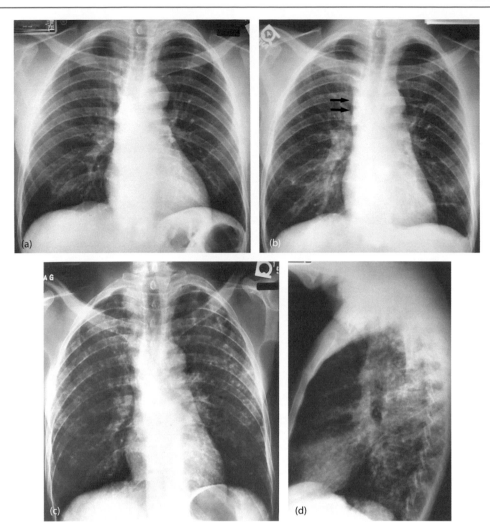

Figure 8.5 (a–d) A 25-year-old male with cough and fever. There is right paratracheal, right hilar, and aortopulmonary adenopathy as well as a left pleural effusion (b). A chest radiograph 4 months earlier (a) shows that these findings are new. All of these findings favor primary infection. The patient was lost to follow-up until he returned 2 months later with continued fever and a 30 lb. weight loss. The adenopathy and pleural effusion resolved, but there are nodules disseminated throughout both lungs (c, d); the sputum was positive for acid-fast bacilli (AFB). No apparent cavitary focus is present and the nodules, now larger than 3 mm, are too big to be considered miliary. Presumably, this represents progression of the hematogenously disseminated primary disease, or primary progressive tuberculosis.

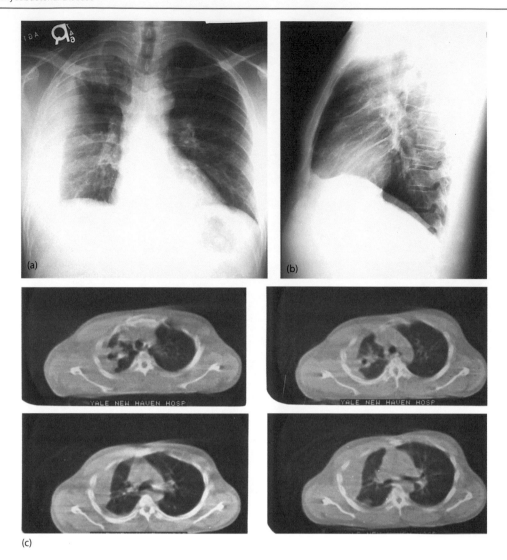

Figure 8.6 (a–c) A 32-year-old male with an asymptomatic routine chest radiograph. No parenchymal focus is evident on posteroanterior and lateral chest radiographs in the presence of a large effusion (a, b). Computed tomography of the chest shows an apical focus of parenchymal disease (c). *Mycobacterium tuberculosis* was found on pleural biopsy and culture. In cases of pleural effusion, a parenchymal lesion that ruptures into the pleural space to produce the effusion usually may be found on computed tomography. Effusions are more frequent with primary infection.

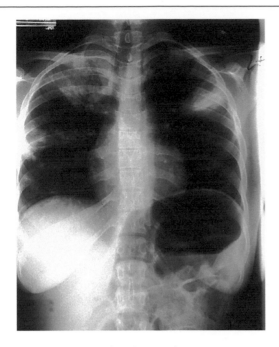

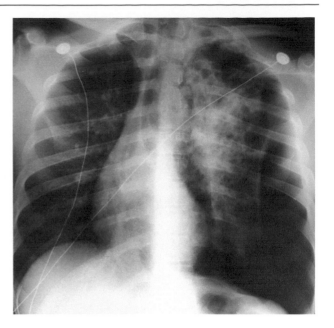

Figure 8.7 A 23-year-old female, 7 weeks postpartum, presented with fever. Bilateral cavitary opacities are present in the upper lobes. The tuberculin skin test was negative and septic emboli were suspected. Angiography was negative. An open lung biopsy demonstrated *M. tuberculosis*. The skin test converted 6 weeks after admission.

Figure 8.8 A 32-year-old male presented with chest pain, fever, and a 20 lb weight loss the day his sister was discharged from the hospital for treatment of active pulmonary tuberculosis. Multiple areas of cavitation are noted in the left lung, which is partially collapsed in the presence of a pneumothorax. The pneumothorax probably resulted from rupture of a necrotic focus into the pleural space. Smear and culture were positive for *M. tuberculosis*.

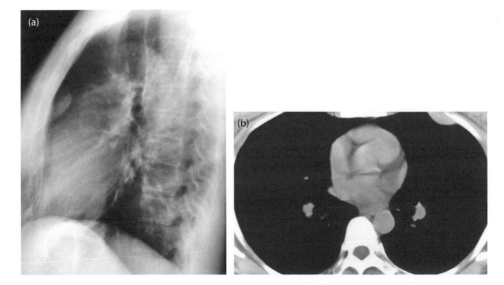

Figure 8.9 (a, b) Residual pleural focus. A 45-year-old female with a history of fever and pleurisy 7 years earlier treated in China for 3 months with streptomycin, isoniazid, and penicillin. A lateral chest film and computed tomography show a pleural-based soft-tissue mass without evidence of bony destruction. No parenchymal lesions or adenopathy were evident. A needle biopsy was negative; caseating granulomas were found at surgery, and *M. tuberculosis* was cultured. The differential diagnosis includes pleural tumors, both benign and malignant.

REACTIVATION TUBERCULOSIS

PULMONARY

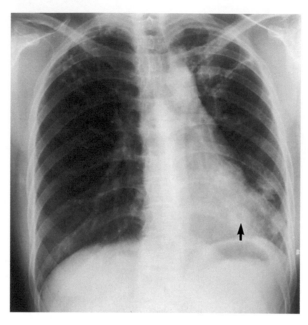

Figure 8.10 A 28-year-old laboratory worker with chronic cough. Bilateral upper lobe volume loss with nodular opacities of varying sizes are seen. Poorly marginated larger opacities are noted in the left lower lobe with a central lucency (arrow) representing cavitation. This is an example of bronchogenic spread.

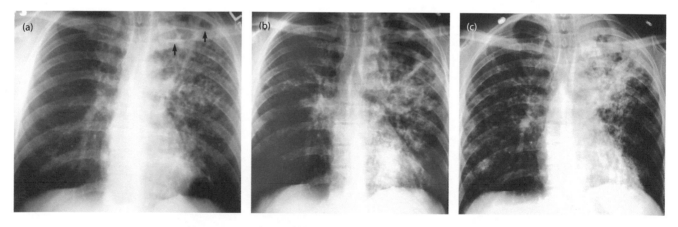

Figure 8.11 (a–c) Bronchogenic spread. A 31-year-old male with fever and cough. Cavities at the left apex (arrow) were not observed initially and the patient was treated for a presumed community acquired infection (a). Progressive cavitation developed with bronchogenic spread to both lungs (b, c). The sputum smear was markedly positive for *M. tuberculosis*. This patient is the contact for Figure 8.4.

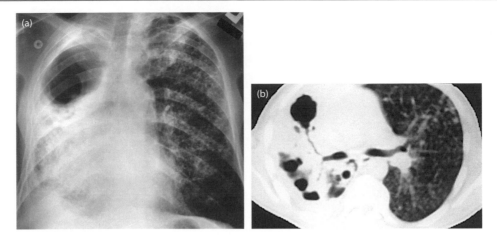

Figure 8.12 (a, b) Multiple cavities with bronchogenic spread. A 52-year-old alcoholic male with cough and weight loss. The sputum smear was markedly positive for *M. tuberculosis*. There is extensive destruction of the right upper lobe with consolidation of the rest of the right lung and bronchogenic spread to the left lung (a). Computed tomography demonstrates much more destruction with multiple irregular cavities in the right lung, as well as tree-in-bud pattern in the left upper lobe, characteristic of bronchogenic spread (b).

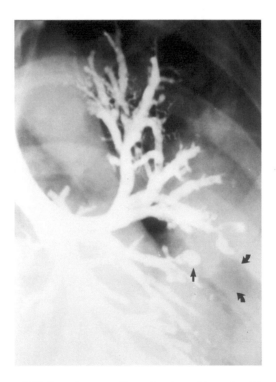

Figure 8.13 Bronchogram. Extensive bronchiectasis with small cavity formation (arrows). Note the lucency peripherally which represents a cavity that did not fill (curved arrows) at bronchography. The smear was markedly positive for *M. tuberculosis*.

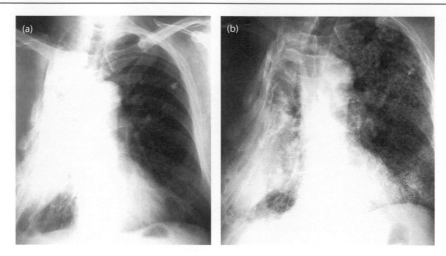

Figure 8.14 (a, b) A 60-year-old male who had had a thoracoplasty for tuberculosis 30 years earlier (a). He presented with a fever and chest radiograph shows miliary dissemination (b).

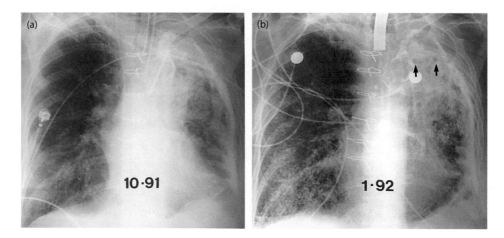

Figure 8.15 (a, b) A 55-year-old female with diabetes who underwent a therapeutic pneumothorax for tuberculosis in 1944. Multiple complications followed a coronary artery bypass graft in October 1991 (a). In January 1992, the patient developed a relentless fever and the sputum was positive for *M. tuberculosis*. On the film of January 1992 (b), lucencies in the left upper lobe represent necrotic foci from which bronchogenic spread occurred (arrow).

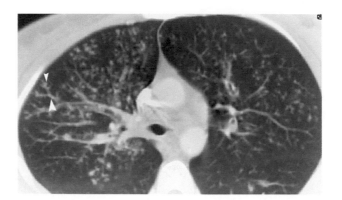

Figure 8.16 Tree-in-bud pattern. A 31-year-old Asian female presented with cough, fever, and a positive smear for *M. tuberculosis*. The buds, or tufts (small arrowhead), represent impacted material in the lobular bronchioles and alveolar ducts, while the stem represents impaction in the last order bronchus of the secondary pulmonary lobule (large arrowhead).

EXTRAPULMONARY

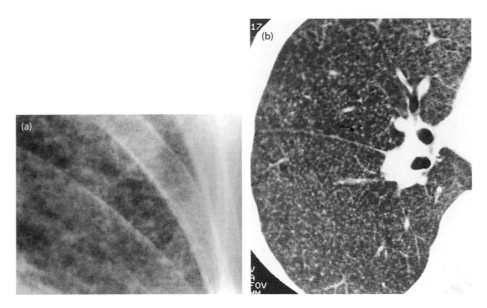

Figure 8.17 (a, b) A 43-year-old male with multiple abdominal fistulae and abscesses as a result of a gunshot wound. One year following the initial injury, he developed miliary lesions in the lung. Bronchoscopy demonstrated caseating granulomas, *M. tuberculosis* was grown from the lungs, and multiple abscesses were visualized in the abdomen. Miliary lesions are seen on a chest radiograph (a) and to better advantage on computed tomography (b).

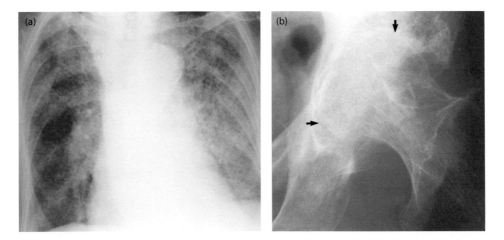

Figure 8.18 (a, b) A 50-year-old female with a history of congestive heart failure and hip pain who was treated with steroids. The chest radiograph initially was thought to suggest congestive heart failure (a). However, typical miliary lesions are noted throughout both lungs. Such miliary spread may occur either in primary or reactivation tuberculosis. The left hip film demonstrates narrowing and destruction of the joint space (arrows) (b). Lack of marginal erosions of the joint are unusual. Aspiration of the hip demonstrated *M. tuberculosis*. Presumably, the steroids led to the breakdown of preexisting tuberculous foci.

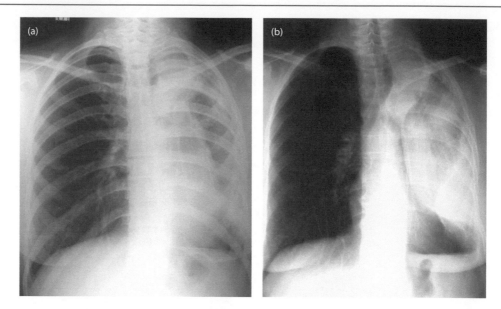

Figure 8.19 (a, b) Progressive fibrothorax. A fibrothorax resulting from a tuberculous empyema is shown with progressive contraction and calcification of the left pleural space over 26 years. Computed tomography occasionally may demonstrate fluid within the "fibrothorax" and viable organisms may be present as well, predisposing to reactivation. Hydropneumothorax (b) resulted from attempted aspiration.

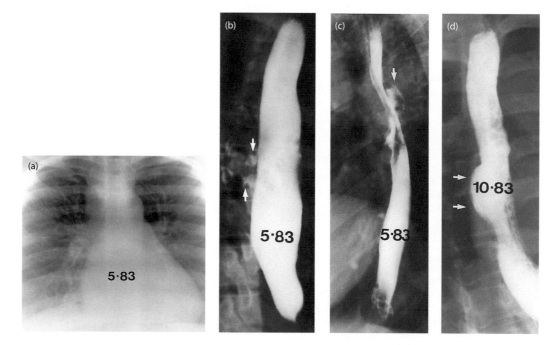

Figure 8.20 (a–d) A 35-year-old female with cough. A chest radiograph in May 1983 demonstrates right paratracheal adenopathy (a). A barium swallow shows ulceration of the esophagus with extravasation of contrast into the tracheobronchial tree at the level of the subcarinal lymph nodes (arrows) (b, c). Follow-up in October demonstrates healing with a residual esophageal diverticulum (arrows) (d). Similar pathology with erosion of tuberculous nodes into the right middle lobe bronchus with resulting stricture was the original cause of the right middle lobe syndrome, i.e., atelectasis with a patent bronchus.

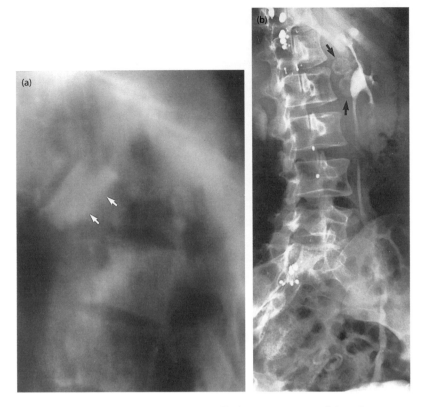

Figure 8.21 (a, b) Tuberculosis of the spine and cavitary tuberculosis of kidney. Destruction of the inferior portion of an upper thoracic vertebral body and complete destruction of the vertebral body below resulted in a gibbus deformity (a). The initial infection usually results from hematogenous spread. Spread from one vertebral body to the next may occur across the disk space or beneath the anterior and posterior longitudinal ligaments. The cavitary lesions in the kidney (arrows) are filled with debris (b). Stricture formation may occur with healing, and careful follow-up with intravenous pyelography is warranted to avoid obstruction. (Photo courtesy of Arthur Rosenfield, MD.)

HEALING

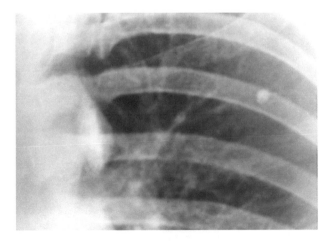

Figure 8.22 Formation of Rhanke complex. Calcified nodule associated with a calcified mediastinal lymph node.

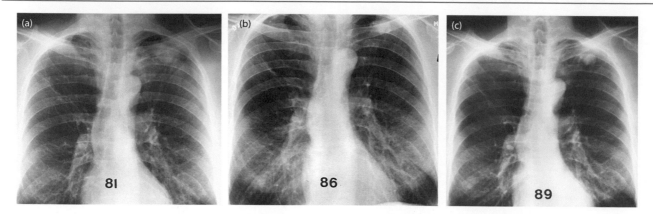

Figure 8.23 (a–c) Tuberculoma formation in a 40-year-old male. A 1981 radiograph shows a poorly marginated opacity in the left upper lobe and some scarring (stable over several years) in the right upper lobe (a). Sputum was positive for *M. tuberculosis*. Films in 1986 (b) and 1989 (c) demonstrate contraction of the left upper lobe nodular opacity with increasing density to form a smooth lobulated mass, typical of a tuberculoma. At autopsy, tuberculomas may contain viable organisms.

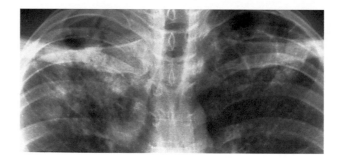

Figure 8.24 Biapical cavities as well as nodules in a 39-year-old alcoholic male. Complete resolution occurred after 1 year of therapy.

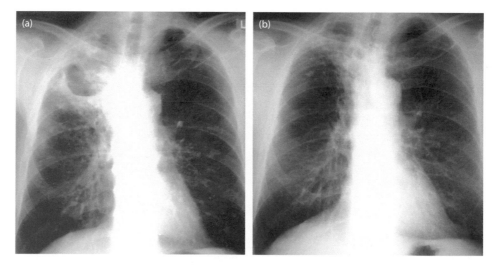

Figure 8.25 (a, b) Healing with cavity closure. A large cavity in the right upper lobe in October has an air fluid level (a). Note the calcified nodule in the left perihilar region. Twelve months following treatment the cavity has closed with right upper lobe volume loss and residual apical nodular opacities (b). In cavitary tuberculosis, air fluid levels are slightly unusual, but do occur. Cavities may or may not close completely. Radiographic stability for 6 months must be documented to describe "inactive" tuberculosis.

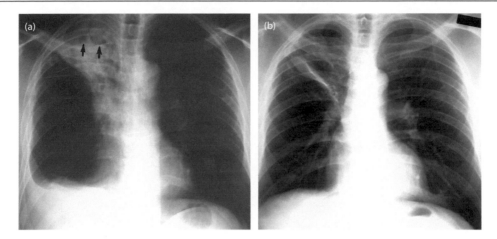

Figure 8.26 (a, b) Incomplete cavity closure. Right upper lobe consolidation, volume loss and multiple lucencies representing cavities are present in association with a pleural effusion (a). Considerable resolution is present after 6 months of treatment with clearing of the pleural effusion. Volume loss persists as well as a cystic space (b). Repeated cultures were negative. Preexisting cystic spaces may simulate cavitary disease where infection occurs with community acquired pneumonia (see Figure 8.27).

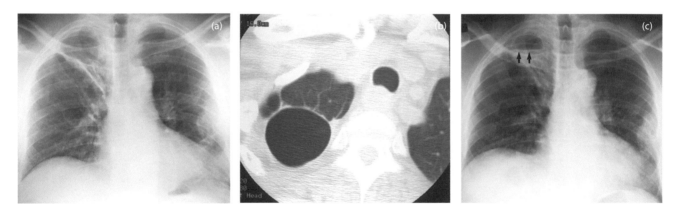

Figure 8.27 (a–c) A 55-year-old male alcoholic with cavitary tuberculosis diagnosed in October 1982 (a) that healed with contraction and residual cystic spaces by April 1983 (b). He presented in December 1992 with weakness, seizures, and vomiting. There is an air-fluid level in the right upper lobe at presentation (c). Although tuberculosis was suspected, it was not found at bronchoscopy and the cavitary opacity healed with nontuberculous antibiotic therapy. This demonstrates that air fluid levels may occur in preexisting spaces and do not necessarily reflect necrosis with cavitation, as would be seen in active tuberculosis.

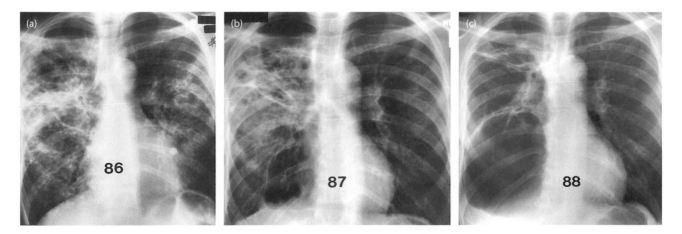

Figure 8.28 (a–c) A 32-year-old male with active tuberculosis and a positive sputum smear. Over a 2-year period, healing occurs with progressive destruction of the parenchyma and extensive bullous formation in the right lung. Minimal nodular changes are seen on the left.

TUBERCULOSIS OR CANCER?

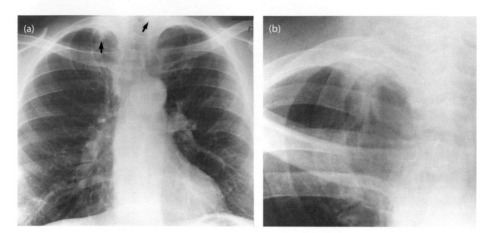

Figure 8.29 (a, b) A 60-year-old male with a 50 pack/year smoking history and an apical density at the right apex. The skin test was negative and old films were not available. The irregular margins of this lesion are highly suspicious for a neoplasm, but at resection the lesion proved to be tuberculous.

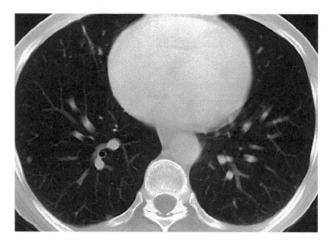

Figure 8.30 CT of a 54-year-old male nonsmoker performed to evaluate the pulmonary hilum, which was normal. Nodular opacities are noted peripherally at both bases. At surgery, multiple subpleural nodules were found that were non-necrotizing granulomas. A lymph node resected at the same time was culture positive for *M. tuberculosis*.

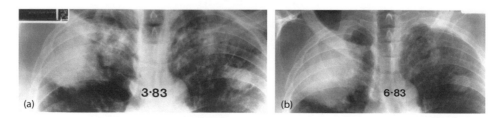

Figure 8.31 (a, b) A 50-year-old male with cough and weight loss whose sputum was positive on culture for *M. tuberculosis* (a). A mass in the right upper lobe continued to enlarge despite response to therapy in the left upper lobe (b), and adenocarcinoma was demonstrated by biopsy.

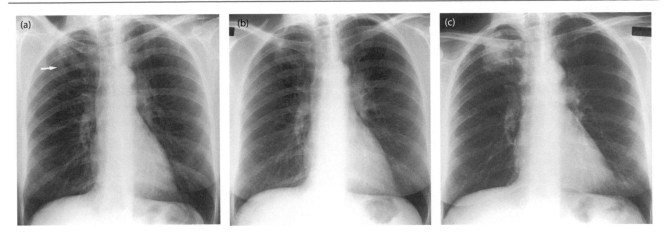

Figure 8.32 (a–c) A 44-year-old white female with a history of incomplete treatment for tuberculosis. The patient was followed for several years, and a growing mass was resected and proved to be an adenocarcinoma. Multiple granulomas were noted in the specimen as well. The patient had a 40 pack/year smoking history, but stopped 6 years before entry into the clinic. Adenocarcinoma is the most frequently associated "scar" carcinoma, but other cell types have been reported as well. It is important when evaluating serial films to compare films widely separated in time (e.g., 2 years) if they are available. Subtle progressive changes over repeated short intervals (e.g., 3–6 months) may be overlooked, as had happened to this patient over a 6-year period.

TUBERCULOSIS AND NON-HIV-RELATED IMMUNOSUPPRESSION

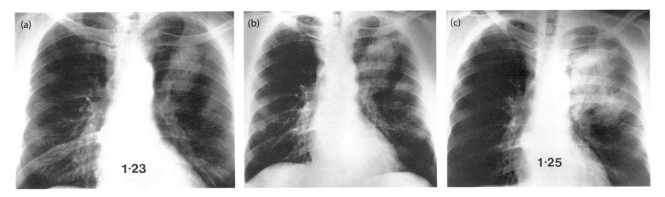

Figure 8.33 (a–c) A 67-year-old male with fever and chronic myelogenous leukemia. Over 3 days, aggressive opacification of the left upper lobe was noted. Sputum smear and culture were positive for *M. tuberculosis*. Rapid progression may be related to immunosuppression.

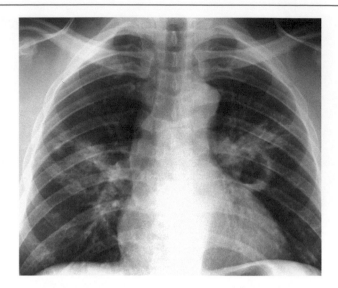

Figure 8.34 A 50-year-old male presenting with fever and nasal stuffiness completed 1 year of treatment with cyclophosphamide for granulomatosis with polyangiitis. Recurrence of granulomatosis with polyangiitis has not been reported once complete remission has occurred in a patient who continues on full doses of chemotherapy. In this case, with a new infiltrate, there was no evidence of relapse, and another cause of cavitary disease was sought. Although tuberculosis is very unusual in patients with granulomatosis with polyangiitis, *M. tuberculosis* was found at bronchoscopy.

HIV-RELATED TUBERCULOSIS

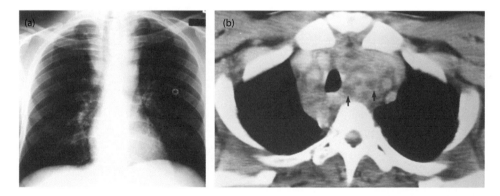

Figure 8.35 (a, b) An HIV-positive intravenous drug abuser with a 3-month history of fever and a mass in the neck. Mediastinal widening extending into the neck with deviation of the trachea to the right is seen on a chest radiograph (a). Computed tomography demonstrates multiple enlarged lymph nodes with low-density centers (arrows) (b). *M. tuberculosis* was obtained at mediastinoscopy. Thoracic adenopathy is not a feature of AIDS-related complex, and an infectious or neoplastic cause should be sought to explain the adenopathy.

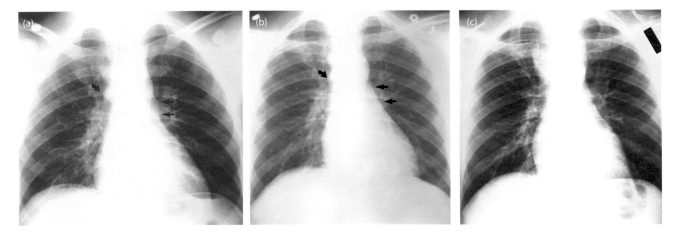

Figure 8.36 (a–c) A 27-year-old HIV-negative intravenous drug abuser, on peritoneal dialysis for 1 year, presented with fevers. Initial chest radiograph (a) shows free intraperitoneal air as well as azygos (curved arrow) and aortopulmonary adenopathy with a convex margin at the main pulmonary outflow tract (straight arrows). Empiric therapy for *M. tuberculosis* was given for 6 weeks. Treatment was discontinued when cultures were negative. The chest radiograph after 6 weeks of treatment shows regression of the aortopulmonary and azygos adenopathy (arrows) (b). A routine chest radiograph 7 months later demonstrates a mediastinal mass, and the patient was noted to have become HIV positive (c). Thoracotomy demonstrated *M. tuberculosis* in the mediastinal nodes. Adenopathy is far more common in patients with tuberculosis who are HIV positive than those who are HIV negative. Careful comparison with a baseline radiograph, if available, is mandatory as the adenopathy may be subtle. Tuberculosis may be the first manifestation of AIDS. (Photo courtesy of Ernest Moritz, MD.)

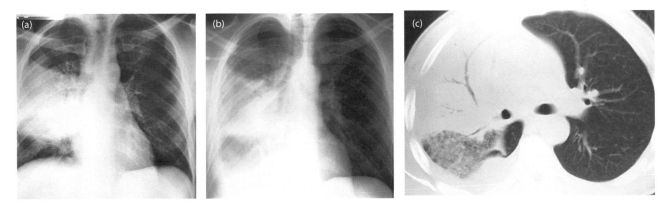

Figure 8.37 (a–c) A 37-year-old HIV-positive male intravenous drug user with fever and cough. Six months before admission, he had been diagnosed with tuberculosis, but discontinued therapy after 4 months. There is consolidation of the right upper lobe with bulging of the fissure, as well as right paratracheal adenopathy (a). A pleural effusion developed 5 days later (b). Computed tomography demonstrates dense consolidation with a bulging fissure, a pleural effusion, and spread to the right lower lobe (c). The sputum was positive for *M. tuberculosis*. Tuberculosis can be very aggressive in immunocompromised patients, particularly those with low CD4 counts. The consolidation in the right upper lobe with a bulging fissure is more typical of staphylococcal and Gram-negative organisms reflecting aggressive infection.

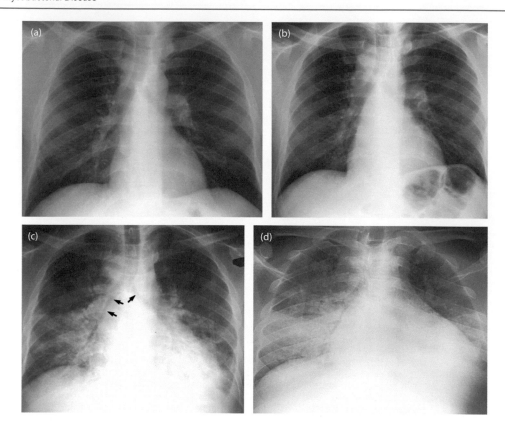

Figure 8.38 (a–d) A 29-year-old intravenous drug abuser with AIDS and a CD4 count of 53 presented with fever and cough. Initial exam demonstrates some hilar adenopathy (a). An exam 1 month later demonstrates progression to right paratracheal adenopathy (b). Two weeks following, there is marked increase in the mediastinal and hilar adenopathy with narrowing of the bronchus intermedius as well as the left main stem bronchus (arrows) (c). Diffuse parenchymal consolidation developed rapidly as well (d). After 12 days, the admission sputum culture was positive for *M. tuberculosis*. The sputum became positive on smear when the parenchymal opacities appeared. Rapid clearing resulted after 2 weeks of therapy. This is an example of extremely rapid progression of both lymphadenopathy and parenchymal consolidation in an immunocompromised patient. This patient typifies what once was called "galloping consumption."

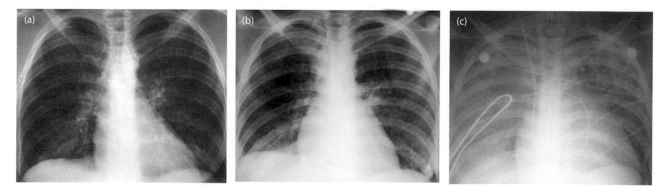

Figure 8.39 (a–c) A 28-year-old HIV-positive female, presenting with cough, fever, abdominal pain, and back pain. Blood cultures were positive for *M. tuberculosis*, and miliary dissemination occurred, followed by acute respiratory distress syndrome (ARDS), shown here with three consecutive daily chest radiographs (a–c). Bronchoscopy following intubation demonstrated AFB on smear. Although unusual, tuberculosis is a well-known cause of ARDS.

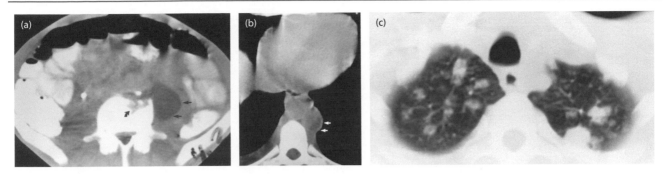

Figure 8.40 (a–c) A 32-year-old HIV-positive male with a history of intravenous drug abuse presented with abdominal pain and was found to have a perforated duodenal ulcer. Computed tomography demonstrates destruction of a vertebral body (curved arrow), with a paraspinal fluid collection (arrow) (a). Similar fluid collections were noted elsewhere in the abdomen. Drainage of the paraspinal collection demonstrated *M. tuberculosis*. Mediastinal computed tomography shows a paravertebral mass extending superiorly from the abdomen, representing a tuberculous abscess (arrow) (b). Chest computed tomography shows parenchymal involvement as well (c).

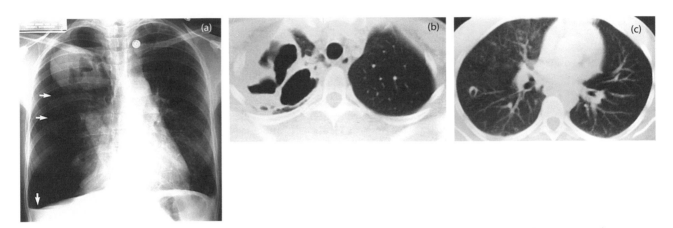

Figure 8.41 (a–c) A 27-year-old HIV-positive female intravenous drug abuser presented with a 1-month history of cough and fever followed by the sudden onset of right-sided chest pain. A hydropneumothorax is demonstrated (arrows) (a). A sharply marginated mass with multiple air fluid levels is seen in the right upper lobe (a). Extensive cavitation ensued (b), and multiple smaller cavitary lesions were noted on computed tomography (c). Resection of the abscess showed *Pneumocystis carinii* on silver stain, and cultures grew *M. tuberculosis*, *M. avium* complex (MAC), *Klebsiella*, and *Enterobacter*. A portion of a resected rib showed necrotizing granulomas in the marrow. This patient responded well to therapy, but died 3 months later with a severe electrolyte disturbance. The chest radiograph during that admission showed no new abnormalities and she was negative for *M. tuberculosis*.

ATYPICAL MYCOBACTERIOSIS: HIV- AND NON-HIV-RELATED

HIV-RELATED

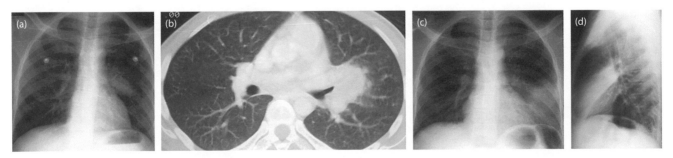

Figure 8.42 (a–d) A 36-year-old HIV-positive male with left hilar adenopathy seen on chest radiography (a) and computed tomography (b), followed by lingular consolidation (c, d). At bronchoscopy, an endobronchial mass was found which occluded the lingular bronchus. This was AFB positive on smear and only MAC was cultured.

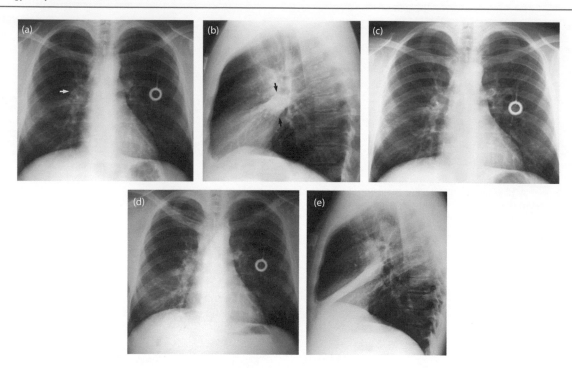

Figure 8.43 (a–e) A 33-year-old HIV-positive male with progressive middle lobe consolidation (a–c) that resulted in complete collapse of the middle lobe (d, e). Adenopathy can be appreciated (arrows) (a, b). Bronchoscopy yielded *M. kansasii*. This is much less frequent than MAC. Consolidation with atelectasis should suggest endobronchial disease and, in the HIV population, mycobacterial disease should be considered strongly.

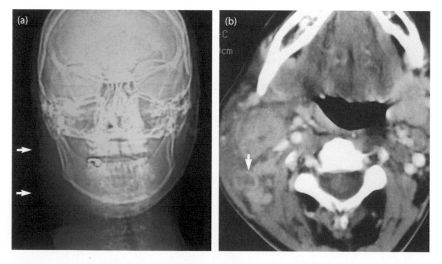

Figure 8.44 (a, b) A 37-year-old male with AIDS and a CD4 count of 16 who presented with fever and neck swelling. A digitized radiograph shows massive swelling in the right neck (a) and computed tomography shows large nodes with low-density central areas typical of tuberculous lymphadenitis (arrow) (b). Culture of the biopsied node was positive for MAC.

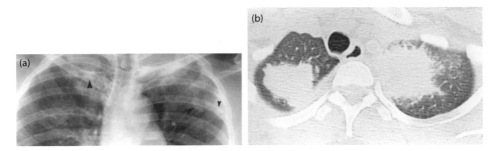

Figure 8.45 (a, b) HIV with reconstituted immunity. A 35-year-old African-American woman diagnosed 2 months previously with AIDS. After 6 weeks of antiviral treatment, she developed a cough and hemoptysis. The CD4 count had risen from 34 to 490, and the PPD had become positive as had the chest radiograph. The open lung biopsy demonstrated MAC. The chest radiograph (a) shows multiple pleural-based poorly marginated apical opacities bilaterally (large arrow) as well as a cavitating parenchymal nodule (small arrow). Computed tomography of the chest shows the poorly marginated pleural-based parenchymal masses (b). Subsequent computed tomography of the abdomen showed necrotic lymph nodes compatible with MAC.

NON-HIV-RELATED

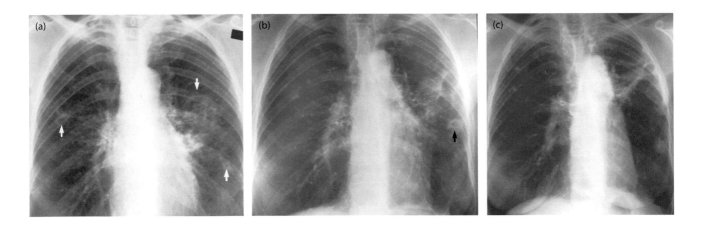

Figure 8.46 (a–c) A 71-year-old female with a history of whooping cough as a child followed by multiple episodes of pneumonia. Bronchiectasis was diagnosed on bronchography in 1977 and, when required, intermittent antibiotics were administered for infection. MAC was seen in increasing concentration in the sputum with the onset of hemoptysis in 1986. A chest radiograph shows cavitary lesions of various sizes in the right and left lungs (a). Over 2 years, the largest cavity on the left has contracted and a new cavity is noted below this (arrow) (b). After 4 years of chemotherapy, the sputum finally became negative and the chest radiograph stabilized (c). Bronchiectasis may be a predisposing factor for infections with atypical mycobacteria.

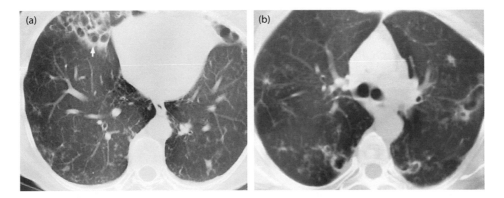

Figure 8.47 (a, b) A 54-year-old female with a history of recurrent pneumonias following an episode of whooping cough as a child. She presented with mild hemoptysis and a positive purified protein derivative (PPD). In 1992 her sputum was positive for AFB, which initially were identified by probe as *M. tuberculosis*, then biochemically as *M. xenopi*, and finally as *M. celatum*. Computed tomography demonstrates an area of cystic bronchiectasis in the right middle lobe (arrow) (a). Elsewhere are cavities of varying sizes, some irregularly shaped (b). Smaller cavitary lesions were present on a computed tomographic examination 7 years previously.

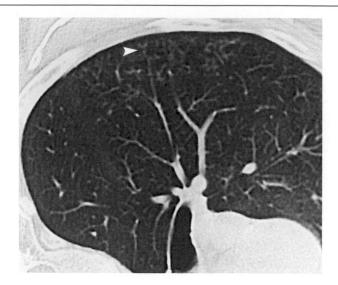

Figure 8.48 Tree-in-bud pattern. A 57-year-old woman with a history of several episodes of hemoptysis, diagnosed with MAC. Peripheral branching and nodular opacities (arrow) represent the tree-in-bud pattern. The tree-in-bud pattern can be seen with a wide variety of pulmonary infections as well as cystic fibrosis, allergic bronchopulmonary aspergillosis, asthma, obliterative bronchiolitis, and panbronchiolitis.

LOOK-ALIKES

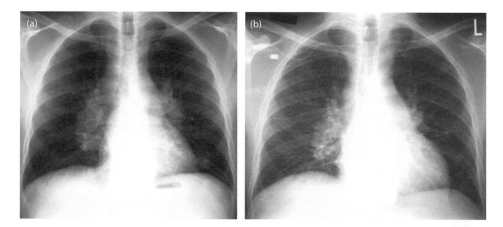

Figure 8.49 (a, b) A 48-year-old HIV-positive male with a history of intravenous drug abuse who presented with a septic groin. A chest radiograph demonstrates extensive bilateral hilar and paratracheal adenopathy (a). A chest radiograph performed 2 years earlier demonstrates that the adenopathy is stable (b). Stable adenopathy is not a feature of tuberculous adenopathy or of HIV disease. A transbronchial biopsy showed noncaseating granulomas compatible with sarcoidosis.

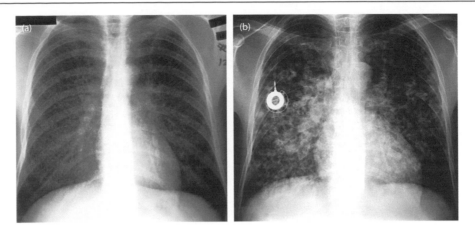

Figure 8.50 (a, b) A 24-year-old HIV-positive Puerto Rican male presented with fevers. A chest radiograph from October 1987 demonstrates typical miliary lesions that are the result of histoplasmosis and not tuberculosis (a). Histoplasmosis is endemic in Puerto Rico and this radiograph is thought to represent endogenous reinfection. The patient responded transiently to antifungal therapy but eventually relapsed (b).

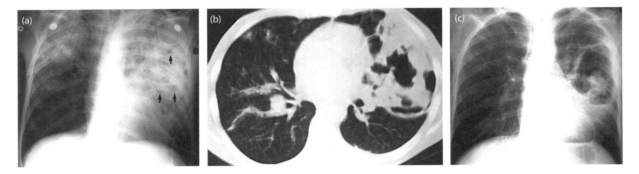

Figure 8.51 (a–c) A 53-year-old HIV-positive male presented with fever. Bilateral consolidation is noted, but there also are areas of lucency (arrows) within the consolidated left lung, suggesting cavitation and necrosis (a). Computed tomography shows extensive cavitation with sloughing of lung on the left (b). A chest radiograph from July 8 demonstrates a large cavity with a central mass (c). This gradually resolved and represents pulmonary gangrene. In this instance, *S. pneumoniae* was obtained. Gangrene most frequently results from *Klebsiella*, and less commonly from *S. pneumoniae* infection. Occasionally, tuberculosis will produce a similar appearance.

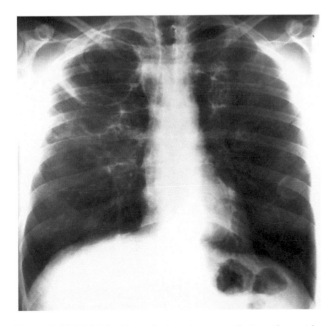

Figure 8.52 Multiple thin-walled cystic spaces that are the residua of a previous *Pneumocystis carinii* infection. These may rupture to produce pneumothoraces. The thin walls are fairly smooth and should not be confused with the cavities of mycobacterial disease.

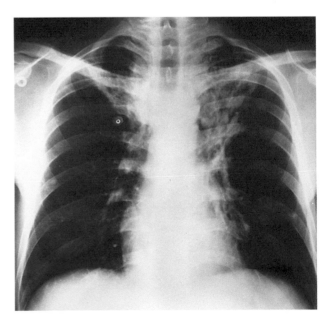

Figure 8.53 Atypical distribution of *P. carinii* pneumonia occurs in patients who are on inhaled pentamidine. This appearance may mimic tuberculosis due to its upper lobe distribution, but the history of prophylactic pentamidine should raise the possibility that this is *P. carinii* pneumonia.

ACKNOWLEDGMENTS

Thanks to Michael Brown for photography and to Louise Leader for preparation of the manuscript.

9

Diagnosis of Latent TB Infection

AJIT LALVANI, CLEMENTINE FRASER, AND MANISH PAREEK

INTRODUCTION

A quarter of the world's population is estimated to be infected with *Mycobacterium tuberculosis* (M.tb),[1] approximately 1.7 billion people.

This provides a very large reservoir for future active tuberculosis. With the implementation of the World Health Organization (WHO) End TB strategy, aiming to reduce tuberculosis (TB) incidence by 90% by 2035, diagnosing and treating latent tuberculosis infection (LTBI) successfully is of paramount importance.

Whether someone develops active TB, LTBI, or clears the infection following exposure is a complex interaction of bacterial, environmental, exposure, and host factors.

Approximately 10% of those with LTBI will progress to active TB. The risk of reactivation and subsequent disease is significantly increased in those with recently acquired LTBI (the majority within the first 2 years post infection),[2] the prevalence of which is estimated to be 0.8% of the global population, amounting to 55.5 million individuals currently at high risk of TB disease.[1] Risk factors for progression from LTBI to active TB are all mediated via immunodeficiency and are outlined in Table 9.1.

Current immunodiagnostic tests for TB encompass humoral and cell-mediated immune-based tests, the widely available tuberculin skin test (TST) and interferon-gamma (IFN-γ) release

Table 9.1 Risk factors for progression of LTBI to active TB

Category	Risk factor
Co-morbidities	HIV, CKD, Diabetes
Drugs	Biologic therapy TNF-α inhibitors, immune regulators used for inflammatory diseases, immunosuppressive therapies for transplant patients
Social	Homelessness, drug and alcohol misuse, malnourishment

Table 9.2 Classes of immunodiagnostic tools available for the diagnosis of TB

Immunodiagnostic tests for TB	Examples
Humoral immunity-based tests	Serology
	Antibodies in lymphocyte supernatant
T-cell-based tests	IGRAs
	Next-generation IGRAs (additional new antigens)
	CTB skin test
	TST
	Multicytokine and multichemokine assays
Measures of host response	Transcriptomics
	Proteomics

assays (IGRAs) as well as other measures of host response (transcriptomics and proteomics) (see Table 9.2).

In the case of LTBI, there are no localizing symptoms, signs, or tissue pathology to target, therefore diagnosis can be challenging. It is in this clinical setting the host response can be used as a marker of infection.

CURRENTLY AVAILABLE IMMUNODIAGNOSTICS

CELL-MEDIATED IMMUNITY-BASED TESTS OF TB INFECTION

Cell-mediated immunity (CMI) in the host response to M.tb is of central importance in the diagnosis of M.tb. All the commercially available platforms exploit the fact that M.tb infection, even at very low bacterial burdens as in LTBI, evokes a strong CMI response to M.tb antigens. TSTs are the oldest CMI-based tests in medicine, with IGRAs being the first antigen-specific T-cell-based diagnostic tests. More recently, a low cost, highly specific C-TB skin test has shown promise.

TST

The TST induces a type IV hypersensitivity reaction when the purified protein derivative (PPD) of several M.tb strains is injected into the sub-dermis of a previously exposed individual (exposure to Bacillus Calmette–Guérin [BCG] vaccine, M.tb, or environmental mycobacteria). Along with the chest x-ray, TST was the mainstay of LTBI diagnosis during the twentieth century and is still widely employed today, especially in high-burden regions. The TST has several disadvantages, which will be discussed later on in this chapter. However, despite its limitations, the TST remains widely used, especially in low-income countries with a high-TB burden. Its relative cheapness and simplicity, combined with years of experience in its use continue to make it an attractive option. Its continued clinical utility has recently been clearly exemplified in a large study from Africa showing the clinical benefit of targeting chemoprophylaxis based on TST results in a population with high burdens of both TB and human immunodeficiency virus (HIV) infection.[3]

IGRA

IGRAs are blood tests, the immunological basis of which involves the *ex vivo* release of the key anti-M.tb cytokine IFN-γ. Purified white blood cells from the test participant are incubated overnight in a laboratory with antigens from M.tb that are not found in the BCG vaccine. IGRAs yield a quantitative readout of IFN-γ secretion, which has a valid basis in our understanding of the immune response to M.tb. Much research over the last decade has shown that M.tb antigen-specific T-cell-derived IFN-γ is a valid and clinically useful biomarker of M.tb infection. Put simply, if the individual has been infected with M.tb then T-cells specific for M.tb antigens will recognize those antigens upon re-encounter *ex vivo* and secrete IFN-γ. Commercially, this is measured using one of two platforms: enzyme-linked immunosorbent assay (ELISA), which measures IFN-γ concentration (QuantiFERON®-TB-Gold In-Tube [QFT-GIT] and more recently QuantiFERON-TB Gold Plus [QFT-Plus], Cellestis, Qiagen, NL), or ELISpot, which measures IFN-γ spot-forming cells (T-Spot.*TB*, Oxford Immunotec, Abingdon, UK) (see Table 9.3 for summary).

Over the last 3–4 years there have been updates to the commercially available immunodiagnostic tests; improvement has been made upon the traditional ELISA and ELISpot methods by allowing the measurement of multiple analytes in one patient sample. The QFT-GIT has been replaced by QuantiFERON Gold Plus (QFT-Plus). This test has two tubes (TB1 and TB2). TB1 includes longer peptides from ESAT-6 and CFP-10 with TB2 including peptides to induce IFN-γ production by both CD4 and CD8 T-cells (TB7.7, present in QFT-GIT, has been removed). The rationale for the inclusion of these new CD8-specific peptides is derived from growing evidence that M.tb-specific CD8+ T-cells are more frequently detected in subjects with active TB disease as opposed

Table 9.3 Summary of characteristics of IGRAs

- IGRAs are based on the *ex vivo* release of the key anti-MTB cytokine interferon gamma (IFN-γ)
- IGRAs are more specific than TST and not affected by previous BCG vaccination
- Sensitivity of IGRAs is at least equivalent to TST
- IGRAs are similar to TST in predicting progression from latent to active TB
- Current IGRAs are unavailable to rule-in/rule-out the diagnosis of active TB
- IGRAs are increasingly incorporated into national guidelines
- IGRAs are unable to differentiate between latent and active TB
- IGRAs should not be used to monitor response to therapy or as a test of cure

to LTBI, or a recent exposure to TB, and decline when patients receive anti-TB treatment. Preliminary data from a multicenter European study suggest that the QFT-Plus retains the same sensitivity as the previous version; however, we are yet to observe any large head to head trials showing superiority.[4–7]

Currently, both assays use the M.tb-specific antigens, early-secreted antigen-6 (ESAT-6), and culture filtrate protein-10 (CFP-10). QFT-GIT additionally includes a third antigen Rv2654 or TB7.7. These antigens confer the high specificity of IGRAs; in contrast, TST utilizes PPD, a highly antigenic but relatively nonspecific mixture of over 200 MTB antigens, many of which are shared with the *Mycobacterium bovis* BCG vaccine leading to false-positive TST results in those who are BCG vaccinated.

ESAT-6 and CFP-10 are proteins encoded in the genomic region of MTB known as region of difference-1 (RD-1). During repeated passages of a virulent strain of *M. bovis in vitro* through ox bile, Calmette and Guérin developed the non-virulent vaccine strain. Exploration of the M.tb genome during the late twentieth century revealed that this process had resulted in the loss of several virulence-encoding genomic regions including RD-1, rendering BCG unable to produce these proteins. ESAT-6 and CFP-10 are the best understood and form a secreted heterodimer that is part of a type VII secretion system.[8,9] Subsequent studies identified them to be highly immunodominant and therefore attractive candidates for a TB blood test.[10,11] Only four species of environmental mycobacteria, *Mycobacterium kansasii*, *M. szulgai*, *M. marinum*, and *M. riyadhense* have RD-1-like regions minimizing false positives. The use of ESAT-6 and CFP-10 has led to the first generation of IGRAs. Over the years, further antigens that are targets of IFN-γ-secreting T-cells in M.tb-infected persons and that are also highly specific for M.tb, either by virtue of being RD1-encoded or RD1-dependent for virulence and secretion have been identified.[12,13]

LATENT TUBERCULOSIS

Latent tuberculosis infection (LTBI) was previously thought to represent a uniform state. However, as research progresses it has become clear that LTBI constitutes a broad spectrum of infection states that differ by the degree of the pathogen replication, host immune response, and inflammation.[14] After initial exposure,

M.tb will either be cleared or individuals will become actively or latently infected. The core concept being that in LTBI, patients remain asymptomatic despite an element of persistent immune response to stimulation by M.tb antigens.

As part of the WHO's aim to eradicate TB strategy there has been a huge research push to understand the natural history and biology of LTBI. Epidemiological studies have shown the majority of reactivated latent disease will do so soon after infection (3–9 months) and almost always within 2 years.[2]

The most important step when diagnosing LTBI is to first ensure that the patient does not have active TB. The diagnostic process for LTBI should begin with a thorough history (to identify risk factors for TB exposure) and examination with the aim being to identify any clinical evidence of active TB. If patients are symptomatic they should be referred for diagnostic evaluation for potential active TB.

LTBI DIAGNOSIS BY IGRA

In parallel with national and international guidelines for TB elimination, awareness, diagnosis, and therefore treatment of LTBI has increased in recent years.[15–19] When investigating patients for possible LTBI, it must first be remembered that one should only investigate those patients in whom a positive result would lead to treatment.

The evidence-base supporting the clinical utility of IGRA is largest in the diagnosis of LTBI in immunocompetent individuals. Generating the evidence base itself has been challenging as the lack of a gold standard test for LTBI makes it impossible to assess any new diagnostic tool with definable certainty as to sensitivity and specificity, because the TST itself is an inadequate reference standard. Studies that evaluate the utility of the IGRA have therefore taken several alternative approaches to substitute LTBI. Active TB has been used as a surrogate as well as the degree of MTB exposure. However, arguably the most pertinent and the new gold standard involves correlating IGRA responses with the subsequent development of disease. To assess IGRA specificity, studies have analyzed the presence of IGRA negativity in healthy BCG-vaccinated individuals at low risk of TB infection due to the absence of epidemiologic risk factors for TB exposure.

IMMUNOCOMPETENT ADULTS

ACTIVE TB AS A SURROGATE MARKER

Results from extensive meta-analyses and systematic reviews conclude that the sensitivity of IGRAs is superior to that of TST. The T-spot has a consistently higher sensitivity than the IGRA or TST in several cohorts (ELISpot 67%–89% vs. ELISA 61%–84% vs. TST 65%–77%).[20–24] Based on published meta-analyses, IGRAs have a specificity for LTBI diagnosis of >95% in settings with a low-TB incidence, with specificity not being affected by BCG vaccination.[20,23,25] Data on the newer QFT-Plus is more limited. However, performance of this assay using active TB as a surrogate appears to be equivalent to that of QFT-GIT with a computed overall sensitivity of 87.9%.[7]

TB EXPOSURE AS A SURROGATE

Exposure studies can take the form of direct contact exposure or the assumption of exposure from countries where TB is endemic. Much of the available data using TB exposure as a surrogate for LTBI in immunocompetent adults come from precise, point source outbreak, and contact-tracing investigations. One of the first studies to use this exposure as a proxy for LTBI looked at adult household contacts of TB patients in the UK. It was shown that IGRA responses were significantly correlated (more so than with TST) with intensity of exposure and not affected by prior BCG vaccination.[10] Subsequently, this has been replicated in recent migrants to the UK. IGRA test positivity was independently associated, on multivariate analysis, with risk factors for TB infection—namely TB incidence in country of origin and age.[26] A recent large prospective study enrolled 10,740 US-based participants at high risk for latent infection (included children, adults, and immunosuppressed). The TST was less specific than either IGRA, particularly among foreign-born populations (TST 70.0% vs. QFT-GIT 98.5% vs. T-SPOT 99.3%), concluding that IGRAs should be strongly preferred over the TST for both foreign-born children and adults.[27]

IMMUNOCOMPROMISED SUBJECTS AND OTHER SPECIAL POPULATIONS

ACTIVE TB AS A SURROGATE FOR LTBI

In general, fewer studies have assessed the performance of IGRAs in HIV-positive individuals who are co-infection with M.tb. The evidence suggests that IGRAs perform better than TST in this population with T-SPOT being superior to QFT-GIT.

Early work from Zambia and South Africa found that the sensitivity of the T-SPOT in HIV-positive adults and children was relatively high and superior to TST.[28–30] Although fewer studies have been conducted in HIV-positive subjects in low-TB burden settings, they have also found the sensitivity of the IGRA to be greater than that observed with the TST.[27,31–33] Studies conducted in HIV-infected subjects in Zambia, Tanzania, and Italy found that the sensitivity of the QFT-GIT in HIV-positive individuals was higher than that of TST but significantly lower than in HIV-negative individuals.[33–35]

Two recent systematic reviews and meta-analyses have computed pooled sensitivity figures for the performance of IGRAs in HIV-positive individuals. Cattamanchi estimated that in HIV-positive individuals with active TB, QFT-GIT sensitivity was 61% (95% confidence interval [CI] 47%–75%) while T-SPOT sensitivity was 72% (95% CI 62–81).[21] Higher sensitivities were reported in high-income countries, i.e., T-SPOT 94% (95% CI 73%–100%) and QFT-GIT 67% (95% CI 47%–83%).[21] By contrast, Santin and colleagues calculated the pooled sensitivities of 61% and 65% for the QFT-GIT and T-SPOT, respectively.[36] Ayubi et al. found that in HIV patients, TST negative/QFT-GIT positive discordance was more commonly observed likely reflecting the lower sensitivity of TST in HIV patients.[37]

The reported effect of CD4 count on IGRA performance is variable. There is some published evidence suggesting that QFT-GIT performance is adversely affected by falling CD4 count.[35] However, in a large study conducted by Clark et al. in a low-TB burden setting they found that T-SPOT results were independent of CD4 cell counts in HIV-positive individuals.[31]

A recent Zambian study of patients with TB–HIV co-infection found an overall sensitivity of 83% for QFT-Plus. Although test sensitivity did not significantly differ according to HIV status, the authors did find that those individuals with a CD4 count <100 were significantly less likely to have a positive result, suggesting that advanced immunosuppression adversely impacts on test performance.[38] A recent systematic review of 4,856 HIV-positive subjects found that both TST and IGRAs (T.SPOT and QFT-GIT) performed similarly, although concordance between the tests varied considerably in certain studies indicating that further research was required.[39]

The consensus of these multiple studies and meta-analyses is that IGRAs perform as well as or better than TST in HIV positive individuals; however they do not perform as well as they do in HIV-negative populations and sensitivity decreases with falling CD4 count.

IGRA has been shown to be more sensitive than TST at diagnosing latent TB in pregnancy. In a pregnant HIV-positive population IGRA has proven superior,[40] having identified >2-fold more women with LTBI compared to TST in one study.[41] This is also true for HIV-negative women in a high-burden setting,[42] and suggests that TST often fails to detect LTBI in pregnant and peripartum women.

The performance of IGRAs is increasingly being evaluated in other special populations—especially in iatrogenically immunosuppressed subjects with immune-mediated inflammatory diseases (IMID). We know that these are a very high risk group for progression to TB.[43] Most studies have been cross-sectional in design and focused on the concordance between TST and IGRAs and correlating IGRA responses with risk factors for LTBI.[44]

Evaluation of T-SPOT responses in individuals with IMID has found that concordance between the IGRA and TST is, in general, moderate to poor.[45,46] In a US study of 200 patients with rheumatoid arthritis, the T-SPOT and TST showed poor concordance; additionally the T-SPOT was not significantly associated with risk factors for LTBI.[47] There is some evidence that the ELISpot (but not TST) is significantly associated with TB exposure.[48–50] As with the T-SPOT, concordance between the QIF-GIT and TST in this population has been moderate/poor.[51–53] Conversely, an Italian study reported high concordance between TST and QIF-GIT. This was likely due to the low proportion of the population previously BCG vaccinated.[54] Two separate studies from Switzerland and Ireland in IMID patients undergoing pre-anti-tumor necrosis factor (TNF) screening found that ELISA positivity was significantly associated with risk factors for LTBI.[48,55]

Although there is no formal meta-analysis in this area, recent work assessing the performance of the IGRAs in patients with end-stage renal failure has found that the T-SPOT, QFT-GIT, and TST were all significantly associated with clinical risk factors for LTBI.[56]

CHILDREN

Children are more likely to progress to active disease following primary infection, and this is especially true for those <2 years and <5 years of age. This is likely to happen in the first 12 months following infection, without significant prior symptoms and be serious in nature.[57]

ACTIVE TB AS A SURROGATE FOR LTBI

Evidence in children is somewhat conflicting. Generally, conclusions are that IGRAs perform better in high-income, low-M. tb burden settings whereas TST performs equally well or slightly superior to IGRA in low-income, high-burden settings. However, results vary depending on which platform is used, the clinical setting, and the inclusion criteria.[58–62] The most recent large meta-analysis conducted by Sollai et al. evaluated 37 studies in high-income countries. QFT-GIT (79%) sensitivity was superior to T-SPOT (67%) and TST in high-income settings. However in low-income settings, although T-SPOT was superior to QFT-GIT, both IGRAs did not perform any better than TST.[58] In a 2011 meta-analysis, both IGRAs had a higher sensitivity than TST, and IGRA performance was superior to TST in high-, rather than low-/middle-income settings (sensitivity of the QFT-GIT and T.SPOT.TB were 83% and 84%, respectively).[59] An Italian meta-analysis found that pooled QFT-GIT sensitivity was higher than that for T-SPOT; however, TST sensitivity was superior to both IGRAs.[62] In combining positive results from TST and either IGRA, over 90% of children with culture-confirmed TB were correctly identified.[62]

TB EXPOSURE A SURROGATE FOR LTBI

In one of the first and largest studies of this type, the T-SPOT was employed in a large school outbreak investigation comprising 535 students.[63] In this study, TST and a pre-commercial T-SPOT were compared and agreement in this principally BCG-vaccinated cohort was high (89% concordance, $\kappa = 0.72$), T-SPOT correlated better with M.tb exposure (based on proximity and duration of exposure to the index case) than TST.[63] Similar findings from other settings have confirmed that the T-SPOT significantly correlates with TB exposure.[64–69] QIF and QIF-GIT have also been found to correlate with exposure to M.tb and be unaffected by the BCG status.[70–74] Similar findings have been found in other high-TB burden settings[73,74] as well as low-TB burden settings.[27,75] A few studies are in conflict with these results—a South African study revealed no significant relationship between the levels of exposure and QIF-GIT positivity in children at high risk of LTBI.[76] In non-BCG-vaccinated children from Australia and Spain (low-TB burden countries), QIF-GIT remained negative in a significant proportion of children with a positive TST, suggesting lower sensitivity than TST in diagnosing LTBI in children.[69,71]

In BCG-vaccinated populations of children, there are lower levels of agreement between IGRAs and TST. This is to be expected as the TST, but not IGRAs, are confounded by BCG vaccination.[63,65,69,77]

SPECIFICITY OF IGRAS IN LTBI DIAGNOSIS

Quantitative estimates of IGRA specificity (for both T-SPOT and QIF-GIT) have been calculated by studying BCG-vaccinated individuals at an ultra-low risk of LTBI due to the absence of epidemiologic risk factors for M.tb exposure. In recent systematic reviews and meta-analyses, the specificity of the QIF-GIT ranged from

96% to 99% and 86% to 93% for the T-SPOT.[23,78] Both IGRAs have consistently been shown to have a higher specificity compared to the TST in the immunodiagnosis of LTBI—particularly in BCG-vaccinated populations. The specificity of the QFT-Plus has been found to be equivalent to that of the QFT-GIT although the evidence base for this test remains limited at present.[79]

THE PREDICTIVE POWER OF IGRAS FOR PROGRESSION TO ACTIVE TB

Clinical benefits from chemoprophylaxis for LTBI can only occur if IGRA-positive contacts are truly at increased risk of subsequently progressing to active TB compared with IGRA-negative contacts. The gold standard marker of LTBI is the correlation with risk of progression to active TB disease. In immunocompetent individuals only a small proportion, approximately 5%–10%, will develop TB disease from a latent infection during their lifetime; nearly all within the 2 years post exposure.[2] If prophylaxis was provided for all those with LTBI, it would result in an enormous waste of resources, increased risks and side effects associated with the medications themselves and increased likelihood of anti-TB drug resistance, especially when the majority of patients would have never developed active TB. An additional caveat is that chemoprophylaxis is not completely effective. Studies have shown that traditional 6–12 month isoniazid regimens as chemoprophylaxis for LTBI (which have the most abundant evidence for clinical efficacy) have a protective effect of 60% when taken correctly,[80] however initiation and completion rates of chemoprophylaxis are frequently suboptimal and vary greatly across different populations.[81]

A more powerfully predictive test to stratify latently infected individuals by progression risk would much improve targeting of preventative treatment.

LOW-TB BURDEN SETTINGS

IMMUNOCOMPETENT ADULTS

Both IGRA platforms were first shown to have prognostic power for subsequent development of active TB in two large longitudinal cohort studies in 2008; since then other studies have confirmed these initial observations.[22,82] However, the size of the prognostic power of IGRAs in comparison with TST until recently has been a key area of uncertainty. One systematic review of 15 studies with 26,680 individuals concluded that the prognostic power of IGRAs and TST were low but broadly equivalent[83] whereas another review of 28 studies including >30,000 individuals found IGRAs to be more predictive than TST.[84] Generally, the studies included were of low numbers and very few individuals progressed to active TB. Similarly, a European study from 26 centers in 10 different European countries tested contacts of TB cases with T-SPOT and QFT-GIT for LTBI. Overall, in the group that received no chemoprophylaxis, 16 people developed active disease of 494 with positive IGRAs, 14/421 (3.3%) QFT-GIT positive contacts and 2/73 (2.7%) T-SPOT positive, over a median follow-up of period of 2.5 years.[85] Until recently, studies have been small scale with many only testing two strategies.[83,84,86–89]

In 2018 the UK PREDICT TB study was published, examining the prognostic value of IGRAs and TST in predicting the development of active TB in those with recent M.tb contacts, arrival to the UK from a high-burden area in the last 5 years, or travel frequently to high-burden countries. It is the largest study to directly compare the predictive power of the two IGRAs and TST for subsequent development of incident TB. This multicenter UK study prospectively compared the predictive value of TST, QFT-GIT, and T-SPOT in almost 9,610 subjects with TB exposure (half contacts and half recent migrants), of whom approximately 20% were deemed to have LTBI at enrollment based on IGRA and TST. They used three different thresholds for positivity of a TST result: TST-5 mm was considered positive if BCG vaccination was absent whereas TST-15 was considered positive if previously vaccinated. During follow-up, 97 incident cases of TB developed. Of those who completed all three tests and follow-up, 77/6,380 patients progressed to active TB; of these 47/77 (61%) had a positive QIF-GIT, 52/77 (68%) a positive T-SPOT, 57/77 (74%) positive TST-15, and 64/77 (83%) a positive TST-5. To identify the most suitable screening test to assess for the progression of disease: a high proportion of tested individuals should be classified as test negative and therefore require no further monitoring; there should be a low rate of progression to TB in those who tested negative, indicating the ability of the test to correctly rule out future disease. All tests had a good negative predictive value (NPV) T-SPOT and TST-15 (99.5%) and QFT (99.4%). The investigators found that the annual incidence of TB in those who tested positive was highest for T-SPOT followed by TST (using a 15 mm cut-off in BCG-vaccinated persons) and then QFT-GIT with positive predictive values (PPVs) of 4.2%, 3.5%, and 3.3% respectively. In total, 1,235 people had a positive T-SPOT of whom 52 went on to develop active TB. This means the number needed to treat (NNT) to prevent one case of TB progression is 24 for T-SPOT-TB, 29 for TST, and 31 for QFT-GIT. All three of these tests were significantly better predictors of progression than using lower TST cut-offs (5 and 10 mm).[90] If the intention is to identify as many individuals as possible with a positive test result in a high risk cohort who will progress to active TB (e.g., among household contacts of patients with smear-positive pulmonary TB), TST-5 is the preferable test (as currently recommended in US Centers for Disease Control and Prevention guidelines).[91] However, although you will then identify the majority of those who go on to develop active TB there will be a huge proportion with a positive test who do not develop active disease.

PREDICT represents the first head-to-head, large-scale comparison of three different testing strategies in a low incidence TB country. It is clear that in immunocompetent adults, when negative, the current IGRAs act as a good rule-out test for the development of TB, however they are still relatively poor at predicting the future development of TB and tests. Higher PPVs are required to affect a step-change in TB control and prevention. Enhancing the prognostic power of IGRAs, finding additional biomarkers or clinical risk scores to identify those that will progress to active TB thereby reducing the NNT to prevent a single case of progression to active TB is therefore an urgent research priority as highlighted by the WHO.[19,92]

INDIVIDUALS WITH HIV

In immunocompromised individuals, especially in patients with HIV infection, the NPV of an immunodiagnostic test is insufficient to rule out the future development of TB.

A systematic review of the predictive power of IGRAs in immunocompromised individuals found that the majority of the immunocompromised cohort that progressed to active TB were HIV-positive, therefore the number of HIV-infected persons with a positive test needed to treat was lower (range 14.0–25.5) and TB cases were only found in patients with ongoing detectable viral loads.[93] It should be noted however that although very few, incident TB cases did occur in individuals with negative test results especially among patients with HIV infection. In all the studies included in the meta-analysis the NPV for both IGRAs was >99%.[85,93,94]

A large study from Europe recruited immunocompromised patients from 17 European healthcare facilities, 10 of 768 HIV-positive individuals progressed to active TB in the time period and this was poorly predicted by TST or IGRAs.[93]

In an Austrian prospective longitudinal study, 830 HIV-1-infected patients underwent testing with the QFT-GIT assay. The cohort was reviewed at 3-month intervals to monitor for any development of active TB. Median follow-up time was 19 months. Active TB occurred in three patients and exclusively in patients with a positive QFT-GIT assay result at a rate of 3/37 (8.1%).[95]

CHILDREN

There are no large studies looking at the use of IGRA to specifically predict progression to active TB in children in low-burden countries. Given the high-risk nature of LTBI in children, if children are found to have a positive IGRA they are offered chemoprophylaxis; therefore, there is very limited available data.

OTHER AT-RISK POPULATIONS

Within immunocompromised groups it is evident that there are different amounts of progression to active TB dependent on numerous clinical and biochemical markers.

Recently, a review of the predictive power of IGRAs in immunocompromised individuals (chronic renal failure, solid organ transplantation, stem cell transplantation, and rheumatoid arthritis) demonstrated with a positive IGRA (n = 1,537) the NNT to prevent one active case ranged from approximately 50 to 80. However, the majority of progression occurred in the HIV-positive cohort. In patients with chronic renal failure, rheumatoid arthritis, stem cell, or solid organ transplant recipients no patients progressed to active TB.[93,96]

The TST and commercial IGRAs have important limitations and poor-predictive value for active TB in patients with advanced chronic kidney disease (CKD). Several studies have explored the diagnostic accuracy of the TST and IGRAs by examining the association between positivity and risk factors for LTBI.[56,97] Although IGRAs perform superiorly to TST in the diagnosis of LTBI in those with diabetes,[98] on immunosuppressive therapy such as anti-TNF-α,[44] transplant and rheumatoid arthritis patients they are not as accurate in immunocompetent individuals.[93]

In three large-scale occupational studies no healthcare workers with LTBI (defined as a positive IGRA) developed active TB during 2 years of follow-up. Therefore, this would suggest they are no longer risk groups in low-incidence countries.[99–101]

HIGH-TB BURDEN SETTING

The predictive value of IGRAs and TST for the development of TB in high-burden countries has been less studied. Studies in different high-risk areas have had conflicting outcomes as to whether IGRAs offer any improvement from the traditional TST testing in the prediction of active TB disease.

IMMUNOCOMPETENT ADULTS

In a recent Indian study, Sharma et al. recruited a large cohort of household contacts of pulmonary TB patients (adults and children). These contacts were prospectively followed-up for 2 years for the development of active TB after getting baseline QFT-GIT assay and TST done. Seventy-six of 1,511 household contacts developed active TB. No significant association of baseline TST and QFT-GIT assay response with subsequent development of active TB was shown.[102]

In a large meta-analysis, Rangaka and colleagues looked at the prognostic ability of the IGRAs. The study included 15 longitudinal studies that mostly took place in high-TB burden settings with a combined sample size of 26,680. In total, 66/601 patients were QIF-GIT positive with 6/41 who received no chemoprophylaxis developing active TB over the study period giving a PPV of 14.6%. No patients with a negative QIF-GIT developed active TB.[83]

One of the first studies in a high-burden setting took place in The Gambia exploring the predictive values of T-SPOT vs. TST in contacts of smear-positive cases of TB. It included a very mixed population (children, adults, and HIV-positive/negative). Initial T-SPOT and TST were each positive in just over half of cases who progressed to active TB (71% were positive in one or other test), concluding that neither TST nor T-SPOT were effective enough at reliably predicting disease progression in this setting.[103]

INDIVIDUALS WITH HIV

TB is the most frequent cause of AIDS-related deaths worldwide; this is despite progress in access to antiretroviral therapy.[104] TB is responsible for approximately 400,000 deaths in people living with HIV in 2016 (one-third of all HIV deaths).[15]

In a study of HIV-infected individuals in Korea (TB rate 110/100,000), 11 patients developed active TB during 238 person-years. Patients with positive T-SPOT responses had a higher TB incidence rate; however, this was not statistically significant (20% [6/30] vs. 6.02% [5/83], p = 0.052). Independent risk factors associated with the progression of TB were low CD4T cell counts, previous history of TB treatment, and positive T-SPOT results. Advanced HIV-infected patients who had a positive T-SPOT had a higher rate of progression to TB in this intermediate TB-endemic area.[105]

In a South African study, the rate of progression to TB in an HIV population who received no chemoprophylaxis did not differ significantly between the IGRA-negative and -positive groups (positive 3.3/100 person-years, negative 3.9/100 person-years).[106]

The WHO currently states people living with HIV who have a positive test for LTBI benefit more from preventive treatment than those who have a negative LTBI test; LTBI testing can be used, where feasible, to identify such individuals. However, prophylactic treatment may be given without LTBI testing for people living with HIV or child household contacts aged <5 years supporting the fact that these tests are generally more unreliable in these cohorts.[15]

PREGNANCY AND HIV INFECTION

Data on HIV, pregnancy, and LTBI progression in high-burden countries is somewhat limited. An Indian study enrolled 252 pregnant HIV-infected women in linked cross-sectional/longitudinal studies: 71 (28%) had a positive QFT-GIT but only 27 (10%) had a positive TST (p < 0.005); 5/252 (2%) women developed active TB, all within 1 year postpartum. All five had a positive QFT-GIT but only one had a positive TST. Based on this, the sensitivity of the QFT-GIT for development of postpartum TB was 100%, but the specificity was 27% and the PPV was only 7%. In those women who developed active TB, three women had samples from pregnancy and delivery showing a 2.9-fold decrease in IFN-γ.[40] These latter findings would support the hypothesis of a weakening of T-cell-mediated immune response in pregnancy thus leading to the higher risk of active TB observed in late pregnancy and postpartum.[107]

A Kenyan study explored the predictive value of T-SPOT in 327 pregnant women with HIV without previous TB of whom nine developed TB within 1 year of delivery. They quantified the positivity of T-SPOT classifying the number of IFN-γ spot forming cells (SFCs). IFN-γ ≥6 SFCs showed a sensitivity (78%) and specificity (55%) with a PPV of 5.9%. In women with CD4 <250 cells/μL, sensitivity and specificity of IFN-γ ≥6 SFCs was 89% and 63%, respectively, with a PPV of 19.2%; however, this study was limited by few cases of active TB, absence of TST for comparison, and absence of TB diagnostic confirmation.[108]

These studies are small and require validation with well-designed, large, prospective studies.

CHILDREN

A number of large studies have been conducted in high-TB burden areas of South Africa examining the predictive value of IGRA vs. TST. In a study of adolescents aged 12–18 years, 5,244 participants were followed-up for a median of 2.4 years. Positive TST and QFT-GIT tests were moderately sensitive predictors of progression to microbiologically confirmed TB disease. There was no significant difference in the predictive ability of the tests.

In a large prospective cohort of young children (2,512 HIV-uninfected young children aged 18–24 weeks were enrolled) from a TB-endemic community in South Africa, they found high rates of QFT-GIT conversion and high incidence of TB disease. The PPVs and NPVs using the manufacturer's cut-off of 0.35 IU/mL were 8% and 99%, respectively. They found an increased risk of incident TB disease following QFT-GIT conversion in those with IFN-γ values (>4.00 IU/mL, >40-fold that of QFT-GIT non-converters and 11-fold that of QFT converters with IFN-γ value between 0.35 and 4.00 IU/mL); however, this then missed a significant proportion of those who went on to develop active TB.[109]

LIMITATIONS OF CURRENT AVAILABLE DIAGNOSTICS

TST

The TST has several disadvantages; it demonstrates poor specificity in BCG-vaccinated populations, gives false positives in patients with non-tuberculous mycobacterium,[110] and has limited sensitivity in immunosuppressed persons and young children. In addition to this, the requirement for two clinical visits (the second to read the result) can make it logistically difficult.

A further factor confounding interpretation of TST results is the phenomenon of potentiation or boosting. This occurs when the skin test is repeated resulting in an amplified response due to progressive sensitization; this complicates interpretation and can lead to false positives in serially tested subjects.

IGRAS

Although both IGRAs have significant advantages over TST, their limitations have driven the research agenda forward to define next-generation IGRAs, T-cell signatures, and novel biomarkers. Although the advent of IGRAs represents a significant advance on the technologies of the twentieth century, they have several limitations, which necessitate further research to improve our ability to diagnose and treat TB.

Although IGRAs have improved diagnostic sensitivity and specificity compared to TST in many populations, IGRAs are not a gold standard test and therefore unable to rule-in or rule-out active TB or LTBI. To date, the magnitude of the IFN-γ responses does not appear to reflect bacillary burden or disease activity. As a result, IGRAs cannot be used to distinguish between active and LTBI, as a tool for monitoring treatment response or as a test of cure following completion of anti-tuberculous therapy.

The use of IGRAs in active TB diagnostics is beyond the scope of this chapter; however, there has been widespread conflicting information regarding this. The recently published large-scale IDEA study has definitively proven that currently available IGRAs as they stand do not have a useful role as rule-in or rule-out tests in routine clinical practice.[111]

IGRAs, as is the case with TST, reflect immune priming and test positivity may remain lifelong due to the presence of long-lived memory T-cells. Therefore, a positive IGRA result is very difficult to interpret in subjects with a past history of active TB and previously treated latent TB.

As discussed extensively currently IGRAs appear to be useful as a rule-out test for the future development of active TB but lack adequate PPV.[90]

KINETICS OF IGRA RESPONSES OVER TIME

CONVERSION

Conversion, when applied to TST and IGRA, is defined as the development of a positive result following new infection.[112] There is no large-scale evidence comparing time to conversion with TST following a point-source exposure precisely defined in time and place. Small studies have suggested that the conversion time is greatly varied between individuals. The majority of contacts who are going to covert do so within 2–7 weeks post exposure[113]; however, it can occur up to 3 months later. An agreement between TST and IGRA results show better concordance after this window period.[114] Clinical guidelines work on the assumption that TST and IGRA conversion happen at similar time periods. Interestingly, there is some recent evidence, however, that responses to certain antigens develop more rapidly than ESAT-6/CFP-10 which opens the possibility of detecting ultra-early responses to MTB infection.[115] Such factors must be considered if an IGRA is used to screen contacts of a TB patient.

SPONTANEOUS REVERSION

Reversion is the process by which a previously positive test result becomes negative. With respect to IGRAs, in untreated exposed individuals, reversion from a baseline positive test could be due to an acute resolving M.tb infection, a phenomenon which was relatively recently described.[116,117] In a UK study, the authors observed similar declines in RD1-specific T-cell responses in TST-positive (who were given chemoprophylaxis) and TST-negative subjects.[116] Given that the TST-negative subjects did not receive chemoprophylaxis, it is possible that the bacterial burden in these untreated contacts may have declined spontaneously and resulted in declining RD1-responses.[116] Spontaneous IGRA reversion occurs almost exclusively in TST-negative exposed contacts and about 50% of such contacts tend to revert.[118,119] This figure of 50% reversion has also been reproduced in the HIV cohort.[120] However, it must be noted that incident TB incidence has been shown to be eight-fold higher in those with reverted QFT-GIT (1.47 cases/100 person-years) than among those with persistently negative QFTs (0.18/100 person-years) ($p = 0.011$), though the numbers of cases were small in both groups.[121]

Other interpretations of IGRA reversion other than bacillary clearance cannot be ignored given the observational nature of current evidence. Peripheral T-cells may migrate to the site of disease over time and be undetectable in the blood IGRA. Alternatively their frequency may wane below the threshold of detection in some individuals despite continued presence of infection. Determining the risk of disease in such individuals over time would aid our understanding of the underlying host–pathogen status it reflects. In untreated survivors of TB from the pre-antibiotic era, both IFN-γ positive and negative responses exist suggesting bacillary clearance at least in some.[122]

SPONTANEOUS FLUCTUATIONS IN IGRA RESPONSE OVER TIME

There is a lack of data regarding the use of IGRAs for serial testing. The small-scale studies that are available all showed large variation in the rates of conversions and reversions.[123] No firm conclusions have been drawn about cut-offs for serial testing. There are case reports of IGRA responses increasing in size prior to individuals with LTBI progressing to active TB, or at the time of reactivation.[124] However, there is no large-scale statistically valid evidence to support the use of longitudinal IGRA fluctuations to monitor latently infected persons for pre-emptive therapy of incipient active TB.

TREATMENT-INDUCED CHANGES IN IGRA RESPONSE

An obvious use for IGRAs is in TB treatment monitoring; if serial IGRA testings were to reflect disease activity or bacillary burden or both, then proof of cure would be possible, a particularly useful tool when testing new antimycobacterials. IGRA reversion has been well documented in a proportion of those adults treated for TB, both active and latent.[125] However, this proportion is insufficient to infer true causality or be generalizable, and very low rates of reversion have been found in children.[126,127] Moreover, a systematic review which summarized studies which had attempted to quantify changes in IGRA response with treatment found wide inter-individual variation in the rate of decline (with responses actually increasing in some patients) and, crucially, these kinetic changes did not correlate with clinical outcomes (such as the rate of response to therapy or future relapse).[128] In summary, current IGRAs cannot be used for treatment monitoring or as a test of cure.

REAPPRAISAL OF THE NATURAL HISTORY OF LTBI IN LIGHT OF STUDIES USING IGRAS

Longitudinal studies which have provided the first evidence of spontaneous IGRA reversion (in other words spontaneous clearance of infection)[116] have advanced our understanding of the natural history of LTBI.

The ability of the IGRA to distinguish between BCG vaccination and M.tb infection has allowed reappraisal of the role of BCG in protection against disease. The effectiveness of BCG against severe childhood TB including meningitis and miliary TB is well accepted.[129] Its ability to protect against adult forms is more controversial[130,131] but was generally believed to be associated with containment of an established infection.[132] TB contact investigations from several different settings have yielded data suggesting that BCG vaccination might also protect against acquisition of M.tb infection.[2,64]

LATENT TB SCREENING

Patients in whom LTBI screening is recommended fall into two groups: those at-risk of new infection due to TB exposure or individuals who are at increased risk of infection and progression to active disease due to host factors (such as age, underlying medical conditions, medications, and social risk factors).

Although TB screening of new migrants arriving in the UK has historically been aimed at identifying active TB disease at the time of their arrival to the UK, data have clearly shown that the prevalence of active TB in migrants is low.[133,134] As the reactivation of LTBI plays a critical role in determining TB epidemiology in low-TB burden settings, screening for LTBI is likely to be of benefit when targeted at high-risk populations including migrants and TB contacts.

In the last few years, a systematic LTBI-screening program has been introduced in the UK, initially in high-risk local authority areas with a high-TB incidence (≥20 per 100,000 population) or a high-TB case burden. Screening is currently being undertaken in those aged 16–35 years who are from or regularly visit high-incidence countries. In 2017/18, 15,102 IGRA tests were carried out,

16.6% (2,507) of these were positive of which 64% (1,605) commenced treatment and 69% (1,107) completed treatment (PHE, unpublished data).

Selection of which adult migrants to screen has been controversial and hampered due to a lack of empirical data. The 2006 NICE guidelines recommended screening adults from countries with TB incidence >500/100,000 and sub-Saharan Africa. However, Pareek and colleagues highlighted that these guidelines were not being closely adhered to; using multicenter screening data and health-economic analysis, Pareek et al. were able to highlight that screening as per the 2006 NICE guidelines would miss the majority of migrants with LTBI and that it would be most cost-effective to screen at an intermediate threshold (150–250/100,000) using single-step IGRAs.[26,68] It is this threshold which has been operationalized in the recent collaborative TB strategy for England.[135]

POLICY AND GUIDELINES FOR THE USE OF IGRAS

Over time, IGRAs have become more routinely used in the UK and elsewhere. As clinical experience and published data have accumulated, international and country-specific guidelines/recommendations on how IGRAs should be used have evolved. Although the target groups remain unchanged (recent migrants from high-TB burden countries, contacts of smear-positive patients and individuals with compromised-immune systems) the role of IGRAs appears to be better understood.

The WHO has now recommended that either TST or IGRA can be used to diagnose LTBI.[15] Unit costs suggest that in resource-limited settings the TST would be used in preference to IGRA. Mirroring the WHO's change in position, other countries including the US, Canada, and UK recommend using either the IGRA or TST to diagnose LTBI. However, it is important to highlight that guidelines in the UK are divergent depending on the population being screened.[18] Although 2016 UK NICE guidelines primarily recommend using TST to identify LTBI in most risk groups (close contacts and healthcare workers), IGRA is the recommended screening tool for migrants being screened as part of the national latent TB screening program.

In HIV-positive individuals, national guidelines on screening for LTBI are different between countries and even within countries. The British HIV Association recently updated its guidance: it previously recommended a complex screening algorithm which required the clinician to use single-step IGRA after taking into consideration the patient's country of origin, duration of anti-retroviral therapy and CD4 count[136]; however, evidence suggested that adherence to this guidance was sub-optimal.[137] New guidance now recommends that single-step IGRA should be used to screen those individuals from medium- and high-TB burden countries or those from a low-TB burden setting with risk factors for TB.[136] Interestingly, 2016 UK NICE guidance recommends that HIV-positive patients who are severely immunosuppressed (CD4 count <200 cells/mm³) should have concurrent TST and IGRA testing whereas all others should be tested using either IGRA alone or concurrent TST and IGRA.[18] This is also supported by the European Centre for Disease Prevention, WHO guidance, and

US guidelines,[15–17,138] although, the WHO guidelines state that isoniazid preventative therapy can be initiated for HIV-positive individuals without undertaking a TST or IGRA.[15]

With respect to iatrogenically immunosuppressed individuals with IMID, although most countries recommend screening for LTBI, guidance is heterogeneous on which specific screening test/strategy to follow (single-step IGRA, TST alone, or both TST and IGRA); dual testing is however widely used aiming to minimize false-negative results given the high risk nature of these patients.[21] In the UK, national guidelines from NICE recommend either using a single-step IGRA or IGRA and TST in parallel.[18] By contrast, the American College of Rheumatology recommends using either TST or IGRA to diagnose LTBI.[139,140]

Guidelines on how best to operationalize IGRAs in children reflect the fact that the evidence supporting their use in children is more limited. UK guidelines recommend age-stratified guidelines where a hybrid TST and IGRA approach is used although the TST is identified as the primary screening tool.[18] Similarly, the US guidelines recommend that children under the age of 5 should have a TST in preference to IGRA.[138]

THE UNMET CLINICAL NEED IN LTBI DIAGNOSTICS

In 2017, the WHO published a target product profile (TPP) of desirable test characteristics. First, for such a test to have utility in high-TB burden and low-income settings, it should ideally be based on a sample type more easily accessible than sputum, with a high PPV for progression from infection to active TB.[92]

It is clear that both the TST and IGRAs that are recommended to diagnose LTBI have a low PPV for the future development of TB, and therefore as they stand are currently insufficient to identify the proportion of people with LTBI who will develop active disease.[85,88,90] Therefore there has been a widespread focus on trying to improve on technologies already available as well as explore the use of other biomarkers, tests, and clinical risk scores.

LIMITATIONS OF IGRA IN LOW-RESOURCE SETTINGS

As previously stated the current IGRAs require specialist lab facilities, not always available in high-TB burden settings. For this reason there has been some research drive toward an IGRA-like test that would be more practical in low-resource, field-based settings. The C-TB skin test has been developed as a replacement for the TST. It uses the same RD1 antigens that are present in the IGRA (ESAT-6 and CFP-10) but importantly these are in a form that can be administered as a skin test, thereby bypassing the need for expensive laboratory processing. It performed similarly to IGRA in terms of specificity with higher positivity observed in those patients with the higher levels of M.tb contact, and outcome was not affected by the BCG status.[141] In the subset of patients with active TB, C-TB test sensitivity (67%) was lower than that observed for both QFT-GIT and T-SPOT.[141] Sensitivity was significantly decreased in HIV-infected patients with CD4 counts <100.[142] Further work is also required to understand how this test performs in different populations and its predictive power for progression from LTBI to active TB disease, and it must also be remembered that the patient must return for the size of induration to be read.[143]

LIMITATIONS OF IGRAS IN A LOW-INCIDENCE TB SETTING

There have been a number of approaches to try and improve upon the already available technologies, including quantification of IFN-γ in the QFT-GIT or the number of IFN-γ SFCs in the T-SPOT, additional antigens and additional secreted markers such as cytokines and chemokines; all of which will be discussed later.

INCREASING SENSITIVITY OF IGRA

Additional cytokines

Although IFN-γ is a fundamental cytokine in the immune response to MTB there has been interest in alternative and additional secreted markers that may improve diagnostic sensitivity and improve the ability to differentiate between active TB and LTBI. Results suggest that different cytokine profiles are associated with different clinical stages of TB infection.[122,144–148]

Downstream chemokines such as inducible protein 10 (IP-10), monocyte chemotactic protein-2 and monokine inducible protein secreted by IFN-γ-activated macrophages (in addition to IFN-γ) have been of particular research interest.[149] It is thought that because they are downstream and induced by IFN-γ these chemokines may serve as a more amplified readout than IFN-γ itself, thereby yielding higher sensitivity.[149]

IP-10 is secreted by multiple different immune cells, and when released acts as a chemoattractant to inflammatory cells.[150] A review of IP-10 concluded that IP-10 was similar to IFN-γ overall but may have improved sensitivity in young children or those with low CD4 counts secondary to HIV-infection.[151] Studies have shown that IP-10 levels are elevated in patients with active TB. The sensitivity of this test either alone or in combination with IFN-γ improves diagnostic accuracy.

In addition to IP-10 and IFN-γ, TNF-α, interleukin (IL)-1ra, IL-2, IL-13, and macrophage inflammatory protein-1β responses have been found to be higher in LTBI and active TB cases than in TB-uninfected children.[152]

Again it must however be noted that these studies are small patient numbers and have yet to be demonstrated in large studies and none as yet are being used in routine clinical evaluation.

Although not a specific secreted marker, the monocyte/lymphocyte ratio in peripheral blood is a readily available biomarker that has been linked to a number of prospective cohort studies in pregnant women and infants in sub-Saharan Africa. Studies have shown that an elevated monocyte/lymphocyte ratio was associated with increased risk of development of TB disease before the appearance of symptoms.[153–155]

Additional antigens

Additional antigens have shown promise not only in increasing sensitivity of IGRA but also distinguishing LTBI from active TB, discriminating recent from remote LTBI, and predicting progression of LTBI to active TB.

Additional antigens increase the sensitivity of the IGRA by improving detection of IFN-γ *in vitro*.[12] In one of the first studies of supplementary antigens, the addition of a new antigen (Rv3879c) improved test sensitivity when compared with the standard T-SPOT; combining the next-generation assay and TST in confirmed and highly probable cases further gave a sensitivity of 99%.[12] Similar improvements have been observed for the QFT-GIT by incorporating a novel antigen (Rv2645).[156]

Recently, a large prospective multicenter study demonstrated that a second-generation IGRA incorporating Rv3615c alongside ESAT-6 and CFP-10 had significantly higher diagnostic sensitivity than T-SPOT.TB and QFT-GIT (in those with suspected active TB). A negative test result was found to reduce the odds of TB post-test 7.7-fold compared to pre-test, thus this could be very useful as a rule-out test for a diagnosis of TB in clinical settings with a low-to-moderate prevalence of TB.[111] This trend toward higher sensitivity of second-generation IGRAs has been referred to as the "first advancement in this field since the introduction of IGRAs."[157] The sensitivity meets the requirement for a triage test, as described by the WHO in a high-priority TPP.[92]

Generally, fewer studies have focused on the ability of using newly identified antigens to aid with the prediction of progression from LTBI to active TB. However, Rv3873 and Rv3879c were found to aid with disease progression prediction. Rv3873 and Rv3879c became positive prior to TST conversion suggesting that they were early markers of progression to active TB disease in children with recent household TB exposure.[115]

Heparin-binding hemagglutinin antigen (HBHA) is an antigen that has a role in maintaining latency; it is located on the surface of mycobacteria and aids with binding to host epithelial cells[158] and inducing apoptosis in infected cells increasing virility, propagation, and facilitating infection.[159,160] A recent review[161] highlighted numerous studies in which LTBI has been associated with larger T-cell responses specific to HBHA, typically absent in active TB and controls.[162–165] These findings have also been observed in HIV-infected individuals.[164,166] HBHA has a key role in maintaining latency and is a correlate of protection to not progress to active TB.

Antigen response has also been successful in discriminating recent from remote LTBI. Higher levels of whole-blood IFN-γ responses to MTB latency antigen Rv2628 have been shown in those with remotely acquired LTBI compared to those with recent LTBI, active TB, and the control group. Remote LTBI had a five-fold increase in IFN-γ response to MTB latency antigen Rv2628 than that in recently infected individuals (p < 0.003).[167] For a list of the most promising antigens linked to latency and the studies' key findings, see Table 9.4.

Characterization of all these additional antigens demonstrate great promise for the future development of more advantageous tests, however it is important to note that these studies have, for the most part, been small-scale and therefore one cannot yet draw any firm conclusions about their clinical utility in routine practice.

INCREASING SPECIFICITY OF IGRAS

Currently, IGRAs are not designed for distinguishing between LTBI and active TB, therefore there has been increasing focus on new cytokine profiles and antigens that may aid us in differentiating between active TB and LTBI (see Table 9.4).

Table 9.4 Summary of findings from studies of latency antigens

MTB antigens	Reference	Main finding(s)
Latency	**Associated antigens**	
Rv0081	Chegou et al.[169]	Higher levels of IFN-γ in HHC vs. aTB
Rv1733c	Chegou et al.[170]	Higher levels of IL-12, IP-10, IL-10, and TNF-α in aTB and HHC
	Chegou et al.[170]	Higher levels of IL-12, IP-10, IL-10, and TNF-α in aTB and HHC
Rv1737c	Commandeur et al.[171]	Higher number of IFN-γ/TNF-α producing CD8 in LTBI vs. aTB
Rv2029c	Arroyo et al.[176]	Higher proportion of IFN-γ and/or TNF-α producing CD4 and CD8T cells in LTBI vs. aTB
	Araujo et al.[177]	Higher levels if IFN-γ in LTBI vs. aTB and healthy controls
	Bai et al.[178]	Higher IFN-γ in LTBI vs. aTB and HC
	Commandeur et al.[171]	Higher number of IFN-γ/TNF-α producing CD8 in LTBI vs. HC
	Hozumi et al.[179]	Induced stronger IFN-γ T-cell responses in LTBI than in aTB
Rv2031c	Araujo et al.[177]	Higher levels if IFN-γ in LTBI vs. aTB and HC
	Belay et al.[180]	Higher levels of IFN-γ, TNF-α and IL-10 in LTBI vs. aTB and HC
	Commandeur et al.[171]	Higher number of IFN-γ/TNF-α producing CD8 in LTBI vs. HC
Rv2645	Harada et al.[156]	Addition of Rv2645 (TB7.7) in QFT-GIT enhanced sensitivity over the QFT-G test in aTB.
Rv2628	Araujo et al.[177]	Higher levels of IFN-γ in LTBI vs. aTB and HC
	Bai et al.[178]	Higher IFN-γ in LTBI vs. aTB and HC
	Goletti et al.[167]	Higher IFN-γ in remote LTBI vs. recent LTBI, aTB and HC. Remotely acquired LTBI ×5 higher than recent LTBI
HBHA	Chiacchio et al.[166]	Higher levels of IFN-γ in aTB and LTBI HIV −ve vs. HIV +ve
	Delogu et al.[164]	Higher levels of IFN-γ in LTBI vs. aTB
	Delogu et al.[181]	Lower IFN-γ responses observed in HIV-LTBI and HIV-TB. None of the six HIV-LTBI responding to HBHA-developed TB
	Dreesman et al.[182]	HBHA-induced IL-17 production by CD4+ T lymphocytes was associated with protection in 3 years higher in LTBI vs. aTB
	Hougardy et al.[163]	Higher concentrations of IFN-γ in LTBI vs. aTB
	Loxton et al.[162]	Induces IFN-γ, IL-2, and IL-17-coexpressing CD4(+) T-cells in HHCs (LTBI) but not in aTB
	Wyndam-Thomas et al.[165]	Higher IFN-γ secreted by CD4+ T lymphocytes in LTBI vs. aTB and HCs
	Wyndam-Thomas et al.[183]	Increased IFN-γ in HIV positive patients with LTBI and aTB
Resuscitation	**Promoting factors**	**(Rpfs)**
Rv0867c	Chegou et al.[169]	Higher levels of IFN-γ in HHC vs. aTB
Rv2389c	Chegou et al.[169]	Higher levels of IFN-γ in HHC vs. aTB
	Arroyo et al.[176]	Higher proportion of IFN-γ and/or TNF-α producing CD4 and CD8T cells in LTBI vs. aTB
	Chegou et al.[170]	Higher levels of IL-12, IP-10, IL-10, and TNF-α in aTB and HHC
Others		
Rv1131	Chegou et al.[170]	Higher levels of IFN-γ in HHC vs. aTB
Ag85 (Rv1886c)	Alvarez-Corrales et al.[173]	Higher concentrations of IFN-γ and Il-17 in exposed vs. aTB
	Schwander et al.[184]	Higher proportion of IFN-γ producing cells secreted Ag 85 in BAC from HHC than in BAC from HC
Rv3615c	Li et al.[185]	Rv3615c as an additional stimulus in IGRA improved the diagnosis efficiency in active TB. No LTBI group
	Millington et al.[13]	Rv3615c was at least as immunodominant as ESAT-6 and CFP-10 in both aTB and LTBI
	Whitworth et al.[111]	Incorporating Rv3615c alongside ESAT-6 and CFP-10, had significantly higher diagnostic sensitivity than T-SPOT.TB and QFT-GIT
Rv3873	Dosanjh et al.[12]	In recently exposed children HHC increasing IFN-γ responses to RV3873 predicted progression to aTB
Rv3879c	Dosanjh et al.[12]	In recently exposed children HHC increasing IFN-γ responses to Rv3879c predicted progression to aTB

Abbreviations: HC, healthy controls; HHC, household contacts; aTB, active TB; BAC, bronchoalveolar cells.

Cytokines

Discrimination between LTBI and active TB has been demonstrated with combinations of TNF-α/IL-1ra and TNF-α/IL-10 achieving correct classification of 95.5% and 100% of cases, respectively.[152] IFN-γ combined with CXCL10 was able to discriminate between active TB and LTBI with a sensitivity of 89.6% and a specificity of 71.1%.[168]

Antigens

A number of studies have highlighted different responses to a number of antigens (RV0081, RV1737, RV0867c, Rv2389c, and Rv1886c), however these studies are all small and are as yet a long way away from being clinically applicable[169–173] (see Table 9.4 for more details).

INCREASING THE PPV OF IGRAS

Quantifying IGRA responses

Studies have explored whether the amount of IFN-γ in the QFT-GIT or the number of IFN-γ SFCs in the T-SPOT that define a positive test result has an influence on the ability to predict TB. The hypothesis being the more positive the IGRA the more likely you are to progress to active TB.

A recent Norwegian study has explored the prognostic value of quantifying the QFT-GIT IFN-γ level response in a low-TB incidence setting.[174] IGRA results from 44,875 individuals were included for prospective analyses. The QFT results were categorized into low-positive (IFN-γ 0.35 to <1.0) medium-positive (IFN-γ 1.0 to <4.0), and high-positive (IFN-γ > 4.0 IU/mL). Incident TB was reported in 257 individuals; of those TB occurred in 219/257 (85%) with positive QFT-GIT (low 17/219 [8%], medium 46/219 [21%], and high 156/219 [71%]), 33/257 (13%) individuals with negative IGRA and 5/257 (2%) individuals with inconclusive results.

Similarly, a European study in 10 different countries explored whether the amount of IFN-γ in the QFT-GIT or the number of SFCs in the T-SPOT that define a positive test result had an influence on the ability to predict TB. The incidence ratio (IR) for a QFT-GIT test result below 0.35 IU/mL IFN-γ was 0.001 suggesting that the current cut-off for positivity is the best predictor for progression and IR of 0.003 for a cut-off less than 5 SFCs/250,000 in the T-SPOT. In using cut-offs at different levels although the NNT came down for both IGRAs, there were a significant proportion who developed TB with a lower quantity of SFC/IFN-γ that were missed.[85]

Recent data from the UK PREDICT cohort has also explored the quantification of IGRA response. Each IGRA-QFT-GIT and T-SPOT was given four levels of strata. Higher quantitative results for both IGRAs were strongly associated with higher TB incidence rates; however, using higher thresholds to aid with the prediction of progression to active TB led to a marked loss in sensitivity across the board in that the majority of the incident TB would be missed if thresholds increased. Even within the highest strata, the PPV was <5%. NPV was good in all positive groups at >99%.[175] These studies highlight the inherent limitation of the IGRA technology currently available.

IMPROVING PPVs REQUIRES NEW TECHNOLOGIES

T-CELL SIGNATURES

Advances in our understanding of the immune response to MTB are helping to profile the cytokine function of predominantly T-lymphocytes to stratify TB-exposed persons into the different clinical stages of infection.

In contrast to IGRAs, which measure IFN-γ responses, a recent study has focused on categorizing CD4$^+$ T-cells into three main subsets: effector T-cells (IFN-γ only), effector-memory T-cells (both IFN-γ and IL-2), and central memory T-cells (IL-2).[144,186]

A number of studies have shown enhanced expression of T-cell activation markers as a correlation of risk prior to developing TB. In recent studies, activated HLA-DR CD4T cells were higher in those infants and adolescents who developed TB disease.[187] These infants were part of a vaccine trial; they were IGRA negative and the results were from baseline. Conversely, in the same study, high levels of Ag85A antibodies and high frequencies of IFN-γ-specific T-cells were associated with a reduced risk of disease.[187,188]

Others have described CD27-IFN-γ^+CD4$^+$ T-cells as predictive markers of TB disease.[189–191] CD27 is expressed on naive T-cells and early effector lymphocytes and appears to decrease as people progress to active TB; this also appears to be true for the HIV-positive population.[192]

Pollock and colleagues found that CD4$^+$ TNF-α-only-secreting T-cells with an effector phenotype accurately distinguished active TB from LTBI.[193] Rozot et al. found that in combining MTB-specific CD4 TNF-α T-cell and MTB-specific CD8 T-cell responses were a potential tool to differentiate active TB and LTBI. Studies from South Africa have also shown that HLA-DR expression is able to differentiate between active and latent TB in a high-HIV burden setting[194] (Table 9.5).

It is well reported that recently infected contacts are at higher risk of progression to active TB and this is the greatest risk factor for progression to TB in immunocompetent individuals.[195,196] Neither IGRA nor TST are capable of discriminating recent from remote infection at present and targeting recently infected persons will continue to depend on epidemiological risk factors until such a test is developed.

The TNF-α-only T$_{EFF}$ signature has been shown to be significantly higher in those with recently acquired LTBI, compared with those with remotely acquired LTBI, with the former's signature

Table 9.5 CD4$^+$ T-cell subset cytokine profiles with clinical correlates

CD4$^+$ T-cell subset	Cytokine profile	Clinical correlates
Effector	IFN-γ only	Higher antigen burden Breakdown of immune control Transition from LTBI to active TB
Effector	TNF-α only	Higher antigen burden Active TB
Effector memory	IFN-γ/IL-2	Persistently low antigen load
Central memory	IL-2 only	Cleared or treated infection; LTBI

being similar to those with active disease. This study was able to discriminate between these groups with high sensitivity and specificity.[197] This suggests that those with LTBI who are at-risk of developing active TB have evidence for subclinical inflammation and/or immune activation that may have the potential for translation into a sensitive and specific test. This may be of great use in risk stratifying those who are IGRA positive and aid with better-directed chemoprophylaxis.

TRANSCRIPTOMICS

Although much of the preceding chapter has focused on T-cell-based immunodiagnostics, research is increasingly focusing on transcriptomics and proteomics as diagnostic tools in LTBI.

Transcriptomics, in general, analyzes changes in genetic expression related to the transcriptome and has been used in studies to differentiate patients with active, latent, and recurrent TB.[198] By contrast, proteomics evaluates changes in the proteins produced from specific tissues and cells. In TB, this concept has been used to identify proteins present in the serum of patients with active TB.[199]

Over the last few years a number of investigators have published whole blood transcriptomic studies. These have predominantly focused on high-TB burden settings to describe the host immune response to M.tb infection.[200–203] Investigators have been able to show that the transcriptomic signature of individuals with LTBI and active TB differ[201,203] and can also give information about the response to treatment.[204,205] However, it is important to note that these studies are highly dependent on accurate clinical phenotyping of patients and host biomarkers may be region/country/strain specific. Although identifying host biomarkers is undoubtedly of clinical utility, a crucial development in TB control would be to be able to identify those individuals with LTBI whose blood profile identifies them at-risk of developing active TB in the future. A recent study from South Africa has been able to identify a gene signature, which predicts the risk of developing future TB although the gene signature only had predictive ability for up to 18 months post infection. The overall sensitivity in two independent cohorts was 53.7% and 66.1%.[200] Further study has identified a polymerase chain reaction (PCR)-based transcriptomic signature, "RISK4," which has been shown to predict the risk of progression to active TB disease in diverse African cohorts of recently exposed household contacts of index TB cases; this four-gene signature predicted risk of progression with similar accuracy in four cohorts from three sub-Saharan African populations with heterogeneous genetic backgrounds, TB epidemiology, and circulating M.tb strains. However, notably, it performed poorly in the Ethiopia group.[201] There has been increasing focus on using transcriptomics in this way with PCR-based versions of published transcriptional signatures, for example "DIAG3," the three-gene diagnostic signature reported by Sweeney and colleagues,[206] and "DIAG4," the four-gene diagnostic signature reported by Maertzdorf and colleagues[207] as further examples.

These tools undoubtedly hold promise but they remain a research tool at present and their position in the clinical diagnostic pathway needs further evaluation and testing. Transcriptional profiling could improve the detection of incipient TB and has the potential to develop into a screening test for risk of progression, for example, during TB contact investigation. The increase in PPV of these tests compared with IGRAs appears small however because of low specificity.[200,208] It is also important to note that the infrastructure required to implement and support such technologies would be difficult in resource limited settings.

CLINICAL RISK SCORES

Until new technologies become validated, approved, and commercially available, exploiting the high NPV of IGRAs and applying clinical risk stratification to those who are IGRA positive would appear to be the best approach; thus, focusing on those at the highest risk of developing TB and prioritizing existing prevention strategies. Evidence suggests strategies should particularly focus on HIV-infected individuals, preferentially with on-going viral replication, and on close contacts of infectious cases of TB.

In the negative HIV cohort clinical scoring systems have been applied in a variety of settings both in adults and children in an attempt to identify those at high risk of progressing to active TB. A recent Peruvian cohort study followed contacts of pulmonary TB cases. Over a 10-year period 65 (3%) of 1,910 contacts developed TB. They found that risk factors for TB were low body-mass index, previous TB, age, sustained exposure to the index case, the index case being in a male patient, lower community household socioeconomic position, indoor air pollution, previous TB among household members, and living in a household with a low number of windows per room.[209]

In children, another simple algorithm focused specifically on the exposure variables in children contacts aged 3 months to 6 years. The 10-point score took into account maternal TB and sleep proximity, index case infectivity, duration of exposure, and exposure to multiple index cases. The odds of being MTB-infected increased by 74% (OR 1.74, 95% CI 1.42–2.12) with each 1-point increase in the contact score.[210] Another 8-point scoring system was developed and validated in child contacts in Taiwan. The score included reaction to TST, smear-positivity, residence in high-incidence areas, and sex of the index case.[211]

These studies show that risk scores could facilitate targeted treatment and resources to those more likely to benefit through the identification of high-risk children and adult contacts. These could be of use as an addition to prioritizing screening, clinical education, and surveillance for all high-risk contacts. In the future, it may also be useful to combine clinical risk stratification within IGRA positive groups and transcriptomics to further try and identify those who will progress to active TB.

CLOSING REMARKS

Over the last 15 years, immunodiagnostics for TB have developed rapidly, especially with respect to IGRAs, for the diagnosis of LTBI. The rapidly expanding evidence base underpinning the use of IGRAs indicates that they are more specific, and of equivalent sensitivity to TST, resulting in their widespread incorporation into national TB control policies. Despite great progress in the field, as yet, no test, biomarker, or signature, has been identified that meets the necessary requirements for a prognostic test. As outlined by the WHO, the field is yearning for a highly predictive test that can help target those who will progress to active TB disease and therefore benefit most from LTBI treatment.

Currently available IGRAs have several limitations and future research is actively seeking to develop next-generation IGRAs, novel T-cell diagnostics, and biomarkers, which are likely to further improve immunodiagnostics for TB. Any test will need to be validated in different populations, geographic locations, and accuracy ensured in varied TB burden settings. Given that a large pool of TB disease is in resource-limited countries, such a test needs to be practical and require minimal infrastructure and follow-up. Addressing the huge latent pool of TB is the only way we are going to make headway in achieving the global end TB strategy.

REFERENCES

1. Houben RMGJ, and Dodd PJ. The global burden of latent tuberculosis infection: A re-estimation using mathematical modelling. *PLoS Med.* 2016;13(10):1–13.

2. Behr MA, Edelstein PH, and Ramakrishnan L. Revisiting the timetable of tuberculosis. *Brit Med J* 2018;2738(August):1–10. doi: 10.1136/bmj.k2738.

3. Samandari T et al. 6-month versus 36-month isoniazid preventive treatment for tuberculosis in adults with HIV infection in Botswana: A randomised, double-blind, placebo-controlled trial. *Lancet* 2011;377(9777):1588–98.

4. Barcellini L, Borroni E, Brown J, Brunetti E, Codecasa L, and Cugnata F. First independent evaluation of QuantiFERON-TB Plus performance. *Eur Respir J.* 2016;47:1587–90.

5. Petruccioli E et al. First characterization of the CD4 and CD8 T-cell responses to QuantiFERON-TB Plus. *J Infect.* 2016;73(6):588–97.

6. Rozot V et al. Combined use of *Mycobacterium tuberculosis*-specific CD4 and CD8 T-cell responses is a powerful diagnostic tool of active tuberculosis. *Clin Infect Dis.* 2015;60(3):432–7.

7. Barcellini L et al. First evaluation of QuantiFERON-TB gold plus performance in contact screening. *Eur Respir J.* 2016;48(5):1411–9.

8. Champion P, Stanley S, Champion M, Brown E, and Cox J. C-terminal signal sequence. *Science (80-).* 2006;313(September):1632–6.

9. Hsu T et al. The primary mechanism of attenuation of bacillus Calmette–Guerin is a loss of secreted lytic function required for invasion of lung interstitial tissue. *Proc Natl Acad Sci.* 2003;100(21):12420–5.

10. Lalvani A et al. Enhanced contact tracing and spatial tracking of *Mycobacterium tuberculosis* infection by enumeration of antigen-specific T cells. *Lancet* 2001;357:2017–2.

11. Mustafa AS, Cockle PJ, Shaban F, Hewinson RG, and Vordermeier HM. Immunogenicity of *Mycobacterium tuberculosis* RD1 region gene products in infected cattle. *Clin Exp Immunol.* 2002;130(1):37–42.

12. Dosanjh DPS et al. UKPMC funders group improved diagnostic evaluation of suspected tuberculosis in routine practice. *Ann Intern Med.* 2009;148(5):325–36.

13. Millington KA et al. Rv3615c is a highly immunodominant RD1 (region of difference 1)-dependent secreted antigen specific for *Mycobacterium tuberculosis* infection. *Proc Natl Acad Sci.* 2011;108(14):5730–5.

14. Esmail H, Barry CE, Young DB, and Wilkinson RJ. The ongoing challenge of latent tuberculosis. *Philos Trans R Soc B Biol Sci.* 2014;369(1645).

15. WHO. Latent Tuberculosis Infection, 2018. Available at: http://apps. who.int/iris/bitstream/handle/10665/260233/9789241550239-eng. pdf?sequence=1.

16. European Centre for Disease Prevention and Control. *Programmatic Management of Latent Tuberculosis Infection in the European Union*, 2018.

17. European Centre for Disease Prevention and Control. *Review of Reviews and Guidelines on Target Groups, Diagnosis, Treatment and Programmatic Issues for Implementation of Latent Tuberculosis Management*, 2018.

18. NICE. Tuberculosis. 2016(January). doi: 10.1038/nrdp.2016.77.

19. WHO. *WHO End TB Strategy*; 2015. Available at: https://www.who. int/tb/post2015_strategy/en/.

20. Sester M et al. Interferon-γ release assays for the diagnosis of active tuberculosis: A systematic review and meta-analysis [*Eur Respir J* (2011) 37, (100–111)]. *Eur Respir J.* 2012;39(3):793.

21. Cattamanchi A et al. Interferon-gamma release assays for the diagnosis of latent tuberculosis infection in HIV-infected individuals: A systematic review and meta-analysis. *J Acquired Immune Defic Syndr.* 2011;56(3):230–8.

22. Diel R, Loddenkemper R, Meywald-Walter K, Niemann S, and Nienhaus A. Predictive value of a whole blood IFN-gamma assay for the development of active tuberculosis disease after recent infection with *Mycobacterium tuberculosis*. *Am J Respir Crit Care Med.* 2008;177(10):1164–70.

23. Pai M, Zwerling A, and Menzies D. Systematic review: T-cell-based assays for the diagnosis of latent tuberculosis infection: An update. *Ann Intern Med.* 2008;149(3):177–84.

24. Menzies D, Pai M, and Comstock G. Meta-analysis: New tests for the diagnosis of latent tuberculosis infection: Areas of uncertainty and recommendations for research. *Ann Intern Med.* 2007;146:340–54.

25. Metcalfe JZ et al. Interferon-γ release assays for active pulmonary tuberculosis diagnosis in adults in low-and middle-income countries: Systematic review and meta-analysis. *J Infect Dis.* 2011;204(4):1120–9.

26. Pareek M et al. Screening of immigrants in the UK for imported latent tuberculosis: A multicentre cohort study and cost-effectiveness analysis. *Lancet Infect Dis.* 2011;11(6):435–44.

27. Stout JE et al. Evaluating latent tuberculosis infection diagnostics using latent class analysis. *Thorax* 2018;73:1062–70.

28. Chapman ALN et al. Rapid detection of active and latent tuberculosis infection in HIV-positive individuals by enumeration of *Mycobacterium tuberculosis*-specific T cells. *AIDS* 2002;16(17):2285–93.

29. Liebeschuetz S, Bamber S, Ewer K, Deeks J, Pathan AA, and Lalvani A. Diagnosis of tuberculosis in South African children with a T-cell-based assay: A prospective cohort study. *Lancet* 2004;364(9452):2196–203.

30. Rangaka M et al. Clinical, immunological, and epidemiological importance of antituberculosis T cell responses in HIV-infected Africans. *Clin Infect Dis.* 2007;44(12):1639–46.

31. Clark SA et al. Tuberculosis antigen-specific immune responses can be detected using enzyme-linked immunospot technology in human immunodeficiency virus (HIV)-1 patients with advanced disease. *Clin Exp Immunol.* 2007;150(2):238–44.

32. Goletti D, Carrara S, Vincenti D, and Girardi E. T cell responses to commercial *Mycobacterium tuberculosis* specific antigens in HIV-infected patients. *Clin Infect Dis.* 2007;45(12):1652–1652.

33. Vincenti D et al. Response to region of difference 1 (RD1) epitopes in human immunodeficiency virus (HIV)-infected individuals enrolled with suspected active tuberculosis: A pilot study. *Clin Exp Immunol.* 2007;150(1):91–8.

34. Raby E et al. The effects of HIV on the sensitivity of a whole blood IFN-γ release assay in Zambian adults with active tuberculosis. *PLOS ONE* 2008;3(6):e2489.

35. Aabye MG et al. The impact of HIV infection and CD4 cell count on the performance of an interferon gamma release assay in patients with pulmonary tuberculosis. *PLOS ONE* 2009;4(1):e4220.

36. Santin M, Muñoz L, and Rigau D. Interferon-γ release assays for the diagnosis of tuberculosis and tuberculosis infection in HIV-infected adults: A systematic review and meta-analysis. *PLOS ONE* 2012;7(3):e32482.

37. Ayubi E, Doosti-Irani A, Moghaddam AS, Sani M, Nazarzadeh M, and Mostafavi E. The clinical usefulness of tuberculin skin test versus interferon-gamma release assays for diagnosis of latent tuberculosis in HIV patients: A meta-analysis. *PLOS ONE* 2016;11(9):e0161983. doi: 10.1371/journal.pone.0161983.

38. Telisinghe L et al. The sensitivity of the QuantiFERON®-TB Gold Plus assay in Zambian adults with active tuberculosis. *Int J Tuberc Lung Dis.* 2017;21(6):690–6.

39. Overton K, Varma R, and Post JJ. Comparison of interferon-gamma release assays and the tuberculin skin test for diagnosis of tuberculosis in human immunodeficiency virus: A systematic review. *Tuberc Respir Dis (Seoul)* 2018;81(1):59–72.

40. Mathad JS et al. Quantitative IFN-γ and IL-2 response associated with latent tuberculosis test discordance in HIV-infected pregnant women. *Am J Respir Crit Care Med.* 2016;193(12):1421–8.

41. LaCourse SM et al. Effect of pregnancy on interferon gamma release assay and tuberculin skin test detection of latent TB infection among HIV-infected women in a high burden setting. *J Acquired Immune Defic Syndr.* 2017;75(1):128–36.

42. Mathad JS et al. Pregnancy differentially impacts performance of latent tuberculosis diagnostics in a high-burden setting. *PLOS ONE* 2014;9:e92308.

43. Zhang Z et al. Risk of tuberculosis in patients treated with TNF-α antagonists: A systematic review and meta-analysis of randomised controlled trials. *BMJ Open* 2017;7(e012567). doi: 10.1136/bmjopen-2016-012567.

44. Lalvani A, and Millington KA. Screening for tuberculosis infection prior to initiation of anti-TNF therapy. *Autoimmun Rev.* 2008;8(2):147–52.

45. Jeong DH et al. Comparison of latent tuberculosis infection screening strategies before tumor necrosis factor inhibitor treatment in inflammatory arthritis: IGRA-alone versus combination of TST and IGRA. *PLOS ONE* 2018;13. doi: 10.1371/journal.pone.0198756.

46. Kwakernaak AJ, Houtman PM, Weel JFL, Spoorenberg JPL, and Jansen TLTA. A comparison of an interferon-gamma release assay and tuberculin skin test in refractory inflammatory disease patients screened for latent tuberculosis prior to the initiation of a first tumor necrosis factor α inhibitor. *Clin Rheumatol.* 2011;30. doi: 10.1007/s10067-010-1550-z.

47. Behar SM, Shin DS, Maier A, Coblyn J, Helfgott S, and Weinblatt ME. Use of the T-SPOT.TB assay to detect latent tuberculosis infection among rheumatic disease patients on immunosuppressive therapy. *J Rheumatol.* 2009;36(3):546–51.

48. Martin J et al. Comparison of interferon γ release assays and conventional screening tests before tumour necrosis factor α blockade in patients with inflammatory arthritis. *Ann Rheum Dis.* 2010;69(1):181–5.

49. Laffitte E et al. Tuberculosis screening in patients with psoriasis before antitumour necrosis factor therapy: Comparison of an interferon-γ release assay vs. tuberculin skin test. *Br J Dermatol.* 2009;161(4):797–800.

50. Bocchino M et al. Performance of two commercial blood IFN-γ release assays for the detection of *Mycobacterium tuberculosis* infection in patient candidates for anti-TNF-α treatment. *Eur J Clin Microbiol Infect Dis.* 2008;27(10):907–13.

51. Cobanoglu N et al. Interferon-gamma assays for the diagnosis of tuberculosis infection before using tumour necrosis factor-alpha blockers. *Int J Tuberc Lung Dis.* 2007;11(11):1177–82.

52. Sellam J et al. Comparison of *in vitro*-specific blood tests with tuberculin skin test for diagnosis of latent tuberculosis before anti-TNF therapy. *Ann Rheum Dis.* 2007;66(12):1610–5.

53. Takahashi H et al. Interferon γ assay for detecting latent tuberculosis infection in rheumatoid arthritis patients during infliximab administration. *Rheumatol Int.* 2007;24(3):188–92.

54. Bartalesi F et al. QuantiFERON-TB Gold and the TST are both useful for latent tuberculosis infection screening in autoimmune diseases. *Eur Respir J.* 2009;33(3):586–93.

55. Matulis G, Jüni P, Villiger PM, and Gadola SD. Detection of latent tuberculosis in immunosuppressed patients with autoimmune diseases: Performance of a *Mycobacterium tuberculosis* antigen-specific interferon γ assay. *Ann Rheum Dis.* 2008;67(1):84–90.

56. Rogerson TE et al. Tests for latent tuberculosis in people with ESRD: A systematic review. *Am J Kidney Dis.* 2013;61:33–43.

57. Marais BJ, Gie RP, Schaaf HS, Hesseling AC, Obihara CC, and Starke JJ. The natural history of childhood intra-thoracic tuberculosis: A critical review of literature from the pre-chemotherapy era. *Int J Tuberc Lung Dis.* 2004;8(4):392–402.

58. Sollai S, Galli L, de Martino M, and Chiappini E. Systematic review and meta-analysis on the utility of Interferon-gamma release assays for the diagnosis of *Mycobacterium tuberculosis* infection in children: A 2013 update. *BMC Infect Dis.* 2014;14(Suppl 1):1–11.

59. Mandalakas AM, Detjen AK, Hesseling AC, Benedetti A, and Menzies D. Interferon-gamma release assays and childhood tuberculosis: Systematic review and meta-analysis. *Int J Tuberc Lung Dis.* 2011;15(8):1018–32.

60. Sun L et al. Interferon gamma release assay in diagnosis of pediatric tuberculosis: A meta-analysis. *FEMS Immunol Med Microbiol.* 2011;63(2):165–73.

61. Machingaidze S, Wiysonge CS, and Hussey GD. Strengthening the expanded programme on immunization in Africa: Looking beyond 2015. *PLoS Med.* 2013;10(3):e1001405.

62. Chiappini E et al. Interferon-γ release assays for the diagnosis of *Mycobacterium tuberculosis* infection in children: A systematic review and meta-analysis. *Int J Immunopathol Pharmacol.* 2012;25(2):335–43.

63. Ewer K et al. Comparison of T-cell-based assay with tuberculin skin test for diagnosis of *Mycobacterium tuberculosis* infection in a school tuberculosis outbreak. *Lancet* 2003;361(9364):1168–73.

64. Soysal A et al. Effect of BCG vaccination on risk of *Mycobacterium tuberculosis* infection in children with household tuberculosis contact: A prospective community-based study. *Lancet* 2005;366(9495):1443–51.

65. Connell TG, Ritz N, Paxton GA, Buttery JP, Curtis N, and Ranganathan SC. A three-way comparison of tuberculin skin testing, QuantiFERON-TB gold and T-SPOT.TB in children. *PLOS ONE* 2008;3(7):e2624.

66. Diel R, Loddenkemper R, Meywald-Walter K, Gottschalk R, and Nienhaus A. Comparative performance of tuberculin skin test, Quanti FERON-TB-Gold in tube assay, and T-SpotTB test in contact investigations for tuberculosis. *Chest* 2009;135(4):1010–8.

67. Nicol MP et al. Comparison of T-SPOT.TB assay and tuberculin skin test for the evaluation of young children at high risk for tuberculosis in a community setting. *Pediatrics* 2009;123(1):38–43.

68. Pareek M et al. Community-based evaluation of immigrant tuberculosis screening using interferon γ release assays and tuberculin skin testing: Observational study and economic analysis. *Thorax* 2013;68:230–9.

69. Domínguez J et al. Comparison of two commercially available gamma interferon blood tests for immunodiagnosis of tuberculosis. *Clin Vaccine Immunol.* 2008;15(1):168–71.

70. Brock I, Weldingh K, Leyten EMS, Arend SM, Ravn P, and Andersen P. Specific T-cell epitopes for immunoassay-based diagnosis of *Mycobacterium tuberculosis* infection. *J Clin Microbiol.* 2004;42(6):2379–87.

71. Connell TG, Curtis N, Rangaka MX, and Wilkinson RJ. QuantiFERON-TB Gold: State of the art for the diagnosis of tuberculosis infection? *Expert Rev Mol Diagn.* 2006;6(5):663–77.

72. Nakaoka H et al. Risk for tuberculosis among children. *Emerging Infect Dis.* 2006;12(9):1383–8.

73. Chun JK et al. The role of a whole blood interferon-γ assay for the detection of latent tuberculosis infection in Bacille Calmette–Guérin vaccinated children. *Diagn Microbiol Infect Dis.* 2008;62(4):389–94.

74. Okada K et al. Performance of an interferon-gamma release assay for diagnosing latent tuberculosis infection in children. *Epidemiol Infect.* 2008;136(9):1179–87.

75. Lighter J, Rigaud M, Huie M, Peng CH, and Pollack H. Chemokine IP-10: An adjunct marker for latent tuberculosis infection in children. *Int J Tuberc Lung Dis.* 2009;13(6):731–6.

76. Tsiouris SJ, Coetzee D, Toro PL, Austin J, Stein Z, and El-Sadr W. Sensitivity analysis and potential uses of a novel gamma interferon release assay for diagnosis of tuberculosis. *J Clin Microbiol.* 2006;44(8):2844–50.

77. Hill PC, Brookes RH, Adetifa IM, Fox A, and Jackson-Sillah DJ. Comparison of enzyme-linked immunospot assay and tuberculin skin test in healthy children exposed to *Mycobacterium tuberculosis. Pediatrics* 2006;117(5):1542–8.

78. Diel R, Loaddenkemper R, and Nienhaus A. Evidence-based comparison of commercial Interferon-γ release assays for detecting active TB a metaanalysis. *Chest* 2010;137(4):952–68.

79. Takasaki J et al. Sensitivity and specificity of QuantiFERON-TB Gold Plus compared with QuantiFERON-TB Gold In-Tube and T-SPOT.TB on active tuberculosis in Japan. *J Infect Chemother.* 2018;24(3):188–92.

80. Smieja M, Marchetti C, Cook D, and Fm S. Isoniazid for preventing tuberculosis in non-HIV infected persons (Review). *Cochrane Database Syst Rev.* 1999;2(1):1–28. doi: 10.1002/14651858. CD001363. Available at: https://www.cochranelibrary.com.

81. Sandgren A, Noordegraaf-schouten MV, Van Kessel F, and Stuurman A. Initiation and completion rates for latent tuberculosis infection treatment: A systematic review. *BMC Infect Dis.* 2016;16(204):1–12.

82. Bakir M et al. Prognostic value of a T-cell-based, interferon-gamma biomarker in children with tuberculosis contact. *Ann Intern Med.* 2008;149(11):777–87.

83. Rangaka M et al. Predictive value of interferon-γ release assays for incident active tuberculosis: A systematic review and meta-analysis. *Lancet Infect Dis.* 2012;12(1):45–55.

84. Diel R, Goletti D, Ferrara G, Bothamley G, Cirillo D, and Kampmann B. Interferon-c release assays for the diagnosis of latent *Mycobacterium tuberculosis* infection: A systematic review and meta-analysis. *Eur Respir J.* 2011;37(1):88–99.

85. Zellweger JP et al. Risk assessment of tuberculosis in contacts by IFN-γ release assays. A tuberculosis network European trials group study. *Am J Respir Crit Care Med.* 2015;191(10):1176–84.

86. Diel R, Loddenkemper R, and Nienhaus A. Predictive value of interferon-γ release assays and tuberculin skin testing for progression from latent TB infection to disease state: A meta-analysis. *Chest* 2012;142:63–75.

87. Altet N et al. Predicting the development of tuberculosis with the tuberculin skin test and QuantiFERON testing. *Ann Am Thorac Soc.* 2015;12(5):680–8.

88. Harstad I, Winje BA, Heldal E, Oftung F, and Jacobsen GW. Predictive values of QuantiFERON (R)-TB Gold testing in screening for tuberculosis disease in asylum seekers. *Int J Tuberc Lung Dis.* 2010;14(9):1209–11.

89. Kik SV et al. Predictive value for progression to tuberculosis by IGRA and TST in immigrant contacts. *Eur Respir J.* 2010;35(6):1346–53.

90. Abubakar I et al. Prognostic value of interferon-γ release assays and tuberculin skin test in predicting the development of active tuberculosis (UK PREDICT TB): A prospective cohort study. *Lancet Infect Dis.* 2018;18(October):1077–87.

91. CDC. *TB Elimination Targeted TB Testing and Interpreting Tuberculin Skin Test Results*, 2016. Available at: http://www.cdc. gov/tb. August.

92. WHO. *Consensus Meeting Report—Development of a Target Product Profile (TPP) and a Framework for Evaluation for a Test for Predicting Progression from Tuberculosis Infection to Active Disease*, 2017. Available at: http://apps.who.int/iris/bitstream/handle/10665/259176/WHO-HTM-TB-2017.18-eng.pdf;jsessionid=99A51E06A68227971366038B51E1C80D?sequence=1

93. Sester M et al. Risk assessment of tuberculosis in immunocompromised patients: A TBNET study. *Am J Respir Crit Care Med.* 2014;190(10):1168–76.

94. Sloot R, Van Der Loeff MFS, Kouw PM, and Borgdorff MW. Risk of tuberculosis after recent exposure: A 10-year follow-up study of contacts in Amsterdam. *Am J Respir Crit Care Med.* 2014;190(9):1044–52.

95. Aichelburg MC et al. Detection and prediction of active tuberculosis disease by a whole-blood interferon-γ release assay in HIV-1-infected individuals. *Clin Infect Dis.* 2009;48(7):954–62.

96. Sester M, Van Leth F, and Lange C. Numbers needed to treat to prevent tuberculosis. *Eur Respir J.* 2015;46:1836–8.

97. Ferguson TW et al. The diagnostic accuracy of tests for latent tuberculosis infection in hemodialysis patients: A systematic review and meta-analysis. *Transplantation* 2015;99:1084–91.

98. Walsh MC et al. The sensitivity of interferon-gamma release assays is not compromised in tuberculosis patients with diabetes. *Int J Tuberc Lung Dis.* 2011;15(2):179–84.

99. Dorman SE et al. Interferon-γ release assays and tuberculin skin testing for diagnosis of latent tuberculosis infection in healthcare workers in the United States. *Am J Respir Crit Care Med.* 2014;189(1):77–87.

100. Schablon A, Nienhaus A, Ringshausen FC, Preisser AM, and Peters C. Occupational screening for tuberculosis and the use of a borderline zone for interpretation of the IGRA in German healthcare workers. *PLOS ONE* 2014;9(12):1–16.

101. Slater ML, Welland G, Pai M, Parsonnet J, and Banaei N. Challenges with QuantiFERON-TB gold assay for large-scale, routine screening of U.S. healthcare workers. *Am J Respir Crit Care Med.* 2013;188(8):1005–10.

102. Sharma SK, Vashishtha R, Chauhan LS, Sreenivas V, and Seth D. Comparison of TST and IGRA in diagnosis of latent tuberculosis infection in a high TB-burden setting. *PLOS ONE* 2017;12(1):1–11.

103. Hill PC et al. Incidence of tuberculosis and the predictive value of ELISPOT and Mantoux tests in Gambian case contacts. *PLOS ONE* 2008;3(1). doi: 10.1371/journal.pone.0001379.

104. Whalen CC et al. Secondary attack rate of tuberculosis in urban households in Kampala, Uganda. *PLOS ONE* 2011;6(2). doi: 10.1371/journal.pone.0016137.

105. Kim YJYR, Kim S Il, Kim YJYR, Wie SH, Park YJ, and Kang MW. Predictive value of interferon-γ ELISPOT assay in HIV 1-infected patients in an intermediate tuberculosis-endemic area. *AIDS Res Hum Retroviruses.* 2012;28(9):120403080225007.

106. Rangaka M et al. Isoniazid plus antiretroviral therapy to prevent tuberculosis: A randomised double-blind placebo-controlled trial Molebogeng. *Lancet* 2014;384(9944):682–90.

107. Zenner D, Kruijshaar ME, Andrews N, and Abubakar I. Risk of tuberculosis in pregnancy: A national, primary care-based cohort and self-controlled case series study. *Am J Respir Crit Care Med.* 2012;185(7):779–84.

108. Jonnalagadda S, Brown E, Lohman Payne B, and Wamalwa D. Predictive value of interferon-gamma release assays for postpartum active tuberculosis in HIV-1 infected women. *Int J Tuberc Lung Dis.* 2013;17(12):1552–7.

109. Andrews JR et al. Serial QuantiFERON testing and tuberculosis disease risk among young children: An observational cohort study. *Lancet Respir Med.* 2017;5(4):282–90.

110. Farhat M, Greenaway C, Pai M, and Menzies D. False-positive tuberculin skin tests: What is the absolute effect of BCG and non-tuberculous mycobacteria ? *Int J Tuberc Lung Dis.* 2006;10(11):1192–204.

111. Whitworth H, Badhan A, Boaky A, Takwoingi Y, Rees-Roberts M, and Partlett C. An observational cohort study to evaluate the clinical utility of current and second-generation interferon-gamma release-assays in diagnostic evaluation of tuberculosis. *Lancet Infect Dis.* 2019;19:193–202.

112. Menzies D. Interpretation of repeated tuberculin tests: Boosting, conversion, and reversion. *Am J Respir Crit Care Med.* 1999;159(1):15–21.

113. Lee SW, Oh DK, Lee SH, and Kang HY. Time interval to conversion of interferon-c release assay after exposure to tuberculosis. *Eur Respir J.* 2011;37:1447–52.

114. Anibarro L, Trigo M, Villaverde C, Pena A, and González-Fernández Á. Tuberculin skin test and interferon-γ release assay show better correlation after the tuberculin "window period" in tuberculosis contacts. *Scand J Infect Dis.* 2011;43:424–9.

115. Dosanjh DPS et al. Novel *M. tuberculosis* antigen-specific T-cells are early markers of infection and disease progression. *PLOS ONE* 2011;6(12). doi: 10.1371/journal.pone.0028754.

116. Ewer K, Millington KA, Deeks JJ, Alvarez L, Bryant G, and Lalvani A. Dynamic antigen-specific T-cell responses after point-source exposure to *Mycobacterium tuberculosis. Am J Respir Crit Care Med.* 2006;174(7):831–9.

117. Nardell EA, and Wallis RS. Here today—gone tomorrow: The case for transient acute tuberculosis infection. *Am J Respir Crit Care Med.* 2006;174(7):734–5.

118. Pai M et al. Serial testing of health care workers for tuberculosis using interferon-γ assay. *Am J Respir Crit Care Med* 2006;174(3):349–55.

119. Franken WPJ et al. Interferon-gamma release assays during follow-up of tuberculin skin test-positive contacts. *Int J Tuberc Lung Dis.* 2008;12(11):1286–94.

120. Ma KC, Mathad JS, Wilkin T, and Wu X. Treat or repeat? Variability of interferon gamma release assays in the detection of latent TB infection among HIV-positive patients. *Open Forum Infect Dis.* 2015;2(Suppl 1):2015.

121. Andrews JR et al. The dynamics of QuantiFERON-TB Gold in-Tube conversion and reversion in a cohort of South African adolescents. *Am J Respir Crit Care Med.* 2015;191(158–591). doi: 10.1164/rccm.201409-1704OC.

122. Millington KAA, Gooding S, Hinks TSCSC, Reynolds DJMJM, and Lalvani A. *Mycobacterium tuberculosis*-specific cellular immune profiles suggest bacillary persistence decades after spontaneous cure in untreated tuberculosis. *J Infect Dis.* 2010;202(11):1685–9.

123. Zwerling A, Van Den Hof S, Scholten J, Cobelens F, Menzies D, and Pai M. Interferon-gamma release assays for tuberculosis screening of healthcare workers: A systematic review. *Thorax* 2011;67:62–70.

124. Richeldi L et al. T-cell-based diagnosis of neonatal multidrug-resistant latent tuberculosis infection. *Pediatrics* 2007;119(1):1–5.

125. Chee CBE, Khinmar KW, Gan SH, Barkham TMS, Pushparani M, and Wang YT. Latent tuberculosis infection treatment and T-cell responses to *Mycobacterium tuberculosis*-specific antigens. *Am J Respir Crit Care Med.* 2007;175(3):282–7.

126. Chiappini E et al. Serial T-Spot.Tb and Quantiferon-TB-gold in-tube assays to monitor response to antitubercular treatment in Italian children with active or latent tuberculosis infection. *Pediatr Infect Dis J.* 2012;31(9):974–7.

127. Nenadić N, Kirin BK, Letoja IZ, Plavec D, Topić RZ, and Dodig S. Serial interferon-γ release assay in children with latent tuberculosis infection and children with tuberculosis. *Pediatr Pulmonol.* 2012;47(4):401–8.

128. Clifford V, He Y, Zufferey C, Connell T, and Curtis N. Interferon gamma release assays for monitoring the response to treatment for tuberculosis: A systematic review. *Tuberculosis* 2015;95(6):639–50.

129. Trunz BB, Fine P, and Dye C. Effect of BCG vaccination on childhood tuberculous meningitis and miliary tuberculosis worldwide: A meta-analysis and assessment of cost-effectiveness. *Lancet* 2006;367(9517):1173–80. doi: 10.1016/S0140-6736(06)68507-3.

130. Colditz GA et al. Efficacy of BCG vaccine in the prevention of tuberculosis: Meta-analysis of the published literature. *JAMA J Am Med Assoc.* 1994;271(9):698–702.

131. Clemens JD, Chuong JJH, and Feinstein AR. The BCG controversy: A methodological and statistical reappraisal. *JAMA J Am Med Assoc.* 1983;249(17):2362–9.

132. Sutherland I, and Lindgren I. The protective effect of BCG vaccination as indicated by autopsy studies. *Tubercle* 1979;60(4):225–31.

133. Erkens C et al. Coverage and yield of entry and follow-up screening for tuberculosis among new immigrants. *Eur Respir J.* 2008;32(1):153–61.

134. Arshad S, Bavan L, Gajari K, Paget SNJ, and Baussano I. Active screening at entry for tuberculosis among new immigrants: A systematic review and meta-analysis. *Eur Respir J.* 2010;35(6):1336–45.

135. PHE. Collaborative Tuberculosis Strategy: Commissioning Guidance. *Public Heal Engl Publ.* 2015;July(January).

136. British HIV Association. *British HIV Association Guidelines for the Management of TB/HIV Co-Infection in Adults 2017 (Consultation),* 2017. doi: 10.1017/S0263593300008038.

137. White HA et al. Latent tuberculosis infection screening and treatment in HIV: Insights from evaluation of UK practice. *Thorax* 2017;72(2):180–2.

138. Lewinsohn DM et al. Official American Thoracic Society/Infectious Diseases Society of America/Centers for Disease Control and Prevention Clinical Practice Guidelines: Diagnosis of tuberculosis in adults and children. *Clin Infect Dis.* 2017;64:111–5.

139. Cush J, Whinthrop K, Dao K, and Chaisson RE. Screening for *Mycobacterium tuberculosis* infection: Questions and answers for clinical practice. *Drug Saf Updat.* 2010;1(2):1–4.

140. Singh JA et al. 2015 American college of rheumatology guideline for the treatment of rheumatoid arthritis. *Arthritis Care Res (Hoboken).* 2016. doi: 10.1002/acr.22783.

141. Ruhwald M et al. Safety and efficacy of the C-Tb skin test to diagnose *Mycobacterium tuberculosis* infection, compared with an interferon γ release assay and the tuberculin skin test: A phase 3, double-blind, randomised, controlled trial. *Lancet Respir Med.* 2017;5(4):259–68.

142. Hoff ST et al. Sensitivity of C-Tb: A novel RD-1-specific skin test for the diagnosis of tuberculosis infection. *Eur Respir J.* 2016;47(3):919–28.

143. Abubakar I, Jackson C, and Rangaka MX. Comment C-Tb: A latent tuberculosis skin test for the 21st century? Management of extensively drug-resistant tuberculosis. *Lancet Respir.* 2017;5(4):236–7.

144. Pantaleo G, and Harari A. Functional signatures in antiviral T-cell immunity for monitoring virus-associated diseases. *Nat Rev Immunol.* 2006;6(5):417–23.

145. Casey R et al. Enumeration of functional T-cell subsets by fluorescence-immunospot defines signatures of pathogen burden in tuberculosis. *PLOS ONE* 2010;5(12):e15619.

146. Day CL et al. Functional capacity of *Mycobacterium tuberculosis*-specific T cell responses in humans is associated with mycobacterial load. *J Immunol.* 2011;187(5):2222–32.

147. Harari A et al. Dominant TNF-α+ *Mycobacterium tuberculosis*-specific CD4+T cell responses discriminate between latent infection and active disease. *Nat Med.* 2011;17(3):372–6.

148. Sester U et al. Whole-blood flow-cytometric analysis of antigen-specific CD4 T-cell cytokine profiles distinguishes active tuberculosis from non-active states. *PLOS ONE* 2011;6(3):2–8.

149. Lalvani A, and Millington KA. T-cell interferon-γ release assays: Can we do better? *Eur Respir J.* 2008;32(6):1428–30.

150. Taub DD et al. Recombinant human interferon-inducible protein 10 is a chemoattractant for human monocytes and T lymphocytes and promotes T cell adhesion to endothelial cells. *J Exp Med.* 1993;177:1809–14.

151. Ruhwald M, Aabye MG, and Ravn P. IP-10 release assays in the diagnosis of tuberculosis infection: Current status and future directions. *Expert Rev Mol Diagn.* 2012;12(2):175–87.

152. Tebruegge M et al. Mycobacteria-specific cytokine responses detect tuberculosis infection and distinguish latent from active tuberculosis. *Am J Respir Crit Care Med.* 2015;192(4):485–99.

153. Naranbhai V et al. Ratio of monocytes to lymphocytes in peripheral blood identifies adults at risk of incident tuberculosis among HIV-infected adults initiating antiretroviral therapy. *J Infect Dis.* 2014;209(4):500–9.

154. Naranbhai V et al. The association between the ratio of monocytes: Lymphocytes at age 3 months and risk of tuberculosis (TB) in the first two years of life. *BMC Med.* 2014;12:120.

155. Rakotosamimanana N et al. Biomarkers for risk of developing active tuberculosis in contacts of TB patients: A prospective cohort study. *Eur Respir J.* 2015;46:1095–103.

156. Harada N et al. Comparison of the sensitivity and specificity of two whole blood interferon-gamma assays for *M. tuberculosis* infection. *J Infect.* 2008;56(5):348–53.

157. Arend SM, and Uzorka JW. New developments on interferon-γ release assays for tuberculosis diagnosis. *Lancet Infect Dis.* 2019;19(2):121–2.

158. Menozzi FD et al. Identification of a heparin-binding hemagglutinin present in mycobacteria. *J Exp Med.* 1996;184:993–1001.

159. Zheng Q et al. Heparin-binding hemagglutinin of *Mycobacterium tuberculosis* is an inhibitor of autophagy. *Front Cell Infect Microbiol.* 2017;7(33):1–11.

160. Pethe K et al. The heparin-binding haemagglutinin of *M. tuberculosis* is required for extrapulmonary dissemination. *Nature.* 2001;412:190–4.

161. Meier NR, Jacobsen M, Ottenhoff THM, and Ritz N. A systematic review on novel *Mycobacterium tuberculosis* antigens and their discriminatory potential for the diagnosis of latent and active tuberculosis. *Front Immunol.* 2018;9(2476). doi: 10.3389/fimmu.2018.02476.

162. Loxton AG, Black GF, Stanley K, and Walzl G. Heparin-binding hemagglutinin induces IFN-γ+IL-2+IL-17+ multifunctional CD4+ T cells during latent but not active tuberculosis disease. *Clin Vaccine Immunol.* 2012;19(5):746–51.

163. Hougardy JM et al. Heparin-binding-hemagglutinin-induced IFN-γ release as a diagnostic tool for latent tuberculosis. *PLOS ONE* 2007;2(10):e926.

164. Delogu G et al. Methylated HBHA produced in *M. smegmatis* discriminates between active and non-active tuberculosis disease among RD1-responders. *PLOS ONE* 2011;21. doi: 10.1371/journal.pone.0018315.

165. Wyndham-Thomas C et al. Key role of effector memory CD4+T lymphocytes in a short-incubation heparin-binding hemagglutinin gamma interferon release assay for the detection of latent tuberculosis. *Clin Vaccine Immunol.* 2014;21:321–8.

166. Chiacchio T et al. Immune characterization of the HBHA-specific response in *Mycobacterium tuberculosis*-infected patients with or without HIV infection. *PLOS ONE* 2017;12:e0183846.

167. Goletti D et al. Response to Rv2628 latency antigen associates with cured tuberculosis and remote infection. *Eur Respir J.* 2010;36(1):135–42.

168. Nonghanphithak D, Reechaipichitkul W, Namwat W, Naranbhai V, and Faksri K. Chemokines additional to IFN-γ can be used to differentiate among *Mycobacterium tuberculosis* infection possibilities and provide evidence of an early clearance phenotype. *Tuberculosis* 2017;105:28–34.

169. Chegou NN et al. Potential of novel *Mycobacterium tuberculosis* infection phase-dependent antigens in the diagnosis of TB disease in a high burden setting. *BMC Infect Dis.* 2012;12. doi: 10.1186/1471-2334-12-10.

170. Chegou NN et al. Potential of host markers produced by infection phase-dependent antigen-stimulated cells for the diagnosis of tuberculosis in a highly endemic area. *PLOS ONE* 2012;7. doi: 10.1371/journal.pone.0038501.

171. Commandeur S et al. Double- and monofunctional CD4+ and CD8+T-cell responses to *Mycobacterium tuberculosis* DosR antigens and peptides in long-term latently infected individuals. *Eur J Immunol.* 2011;41. doi: 10.1002/eji.201141602.

172. Arroyo L, Marín D, Franken KLMC, Ottenhoff THM, and Barrera LF. Potential of DosR and Rpf antigens from *Mycobacterium tuberculosis* to discriminate between latent and active tuberculosis in a tuberculosis endemic population of Medellin Colombia. *BMC Infect Dis.* 2018;18(1):1–9.

173. Alvarez-Corrales N et al. Differential cellular recognition pattern to *M. tuberculosis* targets defined by IFN-γ and IL-17 production in blood from TB+ patients from Honduras as compared to health care workers: TB and immune responses in patients from Honduras. *BMC Infect Dis.* 201313;. doi: 10.1186/1471-2334-13-125.

174. Winje BA et al. Stratification by interferon-γ 3 release assay level predicts risk of incident TB. *Thorax* 2018;73(7):652–61.

175. Gupta RK et al. Quantitative interferon gamma release assays and tuberculin skin test to predict incident tuberculosis: Data from the UK PREDICT Cohort Study. *Am J Respir Crit Care Med.* 2020;201:984–91.

176. Arroyo L, Rojas M, Franken KLMC, Ottenhoff THM, and Barrera LF. Multifunctional T cell response to DosR and Rpf antigens is associated with protection in long-term *Mycobacterium tuberculosis*-infected individuals in Colombia. *Clin Vaccine Immunol.* 2016;23:813–24

177. De Araujo LS, Da Silva NDBM, Da Silva RJ, Leung JAM, Mello FCQ, and Saad MHF. Profile of interferon-gamma response to latency-associated and novel *in vivo* expressed antigens in a cohort of subjects recently exposed to *Mycobacterium tuberculosis*. *Tuberculosis* 2015;95:751–7.

178. Bai XJ et al. Potential novel markers to discriminate between active and latent tuberculosis infection in Chinese individuals. *Comp Immunol Microbiol Infect Dis.* 2016;44:8–13.

179. Hozumi H et al. Immunogenicity of dormancy-related antigens in individuals infected with *Mycobacterium tuberculosis* in Japan. *Int J Tuberc Lung Dis*. 2013;17:818–24.

180. Belay M et al. Pro- and anti-inflammatory cytokines against Rv2031 are elevated during latent tuberculosis: A study in cohorts of tuberculosis patients, household contacts and community controls in an endemic setting. *PLOS ONE* 2015;10. doi: 10.1371/journal.pone.0124134.

181. Delogu G et al. Lack of response to HBHA in HIV-infected patients with latent tuberculosis infection. *Scand J Immunol*. 2016;84:344–52.

182. Dreesman A et al. Age-stratified T cell responses in children infected with *Mycobacterium tuberculosis*. *Front Immunol*. 2017;8. doi: 10.3389/fimmu.2017.01059.

183. Wyndham-Thomas C et al. Contribution of a heparin-binding haemagglutinin interferon-gamma release assay to the detection of *Mycobacterium tuberculosis* infection in HIV-infected patients: Comparison with the tuberculin skin test and the QuantiFERON®-TB Gold In-tube. *BMC Infect Dis*. 2015;15(59). doi: 10.1186/s12879-015-0796-0.

184. Schwander SK et al. Pulmonary mononuclear cell responses to antigens of *Mycobacterium tuberculosis* in healthy household contacts of patients with active tuberculosis and healthy controls from the community. *J Immunol*. 2000;165:1479–85.

185. Li G et al. Evaluation of a new IFN-γ release assay for rapid diagnosis of active tuberculosis in a high-incidence setting. *Front Cell Infect Microbiol*. 2017;7(April):1–9.

186. Wilkinson KA, and Wilkinson RJ. Polyfunctional T cells in human tuberculosis. *Eur J Immunol*. 2010;40(8):2139–42.

187. Fletcher HA et al. T-cell activation is an immune correlate of risk in BCG vaccinated infants. *Nat Commun*. 2016;7(May). doi: 10.1038/ncomms11290.

188. Tameris MD et al. Safety and efficacy of MVA85A, a new tuberculosis vaccine, in infants previously vaccinated with BCG: A randomised, placebo-controlled phase 2b trial. *Lancet* 2013;381:1021–8. doi: 10.1016/S0140-6736(13)60177-4.

189. Petruccioli E et al. Assessment of CD27 expression as a tool for active and latent tuberculosis diagnosis. *J Infect*. 2015;71(526–533). doi: 10.1016/j.jinf.2015.07.009.

190. Portevin D et al. Assessment of the novel T-cell activation marker-tuberculosis assay for diagnosis of active tuberculosis in children: A prospective proof-of-concept study. *Lancet Infect Dis*. 2014;14:931–8.

191. Goletti D, Petruccioli E, Joosten SA, and Ottenhoff THM. Tuberculosis biomarkers: From diagnosis to protection. *Infect Dis Rep*. 2016;8:6568.

192. Schuetz A et al. Monitoring CD27 expression to evaluate *Mycobacterium tuberculosis* activity in HIV-1 infected individuals *in vivo*. *PLOS ONE* 2011;6(11):1–6.

193. Pollock KM et al. T-cell immunophenotyping distinguishes active from latent tuberculosis. *J Infect Dis*. 2013;208(6):952–68.

194. Riou C, Berkowitz N, Goliath R, Burgers WA, and Wilkinson RJ. Analysis of the phenotype of *Mycobacterium tuberculosis*-specific CD$^+$ T cells to discriminate latent from active tuberculosis in HIV-uninfected and HIV-infected individuals. *Front Immunol*. 2017;10(8):968.

195. Parekh MJ, and Schluger NW. Treatment of latent tuberculosis infection. *Ther Adv Respir Dis*. 2013;7(6):351–6.

196. Landry J, and Menzies D. Preventive chemotherapy. Where has it got us? Where to go next? *Int J Tuberc Lung Dis*. 2008;12(12):1352–64.

197. Halliday A et al. Stratification of latent *Mycobacterium tuberculosis* infection by cellular immune profiling. *J Infect Dis*. 2017;215(9):1480–7.

198. Mistry R et al. Gene-expression patterns in whole blood identify subjects at risk for recurrent tuberculosis. *J Infect Dis*. 2007;195(3):357–65.

199. Agranoff D et al. Identification of diagnostic markers for tuberculosis by proteomic fingerprinting of serum. *Lancet* 2006;368:1012–21.

200. Zak DED et al. A blood RNA signature for tuberculosis disease risk: A prospective cohort study. *Lancet* 2016;387(10035):2312–22.

201. Suliman S et al. Four-gene pan-African blood signature predicts progression to tuberculosis. *Am J Respir Crit Care Med*. 2018;197(9):1–4.

202. Mahomed H et al. Predictive factors for latent tuberculosis infection among adolescents in a high-burden area in South Africa. *Int J Tuberc Lung Dis*. 2011;15(3):331–6.

203. Singhania A et al. A modular transcriptional signature identifies phenotypic heterogeneity of human tuberculosis infection. *Nat Commun*. 2018;9(2308):1–17.

204. Dupnik KM et al. Blood transcriptomic markers of *Mycobacterium tuberculosis* load in sputum. *Int J Tuberc Lung Dis*. 2018;22(8):950–8.

205. Thompson EG et al. Host blood RNA signatures predict the outcome of tuberculosis treatment. *Tuberculosis* 2017;107(48–58). doi: 10.1016/j.tube.2017.08.004.

206. Sweeney TE, Braviak L, Tato CM, and Khatri P. Genome-wide expression for diagnosis of pulmonary tuberculosis: A multicohort analysis. *Lancet Respir Med*. 2016;4(3):213–24.

207. Maertzdorf J et al. Concise gene signature for point-of-care classification of tuberculosis. *EMBO Mol Med*. 2016;8(2):86–95.

208. Kik SV, Cobelens F, and Moore D. Predicting tuberculosis risk. *Lancet* 2016;388(10057):2233.

209. Saunders MJ et al. A score to predict and stratify risk of tuberculosis in adult contacts of tuberculosis index cases: A prospective derivation and external validation cohort study. *Lancet Infect Dis*. 2017;17(11):1190–9.

210. Mandalakas AM et al. Well-quantified tuberculosis exposure is a reliable surrogate measure of tuberculosis infection. *Int J Tuberc Lung Dis*. 2012;16(June):1033–9.

211. Chan PC et al. Risk for tuberculosis in child contacts: Development and validation of a predictive score. *Am J Respir Crit Care Med*. 2014;189(2):203–13.

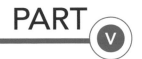

PART V

DRUGS AND VACCINES FOR TUBERCULOSIS

10

Clinical Pharmacology of the Anti-Tuberculosis Drugs

GERRY DAVIES AND CHARLES PELOQUIN

INTRODUCTION

Treatment of active and latent tuberculosis (TB) has evolved steadily over the 70 years since the dawn of the antibiotic era with 25 drugs from many distinct classes now in common use in different clinical situations. This diversity is compounded by the need for combination therapy to avoid the emergence of resistance and to shorten the duration of treatment. Although latent infection can be successfully eradicated with monotherapy, treatment of drug-sensitive disease is typically initiated with four drugs and up to seven drugs may be used together in multidrug-resistant TB. This complexity is almost unique in the treatment of infectious diseases and poses significant problems in the interpretation of efficacy, toxicity, and drug–drug interaction datawithin and between combination regimens. The ability to co-formulate several agents with differing physico-chemical properties has at times proved challenging and fixed-dose combinations are only available for first-line regimens. Finally, the prevalence of human immunodeficiency virus (HIV) co-infection in people with TB and the need for antiretroviral therapy as early as possible mandates consideration of the mutual impact of treatment for each disease on the other, particularly the potential for overlapping toxicities, immune reconstitution inflammatory syndrome, and poorer virological efficacy.

Though a considerable body of evidence from randomized-clinical trials has accumulated over the decades in latent infection and drug-sensitive disease, in multidrug-resistant disease such trials are a recent innovation. Similarly, although millions of patients have been treated with first-line regimens, high-quality observational pharmacovigilance data on the toxicity of these regimens are relatively scarce. After a hiatus of 30 years, the recent resumption of drug development efforts in TB and attempts to re-examine and re-purpose the existing drugs has drawn attention to many gaps in fundamental knowledge about the clinical pharmacology of older agents which are gradually being addressed retrospectively by new studies. This chapter attempts to summarize the current state of knowledge about all the drugs that physicians treating TB may be called upon to prescribe for their patients and to point out how the use of some of them may change in the near future as our understanding of their pharmacokinetics (PK) and pharmacodynamics advances.

ISONIAZID

STRUCTURE AND ACTIVITY

Isoniazid (INH) is a synthetic analog of nicotinamide. It is a highly water-soluble weak acid (log P −0.6, pKa 1.8/3.5/9.5, MW 137.14). INH is a pro-drug which is activated by the mycobacterial catalase-peroxidase enzyme KatG[1] and targets InhA, an NADH-dependent enoyl–acyl carrier protein reductase involved in mycolic acid synthesis.[2] *In vitro* minimum inhibitory concentration (MIC_{99}) for wild-type strains is 0.03–0.25 μg/mL.[3] The spontaneous rate of mutations resulting in resistance is approximately 1 in 10^8.[4] Resistance is conferred by mutations in *katG* (high-level) and/or *inhA* (low-level).[5]

PHARMACOKINETICS/ADME

INH has greater than 90% oral bioavailability and absorption is affected by food which may reduce drug exposure by 12%, but not by antacids.[6] The volume of distribution is typically 0.85–1.2 L/kg and plasma protein binding is 20%.[7] The primary route of metabolism is N-acetylation to the major metabolite acetylisoniazid through the highly polymorphic NAT2 pathway,[8] with numerous

single-nucleotide polymorphisms (SNPs) in the gene resulting in decreased activity.[9] These mutations result in highly variable rates of acetylation and distinct "fast," "intermediate," and "slow" phenotypes, which vary significantly worldwide. Acetylisoniazid undergoes further modification to acetyl- and diacetylhydrazines. However, 40% of each dose is excreted unchanged in the urine. The $t_{1/2}$ ranges from 1 to 3.5 hours, plasma C_{max} ranges from 3 to 5 μg/mL, and area under the curve (AUC) from 15 to 35 μg/mL × hour depending on acetylator status.[10,11] INH accumulates in epithelial lining fluid (1.2–3.2×) and in alveolar macrophages (2.1×)[12] whereas concentrations in pulmonary lesions are similar to plasma.[13] Concentrations in cerebrospinal fluid (CSF) are similar to those in plasma.[14,15]

PHARMACODYNAMICS AND EFFICACY

In monotherapy studies of early bactericidal activity (EBA), INH is the most active anti-TB drug so far evaluated with an EBA_{0-2} of 0.5 log_{10} CFU/mL/day which is both dose and exposure dependent.[16,17] Dose-titration studies suggest that maximal activity is achieved at a dose of approximately 5 mg/kg. In early Phase III clinical trials of INH monotherapy, cure was achieved in 30% after 6 months but the development of resistance was common. Some recent and conflicting data suggest that INH may be antagonistic to the activity of other agents in the first-line regimen but the impact of these findings on long-term treatment outcomes remains unclear.[18–20]

DOSING

The recommended daily dose of INH is 300 mg daily, administered on an empty stomach. For intermittent administration, doses of 15 mg/kg are recommended. Higher doses of up to 20 mg/kg have also been advocated for patients with neurological TB, with *inhA* mutations and in shorter course regimens for MDR-TB.

ADVERSE EFFECTS

Serious drug-induced liver injury occurs in ∼2% of people taking INH monotherapy for chemoprophylaxis at standard doses[21] and has been associated in meta-analyses with NAT2 polymorphisms predicting slow/intermediate acetylator phenotype.[22] The acetyl-hydrazine metabolite has been identified as a candidate toxigen which may generate additional hepatotoxins through the CYP2E1 pathway. Meta-analyses in predominantly Asian populations suggest that polymorphisms in this pathway may be associated with a higher risk of hepatotoxicity.[23] Neurotoxicity of INH is believed to be related to the formation of hydrazones which inhibit enzymes requiring pyridoxal phosphate as a co-factor. The most common manifestation is sensory peripheral neuropathy, which was observed in 2%–12% of patients in early studies and is more common with higher doses, HIV co-infection, and slow acetylator status.[24,25] It is reliably prevented by prophylaxis with small doses of pyridoxine (10–50 mg daily). More serious neurological side effects including encephalopathy may occur in overdose and may be counteracted by much higher doses of pyridoxine. In addition,

INH is structurally related to iproniazid, one of the first mono-amine oxidase inhibitors and can rarely be associated with mood disturbance. INH is also a rare cause of drug-induced systemic lupus erythematosus and of sideroblastic anemia.

DRUG INTERACTIONS

INH is a weak or moderate inhibitor of some CYP isoforms *in vitro* (CYP1A2, CYP2A6, CYP3A4, and CYP2C19)[26] though few confirmed clinically relevant DDIs consistent with these findings have been reported. CYP2B6 slow metabolizers may have clinically important rises in efavirenz plasma concentrations due to INH inhibition of CYP2A6, which is a key accessory metabolic route for these individuals.[27] Drugs that are substrates for CYP3A4 or CYP2C19 including anticonvulsants, coumarins, citalopram, diazepam, and theophylline may have reduced clearance and higher-plasma concentrations. There may also be potential for enhanced hepatotoxicity of paracetamol through undefined mechanisms.

SPECIAL POPULATIONS

INH is not teratogenic but has been associated with embryocidal effects in animal studies and there are no high-quality human data. However, these risks are balanced by long clinical experience with the drug and in practice INH is routinely prescribed for pregnant women with active TB, though delaying chemoprophylaxis is an option in latent tuberculosis infection (LTBI). The relative infant dose during breastfeeding is approximately 1%, though pyridoxine supplementation for the infant is recommended.[28] PK studies in children have resulted in World Health Organization (WHO) recommending that children receive a higher dose of INH (10 mg/kg) to maintain plasma concentrations comparable to adults.[29] In chronic renal failure, changes in dosing are not usually recommended but the half-life may be very variable, possibly due to changes in N-acetylation capacity rather than renal function.[30] Less than 10% of the drug is removed by hemodialysis[31] but INH is usually dosed after a dialysis session. INH should be used with caution and frequent monitoring in patients with liver disease.

RIFAMPICIN

STRUCTURE AND ACTIVITY

Rifampicin (RIF) is a semi-synthetic derivative of Rifamycin SV, a natural product of *Amycolatopsis mediterranei*. It is a moderately lipid-soluble and zwitterionic compound (log P 3.719, pKa 1.7/7.9, MW 822.94). RIF binds to the beta subunit of the mycobacterial DNA-dependent RNA polymerase enzyme, efficiently inhibiting transcription.[32] *In vitro* MIC_{99} for wild-type strains ranges from 0.03 to 0.5 μg/mL.[3] The spontaneous rate of mutation conferring resistance is approximately 1 in 10^{10}.[4] Resistance is conferred by mutations clustered in an 81-bp region of the *rpoB* gene.[5]

PHARMACOKINETICS/ADME

RIF has approximately 70% oral bioavailability and absorption is modestly affected by food which may reduce AUC by up to 6%, but not by antacids.[33] The volume of distribution is typically 0.5 L/kg and protein binding is 80%.[7] At steady state, the $t_{1/2}$ of RIF is 2 hours, plasma C_{max} is approximately 6 μg/mL, and AUC 39 μg/mL $\times$ hour.[34] RIF is a substrate for the hepatic organic anion transporter SLCO1B1 but there are conflicting reports on the clinical significance of polymorphisms in this gene on bioavailability.[35,36] RIF is metabolized by hepatic esterases, possibly arylacetamide deacetylase(AADAC), to the primary metabolites 25-O-desacetyl-rifampicin and 3-formyl-rifampicin.[37] These and many other metabolic pathways including multiple CYP isoforms (CYP3A4) are induced by activation by RIF of several orphan nuclear receptors.[38] Induction appears to be maximal at a dose of approximately 450 mg and 90% complete after 2 weeks of dosing with AUC decreasing by 45% at steady state at doses of 10 mg/kg daily.[39] Non-linear increases in AUC are observed at doses up to 40 mg/kg.[40] RIF and its metabolites are excreted in the bile and may undergo enterohepatic recirculation with only approximately 20% of each dose excreted unchanged in the urine.

RIF concentrations are lower than plasma in epithelial lining fluid (0.2$\times$) but RIF accumulates modestly in alveolar macrophages (1.2$\times$).[41] Penetration into pulmonary lesions is initially only 0.4$\times$ plasma but accumulates with repeated dosing to greater than 9$\times$ in caseum which may explain its unique sterilizing activity.[13] Concentrations in CSF at doses of 10 mg/kg are very low, typically failing to exceed wild-type MICs.[14,15]

PHARMACODYNAMICS/EFFICACY

In EBA studies, activity appears to increase linearly with no maximum effect identified up to doses of 50 mg/kg[42] and doses of up to 35 mg/kg result in more rapid culture conversion.[43] RIF has been identified in meta-analyses of Phase III trials as a key determinant of stable cure, particularly when used throughout the regimen and is largely responsible for the shorter duration of modern regimens.[44]

DOSING

RIF is dosed orally according to weight bands with 600 mg for patients above 50 kg and 450 mg for those below, without food.

The same dose sizes are usually given for intermittent therapy. Higher doses of up to 35 mg/kg have been explored in clinical trials in pulmonary and neurological TB but are not routinely recommended.[43]

ADVERSE EFFECTS

Hepatotoxicity is not common with RIF monotherapy[45] and does not appear to be dose-dependent[46] though transient rises in bilirubin and/or transaminases due to hepatic adaptation may occur in the first 2 weeks of treatment.[47] RIF may be the most common cause of cutaneous hypersensitivity among first-line drugs.[48] Serious hypersensitivity reactions associated with generation of anti-rifamycin antibodies[49] have usually been observed during intermittent dosing and appear to be related to the dosing interval rather than the dose size, generating systemic inflammatory responses resulting in a non-specific flu-like syndrome or rarely respiratory distress.[50] Similar to other rifamycins, hematological toxicities may occur including hemolytic anemia, leukopenia, and severe thrombocytopenia, the last of which mandates permanent discontinuation of the drug.

DRUG–DRUG INTERACTIONS

RIF is a strong inducer of multiple CYP isoforms including CYP3A4, CYP2A6, CYP2B6, CYP2C9, and CYP2C19 but not CYP2D6 in vitro.[51] Induction of metabolism due to RIF therefore results in numerous DDIs because the majority of prescription drugs are metabolized by one or more of these isoforms. Of particular note, efficacy of oral and injectable contraception is impaired and plasma concentrations of azole antifungals, corticosteroids, immunosuppressants such as cyclosporin and tacrolimus, and opiates will be reduced which may impact their efficacy. In HIV-positive people, doses of non-nucleoside reverse transcriptase and integrase-inhibitors may require adjustment whereas most protease inhibitors, boosted or unboosted by ritonavir, are incompatible with RIF therapy.[52,53] Increased doses of PIs have also been associated with unexpectedly high rates of drug-induced liver injury in healthy volunteers, though double doses of lopinavir/ritonavir achieve acceptable plasma concentrations and appear safe in TB patients.[54]

SPECIAL POPULATIONS

RIF is teratogenic in animal models at high doses and there is little reliable human data. In practice however the benefits of RIF in treatment of pregnant patients are usually considered to outweigh these risks. RIF is excreted in breast milk but the relative infant dose has not been defined. RIF treatment may be associated with neonatal hemorrhage due to hypovitaminosis K. The pediatric dose of RIF has recently been adjusted by the WHO to 15 mg/kg to ensure comparable plasma concentrations with adults.[29] No dose adjustments are recommended in renal failure at doses up to 600 mg but saturation of hepatic metabolic pathways at higher doses may lead to accumulation and empirical adjustments may be required. Only 4% of parent drug is dialyzed but RIF is generally dosed after hemodialysis.[31] Caution is necessary when prescribing in those with hepatic disease which may disturb metabolic processing and biliary secretion of the drug.

PYRAZINAMIDE

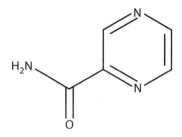

STRUCTURE AND ACTIVITY

Pyrazinamide (PZA) is a synthetic nicotinamide analog which is a pro-drug activated by human and mycobacterial amidases to form pyrazinoic acid (POA). It is a highly water-soluble weak acid (log P −1.88, pKa 0.5, MW 123.11). The mechanism of action remains disputed but it appears that accumulation of protonated POA due to defective efflux mechanisms specific to *Mycobacterium tuberculosis* damages many important cellular processes including fatty acid synthesis, *trans*-translation, and energy metabolism.[55] In vitro MIC_{99}s for wild-type strains range from ≤ 8 to 64 µg/mL.[56] The spontaneous rate of mutations conferring resistance is approximately 1 in 10^5.[57] Resistance is associated with mutations in the *pncA* gene and less commonly in the *rpsA* gene encoding the ribosomal S1 protein.[5]

PHARMACOKINETICS/ADME

Oral bioavailability of PZA in humans has not been determined but it is well-absorbed and not affected by food or antacids.[58] The volume of distribution is 0.7 L/kg and protein binding is 40%.[7] PZA is metabolized by hepatic microsomal deamidase to POA and subsequently to 5-hydroxy-pyrazinoic acid by xanthine oxidase.[59] Only 3% of parent drug is excreted unchanged in the urine. PZA $t_{1/2}$ is 6–7 hours, plasma C_{max} is approximately 35–52 µg/mL, and AUC is 288–386 µg/mL × hour.[10,11] PZA accumulates strongly in epithelial lining fluid (20×) but not in alveolar macrophages (0.8×)[60] whereas penetration into pulmonary lesions of PZA is approximately 0.7×plasma concentrations.[13,61] In animal models, relative penetration of POA into lesions appears 2–3-fold higher than that of PZA.[62] Concentrations in CSF are similar to those in plasma.[14,15]

PHARMACODYNAMICS/EFFICACY

The EBA of PZA over the first 14 days of treatment is 0.036 $\log_{10}$ CFU/mL/day.[63] PZA shortened treatment for DS-TB where its maximum impact appeared to occur within the first 2 months[64] whereas in MDR-TB resistance to PZA is associated with worse outcomes.[65]

DOSING

25 mg/kg once daily or 50–70 mg/kg three times per week. Higher daily doses of 35 mg/kg were also used safely in historical studies.

ADVERSE EFFECTS

In early studies of PZA monotherapy with doses of 50 mg/kg or greater, hepatotoxicity occurred in approximately 6% of patients and available data suggest similar rates at lower doses during combination therapy.[66] However, 2RZ regimens for LTBI with PZA given intermittently at doses of up to 50 mg/kg were associated with discontinuation rates due to drug-induced liver injury of more than 8%, leading to the removal of the regimen from guidelines.[67] Though it can be difficult to judge which individual drug is culpable in combination regimens, current guidelines do not recommend reintroducing PZA after a severe episode of DILI. POA is a high-affinity substrate of the renal organic anion transporter URAT1 (SLC22A12) which stimulates reabsorption of uric acid from the proximal tubule.[68] Increased plasma uric acid concentrations may be associated with arthralgia and pruritis which appears to be dose-related[66] but very rarely results in clinical gout. PZA may also be associated with significant gastrointestinal intolerance.

DRUG INTERACTIONS

PZA is not expected to cause clinically significant drug interactions but should be used with caution with other potentially hepatotoxic drugs and drugs acting on uric acid metabolism.

SPECIAL POPULATIONS

No relevant animal toxicology data or adequate studies of PZA in pregnancy have been conducted but the drug is routinely prescribed for pregnant women with active TB. PZA is excreted in breast milk with an estimated relative infant dose of approximately 1%.[69] Dosing of PZA in children is identical to adults. In chronic kidney disease (CKD) Stage 4, PZA should be dosed thrice weekly to avoid accumulation of POA and uric acid.[70] PZA is significantly removed by hemodialysis (45%)[31,71] and should be dosed after hemodialysis sessions.[72] PZA should be used with caution and enhanced liver enzyme monitoring in patients with liver disease.

ETHAMBUTOL

STRUCTURE AND ACTIVITY

Ethambutol (ETH) is a water-soluble weak acid (log P −0.14, pKa 6.35/9.35, MW 204.31). The D-isomer is an inhibitor of mycobacterial cell wall arabinotransylferases leading to depletion of arabinogalactan and lipoarabinomannan. *In vitro* MIC_{99} for wild-type strains ranges from 0.5 to 4 µg/mL.[3] The spontaneous rate of mutations conferring resistance is 1 in 10^7.[4] Resistance is most commonly associated with mutations in the *embB* gene which codes for the major arabinosyltransferase enzyme and also *embR* and *ubiA* which modulate the activity of the arabinosyltransferase pathway.[5]

PHARMACOKINETICS/ADME

Oral bioavailability is approximately 80% with minimal effect of food or antacids, reducing AUC by 4% and 10%, respectively.[73] The volume of distribution is 0.5–7/kg and protein binding is 12%.[74] ETH undergoes hepatic metabolism to 2,2′-ethylene-diamino-dibutyric acid but 70% is excreted unchanged in the urine and elimination is related to renal function.[75,76] ETH $t_{1/2}$ is 2–3 hours, plasma C_{max} ranges from 2 to 6 µg/mL, and AUC from 20 to 40 µg/mL × hour. ETH does not accumulate in epithelial lining fluid but concentrates 26× in alveolar macrophages.[77] ETH is also strongly concentrated in pulmonary lesions (∼9–12×).[78] Concentrations in CSF are typically 50% or less than those in plasma and frequently below the wild-type MIC.[14]

PHARMACODYNAMICS/EFFICACY

The EBA_{0-2} of ETH is 0.25 log_{10} CFU/mL/day and 0.177 log_{10} CFU/mL/day over the first 14 days of treatment.[79] ETH was used as a companion drug for INH and in retreatment regimens for INH-resistant disease until the mid-1970s. Its addition to the current first-line regimen is intended to prevent emergence of resistance. However, evidence of its independent efficacy is weak and its contribution to outcomes has not been apparent in meta-analyses in MDR-TB.

DOSING

ETH is dosed at 15–25 mg/kg daily or 50 mg/kg thrice weekly.

ADVERSE EFFECTS

The most serious toxicity of ETH is optic neuritis, which occurs in 0.7%–1.2% of adult patients[80,81] and is dose-related.[82] Visual loss is permanent in 50% of patients. Screening of acuity and color vision prior to treatment is therefore essential and the drug should be discontinued as soon as this complication is suspected. ETH may also cause disturbance of liver enzymes, pruritis, arthralgia, gastrointestinal disturbance, headache, and confusion.

DRUG INTERACTIONS

ETH is not expected to cause clinically significant drug interactions. Absorption of ETH may be impacted by antacids and should be avoided for at least 2 hours after dosing.

SPECIAL POPULATIONS

ETH is teratogenic in animals at high doses and there are case reports of ophthalmic abnormalities in neonates. In practice, the drug is often prescribed for short periods in pregnant women pending confirmation of INH sensitivity. ETH is excreted in breast milk with a relative infant dose of about 5%.[83] PK studies suggest that plasma concentrations in children are significantly lower than those in adults but the same mg/kg dose as for adults is usually recommended. The half-life of ETH is prolonged in renal failure[84] and ETH is minimally removed by dialysis (~1%).[31] Three times weekly dosing post-dialysis is recommended with therapeutic drug monitoring to ensure 24-hour trough concentrations are less than 1 µg/mL.[72] Administration during peritoneal dialysis is not recommended. There are no changes in dosing or specific cautions for patients with liver disease.

RIFABUTIN

STRUCTURE AND ACTIVITY

Rifabutin (RBT) is a highly lipid soluble zwitterion (log P 4.8, pKa 7.93/8.62, MW 847.005) which is a synthetic spiropiperidyl derivative of RIF. Similar to RIF, it is an inhibitor of mycobacterial DNA-dependent RNA-polymerase. In vitro MIC_{99}s range from 0.008 to 0.064 µg/mL.[85] Typical mutations in the *rpoB* gene associated with RIF resistance such as S531L are also associated with RBT resistance, whereas even unusual mutations such as A516V clearly raise the MIC outside the wild-type range and close to the plasma C_{max} of RBT, suggesting that such strains are not likely to be more susceptible to RBT compared to RIF.[86]

PHARMACOKINETICS/ADME

Oral bioavailability of RBT is only 20% but AUC is not significantly affected by food (<5%).[87] The volume of distribution is much higher than RIF at 8 L/kg with a lower protein binding of 71%.[88] RBT metabolism is complex: the primary metabolite is 25-O-desacetyl-RBT but there are 20 others including several hydroxylated metabolites (30-, 31-, and 32-OH).[89] Only 5%–10% of a dose is excreted unchanged in the urine. RBT $t_{1/2}$ is 45 hours, plasma C_{max} is 0.3 µg/mL, and AUC 6.1 µg/mL × hour at a dose of 300 mg once daily.[90] No information is available concerning ELF, alveolar macrophage, or lesion penetration.

PHARMACODYNAMICS/EFFICACY

RBT at 300 mg daily showed minimal EBA_{0-2} (0.014 and 0.041 log_{10} CFU/mL/day) in two separate studies.[91,92] However, in Phase III clinical trials, RBT achieved similar rates of stable cure to RIF when substituted into first-line regimens.[93]

DOSING

RBT is dosed at 5 mg/kg once daily up to 300 mg daily, though doses may be adjusted upward when therapeutic drug monitoring is used.

ADVERSE EFFECTS

Similar to RIF, RBT may cause drug-induced liver injury. RBT may also be associated with anterior uveitis, though this side-effect was generally observed at doses of 600–1,200 mg daily used to treat *Mycobacterium avium* infection in HIV-positive individuals in combination with clarithromycin which inhibits RBT metabolism.[94] RBT-associated uveitis usually resolves completely within a few weeks of discontinuation of the drug. At doses of 300 mg or below, reports of uveitis have been uncommon in TB patients.[93] Arthralgia, skin discoloration, and leukopenia have also been reported.

DRUG INTERACTIONS

RBT is a less potent inducer of CYP isoforms compared to RIF[95] and though still prone to the same interactions as RIF, it is often recommended for use with drugs for which RIF would result in unmanageable interactions, particularly HIV protease inhibitors.[96] However, unpredictable bidirectional effects may occur especially when boosted PIs are used, resulting in higher concentrations of RBT and/or the 25-O-desacetyl metabolite.[97] A reduction of the dose of RBT to 150 mg has been suggested[90] and therapeutic drug monitoring is often recommended.

SPECIAL POPULATIONS

RBT is not teratogenic in animal studies but there are no adequate human data on use in pregnancy. No data are available on excretion in breast milk. Doses of 5–10 mg/kg are recommended for children though no PK data are available. The dose of RBT should be reduced by 50% in CKD4 (CrCl <30 mL/min) and it should be used with caution in advanced liver disease.

RIFAPENTINE

STRUCTURE AND ACTIVITY

Rifapentine (RPT) is a highly lipid soluble zwitterionic compound (log P 5.29, pKa 7.01/7.98, MW 877.031). It is a synthetic cyclopentyl derivative of RIF. Similar to RIF, it is an inhibitor of DNA-dependent RNA-polymerase. *In vitro* wild-type MIC_{90}s are lower than those for RIF, ranging from 0.06 to 0.5 μg/mL.[98] The rate of spontaneous mutations resulting in resistance has not been described but is likely to be similar to RIF with a similar distribution of mutations in the *rpoB* gene.

PHARMACOKINETICS/ADME

Oral bioavailability of RPT is 70% and there is an important effect of food, with fat content influencing absorption and resulting in an increase in AUC of 30%–80%.[99] The volume of distribution is 0.9 L/kg and plasma protein binding is 98%–99%.[100] RPT is primarily metabolized to 25-desacetyl-RPT, which is microbiologically active, and subsequently 3-formyl and 3-formyl 25-desacetyl metabolites are formed non-enzymatically in the gut with only 1% excreted unchanged in the urine.[101] The $t_{1/2}$ of RPT is 13 hours, C_{max} is 15 μg/mL, and AUC is 320 μg/mL × hour at a dose of 10 mg/kg. Concentrations in ELF and AM are 0.1–0.2× and 0.2–0.4×, respectively.[102] Though no data on lesion penetration are yet available, unbound concentrations of RPT in *ex vivo* caseum are as low as in plasma.[103]

PHARMACODYNAMICS/EFFICACY

Initial licensing of RPT focused on its use once weekly in the continuation phase of treatment but in recent years daily dosing has been proposed as a route to shortening of first-line therapy. In mouse models, RPT has been associated with a significant shortening of the duration of effective treatment.[104] Human EBA studies did not support the improved activity over RIF that was predicted, possibly due to the high protein binding and lack of penetration of caseous lesions.[105] A Phase II trial of RPT as a replacement for RIF in

the first-line regimen at a dose of 10 mg/kg suggested no benefit in terms of efficacy.[106] Doses of 20 mg/kg however did appear to result in superior culture conversion,[107] and Phase III trials using this dose to shorten the first-line regimen to 4 months will report in 2020.

DOSING

The currently licensed dose of RPT for treatment of active TB is 600 mg twice weekly in the intensive phase of treatment and 600 mg once weekly in the continuation phase. For treatment of LTBI, it is administered once weekly according to weight bands up to a maximum dose of 900 mg.

ADVERSE EFFECTS

Similar to RIF, RPT may be associated with drug-induced liver injury and with severe rifamycin hypersensitivity syndromes. Cytopenias and hypoglycemia have also been reported in 5%–10% of recipients.

DRUG INTERACTIONS

In vitro studies agree that RPT is a less potent inducer of CYP3A4 and ABCB1 then RIF[95] but a clinical study suggested that AUC of CYP3A4 substrates may be reduced at least as much as RIF.[108] For this reason, any CYP-mediated interaction relevant to RIF should be assumed applicable to RPT until further data emerge.

SPECIAL POPULATIONS

RPT is associated with embryopathy in animal models and limited safety data are available from human studies. There are no data on excretion in breast milk. In a recent clinical trial, children were dosed safely at 20–30 mg/kg once weekly for treatment of LTBI.[109] RPT PK have not been studied in chronic renal failure or on dialysis and no dosing adjustments for currently recommended intermittent doses have been suggested. However, for daily dosing, accumulation of the drug or its metabolites is possible in advanced renal disease. Though AUC of RPT has been reported as 19%–25% higher in the presence of liver disease, no dosage adjustment has been proposed in such patients.[110]

MOXIFLOXACIN

STRUCTURE AND ACTIVITY

Moxifloxacin (MFX) is a moderately water-soluble weak acid (log P 0.01, pKa 5.69–9.42, MW 401.43). It is a synthetic fourth-generation fluoroquinolone with an 8-methoxy substitution. Fluoroquinolones inhibit the enzymes DNA gyrase and Topoisomerase IV (though the latter is lacking in *M. tuberculosis*), which are responsible for supercoiling of DNA, resulting in disruption of packing of the bacterial chromosome.[5] *In vitro* MIC_{99}s for wild-type organisms range from 0.03 to 0.5 μg/mL.[111] Spontaneous mutation frequency (determined in *Mycobacterium fortuitum*) is 4×10^{-9} [57] with mutations in both the *gyrA* (particularly codons 90 and 94) and less commonly *gyrB* genes conferring resistance.[5]

PHARMACOKINETICS/ADME

Oral bioavailability of MFX is greater than 90%[112] and is not significantly affected by food.[113] The volume of distribution is 3 L/kg with protein binding of 48%.[114] MFX does not interact with the CYP system but is a substrate of ABCB1. The major route of elimination is N-sulfoconjugation by sulfotransferase 2A1 with a smaller contribution from glucuronidation by UGT 1A1. Approximately 20% of parent drug is eliminated unchanged in the urine.[112] The $t_{1/2}$ of MFX is 7 hours, C_{max} ranges from 2.5 to 4.5 μg/mL, and AUC is 25–40 μg/mL × hour at a dose of 400 mg. MFX concentrates in epithelial lining fluid (1.5–4×) and in alveolar macrophages (9–16×).[115,116] It is also concentrated in pulmonary lesions as measured by microdialysis (3.2×)[117] and matrix-assisted laser desorption/ionization-time-of-flight (MALDI-ToF) imaging (2–3×).[13] CSF penetration was 71%–82% in a small series.[118]

PHARMACODYNAMICS/EFFICACY

MFX at a dose of 400 mg daily has a moderate EBA_{0-2} of 0.33 log_{10} CFU/mL/day[119] and modestly accelerated culture conversion in several Phase IIB studies in DS-TB.[120] However, it was not able to shorten first-line treatment to 4 months in two Phase III trials.[121,122] In MDR-TB, meta-analyses based on individual patient data support the key role of fluoroquinolones in determining outcome.[123,124]

DOSING

The recommended dose of MFX is 400 mg once daily, though higher doses of up to 800 mg have been used in MDR-TB clinical trials.

ADVERSE EFFECTS

MFX prolongs the QT_c interval by 6.4–14.9 mS at C_{max} after a dose of 400 mg[125] and should be used with caution in conjunction with other QT_c-prolonging agents and in patients with proarrhythmic conditions. Similar to other fluoroquinolones, MFX may also be associated with psychiatric disturbances, a lower seizure threshold in epilepsy and tendinopathy. Raised transaminases and drug-induced liver injury have also been described.

DRUG INTERACTIONS

The potential for pathway-mediated drug interactions with MFX is considered low, though two studies have shown a reduction of MFX AUC by 27%–32% when administered with RIF possibly mediated by enhancement of the sulfoconjugation pathway.[126,127] However, use with anti-arrhythmics and other drugs impacting QT_c is usually contraindicated due to additive prolongation, and attention should also be paid to drugs affecting potassium balance. Co-administration with compounds containing di/trivalent cations should also be avoided.

SPECIAL POPULATIONS

Fluoroquinolones have been associated with cartilage defects in animal models though published human data for short-term exposures during early pregnancy are reassuring.[128] However, experience with MFX and with longer exposure is relatively limited.[129] Low concentrations of MFX are present in breast milk. A dose of 5 mg/kg has been suggested for children. Renal failure impacts only on clearance of the minority glucoronidated metabolite and no dosing changes are recommended.[130] MFX is removed by hemodialysis (~30%) and it should therefore be dosed after dialysis.[131] PK are not significantly altered even in patients with severe hepatic impairment, who do not need dose adjustments.[132]

LEVOFLOXACIN

STRUCTURE AND ACTIVITY

Levofloxacin (LFX) is a poorly water-soluble weak acid (log P −0.02, pKa 5.45–6.2) with a MW of 361.37. It is a synthetic second-generation fluoroquinolone with a third morpholine ring and is the (−)-*S* optical isomer of ofloxacin, which is a racemic mixture. Similar to MFX, it inhibits DNA gyrase with wild-type MIC_{99}s ranging from 0.125 to 0.5 μg/mL.[111] Spontaneous mutation frequency (determined in *M. fortuitum*) is 4×10^{-9} [57] with mutations in both *gyrA* and *gyrB* conferring resistance.[5]

PHARMACOKINETICS AND METABOLISM

Oral bioavailability of LFX is 99%–100% with minimal food effect (AUC reduced <10%).[133] The volume of distribution is approximately 1.5 L/kg and protein binding is 24%–38%. In total, 87% of parent drug is excreted unchanged in the urine but two metabolites, desmethyl-levofloxacin and levofloxacin N-oxide have been identified.[134] The $t_{1/2}$ of LFX is 7.4 hours, C_{max} is 15.5 μg/mL, and AUC is 129 μg/mL × hour at a dose of 1,000 mg. LFX concentrations in ELF are approximately 2–3× higher and in alveolar macrophages 4–11× higher compared to plasma.[135,136] LFX accumulates in pulmonary lesions as measured by microdialysis (1.33×)[137] and MALDI-ToF (2×)[138]. CSF penetration has been estimated to be 74%.[139]

PHARMACODYNAMICS/EFFICACY

$EBA_{0–2}$ of LFX at a dose of 1,000 mg was 0.45 $\log_{10}$ CFU/mL/day, slightly higher than that of MFX.[119] LFX at 750 mg daily and MFX produced similar rates of culture conversion at 3 months in a randomized trial of their role in MDR-TB treatment.[140] LFX did not improve culture conversion at 2 months when added to the intensive phase in DS-TB.[141] Individual patient data meta-analyses support the role of fluoroquinolones in treatment of MDR-TB.

DOSING

LFX is dosed at 750–1,000 mg once daily.

ADVERSE EFFECTS

LFX at a dose of 1,000 mg prolongs the QT_c interval by 6 mS at C_{max}.[142] Among the fluoroquinolones, LFX is believed to have the highest risk of tendinopathy and tendon rupture, though this probably does not exceed 0.1% of exposed patients. Patients who are elderly, have renal failure and/or are co-administered corticosteroids are at highest risk.[143] LFX may also be associated with seizures, psychiatric disturbance, peripheral neuropathy, and drug-induced liver injury. It may also cause hemolytic anemia in G6PD deficiency.

DRUG INTERACTIONS

LFX is a weak inhibitor of CYP2C9[144] with potential to affect warfarin metabolism and should be used with caution in conjunction with other drugs that prolong the QT_c interval.

SPECIAL POPULATIONS

LFX, similar to other fluoroquinolones, has been associated with cartilage abnormalities in animal studies. LFX is excreted in breast milk with a relative infant dose of 0.3%.[145] The pediatric dose is 15 mg/kg. The $t_{1/2}$ of LFX increases to 35 hours and the dose size should be reduced when creatinine clearance is less than 20 mL/min but LFX is removed by hemodialysis (20%–30%) and should be dosed after a session.[131] No dosage adjustments are suggested in hepatic impairment.

AMINOGLYCOSIDES

Streptomycin

Kanamycin

Amikacin

STRUCTURE AND ACTIVITY

The aminoglycosides streptomycin (STM), kanamycin (KNM), and amikacin (AMK) are highly water-soluble bases (log P −7.1 to −8.6, pKa 9.75–12.1) with MWs ranging from 581.87 to 585.6. STM and KNM are natural products of *Streptomyces griseus* and *S. kanamyceticus*, respectively, whereas AMK is a semi-synthetic derivative of KNM. Aminoglycosides bind to A site on the 16S RNA of the 30S subunit of the prokaryotic ribosome, though the binding positions of STM and KNM/AMK are distinct.[5] Wild-type MIC_{99}s range from 0.125 to 2 µg/mL for STM, 0.5 to 4 µg/mL for KNM, and 0.25 to 1 µg/mL for AMK.[146] In *M. tuberculosis* resistance is usually mediated by target modification of the ribosomal S12 protein (*rpsL* K43R or K88R associated with STM resistance) or 16S RNA (*rrs* A514C/A908C for STM and A1401G for KAN/AMK resistance). However, mutations in *gidB* may modify the methylation pattern of the 16S RNA leading to low-level resistance to STM whereas the mycobacterial *eis* gene codes for an aminoglycoside acetyltransferase enzyme with highest affinity for KNM which may also affect AMK.[5]

PHARMACOKINETICS/ADME

Aminoglycosides are not orally bioavailable and are administered parenterally. The volume of distribution is approximately 0.2–0.3 L/kg and protein binding is 20% or less. In total, 95% or more of the parent drug is excreted unchanged in the urine and clearance is highly dependent on renal function. The $t_{1/2}$ of all three drugs is 2–3 hours, C_{max} is 35–45 µg/mL for daily dosing at 15 mg/kg and 65–80 at 25 mg/kg.[147,148] Lung penetration of aminoglycosides is generally poor and the ELF/plasma ratio in the only existing study of intrapulmonary PK of AMK was 7%–9%.[149] No information on lesional concentrations is available. Studies of STM suggest the CSF penetration of 7%–21% of plasma concentrations.[150]

PHARMACODYNAMICS/EFFICACY

STM and AMK have weak EBA by comparison with many other agents (0.043 and 0.052 $\log_{10}$ CFU/mL/day, respectively)[151,152] but the clinical efficacy of aminoglycosides in both DS and MDR-TB is supported by meta-analyses of clinical trials and observational data showing their impact on long-term outcomes.

DOSING

A total dose of 15 mg/kg intramuscularly or intravenously is recommended for daily dosing which should not exceed 1 g for STR and 1.5 g for KNM and AMK. A dose of 25 mg/kg is recommended for intermittent dosing.

ADVERSE EFFECTS

Aminoglycosides are associated with nephrotoxicity and ototoxicity which is related to the duration of dosing but not to dose size or interval.[153] High tone hearing loss is common in treatment of MDR-TB[154,155] and is permanent in about two-thirds of cases. A recent systematic review suggested that co-administration of N-acetylcysteine may reduce the risk of ototoxicity.[156] Nephrotoxicity is less common and usually reversible. Hypokalemia and hypomagnesemia due to tubular dysfunction may occur independently of changes in GFR.[157] Therapeutic drug monitoring is helpful where available.[158] Neuromuscular blockade is a rarer side effect, most marked in patients undergoing anesthesia or with myasthenia gravis.

DRUG INTERACTIONS

Though metabolic interactions are not expected, aminoglycosides should be used with caution in conjunction with other drugs that may affect renal function particularly diuretics, calcineurin inhibitors, vancomycin, and amphotericin B.

SPECIAL POPULATIONS

Aminoglycosides have been associated with fetal ototoxicity in human studies. They are excreted in breast milk with a relative infant dose of 0.5% but due to minimal oral bioavailability are considered unlikely to harm the infant.[159] A daily dose of 15–20 mg/kg is recommended for children. The dose of aminoglycosides must be reduced when renal function is altered either by increasing the dosing interval or reducing the dose according to established algorithms. Aminoglycosides are removed by hemodialysis (20+%) and are usually dosed after dialysis.[160,161] No dose modifications are suggested in advanced liver disease though they should be used with caution in this situation.

CAPREOMYCIN

STRUCTURE AND ACTIVITY

Capreomycin (CPR) is a highly water-soluble base ($-\log$ P -11, pKa 10.3–10.62, MW 766.78). It is a macrocyclic polypeptide natural product derived from *Streptomyces capreolus*. CPR binds to a unique site on the 16S RNA and appears to block initiation rather than misreading during translation. Wild-type MIC_{99}s range from 1 to 4 μg/mL[146] and CPR has greater activity against non-replicating organisms *in vitro* than the aminoglycosides.[162] Resistance is mediated by mutations in *rrs* (commonly A1401G) and by mutations in *tlyA*, a ribosomal methyltransferase analogous to *eis*.[5] Hence, cross-resistance with KNM/AMK is common but not with STM.

PHARMACOKINETICS/ADME

CPR is not orally bioavailable and is administered parenterally. No data are available on volume of distribution or protein binding. CPR is excreted unchanged in the urine with no known metabolites. The $t_{1/2}$ is 5.2 hours and C_{max} is 19–44 μg/mL at a dose of 1,000 mg.[163] No data are available for pulmonary, lesion, or CSF penetration.

PHARMACODYNAMICS/EFFICACY

No EBA data are available for CPR. Evidence for the efficacy of CPR rests on historical clinical trials against STR when combined with PAS in new cases or in combination with RIF and ETH for retreatment.[164,165]

DOSING

The recommended dose is 15 mg/kg up to a maximum of 1 g daily or 15–25 mg/kg thrice weekly given intramuscularly.

ADVERSE EFFECTS

Nephro- and oto-toxicity are the most serious side effects of CPR and similar to the aminoglycosides it may also be associated with neuromuscular blockade. Hypokalemia and hypomagnesemia are more common than with the aminoglycosides.[157] Eosinophilia is described on daily dosing and leuko and thromobocytopenia and raised liver enzymes may also occur.

DRUG INTERACTIONS

CPR should be used with caution with drugs known to have synergistic nephro- or oto-toxicity.

SPECIAL POPULATIONS

CPR is teratogenic in animals and human data in pregnancy are limited. There are no data on excretion in breast milk. Children are dosed at 15–30 mg/kg daily up to a maximum of 1 g. The dose size should be reduced at all levels of CKD and therapeutic drug monitoring is recommended. CPR is removed by dialysis and should be dosed after sessions.[166] No dosing adjustment is suggested in liver disease.

*p*ARA-AMINOSALICYLIC ACID

STRUCTURE AND ACTIVITY

para-Aminosalicylic acid (PAS) is a poorly water-soluble weak acid (log P 0.83, pKa 2.19–3.68, MW 153.14). It is a synthetic structural analog of *para*-aminobenzoic acid. PAS is a prodrug activated by the hydropteroate and dihydrofolate synthases and inhibiting dihydrofolate reductase,[167] though it has also been suggested that it may interfere with mycobacterial iron uptake.[168] Wild-type MIC_{99}s range from 0.12 to 4 μg/mL.[169] Resistance is mediated by mutations in the *thyA* locus in about 30% of isolates and *folC* and *ribD in vitro*.[5]

PHARMACOKINETICS/ADME

Absolute bioavailability has not been determined but absorption is improved by food with a higher fat content (50% increase in AUC).[170] The apparent volume of distribution is approximately 1 L/kg and protein binding is 58%–73%.[171] The major metabolites are N-acetyl PAS through the NAT1 pathway and p-aminosalicyluric acid which undergoes glycine conjugation. Both are excreted and secreted into the urine. The NAT1 gene is polymorphic but only one uncommon SNP (*14B) has any important impact on PAS PK.[172] Inhibition of INH acetylation has been observed in patients also taking PAS.[173] The $t_{1/2}$ is 3.9 hours and median C_{max} is approximately 35 μg/mL at a dose of 4 g twice daily.[174] No data are available for pulmonary or lesion distribution but CSF penetration is believed to be less than 50%.[14]

PHARMACODYNAMICS/EFFICACY

PAS at a dose of 15 g once daily had an EBA_{0-2} of 0.26 $\log_{10}$ CFU/mL/day.[79] Randomized trial evidence on the efficacy of PAS in DS-TB is sparse for historical reasons and it has not subsequently been identified in IPD meta-analyses as an independent predictor of outcome in MDR-TB.

DOSING

PAS is dosed at 8–12 g per day in 2–3 divided doses with food.

ADVERSE EFFECTS

Gastrointestinal tolerability is the biggest problem with PAS, despite the introduction of improved formulations and diarrhea with clinically significant malabsorption may occur. PAS also specifically reduces B_{12} uptake, though frank megaloblastic anemia is rare.[175] PAS at high doses has been associated with hypothyroidism and goiter,[176] the risk of which may be exacerbated when used with thioamides. Severe drug-induced liver injury accompanied by signs of systemic hypersensitivity and eosinophilia is also described.

DRUG INTERACTIONS

PAS may reduce acetylation capacity for INH resulting in higher-plasma concentrations when the drugs are used together. Efavirenz co-administration reduces PAS AUC by 30+%.[174] PAS may also affect anticoagulation with vitamin K antagonists.

SPECIAL POPULATIONS

PAS may cause embryopathy in animals and reliable human data are very limited. It is excreted into breast milk with a relative infant dose of 0.01%.[177] The recommended dose in children is 200–300 mg/kg in 2–4 divided doses. No dosage adjustments are suggested in renal failure but PAS is considered relatively contraindicated in severe renal disease due to possible accumulation of the N-acetyl metabolite.[178] Removal of PAS by hemodialysis is only 6%.[179] The drug should also be used with caution in advanced liver disease.

THIOAMIDES

Ethionamide   Prothionamide

STRUCTURE AND ACTIVITY

Ethionamide (ETM) and prothionamide (PTM) are water-insoluble weak acids (log P 1.33/2.22, pKa 5–11.89/7.31, MW 166.24/180.27). ETM is a synthetic structural analog of nicotinamide and PTM is an N-propyl derivative of ETM. Both are prodrugs activated by the mycobacterial mono-oxygenase EthA[180] and target the same enoyl–acyl reductase enzyme InhA as INH, disrupting mycolic acid synthesis.[181] Wild-type MIC_{99}s range from 0.5 to 2 µg/mL for ETM and 0.25 to 1 µg/mL for PTM.[85] High-level resistance is usually mediated by mutations in the *ethA* or *inhA* genes, though *in vitro mshA* mutations also confer resistance.[5]

PHARMACOKINETICS/ADME

Oral bioavailability is believed to be near 100%[182] and is not significantly affected by food (4% change in AUC).[183] The volume of distribution is 3.2 L/kg and protein binding is 10%–30%. Both drugs have a complex metabolic pathway involving sulfoxidation, desulfuration, and deamination followed by methylation, and the sulfoxide metabolites are active. Less than 1% of the drugs are excreted unchanged in the urine. The $t_{1/2}$ of ETH is 1.9 hours and predicted C_{max} is 0.9 µg/mL and AUC 14.4 µg/mL × hour at a dose of 500 mg twice daily.[184] In a recent study of PTH $t_{1/2}$ was 2.7 hours, C_{max} is 2.2 µg/mL and AUC 11 µg/mL × hour at a dose or 250–375 mg twice daily.[185] ETM is concentrated 9.7-fold in epithelial lining fluid though concentrations in alveolar cells are 50% or less of plasma.[102] No information is available on penetration into lesions. CSF concentrations of ETH are approximately 80% of those in plasma.[14] Penetration data are not available for PTM.

PHARMACODYNAMICS/EFFICACY

No EBA data are available for ETH or PTH. Evidence of efficacy is based on randomized trials in new and retreatment patients shortly before the introduction of RIF[186,187] and on evidence of impact on outcomes in individual patient data meta-analyses in MDR-TB.

DOSING

ETH and PTM are dosed at 15–20 mg/kg per day up to a maximum of 1 g. To improve tolerability, the drugs are usually dosed gradually over a period of days. Once daily administration is possible but twice daily dosing is often used because individual doses of greater than 500 mg may not be tolerated.

ADVERSE EFFECTS

Gastrointestinal tolerability of ETH and PTH is poor, though rates of adverse events appear lower with the latter.[188] Central nervous system (CNS) disturbance and peripheral neuropathy are described and may be prevented with pyridoxine prophylaxis. Abnormal thyroid function tests may occur in up to 30% of patients on ETH though the clinical significance of these findings is often unclear and resolves after discontinuation of treatment.[189,190] Gynecomastia may also occur. In diabetics, ETM and PTM have been associated with hypoglycemia.

DRUG INTERACTIONS

Alcohol may increase the risk of psychological/psychiatric problems as may concomitant use of cycloserine.

SPECIAL POPULATIONS

Thioamides are teratogenic in animal studies and few data human data exist. Concentrations in breast milk have not been studied. The recommended dose in children is 10–20 mg/kg per day in 2–3 divided doses. In severe renal impairment (CrCl <30 mL/min) the dose interval should be not more than daily. ETH is not significantly removed by dialysis (2%).[179] Thioamides are contraindicated in severe liver disease.

CYCLOSERINE AND TERIZIDONE

Cycloserine   Terizidone

STRUCTURE AND ACTIVITY

D-Cycloserine (CS) is a water-soluble weak acid (log P −2.4, pKa 4.21–8.36, MW 102.09). Terizidone (TZ) is a condensation product of two CS molecules with terephthalaldehyde, which acts as a pro-drug. CS is a natural product analog of D-alanine originating from *Streptomyces garyphalus*. It is a competitive inhibitor of the enzymes alanine racemase and D-alanine:D-alanine ligase, disrupting peptidoglycan synthesis.[191] Wild-type MIC_{99}s range from 8 to 32 µg/mL.[85] Resistance to CS is uncommon and usually associated with mutations in the *alr* (alanine racemase) locus.[192]

PHARMACOKINETICS/ADME

Oral bioavailability is 65%–90% and absorption is modestly affected by food.[193] The volume of distribution is 0.35 L/kg and protein binding is reported as negligible. A total of 60%–70% of parent drug is excreted unchanged in the urine and metabolites have not been characterized.[194] The $t_{1/2}$ of CS is approximately 13 hours, C_{max} is 20 µg/mL, and AUC 264 µg/mL × hour at a dose of 250 mg.[195] After a dose of 750 mg of TZ, CS median C_{max} was 38 µg/mL and AUC was 319 µg/mL × hour with a $t_{1/2}$ of 14.7 hours.[196] No information is available on pulmonary or lesional concentrations. CSF concentrations are 80%–100% of plasma in meningitis.[14]

PHARMACODYNAMICS/EFFICACY

No EBA studies of CS or TZ are available. Weak evidence for their efficacy derives from combination studies in retreatment from the 1960s.[197,198]

DOSING

The usual starting dose of CS and TZ is 250 mg twice daily, increased after 2 weeks to a maximum of 500 mg twice daily, though once daily dosing is rational for both agents and used in some programs.

ADVERSE EFFECTS

The therapeutic index of CS is low with toxicity associated with a plasma concentration threshold of 30 µg/mL. Neuropsychiatric side-effects are common (~6%) including drowsiness, anxiety, mood disturbance, psychosis, and seizures.[199] Pyridoxine prophylaxis of 50–100 mg is usually suggested and higher doses (200–300 mg) are suggested in counteracting neurotoxicity.[200] Vitamin B_{12} and folate depletion have been reported in patients taking CS which have been associated with megaloblastic or sideroblastic anemia. Rashes due to photosensitivity or hypersensitivity are also described.

DRUG INTERACTIONS

Though potential for metabolic interactions is low, CS should be combined with caution with other medications that may lower seizure threshold, including fluoroquinolones.

SPECIAL POPULATIONS

CS is not teratogenic in animal studies but there is limited experience in pregnancy. It is excreted in breast milk with a relative infant dose of 0.6%.[159] Children are dosed at 10–20 mg/kg in two divided doses. CS is contraindicated in severe renal failure and dosing according to therapeutic drug monitoring is recommended for less severe reductions of GFR. The drug is 56% removed by hemodialysis[179] so should be dosed after sessions. No dose adjustments are suggested in the presence of liver disease.

LINEZOLID

STRUCTURE AND ACTIVITY

Linezolid (LZD) is a water-soluble acid (log P 0.64, pKa −0.66–14.45, MW 337.35). It is a synthetic inhibitor of ribosomal translation which binds to the 23S subunit preventing binding of formyl-methionine tRNA and therefore formation of the initiation complex.[201] Wild-type MIC_{99}s for LZD range from 0.125 to 0.5 μg/mL.[85] Resistance is associated *in vitro* with point mutations in the peptidyl transferase domain of the 23S rRna (*rrs* gene), particularly G2576T and in the gene *rplC* which codes for the L3 protein within the 50S subunit. The latter appears to be more clinically relevant.[202]

PHARMACOKINETICS/ADME

Oral bioavailability is approximately 100% and is not affected by food.[203] The volume of distribution is 0.6 L/kg and protein binding is 31%. Biotransformation by non-enzymatic oxidation of the morpholine ring results in hydroxyethyl and aminoethoxyacetic acid metabolites which are conjugated with glycine and eliminated in the urine. A total of 30% of parent drug is eliminated unchanged in the urine.[204] The $t_{1/2}$ of LZD is 2.9 hours, C_{max} is 10.3 μg/mL, and AUC 66.8 μg/mL × hour at a dose of 600 mg once daily.[205] LZD is concentrated in epithelial lining fluid (4.1–8.4×) but not in alveolar cells (0.14–0.70×).[206,207] Concentrations in lesions determined by *ex vivo* dialysis were 49% of serum.[208] CSF exposure is 57% of plasma.[209]

PHARMACODYNAMICS/EFFICACY

$EBA_{0–2}$ of LZD was 0.18 and 0.26 $\log_{10}$ CFU/mL/day at a dose of 600 mg once and twice daily, respectively.[210] LZD monotherapy achieved 87% culture conversion at 6 months in a small trial of patients with XDR-TB.[211]

DOSING

LZD is usually dosed at 600 mg once daily in TB though higher doses have been used in clinical trials. Twice daily dosing at 300 mg may offer similar efficacy with fewer adverse effects[212] but few comparative clinical data exist.

ADVERSE EFFECTS

LZD inhibits protein synthesis in human mitochondria resulting in clinically significant toxicities including myelosuppression, lactic acidosis, and peripheral and optic neuropathy. With prolonged dosing in MDR-TB more than half of patients will ultimately develop peripheral and/or optic neuropathy and 8% discontinue the drug, despite dose reduction.[211] Trough concentrations of LZD correlate with mitochondrial dysfunction and risk of toxicity and therapeutic drug monitoring may be useful.[213] Sideroblastic anemia has also been described. Nausea and diarrhea are also commonly reported.

DRUG INTERACTIONS

LZD is a weak inhibitor of monoamine oxidase and should usually not be used with MAOIs, selective serotonin reuptake inhibitors, or triptans due to reports of serotonergic syndrome. Tyramine-rich foods (cheese and pickled fish) should also be avoided. LZD does not interact with CYPs *in vitro*. Unexpectedly, a recent study showed that LZD plasma exposure is increased by 44% during co-administration of clarithromycin, possibly through interactions with ABCB1[214] whereas RIF co-administration also reduces LZD AUC 32%.

SPECIAL POPULATIONS

LZD is embryopathic but not teratogenic in animal studies and there are no adequate human data. LZD is excreted in breast milk with a relative infant dose of 16%.[215] Though not recommended by the manufacturer, children have been dosed at 10 mg/kg thrice daily. No dosage adjustment is suggested in mild-moderate renal disease but the drug should be used with caution in severe renal failure (CrCl <30 mL/min) due to accumulation of the major metabolites. LZD and its metabolites are partially removed by hemodialysis (30%–50%).[216] No adjustments are specified for patients with liver disease.

CLOFAZIMINE

STRUCTURE AND ACTIVITY

Clofazimine (CFZ) is a highly water-insoluble cationic amphiphilic compound (log P 7.3, pKa 9.29–16.15, MW 473.40). It is a semi-synthetic riminophenazine derivative of a natural product derived from the lichen *Buella canescens*. The mechanism of action has been postulated to be competitive inhibition of the menaquinone substrate of the NADH:quinone oxidoreductase NDH-2, disrupting electron transport and generating reactive oxygen species.[217] Additional mechanisms have also been suggested including disruption of the membrane potential through inhibition of potassium uptake channels in *M. tuberculosis* and eukaryotic cells, which may also explain the observed anti-inflammatory effects of the drug.[218,219] Wild-type MIC_{99}s to CFZ range from 0.125 to 0.25 μg/mL.[85] The spontaneous rate of mutations associated with resistance *in vitro* is as low as 1 in 10^{26} and these are invariably in the locus *rv0678* which codes for a repressor protein of the membrane transporter MmpS5-MmpL5. However, these mutations have not been observed in clinical isolates to date.[220]

PHARMACOKINETICS/ADME

Oral bioavailability is 45%–62% and is increased 45% by a high-fat meal.[221] The volume of distribution is greater than 12 L/kg suggesting extensive tissue distribution and binding but plasma protein-binding data are not available. Minimal parent drug is excreted unchanged in the urine and the major metabolites are reported to be formed by hydrolytic dehalogenation and deamination, followed by glucoronidation and biliary excretion.[222] After a 200 mg dose, the C_{max} is 0.13–0.37 μg/mL, and AUC 3.6 μg/mL × hour.[221] Though the initial $t_{1/2}$ is 7.8–15.9 hours this reflects distribution, and the terminal elimination $t_{1/2}$ is 70 days. No data are available on concentrations in epithelial lining fluid or alveolar cells but CFZ concentrations in the rim of lesions are 10× higher than in plasma, though similar or lower in caseum.[13]

PHARMACODYNAMICS/EFFICACY

CFZ at a dose of 100 mg (after loading with 300 mg for 3 days) had no appreciable EBA_{0-2}.[63] Though the pooled cure rate of CFZ-containing regimens was 65% in a recent meta-analysis[223] and the drug forms part of the 9-month regimen for MDR-TB,[224] no comparative or controlled clinical data are currently available to support the independent efficacy of CFZ.

DOSING

CFZ is usually dosed at 100 mg daily with food, though 200 mg may be used for short periods in severe disease.

ADVERSE EFFECTS

CFZ crystals are deposited throughout body tissues during treatment and may be associated with side-effects. The major clinical problem is dose-related tissue, epithelial, and body fluid discoloration which may be associated with dry skin, photosensitivity, and corneal deposits. The discoloration is reversible but only after 6 months or more of treatment. Gastrointestinal discomfort is also common and gastrointestinal obstruction and bleeding have been reported. However, the estimated discontinuation rate of CFZ in a recent meta-analysis was only 0.1%.[225] CFZ may also significantly prolong the QT_c interval, with a mean change of 40 mS from baseline in a recent series.[226]

DRUG INTERACTIONS

Very limited clinical data exist on interactions with CFZ but major metabolic interactions are not expected. CFZ should be used with caution with other medications that prolong the QT_c interval.

SPECIAL POPULATIONS

CFZ is not teratogenic but has been associated with embryopathy and fetal loss in animal models. There is no reliable human data in pregnancy. The drug is excreted in breast milk with a relative infant dose of 2%.[227] The drug crosses the placenta and skin discoloration has been reported in offspring of mothers taking the drug.

Children have been dosed at 1 mg/kg. No dosage modifications are suggested in renal failure or liver disease and the drug is not removed by hemodialysis.[179]

BEDAQUILINE

STRUCTURE AND ACTIVITY

Bedaquiline (BDQ) is a highly water-insoluble weak base (log P 7.3, pKa 8.91–13.61, MW 555.505). It is a synthetic diarylquinoline that inhibits the mycobacterial ATP synthase.[228] Wild-type MICs to BDQ range from 0.008 to 0.25 μg/mL.[229] The spontaneous rate of mutations conferring resistance is approximately 1 in 10.[8,57] Mutations in the *atpE* gene selected *in vitro* are clearly associated with high-level resistance whereas SNPs in the gene *rv0678*, a regulator of the MmpL5 efflux pump, are found in 6% of clinical MDR-TB isolates prior to treatment but are inconsistently related to changes in MIC.[230]

PHARMACOKINETICS/ADME

Absolute oral bioavailability has not been determined but is increased two-fold by food.[231] The volume of distribution is greater than 150 L/kg and plasma protein binding is >99%. BDQ is metabolized by CYP3A4, CYP2C8, and 2C19 to N-monodesmethyl and further sequentially demethylated metabolites which are excreted in the feces.[232] Less than 0.001% of the parent compound is excreted unchanged in the urine. Neither metabolite has significant activity. At steady state dosing of 200 mg thrice weekly, the $C_{average}$ is 0.9 μg/mL with a terminal $t_{1/2}$ of 20 weeks.[231,233] No data on intrapulmonary or lesional concentrations are available. A case report suggested that CSF concentrations are undetectable.[234]

PHARMACODYNAMICS/EFFICACY

BDQ exhibits modest EBA over the first 14 days of treatment (0.06–0.11 log_{10} CFU/mL/day).[235,236] Culture conversion at 8 weeks was improved by addition of BDQ to the regimen in a Phase II trial in MDR-TB.[233,237]

DOSING

A loading dose of 400 mg daily is administered for 2 weeks followed by a maintenance dose of 200 mg three times a week with food.

ADVERSE EFFECTS

BDQ at steady state prolongs the QT_c interval by approximately 12 mS[237] but has not been clearly associated with serious dysrhythmias. It may also be associated with gastrointestinal disturbance, arthralgia, headache, and dizziness. Phospholipidosis observed in some preclinical toxicity studies has not been observed in humans to date. The drug currently has a black box warning due to unexplained excess mortality in clinical trials.

DRUG INTERACTIONS

Because it is principally metabolized by CYP3A4, BDQ plasma concentrations may be significantly decreased by inducers of the enzyme (rifamycins, 75% or more for RIF and RPT)[238] and increased by inhibitors (ritonavir, ketoconazole, and clarithromycin).[239] BDQ should be combined with caution and appropriate monitoring with drugs that also prolong the QT_c interval such as MFX and CFZ.

SPECIAL POPULATIONS

No abnormalities have been observed in animal studies with BDQ but there are no relevant human and no data concerning excretion in breast milk. There are no dosing recommendations in children as yet. No dose adjustments are recommended in renal failure or liver disease but BDQ should be used with caution in severe renal or hepatic disease.

DELAMANID

STRUCTURE AND ACTIVITY

Delamanid (DLD) is a highly water-insoluble weak acid (log P 6.14, pKa 5.51, MW 534). It is the *R*-enantiomer of a synthetic nitro-dihydro-imidazo-oxazole derivative which is a prodrug activated by the F_{420} dependent nitroreductases. The mechanism of action remains uncertain but DLD inhibits mycolic acid synthesis and releases reactive oxygen species in mycobacteria.[240] Wild-type MICs range from 0.001 to 0.05 μg/mL.[241] The spontaneous rate of mutation conferring resistance is relatively high at approximately 2 in 10^5 with mutations in any of the F_{420} coenzymes *Rv3547*, *FGD*, *FbiA*, *FbiB*, and *FbiC* associated with *in vitro* resistance.[242]

PHARMACOKINETICS/ADME

Oral bioavailability is estimated to be 25%–47% and is increased three- to four-fold by food. The volume of distribution is 15.5–163.2 L/kg and plasma protein binding is >99.5% to albumin and lipoproteins. The metabolism of DLD is complex. The nitro group of DLD is removed by interactions with albumin and seven other identified metabolites are believed to be subsequently formed by oxidation by CYP3A4 and possibly CYP1A1, CYP2D6, and CYP2E1.[243,244] The C_{max} is 0.41 μg/mL and AUC 7.92 μg/mL × hour with a $t_{1/2}$ of 38 h in MDR-TB patients dosed at 100 mg twice daily.[245] No data are available on intrapulmonary, lesion, or CSF penetration.

PHARMACODYNAMICS/EFFICACY

DLD showed modest EBA over the first 14 days (0.026 log_{10} CFU/mL/day) at a dose of 100 mg twice daily[246] but improved culture conversion at 2 months in MDR-TB patients by 16% compared to placebo.[243] However, evidence of impact on long-term outcomes has been equivocal.

DOSING

DLD is dosed at 100 mg twice daily for 2 months and then 200 mg daily with food.

ADVERSE EFFECTS

DLD prolongs the QT_c interval by 8–12 mS but has not been associated with serious dysrhythmias.[245] Caution should be exercised in patients with hypoalbuminemia. DLD may also be associated with nausea, vomiting, tremor, anxiety, and paraesthesia.

DRUG INTERACTIONS

Co-administration of DLD with RIF leads to a reduction in DLD AUC of 47% whereas ritonavir increases DLD AUC by 25%.[247] These results suggest that DLD will also be impacted by other inducers and inhibitors of CYP3A4. Caution should be used when combining DLD with other drugs that may prolong the QT_c interval.

SPECIAL POPULATIONS

The DLD parent compound did not cause teratogenicity or embryopathy in animals though studies with metabolites resulted in some fetal abnormalities. The drug is likely to be excreted in breast milk and breast feeding is not recommended. No dosing recommendations are available for children as yet. No dosage adjustments are suggested in mild–moderate renal failure but DLD is not recommended for use in severe renal failure and should be avoided in patients with moderate–severe liver impairment.

CLARITHROMYCIN

STRUCTURE AND ACTIVITY

Clarithromycin (CLR, 6-O-methylerythromycin) is a poorly water-soluble weak base (log P 2.69, pKa 8.9, MW 747.95). It is a semi-synthetic derivative of erythromycin, which is a natural product of *Saccharopolyspora erythrea*. Macrolides bind to the 50S subunit of the ribosome, preventing translocation of tRNAs from the A site to the P site by binding in the peptide exit tunnel.[248] Binding of macrolides is affected by the pattern of methylation of 23S rRNA at the target site. Erythromycin ribosome methylase (*erm*) genes code for methylase enzymes that typically target residue A2058 but the *M. tuberculosis* complex has a unique gene *ermMT* (erm37) which also methylates additional adjacent residues, resulting in intrinsic resistance.[249] MICs reported for CLR for *M. tuberculosis* are uniformly >8 μg/mL.[250] Among non-tuberculous mycobacteria, inducible resistance during therapy due to acquisition of *erm* genes has also been described in *M. avium* complex, *Mycobacterium kansasii*, *M. fortuitum*, and *M. chelonae*.[251] The *Mycobacterium abscessus* complex typically exhibits inducible resistance due to the presence of *erm*41 but deletions in the gene confer uniform

susceptibility in *M. massiliense* and rarely in *M. abscessus* sub *abscessus*.[252]

PHARMACOKINETICS/ADME

Absolute bioavailability of CLR is 55% and is not affected by food.[253] The volume of distribution is ~3.5 L/kg and plasma protein binding is 80%. CLR undergoes saturable, extensive first-pass metabolism to the predominant 14-hydroxy metabolite, and also N-demethylation by CYP3A4.[254] Only 18% of parent drug is eliminated in the urine and the majority of excretion is via the biliary route.[255] C_{max} is approximately 2.7 μg/mL, AUC 20 μg/mL × hour, and $t_{1/2}$ 3.6 hours after multiple doses of 500 mg.[256] CLR is concentrated 5× in epithelial lining fluid and more than 90× in alveolar cells, with similar values for the 14-OH metabolite[257] with concentrations in lung tissue 29× and 6× higher than that in plasma, respectively.[258]

PHARMACODYNAMICS/EFFICACY

No studies of EBA have been carried out and observational data in treatment of MDR-TB do not support the efficacy of CLR in *M. tuberculosis*.[250] Recent meta-analyses suggest that CLR is an unreliable agent for treatment of *M. abscessus*[259] but improves culture conversion in treatment of *M. avium* complex.[260]

DOSING

CLR is dosed at 250–500 mg twice daily for most mycobacterial infections though doses of 1,000 mg thrice weekly have been recommended in mild *M. avium* lung disease.[261]

ADVERSE EFFECTS

Similar to other macrolides, the main side effects of CLR are gastrointestinal intolerance, abnormal liver enzymes, and taste disturbance. CLR prolongs the QT_c interval by an average 3 mS but has been associated with torsades de pointes in post-marketing studies, particularly when combined with other QT_c-prolonging drugs.[262]

DRUG INTERACTIONS

CLR is a potent mechanism-based inhibitor of CYP3A4[263] and may cause serious PK interactions with numerous substrates of this enzyme including statins, midazolam, cyclosporin, tacrolimus, carbamazepine, ergot alkaloids, and omeprazole. Because it is also a substrate, plasma concentrations of CLR may also be affected by induction of CYP3A4, for example by rifamycins. CLR should be used with caution with other drugs prolonging the QT interval and in patients with additional risk factors such as electrolyte disturbance.

SPECIAL POPULATIONS

CLR is embryotoxic in several animal species and very limited data are available in humans. CLR is excreted in breast milk with a relative infant dose of 2%.[264] Children are dosed at approximately 8 mg/kg. The dose should be halved in severe renal failure (CrCl <30 mL/min) and CLR is not expected to be removed by hemodialysis. The drug should be used with caution in severe liver disease but no dosage adjustment has been proposed.

THIACETAZONE

STRUCTURE AND ACTIVITY

Thiacetazone (TCZ) is a moderately water-soluble weak acid (log P 1.75, pKa 5.11–5.72, MW 262.293). It is a synthetic thiosemicarbazone. TCZ is a pro-drug, activated similar to ETM by ethA and targets mycolic acid synthesis, principally the FASII β-hydroxyacyl ACP dehydratase, encoded by the *hadABC* operon but also other non-essential mycolic acid-modifying enzymes, including cyclopropane mycolic acid synthases (CmaA2 and PcaA) and the mycolic acid methyltransferases (MMA) (MmaA2 and MmaA4).[265] It is active only against *M. tuberculosis* and *M. kansasii*. Wild-type MIC$_{99}$s range from 0.125 to 2 µg/mL.[85] Spontaneous mutations in *ethA* or *hadABC* conferring resistance occur at a rate of approximately 1 in 10[7].

PHARMACOKINETICS/ADME

Absolute bioavailability of TCZ has not been determined but it is well-absorbed. Metabolism of TCZ has been incompletely studied but the primary route of elimination is believed to be hydroxylation to *para*-aminobenzaldehyde and *para*-acetylaminobenzaldehyde with less than 25% excreted unchanged in the urine.[266] C$_{max}$ is 1.6 µg/mL and t$_{1/2}$ 15 h after a dose of 150 mg once daily.[267] No information is available about intrapulmonary or lesional distribution.

PHARMACODYNAMICS/EFFICACY

EBA$_{0-2}$ of TCZ is weak at 0.067 log$_{10}$ CFU/mL/day.[79] Originally used as a companion drug for INH at durations of 6–18 months

with or without STM, regimens including TCZ even in the continuation phase, were phased out in the 1990s due to inferior efficacy and safety concerns in HIV-positive patients.[268] Observational data on its use in MDR-TB are sparse.

DOSING

TCZ is dosed at 150 mg daily.

ADVERSE EFFECTS

The most serious toxicity of TCZ is its association with severe cutaneous hypersensitivity and Stevens–Johnson syndrome in up to 20% of HIV-co-infected patients.[269] Gastrointestinal intolerance, drug-induced liver injury and blood dyscrasias may also occur.

DRUG INTERACTIONS

Data on interactions with TCZ are scarce but no important contraindications have been described.

SPECIAL POPULATIONS

No data are available on preclinical toxicology or use in pregnancy and it is unknown whether the drug is excreted in breast milk. Children are dosed at approximately 3 mg/kg. No dosing adjustments have been suggested in renal or liver disease and it is not known whether the drug is removed by dialysis.

CARBAPENEMS

Imipenem

Meropenem

STRUCTURE AND ACTIVITY

Imipenem (IMP) and meropenem (MRP) are highly water-soluble weak acids (log P -3.9 and -4.4, pKa 3.2 and 3.47–9.39, MW 299.3 and 383.15). Both are synthetic derivatives of thienamycin, a natural product of *Streptomyces cattleya*. Carbapenems target multiple transpeptidases (penicillin-binding proteins) involved in bacterial cell-wall synthesis including the unique L,D-transpeptidases characteristic of mycobacteria.[270] However, *M. tuberculosis* possesses an extended spectrum class A β-lactamase (BlaC), which must be inactivated for *in vitro* activity of the drugs.[271] Clavulanic acid is the most potent inhibitor of BlaC among licensed β-lactamase inhibitors.[272] MIC_{99}s of meropenem–clavulanate in wild-type MDR and XDR strains range from 0.125 to 2 µg/mL.[273]

PHARMACOKINETICS/ADhME

IMP and MRP are hydrolytically unstable and can only be administered parenterally. They have similar volumes of distribution of approximately 0.2 L/kg.[274] MRP has lower plasma protein binding (2%) compared to IMP (20%). Both drugs are hydrolyzed by renal dehydropeptidase-1 (DHP-1) to a microbiologically active metabolite with approximately 70% of the parent drug excreted unchanged in the urine. IMP has a higher affinity for DHP-1 than MRP and is co-administered with cilastatin, an inhibitor of the enzyme, to prolong the plasma half-life. At a dose of 1,000 mg the C_{max}s of IMP and MRP are 35 and 49 µg/mL and the AUC 96 and 71 µg/mL × hour, respectively. The $t_{1/2}$ of both drugs is about 1 hour.[275] Concentrations of MRP in epithelial lining fluid and alveolar cells are 0.15 and 0.09× plasma, respectively,[276] whereas penetration of ELF for IMP is 0.44×.[277] No data are available on penetration of lesions. Concentrations of IMP and MRP in CSF are 10%–20% of plasma.[278,279]

PHARMACODYNAMICS/EFFICACY

Evidence for the efficacy of carbapenem–clavulanate combinations in TB rests largely on preclinical studies.[280] No comparative or controlled clinical studies have been reported though a meta-analysis of observational studies in MDR-TB observed more favorable response rates with MRP than with IMP.[281]

DOSING

IMP is dosed at 1,000 mg 12 hourly and MRP 1,000 mg 8 hourly intravenously. 125 mg clavulanic acid should be given orally with each dose. Because clavulanate is not currently separately formulated, this is usually given as co-amoxiclav 250/125 mg.

ADVERSE EFFECTS

IMP and MRP may be associated with anaphylaxis and injection site reactions. Both may cause abnormal liver enzymes and drug-induced liver injury. CNS side-effects including seizures may occur in overdose in unrecognized renal failure. MRP may also cause eosinophilia and thrombocythemia.

DRUG INTERACTIONS

Plasma concentrations of sodium valproate are decreased by carbapenems and co-administration should be avoided if possible. Oral anticoagulants should be more frequently monitored.

SPECIAL POPULATIONS

Though neither IMP nor MRP are teratogenic, the former was associated with increased fetal loss in animal studies and data in pregnancy are limited. Both drugs are excreted in breast milk but the relative infant dose is probably less than 1%.[282] The recommended pediatric dose is 25 mg/kg for IMP and 20 mg/kg for MRP. The dose size and/or interval should be reduced in patients with abnormal renal function (<90 mL/min for IMP and <50 mL/min for MRP) and both drugs are removed by hemodialysis (~50%). No dose adjustment is recommended in liver disease.

REFERENCES

1. Lei B, Wei CJ, and Tu SC. Action mechanism of antitubercular isoniazid. Activation by *Mycobacterium tuberculosis* KatG, isolation, and characterization of Inha inhibitor. *J Biol Chem*. 2000 Jan 28;275(4):2520–6.
2. Rawat R, Whitty A, and Tonge P. The isoniazid-NAD adduct is a slow, tight-binding inhibitor of InhA, the *Mycobacterium tuberculosis* enoyl reductase: Adduct affinity and drug resistance. *Proc Natl Acad Sci USA* 2003;100(24):13881–6.
3. Schön T et al. Evaluation of wild-type MIC distributions as a tool for determination of clinical breakpoints for *Mycobacterium tuberculosis. J Antimicrob Chemother*. 2009 Oct;64(4):786–93.
4. David H. Probability distribution of drug-resistant mutants in unselected populations of *Mycobacterium tuberculosis. Appl Microbiol*. 1970;20:810–4.
5. Cohen K, Bishai WR, and Pym AS. Molecular basis of drug resistance in *Mycobacterium tuberculosis*. In: *Molecular Genetics of Mycobacteria*. 2nd ed. American Society of Microbiology; 2014. 413–29.
6. Peloquin CA, Namdar R, Dodge AA, and Nix DE. Pharmacokinetics of isoniazid under fasting conditions, with food, and with antacids. *Int J Tuberc Lung Dis*. 1999 Aug;3(8):703–10.
7. Woo J, Cheung W, Chan R, Chan H, Cheng A, and Chan K. *In vitro* protein binding characteristics of isoniazid, rifampicin and pyrazinamide to whole plasma, albumin and a-1 acid glycoprotein. *Clin Biochem*. 1996;29(2):175–7.
8. Ellard G, and Gammon P. Pharmacokinetics of isoniazid metabolism in man. *J Pharmacokinet Biopharm*. 1976;4:83–113.
9. Sabbagh A, Langaney A, Darlu P, Gérard N, Krishnamoorthy R, and Poloni ES. Worldwide distribution of NAT2 diversity: Implications for NAT2 evolutionary history. *BMC Genet*. 2008;9:21.
10. van Oosterhout JJ et al. Pharmacokinetics of antituberculosis drugs in HIV-positive and HIV-negative adults in Malawi. *Antimicrob Agents Chemother*. 2015 Oct;59(10):6175–80.
11. McIlleron H, Wash P, Burger A, Norman J, Folb P, and Smith P. Determinants of rifampicin, isoniazid, pyrazinamide and ethambutol pharmacokinetics in a cohort of tuberculosis patients. *Antimicrob Agents Chemother*. 2006;50(4):1170–7.

12. Conte JE Jr et al. Effects of gender, AIDS, and acetylator status on intrapulmonary concentrations of isoniazid. *Antimicrob Agents Chemother.* 2002 Aug;46(8):2358–64.

13. Prideaux B et al. The association between sterilizing activity and drug distribution into tuberculosis lesions. *Nat Med.* 2015 Oct;21(10):1223–7.

14. Donald PR. Cerebrospinal fluid concentrations of antituberculosis agents in adults and children. *Tuberc Edinb Scotl.* 2010 Sep;90(5):279–92.

15. Pouplin T et al. Naïve-pooled pharmacokinetic analysis of pyrazinamide, isoniazid and rifampicin in plasma and cerebrospinal fluid of Vietnamese children with tuberculous meningitis. *BMC Infect Dis.* 2016 Apr 2;16:144.

16. Donald P, Sirgel F, Botha F, Seifart H, Parkin D, and Vandenplas M. The early bactericidal activity of isoniazid related to its dose size in pulmonary tuberculosis. *Am J Respir Crit Care Med.* 1997;156:895–900.

17. Donald P et al. The influence of human N-acetyltransferase genotype on the early bactericidal activity of isoniazid. *Clin Infect Dis.* 2004;39:1425–30.

18. Almeida D et al. Paradoxical effect of isoniazid on the activity of rifampin–pyrazinamide combination in a mouse model of tuberculosis. *Antimicrob Agents Chemother.* 2009 Oct;53(10):4178–84.

19. Chigutsa E et al. Impact of nonlinear interactions of pharmacokinetics and MICs on sputum bacillary kill rates as a marker of sterilizing effect in tuberculosis. *Antimicrob Agents Chemother.* 2015 Jan;59(1):38–45.

20. Rockwood N et al. Concentration-dependent antagonism and culture conversion in pulmonary tuberculosis. *Clin Infect Dis.* 2017 May 15;64(10):1350–9.

21. Sterling TR et al. Three months of rifapentine and isoniazid for latent tuberculosis infection. *N Engl J Med.* 2011 Dec 8;365(23):2155–66.

22. Wang P-Y, Xie S-Y, Hao Q, Zhang C, and Jiang B-F. NAT2 polymorphisms and susceptibility to anti-tuberculosis drug-induced liver injury: A meta-analysis. *Int J Tuberc Lung Dis.* 2012 May;16(5):589–95.

23. Wang F-J, Wang Y, Niu T, Lu W-X, Sandford AJ, and He J-Q. Update meta-analysis of the CYP2E1 RsaI/PstI and DraI polymorphisms and risk of antituberculosis drug-induced hepatotoxicity: Evidence from 26 studies. *J Clin Pharm Ther.* 2016 Jun;41(3):334–40.

24. van der Watt JJ, Harrison TB, Benatar M, and Heckmann JM. Polyneuropathy, anti-tuberculosis treatment and the role of pyridoxine in the HIV/AIDS era: A systematic review. *Int J Tuberc Lung Dis.* 2011 Jun;15(6):722–8.

25. van der Watt JJ, Benatar MG, Harrison TB, Carrara H, and Heckmann JM. Isoniazid exposure and pyridoxine levels in human immunodeficiency virus associated distal sensory neuropathy. *Int J Tuberc Lung Dis.* 2015 Nov;19(11):1312–9.

26. Wen X, Wang J-S, Neuvonen PJ, and Backman JT. Isoniazid is a mechanism-based inhibitor of cytochrome P450 1A2, 2A6, 2C19 and 3A4 isoforms in human liver microsomes. *Eur J Clin Pharmacol.* 2002 Jan;57(11):799–804.

27. Court MH et al. Isoniazid mediates the CYP2B6*6 genotype-dependent interaction between efavirenz and antituberculosis drug therapy through mechanism-based inactivation of CYP2A6. *Antimicrob Agents Chemother.* 2014 Jul;58(7):4145–52.

28. Singh N, Golani A, Patel Z, and Maitra A. Transfer of isoniazid from circulation to breast milk in lactating women on chronic therapy for tuberculosis. *Br J Clin Pharmacol.* 2008 Mar;65(3):418–22.

29. World Health Organisation. *Guidance for National Tuberculosis Programmes on the Management of Tuberculosis in Children.* World Health Organization. 2014. Available from: http://www.who.int/tb/publications/childtb_guidelines/en/

30. Kim YG et al. Decreased acetylation of isoniazid in chronic renal failure. *Clin Pharmacol Ther.* 1993 Dec;54(6):612–20.

31. Malone R, Fish D, Spiegel D, Childs J, and Peloquin C. The effect of hemodialysis on isoniazid, rifampicin, pyrazinamide and ethambutol. *Am J Respir Crit Care Med.* 1999;159:1580–4.

32. Campbell E et al. Structural mechanism for rifampicin inhibition of bacterial RNA polymerase. *Cell* 2001;104:901–12.

33. Peloquin C, Namdar R, Singleton M, and Nix D. Pharmacokinetics of rifampin under fasting conditions with food and with antacids. *Chest* 1999;115:12–8.

34. Stott KE et al. Pharmacokinetics of rifampicin in adult TB patients and healthy volunteers: A systematic review and meta-analysis. *J Antimicrob Chemother.* 2018 Apr 26.

35. Chigutsa E et al. The SLCO1B1 rs4149032 polymorphism is highly prevalent in South Africans and is associated with reduced rifampin concentrations: Dosing implications. *Antimicrob Agents Chemother.* 2011 Sep;55(9):4122–7.

36. Sloan DJ et al. Genetic determinants of the pharmacokinetic variability of rifampin in Malawian adults with pulmonary tuberculosis. *Antimicrob Agents Chemother.* 2017;61(7).

37. Nakajima A, Fukami T, Kobayashi Y, Watanabe A, Nakajima M, and Yokoi T. Human arylacetamide deacetylase is responsible for deacetylation of rifamycins: Rifampicin, rifabutin, and rifapentine. *Biochem Pharmacol.* 2011 Dec 1;82(11):1747–56.

38. Martin P, Riley R, Back DJ, and Owen A. Comparison of the induction profile for drug disposition proteins by typical nuclear receptor activators in human hepatic and intestinal cells. *Br J Pharmacol.* 2008 Feb;153(4):805–19.

39. Chirehwa MT et al. Model-based evaluation of higher doses of rifampin using a semimechanistic model incorporating autoinduction and saturation of hepatic extraction. *Antimicrob Agents Chemother.* 2016;60(1):487–94.

40. Svensson RJ et al. A population pharmacokinetic model incorporating saturable pharmacokinetics and autoinduction for high rifampicin doses. *Clin Pharmacol Ther.* 2018 Apr;103(4):674–83.

41. Conte JE, Golden JA, Kipps JE, Lin ET, Zurlinden E. Effect of sex and AIDS status on the plasma and intrapulmonary pharmacokinetics of rifampicin. *Clin Pharmacokinet.* 2004;43(6):395–404.

42. Boeree MJ et al. A dose-ranging trial to optimize the dose of rifampin in the treatment of tuberculosis. *Am J Respir Crit Care Med.* 2015 May 1;191(9):1058–65.

43. Boeree MJ et al. High-dose rifampicin, moxifloxacin, and SQ109 for treating tuberculosis: A multi-arm, multi-stage randomised controlled trial. *Lancet Infect Dis.* 2017 Jan;17(1):39–49.

44. Khan FA et al. Treatment of active tuberculosis in HIV-coinfected patients: A systematic review and meta-analysis. *Clin Infect Dis.* 2010 May 1;50(9):1288–99.

45. Sharma SK, Sharma A, Kadhiravan T, and Tharyan P. Rifamycins (rifampicin, rifabutin and rifapentine) compared to isoniazid for preventing tuberculosis in HIV-negative people at risk of active TB. In: *The Cochrane Library.* John Wiley & Sons, *Ltd*, 2013 [cited 2018 May 8]. Available from: http://cochranelibrary-wiley.com/doi/10.1002/14651858.CD007545.pub2/full

46. Aarnoutse RE et al. Pharmacokinetics, tolerability, and Bacteriological response of rifampin administered at 600, 900, and 1,200 milligrams daily in patients with pulmonary tuberculosis. *Antimicrob Agents Chemother.* 2017 Oct 24 [cited 2018 May 8];61(11). Available from: https://www.ncbi.nlm.nih.gov/pmc/articles/PMC5655063/

47. Acocella G. Clinical pharmacokinetics of rifampicin. *Clin Pharmacokinet.* 1978;3:108–27.

48. Lehloenya RJ, Todd G, Badri M, and Dheda K. Outcomes of reintroducing anti-tuberculosis drugs following cutaneous adverse drug reactions. *Int J Tuberc Lung Dis.* 2011 Dec;15(12):1649–57.

49. Virgilio R. Rifampicin-dependent antibodies during intermittent treatment. *Scand J Respir Dis Suppl.* 1973;84:83–6.

50. Aquinas M et al. Adverse reactions to daily and intermittent rifampicin regimens for pulmonary tuberculosis in Hong Kong. *Br Med J.* 1972 Mar 25;1(5803):765–71.

51. Rae J, Johnson M, Lippmann M, and Flockhart D. Rifampin is a selective, pleiotropic inducer of drug metabolism genes in human hepatocytes: Studies with cDNA and oligonucleotide expression arrays. *J Pharmacol Exp Ther.* 2001;299(3):849–57.

52. Niemi M, Backman J, Fromm M, Neuvonen P, and Kivisto K. Pharmacokinetic interactions with rifampicin; clinical relevance. *Clin Pharmacokinet.* 2003;42(9):819–50.

53. Semvua HH, Kibiki GS, Kisanga ER, Boeree MJ, Burger DM, and Aarnoutse R. Pharmacological interactions between rifampicin and antiretroviral drugs: Challenges and research priorities for resource-limited settings. *Ther Drug Monit.* 2015 Feb;37(1):22–32.

54. Decloedt EH, Maartens G, Smith P, Merry C, Bango F, and McIlleron H. The safety, effectiveness and concentrations of adjusted lopinavir/ritonavir in HIV-infected adults on rifampicin-based antitubercular therapy. *PLOS ONE* 2012 Mar 7 [cited 2018 May 10];7(3). Available from: https://www.ncbi.nlm.nih.gov/pmc/articles/PMC3296695/

55. Zhang Y, and Mitchison D. The curious characteristics of pyrazinamide: A review. *Int J Tuberc Lung Dis.* 2003 Jan;7(1):6–21.

56. Werngren J, Sturegård E, Juréen P, Ängeby K, Hoffner S, and Schön T. Reevaluation of the critical concentration for drug susceptibility testing of *Mycobacterium tuberculosis* against pyrazinamide using wild-type MIC distributions and pncA gene sequencing. *Antimicrob Agents Chemother.* 2012 Mar;56(3):1253–7.

57. McGrath M et al. Mutation rate and the emergence of drug resistance in *Mycobacterium tuberculosis. J Antimicrob Chemother.* 2014 Feb 1;69(2):292–302.

58. Peloquin CA, Bulpitt AE, Jaresko GS, Jelliffe RW, James GT, and Nix DE. Pharmacokinetics of pyrazinamide under fasting conditions, with food, and with antacids. *Pharmacotherapy* 1998 Dec;18(6):1205–11.

59. Lacroix C et al. Pharmacokinetics of pyrazinamide and its metabolites in healthy subjects. *Eur J Clin Pharmacol.* 1989;36(4):395–400.

60. Conte J, Golden J, Duncan S, McKenna E, and Zurlinden E. Intrapulmonary concentrations of pyrazinamide. *Antimicrob Agents Chemother.* 1999;43:1329–33.

61. Kempker RR et al. Lung tissue concentrations of pyrazinamide among patients with drug-resistant pulmonary tuberculosis. *Antimicrob Agents Chemother.* 2017;61(6).

62. Via LE et al. Host-mediated bioactivation of pyrazinamide: implications for efficacy, resistance, and therapeutic alternatives. *ACS Infect Dis.* 2015 May 8;1(5):203–14.

63. Diacon AH et al. Bactericidal activity of pyrazinamide and clofazimine alone and in combinations with pretomanid and bedaquiline. *Am J Respir Crit Care Med.* 2015 Apr 15;191(8):943–53.

64. Fox W, Ellard GA, and Mitchison DA. Studies on the treatment of tuberculosis undertaken by the British Medical Research Council Tuberculosis Units 1946–1986, with subsequent relevant publications. *Int J Tuberc Lung Dis.* 1999;3(10):S231–79.

65. Yuen CM et al. Association between regimen composition and treatment response in patients with multidrug-resistant tuberculosis: A prospective cohort study. *PLoS Med.* 2015 Dec;12(12):e1001932.

66. Pasipanodya JG, and Gumbo T. Clinical and toxicodynamic evidence that high-dose pyrazinamide is not more hepatotoxic than the low doses currently used. *Antimicrob Agents Chemother.* 2010 Jul;54(7):2847–54.

67. Gao XF et al. Rifampicin plus pyrazinamide versus isoniazid for treating latent tuberculosis infection: A meta-analysis. *Int J Tuberc Lung Dis.* 2006 Oct;10(10):1080–90.

68. Mandal AK, and Mount DB. The molecular physiology of uric acid homeostasis. *Annu Rev Physiol.* 2015;77:323–45.

69. Holdiness MR. Antituberculosis drugs and breast-feeding. *Arch Intern Med.* 1984 Sep;144(9):1888.

70. Stamatakis G et al. Pyrazinamide and pyrazinoic acid pharmacokinetics in patients with chronic renal failure. *Clin Nephrol.* 1988 Oct;30(4):230–4.

71. Lacroix C et al. Haemodialysis of pyrazinamide in uraemic patients. *Eur J Clin Pharmacol.* 1989;37(3):309–11.

72. British Thoracic Society Standards of Care Committee and Joint Tuberculosis Committee. Milburn H et al. Guidelines for the prevention and management of *Mycobacterium tuberculosis* infection and disease in adult patients with chronic kidney disease. *Thorax* 2010 Jun;65(6):557–70.

73. Peloquin CA, Bulpitt AE, Jaresko GS, Jelliffe RW, Childs JM, and Nix DE. Pharmacokinetics of ethambutol under fasting conditions, with food, and with antacids. *Antimicrob Agents Chemother.* 1999 Mar;43(3):568–72.

74. Alghamdi WA, Al-Shaer MH, and Peloquin CA. Protein binding of first-line antituberculous drugs. *Antimicrob Agents Chemother.* 2018 May 7;62.

75. Peets EA, Sweeney WM, Place VA, Buyske DA. The absorption, excretion, and metabolic fate of ethambutol in man. *Am Rev Respir Dis.* 1965 Jan;91:51–8.

76. Lee CS, Brater DC, Gambertoglio JG, and Benet LZ. Disposition kinetics of ethambutol in man. *J Pharmacokinet Biopharm.* 1980 Aug;8(4):335–46.

77. Conte JE Jr, Golden JA, Kipps J, Lin ET, and Zurlinden E. Effects of AIDS and gender on steady-state plasma and intrapulmonary ethambutol concentrations. *Antimicrob Agents Chemother.* 2001 Oct;45(10):2891–6.

78. Zimmerman M et al. Ethambutol partitioning in tuberculous pulmonary lesions explains its clinical efficacy. *Antimicrob Agents Chemother.* 2017 Aug 24 [cited 2018 Apr 25];61(9). Available from: https://www.ncbi.nlm.nih.gov/pmc/articles/PMC5571334/

79. Jindani A, Aber V, Edwards E, and Mitchison D. The early bactericidal activity of drugs in patients with pulmonary tuberculosis. *Am Rev Respir Dis.* 1980;121:939–49.

80. Chen S-C, Lin M-C, and Sheu S-J. Incidence and prognostic factor of ethambutol-related optic neuropathy: 10-year experience in southern Taiwan. *Kaohsiung J Med Sci.* 2015 Jul;31(7):358–62.

81. Yang HK, Park MJ, Lee J-H, Lee C-T, Park JS, and Hwang J-M. Incidence of toxic optic neuropathy with low-dose ethambutol. *Int J Tuberc Lung Dis.* 2016 Feb;20(2):261–4.

82. Leibold JE. The ocular toxicity of ethambutol and its relation to dose. *Ann N Y Acad Sci.* 1966 Apr 20;135(2):904–9.

83. Snider DE, and Powell KE. Should women taking antituberculosis drugs breast-feed? *Arch Intern Med.* 1984 Mar;144(3):589–90.

84. Varughese A, Brater DC, Benet LZ, and Lee CS. Ethambutol kinetics in patients with impaired renal function. *Am Rev Respir Dis.* 1986 Jul;134(1):34–8.

85. Schön T et al. Wild-type distributions of seven oral second-line drugs against *Mycobacterium tuberculosis. Int J Tuberc Lung Dis.* 2011 Apr;15(4):502–9.

86. Schön T et al. Rifampicin-resistant and rifabutin-susceptible *Mycobacterium tuberculosis* strains: A breakpoint artefact? *J Antimicrob Chemother.* 2013 Sep;68(9):2074–7.

87. Narang PK, Lewis RC, and Bianchine JR. Rifabutin absorption in humans: Relative bioavailability and food effect. *Clin Pharmacol Ther.* 1992 Oct;52(4):335–41.

88. Gatti G, Di Biagio A, De Pascalis CR, Guerra M, Bassetti M, and Bassetti D. Pharmacokinetics of rifabutin in HIV-infected patients with or without wasting syndrome. *Br J Clin Pharmacol.* 2001 Dec 24;48(5):704–11.

89. Utkin I et al. Isolation and identification of major urinary metabolites of rifabutin in rats and humans. *Drug Metab Dispos Biol Fate Chem.* 1997 Aug;25(8):963–9.

90. Naiker S et al. Randomized pharmacokinetic evaluation of different rifabutin doses in African HIV-infected tuberculosis patients on lopinavir/ritonavir-based antiretroviral therapy. *BMC Pharmacol Toxicol.* 2014 Nov 19;15:61.

91. Chan SL et al. The early bactericidal activity of rifabutin measured by sputum viable counts in Hong Kong patients with pulmonary tuberculosis. *Tuber Lung Dis.* 1992 Feb;73(1):33–8.

92. Sirgel FA et al. The early bactericidal activity of rifabutin in patients with pulmonary tuberculosis measured by sputum viable counts: A new method of drug assessment. *J Antimicrob Chemother.* 1993 Dec;32(6):867–75.

93. Davies G, Cerri S, and Richeldi L. Rifabutin for treating pulmonary tuberculosis. *Cochrane Database Syst Rev Online.* 2007;(4):CD005159.

94. Tseng AL, and Walmsley SL. Rifabutin-associated uveitis. *Ann Pharmacother.* 1995 Nov;29(11):1149–55.

95. Williamson B, Dooley KE, Zhang Y, Back DJ, and Owen A. Induction of influx and efflux transporters and cytochrome P450 3A4 in primary human hepatocytes by rifampin, rifabutin, and rifapentine. *Antimicrob Agents Chemother.* 2013 Dec;57(12):6366–9.

96. Regazzi M, Carvalho AC, Villani P, and Matteelli A. Treatment optimization in patients co-infected with HIV and *Mycobacterium tuberculosis* infections: Focus on drug–drug interactions with rifamycins. *Clin Pharmacokinet.* 2014 Jun;53(6):489–507.

97. Hennig S et al. Population pharmacokinetic drug–drug interaction pooled analysis of existing data for rifabutin and HIV PIs. *J Antimicrob Chemother.* 2016 May;71(5):1330–40.

98. Bemer-Melchior P, Bryskier A, and Drugeon HB. Comparison of the *in vitro* activities of rifapentine and rifampicin against *Mycobacterium tuberculosis* complex. *J Antimicrob Chemother.* 2000 Oct;46(4):571–6.

99. Zvada SP et al. Effect of four different meals types on the population pharmacokinetics of single dose rifapentine in healthy male volunteers. *Antimicrob Agents Chemother.* 2010 Jun 1 [cited 2010 Jun 15]; Available from: http://www.ncbi.nlm.nih.gov.ezproxy.liv.ac.uk/pubmed/20516273

100. Egelund EF et al. Protein binding of rifapentine and its 25-desacetyl metabolite in patients with pulmonary tuberculosis. *Antimicrob Agents Chemother.* 2014 Aug;58(8):4904–10.

101. Reith K, Keung A, Toren P, Cheng L, Eller M, and Weir S. Disposition and metabolism of C14-rifapentine in healthy volunteers. *Drug Metab Dispos.* 1998;26(8):732–8.

102. Conte JE, Golden JA, McQuitty M, Kipps J, Lin ET, and Zurlinden E. Effects of AIDS and gender on steady state plasma and intrapulmonary ethionamide concentrations. *Antimicrob Agents Chemother.* 2000;44(5):1337–41.

103. Sarathy JP et al. Prediction of drug penetration in tuberculosis lesions. *ACS Infect Dis.* 2016 Aug 12;2(8):552–63.

104. Rosenthal IM et al. Daily dosing of rifapentine cures tuberculosis in three months or less in the murine model. *PLoS Med.* 2007 Dec;4(12):e344.

105. Sirgel FA et al. The early bactericidal activities of rifampin and rifapentine in pulmonary tuberculosis. *Am J Respir Crit Care Med.* 2005 Jul 1;172(1):128–35.

106. Dorman SE et al. Substitution of rifapentine for rifampin during intensive phase treatment of pulmonary tuberculosis: Study 29 of the tuberculosis trials consortium. *J Infect Dis.* 2012 Oct 1;206(7):1030–40.

107. Dorman SE et al. Daily rifapentine for treatment of pulmonary tuberculosis. A randomized, dose-ranging trial. *Am J Respir Crit Care Med.* 2015 Feb 1;191(3):333–43.

108. Dooley KE et al. Safety and pharmacokinetics of escalating daily doses of the antituberculosis drug rifapentine in healthy volunteers. *Clin Pharmacol Ther.* 2012 May;91(5):881–8.

109. Weiner M et al. Rifapentine pharmacokinetics and tolerability in children and adults treated once weekly with rifapentine and isoniazid for latent tuberculosis infection. *J Pediatr Infect Dis Soc.* 2014 Jun 1;3(2):132–45.

110. Keung AC, Eller MG, and Weir SJ. Pharmacokinetics of rifapentine in patients with varying degrees of hepatic dysfunction. *J Clin Pharmacol.* 1998 Jun;38(6):517–24.

111. Angeby KA et al. Wild-type MIC distributions of four fluoroquinolones active against *Mycobacterium tuberculosis* in relation to current critical concentrations and available pharmacokinetic and pharmacodynamic data. *J Antimicrob Chemother.* 2010 May;65(5):946–52.

112. Stass H, and Kubitza D. Pharmacokinetics and elimination of moxifloxacin after oral and intravenous administration in man. *J Antimicrob Chemother.* 1999 May;43(Suppl B):83–90.

113. Lettieri J, Vargas R, Agarwal V, and Liu P. Effect of food on the pharmacokinetics of a single oral dose of moxifloxacin 400 mg in healthy male volunteers. *Clin Pharmacokinet.* 2001;40(Suppl 1):19–25.

114. Stass H, Dalhoff A, Kubitza D, and Schühly U. Pharmacokinetics, safety, and tolerability of ascending single doses of moxifloxacin, a new 8-methoxy quinolone, administered to healthy subjects. *Antimicrob Agents Chemother.* 1998 Aug;42(8):2060–5.

115. Soman A, Honeybourne D, Andrews J, Jevons G, and Wise R. Concentrations of moxifloxacin in serum and pulmonary compartments following a single 400 mg oral dose in patients undergoing fibre-optic bronchoscopy. *J Antimicrob Chemother.* 1999 Dec;44(6):835–8.

116. Capitano B et al. Steady-state intrapulmonary concentrations of moxifloxacin, levofloxacin, and azithromycin in older adults. *Chest* 2004 Mar;125(3):965–73.

117. Heinrichs MT et al. Moxifloxacin target site concentrations in patients with pulmonary TB utilizing microdialysis: A clinical pharmacokinetic study. *J Antimicrob Chemother.* 2018 Feb 1;73(2):477–83.

118. Alffenaar JWC et al. Pharmacokinetics of moxifloxacin in cerebrospinal fluid and plasma in patients with tuberculous meningitis. *Clin Infect Dis.* 2009 Oct 1;49(7):1080–2.

119. Johnson JL et al. Early and extended early bactericidal activity of levofloxacin, gatifloxacin and moxifloxacin in pulmonary tuberculosis. *Int J Tuberc Lung Dis.* 2006 Jun;10(6):605–12.

120. Ziganshina LE, Titarenko AF, and Davies GR. Fluoroquinolones for treating tuberculosis (presumed drug-sensitive). *Cochrane Database Syst Rev.* 2013;6:CD004795.

121. Gillespie SH et al. Four-month moxifloxacin-based regimens for drug-sensitive tuberculosis. *N Engl J Med.* 2014 Oct 23;371(17):1577–87.

122. Jindani A et al. High-dose rifapentine with moxifloxacin for pulmonary tuberculosis. *N Engl J Med.* 2014 Oct 23;371(17):1599–608.

123. Falzon D et al. Resistance to fluoroquinolones and second-line injectable drugs: Impact on multidrug-resistant TB outcomes. *Eur Respir J.* 2013 Jul;42(1):156–68.

124. Fox GJ, Benedetti A, Mitnick CD, Pai M, and Menzies D, Collaborative Group for meta-analysis of individual patient data in MDR-TB. Propensity score-based approaches to confounding by indication in individual patient data meta-analysis: Non-standardized treatment for multidrug resistant tuberculosis. *PLOS ONE* 2016;11(3):e0151724.

125. Florian JA, Tornøe CW, Brundage R, Parekh A, and Garnett CE. Population pharmacokinetic and concentration—QTc models for moxifloxacin: Pooled analysis of 20 thorough QT studies. *J Clin Pharmacol.* 2011 Aug;51(8):1152–62.

126. Weiner M et al. Effects of rifampin and multidrug resistance gene polymorphism on concentrations of moxifloxacin. *Antimicrob Agents Chemother.* 2007 Aug;51(8):2861–6.

127. Njiland H et al. Rifampicin reduces plasma concentrations of moxifloxacin in patients with tuberculosis. *Clin Infect Dis.* 2007;45(8):1001–7.

128. Padberg S et al. Observational cohort study of pregnancy outcome after first-trimester exposure to fluoroquinolones. *Antimicrob Agents Chemother.* 2014 Aug;58(8):4392–8.

129. Palacios E et al. Drug-resistant tuberculosis and pregnancy: Management and treatment outcomes of 38 cases in Lima, Peru. *Clin Infect Dis.* 2009 May 15;48(10):1413–9.

130. Stass H, Kubitza D, Halabi A, and Delesen H. Pharmacokinetics of moxifloxacin, a novel 8-methoxy-quinolone, in patients with renal dysfunction. *Br J Clin Pharmacol.* 2002 Mar;53(3):232–7.

131. Czock D et al. Pharmacokinetics of moxifloxacin and levofloxacin in intensive care unit patients who have acute renal failure and undergo extended daily dialysis. *Clin J Am Soc Nephrol CJASN.* 2006 Nov;1(6):1263–8.

132. Barth J, Jäger D, Mundkowski R, Drewelow B, Welte T, and Burkhardt O. Single- and multiple-dose pharmacokinetics of intravenous moxifloxacin in patients with severe hepatic impairment. *J Antimicrob Chemother.* 2008 Sep;62(3):575–8.

133. Lee LJ, Hafkin B, Lee ID, Hoh J, and Dix R. Effects of food and sucralfate on a single oral dose of 500 milligrams of levofloxacin in healthy subjects. *Antimicrob Agents Chemother.* 1997 Oct;41(10):2196–200.

134. Fish DN, and Chow AT. The clinical pharmacokinetics of levofloxacin. *Clin Pharmacokinet.* 1997 Feb;32(2):101–19.

135. Rodvold KA, Danziger LH, and Gotfried MH. Steady-state plasma and bronchopulmonary concentrations of intravenous levofloxacin and azithromycin in healthy adults. *Antimicrob Agents Chemother.* 2003 Aug;47(8):2450–7.

136. Conte JE, Golden JA, McIver M, and Zurlinden E. Intrapulmonary pharmacokinetics and pharmacodynamics of high-dose levofloxacin in healthy volunteer subjects. *Int J Antimicrob Agents.* 2006 Aug;28(2):114–21.

137. Kempker RR et al. Cavitary penetration of levofloxacin among patients with multidrug-resistant tuberculosis. *Antimicrob Agents Chemother.* 2015;59(6):3149–55.

138. Prideaux B, ElNaggar MS, Zimmerman M, Wiseman JM, Li X, and Dartois V. Mass spectrometry imaging of levofloxacin distribution in TB-infected pulmonary lesions by MALDI-MSI and continuous liquid microjunction surface sampling. *Int J Mass Spectrom.* 2015 Feb 1;377:699–708.

139. Thwaites GE et al. Randomized pharmacokinetic and pharmacodynamic comparison of fluoroquinolones for tuberculous meningitis. *Antimicrob Agents Chemother.* 2011 Jul;55(7):3244–53.

140. Koh W-J et al. Comparison of levofloxacin versus moxifloxacin for multidrug-resistant tuberculosis. *Am J Respir Crit Care Med.* 2013 Oct 1;188(7):858–64.

141. el-Sadr WM et al. Evaluation of an intensive intermittent-induction regimen and duration of short-course treatment for human immunodeficiency virus-related pulmonary tuberculosis. Terry Beirn Community Programs for Clinical Research on AIDS (CPCRA) and the AIDS Clinical Trials Group (ACTG). *Clin Infect Dis.* 1998 May;26(5):1148–58.

142. Noel GJ, Goodman DB, Chien S, Solanki B, Padmanabhan M, and Natarajan J. Measuring the effects of supratherapeutic doses of levofloxacin on healthy volunteers using four methods of QT correction and periodic and continuous ECG recordings. *J Clin Pharmacol.* 2004 May;44(5):464–73.

143. Bidell MR, and Lodise TP. Fluoroquinolone-associated tendinopathy: Does levofloxacin pose the greatest risk? *Pharmacotherapy* 2016;36(6):679–93.

144. Zhang L, Wei M, Zhao C, and Qi H. Determination of the inhibitory potential of 6 fluoroquinolones on CYP1A2 and CYP2C9 in human liver microsomes. *Acta Pharmacol Sin.* 2008 Dec;29(12):1507–14.

145. Cahill JB, Bailey EM, Chien S, and Johnson GM. Levofloxacin secretion in breast milk: A case report. *Pharmacotherapy* 2005 Jan;25(1):116–8.

146. Juréen P et al. Wild-type MIC distributions for aminoglycoside and cyclic polypeptide antibiotics used for treatment of *Mycobacterium tuberculosis* infections. *J Clin Microbiol.* 2010 May;48(5):1853–8.

147. Zhu M, Burman WJ, Jaresko GS, Berning SE, Jelliffe RW, and Peloquin CA. Population pharmacokinetics of intravenous and intramuscular streptomycin in patients with tuberculosis. *Pharmacotherapy* 2001 Sep;21(9):1037–45.

148. Dijkstra JA et al. Limited sampling strategies for therapeutic drug monitoring of amikacin and kanamycin in patients with multidrug-resistant tuberculosis. *Int J Antimicrob Agents.* 2015 Sep;46(3):332–7.

149. Najmeddin F et al. Evaluation of epithelial lining fluid concentration of amikacin in critically ill patients with ventilator-associated pneumonia. *J Intensive Care Med.* 2018 Jan 1;885066618754784.

150. Ellard GA, Humphries MJ, and Allen BW. Cerebrospinal fluid drug concentrations and the treatment of tuberculous meningitis. *Am Rev Respir Dis.* 1993 Sep;148(3):650–5.

151. Donald PR et al. The early bactericidal activity of amikacin in pulmonary tuberculosis. *Int J Tuberc Lung Dis.* 2001 Jun;5(6):533–8.

152. Donald PR et al. The early bactericidal activity of streptomycin. *Int J Tuberc Lung Dis.* 2002 Aug;6(8):693–8.

153. Peloquin CA et al. Aminoglycoside toxicity: Daily versus thrice-weekly dosing for treatment of mycobacterial diseases. *Clin Infect Dis.* 2004 Jun 1;38(11):1538–44.

154. Sturdy A et al. Multidrug resistant tuberculosis (MDR-TB) treatment in the UK: A study of injectable use and toxicity in practice. *J Antimicrob Chemother.* 2011 Aug;66(8):1815–20.

155. Harris T, Bardien S, Schaaf HS, Petersen L, De Jong G, and Fagan JJ. Aminoglycoside-induced hearing loss in HIV-positive and HIV-negative multidrug-resistant tuberculosis patients. *South Afr Med J Suid-Afr Tydskr Vir Geneeskd.* 2012 May 8;102(6 Pt 2):363–6.

156. Kranzer K, Elamin WF, Cox H, Seddon JA, Ford N, and Drobniewski F. A systematic review and meta-analysis of the efficacy and safety of N-acetylcysteine in preventing aminoglycoside-induced ototoxicity: Implications for the treatment of multidrug-resistant TB. *Thorax* 2015 Nov;70(11):1070–7.

157. Shin S et al. Hypokalemia among patients receiving treatment for multidrug-resistant tuberculosis. *Chest* 2004 Mar;125(3):974–80.

158. Alsultan A, and Peloquin CA. Therapeutic drug monitoring in the treatment of tuberculosis: An update. *Drugs.* 2014 Jun 1;74(8):839–54.

159. Vorherr H. Drug excretion in breast milk. *Postgrad Med.* 1974 Oct;56(4):97–104.

160. Armstrong DK, Hodgman T, Visconti JA, Reilley TE, Garner WL, and Dasta JF. Hemodialysis of amikacin in critically ill patients. *Crit Care Med.* 1988 May;16(5):517–20.

161. Eschenauer GA, Lam SW, and Mueller BA. Dose timing of aminoglycosides in hemodialysis patients: A pharmacology view. *Semin Dial.* 2016;29(3):204–13.

162. Heifets L, Simon J, and Pham V. Capreomycin is active against non-replicating M tuberculosis. *Ann Clin Microbiol Antimicrob.* 2005;4(6).

163. Black HR, Griffith RS, and Peabody AM. Absorption, excretion and metabolism of capreomycin in normal and diseased states. *Ann N Y Acad Sci.* 1966 Apr 20;135(2):974–82.

164. Schwartz W. Capreomycin compared with streptomycin in original treatment of pulmonary tuberculosis. XVI. A report of the Veterans Administration-Armed Forces Cooperative. Study on the Chemotherapy of Tuberculosis. *Am Rev Respir Dis.* 1966 Dec;94(6):858–64.

165. Aquinas M, and Citron K. Rifampicin, ethambutol and capreomycin in pulmonary tuberculosis, previously treated with first and second line drugs: Results of two years treatment. *Tubercle* 1972;53(153–65).

166. Lehmann CR et al. Capreomycin kinetics in renal impairment and clearance by hemodialysis. *Am Rev Respir Dis.* 1988 Nov;138(5):1312–3.

167. Zheng J et al. Para-Aminosalicylic acid is a prodrug targeting dihydrofolate reductase in *Mycobacterium tuberculosis. J Biol Chem.* 2013 Aug 9;288(32):23447–56.

168. Brown KA, and Ratledge C. The effect of p-aminosalicylic acid on iron transport and assimilation in mycobacteria. *Biochim Biophys Acta.* 1975 Apr 7;385(2):207–20.

169. Mitchison DA, and Monk M. Comparison of solid and liquid medium sensitivity tests of tubercle bacilli to para-aminosalicylic acid. *J Clin Pathol.* 1955 Aug;8(3):229–36.

170. Peloquin CA, Zhu M, Adam RD, Singleton MD, and Nix DE. Pharmacokinetics of para-aminosalicylic acid granules under four dosing conditions. *Ann Pharmacother.* 2001 Nov,35(11):1332–8.

171. Donald PR, and Diacon AH. Para-aminosalicylic acid: The return of an old friend. *Lancet Infect Dis.* 2015 Sep;15(9):1091–9.

172. Hughes NC et al. Identification and characterization of variant alleles of human acetyltransferase NAT1 with defective function using p-aminosalicylate as an *in-vivo* and *in-vitro* probe. *Pharmacogenetics.* 1998 Feb;8(1):55–66.

173. Lauener H, and Favez G. The inhibition of isoniazid inactivation by means of PAS and benzoyl-PAS in man. *Am Rev Respir Dis.* 1959 Jul;80(1, Part 1):26–37.

174. de Kock L et al. Pharmacokinetics of para-aminosalicylic acid in HIV-uninfected and HIV-coinfected tuberculosis patients receiving antiretroviral therapy, managed for multidrug-resistant and extensively drug-resistant tuberculosis. *Antimicrob Agents Chemother.* 2014 Oct;58(10):6242–50.

175. Toskes PP, and Deren JJ. Selective inhibition of vitamin B 12 absorption by para-aminosalicylic acid. *Gastroenterology.* 1972 Jun;62(6):1232–7.

176. Macgregor AG, and Somner AR. The anti-thyroid action of para-aminosalicylic acid. *Lancet (Lond, Engl)* 1954 Nov 6;267(6845):931–6.

177. Tran JH, and Montakantikul P. The safety of antituberculosis medications during breastfeeding. *J Hum Lact.* 1998 Dec;14(4):337–40.

178. Held H, and Fried F. Elimination of para-aminosalicylic acid in patients with liver disease and renal insufficiency. *Chemotherapy* 1977;23(6):405–15.

179. Malone RS, Fish DN, Spiegel DM, Childs JM, and Peloquin CA. The effect of hemodialysis on cycloserine, ethionamide, para-aminosalicylate, and clofazimine. *Chest* 1999 Oct;116(4):984–90.

180. Hanoulle X et al. Selective intracellular accumulation of the major metabolite issued from the activation of the prodrug ethionamide in mycobacteria. *J Antimicrob Chemother.* 2006 Oct;58 (4):768–72.

181. Wang F et al. Mechanism of thioamide drug action against tuberculosis and leprosy. *J Exp Med.* 2007 Jan 22;204(1):73–8.

182. Jenner PJ, Ellard GA, Gruer PJ, and Aber VR. A comparison of the blood levels and urinary excretion of ethionamide and prothionamide in man. *J Antimicrob Chemother.* 1984 Mar;13(3):267–77.

183. Auclair B, Nix DE, Adam RD, James GT, and Peloquin CA. Pharmacokinetics of ethionamide administered under fasting conditions or with orange juice, food, or antacids. *Antimicrob Agents Chemother.* 2001 Mar;45(3):810–4.

184. Zhu M et al. Population pharmacokinetics of ethionamide in patients with tuberculosis. *Tuberc Edinb Scotl.* 2002;82(2–3):91–6.

185. Lee HW et al. Pharmacokinetics of prothionamide in patients with multidrug-resistant tuberculosis. *Int J Tuberc Lung Dis.* 2009 Sep;13(9):1161–6.

186. Schwartz WS. Comparison of ethionamide with isoniazid in original treatment cases of pulmonary tuberculosis. XIV. A report of the Veterans Administration-Armed Forces cooperative study. *Am Rev Respir Dis.* 1966 May;93(5):685–92.

187. Comparison of the clinical usefulness of ethionamide and prothionamide in initial treatment of tuberculosis: Tenth series of controlled trials. *Tubercle* 1968 Sep;49(3):281–90.

188. Scardigli A, Caminero JA, Sotgiu G, Centis R, D'Ambrosio L, and Migliori GB. Efficacy and tolerability of ethionamide versus prothionamide: A systematic review. *Eur Respir J.* 2016;48(3):946–52.

189. Thee S, Zöllner EW, Willemse M, Hesseling AC, Magdorf K, and Schaaf HS. Abnormal thyroid function tests in children on ethionamide treatment. *Int J Tuberc Lung Dis.* 2011 Sep;15(9):1191–3.

190. Munivenkatappa S et al. Drug-induced hypothyroidism during anti-tuberculosis treatment of multidrug-resistant tuberculosis: Notes from the field. *J Tuberc Res.* 2016 Sep;4(3):105–10.

191. Bruning JB, Murillo AC, Chacon O, Barletta RG, and Sacchettini JC. Structure of the *Mycobacterium tuberculosis* D-alanine:D-alanine ligase, a target of the antituberculosis drug D-cycloserine. *Antimicrob Agents Chemother.* 2011 Jan;55(1):291–301.

192. Nakatani Y et al. Role of alanine racemase mutations in *Mycobacterium tuberculosis* D-cycloserine resistance. *Antimicrob Agents Chemother.* 2017 Dec;61(12).

193. Zhu M, Nix DE, Adam RD, Childs JM, and Peloquin CA. Pharmacokinetics of cycloserine under fasting conditions and with high-fat meal, orange juice, and antacids. *Pharmacotherapy* 2001 Aug;21(8):891–7.

194. Baron H, Epstein IG, Mulinos MG, and Nair KG. Absorption, distribution, and excretion of cycloserine in man. *Antibiot Annu.* 1955 1956;3:136–40.

195. Zhou H et al. Pharmacokinetic properties and tolerability of cycloserine following oral administration in healthy Chinese volunteers: A randomized, open-label, single- and multiple-dose 3-way crossover study. *Clin Ther.* 2015 Jun 1;37(6):1292–300.

196. Court R et al. Steady state pharmacokinetics of cycloserine in patients on terizidone for multidrug-resistant tuberculosis. *Int J Tuberc Lung Dis.* 2018 Jan 1;22(1):30–3.

197. Bignall JR. A comparison of regimens of ethionamide, pyrazinamide and cycloserine in re-treatment of patients with pulmonary tuberculosis. *Bull Int Union Tuberc.* 1968 Dec;41:175–7.

198. Zrilić V, Mijatović M, Mirković S, and Muzikravić T. Results of clinical trials of a new antitubercular agent, terizidone (Terivalidine). *Plucne Bolesti Tuberk*. 1972 Jun;24(2):89–98.

199. Hwang TJ, Wares DF, Jafarov A, Jakubowiak W, Nunn P, and Keshavjee S. Safety of cycloserine and terizidone for the treatment of drug-resistant tuberculosis: A meta-analysis. *Int J Tuberc Lung Dis*. 2013 Oct;17(10):1257–66.

200. Cohen AC. Pyridoxine in the prevention and treatment of convulsions and neurotoxicity due to cycloserine. *Ann N Y Acad Sci*. 1969 Sep 30;166(1):346–9.

201. Ippolito JA et al. Crystal structure of the oxazolidinone antibiotic linezolid bound to the 50S ribosomal subunit. *J Med Chem*. 2008 Jun 26;51(12):3353–6.

202. Dookie N, Rambaran S, Padayatchi N, Mahomed S, and Naidoo K. Evolution of drug resistance in *Mycobacterium tuberculosis*: A review on the molecular determinants of resistance and implications for personalized care. *J Antimicrob Chemother*. 2018 May;73(5):1138–51.

203. Welshman IR, Sisson TA, Jungbluth GL, Stalker DJ, and Hopkins NK. Linezolid absolute bioavailability and the effect of food on oral bioavailability. *Biopharm Drug Dispos*. 2001 Apr;22(3):91–7.

204. Stalker DJ, and Jungbluth GL. Clinical pharmacokinetics of linezolid, a novel oxazolidinone antibacterial. *Clin Pharmacokinet*. 2003;42(13):1129–40.

205. McGee B et al. Population pharmacokinetics of linezolid in adults with pulmonary tuberculosis. *Antimicrob Agents Chemother*. 2009 Sep;53(9):3981–4.

206. Conte JE, Golden JA, Kipps J, and Zurlinden E. Intrapulmonary pharmacokinetics of linezolid. *Antimicrob Agents Chemother*. 2002 May;46(5):1475–80.

207. Honeybourne D, Tobin C, Jevons G, Andrews J, and Wise R. Intrapulmonary penetration of linezolid. *J Antimicrob Chemother*. 2003 Jun;51(6):1431–4.

208. Kempker RR et al. A comparison of linezolid lung tissue concentrations among patients with drug-resistant tuberculosis. *Eur Respir J*. 2018 Feb;51(2).

209. Viaggi B et al. Linezolid in the central nervous system: Comparison between cerebrospinal fluid and plasma pharmacokinetics. *Scand J Infect Dis*. 2011 Sep;43(9):721–7.

210. Dietze R et al. Early and extended early bactericidal activity of linezolid in pulmonary tuberculosis. *Am J Respir Crit Care Med*. 2008 Dec 1;178(11):1180–5.

211. Lee M et al. Linezolid for treatment of chronic extensively drug-resistant tuberculosis. *N Engl J Med*. 2012 Oct 18;367(16):1508–18.

212. Millard J et al. Linezolid pharmacokinetics in MDR-TB: A systematic review, meta-analysis and Monte Carlo simulation. *J Antimicrob Chemother*. 2018 Mar 23;

213. Song T et al. Linezolid trough concentrations correlate with mitochondrial toxicity-related adverse events in the treatment of chronic extensively drug-resistant tuberculosis. *EBioMedicine* 2015 Nov;2(11):1627–33.

214. Bolhuis MS et al. Clarithromycin increases linezolid exposure in multidrug-resistant tuberculosis patients. *Eur Respir J*. 2013 Dec;42(6):1614–21.

215. Rowe HE, Felkins K, Cooper SD, and Hale TW. Transfer of linezolid into breast milk. *J Hum Lact*. 2014 Nov;30(4):410–2.

216. El-Assal MI, and Helmy SA. Single-dose linezolid pharmacokinetics in critically ill patients with impaired renal function especially chronic hemodialysis patients. *Biopharm Drug Dispos*. 2014 Oct;35(7):405–16.

217. Yano T et al. Reduction of clofazimine by mycobacterial type 2 NADH:quinone oxidoreductase: A pathway for the generation of bactericidal levels of reactive oxygen species. *J Biol Chem*. 2011 Mar 25;286(12):10276–87.

218. Cholo MC et al. Effects of clofazimine on potassium uptake by a Trk-deletion mutant of *Mycobacterium tuberculosis*. *J Antimicrob Chemother*. 2006 Jan;57(1):79–84.

219. Faouzi M, Starkus J, and Penner R. State-dependent blocking mechanism of Kv 1.3 channels by the antimycobacterial drug clofazimine. *Br J Pharmacol*. 2015 Nov;172(21):5161–73.

220. Cholo MC, Mothiba MT, Fourie B, and Anderson R. Mechanisms of action and therapeutic efficacies of the lipophilic antimycobacterial agents clofazimine and bedaquiline. *J Antimicrob Chemother*. 2017 Feb 1;72(2):338–53.

221. Nix DEDE, Adam RDRD, Auclair B, Krueger TSTS, Godo PGPG, and Peloquin CACA. Pharmacokinetics and relative bioavailability of clofazimine in relation to food, orange juice and antacid. *Tuberc Edinb Scotl*. 2004;84(6):365–73.

222. Holdiness MR. Clinical pharmacokinetics of clofazimine. A review. *Clin Pharmacokinet*. 1989 Feb;16(2):74–85.

223. Gopal M, Padayatchi N, Metcalfe JZ, and O'Donnell MR. Systematic review of clofazimine for the treatment of drug-resistant tuberculosis. *Int J Tuberc Lung Dis*. 2013 Aug;17(8):1001–7.

224. Trébucq A et al. Treatment outcome with a short multidrug-resistant tuberculosis regimen in nine African countries. *Int J Tuberc Lung Dis*. 2018 Jan 1;22(1):17–25.

225. Hwang TJ et al. Safety and availability of clofazimine in the treatment of multidrug and extensively drug-resistant tuberculosis: Analysis of published guidance and meta-analysis of cohort studies. *BMJ Open*. 2014 Jan 2 [cited 2018 May 14];4(1). Available from: https://www.ncbi.nlm.nih.gov/pmc/articles/PMC3902362/

226. Yoon H-Y, Jo K-W, Nam GB, and Shim TS. Clinical significance of QT-prolonging drug use in patients with MDR-TB or NTM disease. *Int J Tuberc Lung Dis*. 2017 Sep 1;21(9):996–1001.

227. Venkatesan K, Mathur A, Girdhar A, and Girdhar BK. Excretion of clofazimine in human milk in leprosy patients. *Lepr Rev*. 1997 Sep;68(3):242–6.

228. Andries K et al. A diarylquinoline drug active on the ATP synthase of *Mycobacterium tuberculosis*. *Science* 2005 Jan 14;307(5707):223–7.

229. Torrea G et al. Bedaquiline susceptibility testing of *Mycobacterium tuberculosis* in an automated liquid culture system. *J Antimicrob Chemother*. 2015 Aug;70(8):2300–5.

230. Villellas C et al. Unexpected high prevalence of resistance-associated Rv0678 variants in MDR-TB patients without documented prior use of clofazimine or bedaquiline. *J Antimicrob Chemother*. 2017 01;72(3):684–90.

231. van Heeswijk RPG, Dannemann B, and Hoetelmans RMW. Bedaquiline: A review of human pharmacokinetics and drug–drug interactions. *J Antimicrob Chemother*. 2014 Sep;69(9):2310–8.

232. Liu K et al. Bedaquiline metabolism: Enzymes and novel metabolites. *Drug Metab Dispos*. 2014 May;42(5):863–6.

233. Diacon AH et al. The diarylquinoline TMC207 for multidrug-resistant tuberculosis. *N Engl J Med*. 2009 Jun 4;360(23):2397–405.

234. Akkerman OW et al. Pharmacokinetics of bedaquiline in cerebrospinal fluid and serum in multidrug-resistant tuberculous meningitis. *Clin Infect Dis*. 2016 Feb 15;62(4):523–4.

235. Rustomjee R et al. Early bactericidal activity and pharmacokinetics of the diarylquinoline TMC207 in treatment of pulmonary tuberculosis. *Antimicrob Agents Chemother*. 2008 Aug;52(8):2831–5.

236. Diacon AH et al. 14-day bactericidal activity of PA-824, bedaquiline, pyrazinamide, and moxifloxacin combinations: A randomised trial. *Lancet* 2012 Sep 15;380(9846):986–93.

237. Diacon AH et al. Multidrug-resistant tuberculosis and culture conversion with bedaquiline. *N Engl J Med*. 2014 Aug 21;371(8):723–32.

238. Svensson EM, Murray S, Karlsson MO, and Dooley KE. Rifampicin and rifapentine significantly reduce concentrations of bedaquiline, a new anti-TB drug. *J Antimicrob Chemother*. 2015 Apr;70(4):1106–14.

239. Svensson EM, Dooley KE, and Karlsson MO. Impact of lopina-vir-ritonavir or nevirapine on bedaquiline exposures and potential implications for patients with tuberculosis-HIV coinfection. *Antimicrob Agents Chemother.* 2014 Nov;58(11):6406–12.

240. Mukherjee T, Boshoff H. Nitroimidazoles for the treatment of TB: Past, present and future. *Future Med Chem.* 2011 Sep;3(11):1427–54.

241. Stinson K et al. MIC of delamanid (OPC-67683) against *Mycobacterium tuberculosis* clinical isolates and a proposed critical concentration. *Antimicrob Agents Chemother.* 2016;60(6):3316–22.

242. Fujiwara M, Kawasaki M, Hariguchi N, Liu Y, and Matsumoto M. Mechanisms of resistance to delamanid, a drug for *Mycobacterium tuberculosis.* *Tuberculosis.* 2018 Jan 1;108:186–94.

243. Sasahara K et al. Pharmacokinetics and metabolism of delamanid, a novel anti-tuberculosis drug, in animals and humans: Importance of albumin metabolism *in vivo.* *Drug Metab Dispos Biol Fate Chem.* 2015 Aug;43(8):1267–76.

244. Shimokawa Y et al. Metabolic mechanism of delamanid, a new anti-tuberculosis drug, in human plasma. *Drug Metab Dispos Biol Fate Chem.* 2015 Aug;43(8):1277–83.

245. Gler MT et al. Delamanid for multidrug-resistant pulmonary tuberculosis. *N Engl J Med.* 2012 Jun 7;366(23):2151–60.

246. Diacon AH et al. Early bactericidal activity of delamanid (OPC-67683) in smear-positive pulmonary tuberculosis patients. *Int J Tuberc Lung Dis.* 2011 Jul;15(7):949–54.

247. Mallikaarjun S et al. Delamanid coadministered with antiretro-viral drugs or antituberculosis drugs shows no clinically relevant drug-drug interactions in healthy subjects. *Antimicrob Agents Chemother.* 2016;60(10):5976–85.

248. Hansen JL, Ippolito JA, Ban N, Nissen P, Moore PB, and Steitz TA. The structures of four macrolide antibiotics bound to the large ribosomal subunit. *Mol Cell.* 2002 Jul;10(1):117–28.

249. Madsen CT, Jakobsen L, Buriánková K, Doucet-Populaire F, Pernodet J-L, and Douthwaite S. Methyltransferase Erm(37) slips on rRNA to confer atypical resistance in *Mycobacterium tuberculosis.* *J Biol Chem.* 2005 Nov 25;280(47):38942–7.

250. van der Paardt A-F et al. Evaluation of macrolides for possible use against multidrug-resistant *Mycobacterium tuberculosis.* *Eur Respir J.* 2015 Aug 1;46(2):444–55.

251. Brown-Elliott BA, Nash KA, and Wallace RJ. Antimicrobial sus-ceptibility testing, drug resistance mechanisms, and therapy of infections with nontuberculous mycobacteria. *Clin Microbiol Rev.* 2012 Jul;25(3):545–82.

252. de Carvalho NFG, Pavan F, Sato DN, Leite CQF, Arbeit RD, and Chimara E. Genetic correlates of clarithromycin susceptibil-ity among isolates of the *Mycobacterium abscessus* group and the potential clinical applicability of a PCR-based analysis of erm(41). *J Antimicrob Chemother.* 2018 Apr 1;73(4):862–6.

253. Chu SY, Deaton R, and Cavanaugh J. Absolute bioavailability of clarithromycin after oral administration in humans. *Antimicrob Agents Chemother.* 1992 May;36(5):1147–50.

254. Rodrigues AD, Roberts EM, Mulford DJ, Yao Y, and Ouellet D. Oxidative metabolism of clarithromycin in the presence of human liver microsomes. Major role for the cytochrome P4503A (CYP3A) subfamily. *Drug Metab Dispos Biol Fate Chem.* 1997 May;25(5):623–30.

255. Ferrero JL et al. Metabolism and disposition of clarithromycin in man. *Drug Metab Dispos Biol Fate Chem.* 1990 Aug;18(4):441–6.

256. Rodvold KA. Clinical pharmacokinetics of clarithromycin. *Clin Pharmacokinet.* 1999 Nov;37(5):385–98.

257. Honeybourne D, Kees F, Andrews JM, Baldwin D, and Wise R. The levels of clarithromycin and its 14-hydroxy metabolite in the lung. *Eur Respir J.* 1994 Jul;7(7):1275–80.

258. Fish DN, Gotfried MH, Danziger LH, and Rodvold KA. Penetration of clarithromycin into lung tissues from patients undergoing lung resection. *Antimicrob Agents Chemother.* 1994 Apr;38(4):876–8.

259. Pasipanodya JG et al. Systematic review and meta-analyses of the effect of chemotherapy on pulmonary *Mycobacterium abscessus* outcomes and disease recurrence. *Antimicrob Agents Chemother.* 2017 Nov;61(11).

260. Pasipanodya JG, Ogbonna D, Deshpande D, Srivastava S, and Gumbo T. Meta-analyses and the evidence base for microbial outcomes in the treatment of pulmonary *Mycobacterium avium-intracellular* complex disease. *J Antimicrob Chemother.* 2017 Sep 1;72(Suppl 2):i3–19.

261. Griffith DE et al. An official ATS/IDSA statement: Diagnosis, treat-ment, and prevention of nontuberculous mycobacterial diseases. *Am J Respir Crit Care Med.* 2007 Feb 15;175(4):367–416.

262. van Haarst AD et al. The influence of cisapride and clarithromycin on QT intervals in healthy volunteers. *Clin Pharmacol Ther.* 1998 Nov;64(5):542–6.

263. Zhou S et al. Mechanism-based inhibition of cytochrome P450 3A4 by therapeutic drugs. *Clin Pharmacokinet.* 2005;44(3):279–304.

264. Sedlmayr T, Peters F, Raasch W, and Kees F. Clarithromycin, a new macrolide antibiotic. Effectiveness in puerperal infections and pharmacokinetics in breast milk. *Geburtshilfe Frauenheilkd.* 1993 Jul;53(7):488–91.

265. Gopal P, and Dick T. The new tuberculosis drug Perchlozone® shows cross-resistance with thiacetazone. *Int J Antimicrob Agents.* 2015 Apr;45(4):430–3.

266. Holdiness MR. Clinical pharmacokinetics of the antituberculosis drugs. *Clin Pharmacokinet.* 1984 Dec;9(6):511–44.

267. Peloquin CA, Nitta AT, Berning SE, Iseman MD, and James GT. Pharmacokinetic evaluation of thiacetazone. *Pharmacotherapy* 1996 Oct;16(5):735–41.

268. Okwera A et al. Randomised trial of thiacetazone and rifampicin-containing regimens for pulmonary tuberculosis in HIV-infected Ugandans. The Makerere University-Case Western University research collaboration. *Lancet* 1994 Nov 12;344(8933):1323–8.

269. Nunn P et al. Cutaneous hypersensitivity reactions due to thi-acetazone in HIV-1 seropositive patients treated for tuberculosis. *Lancet Lond Engl.* 1991 Mar 16;337(8742):627–30.

270. Cordillot M et al. *In vitro* cross-linking of *Mycobacterium tuber-culosis* peptidoglycan by L,D-transpeptidases and inactivation of these enzymes by carbapenems. *Antimicrob Agents Chemother.* 2013 Dec;57(12):5940–5.

271. Hugonnet J-E, Tremblay LW, Boshoff HI, Barry CE, and Blanchard JS. Meropenem-clavulanate is effective against extensively drug-resistant *Mycobacterium tuberculosis.* *Science* 2009 Feb 27;323(5918):1215–8.

272. Hugonnet J-E, and Blanchard JS. Irreversible inhibition of the *Mycobacterium tuberculosis* beta-lactamase by clavulanate. *Biochemistry (Mosc)* 2007 Oct 30;46(43):11998–2004.

273. Davies Forsman L, Giske CG, Bruchfeld J, Schön T, Juréen P, and Ängeby K. Meropenem-clavulanate has high *in vitro* activ-ity against multidrug-resistant *Mycobacterium tuberculosis.* *Int J Mycobacteriol.* 2015;4(Suppl 1):80–1.

274. Nilsson-Ehle I, Hutchison M, Haworth SJ, and Norrby SR. Pharmacokinetics of meropenem compared to imipenem-cilas-tatin in young, healthy males. *Eur J Clin Microbiol Infect Dis.* 1991 Feb;10(2):85–8.

275. Mouton JW, Touzw DJ, Horrevorts AM, and Vinks AA. Comparative pharmacokinetics of the carbapenems: Clinical implications. *Clin Pharmacokinet.* 2000 Sep;39(3):185–201.

276. Conte JE, Golden JA, Kelley MG, and Zurlinden E. Intrapulmonary pharmacokinetics and pharmacodynamics of meropenem. *Int J Antimicrob Agents* 2005 Dec;26(6):449–56.

277 van Hasselt JGC et al. Pooled population pharmacokinetic model of imipenem in plasma and the lung epithelial lining fluid. *Br J Clin Pharmacol.* 2016;81(6):1113–23.

278. Modai J, Vittecoq D, Decazes JM, and Meulemans A. Penetration of imipenem and cilastatin into cerebrospinal fluid of patients with bacterial meningitis. *J Antimicrob Chemother.* 1985 Dec;16(6):751–5.

279. Lu C et al. Population pharmacokinetics and dosing regimen optimization of meropenem in cerebrospinal fluid and plasma in patients with meningitis after neurosurgery. *Antimicrob Agents Chemother.* 2016 Oct 21;60(11):6619–25.

280. England K et al. Meropenem–Clavulanic acid shows activity against *Mycobacterium tuberculosis in vivo. Antimicrob Agents Chemother.* 2012 Jun;56(6):3384–7.

281. Tiberi S et al. Comparison of effectiveness and safety of imipenem/clavulanate- versus meropenem/clavulanate-containing regimens in the treatment of MDR- and XDR-TB. *Eur Respir J.* 2016;47(6): 1758–66.

282. Sauberan JB, Bradley JS, Blumer J, and Stellwagen LM. Transmission of meropenem in breast milk. *Pediatr Infect Dis J.* 2012 Aug;31(8):832–4.

KEY SOURCES NOT SPECIFICALLY CITED

Drugbank, PubChem, Summaries of Product Characteristics, FDA Label, and WHO MDR-TB Companion.

11

New Developments in Drug Treatment

ALEXANDER S. PYM, CAMUS NIMMO, AND JAMES MILLARD

INTRODUCTION

Short-course chemotherapy (SCC) for tuberculosis (TB), using four drugs (isoniazid, rifampicin, pyrazinamide and ethambutol) over 6 months is low cost, highly efficacious, and generally well tolerated. In clinical trial settings, it dependably delivers a cure rate approaching 95% for drug-susceptible TB.[1] Apart from high early mortality rates, good clinical outcomes can also be obtained for HIV co-infected TB patients with 6 months treatment when used with antiretroviral therapy.[2] However, the duration of treatment has proved an insurmountable obstacle to effective implementation of SCC in many areas of the world. Failure of TB programs to ensure patient adherence to therapy and insufficiently optimized regimens has resulted in poor clinical outcomes, ongoing infectiousness, and selection of antibiotic resistance. An ultra-short course of chemotherapy is therefore an urgent priority. While stratification of low-risk patients may allow some reductions in treatment duration[3] to shorten treatment to weeks, new drugs are needed that more effectively target the tiny subpopulations of bacteria that survive the first few bactericidal weeks of SCC, usually referred to as "sterilizing" ability. However formidable challenges remain, as demonstrated by the failure of treatment shortening attempts using fluoroquinolones,[4] as we still do not know the biological basis of persistent organisms in the face of SCC and have no *in vitro* or animal models that confidently replicate persistent organisms.

In contrast to a radical shortening of TB therapy, developing a new generation of drugs for multidrug-resistant tuberculosis (MDR-TB) and extensively drug-resistant tuberculosis (XDR-TB) is more straightforward. While treatment for MDR-TB traditionally required a minimum of 20 months' therapy, the World Health Organization (WHO) drug-resistant TB 2019 guidelines have now incorporated a shorter 9–12-month regimen, which already has been adopted in many countries.[5-7] These regimens consist of repurposed drugs or those rejected for drug-susceptible TB because of their poor efficacy or intolerable toxicity. Traditional MDR-TB regimens are poorly effective, rarely delivering programmatic success rates above 60%, whilst the outcomes of the new shorter regimens, although effective in clinical trial settings, still require further programmatic data.[6,8] Hence, the introduction of several new drugs would have an immediate impact. In fact with the increasing use of bedaquiline since its approval by the US Food and Drug and Administration (FDA) in December 2012, the identification of two other novel classes of anti-TB drugs (DprE1 and MmpL3 inhibitors), appreciation of the mycobacterial action of existing drug classes (oxazolidinones and nitroimidazoles) and better use of currently available drugs (fluoroquinolones and riminophenazines) there is a high probability that significant improvements in MDR-TB and XDR-TB will be achieved relatively soon. This chapter reviews these tangible advances in the development of drugs that are in or shortly to enter clinical development.

FINDING NEW DRUGS

RESPIRATORY CHAIN INHIBITORS

Diarylquinolines (DARQs), a new class of anti-TB compounds were identified in 1996, from a whole-cell screen of 70 000 compounds using *Mycobacterium smegmatis,* a fast-growing non-pathogenic surrogate of *M. tuberculosis.*[9] DARQs are structurally and mechanically different from fluoroquinolones and other quinolines. Subsequent structure—activity studies on leads from the screens resulted in bedaquiline,[10] formerly known as TMC207 and R207910. Bedaquiline is highly active against *M. tuberculosis,* with a minimum inhibitory concentration (MIC) in the range of 0.03–0.12 µg/mL, as well as against a broad range of other mycobacteria.[10] Its mechanism of action was elucidated using whole genome sequencing of drug-resistant mutants that localized resistance to *atpE*. This gene encodes a protein that is part of the F_1F_0 proton ATP synthase, a trans-membrane protein complex that generates ATP from proton translocation. Further functional studies have identified a binding site of drug to ATP synthase, although importantly human mitochondrial ATP synthase is more than 10,000-fold less sensitive than its mycobacterial equivalent, critical for a good safety profile.[11] However, resistant mutants have been identified that do not have any mutations in *atpE*,[12] and *atpE* mutations appear rare in clinical isolates. The majority of bedaquiline resistance in clinical isolates to date has been related to mutations in the *Rv0678* gene, which encodes a negative transcriptional regulator of the MmpL5 efflux pump, which can cause cross-resistance to bedaquiline and clofazimine.[194,195] Loss of function mutations in *pepQ*, which encodes a cytoplasmic peptidase, have also been proposed to caused bedaquiline and clofazimine cross-resistance, although the importance of this in human clinical isolates has yet to be demonstrated.[66]

ATP synthase is an attractive drug target because it is essential, and ATP is required even in persistent bacterial states.[13] Therefore it was not surprising to find that bedaquiline is active on dividing and non-dividing bacteria[14] and displays time-dependent bactericidal activity both *in vitro* and *in vivo*. It has been extensively studied in the murine model and has emerged as a potential key component of new drug regimens.[15] It is highly active given as mono-therapy and can substitute for any of the three first-line drugs,[10,16] exhibits strong synergy with PZA[17] and can shorten MDR-TB treatment.[18] With the aim of developing a universal regimen, active against drug-susceptible and -resistant organisms various combinations of pretomanid (PA-824), clofazimine, sutezolid, bedaquiline, rifapentine and pyrazinamide were evaluated in a long-term mouse model. In terms of relapse-free cure after SCC, only regimens with bedaquiline were successful indicating its importance to new regimens.[15]

In December 2012, the FDA gave expedited approval of bedaquiline for the treatment of MDR-TB in adults with limited options. A phase II clinical study (C208) was conducted in treatment naive MDR-TB patients over two stages in which participants received either placebo or bedaquiline in combination with standard MDR-TB treatment. The first stage involved 2 months of bedaquiline treatment ($n = 47$) and the second stage 6 months of treatment ($n = 160$). For both stages, the time to sputum culture conversion, and proportion of patients culture negative were significantly improved in the bedaquiline arms.[19] In the 6-month stage, the median time to culture conversion was 12 weeks and 18 weeks and the proportion culture converted was 78.8% and 57.6%, in the bedaquiline and placebo arms, respectively. This ingenious two-stage design also allowed for intensive pharmacokinetic analysis in stage I to validate the dosing regimen (400 mg daily for 2 weeks, and then 200 mg thrice weekly) for the larger stage 2 to ensure drug accumulation of bedaquiline (a drug with an extremely long half-life) did not occur.

A follow-on trial (C209) was an open-label single-arm study ($n = 233$) to assess safety in a larger number of patients. It confirms that bedaquiline is generally well tolerated. Of concern is the cumulative effect on the QTc interval, a potentially serious cardiac arrhythmogenic condition. For bedaquiline, relative to the placebo,

there was a modest increase of approximately 12 ms, but this was more than doubled in patients also taking clofazimine. Other drugs such as fluoroquinolones and pretomanid also increase the QTc interval, which might place limitations on combining these drugs. In addition, there was a non-significant increase in mortality in the bedaquiline arm of C208, but this occurred late after bedaquiline had finished, and was not related to cardiac causes of death. While safety data from further phase III studies such as STREAM stage 2 (NCT02409290) are awaited, to date, severe QTc prolongation appears to be an infrequent cause of bedaquiline interruption.[20] Meanwhile, further promising data continue to emerge about the use of bedaquiline for drug-resistant TB in programmatic settings[21–23] and from the Nix-TB clinical trial for XDR-TB treatment.[24]

The imidazopyridine telacebec (Q203) also targets the mycobacterial respiratory chain, inhibiting cytochrome bc1 by binding to its QcrB subunit, leading mycobacteria to switch to the use of cytochrome bd. This induces less efficient respiration and is associated with ATP depletion. Telacebec was discovered using high-throughput phenotypic screening of over 120,000 compounds for activity against *M. tuberculosis* in infected macrophages. The compound has an *M. tuberculosis* MIC <2.5 μg/mL (including MDR strains) and at a dose of 10 mg/kg has an efficacy in a mouse model comparable to isoniazid or bedaquiline over 28 days. In a similar manner to bedaquiline, activity in the murine model is not immediate and this is presumably due to a requirement for cumulative respiratory inhibition to reach a threshold for cell death. Resistance conferring mutations occur in the qcrB gene which encodes the cytochrome bc1 complex.[25,26] The drug has progressed through a phase 2a EBA study and provisional results are available. The drug was tested in doses up to 300 mg and was well tolerated with dose-dependent EBA. Telacebec will now be tested in the adaptive design phase 2c STEP trial in combination with various doses of rifampicin and pyrazinamide.

MYCOBACTERIAL MEMBRANE PROTEIN, LARGE 3 (MMPL3) INHIBITORS

Although SQ109 is indisputably an anti-TB compound with a new mode of action, it was identified through a program to modify ethambutol, the weakest of the four drugs used in SCC.[27,28] Ethambutol was a rational choice as historically its structure—activity relationship had not been exhaustively evaluated. Also there was evidence from early clinical trials that its efficacy was markedly superior when used at high doses, subsequently abandoned because of associated ocular toxicity.[29,30] Using a library of over 60,000 combinatorial compounds, based on the 1,2-ethylenediamine active pharmacophore from ethambutol, researchers identified a diethylamine with promising *in vitro* activity against *M. tuberculosis*.[31] It has an MIC range of 0.11–0.64 μg/mL against *M. tuberculosis*, including MDR-TB strains resistant to ethambutol.[31] It inhibits growth of *M. tuberculosis* in macrophages to a similar extent as isoniazid and to a greater extent than ethambutol.[32]

Ethambutol inhibits the synthesis of arabinogalactan and lipoarabinomannan[33] and probably interacts with three arabinosyltransferases EmbA, EmbB and EmbC. Initial studies showed SQ109 induced a different transcriptional signature from ethambutol in drug-stressed bacteria, indicating a distinct mode of action.[34] Although SQ109-resistant mutants have not been reported, strains resistant to closely related ethylene diamine compounds have been characterized, are cross resistant to SQ109 and have mutations in *mmpl3*,[35] an essential gene.[36] This encodes a transporter of the RND family that is required for the export of trehalose monomycolate (TMM), an essential component of the cell wall,[36] and is compatible with the observation that TMM accumulates in cells treated with SQ109.[35] Intriguingly, other screens have independently selected compounds that appear to target MmpL3. These include AU1235, an adamantyl derivative with structural similarity[36] and two other compounds; a pyrrole derivative,[37,38] and a benzimidazole[39] whose structures bear no resemblance to SQ109. Whole cell screens are not unbiased and perhaps they preferentially select for compounds active against MmpL3. Nevertheless the essentiality of MmpL3, and its key role in cell wall assembly means compounds targeting this transporter could be active clinically, and ultimately it will be interesting to see the head to head comparison of all MmpL3 inhibitors with SQ109 (the only MmpL3 inhibitor in clinical development).

Further characterization of SQ109 has demonstrated it could potentially be combined with a wide range of anti-TB drugs. *In vitro*, at sub-MIC concentrations, SQ109 demonstrates synergy with rifampicin and isoniazid.[40] In murine models of TB the 25 mg/kg dose of SQ109 was found to be equivalent to the 100 mg/kg of ethambutol.[31] This superiority of SQ109 over ethambutol at standard doses was also seen when the two drugs were compared in combination with rifampicin, isoniazid and pyrazinamide in a 2-month treatment model.[41] Pharmacokinetics of SQ109 studied in the mouse suggest the rapid tissue distribution that results in sustained concentrations in lungs (at least 40-fold above the MIC) and spleen may be important for the promising activity seen in the murine model.[32]

SQ109 has also been favorably combined with second-line anti-TB drugs as well as some investigational agents. Activity *in vitro* was either synergistic or additive with a wide range of MDR-TB treatment drugs and the pharmacokinetics in mice of SQ109 were not affected by moxifloxacin.[27] Combinations of SQ109 with bedaquiline were additive with a new oxazolidinone, sutezolid, when tested *in vitro*. Both improved the rate of *M. tuberculosis* killing over individual drugs.[42,43] In a whole blood assay both drugs were found to have an additive affect, but some antagonism with pretomanid was detected.[44] Preliminary studies have recently shown that SQ109, bedaquiline and pyrazinamide combined *in vivo* in a mouse model of TB induced a durable cure of *M. tuberculosis*, and suggested at least equivalence to standard regimens.[27]

In humans, SQ109 appears safe over 14 days' therapy, but the phase 2 trial did not find significant activity as a sole agent or any enhancement of rifampicin efficacy at 150 or 300 mg doses.[45] The SQ109 arms of a multi-arm, multi-stage open-label randomized-controlled trial of rifampicin-susceptible TB substituting ethambutol for SQ109 were stopped early due to failure to meet prespecified efficacy thresholds.[46] However, a phase 2b study in MDR-TB showed an improvement in 6-month culture conversion,[47] suggesting that this drug may still be a useful addition to the armamentarium, at least for drug-resistant TB.

DPRE1 INHIBITORS

Parallel drug discovery efforts have also converged on another essential step in the complex assembly of the mycobacterial cell wall, DprE1, a flavoenzyme responsible for the epimerization of ribose to arabinose. This pathway provides a unique source of arabinose for both lipoarabinomannan and arabinogalactan, building blocks of the cell wall. The benzothiazinone compound BTZ043 was the first from this group to undergo significant development.[48] After nitroreduction by DprE1, BTZ043 covalently binds to a cysteine residue within the active site of DprE1, irreversibly inactivating the enzyme.[49–51] Laboratory-selected spontaneous resistant mutations have been localized to *dprE1* and were uncommon, arising at a frequency of 10^{-8}.[48] Encouragingly, it has a very low MIC (2.3 nM against H37Rv) including against MDR strains.[52] It is principally active against dividing organisms in line with its mode of action against the cell wall, and in short-term mouse studies (28 days of monotherapy) has activity similar to rifampicin.[48] Combination studies conducted *in vitro* show it has synergistic activity against *M. tuberculosis* with bedaquiline and at least additive effects with a range of other first- and second-line anti-TB drugs.[53]

To date 15 new classes of DprE1 inhibitor with antimycobacterial activity have been identified. Six, including BTZ043, form covalent adducts with cysteine 387 in the active site of DprE1, while the other nine are competitive non-covalent inhibitors. Macozinone (previously known as PBTZ169) is another covalent inhibitor that arose from a lead optimization program of BTZ043 and has a very low MIC of 0.6 nM against H37Rv. Like BTZ043, it acts synergistically with bedaquiline[54] as well as clofazimine, delaminid, and sutezolid.[55] It is currently in a phase Ib clinical trial (NCT03776500) by Innovate Medicines for Tuberculosis (Lausanne, Switzerland). It was investigated in parallel in a phase 2a trial (NCT03334734) by Nearmedic Plus in Russia, although this was terminated early due to slow recruitment. Results of this have not been published although the company indicated that it had demonstrated good safety and statistically significant early bactericidal activity (EBA) in seven patients.[56]

From the non-covalent inhibitors identified, the most promising is TCA1 which was identified by screening for inhibitors of *M. tuberculosis* biofilm formation. It is active against two different enzymes: DprE1 and MoeW, which are involved in molybdenum cofactor biosynthesis and are essential for the hypoxic and nitric-oxide stress response. TCA1 resistant mutants remain susceptible to BTZ043 suggesting that it has a different DprE1 binding mechanism. Interestingly, TCA1 also downregulates *fdxA*, a gene associated with persistence, and unlike BTZ is active *in vitro* against both replicating and non-replicating mycobacteria.[57]

The diversity of lead compounds increases the chances of developing a clinically viable drug against the promising DprE1 target.

IMPROVING EXISTING DRUGS

OXAZOLIDINONES

The oxazolidinones are one of a few structurally new classes of antibiotics to be approved in the last 30 years. Currently there is only one oxazolidinone licensed by the US FDA; linezolid, approved in 2000, for the treatment of Gram-positive infections. Many compounds in the class have been evaluated since oxazolidinones were first patented in 1978,[58] the success of linezolid has stimulated the development of newer members of the class, with the aim of improving the safety profile or extending the antibacterial profile.[58] These include three new agents with promising anti-TB activity that have completed at least phase I trials and remain under development; sutezolid (PNU-100480), delpazolid (LCB01–100480) and posizolid (AZD5847).

Linezolid has been recommended for the treatment of all cases of drug-resistant TB,[7] although it is not yet licensed for TB treatment. Its mechanism of action is common to all oxazolidinones but unique amongst anti-TB drugs, ensuring no cross-resistance. It inhibits protein synthesis by binding to 23 s rRNA in the 50 s ribosomal subunit, which is also the site for drug resistance conferring mutations, although other loci might be involved and spontaneous mutations are thought to occur less frequently than for other drugs. Linezolid has high oral bioavailability and an MIC for M. tuberculosis of 0.125–0.5 μg/mL.[59] Its activity evaluated in mouse studies is modest.[60] At 100 mg/kg once daily (a dose equivalent to 600 mg orally in humans) it appeared to be bacteriostatic or weakly bactericidal, causing an approximately 1–1.5 log reduction in bacterial counts over 28 days.[61]

Nonetheless, linezolid has clear clinical efficacy and has become an important anti-tuberculous drug, particularly in the treatment of drug-resistant TB.[62-65] In a recent individual patient data meta-analysis of 12 030 patients with drug-resistant TB, which led directly to the prioritization of linezolid for drug-resistant TB treatment, linezolid was strongly associated with improved outcomes and reduced mortality.[23] However, the use of linezolid for TB treatment is limited by toxicity, principally high rates of myelosuppression and neuropathies.[65,24] Toxicity is thought to be cumulative and side effects are reduced at lower doses, hence doses lower than the licensed 600 mg BD dose are used in many settings, but the implications of these strategies on efficacy and avoidance of the development of resistance are not well characterized.

Results from the open-label Nix-TB trial, combining linezolid with bedaquiline and pretomanid, for patients with difficult-to-treat MDR TB and XDR-TB, demonstrated cure by 6 months in almost all surviving patients, with very low rates of relapse 6 months post treatment completion.[24] The Zenix trial now aims to identify the optimal dose and duration of linezolid within the Nix-TB regimen (NCT03086486). Linezolid also now forms part of treatment shortening trial regimens for drug-sensitive TB (NCT03474198), and drug-resistant TB (NCT02754765, NCT02454205, NCT02589782).

Sutezolid is structurally highly similar to linezolid, differing only by a single sulfur atom, but has superior anti-TB activity.[60] Its MIC is approximately 2–4-fold lower than linezolid for a range of clinical isolates,[67] and in the mouse model it is bactericidal and more active than linezolid.[60,68] Combined with first-line therapy it was able to accelerate the time to culture conversion in the lungs of mice, confirming that it has sterilizing activity.[69] Combining sutezolid with bedaquiline, clofazimine, and pretomanid in a murine model resulted in a regimen that was highly active and achieved low relapse rates after only 3 months of therapy.[15] There was no evidence of antagonism between these agents and this suggests an oxazolidinone could become a key part of a new universal regimen. Sutezolid has now demonstrated EBA over the course of 14 days in humans, a result that was not previously seen with

linezolid and appears to confirm the improved antimycobacterial activity of sutezolid over linezolid. Rates of mitochondrial inhibition are likely to be lower with sutezolid and this is reflected in lower rates of clinical toxicity in limited duration human studies, however, these results need to be replicated over longer treatment periods.[70,71] A phase IIb dose-finding study is now planned (NCT03959566).

Delpazolid (LCB01-0371) appears more potent than linezolid for a range of Gram-positive infections[72] and thus is an attractive candidate for assessment of its potential to treat TB. It has demonstrated activity against clinical drug-resistant Mycobacterium tuberculosis isolates in vitro, albeit with a 2-fold higher MIC_{90} than linezolid.[73] The drug has now gone forward for testing in an EBA study, interim results of which suggest that the drug is well tolerated, with modest EBA.[74-76] Posizolid (AZD5847) appears to have a similar or higher range of Mycobacterium tuberculosis MICs to delpazolid, but improved extra-, and particularly, intracellular killing of Mycobacterium tuberculosis compared to linezolid.[77,78] In a murine chronic infection model, posizolid activity was intermediate between linezolid and sutezolid.[79] However, in a murine model of non-replicating TB, posizolid activity was minimal compared to linezolid and sutezolid.[80] This observation, combined with the relatively high MIC and less favorable pharmacokinetics of posizolid compared to sutezolid and linezolid,[81] may explain the modest activity, which was inferior to that previously described for linezolid, in a recent EBA study.[82] It is unlikely that posizolid will advance further.

NITROIMIDAZOLES

The development of nitroimidazoles to the point where there are two currently in clinical use and clinical trials; delamanid (OPC-67683)[83] and pretomanid (PA-824),[84] is an example of drug development by chemical modification of an existing structure.[85,86] The first clinically active nitroimidazole was metronidazole (MTZ) discovered in the mid-1950s in a screen for drugs active against trichominiasis. MTZ was subsequently found to be effective therapy against a wide range of anaerobes. Since M. tuberculosis anaerobically adapts to survive in hypoxic granulomas,[87] it was rational to try and engineer nitroimidazoles to be more active against mycobacteria. MTZ itself has a maximal effect on M. tuberculosis under anaerobic conditions in vitro,[88] but it exhibits inconsistent activity in animal models of TB.[87,89-91] Some early attempts to develop a new generation of nitroimidazoles were thwarted by problems of mutagenesis.[92] But two independent initiatives succeeded by sidechain modification of the nitroimidazole structure, resulting in a nitroimidazo-oxazine (pretomanid) and a nitroimidazo-oxazole (delamanid). Both of these compounds have good activity against M. tuberculosis grown aerobically and anaerobically, and are active in the mouse and guinea-pig models of TB when given as monotherapy or in combination with other anti-TB drugs.[83,84,93-97]

Pretomanid and delamanid are both pro-drugs, which require nitroreductive activation. The mechanisms of activation, action and resistance are very similar for both compounds. Activation for both drugs is by F(420)-deazaflavin-dependent nitroreductase (Ddn),[98,99] and in the case of pretomanid the active des-nitroimidazole has been shown to act by generating reactive nitrogen species such as nitric oxide (NO).[100] In addition there appears to be a mode of action against mycolic acid synthesis,[84] which probably accounts for the aerobic activity of the drug and has also been seen for delamanid.[83] Spontaneous resistance to pretomanid occurs at a relatively high frequency, similar to that of isoniazid (approximately 1×10^{-6}), in vitro. Mechanisms of resistance have not yet been fully studied in clinical settings.[101] But mutations in *fgd1* (a glucose-6-phosphate dehydrogenase), *fbiA*, *fbiB*, and *fbiC* (cofactor biosynthesis proteins), genes required for cofactor F(420) synthesis needed for a functional nitroreductase as well as in *ddn* that encodes the nitroreductase itself have all been documented in pretomanid- and delamanid-resistant strains[102] selected for in vitro.[103,104] However, there is some evidence that cross-resistance between nitroimidazoles may not be complete.[105] The number of potential drug-resistant conferring genetic loci for pretomanid may partially explain the high spontaneous mutation rate. Thus far, mutations in *fbiA* and *fgd1* have been identified in phenotypically delamanid-resistant clinical isolates.[106,107]

Both pretomanid and delamanid are in clinical development, but currently under different trajectories. Otsuka (https://www.otsuka.co.jp/en/), has focused on evaluating delamanid as a drug for MDR-TB, in contrast to the Global Alliance for Tuberculosis Drug Development (http://www.tballiance.org/), which aims to position pretomanid in an optimized regimen for drug susceptible and now, drug-resistant TB.

Two EBA studies have been completed for delamanid, only one of which has been published to date.[108] It was a 14-day dose ranging study of 100–400 mg given as monotherapy and demonstrated drug activity. The mean fall in bacterial load was less than that seen for rifampicin or isoniazid in a reference study.[109]

The results of a phase IIb study in MDR-TB patients has shown that this modest activity in terms of EBA can translate into significant benefit in terms of culture conversion.[110] In a randomized, multinational clinical trial, 481 patients with pulmonary MDR-TB received either delamanid (at 100 mg or 200 mg twice daily) or placebo for 2 months in combination with a WHO-approved background MDR-TB regimen. The proportion of patients with sputum culture conversion at 2 months was significantly increased in the patients receiving delamanid (41.9% in the 200 mg group in contrast to 29.6% in the placebo group). A proportion of the patients were rolled over to receive a further 6 months of open-label delamanid. Overall, favorable outcomes (a combination of cure and completed treatment) were significantly increased in patients in the long-term (≥6 months) treatment group (74.5%), as compared to those in the short-term (≤2 months) delamanid treatment group (55%). On this basis, the European Medicines Agency (EMA) recommended conditional marketing authorization for delamanid in adults with MDR-TB without other treatment options. Results for the long-awaited phase III, randomized, placebo-controlled trial of delamanid for MDR TB have recently been released.[111] Five hundred and eleven participants were randomized in a 2:1 ratio to either delamanid or placebo in addition to an optimized background regimen. The primary outcome was time to sputum culture conversion over 6 months and hence, only participants who were culture positive at baseline (64%) were assessed in the modified intention-to-treat analysis, leading to imbalances between the delamanid and placebo groups, with

higher rates of bilateral cavitation and resistance beyond MDR in the delamanid group. Even accounting for this, the results were disappointing, no difference in time to stable culture conversion and 87.6 versus 86.1% culture conversion at 6 months in the delamanid and placebo arms, respectively (RR 1.017; 95% CI 0.927–1.115). There were no differences in rates of clinical success or mortality. Whilst these results suggest that delamanid-based regimens will not allow treatment-shortening for MDR TB, it will likely retain a role when resistance or intolerance to other agents precludes building an adequate regimen.[107] Delamanid is known to cause QTc prolongation and hence a key question for its future use has become whether it can safely be used in combination with bedaquiline in order to increase the options for treating MDR TB. A recent phase II trial randomized patients with MDR TB to receive delamanid, bedaquiline, or both as part of their regimen for the first 24 weeks and showed that QTc prolongation from baseline was modest in all arms and was no more than additive when bedaquiline and delamanid were used together. This provides reassurance that these drugs could safely be used together.[112]

In contrast to delamanid, pretomanid has been extensively evaluated in murine models of TB to determine which are its optimal companion drugs. Initial studies demonstrated it had dose-dependent bactericidal activity during both the initial phase and continuation phases of therapy equivalent to rifampicin and isoniazid[113] and could successfully replace isoniazid in combination therapy without showing potential to shorten therapy.[114] However, a series of subsequent studies has suggested pretomanid in various combinations, such as with moxifloxacin–pyrazinamide (PaMZ),[115] moxifloxacin–pyrazinamide–bedaquiline (BPaMZ),[116] bedaquiline–pyrazinamide (BPaZ),[117] bedaquiline–linezolid (BPaL)[118] or bedaquiline–sutezolid[15] could shorten therapy. The latter combination is particularly attractive as it contains no existing first- or second-line drugs, and therefore represents a universal therapy for all forms of susceptible and drug-resistant TB. More recent work has suggested that the addition of pretomanid to the BPaL or BPaMZ regimens independently increased bactericidal activity, prevented emergence of bedaquiline resistance and shortened the duration of treatment needed for relapse-free cure. This suggests that pretomanid may be central to the apparent utility of these regimens.[119]

Experience with rifapentine and fluoroquinolones (described later) suggests that enhanced sterilizing activity seen in the mouse model does not always translate clinically and studies have been initiated to evaluate pretomanid in clinical trials. Two EBA studies with dose ranging pretomanid monotherapy have showed bactericidal activity reaches a plateau above 200 mg daily.[120,121] Using this dose of pretomanid in combination with pyrazinamide and moxifloxacin (PaMZ), it was possible to achieve bactericidal activity over 14 days, although not significantly so given the small numbers of patients.[122] Similarly, in an 8-week phase IIb study of this regimen in participants with both drug-sensitive and MDR TB, bactericidal activity was superior in those with drug-sensitive TB and at least as good in those with MDR TB compared to the RHZE control regimen in drug-sensitive TB patients.[123] The BPaZ and BPaZM regimens were tested amongst patients with drug-sensitive and drug-resistant TB, respectively, in an EBA study (NCT02193776).[124] Validating the murine studies, BPaMZ led to significantly faster mycobacterial clearance than BPaZ and both were superior to the standard regimen. This led to a 8-week phase IIb study, again of BPaZ (with either standard or daily dosing of bedaquiline) in drug-sensitive and BPaZM in drug-resistant TB. Mycobacterial clearance was significantly faster in all investigational arms compared to standard treatment, although higher rates of discontinuation were noted in these arms.[125] The PaMZ regimen was utilized in a phase III treatment shortening trial (NCT02342886) for drug-sensitive and MDR TB. However, this trial had to be stopped early as a result of an unexpectedly high rate of hepatotoxicity. The BPaMZ regimen is also currently being tested in a phase III treatment shortening trial (NCT03338621). Both of these trials aim to reduce drug-sensitive and MDR TB treatment to 4 and 6 months, respectively. The BPaL regimen was assessed in the Nix TB study (see earlier) and this has now led to FDA approval for pretomanid,[24] but only as part of this regimen for XDR TB and difficult to treat MDR TB.[126]

REUSING OLD DRUGS

FLUOROQUINOLONES

Quinolones are synthetic antibiotics originally identified as a by-product of chloroquine synthesis.[127] Since the introduction of nalixidic acid for the treatment of urinary tract infections in 1967, quinolones have been extensively developed to improve their pharmacokinetics, and broaden their spectrum of activity.[128] Lately this focused on developing fluoroquinolones for the treatment of respiratory tract infections caused by *Streptococcus pneumoniae* and other pathogens. Some of these fluoroquinolones were found to have good activity against *M. tuberculosis* and are established as one of the most important drugs in regimens to treat MDR-TB, being consistently and strongly associated with successful treatment outcomes in meta-analyses.[8,23] They now form a core part of WHO-recommended MDR-TB treatment regimens.[7] Their excellent oral bioavailability and bactericidal action, lack of cross-resistance with existing TB drugs and favorable safety profile has also resulted in them being evaluated in the treatment of drug-susceptible TB.

The 8-methoxy-fluoroquinolones, gatifloxacin and moxifloxacin, are two quinolones with the most potent anti-TB activity and were evaluated for their ability to shorten drug-sensitive TB treatment from 6 to 4 months. Compared to the earlier fluoroquinolones such as ciprofloxacin and ofloxacin, gatifloxacin and moxifloxacin have lower MICs[129] and superior activity against non-replicating *M. tuberculosis in vitro*,[130] although gatifloxacin was withdrawn from the market in 2008 as it was associated with a high rate of dysglycemic events.[131] In addition, at clinically recommended doses they have better bioavailability[132] resulting in superior pharmacodynamic parameters such as AUC_{24}/MIC_{90} ratio. This prompted researchers to evaluate whether a fluoroquinolone, such as moxifloxacin, substituted or added to first-line treatment regimens, could shorten therapy by 2 months. Despite impressive results from long-term experiments in the murine model,[133,134] this did not translate to humans in three large phase III clinical trials.[135–137] Although the fluoroquinolone-containing regimens

reported more culture negative results at 2 months, they had higher rates of unfavorable outcome at 18 months largely due to a higher relapse rate. Fluoroquinolones therefore appear not to have sufficient activity against persister bacteria to reduce treatment to less than 6 months and are now only being evaluated as part of treatment regimens for TB resistant to first-line drugs. Current work is now focusing on whether stratification of patients from these trials is able to identify an easy-to-treat phenotype that may be amenable to a 4-month regimen.[3]

The use of fluoroquinolones could be compromised in the future by the emergence of drug resistance. The fluoroquinolones inhibit bacterial topoisomerases, enzymes that regulate DNA coiling. In *M. tuberculosis*, their drug target is DNA gyrase, encoded by *gyrA* and *gyrB*, and resistance conferring mutations often occur in these two genes,[138] although drug efflux is also a mechanism.[139] The widespread use of fluoroquinolones to treat respiratory infections means patients with undiagnosed TB are being treated with fluoroquinolone monotherapy which can select for drug resistance even after limited drug exposure,[140] which was reported soon after the introduction of fluoroquinolones for TB.[141] Among 40 countries with a high TB or MDR-TB burden, fluoroquinolone resistance was detected in 20% of isolates tested.[142] This underlines the importance of developing mycobacterial specific drugs. 8-Methoxy-fluoroquinolones are excellent TB drugs and form a core part of current MDR-TB treatment and are under evaluation in a variety of other combinations (see New Regimens section).

RIFAMYCINS

The use of various rifamycins is currently being reassessed to determine their optimal usage. All rifamycins target the beta subunit of RNA polymerase thereby preventing transcription, and the principal mechanism of resistance is through mutations in *rpoB* that encodes the polymerase. Unlike cell wall inhibitors whose mode of action is dependent on cell division, transcriptional inhibitors should be active even in quiescent states as some degree of transcription will be required for cell viability. It is this activity that is thought to underpin the sterilizing activity that effectively resulted in the shortening of TB therapy from 18 to 9 months with the introduction of rifampicin. Interest has therefore focused on trying to extract the maximal activity out of rifamycins.

In the case of rifampicin, the currently used maximal dose of 600 mg/10 mg/kg per day was introduced for safety and cost reasons and is not at the limit of the dose-response curve.[143] In murine models, higher dose rifampicin regimens demonstrate dose-dependent increases in bactericidal activity and clearance of putative persister organisms, allowing treatment shortening and the prevention of relapse after treatment.[144,145] Several clinical studies have taken these observations forward in an attempt to identify an optimized rifampicin dose that increases efficacy whilst minimizing any additional toxicity and hence may lead to treatment shortening. HIGHRIF 1 compared safety and EBA up to 14 days with doses of rifampicin up to 35 mg/kg and demonstrated no difference in toxicity but improved bactericidal activity at higher doses.[146] HIGHRIF 2 went on to assess 600, 900 and 1200 mg daily dosing alongside standard doses of other first-line drugs during the first 2 months of therapy in a double-blind, randomized, placebo-controlled, phase II clinical trial. Again, this study demonstrated that higher doses of rifampicin are safe but without any statistically significant difference in several measures of antimycobacterial activity between the arms.[147] Similarly, the RIFATOX trial was a non-blinded, randomized, phase II trial comparing 10, 15 and 20 mg/kg rifampicin in combination with standard-dose first-line drugs during the first 4 months of treatment, with no increase in adverse events or efficacy as defined by 2-month culture conversion.[148] The HRIF trial was a randomized phase II trial of doses of 10, 15 and 20 mg/kg rifampicin alongside standard first-line therapy over the course of the first 8 weeks of treatment. A statistically significant improvement in CFU count decline was seen at the 20 mg/kg dose.[149] This is the only one of these studies to examine the effect of rifampicin exposure rather than just dose (defined by area under the time–concentration curve [AUC]) on mycobacterial clearance and identified a faster elimination rate with increased rifampicin exposure in the per-protocol analysis. In the MAMS-TB-01 trial, 20 and 35 mg/kg of rifampicin were combined with various first-line drugs, moxifloxacin and SQ109. There was no difference in adverse events between the arms and only the arm with 35 mg/kg rifampicin had accelerated culture conversion (median 48 vs. 62 days, $p = 0.003$) compared to standard therapy, although this was only seen for liquid and not solid media.[46] Taken together, these results confirm that higher doses of rifampicin, up to 35 mg/kg, are safe, but without clear evidence that this dose of rifampicin will enable treatment shortening. It has been suggested that this dose is still too low and there is evidence that the top of the exposure—response curve has not been obtained at these doses; indeed the lowest dose to achieve relapse-free, shortened treatment in the murine model was 80 mg/kg.[145] To this end, doses of 40 and 50 mg/kg have been recently investigated, with initial reports that the 50 mg/kg dose is associated with unacceptable rates of adverse events, suggesting that 40 mg/kg may be the maximum tolerated dose.[150] Doses of 1200 and 1800 mg of rifampicin are currently being tested as part of an open-label phase III trial aiming to shorten treatment to 4 months (NCT02581527). Higher rifampicin doses may also have a particular role in special situations, for instance, TB meningitis where optimization of CSF exposure may lead to mortality benefits.[151] This was not demonstrated in a recent randomized-controlled trial, although again the rifampicin dose (15 mg/kg) may have been too low to show benefit.[152,153] A potential limitation of this strategy, yet unstudied in detail, are the management of drug—drug interactions (DDIs) that result from cytochrome P450 induction and would likely be increasingly problematic at higher doses of rifampicin.

An alternative approach to increasing rifamycin exposure is through the use of rifapentine, which has a longer half-life of 14–18 hours as well as a lower TB MIC[154] generating a better AUC_{24}/MIC_{90} ratio. Evaluation of rifapentine treatment in combination with moxifloxacin in the murine model suggested this combination given either intermittently or daily could be used to shorten therapy.[155,156] However, the phase III RIFAQUIN study combining twice weekly rifapentine at standard dosing and moxifloxacin for 4 months did not achieve adequate cure rates to allow treatment shortening. Daily dosing of rifapentine has also been assessed. A head to head comparison of daily rifapentine

and rifampicin, both at 10 mg/kg showed no difference in terms of culture conversion at 2 months,[157] Daily 7.5 mg/kg rifapentine and moxifloxacin (replacing rifampicin and ethambutol, respectively) reduced time to stable culture conversion over 8 weeks in liquid (but not solid) media but not rates of culture conversion, compared to standard therapy.[158] Interestingly, in this study moxifloxacin exposures were much lower than those seen in studies combining intermittent rather than daily rifapentine with moxifloxacin and like rifampicin, studies with rifapentine suffer the same limitations in terms of DDIs. Both of these studies of daily rifapentine were initiated on the basis of promising results in mouse models, which failed to translate to findings in humans.[155,156,159] The TBTC study 31 is ongoing and will also test rifapentine with or without moxifloxacin at the higher dose of 1200 mg for the duration of treatment in an attempt to shorten treatment length to 4 months (NCT02410772). In addition to the potential for treatment shortening, these studies are important because if successful they would provide a strong rationale for developing a newer generation of potent and tolerable RpoB inhibitors.

β-LACTAMS

β-Lactam antibiotics form a large bactericidal class, that include penicillins, cephalosporins, monobactams, and carbapenems, whose mode of action is inhibition of transpeptidases which are required for crosslinking (transpeptidation) of the peptidoglycan layer. They have been of little relevance to mycobacterial therapeutics because *M. tuberculosis* has a single, highly active class A β-lactamase, BlaC. This enzyme hydrolyzes a broad spectrum of β-lactams; conferring resistance. Genetically knocking out *blaC* that encodes the β-lactamase,[160] or chemically inhibiting BlaC with the β-lactam inhibitor clavulinic acid does reduce the MIC, but in the case of amoxicillin and ampicillin the MIC remains relatively high in reference strains.[160] For this reason the combination of amoxicillin with clavulinic acid is not classified as a TB drug by WHO, being of questionable benefit.[7]

Carbapenem β-lactam antibiotics, imipenem, ertapenem and meropenem, in combination with the β-lactamase inhibitor clavulinic acid offer a better alternative. Carbapenems bind high-molecular weight penicillin-binding proteins, inactivating the L,D-transpeptidases that form cell wall crosslinks[161] and are less susceptible to BlaC. For example, the MIC for meropenem—clavulinic acid has been reported in a range from 0.32 to 1.28 μg/mL for drug-susceptible reference strains of *M. tuberculosis*.[162,163] There have been some favorable clinical reports with carbapenems[164] but the results from mouse studies have been equivocal with the meropenem—clavulinic acid combination.[165,166] A fall in bacterial counts in treated mice was only seen in one of the studies where the carbapenem was given at a dose of 300 mg/kg. Recently, the currently available formulation of ceftazidime, an older cephalosporin, in combination with avibactam, a potent inhibitor of BlaC, was identified to have anti-mycobacterial activity in an *in vitro* screen which was followed by further evaluation in the hollow fiber system. It demonstrated good sterilization of drug-resistant isolates at clinically achievable concentrations and may offer another option where alternatives are limited.[167]

The development of faropenem, a structurally similar compound that has been modified for oral administration, has displayed bactericidal activity against *M. tuberculosis in vitro* even in the absence of clavulanic acid,[168] and offers a more practical option than other drugs in the class that require parenteral administration.

Interestingly there was greater variability in the MIC for both amoxicillin and carbapenems amongst drug-resistant clinical isolates, with some strains having MICs for amoxicillin−clavulinic acid of less than 1 μg/mL.[162,163] This suggests some drug-resistant strains, including XDR-TB strains, might be hyper-susceptible to β-lactams relative to drug-sensitive *M. tuberculosis*, and therefore more amenable to therapy with them.

The widespread use of β-lactam antibiotics means they have relatively well-established safety profiles and can be used for pediatric MDR-TB, where drug options are far more limited than for adults. However, due to their broad spectrum of action they are at risk of affecting the host microbiome and their common use for other indications means that, as for the fluoroquinolones, there is a risk that undiagnosed patients may be exposed to them as monotherapy, promoting the development of resistance.

CLOFAZIMINE

Clofazimine, a riminophenazine, was initially developed in the 1950s for the treatment of *M. tuberculosis*[164] but found its place in the treatment of leprosy. Its mode of action has only recently been partly elucidated and remains incomplete. Redox cycling is likely to be important, whereby clofazimine undergoes cycles of enzymatic reduction, generating reactive oxygen species that are toxic to the cell.[169] In addition, destabilization and dysfunction of the mycobacterial membrane, perhaps as a consequence of the accumulation of lysophospholipids and interference with potassium ion uptake may be of importance.[170,171] As for bedaquiline, resistance is conferred by mutations in *Rv0678* (which lead to drug efflux) and potentially *pepQ*.[170,171] Additionally, mutations in Rv1979c, which encodes a putative permase, may confer clofazimine monoresistance, although similarly to pepQ, the significance of these mutations in clinical isolates remains undetermined.[196] It is active against persister organisms *in vitro*[172] and has been successfully combined with bedaquiline and pyrazinamide[15] to effectively treat mice in a relapse-free short-course regimen. Perhaps most remarkable are its lipophilic properties that result in massive tissue accumulation in spleen, liver, and other organs.[173] In the lungs of mice chronically treated with clofazimine it can reach tissue concentrations of >100-fold the MIC of 0.5 μg/mL. Part of this accumulation is the formation of crystal-like drug inclusion bodies[174] and accumulation has also been reported in human lung samples.

Interest refocused on its potential as an anti-TB agent after reports of a highly successful short-course treatment for MDR-TB in a cohort of patients from Bangladesh.[5] Using a 9-month treatment protocol a relapse-free cure was obtained in 87% of patients. In combination with clofazimine the regimen included high-dose isoniazid and gatifloxacin alongside other standard MDR-TB drugs. The regimen's success may have been dependent on a high proportion of patients with pyrazinamide-susceptible strains or strains with low-level isoniazid resistance, rather than the activity

of clofazimine alone. However, it did show that even with currently available drugs in select patient groups high success rates can be achieved with short courses of treatment. Subsequently, a meta-analysis of 12 030 patients from 25 countries, used to inform WHO guidelines, identified an adjusted risk difference of 0.06 (95% CI 0.01–0.10) for treatment success versus failure or relapse with the use of clofazimine.[23] This has led to the re-positioning of clofazimine as a priority drug in the treatment of MDR TB.

HOST-DIRECT THERAPY

The challenge to identify and develop sufficient new drugs that are both active against *M. tuberculosis* and have an acceptable human safety profile while attempting to prevent acquisition and spread of resistance has led to increased interest in modulation of the human immune response through host-directed therapies to improve the efficacy of antibiotics and potentially shorten treatment, reduce TB-related immunopathology and enhance immunological memory to prevent relapse.

VITAMIN D

Vitamin D was first identified as a potential treatment for TB through the use of cod liver oil in 1849[175] and has more recently been shown to enhance mycobacterial killing by macrophages and resolution of inflammatory responses during TB treatment.[176] Deficiency has been associated with an increased risk of TB in two meta-analyses,[177,178] although, in one, this relationship was not found in subgroup analyses on African patients and HIV-infected patients.

Despite these associations, no evidence was found to indicate that adding vitamin D to standard TB treatment improves outcomes in a meta-analysis of five studies,[179] a subsequent double-blind placebo controlled trial[180] or Cochrane review of eight studies.[181] A more recent individual patient meta-analysis suggested that vitamin D supplementation did reduce time to sputum culture conversion in patients with MDR-TB but not drug-susceptible TB, although numbers with MDR-TB were small and follow-up was limited to 8 weeks.[182] At present there is little evidence to suggest that any benefit is of clinical relevance.

METFORMIN

Metformin, a synthetically derived biguanide from the *Galega officinalis* plant, was introduced as a glucose-lowering treatment for type 2 diabetes mellitus (T2DM) in the 1950s. In addition to other proposed mechanisms of action, it is known to inhibit the mitochondrial respiratory chain in the human liver by activating AMP-activated protein kinase (AMPK), which switches on catabolic pathways generating cellular ATP and stops those involved in gluconeogenesis, leading to a reduction in glucose. It is of particular interest given that T2DM is associated with both an increased risk of developing active TB[183] and worse outcomes once on treatment.[184]

Metformin-induced AMPK activation has an anti-inflammatory effect through promoting formation of anti-inflammatory M2 macrophages and T-regulatory and CD8 memory T cells and regulation of cellular autophagy, a key mechanism in the control of intracellular pathogens like *M. tuberculosis*.[185] Recent work showed that macrophages exposed to metformin *in vitro* had greater antimycobacterial activity through increased production of reactive oxygen species and promotion of phago-lysosome fusion. In the same study, TB-infected mice treated with metformin had reduced lung pathology and chronic inflammation and enhanced mycobacterial clearance when used in combination with isoniazid or ethambutol.[186] However, another study showed that when metformin was combined with the full four-drug first-line regimen there was no statistically significant increase in bactericidal activity.[187]

Retrospective cohort data from patients with T2DM taking TB treatment has shown that those taking metformin had lower mortality than those not in a mechanism independent of improved blood glucose control.[188] However, these retrospective data may be prone to confounding as metformin is commonly prescribed as a first-line treatment for T2DM, with other treatments such as insulin often added to rather than replacing metformin, and because patients prescribed other medications often have other comorbidities such as renal failure.

In summary, for patients with T2DM and TB co-infection, while retrospective data suggest a benefit to metformin use, pending further prospective clinical studies there remain insufficient data to make any specific recommendations. In patients without diabetes mellitus, it is possible that metformin may have some additive effect to TB treatment through immune modulation, but translation to clinical use will first require a more comprehensive understanding of its action *in vitro* and in the mouse model.[185]

NEW REGIMENS

To prevent resistance development during prolonged therapy and to target differentially metabolically active mycobacterial subpopulations, antituberculous therapy is delivered in multi-drug regimens. However, new drugs are usually either added to, or used to replace, a single drug in existing multi-drug regimens for both drug-sensitive and MDR TB. The characteristics of an "ideal" regimen (or "target regimen profiles", TRPs) for drug-sensitive TB, MDR TB and a "universal" regimen have been outlined by the WHO. Increasingly, potential regimens are identified on the basis of their possible advantages, e.g., all oral treatment, high activity, synergism or lack of use in existing regimens, and then assessed in a systematic fashion using *in vitro*, murine, 14-day phase IIa (of monotherapy or combinations) and 8-week phase IIb combination studies in humans. However, this process is hampered by the lack of a clearly defined optimal pathway whereby these pre-clinical and early-phase clinical studies (and the various measures of anti-mycobacterial activity that come with them) are able to predict clinically important outcomes. Several solutions have been proposed to reduce the risk of phase III trial failures and more efficiently shepherd efficacious regimens into clinical use. There is increasing interest in phase IIc trials in which the same outcomes are measured, with a similar sample size to that in other phase II studies, but the experimental regimen is given for the full duration planned for the phase III trial, and 12-month post-treatment completion outcomes are assessed. These studies

might best be combined with a Bayesian statistical approach in order to provide actionable outcomes, predicting the chances of success if a given regimen was moved into phase III.[189] An alternative or potentially complementary approach is the multi-arm multi-stage (MAMS) trial design where multiple experimental arms are evaluated simultaneously, with poorly performing arms dropped early, minimizing time, expense and sample size, thus advancing the most promising regimens.

CONCLUSIONS

The US FDA approval of Bedaquiline is a milestone in the development of new anti-TB drugs.[10] Bedaquiline is highly selective for mycobacteria, but its target, ATP synthase, is an essential energy-generating mechanism, found throughout all kingdoms of life. Modification of bedaquiline has led to compounds active against other clinically important bacteria,[190,191] so it also represents the discovery of a novel class of antibiotics. It is reminiscent of the discovery of streptomycin in 1943 as part of a search for anti-TB agents, that not only led to the first effective regimen for the treatment of TB in combination with isoniazid and para-aminosalicylic acid, but also spawned a class of antibiotics, aminoglycosides,[192] that have found wide therapeutic applications in infectious diseases. It is plausible that bedaquiline, in combination with other new or repurposed compounds, may herald the beginning of a similar era in the advancement of TB treatment last seen in the 1950s and 1960s.

Even the introduction of a single new drug, such as bedaquiline, into MDR-TB regimens can have a significant impact. It will be particularly useful to patients who have developed treatment-limiting toxicity or have additional resistance, and it is increasingly taking the place of injectable agents in long MDR and XDR-TB treatment regimens around the world, as seen in the recent World Health Organization guidelines. Some countries such as South Africa are already experimenting with it in place of an injectable agent in the short-course MDR-TB regimen, with apparent success, although the effectiveness of this remains to be confirmed by stage 2 of the STREAM trial. The development of bedaquiline, combined with the availability of new and repurposed drugs such as pretomanid, linezolid, and clofazimine, has sparked a series of trials aiming to shorten treatment and improve outcomes for drug-resistant TB, such as ZeNix (NCT03086486) and TB-PRACTECAL (NCT02589782).

Scrutiny of safety will be particularly important where evaluating new regimens in drug-susceptible patients who have a high chance of a favorable outcome with existing SCC. Some regimens with new anti-TB drugs have performed particularly well in the mouse model compared with SCC, and appear to be able to effect relapse-free cure with only 3 months of therapy.[15,193] These need to be tested in clinical trials, but the experience of rifapentine and moxifloxacin suggests that the mouse model may not always be predictive of short-course efficacy in humans. Nevertheless, there are now a sufficient number of drug classes to configure a potentially "universal" regimen, without any cross-resistance to existing agents, that could be evaluated for treatment of all TB patients, regardless of drug susceptibility.

REFERENCES

1. Lienhardt C et al. Efficacy and safety of a 4-drug fixed-dose combination regimen compared with separate drugs for treatment of pulmonary tuberculosis: The Study C randomized controlled trial. *JAMA: J Am Med Assoc.* 2011;305(14):1415–23.

2. Khan FA et al. Treatment of active tuberculosis in HIV-coinfected patients: A systematic review and meta-analysis. *Clini Infec Dis: Off Publ Infec Dis Soc Am.* 2010;50(9):1288–99.

3. Imperial MZ et al. A patient-level pooled analysis of treatment-shortening regimens for drug-susceptible pulmonary tuberculosis. *Nat Med.* 2018;24(11):1708–15.

4. Nimmo C, Lipman M, Phillips PP, McHugh T, Nunn A, and Abubakar I. Shortening treatment of tuberculosis: Lessons from fluoroquinolone trials. *Lancet Infect Dis.* 2015;15(2):141–3.

5. Van Deun A et al. Short, highly effective, and inexpensive standardized treatment of multidrug-resistant tuberculosis. *Am J Respir Crit Care Med.* 2010;182(5):684–92.

6. Nunn AJ et al. A trial of a shorter regimen for rifampin-resistant tuberculosis. *N Engl J Med.* 2019;380(13):1201–13.

7. *WHO Consolidated Guidelines on Drug-Resistant Tuberculosis Treatment.* Geneva: World Health Organization, 2019.

8. Ahuja SD et al. Multidrug resistant pulmonary tuberculosis treatment regimens and patient outcomes: An individual patient data meta-analysis of 9,153 patients. *PLoS Med.* 2012;9(8):e1001300.

9. Guillemont J, Meyer C, Poncelet A, Bourdrez X, and Andries K. Diarylquinolines, synthesis pathways and quantitative structure—activity relationship studies leading to the discovery of TMC207. *Future Med Chem.* 2011;3(11):1345–60.

10. Andries K et al. A diarylquinoline drug active on the ATP synthase of *Mycobacterium tuberculosis. Science.* 2005;307(5707):223–7.

11. Biukovic G et al. Variations of subunit {varepsilon} of the *Mycobacterium tuberculosis* F1Fo ATP synthase and a novel model for mechanism of action of the tuberculosis drug TMC207. *Antimicrob Agents Chemother.* 2013;57(1):168–76.

12. Huitric E, Verhasselt P, Koul A, Andries K, Hoffner S, and Andersson DI. Rates and mechanisms of resistance development in *Mycobacterium tuberculosis* to a novel diarylquinoline ATP synthase inhibitor. *Antimicrob Agents Chemother.* 2010;54(3):1022–8.

13. Rao SP, Alonso S, Rand L, Dick T, and Pethe K. The proton motive force is required for maintaining ATP homeostasis and viability of hypoxic, nonreplicating *Mycobacterium tuberculosis. Proc Natl Acad Sci USA.* 2008;105(33):11945–50.

14. Koul A et al. Diarylquinolines are bactericidal for dormant mycobacteria as a result of disturbed ATP homeostasis. *J Biol Chem.* 2008;283(37):25273–80.

15. Williams K et al. Sterilizing activities of novel combinations lacking first- and second-line drugs in a murine model of tuberculosis. *Antimicrob Agents Chemother.* 2012;56(6):3114–20.

16. Ibrahim M, Truffot-Pernot C, Andries K, Jarlier V, and Veziris N. Sterilizing activity of R207910 (TMC207)-containing regimens in the murine model of tuberculosis. *Am J Respir Crit Care Med.* 2009;180(6):553–7.

17. Ibrahim M et al. Synergistic activity of R207910 combined with pyrazinamide against murine tuberculosis. *Antimicrob Agents Chemother.* 2007;51(3):1011–5.

18. Veziris N, Ibrahim M, Lounis N, Andries K, and Jarlier V. Sterilizing activity of second-line regimens containing TMC207 in a murine model of tuberculosis. *PLOS ONE.* 2011;6(3):e17556.

19. Diacon AH et al. Randomized pilot trial of eight weeks of bedaquiline (TMC207) treatment for multidrug-resistant tuberculosis: Long-term outcome, tolerability, and effect on emergence of drug resistance. *Antimicrob Agents Chemother.* 2012;56(6):3271–6.

20. Cohen K, and Maartens G. A safety evaluation of bedaquiline for the treatment of multi-drug resistant tuberculosis. *Expert Opin Drug Saf.* 2019;18(10):875–82.

21. Ndjeka N et al. High treatment success rate for multidrug-resistant and extensively drug-resistant tuberculosis using a bedaquiline-containing treatment regimen. *Eur Respir J.* 2018;52(6).

22. Borisov SE et al. Effectiveness and safety of bedaquiline-containing regimens in the treatment of MDR- and XDR-TB: A multicentre study. *Eur Respir J.* 2017;49(5).

23. Collaborative Group for the Meta-Analysis of Individual Patient Data in MDRTBt, Ahmad N et al. Treatment correlates of successful outcomes in pulmonary multidrug-resistant tuberculosis: An individual patient data meta-analysis. *Lancet.* 2018;392(10150): 821–34.

24. Conradie F et al. Treatment of highly drug-resistant pulmonary tuberculosis. *N Engl J Med.* 2020 Mar 5;382(10):893–902.

25. Pethe K et al. Discovery of Q203, a potent clinical candidate for the treatment of tuberculosis. *Nat Med.* 2013;19(9):1157–60.

26. Lamprecht DA et al. Turning the respiratory flexibility of *Mycobacterium tuberculosis* against itself. *Nat Commun.* 2016;7:12393.

27. Sacksteder KA, Protopopova M, Barry CE, 3rd, Andries K, and Nacy CA. Discovery and development of SQ109: A new antitubercular drug with a novel mechanism of action. *Future Microbiol.* 2012;7(7):823–37.

28. Lee RE, Protopopova M, Crooks E, Slayden RA, Terrot M, and Barry CE, 3rd. Combinatorial lead optimization of [1,2]-diamines based on ethambutol as potential antituberculosis preclinical candidates. *J Comb Chem.* 2003;5(2):172–87.

29. DeSimoni G. Preliminary observations of ethambutol in pulmonary tuberculosis. *Ann N Y Acad Sci.* 1966;135(2):846–8.

30. Donomae I, and Yamamoto K. Clinical evaluation of ethambutol in pulmonary tuberculosis. *Ann N Y Acad Sci.* 1966;135(2): 849–81.

31. Protopopova M et al. Identification of a new antitubercular drug candidate, SQ109, from a combinatorial library of 1,2-ethylenediamines. *J Antimicrob Chemother.* 2005;56(5):968–74.

32. Jia L et al. Pharmacodynamics and pharmacokinetics of SQ109, a new diamine-based antitubercular drug. *Br J Pharmacol.* 2005;144(1):80–7.

33. Goude R, Amin AG, Chatterjee D, and Parish T. The arabinosyltransferase EmbC is inhibited by ethambutol in *Mycobacterium tuberculosis. Antimicrob Agents Chemother.* 2009;53(10):4138–46.

34. Boshoff HI, Myers TG, Copp BR, McNeil MR, Wilson MA, and Barry CE, 3rd. The transcriptional responses of *Mycobacterium tuberculosis* to inhibitors of metabolism: Novel insights into drug mechanisms of action. *J Biol Chem.* 2004;279(38):40174–84.

35. Tahlan K et al. SQ109 targets MmpL3, a membrane transporter of trehalose monomycolate involved in mycolic acid donation to the cell wall core of *Mycobacterium tuberculosis. Antimicrob Agents Chemother.* 2012;56(4):1797–809.

36. Grzegorzewicz AE et al. Inhibition of mycolic acid transport across the *Mycobacterium tuberculosis* plasma membrane. *Nat Chem Biol.* 2012;8(4):334–41.

37. La Rosa V et al. MmpL3 is the cellular target of the antitubercular pyrrole derivative BM212. *Antimicrob Agents Chemother.* 2012;56(1):324–31.

38. Poce G et al. Improved BM212 MmpL3 inhibitor analogue shows efficacy in acute murine model of tuberculosis infection. *PLOS ONE.* 2013;8(2):e56980.

39. Stanley SA et al. Identification of novel inhibitors of *M. tuberculosis* growth using whole cell based high-throughput screening. *ACS Chem Biol.* 2012;7(8):1377–84.

40. Chen P, Gearhart J, Protopopova M, Einck L, and Nacy CA. Synergistic interactions of SQ109, a new ethylene diamine, with front-line antitubercular drugs *in vitro. J Antimicrob Chemother.* 2006;58(2):332–7.

41. Nikonenko BV, Protopopova M, Samala R, Einck L, and Nacy CA. Drug therapy of experimental tuberculosis (TB): Improved outcome by combining SQ109, a new diamine antibiotic, with existing TB drugs. *Antimicrob Agents Chemother.* 2007;51(4):1563–5.

42. Reddy VM et al. SQ109 and PNU-100480 interact to kill *Mycobacterium tuberculosis in vitro. J Antimicrob Chemother.* 2012;67(5):1163–6.

43. Reddy VM, Einck L, Andries K, and Nacy CA. In vitro interactions between new antitubercular drug candidates SQ109 and TMC207. *Antimicrob Agents Chemother.* 2010;54(7):2840–6.

44. Wallis RS et al. Rapid evaluation in whole blood culture of regimens for XDR-TB containing PNU-100480 (sutezolid), TMC207, PA-824, SQ109, and pyrazinamide. *PLOS ONE.* 2012;7(1):e30479.

45. Heinrich N et al. Early phase evaluation of SQ109 alone and in combination with rifampicin in pulmonary TB patients. *J Antimicrob Chemother.* 2015;70(5):1558–66.

46. Boeree MJ et al. High-dose rifampicin, moxifloxacin, and SQ109 for treating tuberculosis: A multi-arm, multi-stage randomised controlled trial. *Lancet Infect Dis.* 2017;17(1):39–49.

47. Borisov SE et al. Efficiency and safety of chemotherapy regimen with sq109 in those suffering from multiple drug resistant tuberculosis. *Tuberculosis Lung Dis.* 2018;96(3).

48. Makarov V et al. Benzothiazinones kill *Mycobacterium tuberculosis* by blocking arabinan synthesis. *Science.* 2009;324(5928):801–4.

49. Trefzer C et al. Benzothiazinones: Prodrugs that covalently modify the decaprenylphosphoryl-beta-D-ribose 2'-epimerase DprE1 of *Mycobacterium tuberculosis. J Am Chem Soc.* 2010;132(39):13663–5.

50. Neres J et al. Structural basis for benzothiazinone-mediated killing of *Mycobacterium tuberculosis. Sci Trans Med.* 2012;4(150):150ra21.

51. Trefzer C et al. Benzothiazinones are suicide inhibitors of mycobacterial decaprenylphosphoryl-beta-D-ribofuranose 2'-oxidase DprE1. *J Am Chem Soc.* 2012;134(2):912–5.

52. Pasca MR et al. Clinical isolates of *Mycobacterium tuberculosis* in four European hospitals are uniformly susceptible to benzothiazinones. *Antimicrob Agents Chemother.* 2010;54(4):1616–8.

53. Lechartier B, Hartkoorn RC, and Cole ST. In vitro combination studies of Benzothiazinone lead compound BTZ043 against *Mycobacterium tuberculosis. Antimicrob Agents Chemother.* 2012;56(11):5790–3.

54. Makarov V et al. Towards a new combination therapy for tuberculosis with next generation benzothiazinones. *EMBO Mol Med.* 2014;6(3):372–83.

55. Lupien A et al. Optimized background regimen for treatment of active tuberculosis with the next-generation benzothiazinone macozinone (PBTZ169). *Antimicrob Agents Chemother.* 2018;62(11).

56. Macozinone | Working Group on New TB Drugs [Available from: https://www.newtbdrugs.org/pipeline/compound/macozinone-mcz-pbtz-169.

57. Wang F et al. Identification of a small molecule with activity against drug-resistant and persistent tuberculosis. *Proc Natl Acad Sci USA.* 2013;110(27):E2510–7.

58. Shaw KJ, and Barbachyn MR. The oxazolidinones: Past, present, and future. *Ann N Y Acad Sci.* 2011;1241:48–70.

59. Schon T et al. Wild-type distributions of seven oral second-line drugs against *Mycobacterium tuberculosis. Int J Tuberc Lung Dis.* 2011;15(4):502–9.

60. Cynamon MH, Klemens SP, Sharpe CA, and Chase S. Activities of several novel oxazolidinones against *Mycobacterium tuberculosis* in a murine model. *Antimicrob Agents Chemother.* 1999;43(5):1189–91.

61. Fattorini L et al. Activities of moxifloxacin alone and in combination with other antimicrobial agents against multidrug-resistant *Mycobacterium tuberculosis* infection in BALB/c mice. *Antimicrob Agents Chemother.* 2003;47(1):360–2.

62. Cox H, and Ford N. Linezolid for the treatment of complicated drug-resistant tuberculosis: A systematic review and meta-analysis. *Int J Tuberc Lung Dis.* 2012;16(4):447–54.

63. Sotgiu G et al. Efficacy, safety and tolerability of linezolid containing regimens in treating MDR-TB and XDR-TB: Systematic review and meta-analysis. *Eur Respir J.* 2012;40(6):1430–42.

64. Zhang X et al. Systematic review and meta-analysis of the efficacy and safety of therapy with linezolid containing regimens in the treatment of multidrug-resistant and extensively drug-resistant tuberculosis. *J Thorac Dis.* 2015;7(4):603–15.

65. Lee M et al. Linezolid for treatment of chronic extensively drug-resistant tuberculosis. *N Engl J Med.* 2012;367(16):1508–18.

66. Deepak A et al. Mutations in pepQ confer low-level resistance to bedaquiline and clofazimine in *Mycobacterium Tuberculosis. Antimicrob Agents Chemother.* 2016;22;60(8):4590–9.

67. Alffenaar JW et al. Susceptibility of clinical *Mycobacterium tuberculosis* isolates to a potentially less toxic derivate of linezolid, PNU-100480. *Antimicrob Agents Chemother.* 2011;55(3):1287–9.

68. Williams KN et al. Promising antituberculosis activity of the oxazolidinone PNU-100480 relative to that of linezolid in a murine model. *Antimicrob Agents Chemother.* 2009;53(4):1314–9.

69. Williams KN et al. Addition of PNU-100480 to first-line drugs shortens the time needed to cure murine tuberculosis. *Am J Respir Crit Care Med.* 2009;180(4):371–6.

70. Wallis RS et al. Mycobactericidal activity of sutezolid (PNU-100480) in sputum (EBA) and blood (WBA) of patients with pulmonary tuberculosis. *PLOS ONE.* 2014;9(4):e94462.

71. Wallis RS et al. Biomarker-assisted dose selection for safety and efficacy in early development of PNU-100480 for tuberculosis. *Antimicrob Agents Chemother.* 2011;55(2):567–74.

72. Jeong JW et al. In vitro and *in vivo* activities of LCB01-0371, a new oxazolidinone. *Antimicrob Agents Chemother.* 2010;54(12):5359–62.

73. Zong Z et al. Comparison of in vitro activity and MIC distributions between the novel oxazolidinone delpazolid and linezolid against multidrug-resistant and extensively drug-resistant *Mycobacterium tuberculosis* in China. *Antimicrob Agents Chemother.* 2018;62(8).

74. Kim TS et al. Activity of LCB01-0371, a novel oxazolidinone, against *Mycobacterium abscessus. Antimicrob Agents Chemother.* 2017;61(9).

75. A Phase II Clinical Study of LCB01-0371 to Evaluate the EBA, Safety and PK (NCT02836483) [Internet]. Available from: https://clinicaltrials.gov/ct2/show/NCT02836483.

76. Geiter L, ed. Trial of Delpazolid (LCB01-0371) to assess early bactericidal activity and exposure response relationships. *TB Science*; 2019; Hyderabad, India.

77. Balasubramanian V et al. Bactericidal activity and mechanism of action of AZD5847, a novel oxazolidinone for treatment of tuberculosis. *Antimicrob Agents Chemother.* 2014;58(1):495–502.

78. Werngren J et al. In vitro activity of AZD5847 against geographically diverse clinical isolates of *Mycobacterium tuberculosis. Antimicrob Agents Chemother.* 2014;58(7):4222–3.

79. Balasubramanian V et al. Pharmacokinetic and pharmacodynamic evaluation of AZD5847 in a mouse model of tuberculosis. *Antimicrob Agents Chemother.* 2014;58(7):4185–90.

80. Zhang M et al. *In vitro* and *in vivo* activities of three oxazolidinones against nonreplicating *Mycobacterium tuberculosis*. *Antimicrob Agents Chemother*. 2014;58(6):3217–23.

81. Alsultan A et al. Population pharmacokinetics of AZD-5847 in adults with pulmonary tuberculosis. *Antimicrob Agents Chemother*. 2017;61(10).

82. Furin JJ et al. Early bactericidal activity of AZD5847 in patients with pulmonary tuberculosis. *Antimicrob Agents Chemother*. 2016;60(11):6591–9.

83. Matsumoto M et al. OPC-67683, a nitro-dihydro-imidazooxazole derivative with promising action against tuberculosis *in vitro* and in mice. *PLoS Med*. 2006;3(11):e466.

84. Stover CK et al. A small-molecule nitroimidazopyran drug candidate for the treatment of tuberculosis. *Nature*. 2000;405(6789):962–6.

85. Mukherjee T, and Boshoff H. Nitroimidazoles for the treatment of TB: Past, present and future. *Future Med Chem*. 2011;3(11):1427–54.

86. Denny WA, and Palmer BD. The nitroimidazooxazines (PA-824 and analogs): Structure–activity relationship and mechanistic studies. *Future Med Chem*. 2010;2(8):1295–304.

87. Via LE et al. Tuberculous granulomas are hypoxic in guinea pigs, rabbits, and nonhuman primates. *Infect Immun*. 2008;76(6):2333–40.

88. Wayne LG, and Sramek HA. Metronidazole is bactericidal to dormant cells of *Mycobacterium tuberculosis*. *Antimicrob Agents Chemother*. 1994;38(9):2054–8.

89. Driver ER et al. Evaluation of a mouse model of necrotic granuloma formation using C3HeB/FeJ mice for testing of drugs against *Mycobacterium tuberculosis*. *Antimicrob Agents Chemother*. 2012;56(6):3181–95.

90. Klinkenberg LG, Sutherland LA, Bishai WR, and Karakousis PC. Metronidazole lacks activity against *Mycobacterium tuberculosis* in an *in vivo* hypoxic granuloma model of latency. *J Infect Dis*. 2008;198(2):275–83.

91. Lin PL et al. Metronidazole prevents reactivation of latent *Mycobacterium tuberculosis* infection in macaques. *Proc Natl Acad Sci USA* 2012;109(35):14188–93.

92. Ashtekar DR, Costa-Perira R, Nagrajan K, Vishvanathan N, Bhatt AD, and Rittel W. In vitro and *in vivo* activities of the nitroimidazole CGI 17341 against *Mycobacterium tuberculosis*. *Antimicrob Agents Chemother*. 1993;37(2):183–6.

93. Sasaki H et al. Synthesis and antituberculosis activity of a novel series of optically active 6-nitro-2,3-dihydroimidazo[2,1-b]oxazoles. *J Med Chem*. 2006;49(26):7854–60.

94. Saliu OY, Crismale C, Schwander SK, and Wallis RS. Bactericidal activity of OPC-67683 against drug-tolerant *Mycobacterium tuberculosis*. *J Antimicrob Chemother*. 2007;60(5):994–8.

95. Lenaerts AJ et al. Preclinical testing of the nitroimidazopyran PA-824 for activity against *Mycobacterium tuberculosis* in a series of *in vitro* and *in vivo* models. *Antimicrob Agents Chemother*. 2005;49(6):2294–301.

96. Chen X et al. Delamanid kills dormant *Mycobacteria* in vitro and in a guinea pig model of tuberculosis. *Antimicrob Agents Chemother*. 2017;61(6).

97. Stinson K et al. MIC of Delamanid (OPC-67683) against *Mycobacterium tuberculosis* clinical isolates and a proposed critical concentration. *Antimicrob Agents Chemother*. 2016;60(6):3316–22.

98. Cellitti SE et al. Structure of Ddn, the deazaflavin-dependent nitroreductase from *Mycobacterium tuberculosis* involved in bioreductive activation of PA-824. *Structure*. 2012;20(1):101–12.

99. Manjunatha UH et al. Identification of a nitroimidazo-oxazine-specific protein involved in PA-824 resistance in *Mycobacterium tuberculosis*. *Proc Natl Acad Sci USA*. 2006;103(2):431–6.

100. Singh R et al. PA-824 kills nonreplicating *Mycobacterium tuberculosis* by intracellular NO release. *Science*. 2008;322(5906):1392–5.

101. Feuerriegel S et al. Impact of Fgd1 and ddn diversity in *Mycobacterium tuberculosis* complex on *in vitro* susceptibility to PA-824. *Antimicrob Agents Chemother*. 2011;55(12):5718–22.

102. Lee BM et al. Predicting nitroimidazole antibiotic resistance mutations in *Mycobacterium tuberculosis* with protein engineering. *PLoS Pathog*. 2020;16(2):e1008287.

103. Fujiwara M, Kawasaki M, Hariguchi N, Liu Y, and Matsumoto M. Mechanisms of resistance to delamanid, a drug for *Mycobacterium tuberculosis*. *Tuberculosis (Edinb)*. 2018;108:186–94.

104. Haver HL et al. Mutations in genes for the F420 biosynthetic pathway and a nitroreductase enzyme are the primary resistance determinants in spontaneous *in vitro*-selected PA-824-resistant mutants of *Mycobacterium tuberculosis*. *Antimicrob Agents Chemother*. 2015;59(9):5316–23.

105. Hurdle JG et al. A microbiological assessment of novel nitrofuranylamides as anti-tuberculosis agents. *J Antimicrob Chemother*. 2008;62(5):1037–45.

106. Acquired Resistance to Bedaquiline and Delamanid in Therapy for Tuberculosis. *N Engl J Med*. 2015;373(25):e29.

107. Hoffmann H et al. Delamanid and bedaquiline resistance in *Mycobacterium tuberculosis* ancestral Beijing genotype causing extensively drug-resistant tuberculosis in a Tibetan refugee. *Am J Respir Crit Care Med*. 2016;193(3):337–40.

108. Diacon AH et al. Early bactericidal activity of delamanid (OPC-67683) in smear-positive pulmonary tuberculosis patients. *Int J Tuberc Lung Dis*. 2011;15(7):949–54.

109. Jindani A, Dore CJ, and Mitchison DA. Bactericidal and sterilizing activities of antituberculosis drugs during the first 14 days. *Am J Respir Crit Care Med*. 2003;167(10):1348–54.

110. Gler MT et al. Delamanid for multidrug-resistant pulmonary tuberculosis. *N Engl J Med*. 2012;366(23):2151–60.

111. von Groote-Bidlingmaier F et al. Efficacy and safety of delamanid in combination with an optimised background regimen for treatment of multidrug-resistant tuberculosis: A multicentre, randomised, double-blind, placebo-controlled, parallel group phase 3 trial. *Lancet Respir Med*. 2019;7(3):249–59.

112. Dooley KE et al. QT effects of bedaquiline, delamanid or both in MDR-TB patients: The deliberate trial. *Conference on Retroviruses and Opportunistic Infections*, Seattle, Washington, USA, 2019.

113. Tyagi S et al. Bactericidal activity of the nitroimidazopyran PA-824 in a murine model of tuberculosis. *Antimicrob Agents Chemother*. 2005;49(6):2289–93.

114. Nuermberger E et al. Combination chemotherapy with the nitroimidazopyran PA-824 and first-line drugs in a murine model of tuberculosis. *Antimicrob Agents Chemother*. 2006;50(8):2621–5.

115. Nuermberger E et al. Powerful bactericidal and sterilizing activity of a regimen containing PA-824, moxifloxacin, and pyrazinamide in a murine model of tuberculosis. *Antimicrob Agents Chemother*. 2008;52(4):1522–4.

116. Li SY et al. Bactericidal and sterilizing activity of a novel regimen with bedaquiline, pretomanid, moxifloxacin, and pyrazinamide in a murine model of tuberculosis. *Antimicrob Agents Chemother*. 2017;61(9).

117. Tasneen R et al. Sterilizing activity of novel TMC207- and PA-824-containing regimens in a murine model of tuberculosis. *Antimicrob Agents Chemother*. 2011;55(12):5485–92.

118. Tasneen R et al. Contribution of oxazolidinones to the efficacy of novel regimens containing bedaquiline and pretomanid in a mouse model of tuberculosis. *Antimicrob Agents Chemother*. 2016;60(1):270–7.

119. Xu J et al. Contribution of pretomanid to novel regimens containing bedaquiline with either linezolid or moxifloxacin and pyrazinamide in murine models of tuberculosis. *Antimicrob Agents Chemother*. 2019;63(5).

120. Diacon AH et al. Early bactericidal activity and pharmacokinetics of PA-824 in smear-positive tuberculosis patients. *Antimicrob Agents Chemother*. 2010;54(8):3402–7.

121. Diacon AH et al. Phase II dose-ranging trial of the early bactericidal activity of PA-824. *Antimicrob Agents Chemother*. 2012;56(6):3027–31.

122. Diacon AH et al. 14-day bactericidal activity of PA-824, bedaquiline, pyrazinamide, and moxifloxacin combinations: A randomised trial. *Lancet*. 2012;380(9846):986–93.

123. Dawson R et al. Efficiency and safety of the combination of moxifloxacin, pretomanid (PA-824), and pyrazinamide during the first 8 weeks of antituberculosis treatment: A phase 2b, open-label, partly randomised trial in patients with drug-susceptible or drug-resistant pulmonary tuberculosis. *Lancet*. 2015;385(9979):1738–47.

124. Dawson R et al. Efficacy of bedaquiline, pretomanid, moxifloxacin & PZA (BPAMZ) against DS- & MDR-TB. *Conference on Restroviruses and Opportunistic Infections*, Seattle, Washington, USA, 2017.

125. Tweed CD et al. Bedaquiline, moxifloxacin, pretomanid, and pyrazinamide during the first 8 weeks of treatment of patients with drug-susceptible or drug-resistant pulmonary tuberculosis: A multicentre, open-label, partially randomised, phase 2b trial. *Lancet Respir Med*. 2019;7(12):1048–58.

126. FDA approves new drug for treatment-resistant forms of tuberculosis that affects the lungs: Food and Drug Administration; [Available from: https://www.fda.gov/news-events/press-announcements/fda-approves-new-drug-treatment-resistant-forms-tuberculosis-affects-lungs.

127. Lesher GY, Froelich EJ, Gruett MD, Bailey JH, and Brundage RP. 1,8-Naphthyridine derivatives. A new class of chemotherapeutic agents. *J Med Pharm Chem*. 1962;91:1063–5.

128. Andriole VT. The quinolones: Past, present, and future. *Clin Infec Dis: Off Publ Infec Dis Soc Am*. 2005;41(Suppl 2):S113–9.

129. Aubry A, Veziris N, Cambau E, Truffot-Pernot C, Jarlier V, and Fisher LM. Novel gyrase mutations in quinolone-resistant and -hypersusceptible clinical isolates of *Mycobacterium tuberculosis*: Functional analysis of mutant enzymes. *Antimicrob Agents Chemother*. 2006;50(1):104–12.

130. Hu Y, Coates AR, and Mitchison DA. Sterilizing activities of fluoroquinolones against rifampin-tolerant populations of *Mycobacterium tuberculosis*. *Antimicrob Agents Chemother*. 2003;47(2):653–7.

131. Gatifloxacin (marketed as Tequin) Information: Food and Drug Administration; [Available from: https://www.fda.gov/drugs/postmarket-drug-safety-information-patients-and-providers/gatifloxacin-marketed-tequin-information.

132. Lubasch A, Keller I, Borner K, Koeppe P, and Lode H. Comparative pharmacokinetics of ciprofloxacin, gatifloxacin, grepafloxacin, levofloxacin, trovafloxacin, and moxifloxacin after single oral administration in healthy volunteers. *Antimicrob Agents Chemother*. 2000;44(10):2600–3.

133. Nuermberger EL et al. Moxifloxacin-containing regimen greatly reduces time to culture conversion in murine tuberculosis. *Am J Respir Crit Care Med*. 2004;169(3):421–6.

134. Nuermberger EL et al. Moxifloxacin-containing regimens of reduced duration produce a stable cure in murine tuberculosis. *Am J Respir Crit Care Med*. 2004;170(10):1131–4.

135. Jindani A et al. High-dose rifapentine with moxifloxacin for pulmonary tuberculosis. *N Engl J Med*. 2014;371(17):1599–608.

136. Merle CS et al. A four-month gatifloxacin-containing regimen for treating tuberculosis. *N Engl J Med*. 2014;371(17):1588–98.

137. Gillespie SH et al. Four-month moxifloxacin-based regimens for drug-sensitive tuberculosis. *N Engl J Med*. 2014;371(17):1577–87.

138. Malik S, Willby M, Sikes D, Tsodikov OV, and Posey JE. New insights into fluoroquinolone resistance in *Mycobacterium tuberculosis*: Functional genetic analysis of gyrA and gyrB mutations. *PLOS ONE*. 2012;7(6):e39754.

139. Louw GE et al. Rifampicin reduces susceptibility to ofloxacin in rifampicin-resistant *Mycobacterium tuberculosis* through efflux. *Am J Respir Crit Care Med*. 2011;184(2):269–76.

140. Devasia RA et al. Fluoroquinolone resistance in *Mycobacterium tuberculosis*: The effect of duration and timing of fluoroquinolone exposure. *Am J Respir Crit Care Med*. 2009;180(4):365–70.

141. Grimaldo ER et al. Increased resistance to ciprofloxacin and ofloxacin in multidrug-resistant *Mycobacterium tuberculosis* isolates from patients seen at a tertiary hospital in the Philippines. *Int J Tuberc Lung Dis*. 2001;5(6):546–50.

142. *Global Tuberculosis Report*. World Health Organization, 2017.

143. Steingart KR et al. Higher-dose rifampin for the treatment of pulmonary tuberculosis: A systematic review. *Int J Tuberc Lung Dis*. 2011;15(3):305–16.

144. Hu Y, Liu A, Ortega-Muro F, Alameda-Martin L, Mitchison D, and Coates A. High-dose rifampicin kills persisters, shortens treatment duration, and reduces relapse rate *in vitro* and *in vivo*. *Front Microbiol*. 2015;6:641.

145. de Steenwinkel JE et al. Optimization of the rifampin dosage to improve the therapeutic efficacy in tuberculosis treatment using a murine model. *Am J Respir Crit Care Med*. 2013;187(10):1127–34.

146. Boeree MJ et al. A dose-ranging trial to optimize the dose of rifampin in the treatment of tuberculosis. *Am J Respir Crit Care Med*. 2015;191(9):1058–65.

147. Aarnoutse RE et al. Pharmacokinetics, tolerability, and bacteriological response of rifampin administered at 600, 900, and 1200 milligrams daily in patients with pulmonary tuberculosis. *Antimicrob Agents Chemother*. 2017;61(11).

148. Jindani A et al. A randomised Phase II trial to evaluate the toxicity of high-dose rifampicin to treat pulmonary tuberculosis. *Int J Tuberc Lung Dis*. 2016;20(6):832–8.

149. Velasquez GE et al. Efficacy and safety of high-dose rifampin in pulmonary tuberculosis. A randomized controlled trial. *Am J Respir Crit Care Med*. 2018;198(5):657–66.

150. Te Brake L. Increased Bactericidal Activity but Dose-Limiting Tolerability at 50 mg/kg Rifampicin. *TB-PK Meeting*, London, UK, September 2019.

151. Svensson EM et al. Model-based meta-analysis of rifampicin exposure and mortality in Indonesian tuberculosis meningitis trials. *Clin Infec Dis: Off Publ Infec Dis Soc Am*. 2019.

152. Ruslami R et al. Intensified regimen containing rifampicin and moxifloxacin for tuberculous meningitis: An open-label, randomised controlled phase 2 trial. *Lancet Infect Dis*. 2013;13(1):27–35.

153. Heemskerk AD et al. Intensified antituberculosis therapy in adults with tuberculous meningitis. *N Engl J Med*. 2016;374(2):124–34.

154. Bemer-Melchior P, Bryskier A, and Drugeon HB. Comparison of the *in vitro* activities of rifapentine and rifampicin against *Mycobacterium tuberculosis* complex. *J Antimicrob Chemother*. 2000;46(4):571–6.

155. Rosenthal IM et al. Daily dosing of rifapentine cures tuberculosis in three months or less in the murine model. *PLoS Med*. 2007;4(12):e344.

156. Rosenthal IM, Zhang M, Almeida D, Grosset JH, and Nuermberger EL. Isoniazid or moxifloxacin in rifapentine-based regimens for experimental tuberculosis? *Am J Respir Crit Care Med.* 2008;178(9):989–93.

157. Dorman SE et al. Substitution of rifapentine for rifampin during intensive phase treatment of pulmonary tuberculosis: Study 29 of the tuberculosis trials consortium. *J Infect Dis.* 2012;206(7):1030–40.

158. Conde MB et al. A phase 2 randomized trial of a rifapentine plus moxifloxacin-based regimen for treatment of pulmonary tuberculosis. *PLOS ONE.* 2016;11(5):e0154778.

159. Rosenthal IM et al. Dose-ranging comparison of rifampin and rifapentine in two pathologically distinct murine models of tuberculosis. *Antimicrob Agents Chemother.* 2012;56(8):4331–40.

160. Flores AR, Parsons LM, and Pavelka MS, Jr. Genetic analysis of the beta-lactamases of *Mycobacterium tuberculosis* and *Mycobacterium smegmatis* and susceptibility to beta-lactam antibiotics. *Microbiology.* 2005;151(Pt 2):521–32.

161. Dubee V et al. Inactivation of *Mycobacterium tuberculosis* l,d-transpeptidase LdtMt(1) by carbapenems and cephalosporins. *Antimicrob Agents Chemother.* 2012;56(8):4189–95.

162. Hugonnet JE, Tremblay LW, Boshoff HI, Barry CE, 3rd, and Blanchard JS. Meropenem-clavulanate is effective against extensively drug-resistant *Mycobacterium tuberculosis. Science.* 2009;323(5918):1215–8.

163. Gonzalo X, and Drobniewski F. Is there a place for beta-lactams in the treatment of multidrug-resistant/extensively drug-resistant tuberculosis? Synergy between meropenem and amoxicillin/clavulanate. *J Antimicrob Chemother.* 2013;68(2):366–9.

164. Payen MC et al. Clinical use of the meropenem-clavulanate combination for extensively drug-resistant tuberculosis. *Int J Tuberc Lung Dis.* 2012;16(4):558–60.

165. Veziris N, Truffot C, Mainardi JL, and Jarlier V. Activity of carbapenems combined with clavulanate against murine tuberculosis. *Antimicrob Agents Chemother.* 2011;55(6):2597–600.

166. England K et al. Meropenem-clavulanic acid shows activity against *Mycobacterium tuberculosis in vivo. Antimicrob Agents Chemother.* 2012;56(6):3384–7.

167. Deshpande D et al. Ceftazidime-avibactam has potent sterilizing activity against highly drug-resistant tuberculosis. *Sci Adv.* 2017;3(8):e1701102.

168. Dhar N et al. Rapid cytolysis of *Mycobacterium tuberculosis* by faropenem, an orally bioavailable beta-lactam antibiotic. *Antimicrob Agents Chemother.* 2015;59(2):1308–19.

169. Yano T et al. Reduction of clofazimine by mycobacterial type 2 NADH:quinone oxidoreductase: A pathway for the generation of bactericidal levels of reactive oxygen species. *J Biol Chem.* 2011;286(12):10276–87.

170. De Bruyn EE, Steel HC, Van Rensburg EJ, and Anderson R. The riminophenazines, clofazimine and B669, inhibit potassium transport in gram-positive bacteria by a lysophospholipid-dependent mechanism. *J Antimicrob Chemother.* 1996;38(3):349–62.

171. Steel HC, Matlola NM, and Anderson R. Inhibition of potassium transport and growth of mycobacteria exposed to clofazimine and B669 is associated with a calcium-independent increase in microbial phospholipase A2 activity. *J Antimicrob Chemother.* 1999;44(2):209–16.

172. Grant SS, Kaufmann BB, Chand NS, Haseley N, and Hung DT. Eradication of bacterial persisters with antibiotic-generated hydroxyl radicals. *Proc Natl Acad Sci USA.* 2012;109(30):12147–52.

173. Baik J, Stringer KA, Mane G, and Rosania GR. Multiscale distribution and bioaccumulation analysis of clofazimine reveals a massive immune system-mediated xenobiotic sequestration response. *Antimicrob Agents Chemother.* 2013;57(3):1218–30.

174. Baik J, and Rosania GR. Macrophages sequester clofazimine in an intracellular liquid crystal-like supramolecular organization. *PLOS ONE.* 2012;7(10):e47494.

175. Williams CJB. On the use and administration of cod-liver oil in pulmonary consumption. *London J Med.* 1849;1:1–18.

176. Coussens AK et al. Vitamin D accelerates resolution of inflammatory responses during tuberculosis treatment. *Proc Natl Acad Sci USA.* 2012;109(38):15449–54.

177. Nnoaham KE, and Clarke A. Low serum vitamin D levels and tuberculosis: A systematic review and meta-analysis. *Int J Epidemiol.* 2008;37(1):113–9.

178. Huang SJ et al. Vitamin D deficiency and the risk of tuberculosis: A meta-analysis. *Drug Des Devel Ther.* 2017;11:91–102.

179. Xia J, Shi L, Zhao L, and Xu F. Impact of vitamin D supplementation on the outcome of tuberculosis treatment: A systematic review and meta-analysis of randomized controlled trials. *Chin Med J (Engl).* 2014;127(17):3127–34.

180. Daley P et al. Adjunctive vitamin D for treatment of active tuberculosis in India: A randomised, double-blind, placebo-controlled trial. *Lancet Infect Dis.* 2015;15(5):528–34.

181. Grobler L, Nagpal S, Sudarsanam TD, and Sinclair D. Nutritional supplements for people being treated for active tuberculosis. *Cochrane Database Syst Rev.* 2016;(6):CD006086.

182. Jolliffe DA et al. Adjunctive vitamin D in tuberculosis treatment: Meta-analysis of individual participant data. *Eur Respir J.* 2019;53(3).

183. Jeon CY, and Murray MB. Diabetes mellitus increases the risk of active tuberculosis: A systematic review of 13 observational studies. *PLoS Med.* 2008;5(7):e152.

184. Baker MA et al. The impact of diabetes on tuberculosis treatment outcomes: A systematic review. *BMC Med.* 2011;9:81.

185. Restrepo BI. Metformin: Candidate host-directed therapy for tuberculosis in diabetes and non-diabetes patients. *Tuberculosis (Edinb).* 2016;101S:S69–72.

186. Singhal A et al. Metformin as adjunct antituberculosis therapy. *Sci Transl Med.* 2014;6(263):263ra159.

187. Dutta NK, Pinn ML, and Karakousis PC. Metformin adjunctive therapy does not improve the sterilizing activity of the first-line antitubercular regimen in mice. *Antimicrob Agents Chemother.* 2017;61(8).

188. Degner NR, Wang JY, Golub JE, and Karakousis PC. Metformin use reverses the increased mortality associated with diabetes mellitus during tuberculosis treatment. *Clini Infec Dis: Off Publ Infec Dis Soc Am.* 2018;66(2):198–205.

189. Phillips PP et al. A new trial design to accelerate tuberculosis drug development: The Phase IIC Selection Trial with Extended Post-treatment follow-up (STEP). *BMC Med.* 2016;14:51.

190. Bald D, and Koul A. Respiratory ATP synthesis: The new generation of mycobacterial drug targets? *FEMS Microbiol Lett.* 2010;308(1):1–7.

191. Balemans W et al. Novel antibiotics targeting respiratory ATP synthesis in Gram-positive pathogenic bacteria. *Antimicrob Agents Chemother.* 2012;56(8):4131–9.

192. Jones D, Metzger HJ, Schatz A, and Waksman SA. Control of Gram-negative bacteria in experimental animals by streptomycin. *Science.* 1944;100(2588):103–5.

193. Tasneen R, Tyagi S, Williams K, Grosset J, and Nuermberger E. Enhanced bactericidal activity of rifampin and/or pyrazinamide when combined with PA-824 in a murine model of tuberculosis. *Antimicrob Agents Chemother.* 2008;10;9(7):e102135.

194. Koen Andries et al. Acquired resistance of *Mycobacterium Tuberculosis* to Bedaquiline. *PLoS One.* 2014;56(8):4131–9.

195. Villellas C et al. Unexpected high prevalence of resistance-associated Rv0678 variants in MDR-TB patients without documented prior use of clofazimine or bedaquiline. *J Antimicrob Chemother.* 2017;1;72(3):684–90.

196. Zhang S, Chen J, Cui P, Shi W, Zhang W, and Zhang Y. Identification of novel mutations associated with clofazimine resistance in Mycobacterium tuberculosis. *J Antimicrob Chemother.* 2015 Sep;70(9):2507–10.

12

BCG and Other Vaccines

RACHEL TANNER AND HELEN MCSHANE

INTRODUCTION

Prophylactic vaccination is the most effective strategy to control any infectious disease epidemic. It has served to eradicate smallpox and significantly reduce morbidity and mortality due to countless other childhood diseases including polio, pertussis, and measles. Infectious pathogens which induce a latent phase, such as *Mycobacterium tuberculosis* (*M.tb*), will be considerably more difficult to eradicate. All currently licensed vaccines, with the exception of Bacille Calmette–Guérin (BCG), are based on the induction of humoral immunity and protective antibodies. However, for diseases such as tuberculosis (TB), malaria, and human immunodeficiency virus (HIV) where cell-mediated immunity is also important for protection, a different strategy may be required. In TB, the only currently available vaccine, BCG, is effective in some populations some of the time, but overall has failed to control the global TB epidemic. A more effective vaccine regimen is urgently needed. We will review what is known about BCG and the leading approaches currently being developed in an attempt to improve on it in this chapter.

BACILLE CALMETTE–GUÉRIN

DEVELOPMENT OF BCG

BCG is a live attenuated vaccine that was developed at the Institut Pasteur in Lille, France by Albert Calmette and Camille Guérin. Continuous subculture of *Mycobacterium bovis*, the causative agent of bovine TB, led to considerable attenuation. Safety and protective efficacy was demonstrated in animal models followed by the first human immunization in 1921.[1] The initial strain of BCG was widely distributed from Europe to meet growing international demand prior to the introduction of standardized seed stocks. Further culture resulted in the establishment of distinct local strains with sometimes major differences in genetic and antigenic compositions.[2] There are now approximately 13 daughter strains collectively known by the generic term BCG. Initially given by the oral route, BCG is currently administered parenterally throughout most of the world, at or soon after birth.

SAFETY OF BCG

SAFETY PROFILE OF BCG

BCG remains one of the most widely used vaccines globally, having been administered to over 4 billion people. It has a very well-established safety profile with correct intradermal administration on the upper arm generally resulting in a local reaction of a small pustule followed by a small scar. Other possible adverse events include regional lymphadenitis and systemic disease, although the latter is associated almost exclusively with immunosuppression.[3]

As a live vaccine, BCG has always been contraindicated in the immunosuppressed including HIV-infected adults, but until recently has been considered safe for administration in HIV-infected infants. However, recent data from studies in South Africa indicated an increased risk of BCG-osis, leading to a change in the World Health Organization (WHO) recommendations.[4,5] These state that routine BCG vaccination should be withheld in HIV-prevalent regions until the HIV status of the infant is confirmed. As this is not possible until approximately 6 weeks of age, there is a significant delay in the administration of BCG during which time the infant is at risk of acquiring *M.tb* infection and potentially TB disease. Given the considerable overlap in the HIV and TB epidemics, a vaccine that can be safely administered to HIV-infected infants is urgently needed.

When instilled intravesically as immunotherapy for bladder cancer, BCG is tolerated without significant morbidity in 95% of patients.[6] Symptoms associated with the immune stimulation include urinary frequency and burning, mild malaise, and low-grade fever. Pulmonary involvement is a rare complication occurring in 0.3%–0.7% of patients, presenting as interstitial pneumonitis or miliary dissemination.[7,8] Systemic septic and/or hypersensitivity reaction occurs in approximately 1 in 15,000 treated patients.[8] Numerous BCG strains are currently in use, but no differences in side effects were noted in a meta-analysis of 24 trials.[9]

BCG DISEASE

BCG lymphadenitis is characterized by enlarged ipsilateral axillary nodes (although supraclavicular, nuchal, and cervical nodes can also be involved), and is most frequently observed in children under the age of 6 months.[10,11] Non-suppurative lymphadenitis may be considered part of the normal course of BCG vaccination and managed conservatively, usually resolving spontaneously over weeks to months.[11] In cases of suppurative lymphadenitis, nodes can rupture leading to sinus and fistula formation, and may result in residual complications. Treatment approaches include antituberculous therapy, node aspiration, and surgical excision.[12]

Systemic complications can present as osteitis/osteomyelitis or disseminated BCG disease, but are extremely rare and most commonly observed in BCG-vaccinated children with underlying primary immunodeficiency. Osteomyelitis occurs in approximately 1 in 100,000 cases and usually involves epiphysis of long tubular bones.[13] The incidence of disseminated BCG disease in vaccinated children is estimated at 2–3.4 per million with a fatality rate of 80%–85%,[12] whereas 0.4% of bladder cancer patients were reported to develop severe disseminated BCG sepsis following intravesical therapy.[14] The spectrum of symptoms of disseminated BCG disease is similar to that of TB disease, including persistent fever, night sweats, and weight loss. Negative sputum, blood, tissue, or urine cultures and polymerase chain reaction analysis for *M. bovis* are not uncommon. In such cases, a chest radiograph or bone marrow biopsy may permit diagnosis.[15–17]

There are no consensus guidelines for the treatment of systemic BCG disease, although approaches typically include the administration of corticosteroids together with a combination of antituberculous drugs excluding pyrazinamide, to which *M. bovis* is intrinsically resistant.[18] BCG-vaccine strains differ in their drug susceptibilities,[19] and acquired resistances to rifampicin, isoniazid, and ethambutol have been described.[20,21] Higher dosages and prolonged treatment are likely necessary for the management of BCG disease.[10] Immune reconstitution inflammatory syndrome can occur following the initiation of antiretroviral therapy (ART) in HIV-infected BCG-vaccinated children, or following

hematopoietic stem cell transplantation in BCG-infected patients with severe combined immunodeficiency.[22,23]

EFFECT OF BCG ON THE TUBERCULIN SKIN TEST

Despite recent development of the more specific interferon gamma release assays (IGRAs), the tuberculin skin test (TST) is still widely used in the diagnosis of *M.tb* infection; particularly in resource-poor settings. BCG immunization can result in a positive TST, which may persist for up to 25 years and confound diagnosis.[24,25] BCG interference with TST reactivity was part of the rationale for not introducing BCG into routine clinical practice in the United States. Ideally, a new TB vaccine would not interfere with the TST.

BCG EFFICACY

EFFICACY AGAINST TB

EFFICACY AGAINST *M.TB* INFECTION

It was long assumed that BCG was not protective against the establishment of *M.tb* infection, based largely on animal challenge models and autopsy studies showing no difference in incidence of pulmonary foci between the vaccinated and unvaccinated subjects.[26] Furthermore, the incidence of latent *M.tb* infection (LTBI) in endemic countries is very high despite good BCG coverage.[27,28] Opportunities to study this were previously limited by the TST which, due to cross-reactivity, is unable to distinguish between a positive response caused by *M.tb* or BCG vaccination. This is now circumvented by the availability of IGRAs, and several studies have since reported the efficacy of BCG against infection.[29–32] In a recent meta-analysis of 14 retrospective case–control studies in which participants had recent exposure to *M.tb* and had been screened for infection using IGRAs, BCG was significantly associated with protection from infection (overall risk ratio, 0.81; 95% confidence interval [CI] 0.71–0.92).[33]

EFFICACY AGAINST TB DISEASE

When administered at birth, BCG confers consistent, reliable, and cost-effective protection against TB meningitis and disseminated disease.[34–36] Withdrawal of BCG vaccination from Sweden and the former Czechoslovakia was associated with a concomitant increase in the cases of TB meningitis and mycobacterial glandular disease.[37,38] In a meta-analysis of randomized-controlled trials, the summary protective effect against miliary or meningeal TB was 86% (95% CI 65–95).[35] However, the efficacy of BCG against pulmonary disease, the most common form of TB, varies greatly by geographical location.[39] High levels of protection (>70% efficacy) have been reported in schoolchildren in the UK and Denmark, the general population in Norway, and Native Americans in Alaska.[40–43] However, protection has been negligible (<20% efficacy) in studies conducted in Southern India, Malawi, Georgia (US), and Colombia.[44–47] A meta-analysis of 14 prospective trials and 12 case–control studies estimated an overall BCG efficacy of 50%.[36]

DURATION OF PROTECTION

The MRC trial in UK adolescents demonstrated high BCG efficacy for up to 15 years following vaccination.[41] This durability was confirmed to last at least 10 years in observational studies.[48] Although a meta-analysis of 10 randomized trials estimated an average efficacy >10 years post-vaccination of just 14% (95% CI 9–32),[49] studies in Brazil and Norway suggest that protection may extend beyond this period.[50,51] A long-term follow-up study of American Indians and Alaska Natives reported protection for up to 60 years.[52] A recent case–control study in children given BCG at 12–13 years of age reported 57% protection (95% CI 33–72) at 15–20 years post-vaccination which waned between 20 and 29 years.[53]

BCG REVACCINATION

Several studies have indicated that revaccination with BCG confers no additional protection to neonatal vaccination.[54–56] However, a recent phase II placebo-controlled prevention-of-infection trial conducted in South African adolescents found that although BCG revaccination did not demonstrate efficacy in preventing initial infection, it did result in significantly reduced rates of sustained *M.tb* infection.[57]

EFFICACY AGAINST OTHER MYCOBACTERIAL DISEASES

Vaccination with BCG may confer protection against non-tuberculous mycobacterial species due to cross-reactivity with conserved, often immunodominant, antigens.[58] The estimates of protective efficacy against leprosy, caused by *Mycobacterium leprae*, vary from 20% to 90%.[45,59] Although one meta-analysis determined an overall BCG-vaccine protective effect of 41% (95% CI 16–66) for trials and 60% (95% CI 51–70) for observational studies,[60] another analysis reported just 26% (95% CI 14–37) and suggested that protection had been overestimated in observational studies.[61] Cross-protection of BCG against Buruli ulcer disease has been reported in some studies[62,63] but not in others.[64,65] Murine studies have demonstrated a protective effect of BCG against infection with *Mycobacterium avium* and *Mycobacterium kansasii*.[66] A study of neonates in the Czech Republic found that *M. avium intracellulare* complex-associated lymphadenitis was lower in BCG-vaccinated compared with unvaccinated children.[38]

EFFICACY AGAINST NON-MYCOBACTERIAL DISEASES

ALL-CAUSE MORTALITY IN INFANTS

There is evidence, predominantly from observational studies in West Africa, to suggest that BCG may have a non-specific effect on all-cause infant mortality[67–71] which is most pronounced among girls.[72,73] Protection beyond the target pathogen could be promoted by heterologous lymphocyte activation and innate immune memory,[74] as supported by recent *in vitro* studies.[75,76] However, studies in Greenland and Denmark did not identify reduced hospitalization rates due to infectious diseases other than TB in children BCG-vaccinated at birth.[77,78] Such discrepancies may

be associated with geographical differences thought to influence immunity and BCG-vaccine efficacy, as described later. A systematic review found that the receipt of BCG vaccine was associated with reduction in all-cause mortality, but reported a high risk of bias in a number of the published studies and stated uncertainty toward evidence.[79] If a non-specific effect is found to be reproducible and widely applicable in high-quality randomized-controlled trials, this must be taken into consideration when evaluating non-inferiority of BCG replacement vaccine candidates.

BLADDER CANCER THERAPY

The relationship between mycobacteria and cancer was first recognized almost a century ago.[80] Early animal studies demonstrated that BCG-infected mice were resistant to transplantation of tumor cells, leading to the discovery of tumor necrosis factor (TNF).[81,82] Intravesical BCG therapy is now the standard of care for high-risk, non-muscle-invasive bladder cancer,[83,84] demonstrating superiority over other intravesical agents.[85,86] The mechanism of action remains unclear but it has been suggested that BCG may be internalized by bladder cancer cells due to oncogenic aberrations that activate micropinocytosis, leading to recruitment of immune cells to the site and subsequent cytotoxicity and targeted killing of cancer cells.[87]

INFLAMMATORY AND AUTOIMMUNE DISEASES

As a strong inducer of Th1 immunity, BCG may confer efficacy against inflammatory and autoimmune diseases. This hypothesis has been supported by preclinical studies demonstrating protection against allergic asthma, multiple sclerosis, and insulin-dependent diabetes. Although some observational or intervention studies in humans have also indicated a beneficial effect, robust controlled prospective studies are required.[88] In a recent randomized 8-year prospective study of type 1 diabetic subjects with long-term disease, two doses of BCG resulted in stable and long-term reductions in blood sugar in a small number of diabetic subjects.[89]

REASONS FOR VARIABILITY IN BCG EFFICACY

The variability in BCG efficacy against TB disease poses the greatest challenge to new TB vaccine development. Understanding the underlying causes will be essential if we are to avoid a new generation of vaccines being subject to the same pitfall. Several hypotheses, which are not mutually exclusive, have been proposed as described next and summarized in Table 12.1.

DIFFERENCES IN BCG STRAINS

Distinct local strains of BCG show considerable variation in genetic and antigenic compositions,[2] and *in vitro* T-cell responses vary when peripheral blood mononuclear cells (PBMCs) are taken from individuals vaccinated with different strains.[90] However, the impact of these changes on protective efficacy remains unclear. Although some preclinical studies indicate a divergence of protective immunity conferred by different BCG strains,[91] others suggest comparable potency.[92] In humans, similar levels of protection were observed with BCG or an attenuated strain of *Mycobacterium microti*, suggesting that strain differences may not play a major

Table 12.1 Potential reasons for variability in BCG efficacy

Hypothesis	Related literature
Differences in BCG strains	41,48,54,90–93
Exposure to NTM	44,95–100,244
Blocking	
Masking	
Differences between host populations	39,101–104,245
Genetic	
Nutritional	
Co-infections (viral, helminth)	
Environmental influences	39,245
Sunlight exposure	
Variability in cold-chain maintenance	
Differences in circulating M.tb strains	

role in variable levels of efficacy.[41] Furthermore, the same strain of BCG has been found to be effective in some populations but not in others.[48,54] A critical review of animal and human studies found evidence to support the notion that protection afforded against TB differs between BCG-vaccine strains, but concluded that there are insufficient data to recommend one particular strain.[93]

EXPOSURE TO NON-TUBERCULOUS MYCOBACTERIA

Non-tuberculous mycobacteria (NTM) are saprophytic organisms which live in soil or water and do not cause disease except in immunosuppressed individuals. Exposure to both M.tb and NTM is greater in tropical regions, and several epidemiological observations have linked mycobacterial sensitization to the geographically associated reduction in BCG efficacy. BCG vaccination conferred effective protection in trials from which TST-positive (and therefore sensitized) donors were excluded,[41,42] whereas in populations where BCG did not perform well, in Alabama and India, greater than 68% and 95% of individuals, respectively, were purified protein derivative positive by 15–20 years of age.[44,94] In a comparative immunogenicity study, children from the UK had very low levels of baseline anti-mycobacterial immunity which were significantly increased following BCG vaccination, consistent with the known high efficacy of BCG in the UK.[41] In contrast, in Malawi, where BCG does not protect, children had high baseline levels which were not boosted by BCG.[95] A further study in Malawi found that individuals with lower immune responses to NTM showed greater interferon (IFN)-γ responses to BCG.[96] The very cross-reactivity that allows BCG to impart protection against other mycobacteria such as M. leprae may be a double-edged sword.

Palmer and colleagues proposed that exposure to environmental mycobacteria offers some level of protective immunity to TB that BCG can do little to improve on. This "masking hypothesis" is supported by guinea-pig experiments in which animals immunized with various NTM demonstrated immunity to M.tb and a reduction in the protective efficacy of a subsequent BCG vaccination.[97] Alternatively, according to the "blocking hypothesis," pre-existing immunity to antigens common across mycobacterial species may block the ability of BCG to replicate and induce a protective immune response. In a murine study, prior exposure to NTM resulted in a broad immune response that was recalled rapidly after BCG

vaccination and restricted BCG multiplication, with no protective immunity mounted against M.tb; the efficacy of non-replicating subunit vaccines was unaffected.[98] In human trials, accelerated waning of skin-test responses has been observed in Malawi and India, suggesting transient secondary responses recalled from sensitization to NTM or latent M.tb infection.[44,99] Masking and blocking are not mutually exclusive and may work together to interfere with BCG efficacy in high NTM endemic areas.

Interestingly, there is also some evidence from murine experiments that exposure to NTM can induce opposite effects on BCG efficacy depending on the route of exposure and viability of NTM.[100] Further studies applying reproducible preclinical models of NTM exposure and relating quantitative measures of NTM responses to BCG efficacy in humans are required to evaluate the role of anti-mycobacterial immunity in BCG interference. However, such assessment is hampered by the lack of sufficiently immunogenic NTM-specific antigens, with studies to date relying on the use of differential responses to purified protein derivatives from NTM and M.tb.[95]

OTHER FACTORS

The variability in BCG efficacy has also been attributed to genetic or nutritional differences between host populations, environmental influences such as sunlight exposure, variability in cold-chain maintenance, and differences in circulating M.tb strains. However, there is no convincing evidence of a major role for these factors; in particular, the finding that BCG can protect against leprosy where it fails against TB throws into question many of these hypotheses.[39]

Recent evidence from a case–control correlates of risk study found that activated T-cells, driven in part by cytomegalovirus (CMV) infection, were associated with an increased risk of TB disease in BCG-vaccinated South African infants.[101] It is possible that viral infections during the development of the BCG-specific immune response impair the development of protective immunity, as supported by previous studies in Malawi and the Gambia.[102,103] Helminth infections, which are more prevalent in tropical and subtropical regions, may also reduce the immunogenicity of BCG.[104]

PROTECTIVE IMMUNITY AGAINST MYCOBACTERIUM TUBERCULOSIS

Rational design of a more effective TB vaccination regimen relies upon an understanding of the immune mechanisms of protective immunity. In other diseases, such as meningococcal disease, the existence of a validated immunological correlate of protection greatly facilitates vaccine development.[105] There is no clear correlate of protection for TB, but we do have some understanding of immune responses that are necessary and important.

CELLULAR IMMUNITY

Due to the intracellular nature of mycobacteria, cell-mediated immunity is central to protection against M.tb and control of infection. Mice deficient in CD4+ T-cells or major histocompatibility complex class II are unable to control bacterial growth and rapidly succumb to disease.[106,107] Depletion of CD4+ T-cells causes reactivation of latent infection in mice,[107] and increased pathology and bacterial burden during the first 8 weeks of infection in non-human primates (NHPs).[108] The increased risk of TB disease due to decreased CD4+ T-cell number and function associated with HIV provides further evidence of a critical role for this cell type.[109] CD8+ T-cells contribute to protective immunity through secretion of pro-inflammatory cytokines such as IFN-γ or by direct killing of M.tb-infected cells via granule-mediated functions.[110] M.tb lipid antigens can also be presented to unconventional T-cells such as γδ T-cells, natural killer T cells, and mucosal-associated invariant T cells, stimulating effector functions that may be of importance.[111]

Upon recognition of M.tb-infected antigen presenting cells, CD4+ T-cells are primed as Th1 cells and become a primary source of IFN-γ, TNF-α, and interleukin (IL)-2. A central role for IFN-γ in activating macrophages to kill intracellular mycobacteria is well-established. Murine experiments demonstrated that IFN-γ KO mice are extremely susceptible to M.tb infection,[112] and genetic studies of Mendelian susceptibility to mycobacterial disease have indicated defects in the IFN-γ/IL-12 signaling pathway.[113] TNF-α, like IFN-γ, is involved in activation of bactericidal activity in infected macrophages. Treatment of mice with anti-TNF antibody results in fatal reactivation of persistent M.tb infection[114]; and the use of anti-TNF agents for inflammatory conditions such as rheumatoid arthritis has led to reactivation of LTBI.[115] IL-2 directly promotes T-cell expansion and survival, whereas granulocyte-macrophage colony-stimulating factor does so via the modification of dendritic cell function; increasing IL-12 production, and expression of co-stimulatory molecules on the cell surface.[116]

Humoral immunity

The role of B-cells and antibodies in the immune response to M.tb has been elusive; recent evidence suggests they play a greater role than previously thought.[117,118] Although M.tb studies in B-cell-deficient mice have had variable outcomes,[119-121] B-cells are now thought to influence cytokine production, bacillary containment, and immunopathologic progression during M.tb infection. B-cells may modulate the T-cell response, participating in T-cell priming through antigen capture and presentation.[122,123] Variable results from early serum therapy experiments led to a perceived minor role for antibodies. However, more recently monoclonal antibodies specific for mycobacterial components have been shown to protect mice against M.tb.[124,125] Children with low levels of specific immunoglobulin G (IgG) were found to be at greater risk from disseminated TB, and low antibody titers to Ag85 complex antigens have been associated with a poor disease outcome.[126,127] High titers of IgG against Ag85A were associated with reduced risk of developing TB disease in a case–control study in South African infants.[128] Potential mechanisms of antibody-mediated immunity include modulation of the macrophage–pathogen interaction via FcR-mediated phagocytosis, augmentation of complement-induced killing, antibody dependent cell-mediated cytotoxicity, and mucosal protection.[129]

Correlates of protection studies have cast doubt on the sufficiency of the cell-mediated immune response to confer protection by vaccination.[130] Although the vaccine candidate MVA85A was immunogenic, inducing a robust and durable polyfunctional CD4+ T-cell response, it did not demonstrate protective efficacy in a recent phase IIb trial.[131] The key to a successful TB vaccine may lie in the harnessing of humoral immunity in concert with a more potent cell-mediated response.

TARGET POPULATIONS FOR AN IMPROVED TB VACCINE

The populations most in need of a protective TB vaccine are those in which the burden of disease is highest and the public health impact of effective vaccination greatest. This includes infants, adolescents/young people, and HIV-infected adults. In high-burden countries, children contribute greater than 20% of the TB case load.[132] They are at higher risk of developing TB disease after exposure compared with adults, with the greatest risk in those aged less than 2 years.[133] In a study of age-related TB incidence in children in South Africa, TB incidence in children under 5 years of age was high (2.9%), and peaked at 12–23 months.[28] Interestingly, TB disease is relatively uncommon in children aged 5–12 years, but the incidence rises again sharply in adolescence.[134] Rates of smear-positive disease are highest in adolescents and young adults, and this is where the burden of transmission lies. This incidence peak also coincides with the most economically productive age, resulting in high-economic impact for endemic countries. Infection with HIV increases the risk of both new infections with M.tb and reactivation of latent M.tb infection by as much as 20% in high-burden countries.[109,135] Treatment with anti-retroviral therapy reduces this risk but not to the levels observed in HIV-negative individuals.[136]

In the adolescent/young adult and HIV-infected populations, a proportion of individuals will already be latently infected with M.tb. Thus a post-exposure vaccine designed to prevent reactivation of infection, and potentially eradicate it, would be highly desirable. It is unclear whether a vaccine designed to prevent primary disease would also be effective in this setting. Vaccines may also be designed as an immunotherapeutic to be administered as an adjunct to chemotherapy in patients with active disease, particularly in cases of drug-resistant TB. Several candidates in the current TB vaccine pipeline have been developed with this aim.[137,138]

NEW VACCINE APPROACHES

Given the protection conferred by BCG against severe and disseminated disease,[34,35] there are significant ethical issues around withholding routine BCG immunization. This provides logistical challenges in the conduct of efficacy trials of new TB vaccines, particularly those designed to replace BCG. The two main approaches are to improve on BCG through genetic engineering of BCG or another mycobacteria (including M.tb itself), or a prime-boost strategy in which a new vaccine is given at a later stage as a booster to BCG. Despite scientific progress and over a dozen

Table 12.2 Candidate TB vaccines currently in clinical development

Strategy	Vaccine	Description	Phase	Ref.
Replacing BCG				
Recombinant BCG strains	VPM1002	BCG expressing listeriolysin and lacking urease C	III	142
Attenuated *M.tb* strains	MTBVAC	*M.tb* with deletion mutations in the virulence genes *phoP* and *fadD26*	IIa	146–148
Other attenuated whole organism mycobacteria	DAR-901	*M. obuense*	IIb	154
	RUTI	Fragmented *M.tb*; immunotherapeutic	IIa	137
	MIP	Heat-inactivated *M. indicus pranii*; immunotherapeutic	III	138,155,156
Boosting BCG with a subunit vaccine				
Protein/adjuvant candidates	M72/AS01	Fusion protein of Mtb39a and Mtb32a with AS01 adjuvant	IIb	157,160–164
	H4/IC31 (AERAS-404)	Fusion protein of Ag85B and TB10.4	IIa	57,168,169
	H56/IC31 (AERAS-456)	Fusion protein of Ag85B and ESAT-6 and the latency antigen Rv2660	IIb	170,171
	ID93+GLA-SE	Fusion protein of Rv2608, Rv3619, Rv1813 and Rv3620 formulated GLA-SE adjuvant	IIa	172,173
Recombinant viral vectors	MVA85A	MVA vector expressing AgA5A delivered by aerosol	I	185
	ChAdOx1.85A/ MVA85A	Chimpanzee adenovirus 5 expressing Ag85A prime, with an MVA85A boost	I	
	Ad5Ag85A	Human adenovirus 5 expressing Ag85A	I	174,186,187,246
	TB/FLU-04L	Live attenuated influenza A virus vector expressing ESAT-6 and Ag85A	IIa	

vaccine candidates in the current clinical pipeline, few have progressed to efficacy trials and few new vaccines have been added in the last 5 years. The current lead candidates are reviewed later and summarized in Table 12.2.

REPLACING BCG

Live attenuated whole-cell vaccines have the potential advantages over protein-adjuvant and viral-vectored subunit vaccines of a comprehensive antigen repertoire and greater similarity to natural infection. Such BCG replacements aim to improve on both efficacy (particularly in the developing world) and safety, permitting use in infants with HIV infection. Any BCG replacement must demonstrate non-inferiority to BCG in protection against other mycobacterial infections such as leprosy, and potential non-specific effects in reducing all-cause mortality in infants, as well as efficacy against severe forms of TB and pulmonary disease.

RECOMBINANT BCG STRAINS

The two approaches for generating a genetically improved BCG strain are overexpression of immunodominant antigens and manipulation of antigen processing. The first strategy involves addition of antigens which BCG already expresses at a low level such as Ag85B in rBCG30,[139] or addition of antigens that BCG does not currently express such as RD1 in BCG::RD1-2FG.[140] rBCG VPM1002 employs the second strategy, expressing listeriolysin from *Listeria monocytogenes* and lacking urease C, with the aim of increasing acidification of the phagosome to enable enhanced membrane-perforating action of the listeriolysin. This is designed to increase endosomal escape of antigen, thus facilitating cross-priming and induction of a class I-restricted CD8+ T-cell response.[141] VPM1002 has demonstrated clinical safety and

immunogenicity,[142] and has entered into phase II clinical trials evaluating safety and immunogenicity in HIV-exposed infants, and as a method for preventing recurrence after initial successful TB treatment (NCT02391415 and NCT03152903).

AERAS-422 was designed to combine the two strategies, overexpressing Ag85A, Ag85B, and Rv3407, while also expressing perfringolysin (with the same aim as listeriolysin in VPM1002). Further development of this vaccine was terminated due to the reactivation of latent Varicella zoster infection in two subjects during phase I clinical trials.[143] Of the three rBCG vaccines that have entered phase I trials (rBCG30, AERAS-422, and VPM1002), only VPM1002 remains in active development.

ATTENUATED *M.TB* STRAINS

An alternative approach is to use attenuated *M.tb* in which virulence-related genes have been deleted while conserving major immunodominant antigens such as early-secreted antigen-6 (ESAT-6) and culture filtrate protein-10 (CFP-10) that are absent in BCG. In light of safety concerns regarding advancing attenuated strains of *M.tb* to clinical evaluation (particularly in immunocompromised populations), two international meetings with regulators and vaccine developers coordinated by the WHO led to a set of recommendations on the construction and preclinical safety testing of these vaccines.[144,145] MTBVAC, which contains two independent deletion mutations in the virulence genes *phoP* and *fadD26*, fulfills the Geneva consensus safety requirements and is the first of its kind to enter clinical trials. This vaccine demonstrated superior protection to BCG in guinea pigs and NHPs,[146,147] and in a recent phase I clinical trial was found to be as safe as BCG, and comparably immunogenic.[148] A phase Ib/IIa trial in adults with and without LTBI is underway (NCT02933281).

OTHER ATTENUATED WHOLE ORGANISM MYCOBACTERIAL VACCINE CANDIDATES

SRL-172 is an inactivated whole cell non-tuberculous mycobacterial vaccine that has been evaluated in several clinical trials as an immunotherapeutic agent in combination with drug therapy.[149] It was originally designated *Mycobacterium vaccae* by phenotypic methods, but has since been identified as *Mycobacterium obuense*. SRL-172 was shown to be safe and immunogenic in phase I and II studies in HIV-infected adults in Finland and Zambia.[150,151] Although a phase III trial in South Africa found no efficacy in patients with newly diagnosed pulmonary TB,[152] a trial in Tanzania indicated that boosting childhood BCG with five doses of *M. vaccae* provided 39% protection against definite TB in HIV-infected adults.[153] However, there was no protection against clinical/probable TB and insufficient numbers of volunteers reached the primary endpoint of disseminated TB to power a comparison between the vaccine and placebo arms. DAR-901 is a new BCG booster vaccine manufactured from the same seed strain as SRL-172 using a new scalable method. In a phase I dose-escalation trial, DAR-901 was safe and well-tolerated at all dose levels and did not result in IGRA conversion.[154] A phase IIb trial for the prevention of infection (POI) in adolescents is underway in Tanzania (NCT02712424).

RUTI is a polyantigenic liposomal vaccine made of detoxified fragmented *M.tb* cells that aims to improve outcomes in the treatment of both LTBI and TB disease and reduce antibiotic exposure. A phase IIa trial in South Africa demonstrated acceptable tolerability and good immunogenicity in HIV-infected and -uninfected subjects with LTBI following 1 month of isoniazid treatment.[137] A phase IIa trial will assess safety and immunogenicity in patients with MDR-TB. *Mycobacterium indicus pranii* (MIP) (previously *Mw*) is another heat-inactivated mycobacterial strain being tested as a therapeutic agent. Although preclinical studies were promising,[155] MIP had no immunotherapeutic effect on patients with tuberculosis pericarditis in a phase III clinical trial.[138] However, the use of MIP in sepsis was associated with improved outcomes in a recent randomized trial[156] and this vaccine has now progressed to a phase IIb trial in patients with severe sepsis (NCT02330432).

BOOSTING BCG WITH A SUBUNIT VACCINE

An alternative approach to replacing BCG is to continue its administration at birth and develop a heterologous vaccine to be given at a later time with the aim of boosting the primed immune response. This would allow the benefits of BCG to be retained while increasing efficacy and durability. Such a vaccine could be given in infancy soon after BCG vaccination, in adolescence before the rise in TB incidence that occurs in young adults, or to HIV-infected adults at the time of diagnosis prior to the development of immunosuppression. A booster vaccine consists of one or more *M.tb* protein antigens (which must also be expressed in all strains of BCG) together with either an adjuvant or a recombinant viral vector delivery system.

PROTEIN/ADJUVANT VACCINE CANDIDATES

The most advanced protein/adjuvant candidate is M72/AS01; a fusion protein of the Mtb39a and Mtb32a antigens administered with the GSK proprietary AS01 adjuvant, which includes the immunostimulants MPL and the saponin QS21 combined with liposomes.[157] M72 administered with AS02 (a squalene-containing emulsion formulation of the same immunostimulants as AS01) improved survival after *M.tb* challenge when co-administered with BCG in guinea pigs, enhanced immunogenicity but not efficacy in mice, and enhanced survival after challenge in BCG-vaccinated NHPs.[158,159] Clinical trials found that AS01 facilitated greater Th1 responses against both *M.tb* antigens than AS02 and this adjuvant was thus taken forward.[157] M72/AS01 was well-tolerated and induced robust polyfunctional M72-specific CD4+ T-cell and antibody responses in healthy adults, adolescents and BCG-vaccinated infants.[157,160–162] It was also safe and immunogenic in ART-stable and ART-naïve HIV-positive and HIV-negative adults in India.[163] M72/AS01 has recently been evaluated in a phase IIb efficacy trial in Kenya, South Africa, and Zambia, and was found to provide 54% protection for latently infected adults against active TB disease.[164]

Three fusion protein/adjuvant vaccine candidates: Hybrid 1/IC31, Hybrid 4/IC31, and Hybrid 56/IC31 were designed by the Statens Serum Institut (SSI) in Copenhagen. H1/IC31 contains the fusion protein of Ag85B and ESAT-6 adjuvanted to a system combining the antibacterial peptide KLK with a synthetic Toll-like receptor (TLR)-9 agonist (ODN1a). This vaccine was safe in healthy, prior, or latently TB-infected and HIV-infected adults, and induced a robust and durable CD4+ T-cell response.[165–167] However, the inclusion of ESAT-6 potentially confounds the IGRA diagnostic assay which uses a T-cell response to ESAT-6 and CFP-10 as evidence of *M.tb* infection. Indeed, a recent study found that 17% of participants receiving high-dose H1/IC31 developed a positive response to the QuantiFERON TB Gold in-tube assay.[165] H4/IC31 (AERAS-404) circumvents this issue by replacing ESAT-6 with TB10.4, while still demonstrating moderate protective efficacy in preclinical models.[168,169] In a recent phase II trial conducted in South African adolescents, H4/IC31 showed no protection against initial infection, and a non-statistically significant trend toward reduced sustained *M.tb* infections.[57]

H56/IC31 is the newest candidate from this group, and contains the latency-associated antigen Rv2660 in addition to Ag85B and TB10.4. This vaccine is designed to also enhance protective immunity in individuals already latently infected with *M.tb*, to prevent reactivation and facilitate clearance of infection. H56/IC31 was well-tolerated and immunogenic in NHP studies and showed protective efficacy against active TB disease and reactivation of latent infection.[170] Phase I/IIa trials in healthy adults without or with LTBI demonstrated safety and immunogenicity. Interestingly, low-dose vaccination induced more polyfunctional and higher frequencies of specific CD4+ T-cells compared with high-dose vaccination.[171] A phase II prevention-of-recurrence study is planned (NCT03512249).

ID93+GLA-SE consists of a fusion protein of four antigens (Rv2608, Rv3619, Rv1813, and Rv3620) formulated with the TLR adjuvant GLA-SE. This vaccine demonstrated protective immunity in mice and guinea pigs[172] and was well-tolerated and immunogenic in a recent phase I dose-escalation study in healthy adults.[173] Escalating doses induced similar antigen-specific CD4+ T-cell and humoral responses and showed an acceptable safety profile in BCG-vaccinated *M.tb*-infected individuals.[173]

RECOMBINANT VIRAL VECTORS

Live attenuated non-replicating viruses can be genetically engineered to deliver foreign antigens, and have the potential to engage the innate immune system and boost cellular immunity without the need for additional adjuvants. Most of the advanced vectored TB vaccine candidates are based on recombinant adenovirus or vaccinia virus. Other novel viral vectors include Sendai virus, lentivirus, parainfluenza virus 2, and influenza virus.

A recombinant modified vaccinia Ankara (MVA) vector expressing Ag85A was the first new subunit vaccine to enter clinical trials in 2002 and has been a leading candidate in the field for over a decade. MVA85A showed modest protection in preclinical animal models,[147,175–177] and demonstrated safety and immunogenicity in phase I/IIa clinical trials.[178–182] However, no improvement on protection provided by BCG alone was observed in a preventative pre-exposure phase IIb trial in South African infants.[131] Preclinical studies have since demonstrated enhanced immunogenicity and/or protection when Ag85A is delivered intranasally or by aerosol.[183,184] Clinical trials are now assessing the aerosol route of delivery of MVA85A with the aim of enhancing local protective immune responses at the primary site of infection. A phase I trial found that MVA85A delivered by aerosol was well-tolerated and elicited an immune response in the lungs that was superior to that induced by ID administration.[185]

Human adenovirus 5 (AdHu5) engineered to express Ag85A was found to be robustly protective against M.tb challenge in preclinical models, particularly when given via the intranasal route.[186] It was also evaluated in a phase I clinical study and shown to be safe and immunogenic.[187] However, one of the limitations of some virus-vectored vaccines is the presence of pre-existing antibodies induced by natural exposure which may compromise the potency of the vaccine and pose a safety concern when given to high-risk HIV-infected populations. In total, 45%–80% of adults have neutralizing antibody responses to AdHu5, depending on the region.[188,189] One strategy to overcome anti-Ad immunity is the use of replication-defective chimpanzee-derived adenoviruses (AdCh), because neutralizing antibodies against these vectors are rarely found in humans[190] and immunogenicity is comparable with that induced by human adenoviruses.[191,192] In murine studies, AdCh68Ag85A induced superior T-cell responses and immune protection compared with its AdHu5 counterpart.[193] An AdCh vector expressing Ag85A (ChAdOx1.85A) is currently being assessed in a prime-boost regimen with MVA85A in phase I trials (NCT01829490).

Antibodies to the less common AdHu35 virus are detected in just ~5%–15% of adults.[189] AERAS-402 is an AdHu35-vectored vaccine expressing a fusion protein of Ag85A, Ag85B, and TB10.4 which has demonstrated protective immune responses in mice.[194] Safety and immunogenicity has also been assessed in clinical trials of healthy adults, adults with previous or active TB- and HIV-infected adults.[195–200] The vaccine was found to induce polyfunctional CD4$^+$ T-cells and a potent CD8$^+$ T-cell response, although recent analysis suggests that the polyfunctional T-cells do not necessarily recognize M.tb-infected targets.[201] A phase IIb trial in BCG-vaccinated infants demonstrated an acceptable safety profile, but the trial was modified to remove the efficacy objective when the predefined immunogenicity target was not met.[199]

More recent studies have focussed on administering AERAS-402 by the aerosol route,[202] and incorporating the vaccine in a prime-boost strategy with MVA85A which has demonstrated increased frequency and durability of antigen-specific T-cell responses in phase I trials.[203,204]

TB/FLU-04L is a live-attenuated influenza A virus vector expressing the M.tb antigens ESAT-6 and Ag85A which is administered by the intranasal route. Preclinical studies have demonstrated safety, immunogenicity, and efficacy. In a phase I trial in BCG-vaccinated healthy volunteers, the vaccine was well-tolerated and immunogenic with no infectious virus detected in nasal swabs by 5 days post-vaccination (NCT02501421).

CMV has recently been identified as a promising live attenuated viral vector due to its natural periodic reactivation, leading to intermittent re-stimulation of specific T-cells and maintenance of the effector cell population. The CMV/TB vaccine candidate expresses nine M.tb proteins representative of the acute-phase, latency, and resuscitation antigen classes. Preclinical studies in rhesus macaques demonstrated a 68% reduction in extent of M.tb infection and disease in the vaccinated animals compared with unvaccinated controls following M.tb challenge, with 14 out of 34 vaccinated animals showing no evidence of TB disease.[205]

CHALLENGES IN VACCINE DEVELOPMENT

As the pathway for clinical development of new TB vaccines has become clearer, so have the challenges ahead. Major issues for the field over the next decade are the lack of validated immunological correlates of protection for down-selection of candidates going forward to efficacy testing, uncertainty regarding the predictive value of animal models, lack of a human challenge model, and lack of capacity to do and to fund phase IIb/III efficacy trials. Each of these issues is discussed briefly next.

LACK OF A VALIDATED IMMUNOLOGICAL CORRELATE OF PROTECTION

One of the greatest impediments to TB vaccine development is the lack of a validated immune correlate that reliably predicts vaccine efficacy. Such a biomarker would allow down-selection of candidates prior to entry into clinical trials and provide an alternative to clinical disease endpoints, shortening trials, and expediting vaccine development. The lack of an efficacious vaccine makes identification of a correlate of protection extremely challenging. However, biomarkers of reduced disease risk, for example in those who do not relapse after treatment or remain healthy with longstanding LTBI are important indicators of protective immunity and may aid in reducing the size and duration of clinical trials.

T-CELL AND B-CELL RESPONSES

IFN-γ has been widely used as the primary immunological readout in human trials, but studies in recent years have challenged the dogma of "the more IFN-γ the better."[206–209] In a 2-year follow-up study of BCG-immunized infants, the frequency and cytokine profile of mycobacteria-specific T-cells did not correlate with protection against TB.[130] Despite promising results from other disease models and preclinical TB studies,[210-213] polyfunctional T-cells also failed to associate with protective efficacy in this study.[130] Interestingly, BCG-induced IFN-γ producing T-cells were associated with a reduced risk of TB disease in a recent case–control study in BCG-vaccinated South African infants, whereas activated CD4+ T-cells (expressing HLA-DR) were associated with increased risk.[128] The causes of T-cell activation and impact on disease risk should be considered when designing and testing TB-vaccine candidates. B-cell correlates are understudied, but specific memory B-cells were found to be higher in BCG-vaccinated compared with BCG-unvaccinated individuals,[214] and higher concentrations of Ag85-specific IgG were associated with a reduced risk of TB in the infant case–control study.[128]

FUNCTIONAL MYCOBACTERIAL GROWTH INHIBITION ASSAYS

One alternative to hypothesis-driven measurement of predefined immune parameters is the use of unbiased in vitro mycobacterial growth inhibition assays (MGIAs). These are functional assays that take into account a range of immune mechanisms and their interactions.[215] Early assays involved the use of whole blood inoculated with a luciferase-transfected BCG reporter strain,[216] or co-cultures of stimulated or unstimulated lymphocytes added to infected monocytes.[217-219] More recently, a simplified model based on direct infection of PBMC detected a BCG-induced improvement in control of mycobacterial growth in both UK adults and infants.[220,221] Although growth inhibition was not associated with a reduced risk of TB disease in the South African infant case–control study,[128] recent studies have demonstrated a correlation with protection from in vivo mycobacterial challenge in both humans and NHPs.[247] Such assays also offer tractable systems for the investigation of underlying immune mechanisms, and to date control of mycobacterial growth in the direct PBMC MGIA has been associated with polyfunctional T-cells[221] and trained innate immunity.[222]

GENE EXPRESSION SIGNATURES

Other unbiased approaches include global immune, gene expression, and proteomic profiling assays. Previous systems biology studies have reported signatures that discriminate TB disease from LTBI and other disease states.[223-228] A study of latently infected South African adolescents with a 2-year follow-up identified a prospective 16-gene signature of risk of TB disease.[229] This signature was validated in two independent cohorts of LTBI South African and Gambian adults, in which it predicted TB progression with a sensitivity of 53.7% (95% CI 42.6–64.3) and a specificity of 82.8% (95% CI 76.7–86).[229] More recently, a four-gene signature derived from the samples in a South African and Gambian training set predicted progression up to 2 years before onset of disease in blinded test set samples, and was further validated in a cohort of adolescents with latent M.tb infection.[230] A case–control study of more than 5,000 BCG vaccinated infants identified distinct host responses to vaccination observed, with two major clusters of gene expression demonstrating different myeloid and lymphoid activation and inflammatory patterns.[231] This diversity should be taken into account in future vaccine development.

PREDICTIVE VALUE OF PRECLINICAL ANIMAL MODELS

New candidate TB vaccines are currently evaluated using preclinical animal models; typically mice, guinea pigs, NHPs, and cattle. However, the relevance of these models in terms of predicting efficacy in humans is unclear. Vaccine efficacy in animal models, as determined by M.tb challenge studies, is defined as an improvement compared with control groups in a disease-related readout such as bacterial load, pathology score, or long-term survival. A vaccine may be considered to provide protection even if there are measurable bacteria or pathology in the organs or some animals do not survive. In humans, however, efficacy is defined as the prevention of TB disease using clinical endpoints.[232] Furthermore, an artificial aerosol challenge is very different to natural transmission in humans, and the laboratory strains of M.tb commonly used are genetically dissimilar to clinical isolates,[233] with much higher challenge doses employed. In addition to these fundamental differences in experimental design, animals are genetically distinct from humans, and the widely used mouse strains do not exhibit caseating granuloma formation: the hallmark of human disease.[234] Cattle and NHPs are considered better models for human TB but their use is limited by cost and availability of animals and reagents.

There is yet to be an established link between a vaccine effect observed in animal models and human protection; recently, the modest protection conferred by MVA85A in preclinical studies did not translate into efficacy in humans.[131,147,175,176] Only once we have an efficacious vaccine will it be possible to understand which animal models predict human efficacy, allowing those models to be optimized and best applied for subsequent development.

LACK OF A HUMAN CHALLENGE MODEL

Development and utilization of human challenge models has significantly accelerated vaccine development for a range of diseases including malaria, cholera, and typhoid.[235-237] Such models offer the potential to down-select vaccine candidates at an early stage and to identify correlates of protective immunity. Although it is ethically unacceptable to infect volunteers with virulent M.tb, a live attenuated replicating mycobacterial strain such as BCG could offer a safe surrogate. Studies applying an intradermal BCG challenge model and quantifying mycobacteria from skin biopsies have demonstrated the ability to detect a degree of mycobacterial immunity in previously BCG-vaccinated individuals.[238,239] A recent pilot study assessed a less invasive model measuring mycobacterial burden in swab specimens collected from the vaccination site.[240] Further studies are underway, including the development of an aerosol BCG challenge model more representative of natural infection (NCT02709278). Fortune and colleagues are exploring strategies to generate a safe attenuated strain of M.tb that can be reproducibly cleared and not transmitted, and is detectable and quantifiable in vivo.[241]

INADEQUATE CAPACITY TO DO AND TO FUND PHASE IIB/III EFFICACY TRIALS

The implementation of clinical trial sites for TB vaccine efficacy testing poses a major challenge to investigators. The requirements include a robust clinical and laboratory infrastructure, established field resources, human skills and expertise, and known epidemiological data with which to power trials.[242] There are currently very few sites worldwide that fulfill these criteria. The first site specifically developed for the evaluation of TB vaccines was the South African TB Vaccine Initiative (SATVI) site in Worcester, South Africa run jointly by the University of Cape Town. This was followed by a site at the Kenya Medical Research Institute/CDC field station. However, phase III trials will need to extend beyond the African subcontinent, and there is a major requirement for new sites in other TB-endemic regions such as Asia to allow multicenter licensure trials. Once sites have been established, expertise, capacity, and funding must be maintained between clinical trials to ensure that robust efficacy testing can commence without delay as soon as a candidate advances to this stage.

ALTERNATIVE ENDPOINTS

TB case accrual rates are the primary driver of the large size, duration, and cost of clinical efficacy trials. Trials designed with alternative, yet biologically meaningful endpoints that occur at higher rates than TB disease would allow smaller proof-of-concept trials to be conducted. Positive outcomes could then be used to justify subsequent acceleration into classical phase IIb and III prevention of disease trials. Such endpoints include POI and prevention of disease recurrence (POR). As described, recent studies suggest that

POI is feasible in principle,[33] although one limitation is the lack of a gold standard for detecting *M.tb* infection. A recent trial of the AERAS-404 candidate employed an IGRA conversion POI primary endpoint, but did not demonstrate efficacy (NCT02075203). The high rate of TB disease recurrence and short time-frame (91% of relapses occur within the first year after completion of TB treatment[243]) would reduce follow-up time considerably in POR studies. Such studies would also establish proof of concept for vaccination as an adjunct to TB treatment, but perhaps set an unreasonably high bar for a prevention-of-disease vaccine and risk missing an impact on initial infection. The use of LTBI or other high risk volunteers would also accelerate clinical development; an approach currently being taken to evaluate the aforementioned M72/AS01 candidate (NCT01755598). The advantages and disadvantages of different clinical trial endpoints are summarized in Table 12.3.

CONCLUSIONS

After decades of neglect, TB vaccine development gained momentum in the 2000s but progress has slowed in recent years. It is hoped that the considerable advances made in discovery research and experimental medicine studies will feed into an improved pipeline in the future. However, the predictive value of animal models, correlates of protection, and human challenge models can only be

Table 12.3 Advantages and disadvantages of different clinical trial endpoints

Endpoint	Advantages	Disadvantages
Prevention of disease (POD)	Large public health impact by interrupting transmission	Large sample sizes required
	Most widely accepted endpoint for TB vaccine registration	Long duration due to slow accrual of disease endpoints
	Microbiologically confirmed TB disease endpoint accepted gold standard	Costly
		Ability to prevent disease in uninfected and LTBI individuals may differ
		Pre-existing anti-mycobacterial immunity may block vaccine effects in adult POD studies
Prevention of infection (POI)	Infection rates higher than disease making trials smaller and shorter in duration	Lack of gold standard for detecting *M.tb* infection
	Potential marker of biological activity and gating strategy for advancement to POD trials	POD trial still required
	Ability to utilize existing infant vaccination programs for delivery	Phenomenon of reversion; need to capture sustained converters
		Possibility that infection only prevented in those who would not otherwise progress to disease
		POI may have smaller public health impact than POD
		Inadequate animal models to evaluate infection endpoint; limits advancement of POI candidates
Prevention of disease recurrence (POR)	Disease endpoint accrual higher than in POD studies making trials smaller and shorter in duration	POD trial still required
	Potential marker of biological activity and gating strategy for advancement to POD trials	Risk of missing an impact on reducing initial infection
	May establish proof of concept for vaccination as adjunct to therapy	

validated by human efficacy data. The findings of the correlates of risk analysis using samples from the MVA85A phase IIb trial demonstrate how much can be learnt from such studies, regardless of efficacy outcome. It is essential to maintain momentum and funding if we are to attain the goals set out in the Global Plan to Stop TB and to significantly reduce the incidence of this devastating disease.

REFERENCES

1. Calmette A. Preventive vaccination against tuberculosis with BCG. *Proc R Soc Med.* 1931;24(11):1481–90.

2. Oettinger T, Jorgensen M, Ladefoged A, Haslov K, and Andersen P. Development of the *Mycobacterium bovis* BCG vaccine: Review of the historical and biochemical evidence for a genealogical tree. *Tuber Lung Dis.* 1999;79(4):243–50.

3. Casanova J-L, Jouanguy E, Lamhamedi S, Blanche S, and Fischer A. Immunological conditions of children with BCG disseminated infection. *Lancet* 1995;346(8974):581.

4. Hesseling AC et al. Bacille Calmette–Guérin vaccine-induced disease in HIV-infected and HIV-uninfected children. *Clin Infect Dis.* 2006;42(4):548–58.

5. Talbot EA, Perkins MD, Silva SF, and Frothingham R. Disseminated bacille Calmette–Guérin disease after vaccination: Case report and review. *Clin Infect Dis.* 1997;24(6):1139–46.

6. Lamm DL et al. Incidence and treatment of complications of bacillus Calmette–Guérin intravesical therapy in superficial bladder cancer. *J Urol.* 1992;147(3):596–600.

7. Brausi M et al. Side effects of Bacillus Calmette–Guérin (BCG) in the treatment of intermediate- and high-risk Ta, T1 papillary carcinoma of the bladder: Results of the EORTC genito-urinary cancers group randomised phase 3 study comparing one-third dose with full dose and 1 year with 3 years of maintenance BCG. *Eur Urol.* 2014;65(1):69–76.

8. Lamm DL. Efficacy and safety of Bacille Calmette–Guérin immunotherapy in superficial bladder cancer. *Clin Infect Dis.* 2000;31(Suppl 3):S86–90.

9. Sylvester RJ, van der MA, and Lamm DL. Intravesical bacillus Calmette–Guérin reduces the risk of progression in patients with superficial bladder cancer: A meta-analysis of the published results of randomized clinical trials. *J Urol.* 2002;168(5):1964–70.

10. Nicol M, Eley B, Kibel M, and Hussey G. Intradermal BCG vaccination—adverse reactions and their management. *S Afr Med J.* 2002;92(1):39–42.

11. Riordan A, Cole T, and Broomfield C. Fifteen-minute consultation: Bacillus Calmette–Guérin abscess and lymphadenitis. *Arch Dis Child Educ Pract Ed.* 2014;99(3):87–9.

12. Venkataraman A, Yusuff M, Liebeschuetz S, Riddell A, and Prendergast AJ. Management and outcome of Bacille Calmette–Guérin vaccine adverse reactions. *Vaccine* 2015;33(41):5470–4.

13. Gharehdaghi M, Hassani M, Ghodsi E, Khooei A, and Moayedpour A. Bacille Calmette–Guérin Osteomyelitis. *Arch Bone Jt Surg.* 2015;3(4):291–5.

14. Macleod LC, Ngo TC, and Gonzalgo ML. Complications of intravesical Bacillus Calmette–Guérin. *Can Urol Assoc J.* 2014;8(7–8):E540–E4.

15. Eccles SR, and Mehta R. Disseminated BCG disease: A case report. *Respir Med CME* 2011;4(3):112–3.

16. Elkabani M, Greene JN, Vincent AL, Vanhook S, and Sandin RL. Disseminated *Mycobacterium bovis* after intravesicular Bacillus Calmette–Guérin treatments for bladder cancer. *Cancer Control* 2000;7(5):476–81.

17. Kesten S, Title L, Mullen B, and Grossman R. Pulmonary disease following intravesical BCG treatment. *Thorax* 1990;45(9):709–10.

18. Wayne LG. Microbiology of tubercle bacilli. *Am Rev Respir Dis.* 1982;125(3 Pt 2):31–41.

19. Ritz N, Tebruegge M, Connell TG, Sievers A, Robins-Browne R, and Curtis N. Susceptibility of *Mycobacterium bovis* BCG vaccine strains to antituberculous antibiotics. *Antimicrob Agents Chemother.* 2009;53(1):316–8.

20. Hesseling AC et al. Resistant *Mycobacterium bovis* Bacillus Calmette–Guérin disease: Implications for management of Bacillus Calmette–Guérin disease in human immunodeficiency virus-infected children. *Pediatr Infect Dis J.* 2004;23(5).

21. Sicevic S. Generalized BCG tuberculosis with fatal course in two sisters. *Acta Paediatr Scand.* 1972;61(2):178–84.

22. Boulware DR, Callens S, and Pahwa S. Pediatric HIV immune reconstitution inflammatory syndrome. *Curr Opin HIV AIDS* 2008;3(4):461–7.

23. Smith LL, Wright BL, and Buckley RH. Successful treatment of disseminated BCG in a patient with severe combined immunodeficiency. *J Allergy Clin Immunol Pract.* 2015;3(3):438–40.

24. Miret-Cuadras P, Pina-Gutierrez JM, and Juncosa S. Tuberculin reactivity in Bacillus Calmette–Guérin vaccinated subjects. *Tuber Lung Dis.* 1996;77(1):52–8.

25. Burl S et al. The tuberculin skin test (TST) is affected by recent BCG vaccination but not by exposure to non-tuberculosis mycobacteria (NTM) during early life. *PLOS ONE* 2010;5(8):e12287.

26. Sutherland I, and Lindgren I. The protective effect of BCG vaccination as indicated by autopsy studies. *Tubercle* 1979;60(4):225–31.

27. Mahomed H et al. The impact of a change in bacille Calmette–Guérin vaccine policy on tuberculosis incidence in children in Cape Town, South Africa. *Pediatr Infect Dis J.* 2006;25(12):1167–72.

28. Moyo S et al. Age-related tuberculosis incidence and severity in children under 5 years of age in Cape Town, South Africa. *Int J Tuberc Lung Dis.* 2010;14(2):149–54.

29. Soysal A et al. Effect of BCG vaccination on risk of *Mycobacterium tuberculosis* infection in children with household tuberculosis contact: A prospective community-based study. *Lancet* 2005;366(9495):1443–51.

30. Eisenhut M et al. BCG vaccination reduces risk of infection with *Mycobacterium tuberculosis* as detected by gamma interferon release assay. *Vaccine* 2009;27(44):6116–20.

31. Eriksen J et al. Protective effect of BCG vaccination in a nursery outbreak in 2009: Time to reconsider the vaccination threshold? *Thorax* 2010;65(12):1067.

32. Michelsen SW et al. The effectiveness of BCG vaccination in preventing *Mycobacterium tuberculosis* infection and disease in Greenland. *Thorax* 2014;69(9):851–6.

33. Roy A et al. Effect of BCG vaccination against *Mycobacterium tuberculosis* infection in children: Systematic review and meta-analysis. *BMJ: Br Med J.* 2014;349.

34. Trunz BB, Fine P, and Dye C. Effect of BCG vaccination on childhood tuberculous meningitis and miliary tuberculosis worldwide: A meta-analysis and assessment of cost-effectiveness. *Lancet* 2006;367(9517):1173–80.

35. Rodrigues LC, Diwan VK, and Wheeler JG. Protective effect of BCG against tuberculous meningitis and miliary tuberculosis: A meta-analysis. *Int J Epidemiol.* 1993;22(6):1154–8.

36. Colditz GA et al. Efficacy of BCG vaccine in the prevention of tuberculosis. Meta-analysis of the published literature. *JAMA* 1994;271(9):698–702.

37. Romanus V, Svensson A, and Hallander HO. The impact of changing BCG coverage on tuberculosis incidence in Swedish-born children between 1969 and 1989. *Tuber Lung Dis.* 1992;73(3):150–61.

38. Trnka L, Dankova D, and Svandova E. Six years' experience with the discontinuation of BCG vaccination. 4. Protective effect of BCG vaccination against the *Mycobacterium avium* intracellulare complex. *Tuber Lung Dis.* 1994;75(5):348–52.

39. Fine PE. Variation in protection by BCG: Implications of and for heterologous immunity. *Lancet* 1995;346(8986):1339–45.

40. Tverdal A, and Funnemark E. Protective effect of BCG vaccination in Norway 1956–73. *Tubercle* 1988;69(2):119–23.

41. Hart PD, and Sutherland I. BCG and vole bacillus vaccines in the prevention of tuberculosis in adolescence and early adult life. *Br Med J.* 1977;2(6082):293–5.

42. Aronson JD. Protective vaccination against tuberculosis, with special reference to BCG vaccine. *Minn Med.* 1948;31(12):1336.

43. Hyge TV. The efficacy of BCG-vaccination; epidemic of tuberculosis in a State School, with an observation period of 12 years. *Acta Tuberc Scand.* 1956;32(2):89–107.

44. Baily GV. Tuberculosis prevention trial, Madras. *Indian J Med Res.* 1980;72(Suppl):1–74.

45. Ponnighaus JM et al. Efficacy of BCG vaccine against leprosy and tuberculosis in northern Malawi. *Lancet* 1992;339(8794):636–9.

46. Comstock GW, Woolpert SF, and Livesay VT. Tuberculosis studies in Muscogee County, Georgia. Twenty-year evaluation of a community trial of BCG vaccination. *Public Health Rep.* 1976;91(3):276–80.

47. Shapiro C et al. A case-control study of BCG and childhood tuberculosis in Cali, Colombia. *Int J Epidemiol.* 1985;14(3):441–6.

48. Sutherland I, and Springett VH. Effectiveness of BCG vaccination in England and Wales in 1983. *Tubercle* 1987;68(2):81–92.

49. Sterne JA, Rodrigues LC, and Guedes IN. Does the efficacy of BCG decline with time since vaccination? *Int J Tuberc Lung Dis.* 1998;2(3):200–7.

50. Nguipdop-Djomo P, Heldal E, Rodrigues LC, Abubakar I, and Mangtani P. Duration of BCG protection against tuberculosis and change in effectiveness with time since vaccination in Norway: A retrospective population-based cohort study. *Lancet Infect Dis.* 2016;16(2):219–26.

51. Barreto ML et al. Neonatal BCG protection against tuberculosis lasts for 20 years in Brazil. *Int J Tuberc Lung Dis.* 2005;9(10):1171–3.

52. Aronson NE et al. Long-term efficacy of BCG vaccine in American Indians and Alaska Natives: A 60-year follow-up study. *JAMA* 2004;291(17):2086–91.

53. Mangtani P et al. The duration of protection of school-aged BCG vaccination in England: A population-based case–control study. *Int J Epidemiol.* 2018;47(1):193–201.

54. Karonga Prevention Trial Group. Randomised controlled trial of single BCG, repeated BCG, or combined BCG and killed *Mycobacterium leprae* vaccine for prevention of leprosy and tuberculosis in Malawi. *Lancet* 1996;348(9019):17–24.

55. Rodrigues LC et al. Effect of BCG revaccination on incidence of tuberculosis in school-aged children in Brazil: The BCG-REVAC cluster-randomised trial. *Lancet* 2005;366(9493):1290–5.

56. Leung CC, Tam CM, Chan SL, Chan-Yeung M, Chan CK, and Chang KC. Efficacy of the BCG revaccination programme in a cohort given BCG vaccination at birth in Hong Kong. *Int J Tuberc Lung Dis.* 2001;5(8):717–23.

57. Nemes E et al. Prevention of *M. tuberculosis* infection with H4:IC31 vaccine or BCG revaccination. *N Engl J Med.* 2018;379(2):138–49.

58. Harboe M, Mshana RN, Closs O, Kronvall G, and Axelsen NH. Cross-reactions between mycobacteria. II. Crossed immunoelectrophoretic analysis of soluble antigens of BCG and comparison with other mycobacteria. *Scand J Immunol.* 1979;9(2):115–24.

59. Lombardi C, Pedrazzani ES, Pedrazzani JC, Filho PF, and Zicker F. Protective efficacy of BCG against leprosy in Sao Paulo. *Bull Pan Am Health Organ.* 1996;30(1):24–30.

60. Merle CS, Cunha SS, and Rodrigues LC. BCG vaccination and leprosy protection: Review of current evidence and status of BCG in leprosy control. *Expert Rev Vaccines* 2010;9(2):209–22.

61. Setia MS, Steinmaus C, Ho CS, and Rutherford GW. The role of BCG in prevention of leprosy: A meta-analysis. *Lancet Infect Dis.* 2006;6(3):162–70.

62. Smith PG, Revill WD, Lukwago E, and Rykushin YP. The protective effect of BCG against *Mycobacterium ulcerans* disease: A controlled trial in an endemic area of Uganda. *Trans R Soc Trop Med Hyg.* 1976;70(5–6):449–57.

63. Noeske J et al. Buruli ulcer disease in Cameroon rediscovered. *Am J Trop Med Hyg.* 2004;70(5):520–6.

64. Nackers F et al. BCG vaccine effectiveness against Buruli ulcer: A case-control study in Benin. *Am J Trop Med Hyg.* 2006;75(4):768–74.

65. Raghunathan PL et al. Risk factors for Buruli ulcer disease (*Mycobacterium ulcerans* infection): Results from a case-control study in Ghana. *Clin Infect Dis.* 2005;40(10):1445–53.

66. Orme IM, and Collins FM. Prophylactic effect in mice of BCG vaccination against non-tuberculous mycobacterial infections. *Tubercle* 1985;66(2):117–20.

67. Vaugelade J, Pinchinat S, Guiella G, Elguero E, and Simondon F. Non-specific effects of vaccination on child survival: Prospective cohort study in Burkina Faso. *BMJ* 2004;329(7478):1309.

68. Aaby P et al. Randomized trial of BCG vaccination at birth to low-birth-weight children: Beneficial nonspecific effects in the neonatal period? *J Infect Dis.* 2011;204(2):245–52.

69. de Castro MJ, Pardo-Seco J, and Martinon-Torres F. Nonspecific (heterologous) protection of neonatal BCG vaccination against hospitalization due to respiratory infection and sepsis. *Clin Infect Dis.* 2015;60(11):1611–9.

70. Garly ML et al. BCG scar and positive tuberculin reaction associated with reduced child mortality in West Africa. A non-specific beneficial effect of BCG? *Vaccine* 2003;21(21–22):2782–90.

71. Nankabirwa V, Tumwine JK, Mugaba PM, Tylleskär T, and Sommerfelt H. Child survival and BCG vaccination: A community based prospective cohort study in Uganda. *BMC Public Health* 2015;15(1):175.

72. Roth A et al. Tuberculin reaction, BCG scar, and lower female mortality. *Epidemiology* 2006;17(5):562–8.

73. Aaby P et al. Sex differential effects of routine immunizations and childhood survival in rural Malawi. *Pediatr Infect Dis J.* 2006;25(8):721–7.

74. Goodridge HS et al. Harnessing the beneficial heterologous effects of vaccination. *Nat Rev Immunol.* 2016;16(6):392–400.

75. Kleinnijenhuis J et al. Long-lasting effects of BCG vaccination on both heterologous Th1/Th17 responses and innate trained immunity. *J Innate Immunity.* 2014;6(2):152–8.

76. Bekkering S, Blok BA, Joosten LA, Riksen NP, van Crevel R, and Netea MG. *In vitro* experimental model of trained innate immunity in human primary monocytes. *Clin Vaccine Immunol.* 2016;23(12):926–33.

77. Haahr S et al. Non-specific effects of BCG vaccination on morbidity among children in Greenland: A population-based cohort study. *Int J Epidemiol.* 2016;45(6):2122–30.

78. Stensballe LG et al. BCG vaccination at birth and early childhood hospitalisation: A randomised clinical multicentre trial. *Arch Dis Child.* 2017;102(3):224.

79. Higgins JPT et al. Association of BCG, DTP, and measles containing vaccines with childhood mortality: Systematic review. *BMJ* 2016;355.

80. Raymond P. On the pathological relations between cancer and tuberculosis. *Proc Soc Exp Biol Med*. 1928;26(1):73–5.

81. Old LJ, Clarke DA, and Benacerraf B. Effect of Bacillus Calmette–Guérin infection on transplanted tumours in the mouse. *Nature* 1959;184(Suppl 5):291–2.

82. Carswell EA, Old LJ, Kassel RL, Green S, Fiore N, and Williamson B. An endotoxin-induced serum factor that causes necrosis of tumors. *Proc Natl Acad Sci USA* 1975;72(9):3666–70.

83. Hall MC et al. Guideline for the management of nonmuscle invasive bladder cancer (stages Ta, T1, and Tis): 2007 update. *J Urol*. 2007;178(6):2314–30.

84. Babjuk M et al. EAU guidelines on non-muscle-invasive urothelial carcinoma of the bladder, the 2011 update. *Eur Urol*. 2011;59(6):997–1008.

85. de Reijke TM et al. Bacillus Calmette–Guérin versus epirubicin for primary, secondary or concurrent carcinoma *in situ* of the bladder: Results of a European Organization for the Research and Treatment of Cancer-Genito-Urinary Group Phase III Trial (30906). *J Urol*. 2005;173(2):405–9.

86. Shelley MD, Court JB, Kynaston H, Wilt TJ, Coles B, and Mason M. Intravesical bacillus Calmette–Guérin versus mitomycin C for Ta and T1 bladder cancer. *Cochrane Database Syst Rev*. 2003;(3):Cd003231.

87. Redelman-Sidi G, Glickman MS, and Bochner BH. The mechanism of action of BCG therapy for bladder cancer—a current perspective. *Nat Rev Urol*. 2014;11:153.

88. Kowalewicz-Kulbat M, and Locht C. BCG and protection against inflammatory and auto-immune diseases. *Expert Rev Vaccines* 2017;16(7):1–10.

89. Kühtreiber WM et al. Long-term reduction in hyperglycemia in advanced type 1 diabetes: The value of induced aerobic glycolysis with BCG vaccinations. *NPJ Vaccines* 2018;3(1):23.

90. Ritz N et al. The influence of bacille Calmette–Guérin vaccine strain on the immune response against tuberculosis: A randomized trial. *Am J Respir Crit Care Med*. 2012;185(2):213–22.

91. Kozak R, and Behr MA. Divergence of immunologic and protective responses of different BCG strains in a murine model. *Vaccine* 2011;29(7):1519–26.

92. Horwitz MA, Harth G, Dillon BJ, and Maslesa-Galic S. Commonly administered BCG strains including an evolutionarily early strain and evolutionarily late strains of disparate genealogy induce comparable protective immunity against tuberculosis. *Vaccine* 2009;27(3):441–5.

93. Ritz N, Hanekom WA, Robins-Browne R, Britton WJ, and Curtis N. Influence of BCG vaccine strain on the immune response and protection against tuberculosis. *FEMS Microbiol Rev*. 2008;32(5):821–41.

94. Edwards LB, Acquaviva FA, Livesay VT, Cross FW, and Palmer CE. An atlas of sensitivity to tuberculin, PPD-B, and histoplasmin in the United States. *Am Rev Respir Dis*. 1969;99(4 Suppl):1–132.

95. Black GF et al. BCG-induced increase in interferon-gamma response to mycobacterial antigens and efficacy of BCG vaccination in Malawi and the UK: Two randomised controlled studies. *Lancet* 2002;359(9315):1393–401.

96. Black GF et al. Patterns and implications of naturally acquired immune responses to environmental and tuberculous mycobacterial antigens in northern Malawi. *J Infect Dis*. 2001;184(3):322–9.

97. Palmer CE, and Long MW. Effects of infection with atypical mycobacteria on BCG vaccination and tuberculosis. *Am Rev Respir Dis*. 1966;94(4):553–68.

98. Brandt L et al. Failure of the *Mycobacterium bovis* BCG vaccine: Some species of environmental mycobacteria block multiplication of BCG and induction of protective immunity to tuberculosis. *Infect Immun*. 2002;70(2):672–8.

99. Floyd S et al. Kinetics of delayed-type hypersensitivity to tuberculin induced by Bacille Calmette–Guérin vaccination in northern Malawi. *J Infect Dis*. 2002;186(6):807–14.

100. Poyntz HC, Stylianou E, Griffiths KL, Marsay L, Checkley AM, and McShane H. Non-tuberculous mycobacteria have diverse effects on BCG efficacy against *Mycobacterium tuberculosis*. *Tuberculosis (Edinburgh, Scotland)* 2014;94(3):226–37.

101. Muller J et al. Cytomegalovirus infection is a risk factor for TB disease in infants. *JCI Insight*. 2019;4(23):e130090.

102. Ben-Smith A et al. Differences between naive and memory T cell phenotype in Malawian and UK adolescents: A role for cytomegalovirus? *BMC Infect Dis*. 2008;8:139.

103. Miles DJC, Gadama L, Gumbi A, Nyalo F, Makanani B, and Heyderman RS. Human immunodeficiency virus (HIV) infection during pregnancy induces CD4 T-cell differentiation and modulates responses to Bacille Calmette–Guérin (BCG) vaccine in HIV-uninfected infants. *Immunology* 2010;129(3):446–54.

104. Elias D, Britton S, Aseffa A, Engers H, and Akuffo H. Poor immunogenicity of BCG in helminth infected population is associated with increased *in vitro* TGF-beta production. *Vaccine* 2008;26(31):3897–902.

105. Black S et al. Efficacy, safety and immunogenicity of heptavalent pneumococcal conjugate vaccine in children. Northern California Kaiser Permanente Vaccine Study Center Group. *Pediatr Infect Dis J*. 2000;19(3):187–95.

106. Caruso AM, Serbina N, Klein E, Triebold K, Bloom BR, and Flynn JL. Mice deficient in CD4 T cells have only transiently diminished levels of IFN-gamma, yet succumb to tuberculosis. *J Immunol*. 1999;162(9):5407–16.

107. Scanga CA et al. Depletion of CD4(+) T cells causes reactivation of murine persistent tuberculosis despite continued expression of interferon gamma and nitric oxide synthase 2. *J Exp Med*. 2000;192(3):347–58.

108. Lin PL et al. CD4 T cell depletion exacerbates acute *Mycobacterium tuberculosis* while reactivation of latent infection is dependent on severity of tissue depletion in cynomolgus macaques. *AIDS Res Hum Retroviruses* 2012;28(12):1693–702.

109. Geldmacher C, Zumla A, and Hoelscher M. Interaction between HIV and *Mycobacterium tuberculosis*: HIV-1-induced CD4 T-cell depletion and the development of active tuberculosis. *Curr Opin HIV AIDS* 2012;7(3):268–75.

110. Lin PL, and Flynn JL. CD8 T cells and *Mycobacterium tuberculosis* infection. *Semin Immunopathol*. 2015;37(3):239–49.

111. Huang S. Targeting innate-like T cells in tuberculosis. *Front Immunol*. 2016;7:594.

112. Flynn JL, Chan J, Triebold KJ, Dalton DK, Stewart TA, and Bloom BR. An essential role for interferon gamma in resistance to *Mycobacterium tuberculosis* infection. *J Exp Med*. 1993;178(6):2249–54.

113. Bustamante J, Boisson-Dupuis S, Abel L, and Casanova JL. Mendelian susceptibility to mycobacterial disease: Genetic, immunological, and clinical features of inborn errors of IFN-γ immunity. *Semin Immunol*. 2014;26(6):454–70.

114. Mohan VP et al. Effects of tumor necrosis factor alpha on host immune response in chronic persistent tuberculosis: Possible role for limiting pathology. *Infect Immun*. 2001;69(3):1847–55.

115. Lin PL, Plessner HL, Voitenok NN, and Flynn JL. Tumor necrosis factor and tuberculosis. *J Investig Dermatol Symp Proc*. 2007;12(1):22–5.

116. Nambiar JK, Ryan AA, Kong CU, Britton WJ, and Triccas JA. Modulation of pulmonary DC function by vaccine-encoded GM-CSF enhances protective immunity against *Mycobacterium tuberculosis* infection. *Eur J Immunol*. 2010;40(1):153–61.

117. Li H et al. Latently and uninfected healthcare workers exposed to TB make protective antibodies against *Mycobacterium tuberculosis*. *Proc Natl Acad Sci USA* 2017;114(19):5023–8.

118. Lu LL et al. A functional role for antibodies in tuberculosis. *Cell* 2016;167(2):433–43e14.

119. Turner J, Frank AA, Brooks JV, Gonzalez-Juarrero M, and Orme IM. The progression of chronic tuberculosis in the mouse does not require the participation of B lymphocytes or interleukin-4. *Exp Gerontol*. 2001;36(3):537–45.

120. Vordermeier HM, Venkataprasad N, Harris DP, and Ivanyi J. Increase of tuberculous infection in the organs of B cell-deficient mice. *Clin Exp Immunol*. 1996;106(2):312–6.

121. Maglione PJ, Xu J, and Chan J. B cells moderate inflammatory progression and enhance bacterial containment upon pulmonary challenge with *Mycobacterium tuberculosis*. *J Immunol*. 2007;178(11):7222–34.

122. Lund FE, and Randall TD. Effector and regulatory B cells: Modulators of CD4$^+$ T cell immunity. *Nat Rev Immunol*. 2010;10(4):236–47.

123. Kurt-Jones EA, Liano D, HayGlass KA, Benacerraf B, Sy MS, and Abbas AK. The role of antigen-presenting B cells in T cell priming *in vivo*. Studies of B cell-deficient mice. *J Immunol*. 1988;140(11):3773–8.

124. Teitelbaum R et al. A mAb recognizing a surface antigen of *Mycobacterium tuberculosis* enhances host survival. *Proc Natl Acad Sci USA* 1998;95(26):15688–93.

125. Hamasur B, Haile M, Pawlowski A, Schroder U, Kallenius G, and Svenson SB. A mycobacterial lipoarabinomannan specific monoclonal antibody and its F(ab') fragment prolong survival of mice infected with *Mycobacterium tuberculosis*. *Clin Exp Immunol*. 2004;138(1):30–8.

126. Costello AM et al. Does antibody to mycobacterial antigens, including lipoarabinomannan, limit dissemination in childhood tuberculosis? *Trans R Soc Trop Med Hyg*. 1992;86(6):686–92.

127. Sanchez-Rodriguez C et al. An IgG antibody response to the antigen 85 complex is associated with good outcome in Mexican Totonaca Indians with pulmonary tuberculosis. *Int J Tuberc Lung Dis*. 2002;6(8):706–12.

128. Fletcher HA et al. T-cell activation is an immune correlate of risk in BCG vaccinated infants. *Nat Commun*. 2016;7:11290.

129. Jacobs AJ, Mongkolsapaya J, Screaton GR, McShane H, and Wilkinson RJ. Antibodies and tuberculosis. *Tuberculosis (Edinb)* 2016;101:102–13.

130. Kagina BM et al. Specific T cell frequency and cytokine expression profile do not correlate with protection against tuberculosis after Bacillus Calmette–Guérin vaccination of newborns. *Am J Respir Crit Care Med*. 2010;182(8):1073–9.

131. Tameris MD et al. Safety and efficacy of MVA85A, a new tuberculosis vaccine, in infants previously vaccinated with BCG: A randomised, placebo-controlled phase 2b trial. *Lancet* 2013; 381(9871):1021–8.

132. Donald PR, Maher D, and Qazi S. A research agenda to promote the management of childhood tuberculosis within national tuberculosis programmes. *Int J Tuberc Lung Dis*. 2007;11(4):370–80.

133. Marais BJ et al. The natural history of childhood intra-thoracic tuberculosis: A critical review of literature from the pre-chemotherapy era. *Int J Tuberc Lung Dis*. 2004;8(4):392–402.

134. Geldenhuys H et al. Risky behaviour and psychosocial correlates in adolescents—is there a link with tuberculosis? *Afr J Psychiatry (Johannesbg)* 2011;14(5):383–7.

135. Getahun H, Gunneberg C, Granich R, and Nunn P. HIV infection-associated tuberculosis: The epidemiology and the response. *Clin Infect Dis*. 2010;50(Suppl 3):S201–7.

136. Suthar AB et al. Antiretroviral therapy for prevention of tuberculosis in adults with HIV: A systematic review and meta-analysis. *PLoS Med*. 2012;9(7):e1001270.

137. Nell AS et al. Safety, tolerability, and immunogenicity of the novel antituberculous vaccine RUTI: Randomized, placebo-controlled phase II clinical trial in patients with latent tuberculosis infection. *PLOS ONE* 2014;9(2):e89612.

138. Mayosi BM et al. Prednisolone and *Mycobacterium indicus pranii* in tuberculous pericarditis. *N Engl J Med*. 2014; 371(12):1121–30.

139. Horwitz MA, Harth G, Dillon BJ, and Maslesa-Galic S. Recombinant bacillus Calmette–Guérin (BCG) vaccines expressing the *Mycobacterium tuberculosis* 30-kDa major secretory protein induce greater protective immunity against tuberculosis than conventional BCG vaccines in a highly susceptible animal model. *Proc Natl Acad Sci USA* 2000;97(25):13853–8.

140. Pym AS et al. Recombinant BCG exporting ESAT-6 confers enhanced protection against tuberculosis. *Nat Med*. 2003;9(5):533–9.

141. Grode L et al. Increased vaccine efficacy against tuberculosis of recombinant *Mycobacterium bovis* bacille Calmette–Guérin mutants that secrete listeriolysin. *J Clin Invest*. 2005; 115(9):2472–9.

142. Grode L, Ganoza CA, Brohm C, Weiner J 3rd, Eisele B, and Kaufmann SH. Safety and immunogenicity of the recombinant BCG vaccine VPM1002 in a phase 1 open-label randomized clinical trial. *Vaccine* 2013;31(9):1340–8.

143. Kupferschmidt K. Infectious disease. Taking a new shot at a TB vaccine. *Science* 2011;334(6062):1488–90.

144. Walker KB et al. The second Geneva Consensus: Recommendations for novel live TB vaccines. *Vaccine* 2010;28(11):2259–70.

145. Kamath AT et al. New live mycobacterial vaccines: The Geneva consensus on essential steps towards clinical development. *Vaccine* 2005;23(29):3753–61.

146. Martin C et al. The live *Mycobacterium tuberculosis* phoP mutant strain is more attenuated than BCG and confers protective immunity against tuberculosis in mice and guinea pigs. *Vaccine* 2006;24(17):3408–19.

147. Verreck FA et al. MVA.85A boosting of BCG and an attenuated, phoP deficient *M. tuberculosis* vaccine both show protective efficacy against tuberculosis in rhesus macaques. *PLOS ONE* 2009;4(4):e5264.

148. Spertini F et al. Safety of human immunisation with a live-attenuated *Mycobacterium tuberculosis* vaccine: A randomised, double-blind, controlled phase I trial. *Lancet Respir Med*. 2015;3(12):953–62.

149. Stanford J, Stanford C, and Grange J. Immunotherapy with *Mycobacterium vaccae* in the treatment of tuberculosis. *Front Biosci*. 2004;9:1701–19.

150. Waddell RD et al. Safety and immunogenicity of a five-dose series of inactivated *Mycobacterium vaccae* vaccination for the prevention of HIV-associated tuberculosis. *Clin Infect Dis*. 2000;30(Suppl 3):S309–S15.

151. Vuola JM et al. Immunogenicity of an inactivated mycobacterial vaccine for the prevention of HIV-associated tuberculosis: A randomized, controlled trial. *AIDS* 2003;17(16):2351–5.

152. Durban Immunotherapy Trial Group. Immunotherapy with *Mycobacterium vaccae* in patients with newly diagnosed pulmonary tuberculosis: A randomised controlled trial. *Lancet* 1999;354(9173):116–9.

153. von Reyn CF et al. Prevention of tuberculosis in Bacille Calmette–Guérin-primed, HIV-infected adults boosted with an inactivated whole-cell mycobacterial vaccine. *AIDS* 2010;24(5):675–85.

154. von Reyn CF et al. Safety and immunogenicity of an inactivated whole cell tuberculosis vaccine booster in adults primed with BCG: A randomized, controlled trial of DAR-901. *PLOS ONE* 2017;12(5):e0175215.

155. Gupta A et al. Protective efficacy of *Mycobacterium indicus pranii* against tuberculosis and underlying local lung immune responses in guinea pig model. *Vaccine* 2012;30(43):6198–209.

156. Sehgal IS, Agarwal R, Aggarwal AN, and Jindal SK. A randomized trial of *Mycobacterium* w in severe sepsis. *J Crit Care* 2015;30(1):85–9.

157. Leroux-Roels I et al. Improved CD4(+) T cell responses to *Mycobacterium tuberculosis* in PPD-negative adults by M72/AS01 as compared to the M72/AS02 and Mtb72F/AS02 tuberculosis candidate vaccine formulations: A randomized trial. *Vaccine* 2013;31(17):2196–206.

158. Brandt L et al. The protective effect of the *Mycobacterium bovis* BCG vaccine is increased by coadministration with the *Mycobacterium tuberculosis* 72-kilodalton fusion polyprotein Mtb72F in *M. tuberculosis*-infected guinea pigs. *Infect Immun.* 2004;72(11):6622–32.

159. Reed SG et al. Defined tuberculosis vaccine, Mtb72F/AS02A, evidence of protection in cynomolgus monkeys. *Proc Natl Acad Sci USA* 2009;106(7):2301–6.

160. Penn-Nicholson A et al. Safety and immunogenicity of candidate vaccine M72/AS01E in adolescents in a TB endemic setting. *Vaccine* 2015;33(32):4025–34.

161. Montoya J et al. A randomized, controlled dose-finding Phase II study of the M72/AS01 candidate tuberculosis vaccine in healthy PPD-positive adults. *J Clin Immunol.* 2013;33(8):1360–75.

162. Idoko OT et al. Safety and immunogenicity of the M72/AS01 candidate tuberculosis vaccine when given as a booster to BCG in Gambian infants: An open-label randomized controlled trial. *Tuberculosis (Edinb)* 2014;94(6):564–78.

163. Kumarasamy N et al. A randomized, controlled safety, and immunogenicity trial of the M72/AS01 candidate tuberculosis vaccine in HIV-positive Indian adults. *Medicine (Baltim)* 2016;95(3):e2459.

164. Van Der Meeren O et al. Phase 2b controlled trial of M72/AS01E vaccine to prevent tuberculosis. *N Engl J Med.* 2018;379(17):1621–34.

165. van Dissel JT et al. Ag85B-ESAT-6 adjuvanted with IC31® promotes strong and long-lived *Mycobacterium tuberculosis* specific T cell responses in volunteers with previous BCG vaccination or tuberculosis infection. *Vaccine* 2011;29(11):2100–9.

166. Reither K et al. Safety and immunogenicity of H1/IC31(R), an adjuvanted TB subunit vaccine, in HIV-infected adults with CD4+ lymphocyte counts greater than 350 cells/mm³: A phase II, multicentre, double-blind, randomized, placebo-controlled trial. *PLOS ONE* 2014;9(12):e114602.

167. Ottenhoff TH et al. First in humans: A new molecularly defined vaccine shows excellent safety and strong induction of long-lived *Mycobacterium tuberculosis*-specific Th1-cell like responses. *Hum Vaccine* 2010;6(12):1007–15.

168. Skeiky YA et al. Non-clinical efficacy and safety of HyVac4:IC31 vaccine administered in a BCG prime-boost regimen. *Vaccine* 2010;28(4):1084–93.

169. Billeskov R, Elvang TT, Andersen PL, and Dietrich J. The HyVac4 subunit vaccine efficiently boosts BCG-primed anti-mycobacterial protective immunity. *PLOS ONE* 2012;7(6):e39909.

170. Lin PL et al. The multistage vaccine H56 boosts the effects of BCG to protect cynomolgus macaques against active tuberculosis and reactivation of latent *Mycobacterium tuberculosis* infection. *J Clin Invest.* 2012;122(1):303–14.

171. Luabeya AK et al. First-in-human trial of the post-exposure tuberculosis vaccine H56:IC31 in *Mycobacterium tuberculosis* infected and non-infected healthy adults. *Vaccine* 2015;33(33):4130–40.

172. Baldwin SL, Bertholet S, Reese VA, Ching LK, Reed SG, and Coler RN. The importance of adjuvant formulation in the development of a tuberculosis vaccine. *J Immunol.* 2012;188(5):2189–97.

173. Penn-Nicholson A et al. Safety and immunogenicity of the novel tuberculosis vaccine ID93+ GLA-SE in BCG-vaccinated healthy adults in South Africa: A randomised, double-blind, placebo-controlled phase 1 trial. *Lancet Respir Med.* 2018;6(4):287–98.

174. Santosuosso M, McCormick S, Zhang X, Zganiacz A, and Xing Z. Intranasal boosting with an adenovirus-vectored vaccine markedly enhances protection by parenteral *Mycobacterium bovis* BCG immunization against pulmonary tuberculosis. *Infect Immun.* 2006;74(8):4634–43.

175. Vordermeier HM et al. Viral booster vaccines improve *Mycobacterium bovis* BCG-induced protection against bovine tuberculosis. *Infect Immun.* 2009;77(8):3364–73.

176. Goonetilleke NP, McShane H, Hannan CM, Anderson RJ, Brookes RH, and Hill AV. Enhanced immunogenicity and protective efficacy against *Mycobacterium tuberculosis* of bacille Calmette–Guérin vaccine using mucosal administration and boosting with a recombinant modified vaccinia virus Ankara. *J Immunol.* 2003;171(3):1602–9.

177. Williams A et al. Boosting with poxviruses enhances *Mycobacterium bovis* BCG efficacy against tuberculosis in guinea pigs. *Infect Immun.* 2005;73(6):3814–6.

178. McShane H et al. Recombinant modified vaccinia virus Ankara expressing antigen 85A boosts BCG-primed and naturally acquired antimycobacterial immunity in humans. *Nat Med.* 2004;10(11):1240–4.

179. Whelan KT et al. Safety and immunogenicity of boosting BCG vaccinated subjects with BCG: Comparison with boosting with a new TB vaccine, *MVA85A*. *PLOS ONE* 2009;4(6):e5934.

180. Beveridge NE et al. Immunisation with BCG and recombinant MVA85A induces long-lasting, polyfunctional *Mycobacterium tuberculosis*-specific CD4+ memory T lymphocyte populations. *Eur J Immunol.* 2007;37(11):3089–100.

181. Scriba TJ et al. Dose-finding study of the novel tuberculosis vaccine, *MVA85A*, in healthy BCG-vaccinated infants. *J Infect Dis.* 2011;203(12):1832–43.

182. Scriba TJ et al. A phase IIa trial of the new tuberculosis vaccine, *MVA85A*, in HIV- and/or *Mycobacterium tuberculosis*-infected adults. *Am J Respir Crit Care Med.* 2012;185(7):769–78.

183. Tchilian E, Ahuja D, Hey A, Jiang S, and Beverley P. Immunization with different formulations of *Mycobacterium tuberculosis* antigen 85A induces immune responses with different specificity and protective efficacy. *Vaccine* 2013;31(41):4624–31.

184. White AD et al. Evaluation of the safety and immunogenicity of a candidate tuberculosis vaccine, *MVA85A*, delivered by aerosol to the lungs of macaques. *Clin Vaccine Immunol.* 2013;20(5):663–72.

185. Satti I et al. Safety and immunogenicity of a candidate tuberculosis vaccine MVA85A delivered by aerosol in BCG-vaccinated healthy adults: A phase 1, double-blind, randomised controlled trial. *Lancet Infect Dis.* 2014;14(10):939–46.

186. Wang J et al. Single mucosal, but not parenteral, immunization with recombinant adenoviral-based vaccine provides potent protection from pulmonary tuberculosis. *J Immunol.* 2004;173(10):6357–65.

187. Smaill F et al. A human type 5 adenovirus-based tuberculosis vaccine induces robust T cell responses in humans despite preexisting anti-adenovirus immunity. *Sci Transl Med.* 2013;5(205):205ra134.

188. Farina SF et al. Replication-defective vector based on a chimpanzee adenovirus. *J Virol.* 2001;75(23):11603–13.

189. Vogels R et al. Replication-deficient human adenovirus type 35 vectors for gene transfer and vaccination: Efficient human cell infection and bypass of preexisting adenovirus immunity. *J Virol.* 2003;77(15):8263–71.

190. Xiang Z et al. Chimpanzee adenovirus antibodies in humans, sub-Saharan Africa. *Emerging Infect Dis.* 2006;12(10):1596–9.

191. Quinn KM et al. Comparative analysis of the magnitude, quality, phenotype, and protective capacity of simian immunodeficiency virus gag-specific CD8+ T cells following human-, simian-, and chimpanzee-derived recombinant adenoviral vector immunization. *J Immunol.* 2013;190(6):2720–35.

192. Colloca S et al. Vaccine vectors derived from a large collection of simian adenoviruses induce potent cellular immunity across multiple species. *Sci Transl Med.* 2012;4(115):115ra2.

193. Jeyanathan M et al. Novel chimpanzee adenovirus-vectored respiratory mucosal tuberculosis vaccine: Overcoming local anti-human adenovirus immunity for potent TB protection. *Mucosal Immunol.* 2015;8(6):1373–87.

194. Radosevic K et al. Protective immune responses to a recombinant adenovirus type 35 tuberculosis vaccine in two mouse strains: CD4 and CD8 T-cell epitope mapping and role of gamma interferon. *Infect Immun.* 2007;75(8):4105–15.

195. Abel B et al. The novel tuberculosis vaccine, *AERAS*-402, induces robust and polyfunctional CD4+ and CD8+ T cells in adults. *Am J Respir Crit Care Med.* 2010;181(12):1407–17.

196. van Zyl-Smit RN et al. Safety and immunogenicity of adenovirus 35 tuberculosis vaccine candidate in adults with active or previous tuberculosis. A randomized trial. *Am J Respir Crit Care Med.* 2017;195(9):1171–80.

197. Churchyard GJ et al. The safety and immunogenicity of an adenovirus type 35-vectored TB vaccine in HIV-infected, BCG-vaccinated adults with CD4(+) T cell counts >350 cells/mm³. *Vaccine* 2015;33(15):1890–6.

198. Walsh DS et al. Adenovirus type 35-vectored tuberculosis vaccine has an acceptable safety and tolerability profile in healthy, BCG-vaccinated, QuantiFERON((R))-TB Gold (+) Kenyan adults without evidence of tuberculosis. *Vaccine* 2016;34(21):2430–6.

199. Tameris M et al. A double-blind, randomised, placebo-controlled, dose-finding trial of the novel tuberculosis vaccine AERAS-402, an adenovirus-vectored fusion protein, in healthy, BCG-vaccinated infants. *Vaccine* 2015;33(25):2944–54.

200. Kagina BM et al. The novel tuberculosis vaccine, AERAS-402, is safe in healthy infants previously vaccinated with BCG, and induces dose-dependent CD4 and CD8 T cell responses. *Vaccine* 2014;32(45):5908–17.

201. Nyendak M et al. Adenovirally-induced polyfunctional T cells do not necessarily recognize the infected target: Lessons from a phase I trial of the AERAS-402 vaccine. *Sci Rep.* 2016;6:36355.

202. Darrah PA et al. Aerosol vaccination with AERAS-402 elicits robust cellular immune responses in the lungs of rhesus macaques but fails to protect against high-dose *Mycobacterium tuberculosis* challenge. *J Immunol.* 2014;193(4):1799–811.

203. Hokey D et al. Heterologous prime-boost with Ad35/AERAS-402 and MVA85A elicits potent CD8+ T cell immune responses in a phase I clinical trial (VAC7P.969). *J Immunol.* 2014;192(Suppl 1):141.14.

204. Sheehan S et al. A Phase I, Open-Label Trial, evaluating the safety and immunogenicity of candidate tuberculosis vaccines AERAS-402 and MVA85A, administered by prime-boost regime in BCG-vaccinated healthy adults. *PLOS ONE* 2015;10(11):e0141687.

205. Hansen SG et al. Prevention of tuberculosis in rhesus macaques by a cytomegalovirus-based vaccine. *Nat Med.* 2018;24(2):130–43.

206. Elias D, Akuffo H, and Britton S. PPD induced *in vitro* interferon gamma production is not a reliable correlate of protection against *Mycobacterium tuberculosis*. *Trans R Soc Trop Med Hyg.* 2005;99(5):363–8.

207. Mittrücker HW et al. Poor correlation between BCG vaccination-induced T cell responses and protection against tuberculosis. *Proc Natl Acad Sci USA* 2007;104(30):12434–9.

208. Lazarevic V, Nolt D, and Flynn JL. Long-term control of *Mycobacterium tuberculosis* infection is mediated by dynamic immune responses. *J Immunol.* 2005;175(2):1107–17.

209. Mattila JT, Diedrich CR, Lin PL, Phuah J, and Flynn JL. Simian immunodeficiency virus-induced changes in T cell cytokine responses in cynomolgus macaques with latent *Mycobacterium tuberculosis* infection are associated with timing of reactivation. *J Immunol.* 2011;186(6):3527–37.

210. Darrah PA et al. Multifunctional TH1 cells define a correlate of vaccine-mediated protection against *Leishmania major. Nat Med.* 2007;13(7):843–50.

211. Boaz MJ, Waters A, Murad S, Easterbrook PJ, and Vyakarnam A. Presence of HIV-1 Gag-specific IFN-gamma+IL-2+ and CD28+IL-2+ CD4 T cell responses is associated with nonprogression in HIV-1 infection. *J Immunol.* 2002;169(11):6376–85.

212. Lindenstrøm T et al. Tuberculosis subunit vaccination provides long-term protective immunity characterized by multifunctional CD4 memory T cells. *J Immunol.* 2009;182(12):8047–55.

213. Derrick SC, Yabe IM, Yang A, and Morris SL. Vaccine-induced anti-tuberculosis protective immunity in mice correlates with the magnitude and quality of multifunctional CD4 T cells. *Vaccine* 2011;29(16):2902–9.

214. Sebina I et al. Long-lived memory B-cell responses following BCG vaccination. *PLOS ONE* 2012;7(12):e51381.

215. Tanner R, O'Shea MK, Fletcher HA, and McShane H. *In vitro* mycobacterial growth inhibition assays: A tool for the assessment of protective immunity and evaluation of tuberculosis vaccine efficacy. *Vaccine* 2016;34(39):4656–65.

216. Kampmann B, Gaora PO, Snewin VA, Gares MP, Young DB, and Levin M. Evaluation of human antimycobacterial immunity using recombinant reporter mycobacteria. *J Infect Dis.* 2000;182(3):895–901.

217. Cheng SH et al. Demonstration of increased anti-mycobacterial activity in peripheral blood monocytes after BCG vaccination in British school children. *Clin Exp Immunol.* 1988;74(1):20–5

218. Worku S, and Hoft DF. *In vitro* measurement of protective mycobacterial immunity: Antigen-specific expansion of T cells capable of inhibiting intracellular growth of bacille Calmette–Guérin. *Clin Infect Dis.* 2000;30(Suppl 3):S257–61.

219. Silver RF, Li Q, Boom WH, and Ellner JJ. Lymphocyte-dependent inhibition of growth of virulent *Mycobacterium tuberculosis* H37Rv within human monocytes: Requirement for CD4+ T cells in purified protein derivative-positive, but not in purified protein derivative-negative subjects. *J Immunol.* 1998;160(5):2408–17.

220. Fletcher HA et al. Inhibition of mycobacterial growth *in vitro* following primary but not secondary vaccination with *Mycobacterium bovis* BCG. *Clin Vaccine Immunol.* 2013;20(11):1683–9.

221. Smith SG, Zelmer A, Blitz R, Fletcher HA, and Dockrell HM. Polyfunctional CD4 T-cells correlate with *in vitro* mycobacterial growth inhibition following *Mycobacterium bovis* BCG-vaccination of infants. *Vaccine* 2016;34(44):5298–305.

222. Joosten SA et al. Mycobacterial growth inhibition is associated with trained innate immunity. *J Clin Invest.* 2018;128(5):1837–51.

223. Berry MP et al. An interferon-inducible neutrophil-driven blood transcriptional signature in human tuberculosis. *Nature* 2010;466(7309):973–7.

224. Bloom CI et al. Transcriptional blood signatures distinguish pulmonary tuberculosis, pulmonary sarcoidosis, pneumonias and lung cancers. *PLOS ONE* 2013;8(8):e70630.

225. Cliff JM et al. Distinct phases of blood gene expression pattern through tuberculosis treatment reflect modulation of the humoral immune response. *J Infect Dis.* 2013;207(1):18–29.

226. Maertzdorf J et al. Common patterns and disease-related signatures in tuberculosis and sarcoidosis. *Proc Natl Acad Sci USA* 2012;109(20):7853–8.

227. Maertzdorf J et al. Human gene expression profiles of susceptibility and resistance in tuberculosis. *Genes Immun.* 2011;12(1):15–22.

228. Maertzdorf J et al. Functional correlations of pathogenesis-driven gene expression signatures in tuberculosis. *PLOS ONE* 2011;6(10):e26938.

229. Zak DE et al. A blood RNA signature for tuberculosis disease risk: A prospective cohort study. *Lancet* 2016;387(10035):2312–22.

230. Suliman S et al. Four-gene Pan-African blood signature predicts progression to tuberculosis. *Am J Respir Crit Care Med.* 2018;197(9):1198–208.

231. Fletcher HA et al. Human newborn bacille Calmette–Guérin vaccination and risk of tuberculosis disease: A case-control study. *BMC Med.* 2016;14:76.

232. McShane H, and Williams A. A review of preclinical animal models utilised for TB vaccine evaluation in the context of recent human efficacy data. *Tuberculosis (Edinb)* 2014;94(2):105–10.

233. Niemann S, and Supply P. Diversity and evolution of *Mycobacterium tuberculosis*: Moving to whole-genome-based approaches. *Cold Spring Harb Perspect Med.* 2014;4(12):a021188.

234. Orme IM, and Basaraba RJ. The formation of the granuloma in tuberculosis infection. *Semin Immunol.* 2014;26(6):601–9.

235. Dunachie S, Hill AV, and Fletcher HA. Profiling the host response to malaria vaccination and malaria challenge. *Vaccine* 2015;33(40): 5316–20.

236. Shirley DA, and McArthur MA. The utility of human challenge studies in vaccine development: Lessons learned from cholera. *Vaccine (Auckl)* 2011;2011(1):3–13.

237. McArthur MA et al. Activation of *Salmonella* Typhi-specific regulatory T cells in typhoid disease in a wild-type *S. Typhi* challenge model. *PLoS Pathog.* 2015;11(5):e1004914.

238. Minassian AM, Satti I, Poulton ID, Meyer J, Hill AV, and McShane H. A human challenge model for *Mycobacterium tuberculosis* using *Mycobacterium bovis* bacille Calmette–Guérin. *J Infect Dis.* 2012;205(7):1035–42.

239. Harris SA et al. Evaluation of a human BCG challenge model to assess antimycobacterial immunity induced by BCG and a candidate tuberculosis vaccine, MVA85A, alone and in combination. *J Infect Dis.* 2014;209(8):1259–68.

240. Blazevic A, Xia M, Turan A, Tennant J, and Hoft DF. Pilot studies of a human BCG challenge model. *Tuberculosis (Edinb)* 2017;105:108–12.

241. Kaufmann SHE, Fortune S, Pepponi I, Ruhwald M, Schrager LK, and Ottenhoff THM. TB biomarkers, TB correlates and human challenge models: New tools for improving assessment of new TB vaccines. *Tuberculosis.* 2016;99:S8–S11.

242. Brennan MJ, Fruth U, Milstien J, Tiernan R, de Andrade Nishioka S, and Chocarro L. Development of new tuberculosis vaccines: A global perspective on regulatory issues. *PLoS Med.* 2007;4(8):e252.

243. Nunn AJ, Phillips PPJ, and Mitchison DA. Timing of relapse in short-course chemotherapy trials for tuberculosis. *Int J Tuberc Lung Dis.* 2010;14(2):241–2.

244. Lalor MK et al. Population differences in immune responses to Bacille Calmette–Guérin vaccination in infancy. *J Infect Dis.* 2009;199(6):795–800.

245. Wilson ME, Fineberg HV, and Colditz GA. Geographic latitude and the efficacy of Bacillus Calmette–Guérin vaccine. *Clin Infect Dis.* 1995;20(4):982–91.

246. Xing Z, and Lichty BD. Use of recombinant virus-vectored tuberculosis vaccines for respiratory mucosal immunization. *Tuberculosis (Edinb)* 2006;86(3–4):211–7.

247. Tanner R et al. Tools for assessing the protective efficacy of TB vaccines in humans: *In vitro* mycobacterial growth inhibition predicts outcome of *in vivo* mycobacterial infection. *Front. Immunol.* 2020;10:2983. doi: 10.3389/fimmu.2019.02983.

CLINICAL ASPECTS AND TREATMENT

13

Pulmonary Tuberculosis

CHARLES S. DELA CRUZ, BARBARA SEAWORTH, AND GRAHAM BOTHAMLEY

PROGRESSIVE PRIMARY TUBERCULOSIS

EPIDEMIOLOGY

Primary tuberculosis (TB) is the disease that occurs when there is no existing immune response to *Mycobacterium tuberculosis*. These forms of TB occur, therefore, in children who have been recently exposed to an infectious case,[1,2] in adults with immunosuppression, for example due to HIV[3] and the use of anti-TNF inhibitors,[4] and in the elderly where there is waning immunity.[5] They may also occur in the rare and atypical forms of TB in those with deficiencies in interferon-γ and IL-12 and their receptors and pathways.[6]

PATHOGENESIS (SEE ALSO CHAPTER 4)

An infectious particle is inhaled. The size of the tubercle bacillus ($2–4 \times 0.2–0.5\,\mu$m) is such that it can reach the alveolus. Early defense mechanisms such as mucus, the mucociliary escalator and cough likely remove larger infectious particles. In the alveolus, alveolar macrophages phagocytose the bacilli, which replicate within the cytoplasm (phagosome–lysosome fusion is inhibited[7]). After bursting this cell, other phagocytes enter from the blood and ingest the extracellular bacilli. This collection of cells forms the "primary focus." As with most inhaled particles, 60% occur within the right lower lobe and 40% within the left lower lobe (Figure 13.1). At this stage, there are no antigen-specific immune cells and the lesion is not visible on the chest radiograph. There may be non-specific inflammation and immune responses, of which the type I interferons have been implicated in a measurable response,[8] whereas the roles of lysozyme,[9] defensins,[10] lactoferrin,[11] complement[12] and natural antibodies[13] are unclear. A non-specific cellular response, consisting of neutrophils, natural killer cells and $\gamma\delta$ cells may also take part if there is sufficient inflammation. Such a collection of cells can be termed an "early" granuloma and has been seen in animal models such as the zebrafish.[14] Video footage of this model suggests that such granulomas "metastasize," causing both hematogenous and lymphatic dissemination.

Material from the primary focus may then reach draining mediastinal lymph nodes, where mycobacterial antigens can be presented by dendritic cells to engage specific immunity. Such immunity can be detected by the tuberculin response 3–6 weeks after infection. These immune cells then circulate and, through chemotaxis, enter the early granuloma, which enlarges and where the specific immune response may either contain the lesion or cause further tissue damage. The combination of the primary focus and an enlarged mediastinal lymph node, containing the germinal centers where T and B cells proliferate, is termed the primary (Ghon) complex. Both the primary (Ghon) focus and lymph nodes are now visible on a chest radiograph. The primary focus may have indistinct edges; subsequent healing with calcification leads to a clearly defined small nodule. The effectiveness of this primary immune response determines whether progressive primary TB will occur, or whether the disease will be contained at this stage.

CLINICAL FEATURES

The salient features of progressive primary TB were defined by studies of TB in children at the beginning of the last century.[15] Most patients with TB infection do not notice any symptoms.[16] The earliest stages include fever and, rarely, there may be erythema nodosum (Figure 13.2) and phlyctenular keratoconjunctivitis (Figure 13.3). Then follows mediastinal lymph node TB as noted earlier. Endoscopic biopsy under ultrasound can make the diagnosis using both mycobacterial culture and histology.[17] Large mediastinal lymph nodes can compress an airway (see Complications section); this is an indication for steroids in addition to standard TB treatment. Rarely, these lymph nodes may

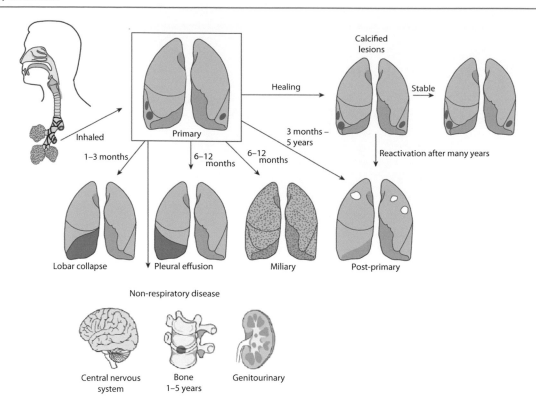

Figure 13.1 Diagram of the development of TB disease and its spread through the body.

contain caseating granulomas, which may then erode into a bronchus and cause tuberculous pneumonia; the sputum smear is positive and the prognosis is poor.

Pleural effusions are related to a primary focus close to the pleura, such that the inflammatory response causes fluid to accumulate within the pleural space. As such, the bacterial load is low (below the limit of 10⁴/mL, at which point bacilli can be seen under the microscope[18]) and cultures for TB are rarely positive.[19] Blind pleural biopsies can increase the likelihood of making the diagnosis from 60% to 90%.[20,21] Video-assisted thoracoscopy may show a characteristic appearance of granulomas, if seeding of TB has occurred, and biopsies will then confirm the diagnosis by mycobacterial culture.[22] In many cases, pleural effusions may resolve spontaneously, but infectious post-primary TB is then likely to occur within the next 5 years if no treatment is given.[23,24]

Hematogenous spread without bacterial containment results in miliary TB and TB meningitis. These occur within 12 months of infection.[15] The chest radiograph in the former shows a haze

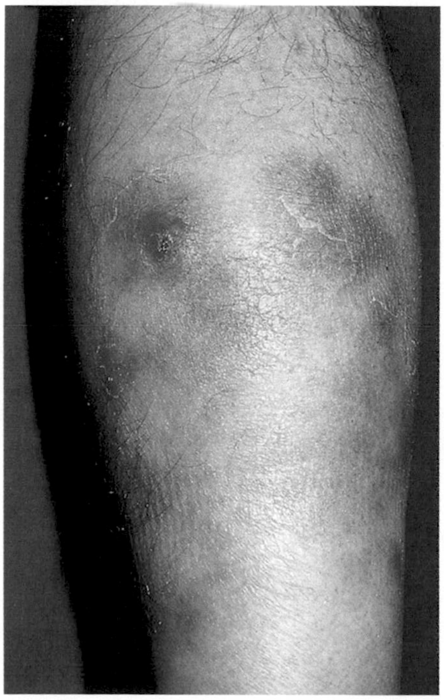

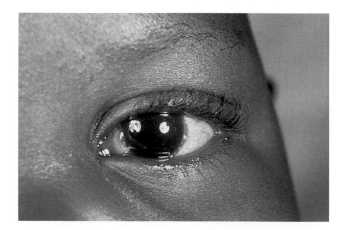

Figure 13.2 View of patient's shins showing erythema nodosum.

Figure 13.3 Phlyctenular conjunctivitis in an African infant.

of small nodules 2–3 mm in size. The diagnosis is often missed due to the symmetrical appearance of the chest x-ray; a CT scan, however, is diagnostic.[25,26] Approximately half of those with miliary TB develop acute respiratory distress syndrome (ARDS), characterized by interstitial pulmonary edema in the absence of heart failure.[27]

Later forms of progressive primary TB include bone disease (within 3 years) and renal or skin disease (>3 years). Thus, the majority of the forms of progressive primary TB are extra-pulmonary and, without bronchial erosion, are non-infectious. These are the forms of TB against which BCG vaccination has been shown to have the greatest and a significant effect.[28]

POST-PRIMARY TB

Post-primary TB is defined by the presence of an antigen-specific immune response at the start of the disease process. As such, it can occur in those with self-healed infections (latent TB infection or long-lasting TB immunity—LTBI[29]), either due to reactivation or re-infection, or in those whose initial primary immune response is followed rapidly by the post-primary response.

EPIDEMIOLOGY

Post-primary TB is the most common form of adult TB that is responsible for transmission of the disease. Approximately half of those with post-primary TB have a positive sputum smear.[30] Those with a positive sputum smear are infectious and those with a negative sputum smear but a positive culture less so.[31] Unlike primary TB, there is a gender bias toward males for post-primary TB.[32] Patients are most commonly adults in their economically productive years, aged between 20 and 35 years.[33] The main risk factors require the release of infectious droplets and time for them to survive until the next human host breathes them in. Other risk factors relate to the likelihood of infection (see Chapter 6) and include individuals with either a greater risk of having TB due to their previous life experiences such as living in a high burden country or associating with those with a high incidence of TB. However, even a person with sputum smear-positive disease releases few infectious particles.[34] Close contact is needed (overcrowding, associated with social deprivation, and poor ventilation).[35,36] The tubercle bacillus is killed by exposure to daylight within 30 minutes (overcrowding and lack of natural light) and by desiccation (more transmission in humid environments). There is a small element of genetic susceptibility (family members of an infectious case are especially susceptible).[37]

The higher incidence and mortality in HIV infection is associated with progressive primary TB and lower CD4 cell counts.[3] Whether HIV infection increases the risk of sputum smear- and culture-positive pulmonary TB remains an open question without case-control studies that take account of the denominator population and its risk of TB, the enhanced screening associated with a diagnosis of HIV as well as the CD4 count.[38] In the same way, other risk factors for TB may not withstand the scrutiny of case-control studies, which account for the likelihood of previous infection (see later).

PATHOGENESIS

Post-primary TB is dependent on the presence of a functioning, and perhaps over-active, immune response (see also Chapter 4). This means that bacilli seeded through hematogenous spread are associated with "late" granulomas, containing immune cells. Unlike progressive primary TB, the lung is favored as the place for TB multiplication due to its high oxygen rather than anoxic environment.[39] Thus, TB in the lung is located predominantly in the upper lobes or in the apical segments of the lower lobes[40] (see also Chapter 8). The importance of a pneumonic and endobronchial phase has gained recent attention through careful pathological studies correlated with computed tomography images.[41] The immune response is vigorous and leads to cell death within the granuloma (caseation).[42] Tissue destruction may then lead to connection of the granuloma with a blood vessel and result in hemoptysis. If the caseum connects with an alveolus, further lung destruction causes a cavity. These cavities are lined by a biofilm of tubercle bacilli, which are no longer contained within a granuloma.[43] This pathology explains how bacilli can then enter the sputum to give a positive sputum smear. Thus, the presence of a positive sputum smear implies cavitation, even if this is not visible on a chest x-ray. Healing can be accompanied by parenchymal lung fibrosis.

CLINICAL FEATURES

Patients with infectious TB are surprisingly well. This accounts for their often late presentation and longer period of infectiousness, allowing for transmission.[44] Regular screening in the Netherlands after World War II showed that a normal chest radiograph could be followed by extensive disease in less than 3 months.[45] Most studies indicate that the period of symptoms before first presentation is about 2 months.[2,46]

The symptoms of post-primary TB with the highest sensitivity and specificity include hemoptysis, night sweats (by definition, soaking of pyjamas and bed linen) and unexplained weight loss. Other symptoms such as cough, cough with sputum, fever, loss of appetite and general malaise are non-specific, although have a high sensitivity in areas where TB is endemic.[47] Breathlessness is rare, unless there has been a long time between the onset of symptoms and the start of effective treatment, when fibrosis can predominate. There is little inflammation and so the ventilation-perfusion mismatch found in pneumonia is not a significant feature of pulmonary TB. If access to health services and treatment is poor, then the features of "consumption" with weight loss and lethargy ensue.

There are few clinical signs of pulmonary TB. The cavitation obscures any sign of consolidation due to infiltration of the lung parenchyma. Crackles are rarely audible compared to normal breath sounds. Cavities cannot be demonstrated by percussion and auscultation unless huge.

The chest radiograph is the most helpful initial investigation in terms of diagnosis (see Chapter 8), as it leads to requests for a sputum smear and mycobacterial culture (see Chapter 7) (Figure 13.4). Screening of patients with a cough using a molecular test such as Xpert® MTB/RIF has been recommended by WHO,[48] as

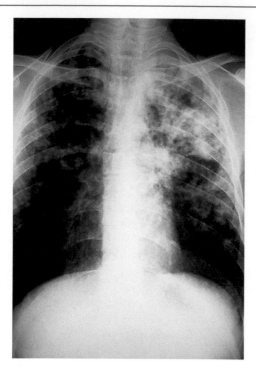

Figure 13.4 Chest x-ray of 40-year-old man showing characteristic changes of post-primary TB with soft cavitating lesions in the upper zones, particularly the left.

this will also detect those with sputum smear-negative culture-positive disease. A full blood count is usually helpful by showing a normal neutrophil count and thereby excluding other bacterial infections as the cause of the chest x-ray appearance. Raised inflammatory markers (C-reactive protein, erythrocyte sedimentation rate) and a high globulin with a low albumin can often alert the attending physician to the possibility of pulmonary TB.

Fibrosis is a late feature of pulmonary TB, although the prevalence is probably overestimated due to selective reporting.[49,50] Untreated, smear-positive pulmonary TB has a case fatality rate of 0.34, with an average duration of 3 years and a 10-year mortality of 70% (range 58%–80%), as has been estimated in a review of TB epidemiology in the pre-antibiotic era.[51] Considerable individual variation existed and persistently sputum smear-positive individuals constitute a sizeable proportion (13%) even in the antibiotic era.[52]

COMPLICATIONS

MASSIVE HEMOPTYSIS

Massive hemoptysis is defined as expectoration of approximately 150 mL of blood or more. The choice of this relatively small amount, compared to blood loss from the gastro-intestinal tract, is that it is sufficient to cause clotting of the central airways and death by asphyxiation rather than exsanguination. Before antibiotic treatment, it was the commonest cause of death from TB.

The tissue destruction associated with cavitating post-primary TB, e.g., bronchiolar erosion with necrosis of adjacent blood

vessels,[53] Rasmussen's aneurysm[54,55] and post-tuberculous bronchiectasis[56] may cause massive hemoptysis, as can an aspergilloma (see later). The vascular supply of the lung consists of the low-pressure pulmonary circulation and the high-pressure bronchial circulation, from which most significant hemoptyses arise.[57]

An urgent chest x-ray may localize the lung from which bleeding is occurring. CT scans replace an urgent chest x-ray where possible.[58] The patient can then be placed with the affected lung downwards, whilst localizing the source of bleeding more accurately. Intubation may be required in order to remove blood from the main airways and can be used to block off the lung from which bleeding arises by placing the endotracheal tube beyond the carina. Bronchoscopy will define the site of bleeding and a rigid bronchoscope permits more effective suction to remove blood and clot if there is danger of asphyxia; otherwise the blood should be allowed to clot in order to arrest further bleeding. Irrigation with cold saline can reduce the bleeding. If bronchoscopy is unsuccessful angiography can localize the source of bleeding.

Bronchial artery embolization is the first mode of treatment where conservative measures fail to halt the hemoptysis.[59] Cannulation of bronchial arteries is technically difficult and requires an experienced interventional radiologist.

If the bleeding fails to stop, surgery is required (see Chapter 17). Lobectomy is to be preferred to pneumonectomy to reduce post-surgical morbidity. As noted later post-tuberculous bronchiectasis is most commonly confined to the right middle lobe, and removal of this lobe has the least mortality and post-operative morbidity.

ASPERGILLOMA

Aspergillus fumigatus colonizes lung cavities and this is especially the case in large cavities related to previous pulmonary TB.[60] Fungal balls (aspergillomas) can be seen on chest radiographs within a cavity (Figure 13.5). CT appearances are characterized by a dependent mycetoma with surrounding air in the form of a crescent. Most are coincidental findings and cause no problems. Treatment with anti-fungal agents, such as itraconazole, has been suggested,[61] but no randomized-controlled trial comparing such treatment with observation has been conducted. Some aspergillomas cause erosion of the cavity wall and significant hemoptysis.[62]

As with massive hemoptysis (see earlier), the treatment of choice is bronchial artery embolization.[5,63] Some have used radiotherapy to induce hemostasis.[64] Surgical series show significant post-surgical morbidity (16%–30%) and mortality (1.2%–3.3%).[57,65–67]

BRONCHIECTASIS

Bronchiectasis was originally defined as the production of more than a cupful of purulent sputum daily, usually with finger clubbing to indicate chronic sepsis. A radiological definition correlating with the pathological finding of dilated bronchial tubes was achieved by lipoidal bronchography.[68] As high-resolution CT scanning with 1–3 mm sections became more widespread, a radiological definition of an airway greater than the accompanying pulmonary artery became the standard,[69] usually with bronchial wall thickening, air-fluid levels or mucus impaction,

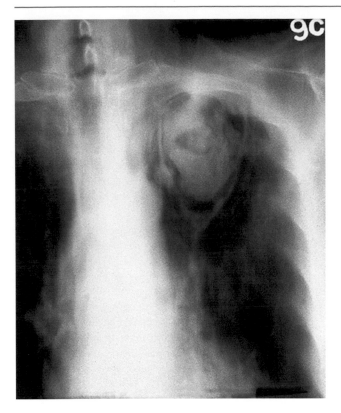

Figure 13.5 Posteranterior chest x-ray showing an aspergilloma in the left apex.

loss of definition of blood vessels due to peri-bronchial fibrosis and evidence of infection.[70] Most CT scans were performed for minor hemoptysis or a persistent cough. Transitory bronchiectasis in pneumonia and atelectasis occurs, so that a single CT scan may over-estimate the presence of bronchiectasis. The cause of bronchiectasis appears to be obstruction of the airway such that infected mucus cannot be expectorated, leading to a cycle of chronic inflammation. The relative contribution of TB to bronchiectasis varies according to its local incidence.[71]

Tuberculous bronchiectasis, thus, has several forms. In focal TB, the areas of pneumonic consolidation may be accompanied by local bronchiectasis; this is considered temporary, but long-term bronchiectasis may occur if bronchial obstruction by caseous material is prolonged.[72] Fibrosis in self-healed TB may cause traction bronchiectasis. Obstruction of airways by enlarged mediastinal lymph nodes may prevent removal of infected mucus. As the entrance to the right middle lobe is the smallest in size of all the lobes and there is little collateral aeration, the "middle lobe syndrome" (Brock's syndrome) with lobar bronchiectasis is a common cause of post-tuberculous bronchiectasis.[73] Prevention can be achieved by early diagnosis and treatment of TB.

PNEUMOTHORAX

Pneumothorax may be due to either active or healed TB, with rupture of a cavity into the pleural space. If there is sufficient caseous material, a tuberculous empyema and a bronchopleural fistula can result (see later). Self-healed TB, before the advent of specific treatment, was considered to be one of the commonest causes

of pneumothorax. TB remains a significant cause of spontaneous pneumothorax in children[74] and adults[75] in high incidence areas. The time required to achieve resolution of a pneumothorax appeared higher in those with TB than in others, but this could be an age-related phenomenon.[76] If the lung fails to inflate, a broncho-pleural fistula is suspected (see next).

Artificial pneumothoraces were prescribed as treatment for TB before the antibiotic era, in an attempt to "rest" the lung and were probably effective by reducing oxygen levels close to dividing tubercle bacilli.[77]

BRONCHOPLEURAL FISTULA

Most bronchopleural fistulae occur after surgery (see Chapter 17). Anatomical delineation by CT scanning is essential before making the diagnosis of a spontaneous bronchopleural fistula as large cavities with fluid levels can give the same radiographic appearance, but attempts to drain such a cavity will cause an iatrogenic bronchopleural fistula.[78] Surgical management (Chapter 17) of persistent bronchopleural fistulae, despite intercostal drainage and antibiotic treatment, has improved greatly since the times of thoracoplasty, omental flaps and muscle flaps. Glues, coils and sealants via endoscopic procedures are effective and have much less post-operative morbidity.[79]

TUBERCULOUS EMPYEMA

The connection of a tuberculous cavity in the lung parenchyma with the pleural space can lead to empyema and a persisting connection between the airways and the pleural space. Empyema is diagnosed by aspiration of pleural fluid showing a significant cellular content. Bacterial causes are common and placement of an intercostal drain is required in order to remove the pus and prevent the need for later surgical decortication. A diagnosis of tuberculous empyema usually occurs *after* placement of the drain. There are therefore no studies to indicate whether, unlike other bacterial infections, antibiotic treatment for TB might be sufficient of itself, as it is in those with a primary tuberculous pleural effusion. The lack of an inflammatory response and the slower response to treatment means that an intercostal drain is required for longer in those with a tuberculous etiology.[80,81] Even after drainage, pleural fibrosis, and later calcification, can be significant (Figure 13.6).

ENDOBRONCHIAL TB AND BRONCHIAL STENOSIS

Rarely, TB may present at bronchoscopy as a nodule or caseating lesion in the bronchial airways, due to tissue necrosis either from a mediastinal lymph node, adjacent lung parenchyma or in relation to hematogenous spread. The diagnosis is made by biopsy and mycobacterial culture. Bronchial stenosis used to be a common outcome, and corticosteroids with standard TB treatment are often recommended to prevent this (see Treatment section).[82] Stenting or sleeve resection (see Chapter 17) may be required.

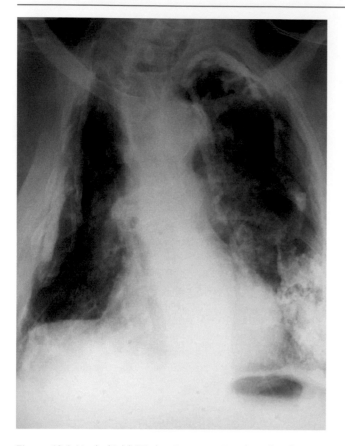

Figure 13.6 Healed (old) TB showing extensive pleural and parenchymal calcification.

CHRONIC LUNG FUNCTION IMPAIRMENT

Smoking is the commonest cause of chronic obstructive pulmonary disease (COPD), but an independent association with previous TB has been observed.[83] In the absence of pneumoconiosis (see later), TB in South African miners reduced forced expiratory volume (FEV1) and forced vital capacity (FVC) with a dose effect for the number of episodes; both restrictive and obstructive defects were observed.[84] Case-control studies, especially in sub-Saharan Africa, need to exclude wood burning stoves as a feature of poorer communities with a higher incidence of TB. In Texas, patients seen 6 months after completing TB treatment were more likely to have lung impairment than those with LTBI, with a lesser effect of smoking and younger age.[85] In a cohort of patients with COPD, those with previous TB were more likely to have bronchiectasis and more severe emphysema.[86] The most frequently missed variable was the time to diagnosis of TB—more lung destruction would be expected the longer the period of time before adequate treatment. Unilateral tuberculous lung destruction is a known feature of chronic TB with significantly delayed treatment.[87]

NON-TUBERCULOUS MYCOBACTERIAL DISEASE

Non-tuberculous mycobacterial diseases (NTMDs) can affect patients who have had TB. The diagnosis of NTMD requires symptoms, the isolation of the same species of mycobacteria on two or more occasions (or one from a protected bronchoalveolar lavage) with radiological evidence of disease, other diseases being excluded.[88] The difficulty in making the diagnosis is that a substantial minority of patients with TB will have radiological abnormalities and that atypical mycobacteria are frequently cultured in the absence of disease.[89] Equally, NTMD is often found where the anatomy of the lung has been distorted, e.g. by bronchiectasis or fibrosis. The development of 16S rRNA species identification without the need for culture has permitted identification of the "lung microbiome."[90] Such techniques will likely play an important role in defining the role of non-tuberculous mycobacteria after successful treatment of TB.

GOALS OF TREATMENT

Providers and programs which treat persons with TB are responsible for both the care of the patient and public health outcomes. They must aim to (1) cure the individual while providing patient-centered therapy and (2) prevent transmission in the community by rapidly rendering them non-infectious. These are the dual charges for all TB programs and providers who accept the responsibility for treatment of TB.

Treatment regimens are designed to provide a rapid clinical and bacteriological response which limits lung damage, prevents death, and ensures a lasting cure. Multi-drug regimens are needed to prevent acquisition of drug resistance, treatment failure, and relapse.[91]

The globally recommended initial treatment regimen for all forms of drug-susceptible TB includes four drugs: isoniazid (INH), rifampin (RMP), ethambutol (EMB), and pyrazinamide (PZA). Each has a specific indication. INH has excellent early bactericidal activity, it is primarily active against rapidly dividing bacteria such as those in the walls of cavitary lesions. Rapidly decreasing the size of the bacterial population limits infectiousness and the risk of acquired resistance. Persons with isolates that are susceptible to INH are reported to have a >90% decrease in the concentration of viable bacilli in the sputum after 2 days of treatment.[92] Further reports suggest that after the first 2–3 weeks of treatment that the degree of infectiousness is <1% of the original level. This is also attributed to the effects of rifampin.[93] Rifampin is both a strong bactericidal drug and the key sterilizing drug in the standard regimen through its activity against both rapidly dividing mycobacteria and persisters.[94] The action of anti-TB drugs in short-course chemotherapy.[94] Ethambutol is added to the regimen pending drug susceptibility tests to prevent the development of resistance should the isolate be resistant to either INH or RMP. Ethambutol has little bactericidal activity but can protect against acquired resistance during the early weeks of treatment.[93] PZA targets slowly growing or semi-dormant bacilli especially in acidic environments and is responsible for decreasing the risk of relapse.[95]

TREATMENT REGIMENS

Treatment consists of two phases: the initial (intensive) phase and the continuation phase. The initial phase includes INH, RIF, EMB and PZA. If the tuberculous isolate is already known to be susceptible to both INH and rifampin then ethambutol does not need to be included. The initial phase is given for the first 2 months. The continuation phase includes INH and RMP and is usually given for another 4 months; a total of 6 months of treatment (see also Chapter 21).[96,97] Treatment should be supplemented with pyridoxine at 25–50 mg daily for all patients with a risk of neuropathy due to dietary deficiency (diabetics, pregnant women, breastfeeding infants, and individuals with HIV, chronic renal disease, alcoholism, and malnutrition). Pyridoxine may be increased to 100 mg daily in people with the previously listed medical conditions.[98,99]

Following the initial phase, PZA is stopped and if drug susceptibility is known then ethambutol can also be stopped.[96] In the United States, if drug susceptibility test results are delayed, ethambutol should be continued into the second phase and many experts would also continue the PZA pending receipt of susceptibility reports. This is done to limit the possibility of rifampin monotherapy in persons with unknown INH resistance which could lead to acquisition of rifampin resistance, hence acquired multiple drug-resistant TB (MDR-TB). WHO guidelines allow for the continued use of ethambutol in the continuation phase of treatment when there is a suspicion of INH resistance or in populations with known or suspected elevated levels of INH resistance in new patients. In patients with prior treatment, susceptibility testing should be done to guide treatment.[97]

Treatment completion is determined by the number of directly observed therapy (DOT) doses taken by the patient within a given time. In general, to complete the 6-month standard regimen (often given 5 days per week, Monday through Friday) requires a minimum of 40 doses of daily PZA and 130 doses of medication in total. The 6-month regimen should be completed in 9 months. Poor adherence is associated with a significantly increased likelihood of relapse.[100]

When PZA is not tolerated, patients whose isolates are susceptible to both INH and RMP can be successfully treated with these two drugs but treatment must be continued for 9 months. Ethambutol is added until drug susceptibility is confirmed. This alternate regimen is recommended by the ATS/CDC/IDSA for most persons 70 and over to avoid the toxicity from PZA.

When RMP cannot be tolerated or cannot be used due to drug interactions, treatment must include additional drugs and the duration extended to 12–18 months or longer (see Chapter 16).

Treatment is usually completed after a total of 6 months but in the event of cavitary disease and/or a delayed response (described later), treatment should be extended for an additional 3 months or a total duration of 9 months.[96] Treatment can be completed in 6 months when INH is not included due to either resistance or intolerance if RMP, ETH and PZA are given daily for 6 months or if a fluoroquinolone is added to the regimen and PZA is given daily for at least 3–4 months.[101]

DELIVERY OF TREATMENT

Treatment often requires cooperation between the provider and a public health agency. Responsibility for coordination between these sectors and the patient is needed, and is often given to the patient's case manager, who seeks to ensure that treatment is individualized and patient centered. The least restrictive public health interventions needed to assure adherence are preferred.[102] DOT, the practice of observing the patient swallow anti-TB medication, is the standard of care in the United States,[96,103,104] Europe,[105] and many other countries. DOT is endorsed by the World Health Organization (WHO).[97] DOT rather than self-administered therapy (SAT) is suggested for the routine treatment of patients with all forms of TB along with case management interventions during treatment by the American Thoracic Society (ATS), Centers for Disease Control and Prevention (CDC) and Infectious Disease Society of American's (IDSA) guidelines for drug-susceptible pulmonary TB.[96] Although a systematic review did not identify a significant difference between SAT and DOT for mortality, treatment completion or relapse, DOT was significantly associated with improved treatment success and with increased sputum smear conversion during treatment, when compared to SAT.[96] Resource limits may dictate patient populations prioritized for DOT such as those with drug resistance, extensive disease, at risk for toxicity, poor adherence or poor outcomes and children. Although no controlled studies exist, extensive programmatic experience in the United States supports the use of 5 times per week daily DOT.

Treatment should be given on an empty stomach. If the patient has difficulty taking medications when fasting, a small snack can be given such as toast, a piece of fruit, tea, crackers or a similar food which is culturally appropriate. The entire dose of the medications should be given at once. Doses of individual first-line medications used in treatment of drug-susceptible TB cannot not be split. If the patient is not able to tolerate all medications taken at once, individual medications can be separated, with the entire dose of each medication taken at one time, if DOT can be arranged twice daily.

INTENSITY OF DOSING

Both the WHO and ATS/CDC/IDSA guidelines recommend daily dosing throughout treatment as the preferred approach.[96,97] Daily dosing during the intensive period improves all treatment outcomes. These recommendations are based on a systematic review commissioned for the 2010 WHO guidelines and updated for the 2017 document.[97,106] The recommendation from WHO is conditional but leaves little room for alternate approaches. ATS/CDC/IDSA's recommendation is categorized as "strong with moderate certainty in the evidence" but notes subgroups who may be considered for the three times per week treatment, even in the initiation phase, after several weeks of daily treatment and during the continuation phase for those with good prognostic indicators when programmatic or patient factors do not allow daily dosing.

Patients who may be considered for three times per week dosing should have excellent adherence, be HIV-uninfected, noncavitary and/or be smear negative, and have drug-susceptible TB.[96] The WHO notes that with three times per week intermittent dosing during the continuation phase "no doses must be missed because the rates of unfavorable outcomes then rise."[97]

Three times per week dosing throughout treatment was associated with a higher rate of treatment failure, relapse and acquired drug resistance when compared to daily treatment in patients both with known drug susceptibility and those with unknown strain susceptibility.[107,108] Poor outcomes were higher in HIV-infected persons, especially those not on highly active antiretroviral therapy (ART), those with cavitary disease or baseline drug resistance.[109-112]

Twice weekly dosing is generally not recommended in either the initial or continuation phase. When compared to three times per week dosing it is associated with higher rates of treatment failure, relapse, and acquired drug resistance. The WHO notes that "twice-weekly dosing should never be used during any part of TB therapy."[106]

LENGTH OF TREATMENT

Six months remain the minimum duration of treatment for TB disease. The success of the 6-month regimen depends on the presence of a rifamycin throughout and PZA for the initial 2 months of treatment. Treatment can be completed in 6 months when the patient cannot tolerate INH, or is resistant, if a rifamycin, PZA and ethambutol are given daily for 6 months. New guidelines from WHO recommend using 6 months of either levofloxacin or moxifloxacin along with RMP, PZA and ethambutol.[101] Four-month treatment regimens employing a second-generation fluoroquinolone, either levofloxacin or moxifloxacin, substituted for either ethambutol or INH, with or without rifapentine substituted for RMP have had unacceptable relapse rates.[112-116] With a fluoroquinolone in the regimen culture conversion occurs earlier but this has not translated to the long-term good outcomes seen in the 6-month standard regimen described previously.

Reanalysis of studies of 4-month regimens shows that some groups of low-risk individuals can be identified that have a good response. These include those who have non-cavitary disease, are smear negative and, are HIV negative.[100]

Treatment extension is recommended when those with cavitary disease have positive sputum cultures after completing 2 months of the initiation phase of treatment. These individuals with both cavitary disease and a culture that remains positive at 2 months of treatment have rates of relapse of approximately 20% compared with 2% among persons with neither factor.[109-117] Treatment should be extended in these persons. After the initial phase of daily INH, RMP, PZA and ETH, INH and RMP should continue daily for an additional 7 months. The total treatment duration will be 9 months.[105,106] Cavitation on the initial chest radiograph (CXR) is itself a risk factor for relapse even with culture conversion by the end of the second month of treatment.[118] A meta-analysis to assess the sensitivity of sputum smear and culture alone at 2 months had a relatively low sensitivity to predict treatment failure or relapse.[119]

There are limited data to identify the duration of treatment in HIV-infected individuals who are receiving ART but the ATS/CDC/ISDA guidelines note "it is widely believed that the standard 6-month regimen is effective and achieves TB cure rates comparable to those reported for HIV-uninfected patients."[96] They further recommend that in the rare situation where the individual is not receiving ART, the continuation phase of treatment should be extended by 3 months for a total of 9 months. The WHO also recommends a standard duration of treatment for those with TB and HIV.[97]

Treatment extension is not routinely recommended for adults with non-CNS extra-pulmonary or disseminated disease. Many experts extend treatment where the extra-pulmonary site includes the central nervous system. Clinical assessment of a slow or delayed response, especially in persons with extensive disease and other risk factors associated with a poor outcome (smokers, diabetes, chronic kidney disease, and other immune suppression) should prompt consideration of treatment extension. Other factors associated with a delayed response should also be investigated including an assessment of adherence, absorption, and drug susceptibility. If poor absorption is identified, treatment may be extended once the situation is resolved.

CULTURE-NEGATIVE TB

Patients who present with classical symptoms of TB, who have an abnormal CXR consistent with TB disease and have a positive interferon gamma release assay (IGRA) but have negative acid-fast bacilli (AFB) smears and a negative nucleic amplification test (NAAT) should be evaluated for clinical TB. If there is not another diagnosis, the standard treatment for TB should be started. After 2 months of treatment, they should be monitored for evidence of clinical improvement (decreased cough, increased energy, increased appetite, and weight) and radiographic improvement. A repeat CXR done at 2 months and compared to baseline film is key to the diagnosis of culture negative TB. If either clinical or radiographic improvement is noted, the diagnosis should be confirmed. Treatment for a total of 4 months is adequate. The full four drug regimen may be continued for 4 months if there is a possibility of undetected INH resistance.[96]

ADJUNCTIVE CORTICOSTEROIDS

Adjunct corticosteroid use has not been shown to reduce all-cause mortality or result in higher sputum conversion in patients with pulmonary TB.[120] However, the addition of corticosteroid therapy to anti-mycobacterial treatment has been considered for some HIV-infected patients who develop clinical manifestations suggestive of an immune reconstitution inflammatory syndrome (IRIS) after treatment with anti-TB and antiretroviral medications. Signs and symptoms include high fevers, new or worsening pulmonary and pleural disease, lymphadenopathy and/or CNS manifestations. These reactions are felt to develop due to the reconstitution of the immune response from the antiretroviral treatment.[121] For patients with TB, IRIS is more commonly seen in patients with a CD4 cell count of less than 50 cell/mm^3 early on during their antiretroviral treatment.

Treatment with adjunctive corticosteroids for IRIS-related TB manifestations is considered only after other possible causes such as treatment failure from drug-resistant TB or other opportunistic infections or non-infectious disease such as lymphoma. For most patients with mild IRIS, treatment for both TB and HIV can be continued with the addition of non-steroidal anti-inflammatory drugs.

For more severe cases of IRIS, it has been suggested that prednisone at the dose of 1.25 mg/kg/day or 50–80 mg/day can be used for patients who develop IRIS. Typically, prednisone is used for 2–4 weeks with the goal for tapering of dose over 6–12 weeks or longer.[96] In the absence of HIV co-infection, corticosteroids are used if there is lobar collapse due to paradoxical enlargement of mediastinal lymph nodes to prevent loss of function or bronchiectasis, as well as in some forms of extrapulmonary TB (see Chapter 14).[120,122]

BASELINE ASSESSMENT AND MONITORING DURING TREATMENT

Initial assessment of the newly diagnosed patient with TB should include a medical assessment which identifies risk factors for a poor or delayed outcome, weight should be recorded at baseline and repeated at least monthly. If significant changes occur doses may need to be changed. Visual acuity testing and assessment of Ishihara Plates is done prior to initiation of treatment and repeated monthly while the patient is on ethambutol. Baseline assessment of neuropathy should be documented and repeated monthly while the patient is on INH.

All patients, even those thought to have only extrapulmonary disease, should have an initial CXR. The radiograph should be repeated at 2 months, especially in those with a negative culture. Many experts obtain a CXR at the end of treatment. Prior to starting treatment three sputum specimens should be collected at least 8 hours apart, one of which should be a first morning and preferably one induced and/or observed.[123] A NAAT should be done on one of the specimens, AFB smears and culture should be done on all three. Molecular testing for rifampin resistance should be done on the initial specimen if the NAAT is positive and is a routine part of some NAAT tests. Sputum should be collected monthly during treatment for AFB smear and culture until two consecutive cultures are negative. If a culture is positive after completing 3 months of treatment, culture with susceptibility testing should be repeated; earlier if there is concern regarding possible treatment failure.

Initial laboratory testing should include an HIV test, complete blood count (CBC), liver enzymes, total bilirubin, glucose, and serum creatinine. If the patient is at risk of hepatitis, a baseline hepatitis panel should be included. If the initial glucose is high, a baseline hemoglobin A1c is helpful. Repeat liver enzymes should be done at least monthly in persons with abnormal enzymes at baseline and those who are pregnant, HIV infected, are heavy users of alcohol, have underlying liver disease, other chronic medical problems or taking medication with potential for drug-induced liver toxicity.

Some experts recommend doing therapeutic serum drug level testing for persons at risk of poor absorption, especially those with HIV infection, poorly controlled diabetes, other gastrointestinal diagnosis and persons with delayed response to treatment.

Drug interactions with the patients' other medications should be assessed and, if present, discussed with the primary care provider. Most interactions are related to RMP's effect on the cytochrome P450 metabolic pathway in the liver. A list of common drug interactions can be found in the ATS/CDC/IDSA guidelines[96] and a variety of drug interaction checkers are available on various websites. In many situations where RMP causes significant enhanced metabolism of a needed medication, it can be replaced in the standard regimen with rifabutin 300 mg daily.

ADVERSE EVENTS

Patients should be encouraged to identify difficulties with the medical regimen and discuss them with their case manager or provider. Rashes are the most common adverse effect. A flush after the first dose of PZA is frequent, but not repeated. Antihistamines are usually effective in controlling rashes, other than those associated with Stevens-Johnson syndrome, most commonly due to RMP.

Gastrointestinal upset is the next most common problem. The patient should be educated that this is quite common in the initial weeks but usually improves. The most important thing is to exclude drug-induced liver toxicity. Whenever this is a consideration, medication should be withheld until liver enzymes are documented to be less than twice the upper limit of normal.

If elevated liver enzymes ≥3 times the upper limit of normal in the presence of symptoms or ≥5 times the upper limit of normal in the absence of symptoms and/or a total bilirubin >2 are found, anti-TB medications should be stopped. Other causes of liver disease should be excluded (biliary disease, pancreatitis, gastritis, infectious hepatitis), but often drug-induced hepatitis from one of the anti-TB medications is likely. Treatment with drugs which are hepatotoxic should be held until liver enzymes return to less than twice the upper limit of normal at which time they can be re-introduced simultaneously with careful follow up of liver enzymes for 5–7 days.[124] In 90%, there is no repeated rise in liver enzymes. For the 10% who have repeated hepatotoxicity, a predominant hepatitis picture is associated with INH and a predominant obstructive picture, especially with a raised bilirubin, is associated with RMP. Patients may prefer the shortest course possible and therefore wish for a re-challenge with PZA to limit treatment to 6 months, rather than take a 9-month course without PZA. Using an injectable drug and ethambutol can protect against drug resistance when re-introducing a single drug. The order of introduction of an individual drug varies widely among different guidelines and none has an evidence base.

Once liver toxicity is excluded as the cause of gastrointestinal upset, a variety of approaches can be used. Patients can be encouraged to take a short nap after the medication as most often they are still on home isolation when initially starting medication. Changing the time of the dose may be helpful for some patients. An antacid may be helpful for some patients, especially those with reflux (antacids cannot be given within two hours of the fluoroquinolone dose; aluminum hydroxide reduces the effective RMP dose; proton pump inhibitors may reduce the conversion of PZA to its effective metabolite pyrazinoic acid). Alternatively, medications can be given with a small snack such as toast without butter or margarine, crackers, or a small piece of fruit. When these simple measures fail, an antiemetic can be given ½ hour prior to the medication dose. Usually patients become more tolerant of medication after several weeks. PZA often is the drug most likely to be responsible for gastrointestinal complaints and the patient may improve after the initiation phase of treatment with PZA is completed.[125]

Patients on EMB must have baseline vision assessments including visual acuity and testing for red-green color blindness for each eye. This testing should be repeated monthly while they are receiving EMB. If changes in vision occur, EMB should be stopped and the patient should be referred to an ophthalmologist. Visual changes are reversible when recognized early and the offending drug is discontinued.

Other common adverse effects with the first-line medications include arthralgia with PZA. Hematologic abnormalities and neuropathy are important to recognize and address. An extensive approach to the evaluation and management of adverse effects and drug toxicities is available from the Curry International TB Center's "Drug-Resistant Tuberculosis: A Survival Guide for Clinicians, 3rd edition," Chapter 8.[126]

REFERENCES

1. Marais BJ et al. The spectrum of disease in children treated for tuberculosis in a highly endemic area. *Int J Tuberc Lung Dis.* 2006;10(7):732–8.

2. Wallgren A. The time-table of tuberculosis. *Tubercle* 1948;29:245–51.

3. Jones BE et al. Relationship of the manifestations of tuberculosis to CD4 cell counts in patients with human immunodeficiency virus infection. *Am Rev Respir Dis.* 1993;148:1292–7.

4. Keane J et al. Tuberculosis associated with infliximab, a tumor necrosis factor α-neutralizing agent. *New Engl J Med.* 2001;345(15):1098–104.

5. Perez-Guzman C et al. progressive age-related changes in pulmonary tuberculosis images and the effect of diabetes. *Am J Respir Crit Care Med.* 2000;162:1738–40.

6. Boisson-Dupuis S et al. Inherited and acquired immunodeficiencies underlying tuberculosis in childhood. *Immunol Rev.* 2015;264(1):103–20.

7. Armstrong JA, and Hart PD. Responses of cultured macrophages to *Mycobacterium tuberculosis*, with observations on fusion of lysosomes with phagosomes. *J Exp Med.* 1971;134(3 Pt 1):713–40.

8. Cliff JM et al. The human immune response to tuberculosis and its treatment: A view from the blood. *Immunol Rev.* 2015;264(1):88–102.

9. Malm S et al. In vivo virulence of *Mycobacterium tuberculosis* depends on a single homologue of the LytR-CPs-A-Psr proteins. *Sci Rep.* 2017;8(1):3936.

10. Jacobsen M et al. Candidate biomarkers for discrimination between infection and disease caused by *Mycobacterium tuberculosis*. *J Mol Med.* 2007;85(6):613–21.

11. Malhotra H et al. *Mycobacterium tuberculosis* glyceraldehyde-3-phosphate dehydrogenase (GAPDH) functions as a receptor for human lactoferrin. *Front Cell Infect Microbiol.* 2017;7:245.

12. Azad AK, Sadee W, and Schlesinger LS. Innate immune gene polymorphisms in tuberculosis. *Infect Immun.* 2012;80(10):3343–59.

13. Bardana EJ et al. Universal occurrence of antibodies to tubercle bacilli in sera from non-tuberculous and tuberculous individuals. *Clin Exp Immunol.* 1973;13:65–77.

14. Davis JM et al. Real-time visualization of mycobacterium macrophage interactions leading to initiation of granuloma formation in zebrafish embryos. *Immunity.* 2002;17(6):693–702.

15. Miller FJW. The evolution of primary infection with *Mycobacterium tuberculosis*. In: Miller FJW (ed.). *Tuberculosis in Children.* Edinburgh: Churchill Livingstone, 1981, 1–17.

16. Zak DE et al. A blood RNA signature for tuberculosis disease risk: A prospective cohort study. *Lancet.* 2016;387(10035):2312–22.

17. Tomlinson G et al. Transcriptional profiling of endobronchial ultrasound-guided lymph node samples aids diagnosis of mediastinal lymphadenopathy. *Chest.* 2016;149(2):535–44.

18. Toman K. How many bacilli are present in a sputum smear specimen found positive by smear microscopy? In: Frieden T (ed.). *Toman's Tuberculosis Case Detection, Treatment and Monitoring: Questions and Answers.* 2nd ed. Geneva: WHO, 2004, 11–3.

19. Light RW. Pleural effusion. *N Engl J Med.* 2002;346(25):1971–7.

20. Levine H et al. Diagnosis of tuberculous pleurisy by culture of pleural biopsy specimen. *Arch Intern Med.* 1970;126:269–71.

21. Scharer L, and McClement JH. Isolation of tubercle bacilli from needle biopsy specimens of the parietal pleural. *A, Rev Respir Dis.* 1968;97:466–8.

22. Sihoe AD, Shiraishi Y, and Yew YY. The current role of thoracic surgery in tuberculosis management. *Respirology.* 2009;14(7):954–68.

23. Roper WH, and Waring JJ. Primary serofibrinous pleural effusion in military personnel. *Am Rev Tuberc.* 1955;71:616–34.

24. Patiala J, and Matilla M. Effect of chemotherapy of exudative tuberculous pleurisy on the incidence of post-pleuritic tuberculosis. *Acta Tuberc Scand.* 1964;44:290–6.

25. McGuinness G et al. High resolution CT findings in miliary lung disease. *J Coumput Assist Tomogr.* 1992;16(3):384–90.

26. Sharma SK et al. Computed tomography in miliary tuberculosis: Comparison with plain films, bronchoalveolar lavage, pulmonary functions and gas exchange. *Australs Radiol.* 1996;40(2):113–8.

27. Maartens G, Willcox PA, and Benatar SR. Miliary tuberculosis: Rapid diagnosis, hematologic abnormalities, and outcome in 109 treated adults. *Am J Med.* 1990;89:291–6.

28. Colditz GA et al. Efficacy of BCG vaccine in the prevention of tuberculosis: Meta-analysis of the published literature. *JAMA.* 1994;27(9):698–702.

29. Mack U et al. LTBI: Latent tuberculosis infection or lasting tuberculosis immune responses? *Eur Resp J.* 2009;33:956–73.

30. Public Health England. *Tuberculosis in England: 2017.* London: Public Health England, 2017, 29–32.

31. Tostman A et al. Tuberculosis transmission by patients with smear-negative pulmonary tuberculosis in a large cohort in the Netherlands. *Clin Infect Dis.* 2008;47:1135–42.

32. Horton KC et al. Sex differences in tuberculosis burden and notification in low- and middle-income countries: A systematic review and meta-analysis. *PLoS Med.* 2016;13(9):e1002119.

33. Murray CJ et al. Global, regional and national incidence and mortality of HIV, tuberculosis, and malaria during 1990–2013: A systematic analysis for the Global Burden of Disease Study 2013. *Lancet.* 2014;384(9947):1005–70.

34. Riley RL et al. Aerial dissemination of pulmonary tuberculosis: A two-year study of contagion in a tuberculosis ward. *Am J Hyg.* 1959;70:185–96. (reprinted *Am J Epidemiol.* 1995; 142(1):3–14).

35. Houk VN et al. The epidemiology of tuberculosis in a closed environment. *Arch Environ Health.* 1968;16:26–35.

36. Escombe AR et al. Natural ventilation for the prevention of airborne contagion. *PLoS Med.* 2007;4(2):e68.

37. Lalor MK et al. Recent household transmission of tuberculosis in England, 2010–12: Retrospective national cohort study combining epidemiological and molecular strain typing data. *BMC Med.* 2017;15:105.

38. Mukadi Y et al. Spectrum of immunodeficiency in HIV-1 infected patients with pulmonary tuberculosis in Zaire. *Lancet.* 1993;342(8864):143–6.

39. Balusubramanian V, Wiegeshaus EH, Taylor BT, and Smith DW. Pathogenesis of tuberculosis: Pathway to apical localization. *Tubercle Lung Dis.* 1994;75:168–78.

40. Aktoğu S et al. Clinical spectrum of pulmonary and pleural tuberculosis: A report of 5,480 cases. *Eur Respir J.* 1996;9:2031–5.

41. Hunter RL. Tuberculosis, as a three-act play: A new paradigm for the pathogenesis of pulmonary tuberculosis. *Tuberculosis* 2016;97:8–17.

42. Dorhoi A, and Kaufmann SH. Pathology and immune reactivity: Understanding multidimensionality in pulmonary tuberculosis. *Semin Immunopathol.* 2016;38(2):153–66.

43. Hunter RL. Pathology of post primary tuberculosis of the lung: An illustrated critical review. *Tuberculosis* 2011;91(6):497–509.

44. Toman K. How does pulmonary tuberculosis develop and how can it be detected at an early stage. In: Frieden T (ed.). *Toman's Tuberculosis.* 2nd ed. Geneva: WHO (WHO/HTM/TB/2004.334), 2004, 66–71.

45. Rieder H. What is the role of case detection by periodic mass radiographic examination in tuberculosis control. In: Frieden T (ed.). *Toman's Tuberculosis.* 2nd ed. Geneva: WHO (WHO/HTM/TB/2004.334), 2004, 72–8.

46. Getnet F et al. Delay in diagnosis of pulmonary tuberculosis in low- and middle-income settings: Systematic review and meta-analysis. *BMC Pulm Med.* 2017;17(1):202.

47. Field SK et al. Cough due to TB and other chronic infections: CHEST guideline and expert panel report. *Chest.* 2018;153(2):467–97.

48. World Health Organization. Automated real-time nucleic acid amplification technology for rapid and simultaneous detection of tuberculosis and rifampicin resistance: Xpert MTB/RIF assay for the diagnosis of pulmonary and extrapulmonary TB in adults and children. Policy update. World Health Organization, Geneva, 2013, and The use of Xpert MTB/RIF assay for the diagnosis of TB Meeting Report 2016.

49. Meghji J, Simpson H, Squire SB, and Mortimer K. A systematic review of the prevalence and pattern of imaging post-TB lung disease. *PLOS ONE* 2016;11(8):e0161176.

50. Hatipoglu ON et al. High resolution computed tomographic findings in pulmonary tuberculosis. *Thorax.* 1996;51:397–402.

51. Tiemersma EW et al. Natural history of tuberculosis: Duration and fatality of untreated pulmonary tuberculosis in HIV negative patients: A systematic review. *PLOS ONE* 2011;6(4):e17601.

52. Mlotshwa M et al. Risk factors for tuberculosis smear non-conversion in Eden district, Western Cape, South Africa, 2007–13: A retrospective cohort study. *BMC Infect Dis.* 2016;16:365.

53. Cahill BC, and Ingbar DH. Massive hemoptysis: Assessment and management. *Clin Chest Med.* 1994;15:147–67.

54. Rasmussen V. On hemoptysis, especially when fatal, in its anatomical and clinical aspects. *Edinburgh Med J.* 1868;14:385–401.

55. Bartter T, Irwin RS, and Nash G. Aneurysms of the pulmonary arteries. *Chest.* 1988;94:1065–75.

56. Fartoukh M et al. Early prediction of in-hospital mortality of patients with hemoptysis: An approach to defining severe hemoptysis. *Respiration.* 2012;83:106–14.

57. Radchenko C, Alraiyes AH, and Shojaee S. A systematic approach to the management of massive hemoptysis. *J Thorac Dis.* 2017;9(Suppl 10):S1069–86.

58. Revel MP et al. Can CT replace bronchoscopy in the detection of the site of bleeding in patients with large or massive hemoptysis? *Am J Roentgenol.* 2002;179:1217–24.

59. Panda A, Bhalla AS, and Goyal A. bronchial artery embolization in hemoptysis: A systematic review. *Diagn Interv Radiol.* 2017;23(4):307–17.

60. Dhooria S et al. Prevalence of *Aspergillus* sensitization in pulmonary-tuberculosis-related fibrocavitary disease. *Int J Tuberc Lung Dis.* 2014;18(7):850–5.

61. Campbell JH et al. Treatment of pulmonary aspergilloma with itraconazole. *Thorax.* 1991;46:839–41.

62. Lee JK et al. Clinical course and prognostic factors of pulmonary aspergilloma. *Respirology.* 2014;19(7):1066–72.

63. He G et al. Intervention treatment on massive hemoptysis of pulmonary aspergilloma. *Exp Ther Med.* 2017;13(5):2259–62.

64. Sapienza LG, Gomes MJ, Maliska C, and Norberg AN. Hemoptysis due to fungus ball after tuberculosis: A series of 21 cases treated with hemostatic radiotherapy. *BMC Infect Dis.* 2015;15:546.

65. Brik A et al. Surgical outcome of pulmonary aspergilloma. *Eur J Cardiothorac Surg.* 2008;34(4):882–5.

66. Chen QK, Jiang GN, and Ding JA. Surgical treatment for pulmonary aspergilloma: A 35-year experience in the Chinese population. *Interact Cardiovasc Thorac Surg.* 2012;15(1):77–80.

67. Muniappan A et al. Surgical therapy of pulmonary aspergillomas: A 30-year North American experience. *Ann Thorac Surg.* 2014;97(2):432–8.

68. Sicard JA, and Forestier J. General method of radiologic exploration with iodized oil. *Bull Med Soc Hop Paris* 1922;46:463–8.

69. Heard BE et al. The morphology of emphysema, chronic bronchitis, and bronchiectasis: Definition, nomenclature, and classification. *J Clin Pathol.* 1979;32:882–92.

70. Naidich DP et al. Computed tomography of bronchiectasis. *J Comput Assist Tomogr.* 1982;6:437–44.

71. Gao Y et al. Aetiology of bronchiectasis in adults: A systematic literature review. *Respirology.* 2016;21(8):1376–83.

72. Ko JM, Kim KJ, Park SH, and Park HJ. Bronchiectasis in active tuberculosis. *Acta Radiol.* 2013;54(4):412–7.

73. Graham EA, Burford TH, and Mayer JH. Middle lobe syndrome. *Postgrad Med.* 1948;4(1):29–34.

74. Beg MH et al. Spontaneous pneumothorax in children—A review of 95 cases. *Ann Trop Paediatr.* 1988;8(1):18–21.

75. Hussain SF, Aziz A, and Fatima H. Pneumothorax: A review of 146 adult cases admitted at a university teaching hospital in Pakistan. *J Pak Med Assoc.* 1999;49(10):243–6.

76. Lee SC, and Lee DH. Influence of old pulmonary tuberculosis on the management of secondary spontaneous pneumothorax in patients over the age of 70. *J Thorac Dis.* 2016;8(10):2903–10.

77. Allinson JP, Mackay AJ, and Shah PL. AJRCCM: 100-year anniversary, special historical image section: Tuberculosis then and now. *Am J Respir Crit Care Med.* 2017;195(9):1118–23.

78. Tam JK, and Lim KS. Massive pulmonary tuberculosis cavity misdiagnosed as pneumothorax. *Respirol Case Rep.* 2013;1(2):23–5.

79. Lois M, and Noppen M. Bronchopleural fistulas: An overview of the problem with special focus on endoscopic management. *Chest.* 2005;128(6):3955–65.

80. Kundu S, Mitra S, Mukherjee S, and Das S. Adult thoracic empyema: A comparative analysis of tuberculous and nontuberculous etiology in 75 patients. *Lung India* 2010;27(4):196–201.

81. Malhotra P et al. Clinical characteristics and outcomes of empyema thoracis in 117 patients: A comparative analysis of tuberculous vs. non-tuberculous aetiologies. *Respir Med.* 2007;101(3):423–30.

82. Slow WT, and Lee P. Endobronchial tuberculosis: A clinical review. *J Thorac Dis.* 2017;9(1):E71–7.

83. Allwood BW, Myer L, and Bateman ED. A systematic review of the association between pulmonary tuberculosis and the development of chronic airflow obstruction in adults. *Respiration.* 2013;86(1):76–85.

84. Hnizdo E, Singh T, and Churchyard G. Chronic pulmonary function impairment caused by initial and recurrent pulmonary tuberculosis following treatment. *Thorax.* 2000;55:32–8.

85. Pasipanodya JG et al. Pulmonary impairment after tuberculosis. *Chest.* 2007;131(6):1817–24.

86. Jin J et al. Emphysema and bronchiectasis in COPD patients with previous tuberculosis: Computed tomography features and clinical implications. *Int J Chron Obstruct Pulmon Dis.* 2018;13:375–84.

87. Varona Porreas D et al. Radiological findings of unilateral tuberculous lung destruction. *Insights Imaging* 2017;8(2):271–7.

88. Griffith DE et al. An official ATS/IDSA statement: Diagnosis, treatment, and prevention of nontuberculous mycobacterial diseases. *Am J Respir Crit Care Med.* 2007;175:367–416.

89. Tsukamura M. Diagnosis of disease caused by *Mycobacterium avium* complex. *Chest.* 1991;99:667–9.

90. O'Dwyer D, Dickson RP, and Moore BB. The lung microbiome, immunity, and the pathogenesis of chronic lung disease. *J Immunol.* 2016;196(12):4839–47.

91. Fox W, Ellard GA, and Mitchison DA. Studies on the treatment of tuberculosis undertaken by the British Medical Research Council tuberculosis units, 1946–1986, with relevant subsequent publications. *Int J Tuberc Lung Dis.* 1999;3(10 Suppl 2):S231–79.

92. Jindani A, Aber VR, Edwards EA, and Mitchison DA. The early bactericidal activity of drugs in patients with pulmonary tuberculosis. *Am Rev Respir Dis.* 1980;121(6):939–49.

93. Jindani A, Dore CJ, and Mitchison DA. Bactericidal and sterilizing activities of antituberculosis drugs during the first 14 days. *Am J Respir Crit Care Med.* 2003;167(10):1348–54.

94. Mitchison DA. The action of antituberculosis drugs in short-course chemotherapy. *Tubercle.* 1985 Sep;66(3):219–25.

95. Mitchison DA, and Dickinson JM. Bactericidal mechanisms in short course chemotherapy. *Proceedings of the XXIV International Tuberculosis.*

96. Nahid P et al. Official American Thoracic Society/Centers for Disease Control and Prevention/Infectious Diseases Society of America Clinical Practice Guidelines: Treatment of drug-susceptible tuberculosis. *Clin Infect Dis.* 2016;63(7):e147–e95.

97. Guidelines for treatment of drug susceptible tuberculosis and patient care, 2017 update. Geneva. World Heatlh Organization, 2017. License CC B&-NC-SA 3.0 IGO: CDC, 2014.

98. Snider DE, Jr. Pyridoxine supplementation during isoniazid therapy. *Tubercle.* 1980;61(4):191–6.

99. Visser ME, Texeira-Swiegelaar C, and Maartens G. The short-term effects of anti-tuberculosis therapy on plasma pyridoxine levels in patients with pulmonary tuberculosis. *Int J Tuberc Lung Dis.* 2004;8(2):260–2.

100. Imperial MZ et al. A patient-level pooled analysis of treatment-shortening regimens for drug-susceptible pulmonary tuberculosis. *Nat Med.* 2019;24(11):1708–15.

101. Organization WH. Guidelines for INH resistant tuberculosis, Geneva. 2018.

102. Prevention CfDCa. *Managing Tuberculosis Patients and Improving Adherence.* Atlanta, GA: CDC, 2014.

103. Chaulk CP, and Kazandjian VA. Directly observed therapy for treatment completion of pulmonary tuberculosis: Consensus Statement of the Public Health Tuberculosis Guidelines Panel. *JAMA.* 1998;279(12):943–8.

104. Stop TB USA Tuberculosis Elimination Plan Committee A call for action on the tuberculosis elimination plan for the United States. Available at: http://wwwthoracicorg/advocacy/stop-tb/eliminate_TB_USApdf. 2010.

105. Migliori GB et al. European Union standards for tuberculosis care. *Eur Respir J.* 2012;39(4):807–19.

106. *Guidelines for Treatment of Tuberculosis,* 4th ed. Geneva: World Health Organization, 2010. Available at: http://who.int/tb/publi cations/2010/97892415478833/en/

107. Menzies D et al. Effect of duration and intermittency of rifampin on tuberculosis treatment outcomes: A systematic review and meta-analysis. *PLoS Med.* 2009;6(9):e1000146.

108. Chang KC, Leung CC, Yew WW, Chan SL, and Tam CM. Dosing schedules of 6-month regimens and relapse for pulmonary tuberculosis. *Am J Respir Crit Care Med.* 2006;174(10):1153–8.

109. Benator D et al. Rifapentine and isoniazid once a week versus rifampicin and isoniazid twice a week for treatment of drug-susceptible pulmonary tuberculosis in HIV-negative patients: A randomised clinical trial. *Lancet.* 2002;360(9332):528–34.

110. Vernon A, Burman W, Benator D, Khan A, and Bozeman L. Acquired rifamycin monoresistance in patients with HIV-related tuberculosis treated with once-weekly rifapentine and isoniazid. Tuberculosis Trials Consortium. *Lancet.* 1999;353(9167):1843–7.

111. Burman W et al. Acquired rifamycin resistance with twice-weekly treatment of HIV-related tuberculosis. *Am J Respir Crit Care Med.* 2006;173(3):350–6.

112. Narendran G et al. Acquired rifampicin resistance in thrice-weekly antituberculosis therapy: Impact of HIV and antiretroviral therapy. *Clin Infect Dis.* 2014;59(12):1798–804.

113. Gillespie SH et al. Four-month moxifloxacin-based regimens for drug-sensitive tuberculosis. *N Engl J Med.* 2014;371(17):1577–87.

114. Merle CS et al. A four-month gatifloxacin-containing regimen for treating tuberculosis. *N Engl J Med.* 2014;371(17):1588–98.

115. Jindani A et al. High-dose rifapentine with moxifloxacin for pulmonary tuberculosis. *N Engl J Med.* 2014;371(17):1599–608.

116. Jawahar MS et al. Randomized clinical trial of thrice-weekly 4-month moxifloxacin or gatifloxacin containing regimens in the treatment of new sputum positive pulmonary tuberculosis patients. *PLOS ONE* 2013;8(7):e67030.

117. Jo KW et al. Risk factors for 1-year relapse of pulmonary tuberculosis treated with a 6-month daily regimen. *Respir Med.* 2014;108(4):654–9.

118. Chang KC, Leung CC, Yew WW, Ho SC, and Tam CM. A nested case-control study on treatment-related risk factors for early relapse of tuberculosis. *Am J Respir Crit Care Med.* 2004;170(10):1124–30.

119. Horne DJ et al. Sputum monitoring during tuberculosis treatment for predicting outcome: Systematic review and meta-analysis. *Lancet Infect Dis.* 2010;10(6):387–94.

120. Critchley JA, Orton LC, and Pearson F. Adjunctive steroid therapy for managing pulmonary tuberculosis. *Cochrane Database Syst Rev.* 2014.

121. Meintjes G et al. Tuberculosis-associated immune reconstitution inflammatory syndrome: Case definitions for use in resource-limited settings. *Lancet Infect Dis.* 2008;8(8):516–23.

122. Prasad K, and Singh MB. Corticosteroids for managing tuberculous meningitis. *Cochrane Database Syst Rev.* 2008;(1):CD002244.

123. Lewinsohn DM et al. Official American Thoracic Society/Infectious Diseases Society of America/Centers for Disease Control and Prevention Clinical Practice Guidelines: Diagnosis of Tuberculosis in Adults and Children. *Clin Infect Dis.* 2017;64(2):111–5.

124. Sharma SK, Singla R, Sarda P, Mohan A, Makharia G, Jayaswal A, Sreenivas V, and Singh S. Safety of three different re-introduction regimens compared with separate drugs for treatment of pulmonary tuberculosis: A randomised controlled trial. *Clin Infect Dis.* 2010 Mar 15;50(6):833–9.

125. Saukkonen JJ et al. An official ATS statement: Hepatotoxicity of antituberculosis therapy. *Am J Respir Crit Care Med.* 2006;174(8):935–52.

126. http://wwwcurrytbcenterucsfedu/proucts/drug-resistant-tuber culosis-survival-guide-clinicians-3rd-edition/chapter-8-moni toring-case.

14

Extrapulmonary Tuberculosis

CHARLES L. DALEY

INTRODUCTION

Mycobacterium tuberculosis can infect and cause disease at any site in the body. When tuberculosis (TB) occurs outside of the lung parenchyma, it is referred to as extrapulmonary TB, and results from the spread of tubercle bacilli throughout the body during the initial tuberculous infection. Approximately 20% of HIV-uninfected patients with TB have an extrapulmonary form of disease only, although the frequency varies between geographic areas and different populations.[1,2] HIV-infected patients may be more likely to have an extrapulmonary site of disease than HIV-uninfected persons, and the risk of extrapulmonary TB increases as the CD4 lymphocyte count decreases.[3,4] The two most commonly involved extrapulmonary sites are peripheral lymph nodes and the pleura, but any site or organ can be involved.[5,6] Other common sites for extrapulmonary TB are those in well-vascularized areas such as the kidney, the meninges, the spine, and the growing ends of long bones.

Diagnosis of extrapulmonary TB can be challenging given the nonspecific clinical presentations, difficulty in obtaining specimens for testing, and variable sensitivity and specificity of diagnostic tests. Treatment can also be challenging but the general principles for treatment of pulmonary TB are still followed with extrapulmonary disease although treatment durations may be longer and use of corticosteroids adjunctively are recommended in some settings, such as TB involving the central nervous system (CNS). This chapter reviews the clinical presentation, diagnosis, and treatment of the more common forms of extrapulmonary TB.

EPIDEMIOLOGY

The World Health Organization reported that 14% of incident cases of TB (new and relapses) reported in 2017 were due to extrapulmonary disease.[2] The percentage of extrapulmonary TB cases varied significantly across regions and countries (Figure 14.1) ranging from 8% in the WHO Western Pacific Region to 24% in the Eastern Mediterranean Region. Some of the variations in prevalence are due to the large number of undiagnosed cases in many developing countries and large variation in HIV prevalence.

TB has been declining in the United States but the proportion of TB due to extrapulmonary TB has increased (Figure 14.2). Among the 253,299 reported TB cases in the United States between 1993 and 2006, extrapulmonary TB increased from 15.7% of TB cases in 1993 to 21.0% in 2006. During the study period, 73.6% had pulmonary TB and 18.7% had extrapulmonary TB: 40.4% lymphatic, 19.8% pleural, 11.3% musculoskeletal, 6.5% genitourinary, 5.4% meningeal, 4.9% peritoneal, and 11.8% unclassified.[6] Extrapulmonary TB was associated with female sex, foreign birth, was almost equal for HIV infection, and was negatively associated with multidrug-resistant TB (MDR-TB), homelessness, and excess alcohol use. In 2017, the CDC (Centers for Disease Control and Prevention) reported 9105 cases of TB in the United States of whom 6271 (68.9%) had pulmonary TB, 1887 (20.7%) had extrapulmonary TB, and 933 (10.2%) had both (Table 14.1).[1] The proportion of extrapulmonary cases varied significantly by state. More recently, the CDC reported a total of 1828 cases of extrapulmonary TB which represents 20.3% of all TB cases in the United States.[7]

Of 55,337 TB cases notified in the European Union and European Economic Area in 2017, 68.8% were diagnosed with pulmonary disease, 22.6% with extrapulmonary disease, and 7.8% with both.[8] Eight countries reported over 30% of their TB cases having extrapulmonary disease and the proportion was highest in the Netherlands (41.7%), Norway (39.5%), and the United Kingdom (45.0%), and lowest in Hungary (3.9%) and Liechtenstein (0%). In a study reporting extrapulmonary disease between 2002 and 2011, the most frequent sites of extrapulmonary disease were pleural (36.7%) and peripheral lymphatic (20.1%).[5] In another study including over

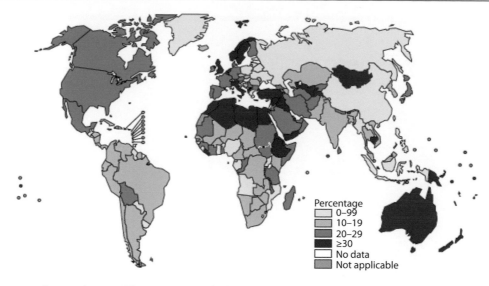

Figure 14.1 Percentage of extrapulmonary TB among new and relapse TB case, 2017. (From World Health Organization. Global Tuberculosis Report, 2018. Permission granted from WHO: https://apps.who.int/iris/bitstream/handle/10665/274453/9789241565646-eng.pdf.)

500,000 cases of extrapulmonary TB reported between 2003 and 2014 in Europe, extrapulmonary disease was associated with age <15 years, female sex, no previous TB treatment, and geographic origin; origin from the Indian subcontinent or Africa was associated with lymphatic, osteoarticular, and peritoneal/digestive disease, and age <15 years with lymphatic and CNS disease.[9]

In areas with higher burdens of TB, the reported frequency and sites of disease have varied significantly. In Tianjin, China between 2006 and 2011, only 10% of the reported 14,561 adult TB patients had extrapulmonary disease of which approximately two-thirds had pleural disease.[10] Patients with extrapulmonary TB were more likely to be 65 years and older and to live in urban areas. In Ghana, among 3342 patients ≥15 years of age, 728 (21.8%) had extrapulmonary disease but the most common forms were disseminated (32.8%), pleural (21%), spine (13%), and CNS (11%). HIV positivity and female sex were significantly associated with extrapulmonary TB, and older age, HIV positivity, and

CNS disease were associated with mortality.[11] A recent study from South Africa described a 13% decrease in TB cases overall between 2009 and 2013, however, TB meningitis and bone and joint TB increased whereas TB pleuritis and lymph node disease remained stable, and miliary/disseminated disease declined.[12]

Extrapulmonary TB has been reported to be more common in HIV-infected patients, and the risk increases as the CD4 count decreases.[3] A systematic review evaluated 16 studies (15 cross-sectional and 1 case–control) conducted from 1984 to 2016.[13] Most of the individual studies showed increased odds of extrapulmonary TB compared with pulmonary TB alone among HIV-infected individuals although a pooled estimate was not provided. In another systematic review that included 19 studies (7 case–control and 12 cohort studies), the authors reported a significant association between HIV and extrapulmonary TB.[3]

Risk factors for extrapulmonary disease have varied across studies. Untreated HIV infection, infancy, corticosteroids or other

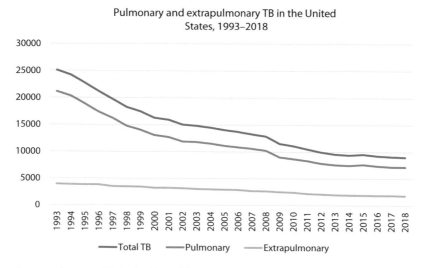

Figure 14.2 Pulmonary and extrapulmonary TB in the United States, 1993–2017. (Centers for Disease Control and Prevention Annual TB Reports.)

Table 14.1 Percentage of extrapulmonary TB sites, United States and Europe

Site of disease	United States, 2018	European Union, European Economic Area (2003–2014)[a]
Total	20.4%	16.8%
Lymph node/lymphatic	36.9%	29.5%
Pleural	16.9%	40.0%
Bone and joint/ osteoarticular	9.6%	8.7%
Urogenital	4.8%	6.3%
Peritoneal/digestive	5.8%	2.9%
Meningeal/CNS	3.8%	3.3%
Disseminated	—[b]	1.3%
Other	22.1%	8.0%

Source: Centers for Disease Control and Prevention. Reported tuberculosis in the United State, 2018. https://www.cdc.gov/tb/statistics/reports/2018/default.htm; Sotgiu G et al. *PLOS ONE.* 2017;12(11): e0186499.
[a] Includes 27 countries.
[b] Included in "other."

forms of immunosuppression, and female sex have been identified in several studies.[14] A study that evaluated 10,152 and 277,013 extrapulmonary TB cases from the United Kingdom and United States, respectively, reported that local-born white individuals had a lower frequency of extrapulmonary TB than local-born nonwhites and both groups had a lower proportion of extrapulmonary disease than foreign-born nonwhites.[14] Vitamin D deficiency was strongly associated with extrapulmonary disease independent of ethnicity, sex, or other factors.

The impact of extrapulmonary TB on mortality has varied between studies although on average pulmonary TB has been associated with a higher all-cause case fatality rate than extrapulmonary TB.[15] A study from the United Kingdom followed 571 cases of TB and assessed outcomes 1 year after initiating therapy.[16] Age at diagnosis and pulmonary TB were independently associated with death. In a retrospective study from Singapore, having both pulmonary and extrapulmonary disease was associated with a higher mortality than pulmonary disease alone.[17] In that study, extrapulmonary TB alone trended toward lower mortality. In Texas, age ≥45 years, HIV infection, excessive alcohol use within the past 12 months, end-stage renal disease, and abnormal chest radiographs were independent predictors of mortality during TB treatment.[18]

There are few studies addressing long-term mortality in patients with TB. A nationwide cohort study in Denmark from 1997 to 2008 reported that all-cause and cause-specific mortality were higher among adults with pulmonary and extrapulmonary TB than the general population.[19] A total of 8291 patients were assessed including 6402 with pulmonary TB and 1889 (22.8%) with extrapulmonary disease. The mortality rate ratio was 1.86 and 1.24 for pulmonary and extrapulmonary TB, respectively. The increased risk of death in both groups was related to infectious diseases and diabetes mellitus. Additionally, the increased mortality in those with pulmonary TB was associated with cancers (primarily respiratory and gastrointestinal), liver and respiratory system diseases, and alcohol and drug abuse.

PATHOGENESIS OF EXTRAPULMONARY DISEASE

Most extrapulmonary TB arises from the hematogenous spread of tubercle bacilli throughout the body during the initial tuberculous infection. Despite this presumably universal phenomenon, only about 20% of all patients with TB develop extrapulmonary disease as the only site of disease.[5,6,20] Why some individuals present with extrapulmonary TB and others with pulmonary disease only is not clear although immune defects appear to play a role. Previous studies have reported higher rates of extrapulmonary TB in HIV-infected persons and the rate increases as the CD4 lymphocyte decreases.[3,4] Young children also have an increased incidence of extrapulmonary disease presumably because of an immature immune system.[21]

HIV-uninfected patients who have previously had extrapulmonary TB have been shown to have reduced peripheral blood mononuclear cell cytokine production and CD4 lymphocytes compared with those with previous pulmonary TB or latent TB infection.[22,23] In an *in vitro* model, persons with previous extrapulmonary TB had decreased production of several cytokines (interferon [IFN]-γ, tumor necrosis factor [TNF]-alpha, IL-6 [interleukin-6]), both at rest and after stimulation with *M. tuberculosis,* suggesting a global immune defect that affects the response to *M. tuberculosis* infection.[24] Extrapulmonary TB has been associated with genetic polymorphisms in the vitamin D receptor (VDR) and toll-like receptor (TLR)-2,[25,26] and increased macrophage expression of VDR after stimulation with live *M. tuberculosis* has been reported in persons with previous extrapulmonary TB compared with those with previous pulmonary TB, LTBI, and uninfected controls.[27]

In addition to disease resulting from lymphohematogenous spread, TB can occur rarely at sites of skin puncture, such as in the case of direct inoculation of *M. tuberculosis* into the skin, referred to as "prosector's wart,"[28] or through mucosal inoculation in the case of laryngeal TB or gastrointestinal TB.

CLINICAL MANIFESTATIONS AND DIAGNOSIS: GENERAL COMMENTS

Diagnosis of extrapulmonary TB can be challenging due to the nonspecific symptoms and signs of disease, the challenge of obtaining appropriate fluid and tissue for diagnostic testing, and variable sensitivities and specificities of diagnostic tests. Acid-fast bacillus (AFB) smear microscopy and mycobacterial cultures remain critical in the diagnosis of TB and should be pursued in all patients suspected of having extrapulmonary disease.[29] Although the sensitivity of AFB smear microscopy is relatively low (<50%), the specificity is typically over 90%. For mycobacterial cultures, the sensitivity varies significantly by site of disease with a sensitivity 80%–90% for urine cultures in genitourinary TB to 23%–58% for pleural TB.[29] In some areas of the world, drug-resistant TB is common so obtaining appropriate specimens for culture and drug susceptibility testing is critical. For example, over a 6-year period (2005–2012) in New Delhi, India, over 30% of extrapulmonary isolates were found to harbor drug resistance to isoniazid (INH) and approximately 20%

Table 14.2 Meta-analysis of the sensitivity and specificity of Xpert MTB/RIF in diagnosing extrapulmonary TB and RIF resistance in adults and children

Specimen type	No. studies, samples	Pooled sensitivity median (95% CI)	Pooled specificity median (95% CI)
Lymph node tissue and aspirate	14 studies, 849 samples	84.9 (72–92)	92.5 (80–97)
Cerebrospinal fluid	16 studies, 709 samples	79.5 (62–90)	98.6 (96–100)
Pleural fluid	17 studies, 1385 samples	43.7 (25–65)	98.1 (95–99)
Gastric lavage and aspirate	12 studies, 1258 samples	83.8 (66–93)	98.1 (92–100)
Other tissues	12 studies, 699 samples	81.2 (68–90)	98.1 (87–100)

Source: World Health Organization. Automated real-time nucleic acid amplification technology for rapid and simultaneous detection of tuberculosis and rifampicin resistance: Xpert MTB/RIF assay for the diagnosis of pulmonary and extrapulmonary TB in adults and children. Policy update. Geneva, 2011.

had multidrug-resistant TB (MDR-TB).[30] Similarly, among inpatients with extrapulmonary TB in China, the frequency of MDR-TB increased from 17.3% in 2008 to 35.7% in 2017.[31]

Newer, rapid molecular tests, such as Xpert MTB/RIF which can identify *M. tuberculosis* and the presence of rifampicin resistance, allow for more rapid diagnosis and treatment of extrapulmonary TB and are recommended by the World Health Organization in some settings (Table 14.2).[32] However, there are limited data available for many extrapulmonary sites. Cell counts and chemistries should be performed on appropriate fluids collected from sites of extrapulmonary TB such as pleural, CSF, ascites, and joint fluids.[29] Measurement of adenosine deaminase (ADA) levels is recommended in suspected pleural, CNS, peritoneal, or pericardial TB, and INF-γ levels are recommended to be measured in suspected pleural or peritoneal TB.[29] Although elevation of these levels in fluid does not provide a definitive diagnosis, they provide supportive evidence that may be helpful for the treating provider in the right clinical context.

TREATMENT: GENERAL COMMENTS

The principles underlying the treatment of pulmonary TB also apply to extrapulmonary disease although the duration of therapy can vary depending on the site of infection. A four-drug initial phase including INH, rifampicin (RIF), pyrazinamide (PZA), and ethambutol (EMB) is administered for the first 2 months. After 2 months, PZA and EMB may be discontinued, and INH and RIF continued during a 4-month continuation phase. The exceptions are TB meningitis and bone and joint infection where most experts and society guidelines recommend 12 months and 6–9 months of treatment, respectively (Table 14.3).[33–36] Most experts recommend daily dosing for extrapulmonary TB for both the intensive and continuation phases.[36] Corticosteroids are recommended, in addition to antimicrobial therapy, in the setting of TB meningitis.[36] In regard to treatment monitoring, bacteriologic evaluation is often limited by the difficulty in obtaining follow-up specimens. Sputum specimens are obtained when there is concurrent pulmonary involvement, otherwise, response to treatment in extrapulmonary TB is often judged on the basis of clinical and radiographic findings.

EXTRAPULMONARY TB: SPECIFIC SITES OF DISEASE (ALPHABETICAL ORDER)

BONE AND JOINT TB

EPIDEMIOLOGY

Musculoskeletal involvement accounts for approximately 10% of extrapulmonary TB in the United States,[1,6] however, significantly

Table 14.3 Treatment duration and use of adjunctive corticosteroids by site if disease

Site of disease	Treatment duration (months)		Adjunctive corticosteroids		Comments
	CDC	WHO	CDC	WHO	
Bone/joint/spine	6–9	6	No	No	
Meningitis/CNS	9–12	12	Yes	Yes	In some cases, steroids must be given for a prolonged period
Disseminated	6	6	No	No	Steroids are sometimes given to patients with acute lung injury
Gastrointestinal	6	6	No	No	
Lymph nodes	6	6	No	No	Steroids have been used in selected cases to decrease swelling
Pericardial	6	6	Maybe	Maybe	Steroids are considered in those at highest risk for inflammatory complications
Pleural	6	6	No	No	Steroids have been used in selected cases with large or particularly painful effusions
Urogenital	6	6	No	No	

Source: Nahid P et al. *Clin Infect Dis.* 2016;63(7):e147–95.

higher rates have been described in South Asian ethnic immigrants in the United Kingdom[37] and those from Africa in France.[38] Although weight-bearing bones are the most likely to be affected, any bone or joint may be involved. In most series, TB of the spine, or Pott's disease, makes up more than 50% of cases.[39–42] A study from 1996 reported that spinal involvement occurred in 50% of patients (50% thoracic, 25% cervical, 25% lumbar), pelvic involvement in 12%, hip/femur in 10%, rib in 7%, other joints in 2%, and multiple joints in 3% of patients.[42]

CLINICAL PRESENTATION

Most patients present with pain in the involved joint. Systemic symptoms such as fever, chills, and weight loss are present in <40% of patients with skeletal TB, and delays in diagnosis are common.[41,43–46] Concomitant pulmonary disease has varied[38,45,47] but the largest study noted the lowest reported rate (2.7%).[47] Typical radiographic findings include metaphyseal erosion and cysts, loss of cartilage, and narrowing of the joint space (Figure 14.3). In Pott's disease, two vertebral bodies and the intervening joint space are usually involved. Infection is thought to begin in the

disc and then spreads along the longitudinal and anterior spinal ligaments to involve the inferior and superior borders of the adjacent vertebral bodies (Figure 14.4). In children, the upper thoracic spine is the most frequent site, whereas in adults, the lower thoracic and upper lumbar vertebrae are usually involved.[43,48] Where available, CT (computed tomography) and/or MRI (magnetic resonance imaging) should be obtained to better define the pattern and extent of involvement. Metastatic malignant disease can present with similar radiographic findings; however, in metastatic disease, the disc space is preserved and there may be erosion of the vertebral bodies and pedicles.

TB arthritis is usually monoarticular; however, 10%–15% of cases in developing countries have been reported to have multiple joints involved.[49] Hip involvement is most common and may present with pain, swelling, and decreased function.[50] With more advanced disease, sinus formation may occur. TB osteomyelitis can involve any bone and with arthritis typically involves a single site. The presentation is variable depending on the site and the duration of infection.

DIAGNOSIS

Early diagnosis is important in order to preserve cartilage and joint space and avoid loss of function. Unfortunately, delays in diagnosis of months to years are common due to the subacute course.[51] Chest radiographs are normal in half of the patients.[52] CT or MRI is more likely than plain radiographs to identify vertebral involvement as well as psoas and paraspinous abscesses.[52–54] Confirmation of the diagnosis requires aspiration of joint fluid or periarticular abscesses or biopsy of the affected bone or synovium. AFB smears are positive in 20%–25% of joint fluid aspirates, with mycobacteria being isolated in 60%–80%.[29] Histopathologic evidence of granulomatous inflammation is almost always present in bone and synovial biopsies. The role of GeneXpert has not been defined.

TREATMENT

A 6–9-month regimen is recommended for patients with musculoskeletal TB based on randomized controlled trials.[36] Longer durations may be indicated in extensive disease or where hardware

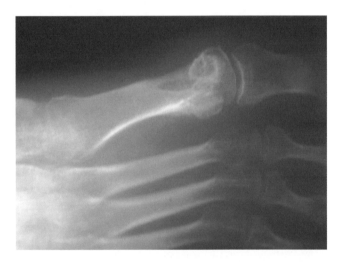

Figure 14.3 Tuberculous osteomyelitis of the metatarsal bone. Note the osteolytic lesion in the distal metatarsal.

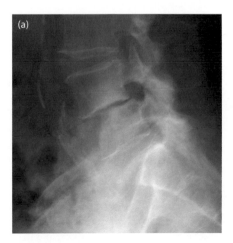
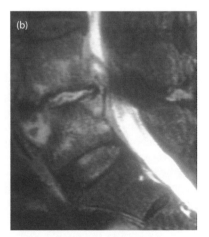

Figure 14.4 Pott's disease involving the lumbar vertebra in a patient with disseminated TB. (a) A radiograph demonstrating erosion of the anterior vertebral body. (b) An MRI demonstrating compression of the spinal cord.

is in place. Six- to nine-month regimens containing RIF are effective[55–57] and several trials found no additional benefit of surgical debridement in combination with chemotherapy compared with chemotherapy alone for spinal TB.[56–59] However, surgery should be considered in situations in which (1) there is poor response to chemotherapy with evidence of ongoing infection or ongoing deterioration; (2) relief of cord compression is needed in patients with persistence or recurrence of neurologic deficits; or (3) there is instability of the spine.[36,60] In addition, large psoas abscesses may be present and require drainage. Complications of spinal TB include kyphoscoliosis with gibbus formation, myelopathy, "cold" abscesses, fistulas, and spinal cord compression with radiculopathy and paralysis.[43,48,51]

CENTRAL NERVOUS SYSTEM TB

EPIDEMIOLOGY

CNS disease makes up about 5% of cases in the United States.[6] Meningitis is the most common form of CNS TB and remains a potentially devastating disease associated with high morbidity and mortality in children and adults. In high prevalence areas, TB meningitis is more likely to occur in children whereas in low prevalence areas most cases occur in adults. Approximately one-third of patients with TB meningitis have disseminated disease. Predisposing conditions include untreated HIV infection, and other forms of immunosuppression including corticosteroids, alcoholism, substance abuse, and head trauma.[61,62]

CLINICAL PRESENTATION

The clinical presentation of TB meningitis is variable and often associated with an insidious onset. Classically, the disease has been described in three phases: (1) prodromal phase of 2–3 weeks with malaise, headache, low grade fever, and possible change in personality; (2) meningitis phase associated with neurologic features such as meningismus, protracted headache, emesis, lethargy, confusion, and focal CNS signs; (3) paralytic phase associated with confusion, stupor, coma, seizures, hemiparesis, and death.[63,64] Mortality increases as patients progress through the clinical stages, and during the pre-chemotherapy era mortality was 45% in stage 1, 70% in stage 2, and 90% in stage 3.[63,64]

DIAGNOSIS

CT and MRI studies may demonstrate basilar meningitis, hydrocephalus, or show evidence of tuberculous abscesses (Figure 14.5). However, to confirm the diagnosis, CSF must be sampled for examination and culture. CSF protein is usually elevated ranging from 100 to 500 mg/dL but may be higher when spinal block is present.[63,65] Very high protein concentrations are associated with a worse prognosis but increasing concentrations during treatment does not necessarily represent treatment failure.[66] CSF glucose is usually below 40 mg/dL and the CSF/blood glucose ratio is below 0.5 in most patients.[64,66] White blood cell counts are elevated with values of 100–1000 cells/μL, most of which are lymphocytes, although polymorphonuclear cells may predominate early in the disease.[64] AFB smears of CSF are positive in only 10%–30% of cases, and cultures are positive in approximately 45%–70%.[29] Two meta-analyses estimated the test characteristics of ADA in CSF.

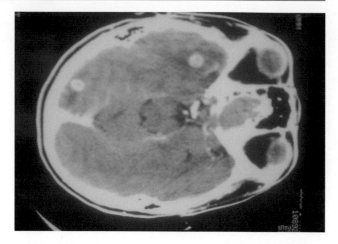

Figure 14.5 A CT of the brain demonstrating two enhancing lesions in an HIV-infected patient with disseminated TB.

One included 10 studies and reported a sensitivity and specificity of 79% and 91%, respectively.[67] The second meta-analysis included 13 studies and noted that the test characteristics were very sensitive to the threshold used to define an elevated ADA level.[68] If a 4 U/L threshold was used, the sensitivity and specificity were >93% and <80%, respectively. In a retrospective study from South Africa, the optimum threshold was calculated to be 2 U/L which gave a sensitivity of 86% and specificity of 78%.[69] However, using this threshold, 13 cases of TB meningitis were missed.

The WHO recommends that Xpert MTB/RIF be used in preference to conventional microscopy and culture as the initial diagnostic test for CSF specimens from patients suspected of having TB meningitis.[32] A systematic review commissioned by the WHO identified 16 studies where CSF samples were tested with Xpert MTB/RIF and the results were compared against culture.[32] Estimates of sensitivity varied widely and ranged from 51% to 100%. The pooled sensitivity across studies was 79.5% (95% CI 62.0%–90.2%) and the pooled specificity was 98.6% (95% CI 95.8%–99.6%), suggesting good performance of Xpert MTB/RIF in detecting *M. tuberculosis* in CSF.[32]

Ten of the 16 studies comparing Xpert MTB/RIF with culture as a reference standard used a concentration step in processing the sample. A concentration step appeared to increase the sensitivity of Xpert MTB/RIF (82%; 95% CI 71%–93% for concentrated samples vs. 56%; 95% CI 36%–77% for unconcentrated samples), although the confidence intervals overlapped.[32] The use of a concentration step did not affect the specificity.

TREATMENT

The ATS (American Thoracic Society)/IDSA (Infectious Diseases Society of America)/CDC recommend treatment be initiated with INH, RIF, PZA, and EMB for a 2-month initial phase.[36] After 2 months of therapy, PZA and EMB may be discontinued, and INH and RIF continued for an additional 7–10 months.[36] The American Academy of Pediatrics recommends an initial four-drug regimen of INH, RIF, PZA, and an aminoglycoside or ethionamide for 2 months followed by 7–10 months of INH and RIF.[36] Repeated lumbar punctures should be performed to monitor changes in CSF cell count, glucose, and protein, especially early in the course of therapy.[77]

There have been several attempts to improve treatment outcomes by introducing short intensified regimens for treatment of drug-susceptible TB meningitis. The first such study was a randomized, controlled, open label study that evaluated a 9-month regimen in persons >14 years of age in Indonesia.[70] Patients were randomized to receive either oral RIF (450 mg) or intravenous RIF (600 mg) plus no moxifloxacin, moxifloxacin (400 mg), or moxifloxacin (800 mg) along with INH and PZA. The "higher" dose RIF regimen lowered mortality but there were no differences in mortality by moxifloxacin arms. Another study randomized adults with TB meningitis in Vietnam to receive INH, RIF (10 mg/kg), EMB, and PZA or INH, RIF (15 mg/kg), EMB, PZA, and levofloxacin (20 mg/kg) for 3 months followed by INH and RIF for 6 months.[71] There was no significant difference in the primary outcome (death) between arms including in HIV-infected patients. There was a trend toward better outcomes in INH-resistant cases although the study was underpowered to address this.

A systematic review and meta-analysis of childhood TB meningitis reported that the risk of death was 19%.[72] The probability of survival without neurologic deficits was only 37% and among survivors the risk of neurologic sequelae was approximately 54%. There are limited data on how to improve this high mortality rate although a four-drug regimen substituting ethionamide for EMB reported a relatively low mortality rate when TB meningitis was diagnosed early in the course of disease. In that study, children (n=184) with TB meningitis were treated with a four-drug regimen including INH (10–15 mg/kg), RIF (20 mg/kg), PZA (40 mg/kg), and ethionamide (20 mg/kg) for 6 months with HIV-infected children treated for 9 months.[73] Eighty percent of the children had stage 2–3 disease. Overall the mortality was 3.8%. All children with stage 1 TB meningitis had a good outcome compared with 97% with stage 2 disease and 47% with stage 3 disease.

Several studies have examined the role of adjunctive corticosteroid therapy in the treatment of TB meningitis.[74–86] Evidence from randomized controlled trials (39–43) have shown lower rates of mortality, severe disability, and disease relapse when patients were treated with steroids in addition to anti-TB treatment. The mortality benefit increased with increasing TB meningitis stage (i.e., increasing severity of disease). Additionally, rates of adverse events and severe adverse events, including severe hepatitis, were lower in the patients receiving steroids. Based on these studies, the ATS/IDSA/CDC and WHO recommend adjunctive corticosteroid therapy with dexamethasone or prednisolone tapered over 6–8 weeks for patients with TB meningitis.[36] Steroids should be given regardless of the severity of meningitis and it is not uncommon to have to restart steroids if neurologic symptoms and/or signs reappear.

DISSEMINATED (MILIARY) TB

EPIDEMIOLOGY

Disseminated, or miliary TB, occurs when tubercle bacilli spread through the bloodstream resulting in small (approximately 1–2 mm) granulomatous lesions. The term "miliary" was proposed by John Jacob Manget to describe the gross appearance of pathological findings that were similar in size and appearance to millet seeds.[87] Disseminated disease is defined as involvement of two or more noncontiguous sites or the presence of bacteremia.

Disseminated TB has been reported to occur in approximately 1% of TB patients from Europe,[9] but has been reported to account for 6%–8% of extrapulmonary TB in England and Wales[88] and 11.2%–12.2% of cases in the United States.[89] Historically, disseminated TB has been seen more commonly in infants and children <4 years old,[90,91] however, disease also occurs in older individuals. There are now two peaks, one involving adolescents and young adults and the other among elderly individuals.[90] In fact, the "cryptic" variety typically occurs in individuals older than 60 years of age.[92] Males are more frequently affected in some series and females in others. Medical risk factors for disseminated TB include malnutrition, immunosuppression, alcoholism, diabetes mellitus, and chronic hemodialysis.[93,94] Disease can result from early dissemination after infection or later after reactivation.[95,96] Factors associated with an increased mortality include older age, lymphopenia, hypoalbuminemia, elevated transaminases, altered mental status, HIV infection, and delay in therapy.[95]

CLINICAL PRESENTATION

Disseminated TB usually develops insidiously with systemic symptoms such as fever, weakness, weight loss, fatigue, and anorexia. Cough and dyspnea may also be prominent symptoms. Choroidal tubercles may be present and can provide an early clue in the diagnosis of disseminated mycobacterial disease.[90,91] The mean duration of symptoms approaches 16 weeks, but some patients may go undiagnosed for more than 2 years. Remarkably, of all patients with disseminated TB noted on autopsy, 33%–80% were unsuspected premortem.[97] Disseminated TB can also present acutely which can be rapidly progressive with wide dissemination. The chest radiograph typically shows the classic "miliary" pattern of diffuse small nodules and with severe disease, acute lung injury may occur resulting in acute respiratory distress syndrome.[98] Chronic or cryptic disseminated TB does not usually present with a typical miliary radiographic pattern.[97] Importantly, CNS involvement may complicate disseminated TB in 10%–30% or more of adult cases.[87,96,99,100]

DIAGNOSIS

Chest radiographs may be the first clue to the diagnosis but the findings are nonspecific and the radiograph may be normal in 25%–50% of patients.[95,101] Chest CT scans are more sensitive than chest radiographs and may detect intrathoracic adenopathy.[101] Sputum AFB smears are positive in 20%–25% of cases and sputum is culture-positive for *M. tuberculosis* in up to 65% of cases.[95,102,103] Bronchoscopy should be considered in patients who are unable to produce sputum or who have produced negative sputum smears.[29] Studies have reported immediate presumptive diagnosis of miliary TB by histopathology and/or AFB smears in up to 80% of patients with an additional 45%–100% yield with cultures.[95,104,105] Other potential sources include urine, which is culture-positive in up to 30% of patients, and liver and bone marrow, which are culture-positive in up to 25%–67%.[87] Blood cultures have been reported to be positive in up to 40% of HIV-infected patients with disseminated TB but rarely so in HIV-uninfected patients.[106–108]

TREATMENT

A 6-month regimen is recommended for disseminated drug-susceptible TB (miliary or multiple sites) based on limited data.[36]

Although the role of adjunctive corticosteroids is unclear, some experts believe corticosteroid therapy is indicated for treating severe respiratory failure or adrenal insufficiency caused by disseminated TB.[109,110] Even with appropriate therapy, mortality remains high ranging from 16% to 24%.[95,100,102,103]

GASTROINTESTINAL TB

EPIDEMIOLOGY

Gastrointestinal disease is a relatively uncommon manifestation of extrapulmonary TB accounting for approximately 5% of cases worldwide.[50] In the United States, peritoneal TB was reported in 6.2% of reported extrapulmonary cases in 2017.[20] However, the frequency of gastrointestinal TB appears to be more common in developing countries. TB peritonitis and ileocecal involvement are the most common forms of disease although TB can affect any abdominal organ including the liver. In a study from 1969 to 1973, peritoneal TB was five times more common than all other forms of abdominal TB combined.[111] Approximately half of all ascites in developing countries has been attributed to TB.[112] Peritoneal TB typically affects young adults in the third and fourth decades of life.[113,114] Ileocecal disease is the most common site of disease (21%) within the intestinal tract followed by anorectal (20%) and sigmoid disease (1%).[115]

CLINICAL PRESENTATION

In patients with peritoneal TB, ascites (93%), abdominal pain (73%), and fever (58%) are common and symptoms may persist for weeks to months before diagnosis.[116] In more advanced disease, the classic "doughy" abdomen may be present in approximately 10% of patients.[117,118] A pleural effusion has been reported to be present in 22%–32% of patients.[112,115,119]

The clinical presentation of TB enteritis may be quite variable from acute onset of symptoms to chronic to asymptomatic.[112] Patients with ileocecal involvement, the most common site of intestinal involvement, may present initially with abdominal pain simulating appendicitis or intestinal obstruction.[119] Diagnosis of ileocecal TB can be difficult given the nonspecific clinical features resulting in substantial delays and often is made at the time of surgery.

Hepatic involvement can occur in the setting of pulmonary TB, miliary disease, or focal hepatic disease. Noncaseating hepatic granulomas have been reported in 25% of patients with pulmonary TB[120] and 50%–100% of patients with miliary TB.[95,121] Focal hepatic disease may be symptomatic or associated with fever, right upper quadrant pain, or jaundice.

DIAGNOSIS

Patients with suspected gastrointestinal TB should undergo CT imaging and paracentesis to sample ascitic fluid, if present (Figure 14.6). Ultrasound may facilitate aspiration of loculated ascites. Ascitic fluid is usually exudative with typically 500–1000 cells/mm³ with a lymphocytic predominance (40%–92%).[122] The serum-ascites albumin gradient (SAAG) is <1.1 g/dL and the peritoneal fluid protein concentration >3 g/dL in those without cirrhosis.[117] The ascitic fluid/blood glucose ratio is below 1.0 in approximately 80% of patients.[119] AFB smears of ascitic fluid are usually negative, but cultures are positive in approximately

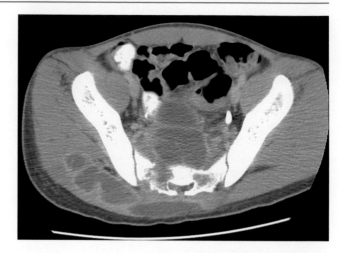

Figure 14.6 Abdominal TB with a large peritoneal fluid collection and erosion into bone and soft tissues posteriorly.

45%–69% of cases[123]; the higher yield has been reported when 1 L of fluid was cultured.[119] A meta-analysis of four studies estimated that the sensitivity and specificity of an elevated ADA level in peritoneal fluid was 100% and 97%, respectively, with a threshold to define an elevated level of 36–40 U/L.[123] The sensitivity and specificity of IFN-γ levels is estimated to be 93% and 99%, respectively.[124]

Laparoscopic biopsy is usually required to make the diagnosis of peritoneal TB. A systematic review that included 402 patients reported that the sensitivity and specificity of laparoscopic examination for making the diagnosis of peritoneal TB were 93% and 98%, respectively.[117] Culture of the biopsy is positive in 38%–78% of specimens.[29] A blind peritoneal biopsy has a diagnostic yield of about 65% but is associated with more complications than when guided laparoscopically.

For enteric disease, endoscopy often is required to identify areas consistent with TB such as ulcerations, strictures, nodules, pseudo-polyps, fistulas and fibrotic areas. Biopsy of these lesions may demonstrate characteristic histopathologic findings of TB. Unfortunately the sensitivity of AFB smear and mycobacterial cultures are <50%. Culture confirmation is important as *Mycobacterium bovis* can be the causative agent and this organism is resistant to PZA.[125] Of note, as much as 45% of patients with smear-positive pulmonary TB have gastrointestinal disease by colonoscopy.[126]

Hepatic disease can be diagnosed with ultrasound guided liver biopsy or laparoscopy in 70% and 90% of patients, respectively.[127] Histopathology typically demonstrates a variety of pathology including granuloma formation. AFB smears are negative in 50%–90% of patients.

TREATMENT

A 6-month regimen is recommended for patients with peritoneal or intestinal TB caused by *M. tuberculosis*[36] based on small nonrandomized studies.[128–130] Treatment of disease caused by *M. bovis* should include INH, RIF, and EMB administered for 9 months. Adjunctive corticosteroid therapy in the treatment of TB peritonitis is not recommended.[131] Delays in treating patients with gastrointestinal TB have resulted in complications including perforation, adhesions, intestinal obstruction, fistulae, abscesses, and hemorrhage.[122,132,133] In one series, 80% of patients deteriorated clinically and 35% died while waiting to begin treatment.[116] Patients with ascites usually respond within a few weeks of starting therapy.[129] In enteric disease, ulcers and erosions were completely healed within 2–3 months of starting anti-TB therapy.[134]

Lymph node TB (scrofula)

EPIDEMIOLOGY

Lymphadenitis is the most common form of extrapulmonary TB, accounting for up to 40% of extrapulmonary disease in the United States.[6] TB lymphadenitis is often thought of as a disease of children, however, studies have reported the peak incidence is in young adults between 20 and 40 years of age.[135–137] Sex, ethnicity, and immune status are associated with the development of TB lymphadenitis with studies showing a 2:1 female to male predominance which is the opposite of pulmonary TB.[138,139] In developed countries, Indian, Asian, and Blacks have been reported to have higher rates than Caucasians.[135,140,141] TB lymphadenitis is particularly common in persons with HIV coinfection with reports of peripheral TB lymphadenitis of 22%–31% in patients with AIDS.[107,142–144]

CLINICAL MANIFESTATIONS

Most lymphadenitis involves cervical lymph nodes and presents with a painless, erythematous, firm mass (or masses) most commonly involving the anterior and posterior cervical nodes or supraclavicular fossa. Among the 10,496 reported TB cases in Texas between 2009 and 2016, 547 (5.2%) had head and neck TB and cervical adenopathy occurred in 97% of the patients.[145] In HIV-uninfected individuals, the mass is usually unilateral, not associated with other sites, and systemic symptoms are absent. However, bilateral disease has been reported in up to 26% of patients.[146,147] Progression of disease may be associated with significant swelling and fluctuance with sinus formation developing in <10% of patients.[135,138,140,148] In HIV-infected patients, TB lymphadenitis often is associated with multifocal disease and systemic symptoms.[107]

DIAGNOSIS

Diagnosis of TB lymphadenitis usually involves fine-needle aspiration (FNA) or excisional biopsy with histopathologic examination, examination for acid-fast organisms, and culture for mycobacteria. Histologic evidence of mycobacterial infection, including caseating granulomas, are seen in nearly all cases, but the AFB smear is positive in only approximately 25%–50% of cases and the culture in approximately 70%–80%.[29] When FNA is not diagnostic, excisional biopsy is recommended. In a small series of 47 patients who underwent FNA and excisional biopsy, the diagnosis of TB was established in all patients with excisional biopsy but only 62% of those by FNA.[149]

New rapid diagnostic tests, such as Xpert MTB/RIF can also be used to diagnose TB lymphadenitis. A systematic review and meta-analysis that contained 18 studies assessed the accuracy of Xpert MTB/RIF on samples from lymph node biopsies or FNA compared against culture. The estimates for sensitivity and specificity were 83% and 94%, respectively.[150]

Chest radiographs should be obtained in all patients with suspected or culture confirmed TB. Although most patients with TB lymphadenitis have no evidence of pulmonary TB,[151,152] the frequency of concurrent pulmonary disease increases in TB endemic countries and in patients coinfected with HIV.[153] Ultrasound may be used to guide FNA in some cases and either CT or MRI may be indicated in cases where vital structures are being compressed.

TREATMENT

A 6-month regimen is recommended for initial treatment of all patients with drug-susceptible TB lymphadenitis.[36] This recommendation is based on both observational and randomized studies, the latter of which compared treatment outcomes of 6 versus 9 months of therapy.[154–159] For example, in a randomized trial comparing a three times weekly, 6-month standard four-drug regimen with the same regimen administered for 9 months, there was no difference in treatment failure or recurrence at 5 years.[159] It is important to note that response to treatment may be slow and affected lymph nodes may enlarge and new nodes can appear during or after therapy without any evidence of bacteriological relapse.[154,156,157,160] These "paradoxical" reactions have been reported to occur in up to 23% of HIV-uninfected patients.[161,162] In HIV-infected patients, paradoxical reactions are often associated with initiation of antiretroviral therapy.[163,164] Spontaneous resolution occurs in most patients. Anti-inflammatory medications such as nonsteroidal agents and corticosteroids have been used to treat milder paradoxical reactions.

For patients with more severe reactions, aspiration of large fluctuant lymph nodes that are about to drain may be beneficial but lymph node excision is not indicated except in unusual circumstances. When surgical excision is performed, complete excision is recommended. In a study of 40 patients with cervical lymphadenitis, 17 (77%) of 22 patients who underwent a simple drainage procedure required a second drainage procedure because of sinus tract formation, but 17 (94%) of 18 patients who underwent complete excision required no further surgery.[165]

Pericardial TB

EPIDEMIOLOGY

TB pericarditis is a relatively uncommon manifestation of extrapulmonary TB that occurs in approximately 1%–2% of patients with pulmonary TB.[166] The prevalence is higher in developing countries, particularly those with a high prevalence of HIV.[167] TB pericarditis was the leading cause of pericarditis in AIDS patients at one hospital in New York City in the late 1980s.[168] TB pericarditis typically occurs during middle age[166] but can affect any age group.

CLINICAL PRESENTATION

The clinical presentation is quite variable and determined by the stage of presentation: (1) fibrinous exudation with polymorphonuclear leukocytes, large number of mycobacteria, and early granuloma formation; (2) serosanguinous effusion with lymphocytic exudate, high protein concentration, and low number of mycobacteria; (3) granulomatous caseation, pericardial thickening; and (4) fibrosis with constriction. Most patients present early in the course of disease with fever and chest pain. Cough, weight loss, dyspnea, and orthopnea also are possible. Patients may present with tachycardia, cardiomegaly, and elevated jugular venous pressure and approximately 50% have a pericardial friction rub.[169] Cardiomegaly is almost universally present on chest radiograph.[170] EKG (electrocardiogram) may demonstrate ST segment and T wave depression.[171] Some patients present with large volume pericardial effusions and signs and symptoms of tamponade. Other patients may present with constrictive pericarditis. Pulmonary opacities or pleural effusions are seen in 32% and 36% of patients, respectively.[169,172] Constrictive pericarditis occurs in approximately 20% of patients, and calcification in 50%.[172]

DIAGNOSIS

Pericardiocentesis should be performed in order to sample pericardial fluid. In most situations, ultrasound is used to safely guide the procedure. The pericardial fluid is usually serosanguineous and occasionally grossly bloody.[173,174] The fluid is typically a lymphocytic exudative fluid with white blood cell counts in the 5,000–7,000 cells/μL range, although counts up to 50,000 have been reported.

AFB smears of the pericardial fluid are positive in 0%–42% and cultures in 50%–65% of cases, so a negative culture result does not rule out disease.[29] Pericardial biopsy samples show histologic evidence consistent with a mycobacterial infection in 73%–100% of cases. As with pleural TB, ADA and IFN-γ may provide evidence supporting a diagnosis of pericardial TB. ADA (>35 IU/L) has a sensitivity of 95.7% and specificity of 84% whereas IFN-γ (>44 μg/mL) has the same sensitivity but higher specificity of 96.3%.[29] Gene Xpert MTB/RIF has a sensitivity of 63.8% and specificity of 100%.[175]

TREATMENT

A 6-month regimen is recommended for patients with drug-susceptible pericardial TB.[36] The 2003 ATS/IDSA/CDC guidelines recommended that patients with TB pericarditis receive adjunctive corticosteroids based on small studies that reported mortality and morbidity benefits.[170,176–178] A subsequent systematic review that included five clinical trials showed a benefit to steroid treatment with regard to death, constrictive pericarditis, and treatment adherence.[36] However, another systematic review,[179] which included six randomized trials, concluded that in HIV-uninfected patients with pericardial TB, corticosteroids probably reduced deaths and need for repeated pericardiocentesis and in HIV-infected patients, the use of corticosteroids may reduce constriction and hospitalization. However, the largest (1400 patients) study showed no benefit of steroids.[180] A subgroup analysis suggested a benefit in preventing constrictive pericarditis. In this study, 67% of subjects were HIV-positive and only 14% were on ART. Among HIV-negative patients, a small mortality benefit was shown with steroid treatment. In another smaller study of 58 subjects, in which all were HIV-positive, steroids were found to reduce mortality.

While adjunctive corticosteroids should not be used routinely in the treatment of patients with pericardial TB, selective use of corticosteroids in patients who are at the highest risk for inflammatory complications, such as those with large pericardial effusions, those with high levels of inflammatory cells or markers in pericardial fluid, or those with early signs of constriction, might be appropriate.[181]

PLEURAL TB

EPIDEMIOLOGY

Pleural TB, which accounts for approximately 20% of extrapulmonary TB cases in the United States,[6] usually represents a manifestation of primary TB,[182] and occurs when a subpleural caseous focus ruptures into the pleural space. The resulting delayed-type hypersensitivity reaction produces pleural liquid that has a high protein concentration. The frequency of pleural TB is higher in Europe, reported in 40% of extrapulmonary disease.[9] Pleural TB typically affects individuals in the 20–40 year age group although any age group can be affected.[183,184] Among HIV-infected patients, TB pleuritis has been reported in 9%–20% with HIV and TB.[107,143,144]

CLINICAL PRESENTATION

The release of tuberculous antigens into the pleural space creates an exudative effusion which often presents abruptly in about two-thirds of patients.[183,185] Most patients are seen initially with chest pain, fever, and a nonproductive cough. Effusions are usually unilateral and small or moderate in size and without clear predilection for one side.[183,184] Massive effusions have been reported in 14%–29% of patients with primary disease.[183] If left untreated, the pleural effusion will resolve spontaneously over 2–4 months; however, the frequency of reactivation is approximately 43%–65% within the next 5–7 years.[186,187]

DIAGNOSIS

Diagnosis of pleural TB begins with sampling of the pleural fluid. Early in the course of disease, the fluid may have a polymorphonuclear predominance, but in almost all cases, mononuclear cells become the majority.[184,188] Cell counts are typically in the 100–5,000 cells/μL range, and the cells are almost all lymphocytes; the presence of mesothelial cells and/or eosinophils makes the diagnosis of TB unlikely.

Pleural fluid AFB smears are positive in only 0%–10% of patients, and pleural fluid cultures are positive in approximately 23%–58% of cases.[29] M. tuberculosis can be isolated from 30% to 50% of induced sputum specimens from patients with TB pleuritis and should be obtained in all patients.[189] Pleural biopsy specimens provide the highest diagnostic yield, with positive culture results in up to 45%–85% of cases when at least three specimens are obtained. Histopathologic evidence of TB can be seen in 69%–97% of patients.[183,184,190] Pleural biopsies are the preferred diagnostic sample given the high diagnostic yield. Thoracoscopy or pleuroscopy provide rapid and safe ways to diagnose pleural TB and are associated with a high yield. In a study of 40 patients with undiagnosed pleural effusions, a diagnosis of TB was made in 42.5% and the yield of TB was 100%.[191,192] In another study, thoracoscopic pleural biopsy had a similarly high yield of 90%.[192]

Other tests that may be helpful in the diagnosis of TB pleuritis are ADA and IFN-γ levels. Six meta-analyses including up to 63 studies estimated the sensitivity of an elevated ADA level to be 89%–99% with a specificity of 88%–97%.[29] The test performance varied in part due to different thresholds for determining an elevated ADA level with most using around 40 U/L (range 10–71 U/L). A recent meta-analysis suggested that pleural fluid IFN-γ concentration has a sensitivity of 89% and specificity of 97% for pleural TB in HIV-uninfected patients.[193]

Gene Xpert MTB/RIF can be used to diagnose pleural TB although the sensitivity is low. Seventeen studies (1385 samples, 217 culture-positive) provided data allowing an estimate of sensitivity and specificity of Xpert MTB/RIF in testing pleural fluid. The pooled sensitivity was low at 43.7% (95% CI 24.8%–64.7%) and the pooled specificity was high at 98.1% (95% CI 95.3%–99.2%).

TREATMENT

A 6-month regimen is recommended for treating drug-susceptible pleural TB.[36] Although some clinicians use adjunctive corticosteroid therapy for tuberculous pleural effusions, there is limited evidence to support the use of corticosteroids in this setting. In four, prospective, double blind, randomized trials,[194–197] the administration of prednisone (or prednisolone) did not confer a beneficial effect on residual pleural thickening or prevention of other long-term pleural sequelae. A systematic review that included six trials was also unable to document significant benefit of corticosteroids.[198] Treatment of tuberculous empyema consists of drainage (often requiring a surgical procedure) and anti-tuberculous chemotherapy.[199]

UROGENITAL TB

EPIDEMIOLOGY

Urogenital disease is responsible for approximately 7%–15% of extrapulmonary cases, with higher rates reported in developing countries, and can affect either the kidneys or genitals. Disease often presents in young adults affecting two males to each female.[200,201] Urogenital TB occurs in 2%–20% of patients with pulmonary TB.[202–205]

CLINICAL PRESENTATION

Renal disease may present with local symptoms that include dysuria, hematuria, urinary frequency, and flank discomfort. However, in many cases, the patient may be asymptomatic. Unilateral involvement is most common. Urine examination may demonstrate sterile pyuria, hematuria, or both.

Genital involvement is common in patients with renal TB. Males usually present with a slowly enlarging mass in the seminal vesicles, prostate, or epididymis. Epididymitis is the most common genital site in males presenting with epididymal swelling or hardening. Bilateral involvement occurs in one-third of patients. Prostatic involvement may present with incidental detection of nodularity on digital rectal examination. TB of the penis is extremely rare and often is initially misdiagnosed as a sexually transmitted disease.[206]

In females, the fallopian tube is the primary site of involvement affecting 90%–100% of cases.[207] Bilateral involvement is typical with lesions occurring in the ampulla followed by isthmus. In approximately half of patients, the infection spreads to the endometrium. Women tend to present with pelvic pain, abnormal uterine bleeding, irregular menses, amenorrhea, or infertility.[208–211] Genital TB has been associated with a 0.2%–21% rate of infertility, primarily among women in resource limited settings.[209,212]

DIAGNOSIS

M. tuberculosis can be isolated from urine in 80%–90% of patients who have three morning urine specimens obtained for culture.[29] In patients with pulmonary TB, urine cultures have been reported to be positive in approximately 5% of cases. In renal TB, urine AFB stains have a sensitivity of approximately 50% and specificity of 97%.[207,213] Urine nucleic acid amplification has a sensitivity of 56%–96% and specificity of 98%.[29] An intravenous pyelogram may show evidence of destructive changes in the kidney or ureteral abnormalities such as strictures and hydronephrosis. CT often demonstrates renal enlargement with abscess formation (Figure 14.7). Ultrasound guided FNA can identify typical histopathological features in 86%–94% of patients and culture is positive in about 45% of samples.[214]

Genital TB in males is usually diagnosed with FNA or urine culture whereas genital TB in women is diagnosed with urine culture and endometrial biopsy or curettage. Curettage cultures are positive in approximately one-third of patients and histology demonstrates typical histopathologic features in 60%–70%.[29,215,216] Rarely, menstrual blood culture will be positive.

TREATMENT

A 6-month regimen is recommended for patients with drug-susceptible urogenital TB[36] based on limited observational studies.[217–219] Dose adjustment may be required in patients with

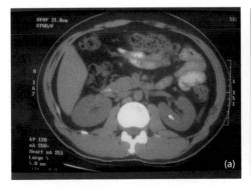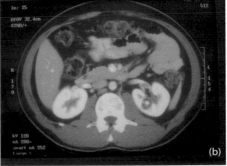

Figure 14.7 Renal TB in a patient with diabetes mellitus. (a) A calcified lesion the left kidney. (b) A renal abscess visible in a contrast enhanced scan.

coexistent renal failure. TB recurrence occurs in 6% of patients with very low recurrence after nephrectomy. Nephrectomy should be considered when there is a nonfunctioning or poorly functioning kidney, particularly in the setting of hypertension, as this can be cured in most patients in this setting.[220,221] If ureteral obstruction occurs, procedures to relieve the obstruction are indicated. In cases of hydronephrosis and progressive renal insufficiency due to obstruction, renal drainage by stenting or percutaneous nephrostomy is advised. In one study of 77 patients with ureteral stricture, the rate of nephrectomy was higher (73% vs. 34%) in those who did not undergo ureteral stenting or nephrostomy in addition to anti-TB therapy.[222] TB of the female or male genital tract responds well to standard chemotherapy, although surgery may be indicated for residual, large, tubo-ovarian abscesses. Unfortunately, infertility is common even after successful treatment.

REFERENCES

1. *Reported Tuberculosis in the United States, 2017*. Atlanta, GA: US Department of Health and Human Services, CDC, 2018.
2. *Global Tuberculosis Report, 2018*. Geneva: World Health Organization. License CC BY-NC-SA 3.0 IGO, 2018.
3. Naing C, Mak JW, Maung M, Wong SF and Kassim AI. Meta-analysis: The association between HIV infection and extrapulmonary tuberculosis. *Lung*. 2013;191(1):27–34.
4. Jones BE, Young SM, Antoniskis D, Davidson PT, Kramer F and Barnes PF. Relationship of the manifestations of tuberculosis to CD4 cell counts in patients with human immunodeficiency virus infection. *Am Rev Respir Dis*. 1993;148(5):1292–7.
5. Sandgren A, Hollo V and van der Werf MJ. Extrapulmonary tuberculosis in the European Union and European Economic Area, 2002 to 2011. *Euro Surveill*. 2013;18(12).
6. Peto HM, Pratt RH, Harrington TA, LoBue PA and Armstrong LR. Epidemiology of extrapulmonary tuberculosis in the United States, 1993–2006. *Clin Infect Dis*. 2009;49(9):1350–7.
7. Talwar A et al. Tuberculosis—United States, 2018. *Am J Transplant*. 2019;19(5):1582–8.
8. World Health Organization. *Tuberculosis Surveillance and Monitoring in Europe 2019-2017 Data*. Copenhagen: WHO Regional Office in Europe, 2019.
9. Holow Sotgiu G et al. Determinants of site of tuberculosis disease: An analysis of European surveillance data from 2003 to 2014. *PLOS ONE*. 2017;12(11):e0186499.
10. Wang X et al. Insight to the epidemiology and risk factors of extrapulmonary tuberculosis in Tianjin, China during 2006–2011. *PLOS ONE*. 2014;9(12):e112213.
11. Ohene SA, Bakker MI, Ojo J, Toonstra A, Awudi D and Klatser P. Extra-pulmonary tuberculosis: A retrospective study of patients in Accra, Ghana. *PLOS ONE*. 2019;14(1):e0209650.
12. Hoogendoorn JC et al. Reduction in extrapulmonary tuberculosis in context of antiretroviral therapy scale-up in rural South Africa. *Epidemiol Infect*. 2017;145(12):2500–9.
13. Shivakoti R, Sharma D, Mamoon G and Pham K. Association of HIV infection with extrapulmonary tuberculosis: A systematic review. *Infection*. 2017;45(1):11–21.
14. Pareek M et al. Vitamin D deficiency and TB disease phenotype. *Thorax*. 2015;70(12):1171–80.
15. Rieder H. *Epidemiologic Basis of Tuberculosis Control*. 1st ed. Paris: Internationa Union Against Tuberculosis and Lung Disease, 1999.
16. Anyama N, Bracebridge S, Black C, Niggebrugge A and Griffin SJ. What happens to people diagnosed with tuberculosis? A population-based cohort. *Epidemiol Infect*. 2007;135(7):1069–76.
17. Low S et al. Mortality among tuberculosis patients on treatment in Singapore. *Int J Tuberc Lung Dis*. 2009;13(3):328–34.
18. Qian X, Nguyen DT, Lyu J, Albers AE, Bi X and Graviss EA. Risk factors for extrapulmonary dissemination of tuberculosis and associated mortality during treatment for extrapulmonary tuberculosis. *Emerging Microbes Infect*. 2018;7(1):102.
19. Christensen AS, Roed C, Andersen PH, Andersen AB and Obel N. Long-term mortality in patients with pulmonary and extrapulmonary tuberculosis: A Danish nationwide cohort study. *Clin Epidemiol*. 2014;6:405–21.
20. Centers for Disease Control and Prevention. *Reported tuberculosis in the United States, 2017*. Atlanta, Georgia: Centers for Disease Control and Prevention, 2017.
21. Lewinsohn DA, Gennaro ML, Scholvinck L and Lewinsohn DM. Tuberculosis immunology in children: Diagnostic and therapeutic challenges and opportunities. *Int J Tuberc Lung Dis*. 2004;8(5):658–74.
22. Antas PR et al. Decreased CD4+ lymphocytes and innate immune responses in adults with previous extrapulmonary tuberculosis. *J Allergy Clin Immunol*. 2006;117(4):916–23.
23. Sterling TR et al. Immune function in young children with previous pulmonary or miliary/meningeal tuberculosis and impact of BCG vaccination. *Pediatrics*. 2007;120(4):e912–21.
24. Fiske CT, de Almeida AS, Shintani AK, Kalams SA and Sterling TR. Abnormal immune responses in persons with previous extrapulmonary tuberculosis in an in vitro model that simulates in vivo infection with *Mycobacterium tuberculosis*. *Clin Vaccine Immunol*. 2012;19(8):1142–9.
25. Wilkinson RJ et al. Influence of vitamin D deficiency and vitamin D receptor polymorphisms on tuberculosis among Gujarati Asians in West London: A case-control study. *Lancet*. 2000;355(9204):618–21.
26. Motsinger-Reif AA, Antas PR, Oki NO, Levy S, Holland SM and Sterling TR. Polymorphisms in IL-1beta, vitamin D receptor Fok1, and Toll-like receptor 2 are associated with extrapulmonary tuberculosis. *BMC Med Genet*. 2010;11:37.
27. Fiske CT et al. Increased vitamin D receptor expression from macrophages after stimulation with *M. tuberculosis* among persons who have recovered from extrapulmonary tuberculosis. *BMC Infect Dis*. 2019;19(1):366.
28. Allen RK, Pierson DL and Rodman OG. Cutaneous inoculation tuberculosis: Prosector's wart occurring in a physician. *Cutis*. 1979;23(6):815–8.
29. Lewinsohn DM et al. Official American Thoracic Society/Infectious Diseases Society of America/Centers for Disease Control and Prevention Clinical Practice Guidelines: Diagnosis of tuberculosis in adults and children. *Clin Infect Dis*. 2017;64(2):e1–e33.
30. Dusthackeer A, Sekar G, Chidambaram S, Kumar V, Mehta P and Swaminathan S. Drug resistance among extrapulmonary TB patients: Six years' experience from a supranational reference laboratory. *Indian J Med Res*. 2015;142(5):568–74.
31. Pang Y et al. Epidemiology of extrapulmonary tuberculosis among inpatients, China, 2008–2017. *Emerg Infect Dis*. 2019;25(3):457–64.
32. Automated real-time nucleic acid amplification technology for rapid and simultaneous detection of tuberculosis and rifampicin resistance: Xpert MTB/RIF assay for the diagnosis of pulmonary and extrapulmonary TB in adults and children. Policy update. Geneva, Switzerland: World Health Organization, 2011.
33. National Institute for Health and Care Excellence. Tuberculosis: Prevention, diagnosis, management and service organization (NICE guideline 33). 2016.

34. Thwaites G et al. British Infection Society guidelines for the diagnosis and treatment of tuberculosis of the central nervous system in adults and children. *J Infect*. 2009;59(3):167–87.

35. Guidelines for treatment of drug-susceptible tuberculosis and patient care, 2017 update. Geneva: World Health Organization, 2017.

36. Nahid P et al. Official American Thoracic Society/Centers for Disease Control and Prevention/Infectious Diseases Society of America Clinical Practice Guidelines: Treatment of drug-susceptible tuberculosis. *Clin Infect Dis*. 2016;63(7):e147–95.

37. National survey of tuberculosis notifications in England and Wales in 1983: Characteristics of disease. Report from the Medical Research Council Tuberculosis and Chest Diseases Unit. *Tubercle*. 1987;68(1):19–32.

38. Pertuiset E et al. Spinal tuberculosis in adults. A study of 103 cases in a developed country, 1980–1994. *Medicine (Baltim)*. 1999;78(5):309–20.

39. Vohra R, Kang HS, Dogra S, Saggar RR and Sharma R. Tuberculous osteomyelitis. *J Bone Joint Surg Br*. 1997;79(4):562–6.

40. Davies PD et al. Bone and joint tuberculosis. A survey of notifications in England and Wales. *J Bone Joint Surg Br*. 1984; 66(3):326–30.

41. Hodgson SP and Ormerod LP. Ten-year experience of bone and joint tuberculosis in Blackburn 1978–1987. *J R Coll Surg Edinb*. 1990;35(4):259–62.

42. Watts HG and Lifeso RM. Tuberculosis of bones and joints. *J Bone Joint Surg Am*. 1996;78(2):288–98.

43. Gorse GJ, Pais MJ, Kusske JA and Cesario TC. Tuberculous spondylitis. A report of six cases and a review of the literature. *Medicine (Baltim)*. 1983;62(3):178–93.

44. Fuentes Ferrer M, Gutierrez Torres L, Ayala Ramirez O, Rumayor Zarzuelo M and del Prado Gonzalez N. Tuberculosis of the spine. A systematic review of case series. *Int Orthop*. 2012;36(2):221–31.

45. Nussbaum ES, Rockswold GL, Bergman TA, Erickson DL and Seljeskog EL. Spinal tuberculosis: A diagnostic and management challenge. *J Neurosurg*. 1995;83(2):243–7.

46. Pigrau-Serrallach C and Rodriguez-Pardo D. Bone and joint tuberculosis. *Eur Spine J*. 2013;22 Suppl 4:556–66.

47. Turgut M. Spinal tuberculosis (Pott's disease): Its clinical presentation, surgical management, and outcome. A survey study on 694 patients. *Neurosurg Rev*. 2001;24(1):8–13.

48. Lifeso RM, Weaver P and Harder EH. Tuberculous spondylitis in adults. *J Bone Joint Surg Am*. 1985;67(9):1405–13.

49. Kumar K and Saxena MB. Multifocal osteoarticular tuberculosis. *Int Orthop*. 1988;12(2):135–8.

50. Sharma SK and Mohan A. Extrapulmonary tuberculosis. *Indian J Med Res*. 2004;120(4):316–53.

51. Walker GF. Failure of early recognition of skeletal tuberculosis. *Br Med J*. 1968;1(5593):682–3.

52. Omari B, Robertson JM, Nelson RJ and Chiu LC. Pott's disease. A resurgent challenge to the thoracic surgeon. *Chest*. 1989;95(1):145–50.

53. Sharif HS et al. Granulomatous spinal infections: MR imaging. *Radiology*. 1990;177(1):101–7.

54. Bell GR, Stearns KL, Bonutti PM and Boumphrey FR. MRI diagnosis of tuberculous vertebral osteomyelitis. *Spine (Phila Pa 1976)*. 1990;15(6):462–5.

55. A controlled trial of six-month and nine-month regimens of chemotherapy in patients undergoing radical surgery for tuberculosis of the spine in Hong Kong. Tenth report of the Medical Research Council Working Party on Tuberculosis of the Spine. *Tubercle*. 1986;67(4):243–59.

56. Controlled trial of short-course regimens of chemotherapy in the ambulatory treatment of spinal tuberculosis. Results at three years of a study in Korea. Twelfth report of the Medical Research Council Working Party on Tuberculosis of the Spine. *J Bone Joint Surg Br*. 1993;75(2):240–8.

57. Five-year assessment of controlled trials of short-course chemotherapy regimens of 6, 9 or 18 months' duration for spinal tuberculosis in patients ambulatory from the start or undergoing radical surgery. Fourteenth report of the Medical Research Council Working Party on Tuberculosis of the Spine. *Int Orthop*. 1999;23(2):73–81.

58. Pattisson PR. Pott's paraplegia: An account of the treatment of 89 consecutive patients. *Paraplegia*. 1986;24(2):77–91.

59. Jutte PC and Van Loenhout-Rooyackers JH. Routine surgery in addition to chemotherapy for treating spinal tuberculosis. *Cochrane Database Syst Rev*. 2006;(1):CD004532.

60. Nene A and Bhojraj S. Results of nonsurgical treatment of thoracic spinal tuberculosis in adults. *Spine J*. 2005;5(1):79–84.

61. Bishburg E, Sunderam G, Reichman LB and Kapila R. Central nervous system tuberculosis with the acquired immunodeficiency syndrome and its related complex. *Ann Intern Med*. 1986;105(2):210–3.

62. Ogawa SK, Smith MA, Brennessel DJ and Lowy FD. Tuberculous meningitis in an urban medical center. *Medicine (Baltim)*. 1987;66(4):317–26.

63. Humphries M. The management of tuberculous meningitis. *Thorax*. 1992;47(8):577–81.

64. Molavi A and LeFrock JL. Tuberculous meningitis. *Med Clin North Am* 1985;69(2):315–31.

65. Dube MP, Holtom PD and Larsen RA. Tuberculous meningitis in patients with and without human immunodeficiency virus infection. *Am J Med*. 1992;93(5):520–4.

66. Berenguer J et al. Tuberculous meningitis in patients infected with the human immunodeficiency virus. *N Engl J Med*. 1992;326(10):668–72.

67. Xu HB, Jiang RH, Li L, Sha W and Xiao HP. Diagnostic value of adenosine deaminase in cerebrospinal fluid for tuberculous meningitis: A meta-analysis. *Int J Tuberc Lung Dis*. 2010;14(11):1382–7.

68. Tuon FF et al. Adenosine deaminase and tuberculous meningitis—A systematic review with meta-analysis. *Scand J Infect Dis*. 2010;42(3):198–207.

69. Ekermans P, Duse A and George J. The dubious value of cerebrospinal fluid adenosine deaminase measurement for the diagnosis of tuberculous meningitis. *BMC Infect Dis*. 2017;17(1):104.

70. Ruslami R et al. Intensified regimen containing rifampicin and moxifloxacin for tuberculous meningitis: An open-label, randomised controlled phase 2 trial. *Lancet Infect Dis*. 2013;13(1):27–35.

71. Heemskerk AD et al. Intensified antituberculosis therapy in adults with tuberculous meningitis. *N Engl J Med*. 2016;374(2):124–34.

72. Chiang SS et al. Treatment outcomes of childhood tuberculous meningitis: A systematic review and meta-analysis. *Lancet Infect Dis*. 2014;14(10):947–57.

73. van Toorn R, Schaaf HS, Laubscher JA, van Elsland SL, Donald PR and Schoeman JF. Short intensified treatment in children with drug-susceptible tuberculous meningitis. *Pediatr Infect Dis J*. 2014;33(3):248–52.

74. Chotmongkol V, Jitpimolmard S and Thavornpitak Y. Corticosteroid in tuberculous meningitis. *J Med Assoc Thai* 1996;79(2):83–90.

75. Critchley JA, Young F, Orton L and Garner P. Corticosteroids for prevention of mortality in people with tuberculosis: A systematic review and meta-analysis. *Lancet Infect Dis*. 2013;13(3):223–37.

76. Girgis NI, Farid Z, Hanna LS, Yassin MW and Wallace CK. The use of dexamethasone in preventing ocular complications in tuberculous meningitis. *Trans R Soc Trop Med Hyg*. 1983;77(5):658–9.

77. Girgis NI, Farid Z, Kilpatrick ME, Sultan Y and Mikhail IA. Dexamethasone adjunctive treatment for tuberculous meningitis. *Pediatr Infect Dis J.* 1991;10(3):179–83.

78. Ashby M and Grant H. Tuberculous meningitis treated with cortisone. *Lancet.* 1955;268(6854):65–6.

79. O'Toole RD, Thornton GF, Mukherjee MK and Nath RL. Dexamethasone in tuberculous meningitis. Relationship of cerebrospinal fluid effects to therapeutic efficacy. *Ann Intern Med.* 1969;70(1):39–48.

80. Escobar JA, Belsey MA, Duenas A and Medina P. Mortality from tuberculous meningitis reduced by steroid therapy. *Pediatrics.* 1975;56(6):1050–5.

81. Kumarvelu S, Prasad K, Khosla A, Behari M and Ahuja GK. Randomized controlled trial of dexamethasone in tuberculous meningitis. *Tuber Lung Dis.* 1994;75(3):203–7.

82. Dooley DP, Carpenter JL and Rademacher S. Adjunctive corticosteroid therapy for tuberculosis: A critical reappraisal of the literature. *Clin Infect Dis.* 1997;25(4):872–87.

83. Schoeman JF, Van Zyl LE, Laubscher JA and Donald PR. Effect of corticosteroids on intracranial pressure, computed tomographic findings, and clinical outcome in young children with tuberculous meningitis. *Pediatrics.* 1997;99(2):226–31.

84. Thwaites GE et al. Dexamethasone for the treatment of tuberculous meningitis in adolescents and adults. *N Engl J Med.* 2004;351(17):1741–51.

85. Prasad K and Singh MB. Corticosteroids for managing tuberculous meningitis. *Cochrane Database Syst Rev.* 2008;(1):CD002244.

86. Malhotra HS, Garg RK, Singh MK, Agarwal A and Verma R. Corticosteroids (dexamethasone versus intravenous methylprednisolone) in patients with tuberculous meningitis. *Ann Trop Med Parasitol.* 2009;103(7):625–34.

87. Sharma SK and Mohan A. Miliary tuberculosis. *Microbiol Spectr.* 2017;5(2).

88. Kumar D, Watson JM, Charlett A, Nicholas S and Darbyshire JH. Tuberculosis in England and Wales in 1993: Results of a national survey. Public Health Laboratory Service/British Thoracic Society/Department of Health Collaborative Group. *Thorax.* 1997; 52(12):1060–7.

89. Centers for Disease Control and Prevention. Reported tuberculosis in the United States, 2017. Available at: https://www.cdc.gov/tb/statistics/reports/2018/default.htm. Accessed September 21.

90. Sharma SK, Mohan A, Sharma A and Mitra DK. Miliary tuberculosis: New insights into an old disease. *Lancet Infect Dis.* 2005;5(7):415–30.

91. Sahn SA and Neff TA. Miliary tuberculosis. *Am J Med.* 1974;56(4):494–505.

92. Proudfoot AT, Akhtar AJ, Douglas AC and Horne NW. Miliary tuberculosis in adults. *Br Med J.* 1969;2(5652):273–6.

93. Kaplan MH, Armstrong D and Rosen P. Tuberculosis complicating neoplastic disease. A review of 201 cases. *Cancer.* 1974; 33(3):850–8.

94. Pradhan RP, Katz LA, Nidus BD, Matalon R and Eisinger RP. Tuberculosis in dialyzed patients. *JAMA.* 1974;229(7):798–800.

95. Maartens G, Willcox PA and Benatar SR. Miliary tuberculosis: Rapid diagnosis, hematologic abnormalities, and outcome in 109 treated adults. *Am J Med.* 1990;89(3):291–6.

96. Slavin RE, Walsh TJ and Pollack AD. Late generalized tuberculosis: A clinical pathologic analysis and comparison of 100 cases in the preantibiotic and antibiotic eras. *Medicine (Baltim).* 1980;59(5):352–66.

97. MacGee W. The frequency of unsuspected tuberculosis found postmortem in a geriatric population. *Z Gerontol.* 1989;22(6):311–4.

98. So SY and Yu D. The adult respiratory distress syndrome associated with miliary tuberculosis. *Tubercle.* 1981; 62(1):49–53.

99. Long R, O'Connor R, Palayew M, Hershfield E and Manfreda J. Disseminated tuberculosis with and without a miliary pattern on chest radiograph: A clinical-pathologic-radiologic correlation. *Int J Tuberc Lung Dis.* 1997;1(1):52–8.

100. Gelb AF, Leffler C, Brewin A, Mascatello V and Lyons HA. Miliary tuberculosis. *Am Rev Respir Dis.* 1973;108(6):1327–33.

101. McGuinness G, Naidich DP, Jagirdar J, Leitman B and McCauley DI. High resolution CT findings in miliary lung disease. *J Comput Assist Tomogr.* 1992;16(3):384–90.

102. Kim JH, Langston AA and Gallis HA. Miliary tuberculosis: Epidemiology, clinical manifestations, diagnosis, and outcome. *Rev Infect Dis.* 1990;12(4):583–90.

103. Munt PW. Miliary tuberculosis in the chemotherapy era: With a clinical review in 69 American adults. *Medicine (Baltim).* 1972;51(2):139–55.

104. Pant K, Chawla R, Mann PS and Jaggi OP. Fiberbronchoscopy in smear-negative miliary tuberculosis. *Chest* 1989;95(5):1151–2.

105. Willcox PA, Potgieter PD, Bateman ED and Benatar SR. Rapid diagnosis of sputum negative miliary tuberculosis using the flexible fibreoptic bronchoscope. *Thorax.* 1986;41(9):681–4.

106. Saltzman BR, Motyl MR, Friedland GH, McKitrick JC and Klein RS. *Mycobacterium tuberculosis* bacteremia in the acquired immunodeficiency syndrome. *JAMA.* 1986;256(3):390–1.

107. Shafer RW, Kim DS, Weiss JP and Quale JM. Extrapulmonary tuberculosis in patients with human immunodeficiency virus infection. *Medicine (Baltim).* 1991;70(6):384–97.

108. Kramer F, Modilevsky T, Waliany AR, Leedom JM and Barnes PF. Delayed diagnosis of tuberculosis in patients with human immunodeficiency virus infection. *Am J Med.* 1990;89(4):451–6.

109. Huseby JS and Hudson LD. Miliary tuberculosis and adult respiratory distress syndrome. *Ann Intern Med.* 1976;85(5):609–11.

110. Murray HW, Tuazon CU, Kirmani N and Sheagren JN. The adult respiratory distress syndrome associated with miliary tuberculosis. *Chest.* 1978;73(1):37–43.

111. Farer LS, Lowell AM and Meador MP. Extrapulmonary tuberculosis in the United States. *Am J Epidemiol.* 1979;109(2):205–17.

112. Fitzgerald JM, Menzies RI and Elwood RK. Abdominal tuberculosis: A critical review. *Dig Dis.* 1991;9(5):269–81.

113. Tan KK, Chen K and Sim R. The spectrum of abdominal tuberculosis in a developed country: A single institution's experience over 7 years. *J Gastrointest Surg.* 2009;13(1):142–7.

114. Chen HL, Wu MS, Chang WH, Shih SC, Chi H and Bair MJ. Abdominal tuberculosis in Southeastern Taiwan: 20 years of experience. *J Formos Med Assoc.* 2009;108(3):195–201.

115. Jakubowski A, Elwood RK and Enarson DA. Clinical features of abdominal tuberculosis. *J Infect Dis.* 1988;158(4):687–92.

116. Chow KM, Chow VC, Hung LC, Wong SM and Szeto CC. Tuberculous peritonitis-associated mortality is high among patients waiting for the results of mycobacterial cultures of ascitic fluid samples. *Clin Infect Dis.* 2002;35(4):409–13.

117. Sanai FM and Bzeizi KI. Systematic review: Tuberculous peritonitis—Presenting features, diagnostic strategies and treatment. *Aliment Pharmacol Ther.* 2005;22(8):685–700.

118. Bhargava DK, Shriniwas, Chopra P, Nijhawan S, Dasarathy S and Kushwaha AK. Peritoneal tuberculosis: Laparoscopic patterns and its diagnostic accuracy. *Am J Gastroenterol.* 1992;87(1):109–12.

119. Singh MM, Bhargava AN and Jain KP. Tuberculous peritonitis. An evaluation of pathogenetic mechanisms, diagnostic procedures and therapeutic measures. *N Engl J Med.* 1969;281(20):1091–4.

120. Bowry S, Chan CH, Weiss H, Katz S and Zimmerman HJ. Hepatic involvement in pulmonary tuberculosis. Histologic and functional characteristics. *Am Rev Respir Dis*. 1970;101(6):941–8.

121. Prout S and Benatar SR. Disseminated tuberculosis. A study of 62 cases. *S Afr Med J*. 1980;58(21):835–42.

122. Vaid U and Kane GC. Tuberculous peritonitis. *Microbiol Spectr*. 2017;5(1).

123. Riquelme A et al. Value of adenosine deaminase (ADA) in ascitic fluid for the diagnosis of tuberculous peritonitis: A meta-analysis. *J Clin Gastroenterol*. 2006;40(8):705–10.

124. Su SB, Qin SY, Guo XY, Luo W and Jiang HX. Assessment by meta-analysis of interferon-gamma for the diagnosis of tuberculous peritonitis. *World J Gastroenterol*. 2013;19(10):1645–51.

125. Veeragandham RS, Lynch FP, Canty TG, Collins DL and Danker WM. Abdominal tuberculosis in children: Review of 26 cases. *J Pediatr Surg*. 1996;31(1):170–5; discussion 5–6.

126. Pettengell KE, Larsen C, Garb M, Mayet FG, Simjee AE and Pirie D. Gastrointestinal tuberculosis in patients with pulmonary tuberculosis. *Q J Med*. 1990;74(275):303–8.

127. Harrington PT, Gutierrez JJ, Ramirez-Ronda CH, Quinones-Soto R, Bermudez RH and Chaffey J. Granulomatous hepatitis. *Rev Infect Dis* 1982;4(3):638–55.

128. Bastani B, Shariatzadeh MR and Dehdashti F. Tuberculous peritonitis—Report of 30 cases and review of the literature. *Q J Med*. 1985;56(221):549–57.

129. Demir K et al. Tuberculous peritonitis—Reports of 26 cases, detailing diagnostic and therapeutic problems. *Eur J Gastroenterol Hepatol*. 2001;13(5):581–5.

130. Singhal A, Gulati A, Frizell R and Manning AP. Abdominal tuberculosis in Bradford, UK: 1992–2002. *Eur J Gastroenterol Hepatol*. 2005;17(9):967–71.

131. Alrajhi AA, Halim MA, al-Hokail A, Alrabiah F and al-Omran K. Corticosteroid treatment of peritoneal tuberculosis. *Clin Infect Dis*. 1998;27(1):52–6.

132. Rasheed S, Zinicola R, Watson D, Bajwa A and McDonald PJ. Intra-abdominal and gastrointestinal tuberculosis. *Colorectal Dis*. 2007;9(9):773–83.

133. Khan AR et al. Tuberculous peritonitis: A surgical dilemma. *South Med J*. 2009;102(1):94–5.

134. Park YS et al. Colonoscopy evaluation after short-term anti-tuberculosis treatment in nonspecific ulcers on the ileocecal area. *World J Gastroenterol*. 2008;14(32):5051–8.

135. Kent DC. Tuberculous lymphadenitis: Not a localized disease process. *Am J Med Sci*. 1967;254(6):866–74.

136. Ord RJ and Matz GJ. Tuberculous cervical lymphadenitis. *Arch Otolaryngol*. 1974;99(5):327–9.

137. Lai KK, Stottmeier KD, Sherman IH and McCabe WR. *Mycobacterial cervical* lymphadenopathy. Relation of etiologic agents to age. *JAMA*.1984;251(10):1286–8.

138. Shikhani AH, Hadi UM, Mufarrij AA and Zaytoun GM. Mycobacterial cervical lymphadenitis. *Ear Nose Throat J*. 1989;68(9):660, 2–6, 8–72.

139. Huhti E, Brander E, Paloheimo S and Sutinen S. Tuberculosis of the cervical lymph nodes: A clinical, pathological and bacteriological study. *Tubercle*. 1975;56(1):27–36.

140. Hooper AA. Tuberculous peripheral lymphadenitis. *Br J Surg*. 1972;59(5):353–9.

141. Cantrell RW, Jensen JH and Reid D. Diagnosis and management of tuberculous cervical adenitis. *Arch Otolaryngol*. 1975;101(1):53–7.

142. Chaisson RE, Schecter GF, Theuer CP, Rutherford GW, Echenberg DF and Hopewell PC. Tuberculosis in patients with the acquired immunodeficiency syndrome. Clinical features, response to therapy, and survival. *Am Rev Respir Dis*. 1987;136(3):570–4.

143. Pitchenik AE, Burr J, Suarez M, Fertel D, Gonzalez G and Moas C. Human T-cell lymphotropic virus-III (HTLV-III) seropositivity and related disease among 71 consecutive patients in whom tuberculosis was diagnosed. A prospective study. *Am Rev Respir Dis*. 1987;135(4):875–9.

144. Modilevsky T, Sattler FR and Barnes PF. Mycobacterial disease in patients with human immunodeficiency virus infection. *Arch Intern Med*. 1989;149(10):2201–5.

145. Qian X et al. An eight-year epidemiologic study of head and neck tuberculosis in Texas, USA. *Tuberculosis (Edinb)*. 2019.

146. Agarwal AK, Sethi A, Sethi D, Malhotra V and Singal S. Tubercular cervical adenitis: Clinicopathologic analysis of 180 cases. *J Otolaryngol Head Neck Surg*. 2009;38(5):521–5.

147. Artenstein AW, Kim JH, Williams WJ and Chung RC. Isolated peripheral tuberculous lymphadenitis in adults: Current clinical and diagnostic issues. *Clin Infect Dis*. 1995;20(4):876–82.

148. Malik SK, Behera D and Gilhotra R. Tuberculous pleural effusion and lymphadenitis treated with rifampin-containing regimen. *Chest*. 1987;92(5):904–5.

149. Lee KC, Tami TA, Lalwani AK and Schecter G. Contemporary management of cervical tuberculosis. *Laryngoscope*. 1992;102(1):60–4.

150. Denkinger CM, Schumacher SG, Boehme CC, Dendukuri N, Pai M and Steingart KR. Xpert MTB/RIF assay for the diagnosis of extrapulmonary tuberculosis: A systematic review and meta-analysis. *Eur Respir J*. 2014;44(2):435–46.

151. Geldmacher H, Taube C, Kroeger C, Magnussen H and Kirsten DK. Assessment of lymph node tuberculosis in northern Germany: A clinical review. *Chest*. 2002;121(4):1177–82.

152. Thompson MM, Underwood MJ, Sayers RD, Dookeran KA and Bell PR. Peripheral tuberculous lymphadenopathy: A review of 67 cases. *Br J Surg*. 1992;79(8):763–4.

153. Shriner KA, Mathisen GE and Goetz MB. Comparison of mycobacterial lymphadenitis among persons infected with human immunodeficiency virus and seronegative controls. *Clin Infect Dis*. 1992;15(4):601–5.

154. Campbell IA and Dyson AJ. Lymph node tuberculosis: A comparison of treatments 18 months after completion of chemotherapy. *Tubercle*. 1979;60(2):95–8.

155. Short course chemotherapy for tuberculosis of lymph nodes: A controlled trial. British Thoracic Society Research Committee. *Br Med J (Clin Res Ed)*. 1985;290(6475):1106–8.

156. Jawahar MS et al. Short course chemotherapy for tuberculous lymphadenitis in children. *BMJ*. 1990;301(6748):359–62.

157. Six-months versus nine-months chemotherapy for tuberculosis of lymph nodes: Preliminary results. British Thoracic Society Research Committee. *Respir Med*. 1992;86(1):15–9.

158. Campbell IA, Ormerod LP, Friend JA, Jenkins PA and Prescott RJ. Six months versus nine months chemotherapy for tuberculosis of lymph nodes: Final results. *Respir Med*. 1993;87(8):621–3.

159. Yuen AP, Wong SH, Tam CM, Chan SL, Wei WI and Lau SK. Prospective randomized study of thrice weekly six-month and nine-month chemotherapy for cervical tuberculous lymphadenopathy. *Otolaryngol Head Neck Surg*. 1997;116(2):189–92.

160. Campbell IA and Dyson AJ. Lymph node tuberculosis: A comparison of various methods of treatment. *Tubercle*. 1977;58(4):171–9.

161. Cho OH et al. Paradoxical responses in non-HIV-infected patients with peripheral lymph node tuberculosis. *J Infect*. 2009;59(1):56–61.

162. Carvalho AC et al. Paradoxical reaction during tuberculosis treatment in HIV-seronegative patients. *Clin Infect Dis*. 2006;42(6):893–5.

163. Narita M, Ashkin D, Hollender ES and Pitchenik AE. Paradoxical worsening of tuberculosis following antiretroviral therapy in patients with AIDS. *Am J Respir Crit Care Med*. 1998;158(1):157–61.

164. Wendel KA, Alwood KS, Gachuhi R, Chaisson RE, Bishai WR and Sterling TR. Paradoxical worsening of tuberculosis in HIV-infected persons. *Chest.* 2001;120(1):193–7.

165. Cheung WL, Siu KF and Ng A. Tuberculous cervical abscess: Comparing the results of total excision against simple incision and drainage. *Br J Surg.* 1988;75(6):563–4.

166. Larrieu AJ, Tyers GF, Williams EH and Derrick JR. Recent experience with tuberculous pericarditis. *Ann Thorac Surg.* 1980;29(5):464–8.

167. Cegielski JP et al. Tuberculous pericarditis in Tanzanian patients with and without HIV infection. *Tuber Lung Dis.* 1994;75(6):429–34.

168. Reynolds MM, Hecht SR, Berger M, Kolokathis A and Horowitz SF. Large pericardial effusions in the acquired immunodeficiency syndrome. *Chest.* 1992;102(6):1746–7.

169. Fowler NO and Manitsas GT. Infectious pericarditis. *Prog Cardiovasc Dis.* 1973;16(3):323–36.

170. Strang JI et al. Controlled clinical trial of complete open surgical drainage and of prednisolone in treatment of tuberculous pericardial effusion in Transkei. *Lancet.* 1988;2(8614):759–64.

171. Fowler NO. The electrocardiogram in pericarditis. *Cardiovasc Clin.* 1973;5(3):255–67.

172. Rooney JJ, Crocco JA and Lyons HA. Tuberculous pericarditis. *Ann Intern Med.* 1970;72(1):73–81.

173. Fowler NO. Tuberculous pericarditis. *JAMA.* 1991;266(1):99–103.

174. Schepers GW. Tuberculous pericarditis. *Am J Cardiol.* 1962;9:248–76.

175. Pandie S et al. Diagnostic accuracy of quantitative PCR (Xpert MTB/RIF) for tuberculous pericarditis compared to adenosine deaminase and unstimulated interferon-gamma in a high burden setting: A prospective study. *BMC Med.* 2014;12:101.

176. Strang JI, Kakaza HH, Gibson DG, Girling DJ, Nunn AJ, and Fox W. Controlled trial of prednisolone as adjuvant in treatment of tuberculous constrictive pericarditis in Transkei. *Lancet.* 1987;2(8573):1418–22.

177. Hakim JG, Ternouth I, Mushangi E, Siziya S, Robertson V and Malin A. Double blind randomised placebo controlled trial of adjunctive prednisolone in the treatment of effusive tuberculous pericarditis in HIV seropositive patients. *Heart.* 2000;84(2):183–8.

178. Blumberg HM et al. American Thoracic Society/Centers for Disease Control and Prevention/Infectious Diseases Society of America: Treatment of tuberculosis. *Am J Respir Crit Care Med.* 2003;167(4):603–62.

179. Wiysonge CS et al. Interventions for treating tuberculous pericarditis. *Cochrane Database Syst Rev.* 2017;9:CD000526.

180. Mayosi BM et al. Prednisolone and *Mycobacterium indicus pranii* in tuberculous pericarditis. *N Engl J Med.* 2014;371(12):1121–30.

181. Chaisson RE and Post WS. Immunotherapy for tuberculous pericarditis. *N Engl J Med.* 2014;371(26):2535.

182. Ong A et al. A molecular epidemiological assessment of extrapulmonary tuberculosis in San Francisco. *Clin Infect Dis.* 2004;38(1):25–31.

183. Berger HW and Mejia E. Tuberculous pleurisy. *Chest.* 1973;63(1):88–92.

184. Epstein DM, Kline LR, Albelda SM and Miller WT. Tuberculous pleural effusions. *Chest.* 1987;91(1):106–9.

185. Levine H, Szanto PB and Cugell DW. Tuberculous pleurisy. An acute illness. *Arch Intern Med.* 1968;122(4):329–32.

186. Roper WH and Waring JJ. Primary serofibrinous pleural effusion in military personnel. *Am Rev Tuberc.* 1955;71(5):616–34.

187. Patiala J. Initial tuberculous pleuritis in the Finnish armed forces in 1939–1945 with special reference to eventual postpleuritic tuberculosis. *Acta Tuberc Scand Suppl.* 1954;36:1–57.

188. Seibert AF, Haynes J, Jr. Middleton R and Bass JB, Jr. Tuberculous pleural effusion. Twenty-year experience. *Chest.* 1991;99(4):883–6.

189. Conde MB et al. Yield of sputum induction in the diagnosis of pleural tuberculosis. *Am J Respir Crit Care Med.* 2003;167(5):723–5.

190. Chan CH, Arnold M, Chan CY, Mak TW and Hoheisel GB. Clinical and pathological features of tuberculous pleural effusion and its long-term consequences. *Respiration.* 1991;58(3–4):171–5.

191. Sarkar SK, Purohit SD, Sharma TN, Sharma VK, Ram M and Singh AP. Pleuroscopy in the diagnosis of pleural effusion using a fiber-optic bronchoscope. *Tubercle.* 1985;66(2):141–4.

192. Boutin C, Astoul P and Seitz B. The role of thoracoscopy in the evaluation and management of pleural effusions. *Lung.* 1990;168 Suppl:1113–21.

193. Jiang J, Shi HZ, Liang QL, Qin SM, and Qin XJ. Diagnostic value of interferon-gamma in tuberculous pleurisy. A meta-analysis. *Chest.* 2007;131:1133–41.

194. Galarza I, Canete C, Granados A, Estopa R and Manresa F. Randomised trial of corticosteroids in the treatment of tuberculous pleurisy. *Thorax.* 1995;50(12):1305–7.

195. Wyser C, Walzl G, Smedema JP, Swart F, van Schalkwyk EM and van de Wal BW. Corticosteroids in the treatment of tuberculous pleurisy. A double-blind, placebo-controlled, randomized study. *Chest.* 1996;110(2):333–8.

196. Elliott AM et al. A randomized, double-blind, placebo-controlled trial of the use of prednisolone as an adjunct to treatment in HIV-1-associated pleural tuberculosis. *J Infect Dis.* 2004;190(5):869–78.

197. Engel MEMP and Volmink J. Corticosteroids for tuberculous pleurisy. *Cochrane Database Syst Rev.* 2007;4:CD001876.

198. Ryan H, Yoo J and Darsini P. Corticosteroids for tuberculous pleurisy. *Cochrane Database Syst Rev.* 2017;3:CD001876.

199. Sahn SA and Iseman MD. Tuberculous empyema. *Semin Respir Infect.* 1999;14(1):82–7.

200. Figueiredo AA and Lucon AM. Urogenital tuberculosis: Update and review of 8961 cases from the world literature. *Rev Urol.* 2008;10(3):207–17.

201. Figueiredo AA, Lucon AM, Junior RF and Srougi M. Epidemiology of urogenital tuberculosis worldwide. *Int J Urol* 2008;15(9):827–32.

202. Psihramis KE and Donahoe PK. Primary genitourinary tuberculosis: Rapid progression and tissue destruction during treatment. *J Urol.* 1986;135(5):1033–6.

203. Alvarez S and McCabe WR. Extrapulmonary tuberculosis revisited: A review of experience at Boston City and other hospitals. *Medicine (Baltim).* 1984;63(1):25–55.

204. Christensen WI. Genitourinary tuberculosis: Review of 102 cases. *Medicine (Baltim).* 1974;53(5):377–90.

205. Gokalp A, Gultekin EY and Ozdamar S. Genito-urinary tuberculosis: A review of 83 cases. *Br J Clin Pract.* 1990;44(12):599–600.

206. Singal A, Pandhi D, Kataria V and Arora VK. Tuberculosis of the glans penis: An important differential diagnosis of genital ulcer disease. *Int J STD AIDS.* 2017;28(14):1453–5.

207. Abbara A, Davidson RN and Medscape. Etiology and management of genitourinary tuberculosis. *Nat Rev Urol.* 2011;8(12):678–88.

208. Figueiredo AA, Lucon AM and Srougi M. Urogenital tuberculosis. *Microbiol Spectr.* 2017;5(1).

209. Aliyu MH, Aliyu SH and Salihu HM. Female genital tuberculosis: A global review. *Int J Fertil Women's Med* 2004;49(3):123–36.

210. Parikh FR, Nadkarni SG, Kamat SA, Naik N, Soonawala SB and Parikh RM. Genital tuberculosis—A major pelvic factor causing infertility in Indian women. *Fertil Steril.* 1997;67(3):497–500.

211. Namavar Jahromi B, Parsanezhad ME and Ghane-Shirazi R. Female genital tuberculosis and infertility. *Int J Gynaecol Obstet.* 2001;75(3):269–72.

212. Mondal SK and Dutta TK. A ten year clinicopathological study of female genital tuberculosis and impact on fertility. *JNMA J Nepal Med Assoc.* 2009;48(173):52–7.

213. Mortier E, Pouchot J, Girard L, Boussougant Y and Vinceneux P. Assessment of urine analysis for the diagnosis of tuberculosis. *BMJ.* 1996;312(7022):27–8.

214. Das KM, Vaidyanathan S, Rajwanshi A and Indudhara R. Renal tuberculosis: Diagnosis with sonographically guided aspiration cytology. *AJR Am J Roentgenol.* 1992;158(3):571–3.

215. Sutherland AM. Tuberculosis of the female genital tract. *Tubercle.* 1985;66(2):79–83.

216. Falk V, Ludviksson K and Agren G. Genital tuberculosis in women. Analysis of 187 newly diagnosed cases from 47 Swedish hospitals during the ten-year period 1968 to 1977. *Am J Obstet Gynecol.* 1980;138(7 Pt 2):974–7.

217. Gow JG. Genito-urinary tuberculosis. A study of the disease in one unit over a period of 24 years. *Ann R Coll Surg Engl.* 1971;49(1):50–70.

218. Simon HB, Weinstein AJ, Pasternak MS, Swartz MN and Kunz LJ. Genitourinary tuberculosis. Clinical features in a general hospital population. *Am J Med.* 1977;63(3):410–20.

219. Skutil V, Varsa J and Obsitnik M. Six-month chemotherapy for urogenital tuberculosis. *Eur Urol.* 1985;11(3):170–6.

220. Cek M et al. EAU guidelines for the management of genitourinary tuberculosis. *Eur Urol.* 2005;48(3):353–62.

221. Fischer M and Flamm J. The value of surgical therapy in the treatment of urogenital tuberculosis. *Urol A.* 1990;29(5):261–4.

222. Shin KY, Park HJ, Lee JJ, Park HY, Woo YN and Lee TY. Role of early endourologic management of tuberculous ureteral strictures. *J Endourol.* 2002;16(10):755–8.

15

Tuberculosis and Human Immunodeficiency Virus Coinfection

CHARISSE MANDIMIKA AND GERALD FRIEDLAND

INTRODUCTION

The syndemics of tuberculosis (TB) and human immunodeficiency virus/acquired immunodeficiency syndrome (HIV/AIDS) have been a dangerous and ongoing collision of one of the oldest and among the newest of human infectious diseases. They have resulted in mutually severe and challenging global consequences. The entry of HIV/AIDS into high-prevalence areas and populations with TB infection and disease has resulted in major secondary TB epidemics and deadly alterations in TB outcomes. Conversely, TB is the most common presenting illness among people living with HIV (PLWH), accelerating HIV disease progression and is the major cause of HIV-related deaths globally. These two epidemic diseases have been joined by an emerging and growing global epidemic of drug-resistant TB, associated with HIV, and threatening many recent exciting and beneficial TB and HIV advances.

We discuss the global and local epidemiology, clinical features, and recent selected advances and challenges in the prevention and treatment of TB/HIV disease. Rather than accepting the traditional separation of TB and HIV, we consider the barriers and challenges in the integration of TB and HIV efforts and, in so doing, the importance and benefit of a person-centered comprehensive approach to integration for individuals and communities impacted by both diseases. We provide evidence for progress in the integration of HIV and TB prevention, diagnosis, care, and treatment, but also identify gaps where more effort is needed. Full implementation of evidence-based components and World Health Organization (WHO) advocated strategies are needed to improve outcomes of TB and HIV and to bring both closer to epidemic elimination.

EPIDEMIOLOGY OF THE CONVERGENT TB AND HIV EPIDEMICS

GLOBAL SCALE AND TENDS

TB is the ninth leading cause of death globally and has surpassed HIV as the leading cause of death from a communicable disease. The epidemiology of these convergent epidemic diseases illustrates their great clinical and public health challenges. TB remains the leading cause of death globally in PLWH. Globally, an estimated 10.0 million (range, 9.0–11.1 million) people fell ill with TB in 2018. A total of 10% of the incident cases of TB were estimated to occur in PLWH. There were an estimated 1.2 million (range, 1.1–1.3 million) TB deaths among HIV-negative people in 2018 (a 27% reduction from 1.7 million in 2000), and an additional 251,000 deaths (range, 223,000–281,000) among HIV-positive people (a 60% reduction from 620,000 in 2000).[1]

The regional and national global distribution of TB- and HIV-coinfection risks and rates vary greatly.

The global geographic and epidemiologic differences in the distribution of TB and of TB/HIV-coinfection are shown in Figures 15.1 and 15.2.

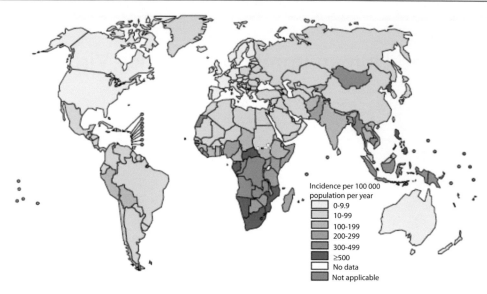

Figure 15.1 Estimated TB incidence rate, 2018.

Sub-Saharan Africa has borne the brunt of the converging epidemics with over 50% of TB incident cases co infected with HIV in many areas and harboring the highest prevalence and proportion of globally coinfected individuals.[1] Sub-Saharan Africa accounts for 72% of new TB cases among PLWH and 84% of global deaths from TB in people living with HIV. South Africa's TB incidence, among the highest in the world, is now estimated as 520 per 100,000, with an estimated HIV prevalence of 60%–80% among newly diagnosed active TB cases.[2] In Zulu speaking rural KwaZuluNatal, the diagnosis TB is so frequently accompanied by a second diagnosis of HIV/AIDS that their relationship is expressed in Zulu as:

"TB is the mother of AIDS"

In contrast to sub-Saharan Africa, India's TB incidence in 2018 was 199 per 10,000, but with a much smaller estimated HIV prevalence of only 6.8%. In the countries of the former Soviet Union, although the TB incidence rates are lower, the proportion of cases that are HIV coinfected is substantially higher. For example, in 2018, the Russian Federation's estimated incidence of TB was 55 per 100,000 with a higher estimated HIV prevalence of 11%. Although these selected estimated global rates have declined compared to the previous year,[2] they remain dangerously high, volatile and challenging. The TB- and HIV–coinfection rates are substantially lower in most countries in Western Europe. The TB incidence in the United States was 52.6/100,000 in 1953, the year national TB incidence surveillance began and steadily declined thereafter, except for a dramatic HIV-associated rise in the 1980s and 1990's, and since has gratifyingly fallen to 2.8 per 100,000 by

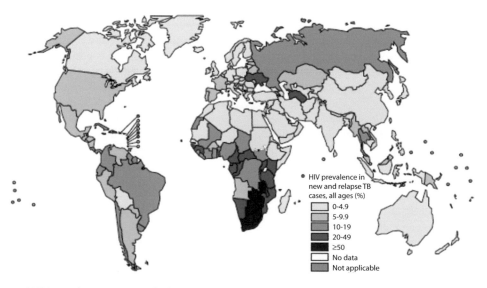

Figure 15.2. Estimated HIV prevalence in new and relapse TB cases, 2018.

2017.[3] Among the 9,093 reported cases in the United States in 2017, HIV status was known for 86.3% and of these 5.6% or 509 had coinfection with HIV[3]

THE EMERGENCE OF DRUG-RESISTANT TB AND HIV

In the past two decades, the global growth of the convergent epidemics of TB and HIV has been joined by the recognition of a third epidemic of drug-resistant TB. In many geographic areas, this has also occurred in close association with HIV and has threatened and confounded advances in both TB and HIV elimination.

MULTIDRUG-RESISTANT AND EXTENSIVELY DRUG-RESISTANT TB AND HIV

Multidrug-resistant TB (MDR-TB) is defined as *Mycobacterium tuberculosis* isolates resistant to at least isoniazid (INH) and rifampin (RIF).[4] MDR-TB is either acquired by direct transmission or develops through incompletely treated or mutated and amplified initially sensitive *M. tuberculosis*. It is particularly problematic in countries of the former Soviet Union and Southeast Asia where populations have been devastated by this third convergent epidemic disease. In areas of sub-Saharan Africa, HIV-coinfection rates among those with MDR-TB are extremely high and mirror those of drug-susceptible TB. The three countries with the highest total burden of MDR-TB disease are China, India, and Russia, although their HIV-coinfection rates do not approach those of sub-Saharan Africa.[1] The proportion of people in Eastern Europe living with MDR-TB and HIV coinfection rose by 40% between 2011 and 2015, driven by a sharp increase in the number of coinfections in Russia and other countries of the former Soviet Union.

Globally, among these populations, on average, an estimated 6.2% of people with MDR-TB have extensively-drug-resistant TB (XDR-TB), defined as MDR-TB plus resistance to any fluoroquinolone and at least one of three injectable second-line drugs (amikacin, kanamycin, or capreomycin).[5] Between 2005 and 2006, the largest known cluster of cases of XDR-TB was identified in a rural hospital in KwaZulu Natal, almost exclusively in PLWH.[6] All patients identified with XDR-TB who were tested were co-infected with HIV, 55% had never been treated for TB, and 67% had previously been hospitalized, suggesting nosocomial transmission. Genotyping of isolates showed that 85% (95% confidence interval [CI]: 74–95) had the similar F15/LAM4/KZN genome, further supporting healthcare facility acquisition. Subsequent studies revealed the presence of XDR-TB in all nine South African provinces and in neighboring countries. A more contemporary study involving patients with XDR-TB from a broader area of KwaZulu Natal, revealed an HIV-coinfection rate in 77% of those with diagnosed XDR-TB and genotypic analysis revealed common cluster strains and person-to-person or epidemiologic links supporting transmission in 30% of participants.[7] By 2016, 123 countries had reported cases meeting the XDR-TB case definition.[8] Among these cases, rates of HIV coinfection varied widely from ~60% in South Africa to fewer than 1% in the United States.

The global distribution and overlap of countries with the highest burden of incident cases and incidence rate/100,000 population

for overall TB and drug-resistant TB and HIV-associated TB are illustrated in Figure 15.3. Forty-eight countries appear in at least one category; there is clear overlap among countries in the three categories, and 14 countries (shown in the central diamond) are high burden in all three categories.

Drug-susceptible and drug-resistant TB and HIV epidemics are a consequence of reactivation of latent TB infection (LTBI), treatment-related amplification of TB resistance mutations, and transmission of both susceptible and resistant TB strains. Each of these is important, adversely influenced by HIV, and their likelihood varies in distribution among different populations related to HIV prevalence and the local force of TB infection and disease as well as the strengths and weaknesses of accompanying social and health systems. As the global distribution of drug-susceptible and drug-resistant TB and HIV varies dramatically and can be characterized as a mosaic of more local epidemics, a combined and integrated comprehensive but site appropriate and flexible approach to both diseases is critically needed.

In addition to the increased risk for transmission-related drug-resistance among PLWH, factors such as malabsorption of anti-TB drugs,[9,10] altered drug metabolism, or drug interactions due to concomitant antiretroviral therapy (ART) may play a role,[11] as may incomplete treatment resulting from unsuccessful medication adherence or system failures (i.e., drug stockouts or poor clinic functioning). Despite these important issues, the accumulating weight of evidence supports the view that the perpetuation and acceleration of drug-resistant TB epidemics is now associated with the transmission of resistant organisms.

Regardless of etiology, mortality among those with advanced MDR-/XDR-TB and untreated HIV is extremely high. Global surveillance data regarding drug-resistant TB outcomes, as well as a retrospective case control study of XDR-TB patients in South Africa,[12] indicates that there are consistently higher death rates among those with both drug-resistant TB and HIV compared to those with drug-resistant TB alone. Furthermore, case control, observational and nested studies of randomized-control trials have demonstrated the great importance of reducing mortality in this population by earlier initiation and administration of ART.[13]

DRUG-RESISTANT TB AND HIV IN THE UNITED STATES

In the United States, a focal MDR-TB epidemic occurred between 1985 and 1992 in several cities. Studies showed that MDR/XDR was being spread in hospitals, jails, prisons, homeless shelters, residential AIDS facilities, and in other congregate settings where PLWH were exposed. A high proportion of MDR-TB cases in New York City and other sites were co-infected with HIV, and transmission was believed to be responsible for most infections. Mortality was exceedingly high, as most cases identified had far advanced TB and HIV disease and effective treatment for HIV had not yet become available.

Rates of drug-resistant TB have fallen steadily since then and remain relatively low in the United States as has the proportion co-infected with HIV. In 2016, MDR-TB drug-susceptibility testing results were reported for 98.3% of culture-confirmed TB cases.[3] Among all 9,256 cases reported, only 97 (1.0%) were MDR-TB, including 78 (80.4%) cases with primary or transmitted

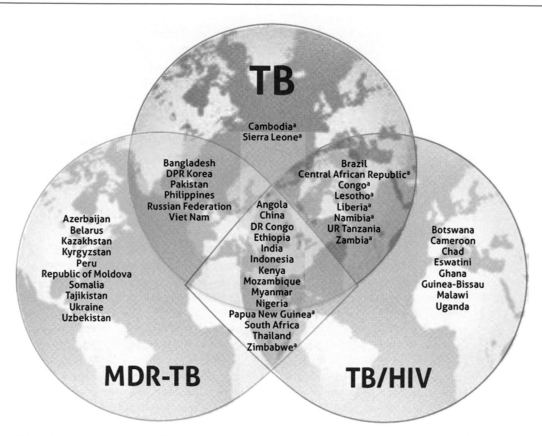

a Indicates countries that are included in the list of 30 high TB burden countries on the basis of the severity of their TB burden (i.e, TB incident cases per 100 000 population per year), as opposed to the top 20, which are included on the basis of their absolute number of incident cases per year.

Figure 15.3 Countries in the three high-burden country lists for TB, TB/HIV, and MDR-TB being used by the WHO during the period 2016–2020, and their areas of overlap.

MDR-TB, 18 (18.6%) with a prior history of TB, and 1 (1.0%) with an unknown history of previous TB diagnosis.[3] Among the 97 MDR-TB cases in 2016, 89 (91.8%) occurred among 6,355 non-US born persons diagnosed with TB, accounting for 1.4% of all TB cases among non-US born persons.[3] Although both MDR- and XDR-TB numbers are rising globally, in the United States, in 2016, only one of the reported cases of MDR-TB in a non-US born person was XDR-TB.[3]

REACTIVATION AND TRANSMISSION OF M. TUBERCULOSIS

REACTIVATION OF LTBI AND THE IMPORTANT ROLE OF HIV

Early studies of PLWH with LTBI clearly demonstrated the power of the interaction between LTBI and HIV.[14] A seminal study performed among people who inject drugs (PWID) in a methadone program in the Bronx, New York City in 1987 defined the consequences of this relationship. The study evaluated the risk of developing active TB among those with LTBI who were living with and without HIV. Prospective follow-up in the two populations revealed a significantly increased risk of developing active TB of 7.9 cases/100 years at-risk in purified protein derivative

(PPD) positive patients who were co-infected with HIV compared to 0 cases/100 years in persons without HIV coinfection (p < 0.002).

This high-annual rate contrasts dramatically with the lifelong risk of TB reactivation of 5%–10% among those with LTBI but without HIV coinfection. The WHO estimates the risk of developing TB to be >20 times higher in PLWH than in people living without HIV.[1,2] Notably, PLWH's annual risk of TB reactivation, equivalent to the lifetime risk of those without HIV far exceeds other co-morbid risks such as diabetes, silicosis, and other immunosuppressive conditions. This increased risk is proportionate to the level of HIV-induced immunosuppression but occurs at any level of CD4 cell count among co-infected individuals. An estimated quarter of the globe's population is estimated to harbor LTBI.[15] Introduction of HIV by either injection drug use or sex in populations with high-baseline prevalence of LTBI inevitably results in secondary TB rate increases and epidemics.

TB preferentially reactivates in PLWH through several mechanisms. One is reduced T-cell response in LTBI through depletion of anti-TB-specific CD4+ memory cells, and enhancement of CXCR3+CCR6+CCR4− memory cells which play a critical role in the control of TB infection.[16] In animal models, in addition, there is a dysregulation of cytokines in HIV infection which mediates several immune responses by activating Toll-like receptors in response to invasion of bacteria or viruses triggering signaling events leading to downstream transcription of genes involved in antiviral and antibacterial responses.[16,17] HIV has also been shown to disrupt macrophage function leading to increased TB growth and dissemination.[17] HIV-infected macrophages are also associated with reduced TB-induced apoptosis compared with macrophages infected with TB alone.

TRANSMISSION OF BOTH SUSCEPTIBLE AND RESISTANT TB STRAINS AND HIV

Conventional belief prior to HIV was that repeated episodes of drug-susceptible and drug-resistant TB were the result only of disease recrudescence secondary to inadequate or lapses in treatment and/or loss to follow-up.

Furthermore, it was felt that drug-resistant organisms had a diminished capability of transmission. However, in the presence of HIV, primary, repeated, and exogenous superinfection of drug-susceptible and drug-resistant TB can occur, including in community congregate and healthcare sites,[18,19] prisons, and other crowded and poorly ventilated areas.[20]

This is a major and ongoing problem in TB- and HIV-endemic areas where the force of infection is great, and continued exposure to active TB cases is inevitable. In low-TB prevalent settings, reactivation of LTBI is more common, whereas in areas of high-TB prevalence, particularly among high-HIV-coinfection populations, although reactivation risk is high, transmission of both drug-susceptible and drug-resistant TB plays a larger role in epidemic propagation.[7]

THE WHO END TB STRATEGY AND NEED FOR SIMULTANEOUSLY ADDRESSING TB AND HIV

In 2012, although not fully recognized in the first decades of the HIV epidemic as central to ending TB, the WHO developed recommendations for TB and HIV collaboration. The importance of Intensified case finding, Initiating TB preventive therapy and ART, and Infection control in healthcare facilities and congregate settings (the "3 I s") was recognized, as well as strategies to reduce the burden of HIV in patients with presumptive and diagnosed TB by HIV testing and counseling, HIV-prevention interventions, co-trimoxazole preventive therapy for PLWH, TB treatment, care for TB in PLWH, and rapid initiation of ART for TB patients living with HIV (Table 15.1).

In 2014, the significance of collaboratively addressing both HIV and TB were incorporated as a central component of the first of the three pillars of the WHO End TB Strategy. Addressing HIV in the context of TB elimination is now firmly established within the End TB strategy affirming the importance of collaborative TB and HIV activities with joint management of these comorbidities.[1] The End TB Strategy was unanimously endorsed in the World Health Assembly by all Member States in 2014 and was embarked upon in 2016 to extend through 2035. The overarching goal of the strategy is to end the global epidemic by achieving specific milestones and targets. The strategy aims to end the global TB epidemic, with targets to reduce TB deaths by 95%, to cut new

cases by 90% between 2015 and 2035, to ensure that no family is burdened with catastrophic expenses due to TB, and to set interim milestones for 2020, 2025, and 2030 (https://www.who.int/tb/post2015_strategy/en/). Historically, this represents the first time governments have set a goal to end TB.

More specifically and broadly, the United Nations (UN) 2016 Political Declaration to Fight Against TB advocates for coordination and collaboration between TB and HIV programs, as well as with other health programs and sectors, to ensure universal access to integrated prevention, diagnosis, treatment, and care services, in accordance with national legislation. This includes testing for HIV among people with TB, screening all PLWH and AIDS regularly for TB, and providing TB preventive treatment (TPT), as well as eliminating the financial burden faced by affected people and addressing the common social, economic, and structural determinants of TB and HIV and the complex biological factors that increase TB incidence and mortality, worsen treatment outcomes, and increase drug resistance.

In September 2018, the United Nations General Assembly held its first-ever high-level meeting on TB to accelerate efforts of ending this global epidemic of TB and reaching all affected people, including those with HIV coinfection, with prevention and care.[21] It acknowledged that current efforts had fallen short, but

Table 15.1 WHO-recommended collaborative TB/HIV activities, 2012

Establish and strengthen the mechanisms for delivering integrated TB and HIV services
1. Set up and strengthen a coordinating body for collaborative TB/HIV activities functional at all levels
2. Determine HIV prevalence among TB patients and TB prevalence among PLWH
3. Carry out joint TB/HIV planning to integrate the delivery of TB and HIV services
4. Monitor and evaluate collaborative TB/HIV activities

Reduce the burden of TB in PLWH and initiate early ART "(the Three I's for HIV/TB)"
1. Intensify TB case-finding and ensure high quality anti-TB treatment
2. Initiate TB prevention with INH preventive therapy and early ART
3. Insure airborne infection control of TB Infection in health care facilities and congregate settings

Reduce the burden of HIV in patients with presumptive and diagnosed TB
1. Provide HIV testing and counseling to patients with presumptive and diagnosed TB
2. Provide HIV prevention interventions for patients with presumptive and diagnosed TB
3. Provide co-trimoxazole preventive therapy for TB patients living with HIV
4. Ensure HIV prevention interventions, treatment, and care for TB patients living with HIV
5. Provide ART for TB patients living with HIV

Source: Taken from WHO policy on collaborative TB/HIV activities: guidelines for national programs and other stakeholders, 2012.

continued toward an ultimate goal of eliminating TB. The specific indicators were affirmed with specific reference to HIV; indicators included documentation of HIV status among 100% of patients with TB, provision of ART to 90% of those, and TPT to 90% of those eligible.

The estimated TB decline since 2010 in several high-burden TB and HIV countries has been over 5%: Zimbabwe—11%, Lesotho—7%, Kenya—6.9%, Ethiopia—6.9%, Tanzania—6.7%, and Namibia—6.0%. Although gratifying in itself, it is important to note that this is largely due to the parallel and more dramatic increased yearly decline in the incidence of HIV, a function of availability of use of ART and concerted public health efforts aimed at both diseases.[1] The WHO estimates that from 2000 to 2017, the high mortality among those with TB and HIV coinfection has decreased globally by 44%.[1] This decline in mortality attributed to TB and HIV has been steady over the past decade (but greater for HIV) (see Figure 15.4) with ART provided to PLWH as the attributed mitigatory factor. As a result, TB has now surpassed HIV as the most frequent cause of death from an infectious disease globally.

An estimated 6.6 million lives among PLWH had been saved through scale-up of TB- and HIV-collaborative activities since 2005.[2] This is largely attributed to the success of ART initiation and implementation of available HIV/TB integration strategies in high-TB burden countries in Asia and Africa.

Great strides have been made between 2010 and 2018 in improving ART coverage among PLWH and linking new co-infected cases to both HIV and TB care, leading to the decline in HIV and TB mortality.[1] Nevertheless, despite the global scale-up of ART, and expanding TB services, the WHO estimates that nearly half of people with HIV-associated TB still fail to receive TB care, and less than one-third of new enrollees in HIV care

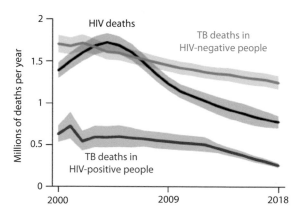

^a For HIV/AIDS, the latest estimates of the number of deaths in 2018 that have been published by UNAIDS are available at http://www.unaids.org/en/ resources/publications/all (accessed 16 August 2019). For TB, the estimates for 2018 are those published in this report.

^b Deaths from TB among HIV-positive people are officially classified as deaths caused by HIV/AIDS in the International Classification of Diseases.

Figure 15.4 Global trends in the estimated number of deaths caused by TB and HIV (in millions), 2000–2018.[a,b] Shaded areas represent uncertainty intervals.

initiated TPT in the subset of countries that reported in 2017. In addition, although ART coverage among PLWH who were *diagnosed* with TB is high, only 41% of PLWH who were *estimated* to actually have TB were receiving ART. These numbers are even lower for children and adolescents. The trajectory of decline established by the WHO for the End of TB by 2035 requires an estimated 17% decline in TB annually. The aforementioned successes still fall far below that aspirational goal. Great challenges remain at all levels to implement and expand the coverage and quality of current collaborative TB and HIV services and to continue to develop new tools and strategies to achieve the WHO End TB strategy in the coming decades. However, this is not likely to be achieved by medical or public health strategies alone and without concerted and successful attention to the underlying social determinants of both TB and HIV.

THE IMPORTANCE OF SOCIAL DETERMINANTS IN ORIGIN AND SPREAD OF CURRENT HIV/TB EPIDEMICS

Socio-economic circumstances including poverty, overcrowding, and malnutrition[22] remain critically important factors underlying community and individual risk for contracting both TB and HIV infection and for poorer outcomes in each. The social determinants that contribute to both TB and HIV risk and poor outcomes are linked both directly and indirectly to social and economic vulnerabilities and human rights abuses and inequities. In low- and middle-income countries and those with concentrated HIV epidemics (>5% of population infected) and in key populations globally, including PWID, and incarcerated and homeless populations, the HIV epidemic has dramatically fueled the increases in TB rates.[20,23] In all of these scenarios, political, financial, and health policies often underlie and have favored the development and perpetuation of the conditions of inequity upon which these two diseases thrive.

It is instructive to characterize the global synergistic HIV/TB socio-economic and structural determinants as the soil into which the two infectious agents have been implanted and then grown to epidemic proportions. We describe three such illustrative and diverse populations, separated by decades and thousands of miles distant from one other: in the Bronx borough of New York City in the 1980s, in young women and men in South Africa in the early 1990s, and in current incarcerated populations in the countries of the former Soviet Union.

First, the HIV/AIDS epidemics in New York City in the 1980s occurred principally in PWID and men who have sex with men (MSM).[24] The dramatic rise in TB was concentrated in the population of PWID and in geographic areas of the city with documented high rates of poverty and homelessness.[23,25–27] These areas, exemplified by the borough of the Bronx, the poorest urban county in the country, had been subjected to planned public social policies of "benign neglect" or "shrinkage" resulting in deliberate economically motivated arson and destroyed housing, with massive increased crowding and homelessness underlying already high rates of LTBI and active TB.[27,28] The intentional policy process also included simultaneous removal of essential safety and health services, including TB services, all setting the stage for the arrival and implantation of HIV and an explosive epidemic of HIV/AIDS and the resurgence of TB and a secondary epidemic of MDR-TB, both with high rates of HIV coinfection. This epidemic scenario was further spread and exacerbated by the initial delayed and incomplete response and the accompanying rise of drug-resistant TB, with rates of TB rising in some areas to >200/100,000.[29] During this period, an estimated 20,000 unanticipated cases of TB were reported in New York.[30]

Second, although geographically distant, separated in time by two decades, and affecting different populations, the intertwined TB and HIV epidemics in South Africa have features that are eerily similar to the TB and HIV epidemics in New York City among PWID. In the case of South Africa, the long history of colonialism, racism, and racial separation, institutionalized in the planned national dehumanizing social and economic policy of Apartheid, resulting destruction of traditional societies, a migrant labor system to provide labor for mines and plantations, the creation of rural African homelands, and removal of urban African populations to rural and urban townships, all resulted in both rural and urban severe poverty and crowding. This occurred in the context of already high-background rates of both latent and active TB and the presence of a weak and poorly functioning TB clinical and public health system.[31,32] Once HIV entered the general population in the 1990s, as documented among young women in public pre-natal clinics, there was an explosive rise in HIV rates from <5% to >30% within 10 years with an associated dramatic increase in TB incidence rates from 200/100,000 to close to 1,000/100,000 in a similar time frame,[33] also accompanied by a

subsequent explosion of MDR-/XDR-TB.[6] The delayed response to these convergent epidemics has likely contributed greatly to their spread and severity (Figure 15.5).[34]

Third, in countries of the former Soviet Union, epidemics of TB and MDR- and XDR-TB, associated with substantial increasing rates of HIV coinfection, are occurring in a pattern again reminiscent of the early HIV/TB epidemic in New York City in the 1980s and early 1990s and the epidemics in South Africa. The spread of HIV and drug-susceptible and drug-resistant TB in the Russian Federation and Eastern Europe has been accelerated by the decline and breakup of the Soviet Union and health service infrastructures. This social and political dislocation severely affected socioeconomic factors which in turn increased unemployment, injection drug use, migration, and incarceration. In prisons where HIV and TB transmission risk are highest, the proportion of prisoners who are affected by drug-resistant TB and HIV coinfection was found to be 24 times higher than the general population.[35]

THE IMPORTANCE OF STIGMA

These socioeconomic similarities are further exacerbated by the social stigma associated with the described social and political soil or root causes of the epidemic as well as the diseases themselves which have flourished in their presence. This accompanying challenge has complicated the lives of PLWH and TB and has complicated the fight against both epidemics, as observed in these specific examples and globally. Stigma is defined as the "social process of devaluing a person or group based on a real or perceived difference."[32,36] The social determinants underlying both HIV and TB, poverty, homelessness, racial, gender, and minority status,

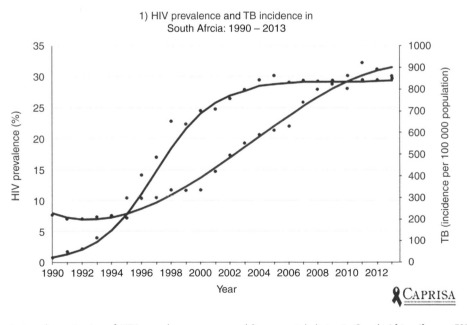

Figure 15.5 Demonstrates dramatic rise of HIV prevalence among public neonatal clinics in South Africa (from <5% in 1990 to 30% by 2002, accompanied by dramatic rise in TB case notifications, rising from 200/100,000 in 1990 to >900/1,000 by 2012. The figure is provided by Professor Salim Abdool Karim, CAPRISA, Durban South Africa Source: Annual point estimates from the South African Department of Health; http://www.tbfacts.org/tb-statistics-south-africa/ and http://data.worldbank.org/indicator/SH.TBS.INCD. (The lines are based on fitted mathematical models developed by E. Gouws [HIV] and A. Grobler [TB]).

and disapproved personal behaviors are themselves stigmatized resulting in people co-infected with HIV and TB experiencing an additional superimposed "double stigma."[37] Stigma regarding both diseases and those suffering from them is present in all aspects of society and continues to be problematic even within healthcare facilities. Such stigma is powerful and pervasive and, in addition to the aforementioned socioeconomic epidemic roots, can negatively impact prevention and care-seeking behaviors and the delivery of health care within the current infrastructures, thereby adversely influencing outcomes and further propagating both HIV and TB transmission.

Remedies are complex and difficult and require "people-first" cultural and systemic solutions. A direct and sensitive approach to clinical and public health humane language can help reduce stigma. A key paradigm shift in the Global Plan to End TB and within the HIV global strategy is "changing the mindset, language, and dialogue on TB and HIV to reduce stigma and to put people with each or both diseases at the center of the global response."[1] This should start with acknowledging that the language commonly used to speak about TB can influence stigma, beliefs, and behaviors, and may determine if a person feels comfortable with getting tested or treated. Just as the HIV/AIDS community would avoid using terms such as "AIDS control" or "AIDS case," preferring, "person living with HIV (PLWH)," the TB community should shift to more empowering, people-centered language to avoid the use of judgmental terms such as "TB suspect" and "TB defaulter" which place blame on the patient for the disease and frequent adverse treatment outcomes, which, in reality, often are attributable to structural and programmatic and not personal deficiencies.[38,39]

CLINICAL FEATURES OF PULMONARY AND EXTRAPULMONARY TB IN PLWH

Despite the favorable epidemiological trends noted earlier, TB with and apart from HIV remains an important global opportunistic illness in all nations. Unlike most HIV-related opportunistic infections, TB is readily transmissible from person to person, particularly to other persons with HIV infection and to those working in healthcare settings. Therefore, all clinicians and particularly those providing care for persons with HIV must remain vigilant in efforts to prevent and diagnose TB, knowledgeable about the clinical presentation and diagnostic challenges of HIV-related TB, and aware of and familiar with the complexities of the co-treatment of HIV and TB.

The symptoms of pulmonary TB are similar in PLWH- and HIV-uninfected persons. These include cough, fever, weight loss, and night sweats. The presence of any one of these four cardinal symptoms should prompt further diagnostic assessment, and consideration of TB. The WHO supports a simple "rule-out" screening algorithm in resource-limited settings whereby the absence of all four of these symptoms portends a low probability of TB in PLWH.[40] A 2010 Vietnamese study evaluating a screening algorithm for TB found that the presence of cough, fever, or night sweats lasting 3 or more weeks in the preceding 4 weeks was 93% sensitive and 36% specific for TB in PLWH.[41] A meta-analysis

found that this rule reliably excluded active TB in 90% to 98% of patients depending on whether the background prevalence of TB was 20% or 5%, respectively. It should be noted that this has limited generalizability to children and adults with extrapulmonary TB (i.e., lymph nodes, bones, liver, kidneys, brain, and blood, all more common in PLWH and advanced immunosuppression), and its efficacy is likely to be more limited in very high-prevalence TB settings where subclinical TB rates are high and the duration of HIV/AIDS-associated symptomatic TB appears to be shorter than the duration of HIV-negative TB with more rapid progression from minimal symptoms to far advanced disease.

LTBI is defined as a state of low level infection by *M. tuberculosis* with a persistent immune response to stimulation by *M. tuberculosis* antigens but without evidence of clinically manifest active disease. Although thought of as part of a binary classification of inactive and active disease, contemporary information supports the view of a dynamic and bidirectional relationship. Latent infection dogma established chronic lung granulomas as the only site where mycobacteria are located, but recent evidence indicates that *M. tuberculosis* can persist intracellularly in pulmonary and extrapulmonary tissues without histological evidence of tuberculous lesions, which have important implications for strategies aimed at the elimination of latent and persistent bacilli. *M. tuberculosis* is located in macrophages and also in other non-phagocytic cells, providing a mechanism of immune evasion.

The estimated 1/4–1/3 of the world's population or approximately 1.7 billion people who harbor LTBI[15] are the major source of future infections and disease. LTBI has a significant impact on the epidemiology and population dynamics of active TB among PLWH, because of significantly higher rates of disease reactivation compared to non-HIV infected populations, and more rapid progression to active disease and represents a huge reservoir of potential disease and ongoing transmission.

Subclinical TB is an important entity characterized by microbiologic and/or radiographic evidence of pulmonary TB in PLWH in the absence of symptoms.[42,43] One study from Durban, South Africa, found that up to 22% of PLWH screened with sputum cultures prior to starting ART had subclinical TB.[44] Clinicians should maintain a high index of suspicion for TB when initiating ART, particularly in high-burden TB settings and in patients with low CD4 cell counts.

RADIOGRAPHIC FEATURES

In PLWH, TB radiologic features vary widely with the degree of immunosuppression. At higher CD4 counts, the pattern tends to mirror both initial and reactivation disease in people without HIV disease with upper lobe infiltrates with or without cavities and associated hilar adenopathy.[45] As the CD4 count decreases, there is less cavitation, a reflection of impaired cell mediated immunity and impaired ability to form necrotic granulomas.[46] In severely immunosuppressed patients (CD4 <200), non-cavitary infiltration and consolidation dominate with either diffuse or middle and lower zone lobe involvement or a hematogenous (miliary) pattern rather than classical upper lobe involvement, again a reflection of impaired immunity.[47] Because cavitation is associated with a greater mycobacterial load and smear positivity, HIV-associated pulmonary TB is more likely to be smear-negative and thus, more difficult to diagnose.[48]

LABORATORY DIAGNOSIS OF TB AND HIV COINFECTION

TB diagnostics for PLWH are similar for persons living without HIV. The sensitivity of TB diagnostics, however, is decreased in PLWH, largely due to paucibacillary disease—most prominently observed as a low burden of *Mycobacterium* bacilli in sputum. Extrapulmonary TB is more frequent in PLWH as is accompanying paucibacillary disease at these sites. In addition, classical TB granulomas, with caseation and multinucleated giant cells are observed less frequently, particularly in advanced HIV disease with severe immunosuppression.

TUBERCULIN SKIN TESTING

Tuberculin skin testing (TST) is still utilized to determine the presence of LTBI and eligibility for isoniazid prevention therapy (IPT) in PLWH. Given that there is a known loss of tuberculin skin test reactivity in PLWH which worsens as CD4 cell count falls, an induration of 5 mm is considered positive. In PLWH, sensitivity is estimated to be between 64% and 71% in those with smear-positive sputum.[49] The loss of sensitivity is secondary to anergy, defined as the absence of delayed type hypersensitivity in sensitized individuals and characterized by a TST reaction <2 mm.

INTERFERON GAMMA RELEASE ASSAY

A variety of interferon gamma release assays (IGRAs) are currently available. A recent meta-analysis suggested that IGRAs perform similarly to TST in PLWH[50] and vary similarly in sensitivity and specificity related to the degree of immunosuppression. There are limited data on the use of IGRA in children under 5 years old and persons recently exposed to TB. Although sensitivity is equivalent to TSTs, IGRAS are preferred in persons who received Bacillus Calmette–Guérin (BCG) because they do not cross react with BCG and in persons who may not be able to return for a TST reading.

SMEAR MICROSCOPY AND CULTURE

Smear microscopy has poor sensitivity in PLWH, ranging from 43% to 51%,[51] a consequence of paucibacillary disease. Sensitivity can be improved up to two-fold by fluorescence microscopy in PLWH compared with conventional microscopy.[52,53] Specificity remains similar in both fluorescence and conventional microscopy in PLWH. Additionally, bleach and concentrating sputum by centrifugation can further increase sensitivity by up to 11%.[54,55] Although still widely used globally, smear microscopy should be replaced by rapid and more sensitive molecular platforms such as Xpert MTB/RIF as the initial diagnostic test in adults and children suspected of having HIV-associated TB or MDR-TB.

GENE XPERT MTB/RIF

The advent of Gene Xpert MTB/RIF developed by Cepheid (Sunnyvale, California, United States) has greatly improved diagnostic abilities in PLWH.[56] Endorsed by the WHO, it provides detection of both *M. tuberculosis* and RIF resistance simultaneously within a 2-hour window. In the 2010 seminal multi-center prospective study in which Gene Xpert MTB/RIF was compared to smear microscopy, 40% of patients were PLWH, and among these, sensitivity was 93.9% (vs. 98.4% in persons without HIV).[57]

In a 2014 meta-analysis of 27 studies in low and middle-income countries, in PLWH, TB detection pooled sensitivity was 79% compared with 86% in people without HIV infection. Among those co-infected with TB/HIV, patients with smear-positive disease were more likely to be diagnosed with the use of Xpert MTB/RIF—97% sensitivity for smear positive, culture positive disease than those with smear-negative disease—61% sensitivity for smear negative, culture positive TB. Similarly when either Xpert MTB/RIF or point-of care light-emitting diode fluorescence microscopy (LED FM) in symptomatic patients were compared, TB was more likely to be detected in patients by Xpert MTB/RF (2.4%) than by LED FM (1.2%).[58]

GENE XPERT MTB/RIF ULTRA

This assay was also developed by Cepheid as the next generation assay in rapid molecular testing and recommended to replace XpertTB/RIF because of increased sensitivity. Sensitivity is improved by the addition of two targets, IS6110 and IS1081, and a larger reaction chamber. Real-time polymerase chain reaction gives way to four probes that identify RIF resistance on the *rpoB* gene using temperature. A multicenter prospective study in low- and middle-income countries in 2016 enrolled patients to compare the efficacy of Xpert Ultra with Xpert.[59] For PLWH, TB detection sensitivity was 90% with Ultra versus 77% with Xpert; compared with 91% and 90%, respectively, in people without HIV infection. Additionally, Ultra has a higher sensitivity in smear-negative, culture positive specimens, and in specimens from PLWH.[60] Modeling of Ultra use in high-burden TB/HIV co-infected areas suggests that there will be a significant beneficial clinical impact on mortality in PLWH.[61]

GENE XPERT OMNI

In 2015, Cepheid announced Gene Xpert Omni, the first "close-to-care" point-of-care (POC) molecular assay for TB, HIV, and Ebola. The Omni is expected to complement existing multimodule GeneXpert instruments, including the GeneXpert Edge® (a single-module GeneXpert instrument connected to a tablet device for transfer of data with an auxiliary battery that allows operation in more decentralized settings at the same level as microscopy in primary care clinics or even community-based settings). Both the Omni and the Edge have been developed to facilitate wider access to rapid molecular testing for TB and rifampicin resistance, and virology parameters for HIV and hepatitis C virus.

A new cartridge built on this platform is able to detect additional mutations that confer resistance to fluoroquinolones, aminoglycosides, and INH. In this cartridge, there are probes to detect approximately 25 mutations in six genes and promoter regions. A prospective study using this cartridge was recently conducted in China and South Korea among adults with symptoms of TB.[62] Although the high sensitivity and specificity is promising, there are no data yet on its performance in PLWH. It is anticipated that there may be sufficient data by 2020 to allow evaluation by the WHO (https://www.who.int/tb/publications/global_report/en/2019).

XPERT PRACTICAL LIMITATIONS

Although a great diagnostic advance, Xpert use is limited by several factors. In low- and middle-income countries, empiric TB treatment based on clinical symptoms is often instituted prior to result availability. Although the test performance only takes 2 hours, it is not a true POC test and communication of results from laboratory to clinical decision-making sites often is substantially delayed. As a consequence, this delay results in treatment decisions often based on clinical judgment alone. Thus, in resource-limited settings with health system weaknesses, early studies indicated that Gene Xpert availability did not impact mortality as large numbers of patient were empirically started on TB therapy while awaiting Xpert results. Newer portable versions, allowing onsite use at clinical sites are now available that can provide close to POC results. Limited Xpert capacity in high-prevalence clinical or screening programs still limits universal utility. With current versions, in areas with substantial rates of MDR-/XDR-TB, treatment institution delay may also occur as performance of additional resistance testing is critical. Despite these limitations, the development and implementation of Xpert has become an extremely valuable tool in settings where systems infrastructure enables timely accurate and effective decision-making regarding treatment initiation for drug-susceptible and MDR-TB.

LINE PROBE ASSAYS

The GenoType MTBDRplus (MTBDR-Plus; Hain Lifesciences GmBH, Nehren, Germany) identifies INH and RIF resistant by mutations in the *rpoB*, *katG*, and *inhA* genes. A multicenter study across seven sites in South America and Southern Africa, exclusively in PLWH, showed detection of 92% of RIF resistance and 71% of INH resistance. In smear-positive specimens, sensitivity was 97%, and in smear-negative specimens, sensitivity was reduced to 75%.[63] However, this test requires sophisticated laboratory treatment and expertise and is not easy to implement in programmatic settings.

LIPOARABINOMANNAN

The TB-urine lipoarabinomannan (LAM) dip stick test has shown particular utility in patients with advanced AIDS with disseminated TB in resource-poor inpatient settings and where patients are unable to produce sputum. As a true POC test, it is especially useful where conventional diagnostics are not readily available or delayed and therapeutic decisions in severely ill patients must be made. This is also of substantial importance with regard to infection control practices and ward isolation. In PLWH, LAM has modest sensitivity (67%) and high specificity (98%) among those with advanced AIDS. Its utility has recently been demonstrated

Table 15.2 Results compared to culture

Diagnostic test	Sensitivity (%)		Specificity (%)
	Smear +	Smear −	
Smear microscopy	51	43	99
Gene Xpert	77	61	98
Gene Xpert Ultra	90	63	96
LAM[a]		67[a]	99
Line Probe Assay	94–97	44–90	100

[a] Urine.

in a large-scale randomized trial of LAM use versus conventional TB diagnostics, including Xpert/TBRIF in hospitalized PLWH in Malawi. Although all-cause mortality did not differ among those with and without LAM use, mortality was significantly lower in the LAM use intervention group than that in the standard-of-care group for those with CD4 counts <100 cells per μL ($p = 0.036$), those with severe anemia (hemoglobin <8 g/dL $p = 0.021$), and those with clinically suspected TB.[64]

LAM testing to diagnose TB among hospitalized or severely immunosuppressed ambulatory PLWH is feasible and accepted. It is a true rapid POC test that requires minimal training and can lead to more widespread implementation. The WHO has now expanded its recommendations for use. In May 2019, the WHO commissioned a systematic review of the use of a lateral flow LAM assay (LF-LAM) (Alere) for the diagnosis of TB in PLWH and convened a Guideline Development Group (GDG) to update the WHO guidance issued in 2015. The key change in the 2015 guidelines is a strengthened indication for the use of LF-LAM among hospitalized HIV-positive patients with signs and symptoms of TB (pulmonary and extrapulmonary); the test is now recommended for all such patients, irrespective of their CD4 count. If the CD4 count is below 100, LF-LAM is recommended even in the absence of TB symptoms. Updated WHO recommended guidelines are in progress (Table 15.2).[65]

Development and deployment of rapid diagnostic tests are essential for achieving earlier identification of active TB disease, institution of therapy, and reduction of morbidity and mortality, particularly among PLWH. All HIV Testing Services in health facilities and community-based settings should integrate screening for TB symptoms into the HIV testing algorithm and correspondingly, TB screening should be accompanied by integrated HIV screening and rapid testing.

INTEGRATED MANAGEMENT OF TB AND HIV INFECTION AND DISEASE

HIV/TB PREVENTION AND TREATMENT INTEGRATION

"Two diseases, one patient, two epidemics, one population"

Although synergistic and co-morbid disastrous epidemics, TB and HIV have been historically and largely approached and managed separately. The logic of integration of treatment is compelling, although it has required overcoming many logistical, structural, and programmatic barriers. A major impediment to the integration of prevention and treatment of the two diseases has also been the divergent cultures associated with the approach and management of each (Figure 15.6).

TB is an ancient disease, present for centuries and stitched into the fabric of history, and has developed, promoted, and implemented a successful global public health "one-size-fits-all" programmatic approach, with program standardized procedures and outcomes. This has achieved great success, with millions of lives restored and saved. However in past decades, the rate of global decline of TB has slowed, drug-resistant TB has emerged and grown, and HIV has added new dramatic growth, complexities, and urgency requiring reassessment and redefinition of the approach to TB prevention and management. Conversely, HIV is historically a new epidemic disease that rapidly adopted an individual patient-centered approach through activism, with new strategies in prevention and treatment and human rights advocacy at its core.

Both diseases originate in and are the product of challenging sociodemographic environments, creating social, economic, and political instability and are cloaked in stigma and isolation. The culture of response and management differences between the two diseases, however, has been difficult to integrate and surmount, particularly in the landscape of largely separate national TB and HIV programs with varying levels of communication.[66] This was initially characterized by the complete separation of TB and HIV programs, funding streams, and personnel from national to local operational levels. More recently and with much effort these barriers to integration have begun to recede.

As the HIV/AIDS epidemic grew, a wave of activism with a revolutionary patient-centered human rights approach engendered a government, foundation, and industry response with an influx of funding, allowing the creation of new infrastructures and an explosion of new drugs and successful treatment strategies for HIV/AIDS whereas TB remained underfunded, and slow to innovate and change. With the resurgence of TB, now surpassing HIV as one of the leading causes of death globally, as the leading cause of death in PLWH, and with the emergence of drug-resistant TB and growing global advocacy, TB has regained deserved and critical attention on the global scene. Although each have markedly different therapeutic paradigms, programs and infrastructures, the collaboration and integration of HIV and TB prevention, diagnosis, and treatment initiation and monitoring to improve outcomes for both diseases has grown and is now advocated by both TB and HIV global and national organizations and programs.[1,3] The details of implementation of integration remains varied and challenging globally though all would agree that "No one living with HIV should die of TB." and "No one with TB and HIV should be without ART."

Past and many current WHO and national TB control programs have relied heavily on passive case finding and directly observed therapy (DOT) as the centerpiece of treatment delivery and treatment success. This strategy has been highly successful in many areas over time, particularly where resources have been sufficient and consistently available, but is incompletely implemented in many settings, particularly where healthcare systems

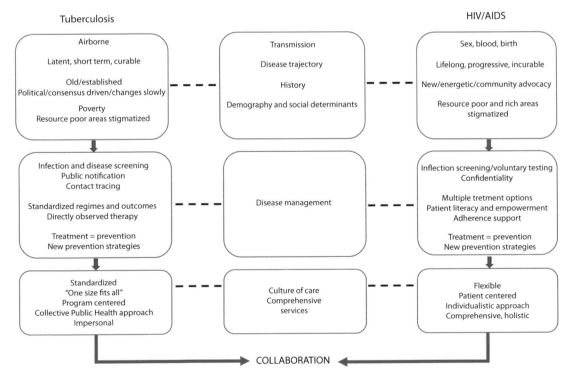

Figure 15.6 Program collaboration amidst the contrasting cultures of TB (left column) and HIV (right column). (Adapted from Daftary A, Calzavara L, Padayatchi N tuberculosis care. AIDS 2015.)

are under-resourced and weak. Medication adherence and care for both drug-susceptible and -resistant TB-HIV could be improved by fully implementing HIV style patient- and community-based education and team-based patient-centered care; empowering patients through education, counseling, and support; maintaining a rights-based approach, whereas acknowledging the responsibility of healthcare systems to provide comprehensive care; and prioritize critical research gaps.

Patient centered, individualistic approach has been a hallmark of HIV care but has not been as strongly articulated as a component of TB care. Driven by activism, HIV programs place enormous emphasis on patient education, confidentiality, and empowerment, and recognize and advocate against stigma and discrimination. In contrast, TB programs have traditionally been more hierarchical, impersonal, and program centered. Patient-centered care respects an individual's right to participate actively as an informed partner in decisions and activities related to TB diagnosis and treatment. The Institute of Medicine defines patient-centered care as "providing care that is respectful of and responsive to individual patient preferences, needs, and values, and ensuring that patient values guide all clinical decisions." Given that TB treatment requires that multiple drugs be given for many months, it is crucial that the patient be involved in a meaningful way in making decisions concerning treatment supervision and overall care. International standards have recently been developed that also support using patient-centered approaches to the management of TB. The culture of TB and global and local leadership has recently added its strength and success by incorporating and advocating for an HIV/AIDS characteristic people first, human rights- and evidence-based approaches to overcome barriers to universal access to TB diagnosis, prevention, treatment, care, and support services.[67] The WHO has now highlighted "patient-centered care and prevention for all people with TB" as the first of the three central pillars of its End TB strategy[68] with collaborative TB/HIV activities and management as one of the crucial components. The global population with and at-risk for both TB and HIV will benefit further from both cultural and programmatic collaboration and, indeed, evidence-based integration of the management of both diseases.

STUDIES SUPPORTING TB/HIV TREATMENT INTEGRATION STRATEGY

TB AND HIV TREATMENT INTEGRATION—EARLY STUDIES

In high-prevalence HIV and TB areas, ART, even if available, was routinely withheld until after completion of TB treatment because of concerns regarding drug–drug interactions, additive toxicity, increased pill burden, adherence challenges, and the immune reconstitution inflammatory syndrome (IRIS).

Starting in 2001, pilot studies of integration of people with smear-positive TB and HIV coinfection were carried out within an urban and public health TB clinics and rural sites in KwaZulu Natal, South Africa and elsewhere. These studies were initially designed to assess the acceptability, feasibility, and effectiveness of integrating HIV/TB care and therapy.[69,70] Patients found to have pulmonary TB and HIV coinfection were placed on standard anti-TB therapy and ART regardless of CD4 count. A once daily ART regimen (efavirenz, didanosine, and emtricitabine [EFV, DDI, and 3TC, respectively]), was chosen to coincide with daily TB dosage and simplify medication adherence. Both studies employed patient treatment literacy and home-based DOT using family, community, and patient treatment supporters. Both DOT and self-administered therapy (SAT) with social support strategies were employed. Medication adherence was excellent and drug adverse toxicity minimal. HIV and TB outcomes were excellent in both mentioned studies and in the presence of effective and supportive treatment, stigma was minimal. Since then, multiple larger studies, including several randomized-controlled trials (RCTs) have examined the relationship between initiation of ART during TB therapy and clinical outcomes, including mortality. Integration of TB and HIV treatment has been convincingly and consistently shown to reduce mortality and improve outcomes of both diseases.[71–74]

RANDOMIZED-CONTROL STUDIES ON WHEN TO INTEGRATE TB AND HIV TREATMENT

The Starting Antiretroviral Therapy at Three Points in Tuberculosis (SAPiT) study was an urban TB clinic RCT in Durban, South Africa which compared the initiation of ART during TB therapy to sequential initiation after completion of standard TB therapy on morbidity and mortality.[71,72] In the SAPiT study, patients with CD4 cell counts <500 cells/mm^3 were randomized to one of three arms—the early integrated arm which initiated ART within 4 weeks of starting TB therapy, the late integration arm which initiated ART within 4 weeks of completing intensive TB treatment, or the sequential treatment arm which initiated ART only after completion of TB treatment. The sequential treatment arm was stopped early because a highly significant (56%) reduction in mortality was found in the integrated arms. The results provided strong evidence to support integration of TB and HIV treatment. SAPiT II consisted of a secondary analysis of the patients in the early integrated therapy group and the late integrated therapy group.[72] The study results supported early initiation in patients with CD4 counts <50 cells/mm^3 given that it increased AIDS-free survival by 68%. It further recommended deferral of treatment in patients with CD4 counts >50 cells/mm^3 but within 8-weeks of TB treatment ART initiation because this reduced the risk of IRIS and adverse events related to ART without increasing mortality.

The Cambodian Early versus Late Introduction of Antiretrovirals (CAMELIA) study in HIV/TB co-infected patients randomized patients to receive ART at either 2 or 8 weeks after starting TB treatment.[73] The results indicated that initiating ART within 2 weeks after starting TB treatment in PLWH with CD4 counts of 200 cells/mm^3 or lower significantly improved survival.

The AIDS Clinical Trials Group Study (ACTG) A5221 STRIDE was a multi-national RCT which evaluated initiation of ART in TB and HIV co-infected patients within 2 weeks versus between 8 and 12 weeks in PLWH with CD4 counts <250 cells/mm^3 and without a previously diagnosed AIDS-defining illness.[74] In the subgroup of patients with CD4 cell counts of <50 cells/mm^3 in whom ART was initiated early, there was significantly greater survival and less progression to AIDS defining illness compared to the group with delayed ART initiation group.

Based on the data acquired from these trials and accumulated clinical studies, the following recommendations can be strongly made regarding the integration and timing of HIV treatment initiation in patients with TB and HIV:

- All PLWH with active TB who are ART-naïve should start ART during treatment for TB in an integrated manner.
- The timing of initiation of ART is influenced by the severity of immune deficiency and severity of both HIV and TB disease.
- If the CD4 count is <50 cells/mm³, ART should be started within 2 weeks after TB treatment initiation.
- If the CD4 count is >CD4 counts >50 cells/mm³, ART should be initiated within 8 weeks of starting TB therapy.
- Although these numerical measures of severity of HIV disease are strongly evidence based, have become generally and widely accepted, and have simplified treatment initiation timing and treatment integration, there is still opportunity for special considerations in individual patients.
  - Many clinicians and experts appreciate that in individual cases, the timing of initiation of ART should be further influenced, beyond the CD4 cell count, by issues of clinical severity of both HIV and TB disease including severe anemia, malnutrition, evidence of organ system failure, and extent of pulmonary or extrapulmonary disease, all of which are independently associated with early mortality[12,75] (https://aidsinfo.nih.gov/guidelines/html/1/adult-and-adolescent-arv/27/tb-hiv).
  - Even if the CD4 cell count is >50 cells/mm³, if these clinical indicators of disease severity are present, they argue for ART initiation closer to or within 2 weeks, as well as aggressive correction of metabolic and hematologic derangements.
  - An important additional exception is HIV-infected patients with TB meningitis, in whom timing of initiation of ART has been controversial and delayed because of dangers of IRIS in the central nervous system. Expert opinion now favors initiating ART within 2–8 weeks of starting anti-TB treatment (within 2 weeks in individuals with CD4 counts <50 cells/mm³, with careful monitoring for central nervous system adverse events, and within 8 weeks for those with CD4 counts >50 cells/mm³) (https://aidsinfo.nih.gov/guidelines/html/1/adult-and-adolescent-arv/27/tb-hiv).
- All pregnant women with HIV and active TB should be started on ART as early as feasible, both for treatment of the person with HIV and to prevent HIV transmission to the infant. The choice of ART should be based on efficacy and safety in pregnancy and should take into account potential drug–drug interactions between ARTs and rifamycins.
- Comprehensively, these observational and randomized-controlled studies represent a body of knowledge that has substantially informed our current treatment strategies and decisions regarding treatment initiation and the integration

and timing of ART therapy to reduce both HIV and TB morbidity and mortality. They have been important in changing and improving the management and outcomes of PLWH with clinically and microbiologically diagnosed TB.

Special issues regarding HIV and TB integration challenges including IRIS, drug–drug interactions, and shared toxicities are discussed in the section "Integrated treatment of TB in PLWH."

Treatment regimens for drug-susceptible and drug-resistant TB and HIV should be harmonized and integrated, depending upon the clinical setting and overall experience with both TB and HIV, in TB-specific healthcare management settings in conjunction with an HIV expert as it is essential to ensure proper ART selection, medication adherence, toxicity monitoring, and monitoring and documentation of HIV treatment outcome success (see section "Utilizing the cascade and continuum of care").

INTEGRATED TREATMENT OF TB IN PLWH

DRUG-SUSCEPTIBLE TB

The treatment of active TB disease in patients with HIV should follow the general principles guiding treatment for individuals without HIV.[76] The standard regimen for the treatment of TB in people with and without HIV caused by organisms that are not known or suspected to be drug-resistant is a regimen consisting of an intensive phase of 2 months of INH, RIF, pyrazinamide (PZA), and ethambutol (EMB) followed by a continuation phase of 4 months of INH and RIF. EMB may be stopped if the organism is found to be pansensitive. This regimen has been preferred and unchanged for over 35 years.

TB treatment has relied on multidrug chemotherapy to achieve three objectives:

1. Rapidly reduce bacterial burden to decrease disease morbidity, mortality, and transmission;
2. Eradicate persistent populations to prevent relapse; and
3. Prevent acquisition of drug resistance.

Both HIV and treatment of TB rely on a synergistic combination of drugs administered for sufficient time and proper dose to result in treatment success. For TB, this goal is cure whereas for HIV, at this point, the goal is lifelong HIV replication suppression and immune reconstitution. Important issues that differentiate TB treatment in PLWH are potential and actual and include IRIS, treatment duration and schedules, medication adherence strategies, pharmacological and pharmacodynamic drug–drug interactions between HIV and TB medications, and overlapping drug side effects and toxicities.

Early ART initiation requires, at the very least, close collaboration between HIV and TB clinicians and clinics with expertise in management of ART regimen selection and close monitoring of treatment success and challenges. This is most confidently done in a setting of site integration of the care of PLWH and TB.

In addition to TB- and HIV-specific medications in PLWH, pyridoxine (vitamin B6) is recommended to be given with INH to all PLWH. Co-trimoxazole (trimethoprim–sulfamethoxazole) prophylaxis has been shown to reduce morbidity and mortality in PLWH with newly diagnosed TB from bacterial infections, malaria, and toxoplasmosis and is recommended by the WHO for all PLWH with active TB disease regardless of the CD4 cell count. In high-income countries, co-trimoxazole is primarily used in HIV-infected patients with CD4 counts <200 cells/μL.

Intermittent dosing (administration less frequent than daily) of TB treatment that included twice- or thrice-weekly dosing during the intensive or continuation phase have been associated with an increased risk of treatment failure or relapse with acquired drug resistance to rifamycins particularly among PLWH. Incomplete absorption of medication among PLWH is well documented and requires daily therapy through the entire course of treatment. Therefore, daily therapy only is recommended.

Treatment duration for TB is recommended beyond the regular 6 months for PLWH. Although the optimal timing of initiation of ART in PLWH patients and TB is well studied and known, as discussed, the optimal duration of TB treatment for PLWH and drug-susceptible TB disease is not known. If drug-susceptibility testing is performed and there is no resistance, EMB may be discontinued prior to 2 months. In general, the outcomes of 6-month regimens (2 months of INH, RIF, EMB, and PZA, followed by 4 months of INH and RIF) given as DOT to patients with HIV have been very good, with cure rates ranging from 70% to 95%, but not universally successful. Extension of therapy to 9 months is currently recommended for all PLWH and TB who have positive sputum culture after 2 months of treatment or severe cavitary or disseminated extrapulmonary disease including tuberculous meningitis, bone, joint, and spinal TB.

A more person centered, though as yet not fully studied way to approaching the issue of treatment duration is by appreciating that "one-size-does-not-fit-all" and to consider personal, clinical, and microbiological characteristics of patients,[77,78] including PLWH, as important determinants of treatment duration. By providing identical dose and duration to all, many with milder disease may be overtreated and others with more severe and advanced disease may be insufficiently treated. Such characteristics as cavitary and 3+ sputum connotes need for longer duration of treatment and conversely, their absence, might only require a shorter course. PLWH are usually automatically placed in the category of more prolonged treatment but by stratifying by CD4 cell count as a measure of disease severity, this issue may be more nuanced than in those with CD4 cell counts >300 cells/mm³, and successful patients on ART might safely reduce treatment duration, whereas in others with more advanced HIV disease, prolonged treatment beyond the standard 9 months may be required. Baseline and treatment markers could be used to select treatment duration with greater precision, providing a programmatically viable alternative to the "one-size-fits-all" paradigm used worldwide. "Patient stratified" medicine principles, however, should be further evaluated in clinical trials of TB and HIV and TB therapeutics.[77]

Medication adherence is a critically important issue which often determines treatment success for both TB and HIV. Although seemingly straightforward, it is actually a complex issue with biological, behavioral, and structural elements.[79] With reliance on DOT for TB treatment alone, medication adherence

has been understudied in high-burden settings among PLWH requiring treatment for both TB and HIV. This is particularly so for patients receiving treatment for drug-resistant TB. Demands of drug-resistant TB/HIV treatment regimens, in particular are daunting, including high-pill burden with the need to initiate a large number of new medications in a short time, adverse effects, lengthy treatment, and stigma. Given these, PLWH and TB should be routinely and consistently offered medication adherence support. Although DOT is recommended for all with HIV-related TB, this issue is still actively debated and often is moot as DOT services are often not fully available or implemented in many low- and middle-income sites. Furthermore, DOT alone does not account for or usually address complex social, behavioral, and structural barriers to treatment which require different approaches, and DOT has not sufficiently addressed issues of ART administration and TB/HIV treatment integration and treatment success. More recently, incorporating a person-centered perspective, DOT has been framed as one type of support among several that are useful and essential and could be combined in different circumstances and patients to address specific treatment barriers. Rather than sole reliance on DOT, many would support a more patient centered flexible approach to ensuring medication adherence, as has been favored with PLWH, emphasizing patient education, social, and community support, mHealth, and other modalities such as specifically addressing alcohol and drug misuse and mental health challenges, as needed.[67,80]

Differential adherence, the presence of adherence to selected but not all prescribed medication is common and often unrecognized. Differential adherence is understudied in high-burden TB/HIV settings. This has been documented for ART among PLWH,[81] but is less likely to occur if fixed dose combination (FDC) ART is available. It is well known but not well documented among people being treated for TB and more recently for those prescribed both TB and HIV medications, with preferential adherence for one or the other. Electronic monitoring of adherence (Wisepill®) as well as self-report, has documented this behavior and has associated it with unsuccessful treatment of TB, HIV, or both.[82] This is of particular concern if TB and HIV medications are separately prescribed and monitored at different clinical sites, an additional strong rational for integration of treatment of both diseases.[83]

IMMUNE RECONSTITUTION INFLAMMATORY SYNDROME

One of the most important clinical issues inhibiting early initiation of ART in people with active TB and remaining problematic has been the concern for increasing rates and seriousness of IRIS, defined as an inflammatory reaction to underlying TB disease with worsening of clinical signs and symptoms of active TB. IRIS can appear in two forms: *paradoxical* or *unmasking*. *Paradoxical* IRIS usually appears with fever and a characteristic worsening disease at the site of known TB disease (i.e., radiological changes on chest X-ray, increased inflammation at extrapulmonary TB sites, including lymph nodes and visceral organs). *Unmasking* IRIS appears when new or previously unrecognized disease becomes apparent after ART is initiated and restoration of immune competence begins. The frequency and severity of IRIS is from 5% to 35% in multiple studies and is correlated with the degree of immunosuppression when ART is initiated. Likelihood of IRIS is inversely correlated with CD4 cell count as a surrogate for severe immunosuppression with the danger and severity occurring at lowest CD4 cell counts. IRIS symptoms usually appear between 1 and 4 weeks after initiation of ART.

IRIS is a clinical diagnosis, as there are no specific diagnostic tests. IRIS is a sign of immune recovery and can usually be managed with non-steroidal inflammatory agents or prednisone, if severe. The typical scenario includes initial improvement of TB and HIV while on treatment followed by clinical deterioration. Differential diagnosis may include drug-resistant TB, other bacterial infections or opportunistic diseases, and inadequate medication adherence or medication toxicity.

Although deferring ART during TB treatment does reduce the occurrence of IRIS, ART deferral needs to be balanced by the high-mortality danger risk when ART initiation is delayed, as well as appreciation that mild IRIS is treatable with anti-inflammatory agents and prednisone. These have been shown to reduce the need for hospitalization and therapeutic procedures and to improve symptoms, performance, and quality of life.[84] In addition, in a recent RCT of patients with TB and HIV with a median CD4 cell count of 39 cells/mm, the frequency of IRIS was significantly reduced by the use of prednisone prophylaxis during the first 4 weeks after initiation ART, without untoward effects.[85]

DRUG–DRUG INTERACTIONS BETWEEN TB AND HIV MEDICATIONS

Drug–drug interactions between TB and HIV medications are among the most important issues that differentiate TB treatment in PLWH from other patients. The ART pharmacopeia is vast, but in clinical use, is relatively restricted to a few regimens, depending on the presence or absence of HIV drug resistance, administration convenience, or side-effect profile. Most of the clinically relevant drug–drug interactions involving TB and HIV medications are due to the effect of rifampin, rifabutin and rifapentine (RIF, RFB, RPT) on specific ART classes as listed later. All rifamycins are inducers of a variety of metabolic pathways, particularly those involving the various isozymes of the cytochrome P450 (CYP) system and drug transporters such as P-glycoprotein. By inducing the activity of metabolic enzymes, rifamycins decrease the serum concentrations of many drugs, including several ARTs metabolized through these pathways. Rifamycins remain the most potent drug class for TB treatment, and RIF, administered daily, is also the most potent, common, and problematic enzyme inducer. Inducer potency of RPT depends on its frequency of administration. Daily RPT is at least as potent an inducer as daily RIF, whereas once-weekly RPT (as used in combination with INH for latent tuberculosis infection) (see section on TPT) has limited effects on other drugs. The complexity and extent of drug–drug interactions between the different rifamycins and many ART drugs can be confusing and daunting. Nevertheless, the rifamycins are critically important in achieving TB-therapeutic success and, unless contraindicated secondary to serious toxicity, should be included.

Nucleoside reverse transcriptase inhibitors including tenofovir and emtricitabine (FTC) or lamivudine (3TC) are not involved in pharmacologic drug–drug interactions with anti-TB therapies.

Nonnucleoside reverse transcriptase inhibitors (NNRTIs) including nevirapine, doravirine, etravirine, and rilpivirine are not recommended for use with RIF because of marked increases in their metabolism induction and subsequent subtherapeutic antiretroviral drug levels. The NNRTI EFV, conversely, is less affected by RIF and has been widely available globally and used extensively with RIF and two nucleoside reverse transcriptase inhibitors (NRTIs tenofovir and emtricitabine) in a FDC single tablet for the treatment of HIV disease and for PLWH receiving TB medication.

HIV protease inhibitors, including, lopinavir and darunavir are metabolized by CYP3A4, and their concomitant administration with RIF leads to >80% reductions in their serum concentrations and loss of therapeutic benefit. RFB can be used in place of RIF with modest decreases in protease inhibitor (PI) exposure but RFB results in additional complicated dose modifications of other drugs.

Integrase strand transfer inhibitors (INSTIs), including dolutegravir (DTG), raltegravir (RAL), and etravirine vary in their susceptibility to RIF metabolism induction. DTG is least affected although its use with RIF requires dose adjustment. Results from the INSPIRE study indicate that DTG 50 mg twice daily is effective and well-tolerated in HIV/TB coinfected adults receiving RIF-based TB therapy.[86] In addition, when used with TB treatment, rates of IRIS were low and there were no new toxicity signals for DTG and no discontinuations. The DOLPHIN TB prevention trial,[87] which tested the safety and pharmacokinetics of DTG with RPT/INH once weekly ×12 doses, showed this combination to be well-tolerated and that DTG at 50 mg daily maintained HIV viral suppression, despite a modest decrease in trough levels, not requiring dose adjustment. DTG is now the global recommended first choice ART for HIV and TB coinfection treatment. Among other INSTIs, both bictegravir and elvitegravir should not be used together with rifamycin-containing TB treatment because of subtherapeutic levels, and RAL requires a substantial dose increase to 800 mg BID when administered with RIF.

Drug–drug interactions can be complex, and side effects, toxicities, and interpreting underlying disease manifestations can be challenging but are usually manageable and part of the care and treatment of drug-susceptible and drug-resistant TB with and without HIV coinfection. The management of HIV-related TB should involve and have available clinicians and clinical services with experience in managing both diseases.

Useful websites regarding drug interactions and shared toxicities and side effects for TB and HIV therapies are available through the following hyperlinks:

- CDC (http://www.cdc.gov/tb/publications/guidelines/TBHIVDrugs/default.htm)
- American Thoracic Society (https://www.atsjournals.org/doi/10.1164/rccm.201909-1874ST)
- AIDSInfo (https://aidsinfo.nih.gov/guidelines)
- University of California San Francisco (http://hivinsite.ucsf.edu/insite?page=ar-00-02)
- University of Liverpool (http://www.hiv-druginteractions.org/), https://www.hivdruginteractionslite.org

Selected side effects and toxicities are summarized in Table 15.3.

Table 15.3 Shared side effects and toxicities between TB and HIV medications

Potential overlapping toxicities and drug–drug interactions	Antiretroviral drugs	TB drugs
GI symptoms	Protease inhibitors	Fluoroquinolones, ethionamide, *para*-aminosalicylic acid, linezolid
Hepatic	Nevirapine, ritonavir	INH, RIF, PZA, ethionamide
Cardiac/QT prolongation	*Note*: PR interval prolongation[a] with atazanavir, lopinavir/ritonavir	Bedaquiline, delamanid
Renal	Tenofovir disoproxil fumarate (TDF)	Aminoglycosides
Rash	Nevirapine, EFV, etravirine, rilpivirine, protease inhibitors, abacavir (hypersensitivity)	All TB drugs skin pigmentation with clofazimine
Peripheral neuropathy	Stavudine and DDI (rarely used)	Linezolid, INH (reduced with B6 administration), ethionamide, aminoglycosides
Neuropsychiatric	EFV (insomnia, dizziness, drowsiness, vivid dreams)	INH, cycloserine, ethionamide
Hematopoietic	Zidovudine (anemia)	Linezolid (myelosuppression)
Sensory/hearing loss/vision loss	None	Aminoglycosides, capreomycin, EMB

Source: Adapted from Nahid, P. et al. Treatment of Drug-Resistant Tuberculosis. An Official ATS/CDC/ERS/IDSA Clinical Practice Guideline (88) (https://www.atsjournals.org/doi/10.1164/rccm.201909-1874ST).
[a] Use with caution in patients with underlying cardiac dysrhythmia.

SELECTING AN ART REGIMEN FOR PLWH AND DRUG-SUSCEPTIBLE TB

The 2019 WHO updated guidelines provide the latest recommendations based on rapidly evolving evidence of safety and efficacy and programmatic experience using DTG and EFV 400 mg in pregnant women and people coinfected with TB. These guidelines are welcome as pretreatment resistance to EFV and other NNRTIs is increasing in low- and middle-income countries, creating demand for access to alternative non-NNRTI ART drugs.[89]

First-line ART regimens

1. *Dolutegravir (DTG)* in combination with a nucleoside reverse-transcriptase inhibitor (NRTI) backbone is recommended as the preferred first-line regimen for PLWH initiating ART and TB treatment. Among PLWH and TB, the dose of DTG needs to be increased to 50 mg twice daily because of drug–drug interactions with rifampicin. This extra dose of DTG is well tolerated, with equivalent efficacy in viral suppression and recovery of CD4 cell count compared with EFV. Compared to EFV, DTG also has lower potential for drug–drug interactions, more rapid viral suppression, and a higher genetic barrier to developing HIV drug resistance. DTG is formulated as a FDC (tenofovir/lamivudine/dolutegravir [TLD]), potentially improving adherence, and is newly available in South Africa and globally. It is proposed as first-line ART for TB/HIV, including DR-TB/HIV, but adherence in this context is not yet well studied. DTG, putatively does not interact with bedaquiline, making it suitable for treatment of drug-resistant TB.
2. *Efavirenz* at low dose (EFV 400 mg) in combination with an NRTI backbone is now recommended as the alternative first-line regimen for adults and adolescents living with HIV initiating ART and TB treatment. EFV 400 mg is better tolerated than EFV in standard dose (EFV 600 mg), with plasma

concentrations maintained above the levels considered to be effective, and reaching comparable viral suppression with lower risk of treatment discontinuation and severe treatment-related adverse events. EFV is not recommended for treatment with bedaquiline because of substantial reduction in bedaquiline levels.

3. *Raltegravir* (RAL)-based regimens may be recommended as the alternative first-line regimen for infants and children for whom approved DTG dosing is not yet available.

Second-line ART regimens

1. *DTG* in combination with an optimized NRTI backbone may be recommended as a preferred second-line regimen for PLWH for whom *non*-DTG-based regimens are failing.
2. *Boosted protease inhibitors* in combination with an optimized NRTI backbone are recommended as a preferred second-line regimen for PLWH for whom DTG-based regimens are failing.

INTEGRATED TREATMENT OF MDR- AND XDR-TB IN PLWH

Issues of diagnosis and treatment of TB with resistance to INH and MDR- and XDR-TB are covered extensively in Chapter 16 and the recent ATS/CDC/ERS/IDSA Clinical Practice Guideline,[88] including those of drug interactions and shared side effects and toxicities of TB medications and antiretroviral therapies. The reader is referred to these sources for more detailed information. In this section, we highlight issues of particular importance related to HIV and drug resistance coinfection and disease.

As with drug-susceptible TB, in co-infected patients, failure to have received ART as well as indicators of far advanced HIV disease (CD4 cell counts <50 cells/mm³) and TB disease (cavities and multilobar disease) are strong independent predictors of high mortality.[12,13] These, in turn, are reflective of late appearance for diagnosis and treatment. Integration of ART and treatment for MDR-TB significantly improves survival. Although the timing of institution of ART in drug-susceptible TB is well studied and known, similar data in drug-resistant TB are not directly available. The timing of ART initiation in this circumstance is recommended to be the same as among PLWH with drug-susceptible TB. Because of the high rate of morbidity and mortality among those with MDR- or XDR-TB, ART should be initiated regardless of CD4 cell count and as soon as anti-TB treatment is tolerated, ideally as early as 2 weeks and no later than 8 weeks after initiation of anti-TB treatment.[11,88,90]

For decades, treatment for MDR-/XDR-TB has been by consensus based on review of largely observational studies. Treatment regimens have consisted of 5–7 drugs from different classes and usually included a 6–8-month intensive phase which included parenteral induction therapy with renal and audio toxic aminoglycosides and with total regimen durations of 18–24 months.

NEW TREATMENT STRATEGIES AND TB MEDICATIONS

The past decade has observed the emergence of several new anti-TB agents, such as bedaquiline, pretomanid, and delamanid, and the repurposing of older agents, such as linezolid for those with these devastating diseases and including PLWH. They have greater potency than most of the older second-line agents, are administered orally, have improved toxicity profiles, and fewer drug–drug interactions. These drugs carry the possibility to transform the treatment of MDR- and XDR-TB in PLWH. The rifamycins, with the possible exception of rifabutin, are not used for treatment of MDR-TB by definition, but interactions of other TB medication classes with ART must be considered. Drug–drug interactions and side effects are problematic for some of the newer or repurposed anti-TB drugs, particularly linezolid, and special attention to this is required when prescribing. Identification and management of drug–drug interactions and overlapping side effects and toxicities must be performed as they can complicate treatment success for both diseases (see Table 15.3).

Further studies are needed to clarify the pharmacokinetic and pharmacodynamic interactions between ARTs and new and old and second-line agents for drug-resistant TB. The NNRTI, EFV, as a metabolic inducer, can produce a decrease in serum bedaquiline concentration and this combination is not recommended. Nevirapine has a less pronounced effect on bedaquiline levels and can be substituted in place of EFV. Nevirapine is not as reliably effective because of side effects and pre-existing levels of resistance. Recent studies have indicated that nevirapine medication adherence as measured by electronic dose monitoring is reduced and inferior to bedaquiline in a substantial proportion of PLWH, with an associated increase in mortality.[83,91]

Other ART drugs, including the protease inhibitors and cobicistat, both inhibitors of bedaquiline metabolism, can result in increased serum bedaquiline levels with concern for prolongation of QT intervals, but the clinical significance of this increase is not yet known. Therapeutic outcomes with bedaquiline and

DTG along with standard second-line TB therapies in PLWH and MDR-/XDR-TB have been greatly improved.

Enhanced attention to the HIV component of HIV-associated MDR-/XDR-TB is critically important to prevent adverse HIV-associated outcomes such as loss of virological control, emergence of drug resistance, and severe toxic effects that can erode gains noted with bedaquiline treatment.[83] To sustain and extend this success, we caution against ART switches that substantively increase patient burden (e.g., multiple pills, multidose regimens as presently required for nevirapine-based therapy). Pharmacovigilance, enhanced treatment support, and increased medication literacy for both TB and HIV medications are required. Development and testing of new companion ART regimens is urgently needed to maximize the benefits of bedaquiline and other newer or repurposed TB medications in patients with HIV who have MDR-/XDR-TB.

In addition to potential TB and HIV drug–drug interactions and shared toxicities, the limited availability of required expertise and infrastructure for DR-TB treatment has been a special challenge. A specific example of MDR-/XDR-TB in South Africa in rural KwaZulu Natal has been the overwhelming number of patients exceeding the capacity of the existing TB care system, with resultant treatment delay and disengagement and propagation of the epidemic. With appropriate efforts in training, treatment and care has been decentralized from the single provincial TB specialty hospital in Durban to rural sites employing a mixture of local designated regional hospital treatment facilities and staff and community based, community healthcare worker (CHW) supported, home care. Patients received the standard 18–24-month regimen. Among 206 patients, 150 (73%) had both MDR-TB and HIV. Overall survival was high (86% and 94%) compared between HIV-infected and -uninfected. CD4 <100 was the strongest predictor of unfavorable outcome, again emphasizing the need for earlier identification of HIV as well as TB disease. This experience, among others from South Africa, have demonstrated high treatment success rates and favorable HIV outcomes when attention is paid to comprehensive concurrent decentralized and community-based patient centered DR-TB and HIV treatment with careful attention to supporting administration of both TB and HIV medications.[92,93]

The WHO, in December 2018, added a series of recommendations supporting patient centered treatment of DR-TB, much of which reflects and benefits from the experience in the treatment of HIV (Figure 15.6) which include:

1. Health education and counseling on the disease and treatment adherence.
2. A package of suitable treatment adherence interventions including one or more:
   a. Tracers and/or digital medication monitor
   b. Material support to the patient
   c. Psychological support to the patient
   d. Staff education.
3. Several treatment administration options may be offered to patients:
   a. Community- or home-based DOT is recommended over health facility-based DOT or unsupervised treatment;

  b. DOT administered by trained lay providers or health-care workers is recommended over DOT administered by family members or unsupervised treatment;

  c. Video-observed treatment (VOT) may replace DOT where available.

4. Patients with MDR-TB treated mainly with ambulatory care rather than mainly with hospitalization.

5. A decentralized model of care is recommended over a centralized model

In the past decade, a series of clinical trials has enabled steady progress in addressing MDR-TB treatment in HIV co-infected patients. In 2016, following reports of the success of "the Bangladesh regimen," that is, a shortened observational study of a 9–12-month course of conventional anti-TB medications (but in a non-HIV co-infected population).[94,95] The WHO issued guidance for programs in resource-limited settings for a standardized shorter-course regimen of 9–12 months with seven anti-TB drugs for selected patients with MDR-TB.

STREAM study

The STREAM study,[96] a randomized non-inferiority designed clinical trial which compared an intensive, shortened, 9-month treatment regimen for MDR-TB using currently available oral medications compared to the standard 20- to 24-month regimen, both still with an injectable aminoglycoside administered for 16 weeks, included enrollees who were PLWH comprising 32.6% of the trial participants. The short-course regimen was non-inferior to the longer regimen (78.8% and 79.8% success, respectively) and a significant improvement compared to historical controls. Although an important step forward, the STREAM trial has left some lingering concerns: first participants still had to tolerate painful daily injections and approximately one-third of patients in each group had a serious adverse event, including major audio toxicity. Second, in terms of HIV, encouragingly, there was no significant difference in outcomes between the HIV-infected and -uninfected enrollees. However, although not significantly different, the mortality outcome among PLWH in the trial the trial was higher than those without HIV. The major comparison was related to the duration of treatment and although CD4 cell counts were balanced in the short and long-term patients, insufficient information was available about ART administration, regimens, and response, and whether mortality occurred in the lowest strata of CD4 cell enrollees, so the larger number of deaths among PLWH may be related to HIV and ART adherence and/or side effects. The recent WHO recommendation of 9-month treatment for MDR-TB also applies to PLWH, but caution in the use of the short-term regimen in PLWH and MDR-TB is recommended until further information is available. Hopefully, the non-significant difference will remain or narrow, particularly if more detailed attention is paid to the HIV disease part of the population. A second stage of the STREAM study is currently evaluating whether a fully oral short-course regimen would be effective and thereby avoid the toxicity.

NIX TB study

On August 14, 2019, the US Food and Drug Administration approved the oral drug pretomanid, a nitroimidazole, together with bedaquiline and linezolid (BPaL), as part of an all oral, 6 month, three-drug regimen for MDR-/XDR-TB. The decision was based on an open-label, uncontrolled, small trial of 107 patients with XDR disease, in which 95 (89%) patients achieved a culture-negative status at 6 months—a remarkable cure rate compared with historical results of 34%–55% with multidrug regimens for 18–24 months. The drug was only the second one approved under the so-called Limited Population Pathway for Antibacterial and Antifungal Drugs and was developed and licensed by the TB Alliance in partnership with Mylan under a public–private partnership model.

Among the study subjects, 56 (51%) were PLWH and results were similar for HIV-negative and -positive patients with 90% of both having a favorable outcome. Patients were treated with a 6-month regimen (9 months in two patients) consisting of 200 mg pretomanid once daily, 400 mg bedaquiline once daily for 2 weeks then 200 mg thrice weekly, and 1,200 mg linezolid daily for 6 months. Patients were followed for 24 months. Successful treatment was defined as a sputum culture-negative status 6 months after the end of treatment. Treatment failure, defined as death, culture conversion to positive status, withdrawal from the study, or loss to follow-up within 6 months post-treatment, occurred in 11% of patients (12/107). The most common adverse reactions observed in patients treated with pretomanid in combination with bedaquiline and linezolid included peripheral neuropathy, acne, anemia, nausea, vomiting, headache, and increased liver enzymes most attributed to linezolid. A caveat in interpreting the results is that as approved only as part of a combined regimen, it is not possible to separate out the specific therapeutic and side-effect profile of pretomanid. Limitations in study design and the small number of participants, with less of an opportunity to observe adverse events (including blood disorders, liver toxicity, and peripheral and optic neuropathy) preclude broad programmatic implementation of the regimen worldwide until additional evidence has been generated. Nevertheless, this study represents an extremely optimistic step forward in the treatment of MDR-/XDR-TB among PLWH. Additional studies are required and are planned. Clinical trials are currently evaluating 15 treatment regimens with a variety of combinations of medications. These will likely result in a variety of shortened all oral regimens, including ones compatible with antiretroviral therapies.[11]

WHO new guidelines

Since The Latest WHO Guidelines were released in December 2018, this and other new evidence relevant to drug-resistant TB treatment has become available and has prompted the WHO to initiate a new guideline update process, including a new GDG expert meeting on November 12–14, 2019. A large dataset comprising both trials and programmatic updated information was reviewed including substantial numbers of PLWH. After the meeting concluded, the WHO provided a Rapid Communication. Key changes to the treatment of drug-resistant TB[97] which concluded that the changes suggested by the current evidence review are:

1. The phasing out of shorter injectable containing regimens and the introduction of a shorter all-oral bedaquiline containing regimen for eligible MDR-/RR-TB patients.

2. In patients with XDR-TB, a shorter regimen, BPaL, with bedaquiline, pretomanid, and linezolid may be used under operational research conditions as an alternative to the longer regimen.

3. Decisions on appropriate regimens should be made according to patient preference and clinical judgment, also considering the results of susceptibility testing, patient treatment history and severity, and site of disease.

4. No distinction was made between those with and without HIV.

Furthermore, multiple clinical trials are underway or in development to explore shortened and all oral active and latent TB treatment and include the participation of PLWH. Critically important in ongoing and future trials is careful attention to the selection, management, and analysis of the antiretroviral components and HIV outcomes in patients treated for TB.

The very bleak recent landscape of DR-TB therapeutics is finally being transforming to one of optimism and hope both for people with this terrible disease and, particularly, for those with HIV coinfection. A hopeful but still cautious transformation is currently underway in drug-resistant TB treatment: new, shorter, less toxic, and more effective drug-regimens can now cure a once barely treatable infection. As in the early, miraculous days of combination ART for HIV, these powerful new therapies offer opportunities for innovations in delivery to make treatment even more effective, efficient, and patient-centered.

PREVENTING TB IN PLWH

TB prevention is crucial, but has been a neglected component of global control of the TB pandemic. For the past 50 years, strategies for controlling TB in high-burden countries have focused on passive case detection and treatment of active disease, despite numerous policy recommendations advocating broader and more comprehensive approaches[98] (https://doi.org/10.1016/S2213-2600(19)30263-2). In addition, for both HIV and TB, there has been a tendency to view prevention and treatment as competing priorities, rather than as essential and mutually reinforcing steps along a continuum.

Multiple strategies are available for preventing TB in PLWH: provision of ART, TPT, enhanced infection control, and addressing and reducing social determinants at the root cause of both epidemic diseases. Each of these, taken together, should be seen as a component of a comprehensive and integrated strategy for the successful prevention and ultimate elimination of both HIV and TB.

ART in PLWH for TB prevention

For PLWH, ART serves as an important and potent TB prevention strategy. Multiple studies have demonstrated a powerful reduction of active TB risk among PLWH who are placed on ART and most notably in settings of high prevalence of both diseases. After initial observations of reduced TB on ART in South Africa,[99] a subsequent modeling study optimistically estimated that if HIV-positive people started ART within 5 years of seroconversion, the incidence of AIDS-related TB in 2015 would have been reduced by 48% (range: 37%–55%). Long-term reductions would depend on the delay to starting ART. If treatment is started 5 years after HIV seroconversion, or as soon as people test positive, the incidence in 2050 was estimated to be reduced by 66% (range: 57%–80%) to over 90%, respectively.[100]

A systematic review analyzed the impact of ART on the incidence of TB in adults through 2012.[101] RCTs, prospective cohort studies, and retrospective cohort studies were included if they compared TB incidence by ART status in HIV-infected adults for a median of over 6 months. Eleven studies met the inclusion criteria. The authors established four categories based on CD4 count strata at ART initiation: (1) <200 cells/μL, (2) 200–350 cells/μL, (3) >350 cells/μL, and (4) any CD4 cell count. ART was strongly associated with a reduction in the incidence of TB in all baseline CD4 count categories: (1) <200 cells/μL (hazard ratio [HR]: 0.16, 95% CI: 0.07–0.36), (2) 200–350 cells/μL (HR: 0.34, 95% CI: 0.19–0.60), (3) >350 cells/μL (HR: 0.43, 95% CI: 0.30–0.63), and (4) any CD4 count (HR: 0.35, 95% CI: 0.28–0.44). Other studies have affirmed the importance of ART in reducing TB incidence, but caution that ART alone would not be sufficient, and a comprehensive strategy of earlier HIV identification and ART initiation as well as TB prevention with INH, would be required to significantly reduce TB incidence.[102]

The benefits of ART in reducing TB incidence have been reported from both high-prevalence HIV and TB countries in sub-Saharan Africa as well as high- and middle-income countries in Europe and the Americas. In the HIV-CAUSAL Collaboration study,[103] 12 cohorts from the United States and Europe of HIV-positive, ART-naive, AIDS-free individuals aged $\geq$18 years were followed from 1996 through 2007. Estimated HRs for ART versus no ART indicated that TB incidence decreased after ART initiation, but not among people >50 years old or with CD4 cell counts of <50 cells/μL, both indications of longstanding HIV disease and marked immunosuppression, arguing for most ART benefits when HIV is diagnosed and ART is initiated early in the course of disease.

The TEMPRANO study,[104] conducted in Côte d'Ivoire, randomized 2,056 participants with ART initiation to one of four study arms: deferred ART (until WHO criteria were met), deferred ART plus IPT, early ART, or early ART plus IPT. Findings showed that early initiation of ART with or without 6 months of IPT reduced the risk of HIV-related illness, the majority of which was TB. The combination of ART and IPT further reduced HIV TB-related illness by 44% and all-cause mortality by 35% compared with deferral of ART and no IPT.

In the START study,[105] 4,685 participants with CD4 counts >500 cells/mm^3 were randomized to receive immediate ART or ART deferred until their CD4 count dropped to 350 cells/mm^3 or until they developed a clinical condition that required ART. TB was one of the three most common clinical events, occurring in 14% of participants in the immediate initiation group and significantly higher at 20% of participants in the deferred initiation group.

Patients initiating ART early in the START and TEMPRANO trials had viral suppression rates exceeding 95% and 80%, respectively. In both trials, a reduced rate of TB after early ART, as compared with deferred ART, was one of the most important contributors to the overall benefits. Collectively, these studies showed that early initiation of ART (with or without IPT) reduced active TB, particularly in countries with a high prevalence of HIV/TB coinfection. Translating early treatment for all PLWH into successful programmatic implementation by weak, underfunctioning, and underfunded healthcare services is, however, a daunting prospect, particularly in areas of the globe with the highest burdens and prevalences of both HIV and TB.

A recent observational study reviewing this issue of poorer standardized programmatic circumstances provide additional support for the role of ART in TB prevention, but also illustrates the limitations of such a strategy under programmatic conditions with weak and challenging healthcare infrastructures.[106] A large study from the Indian private healthcare sector demonstrates that despite ART scale-up and improving life expectancy of PLWH in India, a sizeable proportion of individuals remain susceptible to incident TB. Among close to 2,000 PLWH followed for a median of 57 months from initiation of ART, incident TB cases were associated with a CD4 count <500 cells/mm^3 ($p < 0.0001$), virologic failure on ART (adjusted hazard ratio [aHR]: 3.05 [95% CI: 2.094–4.454], $p < 0.0001$), and receipt of ART without IPT (aHR: 8.24 [95% CI: 3.358–20.204], $p < 0.0001$).

Studies in Africa and India and combined databases in the United States and Canada show an overall decrease in TB incidence on ART, but higher rates in those in subpopulations and groups at increased risk for TB including populations with sociodemographic and behavioral higher baseline rates of TB infection and where issues of inadequate HIV treatment success or newly transmitted TB are more common, including those living in poverty, incarcerated, or recently immigrated from higher TB prevalence countries where such groups have a disproportionately high-TB risk in the general population, irrespective of HIV status.[20,31,103]

Although demonstrably effective in a wide range of studies and environments, this and other studies of ART benefit in reducing active TB demonstrated the need for both TB and HIV integration along the entire cascade of care. This requires: (1) community- and facility-based resources that facilitate access to HIV testing and TB screening, and linkage to care earlier in the course of infection with both pathogens; (2) early initiation of appropriate TB, ART, and IPT at appropriate disease stages; (3) sustained high adherence to ART, IPT, and TB therapy; (4) close monitoring for incident TB in patients with low baseline and time updated CD4 count, and routine virologic monitoring of all TB patients on ART; (5) routine use of IPT with ART in high-TB prevalence areas and populations; and (6) improving long-term retention rates for both diseases (https://aidsinfo.nih.gov/).[67]

Global efforts to provide ART have now reached 20 million PLWH, but another 17–19 million remain untreated and have not received the beneficial effects of ART, including its demonstrated TB incidence reduction. As a consequence, this population remains substantially at-risk for active TB and TB propagation. Continued global identification of PLWH and expansion of ART initiation to 95% by 2030 is a global HIV goal which will contribute to the parallel aim of TB epidemic elimination (*UNAIDS 2019 estimates*, www.who.int/tb/global-report-2019). To fully achieve elimination of both TB and HIV epidemics, this must also be accompanied by the widespread expansion of use of effective TPT to reduce the global reservoir of *M. tuberculosis* infection, particularly among those with HIV and TB coinfection.

TPT for PLWH

ISONIAZID PREVENTION THERAPY (IPT)

TPT, administered as IPT was first shown to be effective in a controlled trial on a population level in a high-TB prevalence area of Alaska 50 years ago. In the final study report, the significant protective effect of IPT administered for 12 months in reducing TB incidence among those with LTBI was shown to persist for more than 19 years.[107] Of note, the magnitude of the effect was related to the amount of INH taken. Over the 6-year period following the controlled trial and after population wide programmatic implementation of the strategy, persons with untreated nonactive TB who were adherent to INH therapy had a reduction of 89% in active TB and 71% less TB than those who were not adherent.[108] The authors presciently suggested that "preventive treatment of previously untreated, nonactive TB can make a major contribution to TB control among populations with a TB problem similar to that among Alaskan natives."[108] Following these landmark trials in Alaska, numerous trials have confirmed IPT effectiveness in many different populations and under a variety of conditions.

It is estimated that currently 25%–33% of the world's population (estimated to be approximately 1.7–2 billion globally)[15] are infected with *M. tuberculosis*. Even improved strategies for TB diagnosis and treatment will not address the large reservoir of latently infected people who might develop TB at any point in their lifetimes. TB control programs have traditionally focused almost exclusively on case finding and treatment. Although this critical activity must continue, it is equally essential to refocus on the vast reservoir of people who are infected, but have not yet progressed to active, reportable, and transmissible disease. Without powerful attempts to deplete this reservoir of *M. tuberculosis* infection, prospects to achieve End TB Goals are scant. To successfully accomplish the End TB Strategy, this latent reservoir of global TB must be incorporated into the elimination strategy. This is particularly pertinent for PLWH and LTBI as HIV infection is the most potent driver of TB reactivation in the global pool of LTBI. Unfortunately, the adoption and implementation of TPT for LTBI in PLWH globally has lagged far behind expected and needed levels. The WHO has recognized this by adding TPT for those at high risk of TB to the first pillar of the End TB strategy.

IPT is one of the three I's of decreasing the impact of TB on populations with HIV. It demonstrates 30%–70% efficacy and has been shown to significantly impact mortality in PLWH independent of ART.[109–111] As noted previously, the value of adding IPT to ART was seen in the TEMPRANO ANRS 12,136 study in Côte d'Ivoire, which showed that using IPT within 1 month of HIV diagnosis and early ART together had an additive impact on severe HIV disease (mostly TB) and mortality. Administration of both ART and IPT resulted in a decrease in the relative risk of a composite outcome of mortality and severe HIV-related disease by 35% and was particularly beneficial to those with CD4 counts below 500.[104] Impressively, long-term follow-up of the TEMPRANO study found that IPT led to a 37% reduction in mortality, independent of ART initiation and CD4 count.[109] Benefit also included a 37% reduction in TB mortality in people living with HIV/AIDS (PLHIV) with high CD4 counts, independent of ART administration. Benefits were sustained through a 6-year follow-up.[104]

A Cochrane review demonstrated that, compared to placebo, INH preventive therapy had a 32% relative reduction in TB disease among HIV patients. The risk reduction almost doubled (62%) when the HIV patient had a positive tuberculin test.

Widespread implementation could favorably impact the global reservoir of LTBI, but despite its promise, many countries have not enacted IPT programs and IPT rates have been variable and disappointing overall. Through 2017, the WHO estimated that fewer than 4 million people with HIV globally have ever received IPT, highlighting the critically important opportunity to substantially scale-up this intervention.[1] For the period 2005–2016, countries were requested to report data for PLHIV newly enrolled in HIV care. In 2005, under 30,000 initiations were reported. Subsequently, countries have been encouraged to report TPT for all PLHIV enrolled in HIV care and the numbers have shown that substantial progress has been made in initial and total enrolment. Another policy change that has accelerated initiation of TPT is to remove the traditional TST or IGRA screening requirement for LTBI as a trigger for TPT. In high-HIV and TB prevalence environments, such as sub-Saharan Africa, the recommendation is now epidemiologically based, because previous exposure to TB has likely occurred on many occasions and LTBI positivity is assumed.

The WHO reported[65] that in 2018, 65 countries reported initiating TPT for 1.8 million PLWH (61% in South Africa), gratifyingly up from just under 1 million in 2017 (Figure 15.7). The 2018 number suggests that the target of 6 million people having received TPT set in the period 2018–2022 in the political declaration at the UN high-level meeting on TB in September 2018 can be achieved. But despite this evidence of progress, substantial gaps

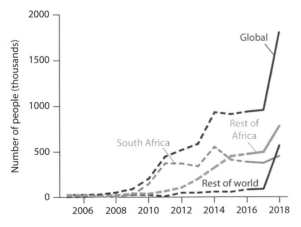

a Prior to 2017, data were collected for PLHIV newly enrolled in HIV care (dotted lines). In 2017 and 2018, data were also collected for PLHIV currently enrolled in HIV care (solid lines).

Figure 15.7 Provision of TB preventive treatment to people enrolled in HIV care,ᵃ 2005–2018.

and challenges with implementation and reporting remain for the provision of TPT to PLHIV. In the 16 high-TB or TB/HIV burden countries that reported providing treatment, coverage was highly variable, ranging from 5% in Eswatini to 10% of PLHIV newly enrolled in care in Indonesia to 97% in the Russian Federation and Haiti. Seven countries did not provide TPT at all to PLHIV in 2018. Overall, in 66 countries for which it could be calculated, coverage was 49%.

Initiation of TPT is the first step to its success, but many additional challenges remain. These include adherence to IPT through the course of therapy and retention in care to completion, as well as well as resolving differences in the recommended duration of therapy in high-prevalence areas where the force of infection and subsequent reinfection is concerning.

A large study of PLWH in Botswana, a high-prevalent HIV and TB environment, sought to evaluate whether there was benefit to extending IPT with continuous therapy (36 months) versus the recommended 6 months.[112] This trial randomized HIV-positive patients to either 6 months of IPT, the standard of care, or continuous therapy, that is, the 36 month duration of the trial. For the first 6 months, the entire cohort—after screening—of 1,995 patients was initiated on open-label 300 mg once-daily INH. After 6 months patients were randomized to either receive placebo or continue receiving INH. There were 989 in the 6-month arm (6H) and 1,006 in the continuous one (36H). Patients also received 25 mg of vitamin B6 daily. There was a significant reduction of active TB in the 6 month compared to placebo groups which persisted for nearly 6 additional months after completion, supporting the use for the 6 months duration. However past this point, TB cases escalated in the 6H arm and rates of TB returned to baseline, strongly supporting continued exogenous superinfection in high-prevalence areas. Overall, there was a 43% reduced incidence of TB in continuous IPT compared with 6-month IPT. In intention-to-treat analysis, there were 34 incident TB cases in the 6H arm and 20 in the 36H arm (HR: 0.57, $p = 0.047$). In a modified intention-to-treat analysis of 1,655 people who were enrolled after 6 months there were 25 TB cases in the 6H arm and 12 on the continued IPT arm (HR: 0.47, $p = 0.033$).

The TB/HIV in Rio de Janeiro (THRio) study published in 2015 evaluated the effectiveness of IPT in PLWH in a medium-burden TB area.[113] Patients were followed for 7 years, and those who received IPT received durable protection. ART was independently associated with reduced TB risk and low CD count with increased risk. There were high levels of adherence in these trials, but programmatic level performance of IPT was shown to be less successful, with only approximately 70% completing a 6- or 9-month course.

Looking more broadly and beyond the growing, but still low rates of enrollment in TPT globally, the next challenge for many enrolled in LTBI treatment is in all subsequent steps in the LTBI cascade of care. This has been well documented in a meta-analysis of studies published between 1946 and 2015, which reported primary data for diagnosis and treatment of LTBI.[114] Among 58 studies, describing 70 distinct cohorts and 748,572 people, multiple steps in the cascade were associated with poor performance at each step resulting in <20% of all candidates for screening completing LTBI treatment (see Figure 15.8).

As with other aspects of TB/HIV integration, IPT implementation and success globally has been compromised by multiple patient-level and systemic barriers along the cascade of care. These include inadequate patient preparation, programmatic commitment and resources, preparation and functioning of sites of initiation and administration, concerns about recognizing active TB disease and reinfection in high-burden settings, unfounded concern of emergence of INH resistance, and the long duration of treatment (6–36 months) with poor levels of medication adherence and treatment completion. Clearly, additional programmatic and technical strategies are needed.

TPT in high-income countries, including United States

Although now thought of as a critical issue at the epicenter of the HIV/TB collision in sub-Saharan Africa, where its greatest impact has been felt, LTBI remains one of substantial importance globally in the United States and other developed countries, where the TB focus has largely been on identifying and treating declining numbers of infectious TB cases.

It is generally well known that there are an estimated 1.2 million Americans living with HIV, but less appreciated that there are an estimated 10–13 million Americans currently living with TB infection. A portion, if not treated for LTBI, will be at continued and increasing risk as they age to progress to active, transmissible TB disease. PLWH are highest among these. Special populations considered to be at increased risk for both LTBI and HIV include PWID, who are incarcerated, immigrants, migrants from high-prevalence areas of both diseases, particularly if subjected to immunosuppressive agents for cancer or inflammatory diseases, and also the aged.

In countries or areas of high-HIV and TB prevalence, TPT should be given to all PLHIV without active TB without need for TST/IGRA. In low-prevalent TB settings, documentation of LTBI via TST or IGRA is recommended.

NEWER, SHORTER TPT REGIMENS, AND HIV COINFECTION

The critical role of elimination of the global reservoir of TB in the End TB Strategy requires increased current and new treatment implementation and completion success through improvements in management of LTBI with current tools and new strategies to address the losses at each step in the cascade. However, additional dramatic new approaches are still needed and these include the exciting new availability of new shortened and effective TPT regimens. A major limitation of IPT is the need for at least 6 months of treatment with subsequent substantial numbers failing to complete therapy. Newer, shorter regimens can address this limitation of IPT and potentially become TPT game-changers[65] (http://stoptb.org/global/advocacy/unhlm_targets.asp).

Prevent TB 3HP

The TBTC Study 26, Prevent TB, was a landmark randomized non-inferiority trial comparing 3 months of weekly rifapentine plus INH (3HP) to 9 months of daily INH (9H).[115] Published in 2011, The trial showed that 3HP administered by DOT was non-inferior and had a higher treatment completion rate, lower TB rate, and less hepatotoxicity compared to 9H in a largely HIV-negative population. This affirmed the efficacy of weekly 3HP as a TPT option. There were very few cases of TB disease in either arm: 7 cases among those taking the 3HP study regimen and 15 cases among those taking the current standard regimen. In addition, there was higher adherence to 3HP with 82% of participants completing the 3-month course of medication, compared to 69% who completed the 9-month IPT course. In 2016, the study was expanded and conducted exclusively in PLWH, and among those with a robust CD4 count (median of 500 cells/μL), 3HP was both effective and non-inferior.[116]

A follow-up study evaluated 3HP for latent TB using DOT versus SAT in a randomized-clinical non-inferiority trial and showed comparable efficacy in high-, middle-, and low-income

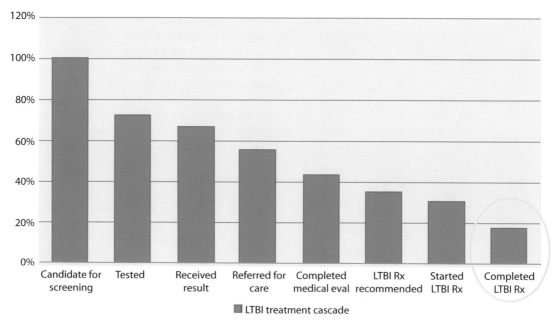

Figure 15.8 LTBI treatment cascade.

countries.[116] Based on data from this and subsequent studies, the WHO 2018 guidelines has endorsed 3HP as an alternative to 6 months of INH monotherapy (6H) as preventative therapy in both adults and children in countries with high-TB incidence.[117,118] Post-marketing surveillance of 3HP in the United States showed that completion of 3HP in routine healthcare settings was greater overall than rates reported from clinical trials, and greater than historical regimens among reportedly nonadherent populations. A systematic review of 3HP safety reviewed 23 RCTs and 55 non-randomized studies. Flu-like reactions were reported with an increased frequency and hepatotoxicity with a lower frequency than standard treatment with INH.

A concern regarding 3HP use in PLWH has been the potential drug–drug interaction between rifapentine (P) and DTG, the integrase strand inhibitor antiretroviral now used widely in the United States and increasingly globally. DTG is metabolized by CYP3A and UGT1A1 which are induced by rifamycins, including rifapentine resulting in concern that this would result in subtherapeutic levels of DTG. This has been resolved by the results of the DOLPHIN pharmacokinetic trial which demonstrated that DTG can be given with short-course TB preventive therapy of 12 once-weekly (3HP) without dose adjustment.[87]

Although DTG area under the curve was reduced by 29% at weeks 3 and 8, the investigators judged DTG levels to be sufficient, based on 96 week outcomes for 10 mg DTG in the original dose finding study. Viral load suppression <40 copies/mL was maintained throughout treatment. The findings mostly put to rest fears of potential deleterious drug interactions with DTG and have paved the way for scale-up of the 3HP regimen in 12 high-burden TB countries across three continents.

3HP has been approved for the treatment of LTBI by the US Food and Drug Administration and is recommended by the WHO and US Centers for Disease Control and Prevention. Regulatory approval of 3HP products is being sought in high-TB and -TB/HIV burden countries.

3HR: Rifampicin plus INH daily for 3 months (available as a fixed-dose combination) has similar efficacy and safety to 3HP and is recommended for children and adolescents less than the age of 15 years.

Further study of 3HP is being introduced in 12 high-burden TB or TB/HIV countries in Africa, Latin America, and Asia which together represent 50% of the global TB burden: Brazil, Ghana, Ethiopia, Kenya, Tanzania, Malawi, Zimbabwe, Mozambique, South Africa, India, Cambodia, and Indonesia. Initially, the safety and drug–drug interactions of 3HP combined with DTG on a larger population basis will be evaluated and then followed by 3HP treatment to 400,000 people. Implementation science projects are planned to determine optimal ways to deliver the regimen with the goal of identifying a generalizable approach to achieve high and successful levels of delivery of TPT during routine care in public clinics.

Brief TB-1HP

Another landmark TPT shortening trial, brief TB (1HP) was reported in 2019. This multicenter RCT in PLWH in high-burden TB settings found that daily INH and rifapentine for 1 month (1HP) was non-inferior to 9H.[119] A total of 3,000 patients were enrolled and followed for a median of 3.3 years. Of these patients, 54% were women, the median CD4+ count was 470 cells/mm³, and half the patients were receiving ART. The primary end point was reported in 32 of 1,488 patients (2%) in the 1-month group and in 33 of 1,498 (2%) in the 9-month group, for an incidence rate of 0.65 per 100 person-years and 0.67 per 100 person-years, respectively The percentage of treatment completion was significantly higher in the 1-month group than in the 9-month group (97% vs. 90%, $p < 0.001$). Additionally, fewer adverse events were noted and patients were more likely to be adherent and thus complete treatment. Serious adverse events occurred in 6% of the patients in the 1-month group and in 7% of those in the 9-month group ($p = 0.07$). The BRIEF-TB study showed that 1HP was non-inferior to 9 months of INH alone for preventing TB in HIV-infected patients and had a higher treatment completion rate and lower rates of adverse events than with 9 months of INH alone (Table 15.4).

Daily RIF-4R

In an open-label trial conducted in nine countries, randomly assigned adults with LTBI received treatment with a 4-month regimen of daily RIF or a 9-month regimen of INH for the prevention of confirmed active TB. Noninferiority and potential superiority were assessed. Secondary outcomes included clinically diagnosed active TB, adverse events of grades 3–5, and completion of the treatment regimen. 4R was non-inferior to 9 months of INH and had higher rates of treatment completion and fewer adverse events.[120] This regimen has not been formally studied in PLWH and is an option for persons who cannot tolerate INH or who have been exposed to INH-resistant TB. Daily RIF will result in a decrease in protease inhibitor and NNRTI antiretrovirals.

These studies provide exciting evidence for shorter TPT regimens. Additional and ongoing implementation research is required to fully realize their benefit and critical role at an individual patient level and in addressing and moving toward HIV/TB elimination.

For exact dosage and patient information refer to http://www.cdc.gov/tb.

Recognizing this slow progress and the need for high-level political commitment, the UNHLM on TB has set ambitious prevention and treatment targets to be achieved by 2022 providing TB preventive therapy for at least 30 million people, including 4 million children under the age of 5, 20 million other household contacts of people affected by TB, and at least 6 million PLWH (http://www.stoptb.org/global/plan/plan2/).

Remaining TPT issues

The success of initial IPT and excitement about short-course TPT regimens has also provided incentive and opportunity for study of additional practical and important implementation issues. These include a collection of ongoing and future additional trials of TPT co-administration with DTG: DOLPHIN TOO study of TPT in ART-naïve patients starting 3HP and DTG, and ACTG A5372 study of ART-naïve patients starting 1HP and DTG. Other studies include TPT regimen use in people with very low CD4 counts, periodic TPT re-administration and the WHIP3TB

Table 15.4 Regimen choices for TB-preventive treatment in PLWH

Regimen	Dose	ART compatibility	Duration	Comments	HIV studied	Success
INH (9H)	Daily 300 mg QD +/− B6	Excellent compatibility with all ART regimens	9–36 months Duration related to local TB prevalence	Standard regimen Inexpensive Poor uptake High non-completion rate	Multiple studies with PLWH	~30%–70% effective in programmatic use
3HP	Weekly INH 900 mg QW Rifapentine 450–900 mg QW Weight-based dosing	EFV and DTG compatible	3 months (12 doses)[a]	Rifapentine[b] Expensive; Limited availability	Multiple studies with PLWH[c]	87% completion Non-inferior to IPT
BRIEF TB 1HP	Daily INH 300 mg + Rifapentine 10 mg/kg ×1 month	DTG and EFV compatible	1 month	Rifapentine Expensive Limited availability	3,000 PLWH enrollees 1:1 comparison with INH	97% completion Non-inferior to IPT 6 months
4R	Daily 10 mg/kg Max: 600 mg	Not tested with ART	4 months	Consider if INH not usable	Not tested in PLWH	High completion Low toxicity

[a] In 2018, based on additional data, the CDC revised recommendation to allow this regimen by SAT.
[b] Recent announcement of rifapentine price drop from $45 to $15 for full course of TPT will increase global availability.
[c] Large-scale multinational programmatic implementation studies underway.

study, Part A comparison of weekly high dose rifapentine plus INH for 3 months (3HP) to 6 months of daily INH (6H), and Part B, a comparison of periodic (one round a year) 3HP (p3HP) to a single round of 3HP.

TPT studies to determine proper use of TPT for critically important populations, pregnant women, and children, are needed and are underway. The IMPAACT P1078 TB APPRISE trial[121] has evaluated the safety and efficacy of initiating IPT in pregnant women living with HIV or delaying IPT until after delivery and has showed no significant difference in TB or maternal safety outcomes between the groups. However, the study did observe a higher incidence of a composite adverse pregnancy outcome (stillbirth, spontaneous abortion, low birth weight, preterm delivery, or major congenital anomalies) in the immediate group, with low-incidence rates of TB in both groups. Currently, the WHO recommends IPT during pregnancy, but these results suggest that the risks may outweigh the benefits in pregnant women living with HIV, and further investigation is warranted to determine the optimal timing of TPT initiation in this population.

Studies in children are needed including use of 3HP and 1HP in children <2 years as well as prevention of MDR-TB.

With improved IPT use and exciting new TPT regimens now available, the next and parallel challenge in the context of TB/HIV integration is to fully roll out and enable widespread global implementation in co-infected populations. Standard INH and newer shorter regimens open many differentiated service delivery (DSD) options for provision of TPT as well as implementation science opportunities to demonstrate in parallel their acceptance, feasibility, and effectiveness. First, TPT must be delivered in a comprehensive patient-centered care model, and initial and ongoing consultation and collaboration with experts in the management of both HIV and TB coinfection should be available.

In high-prevalence settings, as HIV programs shift thousands of people to less-intensive ART provision models, the use of DSD models, coordination, harmonization, and incorporation of TPT into existing HIV programs are essential and could include

- Provision of TPT within HIV/ART and primary care program settings
- Provision of TPT in households and community settings, with enhanced social support
- Use of CHWs and other treatment supporters for treatment support, including weekly DOT as needed and loss to follow-up tracing
- Community adherence clubs for both ART and TPT[122]
- Provision of community-based TPT drug distribution similar to distribution of ART with opt-out addition of TPT to ART at patient pick up sites or use of "Pele-boxes"—a smart box which allows patients to input their cellphone number and a pin code to receive their parcel of medication from inside a locked box to avoid the necessity for standing in lines at pharmacies or clinics (see https://www.pelebox.com)
- Remote adherence monitoring of both ART and TPT via mHealth technologies to reduce the need for frequent clinic visits[123]

MDR-TB TPT

The potential benefit of provision of TPT in the setting of exposure to MDR-TB is a critically important and complex issue but remains undetermined at this time. Three ongoing clinical trials are attempting to guide the choice of latent TB treatment in the setting of MDR-TB exposure. Two trials, V-QUIN MDR and TB-CHAMP, both test a 6-month regimen of levofloxacin with dosing based on weight compared to placebo. The third trial, PHOENIx MDR-TB, has recently started and compares 6 months of INH against 6 months of delamanid. Pending the results of these and other planned trials, the WHO has made the following recommendations (www WHO End TB 2019):[11]

1. Individualize treatment after a careful assessment of the intensity of exposure, the certainty of the source case, reliable information on the drug resistance pattern of the source case, and potential adverse events.
2. In selected high-risk household contacts of patients with MDR-TB, preventive treatment may be considered based on individualized risk assessment and a sound clinical justification.
3. Focus on household contacts at high risk (children, people receiving immunosuppressive therapy, and PLWH).
4. Drugs should be selected according to the drug-susceptibility profile of the source case (many MDR-TB household contacts develop DS TB, so universal preventive regimens are ideal).
5. Confirmation of infection with LTBI tests is required.
6. Strict clinical observation and close monitoring for at least 2 years.
7. Furthermore, these recommendations must not affect ongoing placebo-controlled clinical trials of MDR-TB contacts on ethical grounds. The results of such clinical trials are crucial for updating this recommendation.

NEEDED EARLIER IDENTIFICATION OF PLWH WITH AND AT-RISK FOR TB

New treatment and prevention strategies, tools, policies, and resources have created great progress and an exciting environment for envisioning the end of the TB and HIV epidemics. Nevertheless, unacceptably large numbers of PLWH and TB remain undetected and still appear late in the course of their disease, at a point in the natural history when substantial damage to the immune system or lungs and vital organs has already taken place.[12,13,34,75] This delay in diagnosis and late appearance for care and treatment contribute to the high mortality in PLWH and drug-susceptible and drug-resistant TB. In addition, by the time recognized, undiagnosed disease has likely resulted in unanticipated and unknown transmission to others, estimated to average 15–20 transmissions/case.

Traditionally, both TB and HIV programs have employed separate strategies for diagnosing and treating each disease and predominantly focused within healthcare facilities or on individuals with direct contact with known individuals with either disease. Although this screening and case detection for both TB and HIV remains critical, comprehensive care and treatment success on an individual- and population-based level requires still earlier and broader identification of people living with and at-risk for both diseases. This, in turn, requires work at a wide array of sites at the community level. The success of treatment integration and new diagnostic tools and medications for both diseases have provided additional impetus to consider and implement integration and collaboration of HIV and TB through the entire course in the continuum of care for both diseases. This must extend from screening to prevention to treatment and cure for people at-risk for and with active TB and for decreased mortality and prolongation of life and quality of life of PLWH.

ACTIVE INTENSIVE AND INTEGRATED SCREENING AND CASE FINDING FOR EARLIER DIAGNOSIS OF TB AND HIV INFECTION AND DISEASE

The initial and long-standing WHO-recommended DOTS strategy included case-finding of active TB disease among symptomatic patients presenting to medical services. This strategy is insufficient in high HIV-burdened settings. Passive TB case finding alone will be insufficient to eliminate TB in high-risk HIV co-infected populations. Active and integrated TB and HIV screening and case finding beyond healthcare settings is essential. It is also essential that active case-finding interventions are programmatically inseparable from interventions targeted at preventing TB disease in those latently infected and at greatest risk of developing active disease. In countries with high prevalence of TB and HIV, intensified case finding in PLWH also provides opportunities to identify a high yield of people with TB; the yield is further significantly increased if all such individuals are screened microbiologically without preselection on the basis of the screening of symptoms. Intensified case finding aims to increase case-detection rates and shorten the time to diagnosis of TB, thereby reducing morbidity and mortality and shortening the period of infectiousness. This should, in turn, reduce the risk of transmitting TB in community- and healthcare settings. In community-based intensive case finding (CBICF) studies performed in sub-Saharan Africa, TB and HIV integrated community-based screening has been shown to be feasible, acceptable, and highly productive for both diseases.[124]

One representative study of ongoing integrated TB and HIV screening in community-based congregate settings in a rural South African sub-district illustrates this well. CBICF carried out by trained lay community health workers with nursing supervision accomplished screenings at pension distribution sites, taxi ranks, schools, municipal meetings, so on from March 2010 to June 2012 (before Xpert/TB availability).[19] Community members were offered TB symptom screening based on the WHO standard criteria (cough, fever, night sweats, and weight loss), sputum collection for microbiologic diagnosis, rapid fingerstick HIV testing, and phlebotomy for CD4 cell count. Among 5,615 persons who agreed to be screened for TB at 322 separate community sites, 91.2% also accepted concurrent HIV testing, identifying 510 (9.9%) HIV-positive individuals with a median CD4 count of 382 cells/mm^3 (interquartile range: 260–552), which was substantially higher than those first observed at local healthcare facilities, indicating earlier stage of disease in the community. TB symptoms were reported by 2,049 (36.4%), and sputum was provided by 1,033 (18.4%). Forty-one cases (4.0%) of microbiologically confirmed TB were detected for an extraordinarily high overall case notification rate within the community setting of 730/100,000 population (number needed to screen, NNS = 137).

Of particular additional interest, 11 (28.6%) of TB cases diagnosed were MDR- or XDR-TB. Of further interest, of the 41 cases of TB detected through CBICF, only five (12.2%) were HIV co-infected. All were successfully referred for initiation of TB therapy. This is in contrast to the 64% HIV-coinfection rate among all registered TB cases during the same period, most notified at healthcare facilities ($p < 0.001$) with a significant improvement in treatment linkage. These data illustrate the benefit of earlier time detection in the course both HIV and TB infection during community-based screening, including drug-resistant TB, with an opportunity to improve clinical outcomes and interrupt ongoing community-based transmission.

Multiple additional studies from an array of community settings in sub-Saharan Africa have demonstrated similar acceptance, feasibility, and effectiveness in integrated HIV/TB screening and case finding for HIV and TB in community- and home-based settings. Integration of TB and HIV services have been shown to increase uptake of ART[125] and to reduce the time to ART initiation.[126] Furthermore, TB/HIV service integration of ART and TB treatment among TB/HIV-coinfected patients has been associated with lower mortality during TB treatment.[127] These add to the body of evidence supporting the rapid scale-up of service integration in settings with a high-TB/HIV coinfection burden. Increasing HIV/TB integrated community-based efforts and other integrated strategies directed at both HIV-positive and HIV-negative TB cases may contribute to TB elimination in high-TB/HIV burden regions. Expanding on these data and findings, a dynamic model of HIV and TB transmission over 10 years showed that community-based TB/HIV screening with linkage to care could reduce TB incidence from 868 to 298 per 100,000 population in rural South Africa, and HIV from 1% to 0.8% whereas also decreasing the incidence of MDR- and XDR-TB.[124] This approach was also demonstrated to be cost effective in a formal parallel cost effectiveness study.[128]

ACHIEVING IMPLEMENTATION OF TB AND HIV INTEGRATION

Given the diversity of both epidemics, the WHO 2012 policy emphasized the need to establish generally applicable mechanisms for delivering integrated TB and HIV prevention and treatment services preferably at the same time and location. Integration should permeate and be normalized from the level of national ministries and departments, and on the line facility and community service sites. Implementation, monitoring, and evaluation of collaborative TB/HIV activities should be performed within one national system using standardized indicators, reporting, and recording formats. Setting national and local targets for collaborative and participatory TB/HIV activities should include a process with enhanced community and TB patient and PLWH participation to insure relevance, facilitate implementation, and mobilize political commitment. The components elaborated in 2012 by the WHO on TB/HIV integration remain relevant today, with additional emphasis on person-centered strategies, further health systems strengthening, and research on new differentiated strategies using implementation research to inform the guidelines and promote successful and universal acceptance.[2,129,130]

Community-based strategies for both prevention and treatment success need to be extended and fully supported. Interventions to reduce the burden of TB among PLWH include community-based screening and intensive case finding for both HIV and TB, infection control, and ART in line with the WHO

and national guidelines which now also emphasize TPT, drug-resistant TB, and person-centered strategies for care and prevention. Long-term and medium-term national strategic plans aligned with the health system of individual countries need to be developed to implement scale-up activities nationwide. National HIV programs and TB-control programs should also establish linkage and partnerships with other line ministries and civil society organizations—including nongovernmental and community organizations—for program development, implementation, and monitoring of collaborative TB/HIV activities. HIV programs and TB-control programs should collaborate with other programs to ensure access to integrated and quality-assurance services for women, children, prisoners, and for people who use drugs; this population, where relevant, should also receive harm-reduction services including drug-dependence treatment in in-patient and out-patient settings.

Translation of guidelines and commitments and policies to action remains challenging. These collaborative intentions have been blunted by past and remaining differences in the historical and evolved structures and cultures of the two diseases (Figure 15.6). Importantly, TB research and development and prevention and clinical services have been chronically underfunded. On the ground, successful collaboration and integration of TB and HIV collaborative activities must creatively and tenaciously deal with the realities within existing HIV and TB and health systems and programs that may be overwhelmed by large volumes of patients and limited financial, structural, and human resources. Furthermore, other critical health system components must be strengthened, including well-functioning laboratories for bacteriological and viral studies and DST, secure and reliable access to quality drugs and distribution systems, appropriate training of healthcare workers, functional information systems, and the requisite financial resources and political will.[130]

Notwithstanding these continuing challenges, substantial progress in parts of the integration strategy has been made in the past decade. For example, in association with integration of HIV and TB services, among those diagnosed with TB in 2017 in Africa, HIV status was known in 86%, compared to 14% in 2005 and among notified cases of TB who were living with HIV, 86% of these have been offered ART, a dramatic increase from 36% in 2005[2] and the number of PLWH who received TPT from 2017 to 2018 increased from 1 to 1.8 million.[65] Furthermore, new, innovative and focused implementation strategies have been developed and new medications for both HIV and TB have appeared and are creating new strategies and early successes.

DIFFERENTIATED SERVICE DELIVERY

"One size does NOT fit all"

DSD, is a newly articulated strategy with the potential to streamline implementation of HIV and TB integration. The global HIV and TB epidemics consist of a mosaic of countless smaller epidemics with similarities in social determinants and challenges but also composed of a spectrum of subtle to contextual differences. DSD has been formed in recognition of this global contextual diversity and tailored to the health status and clinical needs of persons living with HIV/AIDS and TB. Originally, DSD was developed and proposed as a strategy for HIV/AIDS care alone to more efficiently utilize limited health system resources to support patient needs, primarily in low-income countries, but is applicable to and now being advocated and employed for TB care and HIV/TB integration.

Although general guidelines for the prevention and management of both HIV and TB informed by rigorous evidence and expert consensus are critically important, the specific components and implementation of programs and services still must consider the local epidemiology of HIV and TB and the sociodemographic, resource, and health-system factors that are specific to individual countries and within country sites. This clearly impacts the configuration of HIV and TB integration. The degree of integration from national program to primary prevention and clinical services, and the mechanisms, structure, facilities, and staff for delivering the integrated services vary and should reflect the preferences and expectations of groups of PLWH and/or TB whereas reducing unnecessary burdens on both clients and the health system.

DSD and medication adherence: DSD strategies can be applied to medication adherence for both TB and HIV. Traditional TB reliance has been centralized globally, and DOT uniformly prescribed and recommended by the WHO is a central feature. Although DOT treatment has achieved great success, this has been spotty and implementation has been incomplete, in part because of the varied nature of TB epidemics and resources to combat them and complicated further by HIV coinfection. Are there alternatives? HIV ART medication adherence has largely been via self administration after providing patient education, assessment of adherence barriers, and counseling, often with social support. Successful required lifelong medication adherence has been accomplished by PLWH and is well documented but is not uniform, and individuals and subpopulations are challenged and struggle with adherence, requiring special attention. Simplification and improvements in regimens have made an enormous difference but structural and personal issues often are central, and "one-size-does-not-fit-all." An array of community-based strategies have evolved to support adherence in general and specifically under these circumstances.[67]

With regard to TB medication adherence, systematic reviews of studies conducted in countries with high, medium, and low burdens of TB have not shown improvement in cure or treatment completion in patients receiving TB treatment by DOT compared with SAT.[131–133] From the existing trials, DOT did not provide a solution to poor adherence in TB treatment. Given the large resource and cost implications of DOT, reconsideration is necessary regarding strategies that depend only on a policy of direct observation. Other options and approaches that motivate patients and staff and defaulter follow-up are needed. DOT remains the standard of practice to support medication adherence advocated by the WHO and in the majority of TB programs in the United States and Europe, but poor resources and structural barriers create implementation issues and challenges and it is not uniformly or successfully practiced in many resource-limited settings. DSD approaches to medication adherence have included much greater flexibility in policies and implementation with patient centered empowerment as a central feature and innovations such as mHealth, and emphasis on social support and other behavioral components, particularly in community-based settings, to support SAT among people being treated for HIV and TB.

As part of a DSD strategy, community health workers, mHealth, ART clubs, and other models of community service delivery are increasingly being used by HIV treatment programs.[134] In these models, participants have been trained to screen for symptoms of TB and other opportunistic infections, refer people for further evaluation, dispense TB preventive therapy, and home-based DOT. This approach has been piloted in several sub-Saharan African settings. In low-incidence countries, studies have shown that video DOT using smartphones is feasible, has high patient uptake, and is associated with similar adherence rates as in-person DOT.[131]

TPT DELIVERY AND DSD CARE FOR PLWH

ART programs are increasingly providing differentiated models of service delivery to deliver patient-centered care more efficiently and effectively. New approaches include initiating ART and IPT simultaneously, with a focus of initiation and monitoring in HIV oriented rather than TB programs, increasing the interval between clinic visits, and aligning ART pickups and IPT for PLHIV deemed to be "stable." As care for PLHIV stable on ART moves increasingly into communities, DSD strategies such as early and increasing use of mHealth, community health workers, and/or ART club members to distribute both ART and TPT and monitor for side effects and/or TB symptoms are being developed and implemented in sites in sub-Saharan Africa.[135]

DSD can also be used to stratify, simplify, and focus on complexities in program design and implementation based on specific patient needs. For example, separating and providing low level care for people who are stable and engaged in HIV treatment, fully medication adherent, and able to manage their own care as compared to a more intensive program for those who are less successful, with severe adherence challenges, and need for more intense and targeted interventions. Developing and implementing these stratifications and flexible treatment models based on person-centered needs is the essence of differentiated care. Differentiated HIV service delivery illustrates how service delivery innovations can improve efficiency and effectiveness, and also how patients and at-risk communities can shape and inform systems. Similar strategies are now necessary to transform TB service delivery.[136]

EXPANSION OF HEALTHCARE WORKFORCE— "TASK SHIFTING/SHARING"

Limited human resources within healthcare systems can impede success along the entire continuum of care for TB and HIV. Expanding and diversifying the healthcare work force is essential for implementation of an expanded and more flexible integrated TB/HIV agenda. This requires redefinition of traditional roles and positions and a more careful and functional matching of work force to needed function. The use of CHWs is an increasingly recognized strategy to accomplish this.[137] CHWs usually lack a formal medical or nursing education, but by receiving focused training can serve as extensions of existing often rigidly defined health systems. They can provide specific diagnostic, preventative, referral, treatment, and follow-up functions within or close to their communities on a volunteer or paid basis and can perform these tasks in a multi disease rather than a single disease-specific fashion. Using a DSD approach, and recognizing that "one-size-does-not-fit–all," DSD creative strategies employing CHWs can be tailored to different contexts based on geography, resource levels, characteristics of the existing healthcare system, and both HIV and TB prevalence. Given the critical need to identify both TB and HIV earlier in the course of natural history[12,13,34,75] for both the benefit of individuals and for stopping epidemic propagation, CHWs have the special cachet of working closest to where the earlier recognition can take place. CHWs have been shown to be able to engage "hard to reach" community members, such as young men, in settings such as alcohol venues, to provide screening and preventive services for HIV and TB.[138] Importantly, CHWs can favorably alter the sometimes unpleasant and impersonal healthcare system-based interactions with individuals and community members by providing a recognizable face, with the requisite sensitivity, skills, and compassion. CHWs have successfully worked in integrated teams with nurses to efficiently and competently screen individuals with both HIV and TB as well as non-communicable diseases through established and ongoing home-based and community-based congregate screenings and are able to do this in a cost-effective manner.[128,139]

UTILIZING THE CASCADE AND CONTINUUM OF CARE

An additional challenge in documenting, analyzing, and utilizing existing and new strategies in addressing both TB and HIV program status and progress is the lack of reliable process and outcome data and uniform measures.[140] The cascade of care (or the care continuum) is a practical and useful program and research tool for evaluating multiple required sequential steps to achieve treatment success. Over the last decade, the cascade has been developed and used extensively to evaluate steps in care delivery for PLWH including screening, case finding, referral, initiation, medication adherence, retention in care and sustained viral suppression, and immune reconstitution, all as part of a patient-centered continuum of care. TB control programs can learn from the HIV systematic use of care cascades and have begun to implement them as well as a technique for delivering and improving comprehensive patient-centered DSD programs. The care cascade analysis facilitates targeted interventions aimed at gaps and points of attrition, enumerating losses at each step across the care continuum. This facilitates planning and implementation of targeted interventions aimed at these points, and assessment of outcomes and temporal changes.[130]

Overall, using continuum of care measures, although improvement over time has been demonstrated, treatment outcomes for PLWH with both drug-susceptible and drug-resistant TB and HIV have remained unacceptable. Gaps in TB and HIV care, demonstrated by the continuum analysis are variable in different settings, but are identified and persist, with more than half of estimated cases not reaching care, and a case fatality ratio that is more than double that of people without HIV.[130] A TB care cascade constructed in South Africa, using data from laboratory services, TB registries and published studies, showed that only 53% of all TB cases were successfully treated[141] (Figure 15.9). Patient attrition occurred along various points of the TB patient care cascade; 5% of individuals did not access TB testing and 13% were lost between TB testing and diagnosis, due largely to failure of healthcare workers to follow the TB diagnostic algorithm. Among known diagnosed TB cases, initial loss to follow-up (i.e., TB diagnosed but treatment not initiated) was 12% (25% in rifampicin-resistant TB, and 11% in drug-susceptible TB), whereas 17% did not successfully complete treatment (Figure 15.9). In an analysis of a subset of those with known TB/HIV coinfection it can be

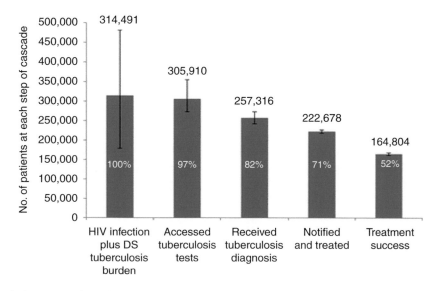

Figure 15.9 Care cascade for HIV-coinfected patients with drug-susceptible TB. The proportion at each step of the cascade is expressed in relation to the estimated burden.

observed that only 52% of those with estimated TB/HIV achieved TB-therapeutic success, and the drop off in steps along the way are identified (Figure 15.9).

Of note, HIV gaps and outcomes are not recorded. Conventionally, programmatic steps and outcomes reported in continuum of care trajectories, when constructed, have been defined separately for each disease and primarily by epidemiological measures.[141] Although themselves of great value, by only recording and analyzing the TB-related outcomes, an incomplete picture of the HIV/TB co-infected patients' and populations' trajectory through the cascade is observed. By integrating cascades of both TB and HIV prevention care and treatment (Figure 15.9), the real world of patients' and populations' experience comes into better view along with the full programmatic needs and gaps.[67]

In the model proposed in Figure 15.10 based on the work of O'Donnell et al.,[67] such an attempt has been made, and proposes to evaluate each step for each disease in a more finely grained integrated manner, representing the development and implementation of well-formulated constructs of care and prevention in an integrated stepwise continuum for both diseases, from screening, engagement in care and prevention, treatment, and treatment outcomes including relapse or reinfection, cure, and lifelong care for TB and HIV, respectively. Ideally, this would function with proper measurement, documentation, and analysis, and by making this an active bidirectional process with local partner's participation in data collection and analysis, the opportunity may exist to develop local corrective or expanded interventions. This process and strategy, integrated across either continuum and utilizing the current and future advances in prevention and treatment for both HIV and TB could improve individual and population health and contribute to reversing and ending the synergistic global HIV and TB syndemics.

CONCLUSION

The syndemics of TB and HIV/AIDS represent a dangerous and ongoing collision of one the oldest and among the newest of human infectious diseases. They have been tragically entwined for 40 decades with global consequences for people and communities living with and at-risk for each and both diseases. There are striking parallels between the two diseases in their social determinant roots, epidemiology, and biologic, prevention, clinical features and in compelling issues of human rights. Given their global nature, it is clear that each is composed of a mosaic of local but connected epidemics with differences reflecting existing geographic, sociodemographic, and political complexities and global historical and cultural differences in approaches. Nevertheless, wherever TB and HIV intersect, the logic and benefit of integration of policies, strategies, and practices is compelling.

TB and HIV together have resulted in the deaths and suffering of many millions of people, but exciting advances in prevention and treatment in the past decade have provided new optimism and signaled a possible turning point in reversing and potentially eliminating both as epidemics in the coming decades. Rather than accepting the traditional separation of TB and HIV, we consider the barriers and challenges in the integration of TB and HIV efforts and, in so doing the importance and benefit of comprehensive and person-centered integration for individuals and communities impacted by both diseases.

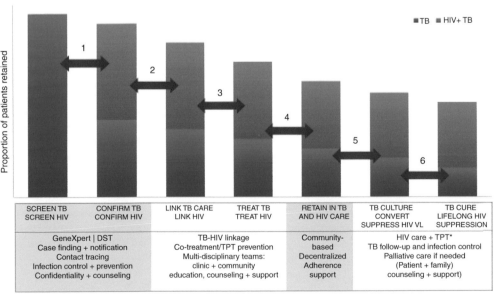

* Duration dependent upon TB prevalence

Figure 15.10 The continuum of TB/HIV care defines the processes and linkages that comprise optimal care for TB/HIV. The y-axis represents patients retained in care, the x-axis represents the stages of the continuum, and the arrows represent the linkages in the continuum. The box below defines tasks and processes that occur at each stage. TB, tuberculosis; HIV, human immunodeficiency virus; VL, viral load; DST, drug-susceptibility testing; TPT, TB preventive treatment.

We provide evidence for progress in new diagnostics and TB prevention particularly among PLWH with both antiretroviral and TB preventive therapies and for new therapies for drug-susceptible and drug-resistant TB among PLWH. Appreciating that the diversity of the TB and HIV epidemics requires that "one-size-does-not-fit-all," we explore new needed strategies for care and treatment where gaps currently exist, including differential service delivery, expanded work force, and propose attention to the continuum of care cascade in an integrated TB and HIV manner.

Elimination of both TB and HIV as clinical and public health global syndemics will require increased and equitable use of and access to existing diagnostics and treatments and innovation in the development and deployment of new technologies for prevention, diagnosis, and treatment. This will best be accomplished with further and sustained integration of TB and HIV throughout the breadth of the prevention and care continuum in strengthened systems of care and with resolute attention and repair of social and human rights inequities at the root of both syndemics.

REFERENCES

1. World Health Organization. *Global Tuberculosis Report 2018.* Geneva, 2019.
2. World Health Organization, Global Tuberculosis Report, 2018, Geneva.
3. Stewart RJ, Tsang CA, Pratt RH, Price SF, and Langer AJ. Tuberculosis—United States, 2017. *MMWR Morb Mortal Wkly Rep.* 2018;67:317–23.
4. Multidrug-resistant Tuberculosis-Fact Sheet. Available from: https://www.cdc.gov/tb/publications/factsheets/drtb/mdrtb.htm.
5. Revised definition of extensively drug-resistant tuberculosis. *MMWR Morb Mortal Weekly Rep.* 2006;55(43):1176.
6. Gandhi NR, Moll A, Sturm AW, Pawinski R, Govender T, Lalloo U, Zeller K, Andrews J, and Friedland G. Extensively drug-resistant tuberculosis as a cause of death in patients co-infected with tuberculosis and HIV in a rural area of South Africa. *Lancet* 2006;368(9547):1575–80.
7. Shah NS et al. Transmission of extensively drug-resistant tuberculosis in South Africa. *N Engl J Med.* 2017;376(3):243–53.
8. [Cited 2019 June 22]. Available from: https://www.who.int/tb/areas-of-work/drug-resistant-tb/global-situation/en/.
9. Gurumurthy P et al. Decreased bioavailability of rifampin and other antituberculosis drugs in patients with advanced human immunodeficiency virus disease. *Antimicrob Agents Chemother.* 2004;48(11):4473–5.
10. Peloquin CA, Nitta AT, Burman WJ, Brudney KF, Miranda-Massari JR, McGuinness ME, Berning SE, and Gerena GT. Low antituberculosis drug concentrations in patients with AIDS. *Ann Pharmacother.* 1996;30(9):919–25.
11. Dheda K et al. The epidemiology, pathogenesis, transmission, diagnosis, and management of multidrug-resistant, extensively drug-resistant, and incurable tuberculosis. *Lancet Respir. Med.* 2017;5(4):235–360.
12. Shenoi SV, Brooks RP, Barbour R, Altice FL, Zelterman D, Moll AP, Master I, van der Merwe TL, and Friedland GH. Survival from XDR-TB is associated with modifiable clinical characteristics in rural South Africa. *PLOS ONE* 2012;7(3).
13. Padayatchi N, Abdool Karim SS, Naidoo K, Grobler A, and Friedland G. Improved survival in multidrug-resistant tuberculosis patients receiving integrated tuberculosis and antiretroviral treatment in the SAPiT trial. *Int J Tuberc Lung Dis.* 2014;18(2):147–54.
14. Selwyn PA, Hartel D, Lewis VA, Schoenbaum EE, Vermund SH, Klein RS, Walker AT, and Friedland GH. A Prospective-study of the risk of tuberculosis among intravenous drug-users with human immunodeficiency virus-infection. *N Engl J Med.* 1989;320(9):545–50.
15. Houben RM, and Dodd PJ. The global burden of latent tuberculosis infection: A re-estimation using mathematical modelling. *PLoS Med.* 2016;13(10):e1002152.
16. Ahmed A, Rakshit S, and Vyakarnam A. HIV-TB coinfection: Mechanisms that drive reactivation of *Mycobacterium tuberculosis* in HIV infection. *Oral Dis.* 2016;22:53–60.
17. Diedrich CR, and Flynn JL. HIV-1/*Mycobacterium tuberculosis* coinfection immunology: How does HIV-1 exacerbate tuberculosis? *Infect Immun.* 2011;79(4):1407–17.
18. Andrews JR, Gandhi NR, Moodley P, Shah NS, Bohlken L, Moll AP, Pillay M, Friedland G, and Sturm AW, Collaboration TFCR. Exogenous reinfection as a cause of multidrug-resistant and extensively drug-resistant tuberculosis in rural South Africa. *J Infect Dis.* 2008;198(11):1582–9.
19. Shenoi SV, Moll AP, Brooks RP, Kyriakides T, Andrews L, Kompala T, Upadhya D, Altice FL, Eksteen FJ, and Friedland G. Integrated tuberculosis/human immunodeficiency virus community-based case finding in rural South Africa: Implications for tuberculosis control efforts. *Open Forum Infect Dis.* 2017;4(3):ofx092.
20. Altice FL, Azbel L, Stone J, Brooks-Pollock E, Smyrnov P, Dvoriak S, Taxman FS, El-Bassel N, Martin NK, Booth R, Stover H, Dolan K, and Vickerman P. The perfect storm: Incarceration and the high-risk environment perpetuating transmission of HIV, hepatitis C virus, and tuberculosis in Eastern Europe and Central Asia. *Lancet* 2016;388(10050):1228–48.
21. United Nations. High level meeting on the fight to end tuberculosis. 2018.
22. Lonnroth K, Castro KG, Chakaya JM, Chauhan LS, Floyd K, Glaziou P, and Raviglione MC. Tuberculosis control and elimination 2010–50: Cure, care, and social development. *Lancet* 2010;375(9728):1814–29.
23. Alland D, Kalkut GE, Moss AR, Mcadam RA, Hahn JA, Bosworth W, Drucker E, and Bloom BR. Transmission of tuberculosis in New York City—An analysis by DNA-fingerprinting and conventional epidemiologic methods. *N Engl J Med.* 1994;330(24):1710–6.
24. The HIV/AIDS epidemic in New York City. In: Jonsen AR SJ (ed.). *The Social Impact of AIDS in the United States.* Washington, DC: National Academies Press, 1993.
25. Friedland GH. A journey through the epidemic. *B New York Acad Med.* 1995;72(1):178–86.
26. Friedman LN, Williams MT, Singh TP, and Frieden TR. Tuberculosis, aids, and death among substance abusers on welfare in New York City. *N Engl J Med.* 1996;334(13):828–33.
27. Wallace, D, and Wallace R. *A Plague on Your Houses.* New York, New York: Verso Books, 2001.
28. Drucker E, Sckell B, Alcabes P, Bosworth W. Childhood tuberculosis in the Bronx, New York. *The Lancet, Public Health.* 1994;343(8911):1482–85.
29. Frieden TR, Sterling T, Pablos-Mendez A, Kilburn JO, Cauthen GM, and Dooley SW. The emergence of drug-resistant tuberculosis in New York City. *N Engl J Med.* 1993;328(8):521–6.
30. Frieden TR, Fujiwara PI, Washko RM, and Hamburg MA. Tuberculosis in New York City—turning the tide. *N Engl J Med.* 1995;333(4):229–33.

31. Coovadia H, Jewkes R, Barron P, Sanders D, and McIntyre D. The health and health system of South Africa: Historical roots of current public health challenges. *Lancet* 2009;374(9692):817–34.

32. Packard R. White Plague, Black Labor 1989.

33. Karim SSA, Churchyard GJ, Karim QA, and Lawn SD. Health in South Africa 3 HIV infection and tuberculosis in South Africa: An urgent need to escalate the public health response. *Lancet* 2009;374(9693):921–33.

34. Basu S, Friedland G, Andrews J, Shah S, Gandhi N, Moll A, Moodley P, Sturm W, Medlock, Galvani A. The emergence and transmission dynamics of XDR-TB in rural KwaZulu Natal, South Africa. *Proc Nat Acad Sci.* 2009;106(18):7672–77.

35. Institute of Medicine (US) Forum on Drug Discovery DaTRAoMS. *The New Profile of Drug-Resistant Tuberculosis in Russia: A Global and Local Perspective: Summary of a Joint Workshop.* Washington, DC: National Academies Press, 2011 Friday, December 21 2018.

36. Stigma and Discrimination [cited 2019 January 8]. Available from: http://www.healthpolicyproject.com/index.cfm?ID=topics-Stigma.

37. Daftary A. HIV and tuberculosis: The construction and management of double stigma. *Soc Sci Med.* 2012;74(10):1512–9.

38. Zachariah R et al. Language in tuberculosis services: Can we change to patient-centred terminology and stop the paradigm of blaming the patients? *Int J Tuberc Lung Dis.* 2012;16(6):714–7.

39. Frick M, von Delft D, and Kumar B. End stigmatizing language in tuberculosis research and practice. *BMJ* 2015;350:h1479.

40. Getahun H et al. Development of a standardized screening rule for tuberculosis in people living with HIV in resource-constrained settings: Individual participant data meta-analysis of observational studies. *PLoS Med.* 2011;8(1).

41. Cain KP et al. An algorithm for tuberculosis screening and diagnosis in people with HIV. *N Engl J Med.* 2010;362(8):707–16.

42. Achkar JM, and Jenny-Avital ER. Incipient and subclinical tuberculosis: Defining early disease states in the context of host immune response. *J Infect Dis.* 2011;204:S1179–S86.

43. Meintjes G, and Wilkinson RJ. Undiagnosed active tuberculosis in HIV-infected patients commencing antiretroviral therapy. *Clin Infect Dis.* 2010;51(7):830–2.

44. Bassett IV, Wang B, Chetty S, Giddy J, Losina E, Mazibuko M, Bearnot B, Allen J, Walensky RP, and Freedberg KA. Intensive tuberculosis screening for HIV-infected patients starting antiretroviral therapy in Durban, South Africa. *Clin Infect Dis.* 2010;51(7):823–9.

45. Greenberg SD, Frager D, Suster B, Walker S, Stavropoulos C, and Rothpearl A. Active pulmonary tuberculosis in patients with AIDS: Spectrum of radiographic findings (including a normal appearance). *Radiology* 1994;193(1):115–9.

46. Jones BE, Young SM, Antoniskis D, Davidson PT, Kramer F, and Barnes PF. Relationship of the manifestations of tuberculosis to CD4 cell counts in patients with human immunodeficiency virus infection. *Am Rev Respir Dis.* 1993;148(5):1292–7.

47. Padyana M, Bhat RV, Dinesha M, and Nawaz A. HIV-tuberculosis: A study of chest X-ray patterns in relation to CD4 count. *N Am J Med Sci.* 2012;4(5):221–5.

48. Perrin FMR, Woodward N, Phillips PPJ, McHugh TD, Nunn AJ, Lipman MCI, and Gillespie SH. Radiological cavitation, sputum mycobacterial load and treatment response in pulmonary tuberculosis. *Int J Tuberc Lung D* 2010;14(12):1596–602.

49. Cobelens FG, Egwaga SM, van Ginkel T, Muwinge H, Matee MI, and Borgdorff MW. Tuberculin skin testing in patients with HIV infection: Limited benefit of reduced cutoff values. *Clin Infect Dis.* 2006;43(5):634–9.

50. Cattamanchi A, Smith R, Steingart KR, Metcalfe JZ, Date A, Coleman C, Marston BJ, Huang L, Hopewell PC, and Pai M. Interferon-gamma release assays for the diagnosis of latent tuberculosis infection in HIV-infected individuals: A systematic review and meta-analysis. *Jaids-J Acq Imm Def.* 2011;56(3):230–8.

51. Cattamanchi A, Dowdy DW, Davis JL, Worodria W, Yoo S, Joloba M, Matovu J, Hopewell PC, and Huang L. Sensitivity of direct versus concentrated sputum smear microscopy in HIV-infected patients suspected of having pulmonary tuberculosis. *BMC Infect Dis.* 2009;9:53.

52. Kivihya-Ndugga LE, van Cleeff MR, Githui WA, Nganga LW, Kibuga DK, Odhiambo JA, and Klatser PR. A comprehensive comparison of Ziehl-Neelsen and fluorescence microscopy for the diagnosis of tuberculosis in a resource-poor urban setting. *Int J Tuberc Lung Dis.* 2003;7(12):1163–71.

53. Steingart KR, Henry M, Ng V, Hopewell PC, Ramsay A, Cunningham J, Urbanczik R, Perkins M, Aziz MA, and Pai M. Fluorescence versus conventional sputum smear microscopy for tuberculosis: A systematic review. *Lancet Infect Dis.* 2006;6(9):570–81.

54. Bruchfeld J, Aderaye G, Palme IB, Bjorvatn B, Kallenius G, and Lindquist L. Sputum concentration improves diagnosis of tuberculosis in a setting with a high prevalence of HIV. *Trans R Soc Trop Med Hyg* 2000;94(6):677–80.

55. Steingart KR, Ng V, Henry M, Hopewell PC, Ramsay A, Cunningham J, Urbanczik R, Perkins MD, Aziz MA, and Pai M. Sputum processing methods to improve the sensitivity of smear microscopy for tuberculosis: A systematic review. *Lancet Infect Dis.* 2006;6(10):664–74.

56. Pathmanathan I, Date A, Coggin WL, Nkengasong J, Piatek AS, and Alexander H. Rolling out Xpert MTB/RIF (R) for tuberculosis detection in HIV-positive populations: An opportunity for systems strengthening. *Afr J Lab Med.* 2017;6(2).

57. Boehme CC et al. Rapid molecular detection of tuberculosis and rifampin resistance. *N Engl J Med.* 2010;363(11):1005–15.

58. Ngwira LG, Corbett EL, Khundi M, Barnes GL, Nkhoma A, Murowa M, Cohn S, Moulton LH, Chaisson RE, and Dowdy DW. Screening for tuberculosis with Xpert MTB/RIF versus fluorescent microscopy among adults newly diagnosed with HIV in rural Malawi: A cluster randomized trial (CHEPETSA). *Clin Infect Dis.* 2019 Mar 19;68(7):1176–83.

59. Dorman SE, Schumacher SG, and Alland D. Xpert MTB/RIF Ultra for detection of *Mycobacterium tuberculosis* and rifampicin resistance: A prospective multicentre diagnostic accuracy study (vol. 18, pg 76, 2018). *Lancet Infect Dis.* 2018;18(4):376.

60. Word Health Organization. WHO Meeting Report of a Technical Expert Consultation: Non-inferiority analysis of Xpert MTB/RIF Ultra compared to Xpert MTB/RIF. 2017.

61. Kendall EA, Schumacher SG, Denkinger CM, and Dowdy DW. Estimated clinical impact of the Xpert MTB/RIF Ultra cartridge for diagnosis of pulmonary tuberculosis: A modeling study. *PLoS Med.* 2017;14(12).

62. Xie YL et al. Evaluation of a rapid molecular drug-susceptibility test for tuberculosis. *N Engl J Med.* 2017;377(11):1043–54.

63. Luetkemeyer AF et al., Adult ACTGAST. Evaluation of two line probe assays for rapid detection of *Mycobacterium tuberculosis*, tuberculosis (TB) drug resistance, and non-TB Mycobacteria in HIV-infected individuals with suspected TB. *J Clin Microbiol.* 2014;52(4):1052–9.

64. Gupta-Wright A et al. Rapid urine-based screening for tuberculosis in HIV-positive patients admitted to hospital in Africa (STAMP): A pragmatic, multicentre, parallel-group, double-blind, randomised controlled trial. *Lancet* 2018;392(10144):292–301.

65. World Health Organization. *Tuberculosis Global Report*. 2019.

66. Tsiouris SJ, Gandhi NR, El-Sadr WM, and Friedland G. Tuberculosis and HIV-needed: A new paradigm for the control and management of linked epidemics. *MedGenMed* 2007;9(3):62.

67. O'Donnell MR et al. Re-inventing adherence: Toward a patient-centered model of care for drug-resistant tuberculosis and HIV. *Int J Tuberc Lung Dis*. 2016;20(4):430–4.

68. World Health Organization. End TB Strategy. 2014.

69. Jack C, Lalloo U, Karim QA, Karim SA, El-Sadr W, Cassol S, and Friedland G. A pilot study of once-daily antiretroviral therapy integrated with tuberculosis directly observed therapy in a resource-limited setting. *Jaids-J Acq Imm Def*. 2004;36(4):929–34.

70. Gandhi NR, Moll AP, Lalloo U, Pawinski R, Zeller K, Moodley P, Meyer E, Friedland G, Tugela Ferry C, and Research C. Successful integration of tuberculosis and HIV treatment in rural South Africa: The Sizonq'oba study. *J Acquired Immune Defic Syndr*. 2009;50(1):37–43.

71. Karim SSA et al. Timing of initiation of antiretroviral drugs during tuberculosis therapy. *N Engl J Med*. 2010;362(8):697–706.

72. Karim SSA et al. Integration of antiretroviral therapy with tuberculosis treatment. *N Engl J Med*. 2011;365(16):1492–501.

73. Blanc FX et al., Team CS. Earlier versus later start of antiretroviral therapy in HIV-infected adults with tuberculosis. *N Engl J Med*. 2011;365(16):1471–81.

74. Havlir DV et al., Study ACTG. Timing of antiretroviral therapy for HIV-1 infection and tuberculosis. *N Engl J Med*. 2011;365(16):1482–91.

75. Gupta-Wright A et al. Tuberculosis in hospitalised patients with HIV: Clinical characteristics, mortality, and implications from the STAMP trial. *Clin Infect Dis*. 2019.

76. Nahid P et al. Official American Thoracic Society/Centers for Disease Control and Prevention/Infectious Diseases Society of America Clinical Practice Guidelines: Treatment of drug-susceptible tuberculosis. *Clin Infect Dis*. 2016;63(7):e147–e95.

77. Imperial MZ et al. A patient-level pooled analysis of treatment-shortening regimens for drug-susceptible pulmonary tuberculosis. *Nat Med*. 2018;24(11):1708–15.

78. Lienhardt C, and Nahid P. Advances in clinical trial design for development of new TB treatments: A call for innovation. *PLoS Med*. 2019;16(3):e1002769.

79. Friedland GH. HIV medication adherence. The intersection of biomedical, behavioral, and social science research and clinical practice. *J Acquired Immune Defic Syndr*. 2006;43(Suppl 1):S3–9.

80. Altice FL, Kamarulzaman A, Soriano VV, Schechter M, and Friedland GH. Treatment of medical, psychiatric, and substance-use comorbidities in people infected with HIV who use drugs. *Lancet* 2010;376(9738):367–87.

81. Gardner EM, Sharma S, Peng G, Hullsiek KH, Burman WJ, Macarthur RD, Chesney M, Telzak EE, Friedland G, and Mannheimer SB. Differential adherence to combination antiretroviral therapy is associated with virological failure with resistance. *AIDS* 2008;22(1):75–82.

82. Bionghi N, Daftary A, Maharaj B, Msibi Z, Amico KR, Friedland G, Orrell C, Padayatchi N, and O'Donnell MR. Pilot evaluation of a second-generation electronic pill box for adherence to bedaquiline and antiretroviral therapy in drug-resistant TB/HIV co-infected patients in KwaZulu-Natal, South Africa. *BMC Infect Dis*. 2018;18(1):171.

83. O'Donnell MR, Padayatchi N, Daftary A, Orrell C, Dooley KE, Rivet Amico K, Friedland G. Antiretroviral switching and bedaquiline treatment of drug-resistant tuberculosis HIV coinfection. *Lancet HIV* 2019;6(3):e201–4.

84. Meintjes G, Wilkinson RJ, Morroni C, Pepper DJ, Rebe K, Rangaka MX, Oni T, and Maartens G. Randomized placebo-controlled trial of prednisone for paradoxical tuberculosis-associated immune reconstitution inflammatory syndrome. *AIDS* 2010;24(15):2381–90.

85. Meintjes G et al., Pred ARTTT. Prednisone for the prevention of paradoxical tuberculosis-associated IRIS. *N Engl J Med*. 2018;379(20):1915–25.

86. Dooley KE, Sayre P, Borland J, Purdy E, Chen S, Song I, Peppercorn A, Everts S, Piscitelli S, and Flexner C. Safety, tolerability, and pharmacokinetics of the HIV integrase inhibitor dolutegravir given twice daily with rifampin or once daily with rifabutin: Results of a phase 1 study among healthy subjects. *J Acquired Immune Defic Syndr*. 2013;62(1):21–7.

87. Dooley KE et al., group Is. Dolutegravir-based antiretroviral therapy for patients co-infected with tuberculosis and HIV: A multicenter, noncomparative, open-label, randomized trial... *Clin Infect Dis*. 2020 Feb 3;70(4):549–56.

88. Nahid P et al. Treatment of drug-resistant tuberculosis. An official ATS/CDC/ERS/IDSA clinical practice guideline. *Am J Respir Crit Care Med*. 2019;200(10):e93–e142.

89. World Health Organization. Update of recommendations on first- and second-line antiretroviral regimens. 2019.

90. WHO consolidated guidelines on drug-resistant tuberculosis treatment. WHO Guidelines Approved by the Guidelines Review Committee. Geneva, 2019.

91. Zelnick J et al. Severe adherence challenges in the treatment of multi- and extensively drug resistant tuberculosis and HIV: Electronic dose monitoring and mixed methods to identify and characterize high-risk subpopulations. *10th International AIDS Conference on HIV Science Mexico City*, Mexico, 2019.

92. Loveday M, Wallengren K, Brust J, Roberts J, Voce A, Margot B, Ngozo J, Master I, Cassell G, and Padayatchi N. Community-based care vs. centralised hospitalisation for MDR-TB patients, KwaZulu-Natal, South Africa. *Int J Tuberc Lung Dis*. 2015;19(2):163–71.

93. Brust JCM et al. Improved survival and cure rates with concurrent treatment for multidrug-resistant tuberculosis-human immunodeficiency virus coinfection in South Africa. *Clin Infect Dis*. 2018;66(8):1246–53.

94. Aung KJM, Van Deun A, Declercq E, Sarker MR, Das PK, Hossain MA, and Rieder HL. Successful "9-month Bangladesh regimen" for multidrug-resistant tuberculosis among over 500 consecutive patients. *Int J Tuberc Lung D* 2014;18(10):1180–7.

95. Van Deun A, Maug AK, Salim MA, Das PK, Sarker MR, Daru P, and Rieder HL. Short, highly effective, and inexpensive standardized treatment of multidrug-resistant tuberculosis. *Am J Respir Crit Care Med*. 2010;182(5):684–92.

96. Nunn AJ et al., Collaborators SS. A trial of a shorter regimen for rifampin-resistant tuberculosis. *N Engl J Med*. 2019;380(13):1201–13.

97. World Health Organization. Rapid Communication: Key changes to the treatment of drug-resistant tuberculosis 2019.

98. Dheda K, Gumbo T, Maartens G, Dooley KE, Murray M, Furin J, Nardell EA, Warren RM, Lancet Respiratory Medicine drug-resistant tuberculosis Commission g. The Lancet Respiratory Medicine Commission: 2019 update: Epidemiology, pathogenesis, transmission, diagnosis, and management of multidrug-resistant and incurable tuberculosis. *Lancet Respir Med*. 2019;7(9):820–6.

99. Badri M, Wilson D, and Wood R. Effect of highly active antiretroviral therapy on incidence of tuberculosis in South Africa: A cohort study. *Lancet* 2002;359(9323):2059–64.

100. Williams BG, Granich R, De Cock KM, Glaziou P, Sharma A, and Dye C. Antiretroviral therapy for tuberculosis control in nine African countries. *Proc Natl Acad Sci USA* 2010;107(45):19485–9.

101. Suthar AB et al. Antiretroviral therapy for prevention of tuberculosis in adults with HIV: A systematic review and meta-analysis. *PLoS Med.* 2012;9(7):e1001270.

102. Lawn SD, Harries AD, Williams BG, Chaisson RE, Losina E, De Cock KM, and Wood R. Antiretroviral therapy and the control of HIV-associated tuberculosis. Will ART do it? *Int J Tuberc Lung Dis.* 2011;15(5):571–81.

103. Sterling TR et al., North American ACCoR, Design of the International Epidemiologic Databases to Evaluate A. Risk factors for tuberculosis after highly active antiretroviral therapy initiation in the United States and Canada: Implications for tuberculosis screening. *J Infect Dis.* 2011;204(6):893–901.

104. Group TAS, Danel C et al. A trial of early antiretrovirals and isoniazid preventive therapy in Africa. *N Engl J Med.* 2015;373(9):808–22.

105. Group ISS, Lundgren JD et al. Initiation of antiretroviral therapy in early asymptomatic HIV infection. *N Engl J Med.* 2015;373(9):795–807.

106. Dravid A et al. Incidence of tuberculosis among HIV infected individuals on long term antiretroviral therapy in private healthcare sector in Pune, Western India. *BMC Infect Dis.* 2019;19(1):714.

107. Comstock GW, Tockman MS, Helsing KJ, and Hennesy KM. Standardized respiratory questionnaires: Comparison of the old with the new. *Am Rev Respir Dis.* 1979;119(1):45–53.

108. Comstock GW, and Woolpert SF. Preventive treatment of untreated, nonactive tuberculosis in an Eskimo population. *Arch Environ Health* 1972;25(5):333–7.

109. Badje A et al., Grp TAS. Effect of isoniazid preventive therapy on risk of death in west African, HIV-infected adults with high CD4 cell counts: Long-term follow-up of the Temprano ANRS 12136 trial. *Lancet Glob Health.* 2017;5(11):E1080–E9.

110. Golub JE, Pronyk P, Mohapi L, Thsabangu N, Moshabela M, Struthers H, Gray GE, McIntyre JA, Chaisson RE, and Martinson NA. Isoniazid preventive therapy, HAART and tuberculosis risk in HIV-infected adults in South Africa: A prospective cohort. *AIDS* 2009;23(5):631–6.

111. Organization WH. *Latent TB Infection: Updated and Consolidated Guidelines for Programmatic Management.* Geneva, 2018.

112. Samandari T, Agizew et al. 6-month versus 36-month isoniazid preventive treatment for tuberculosis in adults with HIV infection in Botswana: A randomised, double-blind, placebo-controlled trial. *Lancet* 2011;377(9777):1588–98.

113. Golub JE, Cohn S, Saraceni V, Cavalcante SC, Pacheco AG, Moulton LH, Durovni B, and Chaisson RE. Long-term protection from isoniazid preventive therapy for tuberculosis in HIV-infected patients in a medium-burden tuberculosis setting: The TB/HIV in Rio (THRio) study. *Clin Infect Dis.* 2015;60(4):639–45.

114. Alsdurf H, Hill PC, Matteelli A, Getahun H, and Menzies D. The cascade of care in diagnosis and treatment of latent tuberculosis infection: A systematic review and meta-analysis. *Lancet Infect Dis.* 2016;16(11):1269–78.

115. Sterling TR et al., Team TBTCPTS. Three months of rifapentine and isoniazid for latent tuberculosis infection. *N Engl J Med.* 2011;365(23):2155–66.

116. Sterling TR et al., Tuberculosis Trials Consortium tACTGftPTBT-TiotTBTC, the Aids Clinical Trials Group for the Prevent Tb Trial are listed in the Supplement I. Three months of weekly rifapentine and isoniazid for treatment of *Mycobacterium tuberculosis* infection in HIV-coinfected persons. *AIDS* 2016;30(10):1607–15.

117. Belknap R et al., Team TBTCiS. Self-administered versus directly observed once-weekly isoniazid and Rifapentine treatment of latent tuberculosis infection: A randomized trial. *Ann Intern Med.* 2017;167(10):689–97.

118. McClintock AH, Eastment M, McKinney CM, Pitney CL, Narita M, Park DR, Dhanireddy S, and Molnar A. Treatment completion for latent tuberculosis infection: A retrospective cohort study comparing 9 months of isoniazid, 4 months of rifampin and 3 months of isoniazid and rifapentine. *BMC Infect Dis.* 2017;17(1):146.

119. Susan Swindells RR et al. . *One month of rifapentine/isoniazid to prevent TB in people with HIV.N Engl J Med* 2019; 380:1001–11.

120. Menzies D et al. Four months of Rifampin or nine months of Isoniazid for latent tuberculosis in adults. *N Engl J Med.* 2018;379(5):440–53.

121. Gupta A et al., Team IPTAS. Isoniazid preventive therapy in HIV-infected pregnant and postpartum women. *N Engl J Med.* 2019;381(14):1333–46.

122. Grimsrud A, Sharp J, Kalombo C, Bekker LG, and Myer L. Implementation of community-based adherence clubs for stable antiretroviral therapy patients in Cape Town, South Africa. *J Int AIDS Soc.* 2015;18:19984.

123. DiStefano MJ, and Schmidt H. mHealth for tuberculosis treatment adherence: A framework to guide ethical planning, implementation, and evaluation. *Global Health Sci Pract.* 2016;4(2):211–21.

124. Gilbert JA, Long EF, Brooks RP, Friedland GH, Moll AP, Townsend JP, Galvani AP, and Shenoi SV. Integrating community-based interventions to reverse the convergent TB/HIV epidemics in rural South Africa. *PLOS ONE* 2015;10(5):e0126267.

125. Pathmanathan I, Pasipamire M, Pals S, Dokubo EK, Preko P, Ao T, Mazibuko S, Ongole J, Dhlamini T, and Haumba S. High uptake of antiretroviral therapy among HIV-positive TB patients receiving co-located services in Swaziland. *PLOS ONE* 2018; 13(5):e0196831.

126. Kerschberger B, Hilderbrand K, Boulle AM, Coetzee D, Goemaere E, De Azevedo V, and Van Cutsem G. The effect of complete integration of HIV and TB services on time to initiation of antiretroviral therapy: A before-after study. *PLOS ONE* 2012;7(10).

127. Burnett SM, Zawedde-Muyanja S, Hermans SM, Weaver MR, Colebunders R, and Manabe YC. Effect of TB/HIV integration on TB and HIV indicators in Rural Ugandan Health Facilities. *J Acquired Immune Defic Syndr.* 2018;79(5):605–11.

128. Gilbert JA, Shenoi SV, Moll AP, Friedland GH, Paltiel AD, and Galvani AP. Cost-effectiveness of community-based TB/HIV screening and linkage to care in Rural South Africa. *PLOS ONE* 2016;11(12):e0165614.

129. Reid MJA et al. Building a tuberculosis-free world: The Lancet Commission on tuberculosis. *Lancet* 2019;393(10178):1331–84.

130. Naidoo K, Gengiah S, Singh S, Stillo J, and Padayatchi N. Quality of TB care among people living with HIV: Gaps and solutions. *J Clin Tuberc Other Mycobact Dis.* 2019;17:100122.

131. Cox HS, Morrow M, and Deutschmann PW. Long term efficacy of DOTS regimens for tuberculosis: Systematic review. *BMJ* 2008;336(7642):484–7.

132. Tian JH, Lu ZX, Bachmann MO, and Song FJ. Effectiveness of directly observed treatment of tuberculosis: A systematic review of controlled studies. *Int J Tuberc Lung Dis.* 2014;18(9):1092–8.

133. Karumbi J, and Garner P. Directly observed therapy for treating tuberculosis. *Cochrane Database Syst Rev.* 2015;(5):CD003343.

134. Seepamore BK et al. Adherence support groups for patients with drug-resistant TB/HIV in South Africa: The Praxis Study Intervention. *50th Union Conference on Lung Health*, Hyderabad, India, 2019.

135. Pathmanathan I, Pevzner E, Cavanaugh J, and Nelson L. Addressing tuberculosis in differentiated care provision for people living with HIV. *Bull World Health Organ.* 2017;95(1):3.

136. Goosby E, Jamison D, Swaminathan S, Reid M, and Zuccala E. The Lancet Commission on tuberculosis: Building a tuberculosis-free world. *Lancet* 2018;391(10126):1132–3.

137. Sinha P, Shenoi SV, and Friedland GH. Opportunities for community health workers to contribute to global efforts to end tuberculosis. *Global Public Health.*, 2020, 15:3, 474–84.

138. Moll A, Choi K, Shenoi SV, and Friedland GH Community-based TB case finding and IPT referrals from alcohol venues in rural South Africa. *50th Union World Conference on Lung Health*, Hyderbad, India, 2019.

139. Howard AA, and El-Sadr WM. Integration of tuberculosis and HIV services in sub-Saharan Africa: Lessons learned. *Clin Infect Dis.* 2010;50(Suppl 3):S238–44.

140. Theron G, Jenkins HE, Cobelens F, Abubakar I, Khan AJ, Cohen T, and Dowdy DW. Data for action: Collection and use of local data to end tuberculosis. *Lancet* 2015;386(10010):2324–33.

141. Naidoo P, Theron G, Rangaka MX, Chihota VN, Vaughan L, Brey ZO, and Pillay Y. The South African Tuberculosis Care Cascade: Estimated Losses and Methodological Challenges. *J Infect Dis.* 2017;216(Suppl_7):S702–S13.

16

Drug-Resistant Tuberculosis

KEERTAN DHEDA, ALIASGAR ESMAIL, ANZAAN DIPPENAAR, ROBIN WARREN,
JENNIFER FURIN, AND CHRISTOPH LANGE

INTRODUCTION

Tuberculosis (TB) is far from eradicated and remains the foremost single infectious disease killer worldwide.[1] TB has killed almost a billion people in the last two centuries and remains out of control in Africa and many parts of Asia. Multidrug-resistant TB (MDR-TB: resistance to rifampicin and isoniazid), and resistance beyond MDR-TB (additional resistance to fluoroquinolones, and other second-line drugs [SLIDs], including injectable drugs) is subverting TB control in several parts of the world through increased mortality and diversion of scarce resources, thus marginalizing TB treatment programs. In 2017 the World Health Organization (WHO) reported that the estimated burden of MDR or rifampicin-resistant TB was ~560,000 cases.[1] Notably, there has been a spike in the detection of TB over the last several years in several high-burden countries including the Russian Federation, South Africa, Congo, India, and China.[1–3] Consequently, the estimated burden of MDR-TB had grown dramatically in terms of the absolute number of cases (from 450,000 cases in 2012 to ~660,000 cases in 2016).[1,3,4] The trend is in keeping with the overall global increase in the burden of antimicrobial resistance (AMR) in general, i.e., to bacteria, fungi, and viruses. Indeed, it is estimated that by 2050 AMR will result in ~10 million deaths annually and will cost the global economy up to $100 trillion.[5] A major contributor to this estimate is drug-resistant TB (DR-TB). Despite the advent of newer drugs, MDR-TB and resistance beyond MDR-TB have been superseded by programmatically incurable TB.

It is critical to prioritize interventions against DR-TB because of its ability to cripple and undermine current programs. MDR- and resistance beyond MDR-TB are associated with considerable morbidity,[1,6,7] high mortality (30%–50%, and thus worse than most cancers),[7–9] and have a deleterious impact on health-care worker recruitment in TB-endemic countries,[7,10] and are extremely costly to the program and to the country. For example, in South Africa in 2012, DR-TB was already consuming 40% of the total TB resources despite forming less than 5% of the total TB case burden.[11] A recent global KPMG report suggested that, in parallel with other African countries, South Africa's GDP was probably impacted by 2%–3% due to TB, equating to ~US$10 billion per annum.[12] Thus, TB and DR-TB have had a massive impact on economic growth, and any cost-effectiveness or affordability of interventions must be interpreted in context.

Encouragingly, there have been a number of advances in new drugs and diagnostic technologies after a dearth of almost 40 years. The term "XDR-TB" (extensively drug-resistant TB) has become a misnomer as SLIDs are no longer part of the frontline regimen (though they may still be useful in selected situations), and a revision of the nomenclature is required.[13] Perhaps, in the future "XDR-TB" will likely be defined by resistance to key second-line drugs including a combination of fluoroquinolones, linezolid, and bedaquiline.

This chapter adopts a clinical perspective and focuses on the clinical and molecular epidemiology, diagnosis, and clinical management of DR-TB. A patient-centered and human rights approach to treatment is also discussed. There are several other important aspects of DR-TB including disease pathogenesis, drug-specific pharmacokinetic and pharmacodynamic aspects, treatment of MDR-TB in children, transmission of MDR-TB, and major research priorities for MDR- and resistance beyond MDR-TB. However, these have recently been covered in detail elsewhere[7] and will not be discussed further due to space constraints. Thus, their exclusion here does not undermine their critical importance in the DR-TB landscape.

CLINICAL AND MOLECULAR EPIDEMIOLOGY

Molecular epidemiology has played an important role in advancing our understanding of DR-TB epidemics (Figure 16.1 and Table 16.1). First, on a population-based level, strain typing provides a means of identifying chains of transmission and providing an indication of how well TB control programs function with respect to transmission control.[1,14,15] Second, on a patient level, strain typing may determine the mechanism whereby DR-TB develops in an individual.[16–19] Third, DNA sequencing, as a molecular tool, increasingly plays a role in the identification of drug resistance in clinical isolates.[20–23]

Numerous molecular epidemiologic studies have conclusively demonstrated that DR-TB is transmitted,[15,17,24–30] albeit to different degrees.[31] On a population level DR-TB develops through: (i) primary infection with a drug-resistant strain[32] (including reinfection with a drug-resistant strain during/after treatment for drug-susceptible TB),[16,17,19,33] or mixed infection with a drug-susceptible and drug-resistant strain with unmasking of the drug-resistant strain during treatment for drug-susceptible TB,[16] or (ii) acquisition of resistance during therapy.[34–37] It is estimated that ~95% of MDR-TB occurring in new TB cases and ~60% in previously treated cases are due to transmission.[38] This contrasts with previous beliefs that suggested that DR-TB was mainly acquired during antibiotic treatment (secondary resistance) and that acquisition of resistance had a fitness cost that limits transmissibility.[39] The restoration of a fitness deficit due to a drug-resistant mutation is thought to occur through epistatic interactions with compensatory mutations in genes encoding in the same or linked pathway(s).[40–42] For example, compensatory mutations of rifampicin conferring resistance mutations in *rpoB* have been described in *rpoA* and *rpoC*.[25,28,41,43]

Molecular epidemiology is now entering a new era where next-generation whole-genome sequencing (WGS) is replacing IS*6110* DNA fingerprinting,[44] MIRU-VNTR (mycobacterial interspersed repetitive unit-variable number tandem repeat) typing,[45,46] and spoligotyping[47] due to its superior resolution to study transmission dynamics[7,48–52] (Table 16.1). Deciphering DR-TB transmission remains crucial for the optimization of local and global control measures and the early detection of MDR and XDR outbreaks.[53–55] Furthermore, the resolution of WGS now provides the opportunity to link genome variants with pathobiology and drug resistance, thereby ensuring a better understanding of factors that drive the DR-TB epidemic as well as providing information to optimize therapy through genetic drug susceptibility testing (DST).[53,56,57]

WGS-based phylogenetic analysis has also enabled the study of the chronology in which resistance is acquired,[25,27,35,58–61] and the factors influencing the emergence of drug resistance.[36,62] Analysis of the LAM4 clone (Tugela Ferry, South Africa) from the first XDR-TB outbreak reported in 2006[15] suggested that development of XDR-TB in KwaZulu-Natal had its roots in drug resistance that arose in the late 1950s, that isoniazid was the first drug resistance acquired, and that MDR-TB emerged in the 1980s, soon after the introduction of rifampicin.[27] Drug resistance is thus driven by cycles of *de novo* drug resistance acquisition, often due to ineffective treatment regimens,[62] diversification, clonal spread, and amplification of resistance.[27] Clones of genetically distinct strains have now evolved to become the dominant circulating DR-TB strains in defined geographical regions that may persist for decades, as observed in Eastern Europe,[25,63,64] Portugal,[65] South Africa,[58,66,67] and South America.[59] WGS will further provide the opportunity to longitudinally measure the impact of policy changes (shortened treatment regimens[68] and implementation of new and repurposed drugs[69,70]) on the trajectory of current DR-TB epidemics, emergence of drug resistance,[35] and past failures of TB control programs. Indeed, it was shown that the mismanagement of even a single TB patient can lead to a public health crisis.[71,72]

WGS is now being used to measure the contribution of transmission driving DR-TB epidemics and in so doing is questioning whether the high resolution of WGS alters our current understanding, which is based on other traditional genotyping techniques.[48] However, interpretation of these early studies is reliant on ill-defined thresholds used to delineate transmission.[29,73,74] Importantly, these studies have concluded that determining the direction of transmission is difficult within the context of institutional or household settings where strain diversity is minimal.[75] Similarly, defining transmission chains in endemic settings will be dependent on the evolutionary rate, which may be strain dependent.[76,77] If the genome of a strain remains stable over many years, this may explain the absence of a direct correlation between clustering (transmission) and epidemiologic links between patients. An alternative explanation is that casual contact is the driver of transmission.[78] The slow evolutionary rate and ability of the bacterium to exist in a dormant state for many years in an individual after initial infection before progressing to disease (known as latent TB) further complicates determining the directionality of transmission.

Despite these limitations, WGS has provided novel insights into mechanisms driving resistance through reinfection,[48,79–82] transmission,[29,30,54,63,73,77,78,83–85] spread of specific drug-resistant strains,[29,30,54,59,74] fatal nosocomial transmission,[86] and incorrect classification of the pathogen causing disease[87] in various global settings.

The global DR-TB epidemic continues to be exacerbated by the movement of people with infectious DR-TB (Figure 16.2),[88–96] which can now be monitored through WGS of the infection-causing *Mycobacterium tuberculosis* strains. These studies show that refugees fleeing from conflict and poverty in high DR-TB incidence countries, or seeking an education, are introducing DR-TB into low incidence settings.[83,88–90,93,96,97] This has prompted the development of assays, based on WGS data, to screen populations at risk of having been exposed to DR-TB in their country of origin, i.e., Russian sex workers in Spain.[97]

Understanding intra-country/community transmission will be critical for directing resources to identified infectious sources and transmission "hot spots,"[88,98] which can now be achieved by combining WGS with geographic information systems (GIS) coordinates.[98] Application of this methodology in South Africa has highlighted the large distance between place of residence and the treatment facility, thereby suggesting how DR-TB can spread through public transport networks ultimately leading to endemic resistance beyond MDR-TB.[98,99]

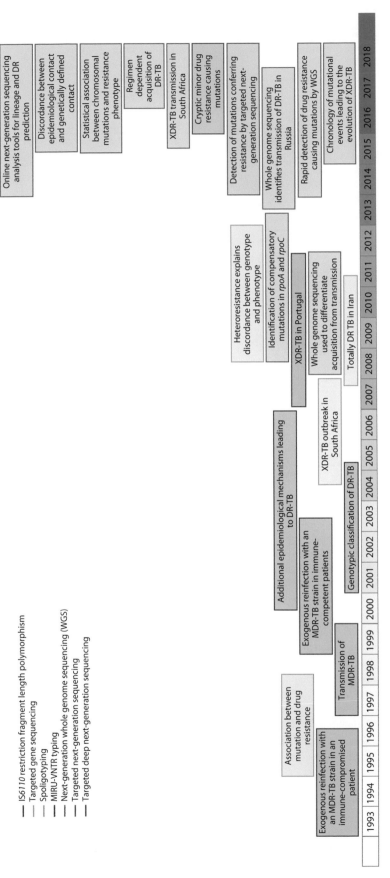

Figure 16.1 Timeline of key molecular epidemiological findings using different genotyping tools. Different colors indicate genotyping tools used for each finding. MDR, multidrug resistant; MIRU-VNTR, mycobacterial interspersed repetitive unit-variable numbers of tandem repeats; XDR, extensively drug-resistant (though this term will likely be redefined soon); DR, drug resistant; TB, tuberculosis. (Adapted from Dheda K et al. *Lancet Respir Med.* 2017.)

Table 16.1 Molecular epidemiological genotyping methods

Method/technique	Advantages	Disadvantages	Applications
Insertion sequence *6110* restriction fragment length polymorphism[44]	High discriminatory index	Requires culture and DNA extraction; cannot differentiate between drug-sensitive and drug-resistant strains; not directly comparable between labs	Identification of transmission chains, and temporal changes in the strain population, reinfection, and strain migration
Spacer oligonucleotide typing[47]	Direct genotyping of clinical specimens; relatively inexpensive; requires few laboratory resources	Low discriminatory index; undergoes homoplasy; cannot differentiate between drug-sensitive and drug-resistant strains	Classification of strains according to lineages, reinfection, and strain migration
Mycobacterial interspersed repetitive unit-variable number tandem repeat (MIRU-VNTR)[65,68,261]	Direct genotyping of clinical specimens; high discriminatory index; global reference database	Undergoes homoplasy; cannot differentiate between drug-sensitive and drug-resistant strains	Identification of transmission chains, and temporal changes in the strain population, reinfection, and strain migration
Targeted Sanger sequencing[20,72]	Direct genotyping of clinical specimens; relatively inexpensive	Information limited to nucleotide variants in a selected set of genes; limited or no strain typing information	Identification of mutations conferring resistance
Targeted deep sequencing[110–112,262,263]	Direct genotyping of clinical specimens	Information limited to nucleotide variants in a selected set of genes; no strain type information; more expensive; requires high-level laboratory infrastructure	Identification of mutations conferring resistance and heteroresistance
Whole-genome sequencing[23,49,57,73,101,102,105,264–266]	Comprehensive analysis of the genome of the pathogen	Requires culture (or specimen enrichment); more expensive; might be computationally demanding or complex	Identification of transmission chains, mutations conferring resistance, heteroresistance (low resolution), mixed infections, specimen heterogeneity, and intrapatient evolution

The phenomenal resolution of WGS also promises to revolutionize the diagnosis of DR-TB.[23,100–103] Guidelines are now being developed on how to interpret WGS data to guide drug choices and to individualize treatment.[23,101,104] A number of countries have initiated WGS for both diagnosis and epidemiological surveillance.[23,80,85,101,102,105–108] Furthermore, it is now possible to use WGS to study the natural history of intrapatient evolution of drug resistance by simultaneously monitoring the sequences of multiple genes conferring resistance.[62,109] However, numerous limitations still exist for the translation of genotypic data into its phenotypic consequences. To address this, large studies (Comprehensive Resistance Prediction for Tuberculosis: An International Consortium [CRyPTIC] and the Relational Sequencing TB Data Platform [ReSeqTB]) have been initiated to establish associations between genotype and phenotype using WGS and culture-based DST.

An alternative to WGS is targeted next-generation deep sequencing.[110,111] This method allows variants to be detected in minor *M. tuberculosis* populations, termed heteroresistance. This has allowed researchers to find resistance at a frequency below the classical 1% proportion method. It is envisaged that targeted deep sequencing may be a replacement for culture-based DST. It also has the potential to identify resistance earlier, thereby allowing

researchers to get a greater understanding of the biology of the evolution of drug resistance. An added advantage is the potential for clinical decisions to be made earlier and for treatment regimens to be individualized based on the comprehensive drug resistance profile of the *M. tuberculosis* isolate infecting the patient, but exactly how this should be implemented remains unclear.[110,112] However, the limited number of genetic targets being evaluated currently precludes targeted deep sequencing as a method to study the epidemiology of DR-TB.

DIAGNOSIS OF MDR-TB AND RESISTANCE BEYOND MDR-TB

The emergence and spread of DR-TB is responsible for destabilizing TB control in high-burden countries.[1,7] Improving TB diagnostics has the potential to improve patient outcomes,[113–116] limit the emergence of resistance,[116,117] and restrict the transmission of DR-TB.[118] However, only two-thirds of the estimated 10 million cases of TB are diagnosed each year and only one-third of the bacteriologically confirmed TB patients are evaluated with phenotypic DST for first-line drugs.[1] The net effect of these "mistreated cases" on transmission is evidenced in countries such as Russia,

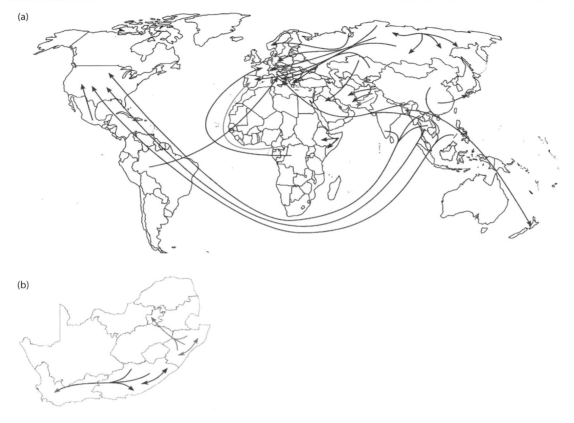

Figure 16.2 Inter-country and intra-country spread of DR-TB according to *M. tuberculosis* genotype. (a) Worldwide spread of drug-resistant strains of *M. tuberculosis*. Red = Beijing strain.[64,94,97,267–274] Green = LAM9 strain.[275] Light blue = Haarlem1 strain.[276] Purple = T1 strain.[277] Orange = S strain[89] Dark blue = untyped strains.[96,278–280] (b) Ongoing intra-country spread of XDR-TB strains in South Africa. Red = atypical Beijing strains. Green = LAM4 strain.[281,282] Intra-country spread has also been reported in Portugal[65] and Spain.[283] (Adapted from Dheda K et al. *Lancet Respir Med.* 2017.)

Ukraine, and Belarus where over 25% of the MDR-TB burden is attributed to person-to-person transmission.[1] This phenomenon is partly responsible for the predicted rise in DR-TB rates high-burden countries.[119]

PHENOTYPIC DST

Phenotypic DST involves incubating a bacterial isolate (grown from a clinical specimen) in the presence and absence of a specific drug and comparing its growth. This method is often the benchmark against which other tests are measured as it directly measures growth and is not reliant on proxies of resistance such as genetic mutations. However, discrepancies between methods are not uncommon and it has been suggested that for rifampicin, genotypic analysis may offer a more reliable reference standard in some contexts but not in others.[120–122] Furthermore, technical difficulties and inconsistent results are common for some drugs.

The first DSTs were developed and validated for solid culture using Lowenstein Jensen slopes or agar plates. However, more rapid commercial versions such as the Bactec MGIT 960 System (Becton Dickinson) are now routinely available, where results may be obtained in 7–12 days.[123] Alternative low-cost DST methods have also been developed that utilize titer plates, microscopic observation of colonies or oxidation–reduction dyes to indicate

growth of bacteria.[123,124] In some circumstances, the minimal inhibitory concentration (MIC) corresponding to resistance is not confidently known and, in these cases, clinicians may choose to treat patients with a higher dose of a particular drug (e.g., isoniazid and moxifloxacin).[123,125,126]

The main disadvantage of using phenotypic testing is the time taken to obtain a result which can range from 3 to 6 weeks, depending on the resources available.[127] This, coupled with demanding technical and infrastructural requirements, makes phenotypic DSTs less useful for patient management except in situations where determination of MICs is required as is the case for low-level fluoroquinolone resistance.[126,128] Another disadvantage of phenotypic DST is that hetero-resistant populations are difficult to quantify using the commonly implemented methods.

GENOTYPIC TESTING

Mutations in the mycobacterial DNA can render bacilli resistant to the action of specific anti-tuberculous drugs. Small nucleotide polymorphisms (SNPs) in genes encoding for drug targets or enzymes are a frequent cause of resistance, although insertions and deletions can also occur.[129,130] The loci implicated in *M. tuberculosis* resistance have been summarized previously.[7] Resistance to rifampicin is mainly is due to alteration in the DNA-dependent

RNA polymerase which is encoded by *rpoB*.[131] Genotypic markers of resistance in the 81 bp rifampicin resistance determining region (RRDR) have a high sensitivity and specificity,[132] resulting in the wide-spread implementation of genotypic rifampicin resistance screening in high TB burden countries.

The main advantage of screening for genotypic markers of resistance is that it is rapid since it does not rely on mycobacterial growth and can go from "specimen in" to "result out" in a few hours. Theoretically this means that patients could present to the clinic, be correctly diagnosed, and be started on effective treatment in a single clinical encounter.[128]

Xpert MTB/RIF is a commercially available quantitative real-time NAAT (nucleic acid amplification test) that diagnoses TB and rifampicin resistance in less than 2 hours.[133] It is an automated, cartridge-based system that can be performed in resourced decentralized locations, outside of reference laboratories and by staff with minimal laboratory training.[133] It has been widely validated, is endorsed by the WHO[134] and the US Federal Drug Administration (FDA)[135] for the initial diagnosis of TB and for the diagnosis of MDR-TB (based on rifampicin resistance), and is increasingly being deployed in high-burden countries. A meta-analysis has reported the sensitivity and specificity for rifampicin resistance to be 95% and 98%, respectively.[136] A new version of the Xpert MTB/RIF (resistance to rifampin) assay cartridge called the Xpert MTB/RIF Ultra was released in 2016. This assay includes multicopy insertion sequence targets (IS*6110* and IS*1081*), which, together with an improved sample volume, allow improved sensitivity in the detection and the differentiation of the *M. tuberculosis complex*.[137] The new cartridges have decreased run-time and improved chemistry, and use probe-based high-resolution melt to determine drug resistance. Its main added value is in the detection of TB in patients with smear negative disease where an increase in sensitivity of ~13% is achieved compared to the Xpert G4 cartridge.[137] Furthermore, Xpert Ultra, based on one preliminary study, may be useful in the diagnosis of TB meningitis when including trace results[138] though further data are awaited. Data on its use in other pauci-bacillary compartments are lacking. A new, point-of-care, portable, battery-operated Xpert Omni platform will likely become available late 2020. This device will use the Xpert Ultra cartridge and will allow for the detection of *M. tuberculosis* and determination of rifampicin resistance in remote locations. Xpert Omni may also prove to be a valuable tool for active case finding.[139]

There are several drawbacks of the Xpert MTB/RIF system. First, it does not detect isoniazid resistance; one in seven TB isolates worldwide is isoniazid mono-resistant (almost a third of TB cases in Eastern Europe).[140,141] Thus, many cases could potentially receive a suboptimal regimen (and effective monotherapy in the continuation phase), which may lead to poor patient outcomes and amplification of resistance.[140] Second, there is a significant false-positive rate for rifampicin resistance in settings with a low prevalence of MDR-TB. However, data on this is conflicting. For example, empiric evidence from Brazil (MDR-TB prevalence ~1%) has suggested the false-positive rates are low when used in programmatic settings (positive predictive value [PPV] ~90%).[142] Last, the assay has a high false-positive rate in patients with a previous history of TB.[137] This could potentially lead to the overtreatment of patients, unnecessarily exposing them to drug toxicity. Collectively, these data suggest that Xpert MTB/RIF may be used as a baseline assay for the diagnosis of TB in most settings. However, clinicians should be aware of the limitations of these assays.

LINE PROBE ASSAYS

Empiric MDR-TB treatment is usually initiated based on an Xpert MTB/RIF result in many high-burden countries like South Africa. However, confirmatory DST for first- and second-line drugs is subsequently performed using phenotypic DST, or often, using a line probe assay (LPA). LPA technology amplifies the target gene of interest followed by the reverse hybridization of the amplicons to a series of oligonucleotide probes immobilized on a membrane.[143] Several assays are available but the most widely used is the Hain GenoType MTBDR*plus* VER 2.0 which detects rifampicin and isoniazid resistance, and the Hain GenoType MTBDR*sl* VER 2.0 which detects fluoroquinolone and aminoglycoside resistance (Hain Lifescience, Germany).[144,145] The Hain MTBDR*plus* can be performed with reasonably high sensitivity and specificity directly on sputa or on a culture isolate.[41,42] It detects rifampicin and isoniazid resistance with a sensitivity of 97.7% and 95.4%, respectively, and a specificity of 91.8% and 89.0%, respectively, using smear positive sputum samples.[146,147] However, its accuracy for detecting rifampicin resistance may be lower in smear negative disease, with sensitivity and specificity of only 77.8% and 97.2%, respectively.[147]

A Cochrane systematic review showed that the Hain MTBDR*sl* assay (version 1.0) had a sensitivity and specificity of 85.1% (95% CI: 71.9, 92.7) and 98.2% (95% CI: 96.8, 99.0), respectively, for the detection of fluoroquinolone resistance using smear positive sputum. The performance was similar in culture isolates with a sensitivity and specificity of 83.1% (95% CI: 78.7, 86.7) and 97.7% (95% CI: 94.3, 99.1), respectively.[148] However, in smear negative samples, the sensitivity was significantly lower at 20.0% for the detection of ofloxacin resistance compared to 85.1% in smear positive samples.[146,149] Indeterminate rates for the detection of fluoroquinolone resistance using MTBDR*sl* is lower when performed on culture isolates than in smear positive sputum and smear negative sputum (0.2% vs. 1.9% vs. 5.1%).[146,149]

For combined SLID (amikacin, kanamycin, and capreomycin) resistance, the sensitivity and specificity of Hain MTBDR*sl* is 94.4% (95% CI: 25.2, 99.9) and 98.2% (95% CI: 88.9, 99.7), respectively, when performed on smear positive sputa. However, the sensitivity of MTBDR*sl* in smear negative sputa was significantly lower at 37.0% for amikacin compared to 94.4% in smear positive samples. The performance of MTBDR*sl* in detecting SLID resistance on culture isolates is best for amikacin 87.9% (95% CI: 82.1, 92.0) compared to capreomycin 79.5% (95% CI: 58.3, 91.4) or kanamycin 66.9% (95% CI: 44.1, 83.8) but retains high specificity for all three injectable drugs (combined SLID specificity of 99.5% [95% CI: 97.1, 99.9]). Indeterminate results for the detection of SLID resistance are lower when performed on culture isolates than in smear positive sputum and smear negative sputum (0.4% vs. 6.1% vs. 13.5%).[146,149,150]

In summary, LPAs have the potential to rapidly detect MDR-TB and resistance beyond MDR-TB, enabling clinicians to initiate appropriate treatment timeously. However, the performance of Hain MTBDR*sl* in smear negative sputum has suboptimal sensitivity for the detection of fluoroquinolone and SLID resistance, which is ~20%–30% with indeterminate rates of 5%–10%.[146] Thus, a negative LPA test result should prompt the clinician to further confirm susceptibility by phenotypic DST.[151]

NEXT-GENERATION WGS

Sequencing has the potential to provide a comprehensive genotypic DST. It facilitates the crafting of individualized treatment regimens, which are more likely to result in cure.[152] However, the clinical impact of this strategy in different settings remains to be established. Targeted next-generation sequencing (NGS) (sequencing of specific genes amplified by polymerase chain reaction [PCR]) is more sensitive and allows for the detection of resistance conferring mutations in sputum samples (see Figure 16.3). It also has the additional advantage of detecting, otherwise undetectable, micro-heteroresistance (emerging low-level drug-specific resistant populations) at diagnosis and during the course of treatment.

Patients with rifampicin resistance detected on Xpert MTB/RIF Ultra usually receive empiric MDR-TB treatment. However, even with regimen modification guided by the LPAs, inadvertent amplification of resistance is promoted due to suboptimal performance of LPA. This would likely be minimized with WGS or targeted NGS, as resistance to multiple drugs are simultaneously detected, thus facilitating precision medicine.[129] However, wide-spread clinical implementation of NGS is dubious since the

M. tuberculosis-specific DNA levels in sputum is below the detection limit of the assay (<1% of sputum DNA from a TB patient's sputa is mycobacterial in origin) and, currently, this test can only be reliably performed on DNA extracted from cultured isolates. The turnaround time for obtaining NGS results may be reduced by the use of "early positive" cultures (2–7 days), though further data about the utility of this approach are awaited.[153] Mutations associated with high confidence drug-specific resistance (including those that portend low- and high-level resistance) have been outlined in detail elsewhere.[7]

In summary, the main advantage of sequencing is its potential for facilitating individualized, effective treatment for patients with DR-TB. However, to achieve this in a clinically useful way, targeted NGS or WGS would need to be performed "directly" on a sputum sample (rather than DNA extracted from a culture isolate) thus allowing for rapid and precise treatment initiation and minimizing the time of exposure of patients to inappropriate empiric regimens. A comparison of WGS with currently available drug resistance tests is presented in Table 16.2.

MANAGEMENT OF MDR- AND RESISTANCE BEYOND MDR-TB

MEDICAL MANAGEMENT OF MDR-TB

The management of MDR- and resistance beyond MDR-TB is complex, and the type of treatment regimen and package chosen will depend on a number of considerations including HIV status,

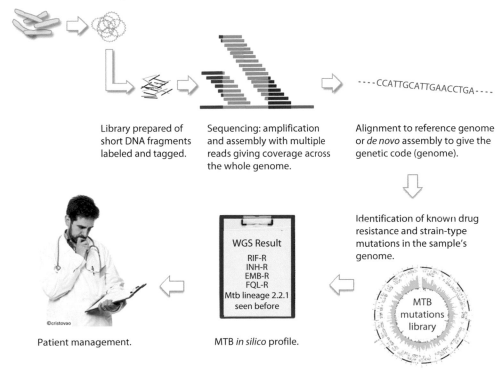

Figure 16.3 Next-generation sequencing. With small bacterial genomes such as *M. tuberculosis* multiple samples can be analyzed within a single run, greatly reducing costs. (Reproduced with permission from *Lancet Respir Med* 2017.)

Table 16.2 Summary comparison of WGS with current drug resistance tests

Test characteristic	Phenotypic tests	Xpert MTB/RIF	Line probe assays	Whole-genome sequencing
Time to result	Slow (weeks/months)	Less than 2 hours	Rapid (hours/days) when performed directly from samples	Rapid (hours/days) if performed directly from samples
Sensitivity for detecting resistance	Sensitivity high	High for rifampicin, zero for other drugs	Sensitivity limited	Sensitivity dependent on knowledge of polymorphisms
Resistance levels	Ability to determine MICs	Does not assess MIC	Limited ability to predict MICs	Ability to predict some MICs
Safety	High safety concerns	Low safety concerns	Reduced safety concerns	Reduced safety concerns
EQA	Quality assurance via WHO/ IUATLD reference lab network	Limited quality assurance schemes	Limited quality assurance schemes	Quality assurance schemes not available
Efficiency	Separate tests for each drug	Detects resistance to one drug only	2–3 drugs per test	Single analysis for all drugs

Source: Reproduced with permission from Dheda K et al. *Lancet Respir Med.* 2017;5:291–360.

CD4 count, degree of organ dysfunction (e.g., renal, liver, etc.), presence of comorbidities, history of previous TB, age, disease severity, the local drug susceptibility profile, resource availability, and access to supportive care, amongst others. Optimal regimen selection for MDR- and resistance beyond MDR-TB is a rapidly changing landscape with the emergence of newer drugs; there are many ongoing clinical trials evaluating new drug combinations and these have been outlined in detail elsewhere.[7] Regimens will also evolve with changing resistance patterns. Thus, clinicians need to be aware of local resistance patterns and the status of access to newer and repurposed drugs. While the focus here is on regimen selection, there are other quintessential aspects of management that include well-functioning laboratories for bacteriological studies and DST, infection control in health-care facilities to minimize transmission, availability, and access to adherence promoting mechanisms, attention to psychosocial factors and financial/resource assistance to patients, access to quality drugs and distribution systems, appropriate training of health-care workers, good systems processes and information systems (to track patients, communicate results, and audit data), and a robust and well-functioning TB program (NTP).

While there are different perspectives about the merits of an empiric PAN TB regimen without the need for prior susceptibility testing, we take the view that this approach is not sustainable nor in the best interests of patients; rather, we subscribe to and support a concept of individualized therapy and precision medicine. Thus, as much information as possible should be obtained through rapid molecular testing in order to, at the least, quasi-individualize regimens. Thus, rifampicin-resistant readouts (typically from Xpert MTB/RIF Ultra in many TB-endemic countries) should be confirmed and clarified with molecular readouts (e.g., LPAs) and extended phenotypic DSTs. Typically, such readouts are obtained within 3–7 days of using LPA (e.g., the Hain MTBDR*plus* and *sl* assay, though other platforms are available). Using such an approach it is feasible to rule-in resistance beyond MDR-TB in a substantial majority of cases within 7–10 days.[132,154–158] Indeed, this approach is the standard of care in South Africa where sputum from patients with rifampicin-resistant TB is subjected to

Hain MTBDR*plus* and *sl* assays. The reality, however, is that in some parts of the country the LPA results are only available in 2–4 weeks, and yield in smear negative patients is lower, limiting the usefulness of the assay. Nevertheless, using this approach ensures that susceptibility to rifampicin, isoniazid, fluoroquinolones, and SLIDs will be ascertained fairly rapidly, as will readouts for ethionamide and high-dose isoniazid (based on the *inhA* and *katG* mutations). Phenotypic DST will still be required given the suboptimal sensitivity and indeterminate rates when using sputum-based LPA testing (discussed in the diagnostics section). Using this approach, resistance profiles for drugs like pyrazinamide, ethambutol, and bedaquiline will still remain unknown (at least given the current format of the LPAs). Although next-generation WGS readouts may address these deficiencies to some extent, the major challenge (as already discussed) is that the results are only available after 6–8 weeks making this a user-unfriendly tool at present, as the lack of a rapid readout fails to prevent resistance amplification. Technology is evolving, but it will take another 5–10 years before WGS directly from the sputum will likely be optimized. However, even with comprehensive WGS readouts, phenotypic susceptibility testing will still be required for drugs such as clofazimine, cycloserine, PAS (para-aminosalicylic acid), and carbapenems. Thus, for the foreseeable future, we will need to rely on a combination of genotypic and phenotypic DST to construct optimal regimens.

The principles to medically managing MDR- and resistance beyond MDR-TB are outlined in Table 16.3. Essentially, a part-individualized and part-empiric MDR-TB regimen should be constructed based on the initial molecular readouts (as outlined earlier) that should comprise a backbone of bedaquiline, fluoroquinolone, and linezolid (group A drugs; see Table 16.4 for the WHO classification of second-line drugs).[159] Other drugs that should likely be added to the regimen after this first step, depending on the DST readouts, would include clofazimine and cycloserine (group B drugs) that will likely make up the five-drug regimen. In the patient meta-analysis, the group A drugs were all associated with substantial mortality reduction (>50%) and treatment success benefit, while the group B drugs showed similar effects but

Table 16.3 Recommended principles to be used when designing a regimen for the medical management of MDR-TB and resistance beyond MDR-TB including in those with pulmonary TB, extra-pulmonary TB, and in children

- *Route of administration*: Use an all oral regimen (ᵃsee note later on WHO-recommended Bangladesh-like shorter course regimen).
- *Number of drugs*: Ideally *use five drugs (minimum four) to which the strain has proven or likely susceptibility* (drugs previously taken for ≥1 month are generally avoided); use at least three (preferably four) likely effective drugs in the continuation phase[b].[288]
- *Individual components of the regimen*:
  i. *Use a backbone of the three Group A drugs*, i.e., a later-generation fluoroquinolone, e.g., levofloxacin (less QT prolongation), linezolid, and bedaquiline.[288] Actively monitor for toxicity especially to linezolid (~30% reduce the dose or stop the drug).[289–291] The optimal duration of individual drugs like linezolid and bedaquiline remains unclear but they are generally used for at least 6 months (in practice extension of bedaquiline to ≥ 9 months may be undertaken, particularly late culture converters and those with poor prognostic features).
  ii. Add additional Group B drugs (e.g., cycloserine/terizidone, and/or clofazimine).
  iii. Add additional Group C drugs, if necessary (based on toxicity and resistance profiles), so that five likely effective drugs make up the regimen.
- *Duration of treatment*: The optimal duration of the multidrug regimen remains unclear. Current practice when treating MDR-TB (using a Group A backbone) varies from 9 to 11 months (e.g., in South Africa) to the WHO-recommended 18–20 months. The optimal duration of treatment will depend on several factors including mycobacterial burden (and time of culture conversion), disease extent, comorbidities (e.g., HIV and diabetes), previous treatment, country setting, local resistance profiles, and patient preference.[292]
- *Empiric versus individualized*: To optimize outcomes and prevent resistance amplification, and loss of newer drugs, drug susceptibility-guided treatment for individual drugs is preferred over empiric treatment regimens. To minimize resistance amplification sputum-based genotypic testing for second-line resistance, particularly FQs, is recommended. Regimens should be further optimized based on drug susceptibility results when they become available.
- Delamanid (Group C) can be used together with bedaquiline, if required, to make up the five-drug regimen (monitor QT interval).[293,294]
- Meropenem or imipenem/cilastin should be administered with clavulanic acid (generally given as oral Augmentin).
- A second-line injectable drug (amikacin or streptomycin; Group C drugs) may be used if an appropriate regimen of four to five likely effective drugs cannot be constructed, provided baseline and follow-up screening for hearing loss and renal toxicity is accessible. We recommend that an intravenous catheter be used for the administration of amikacin and/or a carbapenem. If inaccessible we recommend that amikacin be given intramuscularly together with a local anesthetic agent.[295]
- Psychosocial, adherence, and financial support are critical elements of the treatment package.
- Patients should be actively monitored for adverse drug reactions, which are common.[296]
- A single drug should not be added to a failing regimen.
- The HIV status should be determined, and ART initiated in all HIV-infected patients (within 8 weeks; 2 weeks in advanced HIV).
- Surgical intervention may be offered in appropriate patients who have failed treatment or are at high risk of relapse.
- *Children*: Use the same principles as outlined previously. Bedaquiline can be used from 6 years of age. Delamanid is safe and effective from 3 years of age and prioritized in children. Lack of optimal diagnostics, and child-friendly formulations remain a major challenge.[297]
- ᵃ*WHO-recommended shorter course regimen* (9–11 month Bangladesh-like regimen containing amikacin but not containing bedaquiline or linezolid): While scale up of newer drugs and diagnostics continues, as an interim option, this regimen can be used on a discretionary basis provided there is no proven or likely resistance to any component of the regimen (except isoniazid), there is access to baseline and longitudinal monitoring for hearing loss, and FQ and SLID resistance have been excluded.[159,165] There should be clear plans to transitioning to an oral Group A-based regimen.

Source: Adapted with permission from Dheda K. *Lancet*, 2016; Dheda K. *Lancet Resp Med*, 2017.
Abbreviations: FQ, fluoroquinolone; MDR-TB, multidrug-resistant TB.
ᵃ See main text for the composition of WHO-recommended shorter course regimen.
ᵇ Continuation phase: Some Group A drugs like bedaquiline and/or linezolid may only be given for a limited period (e.g., ~6 months) and thus the period beyond this point may only contain a limited number of drugs. Depending on the length of the regimen and how long each drug is used, in specific instances, there may not be a continuation phase.

reduced in magnitude. Group C drugs did not demonstrate a mortality benefit or data were unavailable.

The optimal duration of linezolid (2–3 vs. ≥6 months) remains unclear. Several other drugs are generally not counted as representing part of the five likely effective drugs. Indeed, in countries like South Africa, there is a ~50% rate of isolate-specific resistance to pyrazinamide and ethambutol in patients with MDR-TB. The rates of isoniazid resistance are region-dependent; for example, in South Africa 40% have *inhA* promoter mutations, and 60% of isolates harbor *katG* mutations, while in Eastern Europe the KatG mutation accounts for over 90%, thus conferring high-level

resistance to isoniazid.[160,161] Thus, ethionamide resistance levels in these, and several other settings, is high (50%–90%); high-dose isoniazid is often used at 10 mg/kg to limit toxicity (resulting in suboptimal drug levels and doubtful effectiveness) and levels are further marginalized in those with high acetylator status. Thus, molecular readouts like the LPA are only a guide and may have limited PPV in the clinical setting. Although the shorter course WHO regimen recommends that both high-dose INH and ethionamide be used concurrently, we recommend that only one of the drugs be used depending on the *inhA* or *katG* mutation available from molecular testing. When using high-dose INH, a dose of

Table 16.4 WHO categorization of second-line anti-tuberculous drugs and recommended treatment for rifampicin-resistant and MDR-TB

WHO Grouping[a]	Anti-tuberculous drug	Key toxicity	Comments
Group A[b]: Include all three medicines (unless they cannot be used)	Levofloxacin or moxifloxacin (Lfx/Mfx)	QTc prolongation (Mfx>Lfx), arthralgia	Lfx should be used in Bdq-containing regimens.
	Bedaquiline (Bdq)[c]	QTc prolongation, arthralgia, hepatitis, and headache	Close monitoring of QTc is recommended especially when using these agents in combination with other QTc-prolonging drugs. EFV should be changed to NVP or a protease inhibitor (may increase Bdq levels ≈ 2-fold with unclear significance[284]), alternatively, an integrase strand transfer inhibitor can be used.
	Linezolid (Lzd)[d]	Peripheral neuropathy, myelosuppression and ocular toxicity	Myelosuppression occurs in the first few months of treatment. Lzd may need to be stopped; transfuse as appropriate; Lzd may be reintroduced at a reduced dose in selected cases. [285,286]
Group B: Add both medicines (unless they cannot be used)	Clofazimine (Cfz)	QTc prolongation, skin and conjunctival pigmentation	Counsel patients on possible skin pigmentation QTc should be monitored when using with FQ, Bdq and Dlm.
	Cycloserine or terizidone (Cs/Trd)	CNS effects including psychosis, confusion, and depression	Should be stopped permanently in patients who develop severe side effects.
Group C[b]: Add to complete the regimen and when medicines from Groups A and B cannot be used	Ethambutol (E)	Ocular toxicity	
	Delamanid (Dlm)	Hypokalemia, nausea, vomiting, dizziness, and QTc prolongation	Close monitoring of QTc is recommended especially when using these agents in combination with other QTc prolonging drugs. No significant anticipated drug-drug interactions with ARVs.[287] Hypoalbuminemia may limit its use in HIV coinfection.
	Pyrazinamide (Z)	Hepatotoxicity, gout	Should be stopped in all patients with significant elevation of liver enzymes.
	Imipenem-cilastin or meropenem[e] (Ipm-Cln/Mpm)	Seizures	Should be administered through a subcutaneous tunneled intravenous catheter where possible. Coadministered with clavulanate usually in form of oral co-amoxyclav.
	Amikacin (or Streptomycin)$^{3\,f}$ (Am (S))	Nephrotoxicity, ototoxicity, electrolyte derangement (K, Mg and Ca)	Use with caution in patients with diabetes mellitus, renal disease, or hearing impairment.
	Ethionamide or prothionamide (Eto/Pto)	Diarrhea, nausea, vomiting and hypothyroidism	With symptoms of nausea and vomiting also consider drug-induced hepatitis or pancreatitis; monitor TSH.
	p-aminosalicylic acid (PAS)	Diarrhea, hypothyroidism, nausea and vomiting	With symptoms of nausea and vomiting also consider drug-induced hepatitis or pancreatitis; monitor TSH.

Source: Adapted; reproduced with permission from the WHO.

a This regrouping is intended to guide the design of conventional regimens.

b Medicines in Groups A and C are shown by decreasing order of usual preference for use.

c There is insufficient evidence to recommend bedaquiline use beyond 6 months.

d Highly effective when used for 6 months, however, toxicity may limit its use.

e Carbapenems and clavulanate are meant to be used together; clavulanate is only available in formulations combined with amoxicillin.

f Streptomycin may substitute other injectable agents under specific conditions and if amikacin is unavailable. Resistance to streptomycin alone does not qualify for the definition of extensively drug-resistant TB (XDR-TB) though this will likely be redefined soon. The use of kanamycin is no longer recommended (low-quality evidence).

10–15 mg/kg daily or 3 times a week is often better tolerated than 16–18 mg/kg per day, and is the practice in South Africa given the high rate of isoniazid-associated hepatoxic and neurotoxic adverse events.[7]

Addition of alternative and other drugs to the regimen will depend on the laboratory-generated susceptibility profile. Ideally at least five likely effective drugs (minimum four), excluding pyrazinamide and ethambutol, should be used in the regimen. However, the precise number that constitutes what is "optimal" remains controversial and will depend on several factors including the efficacy and potency of the drugs being used in the regimen, size and thickness of cavity walls, and disease extent. The PETTS (Preserving Effective Tuberculosis Treatment Study)[162] and the recent patient level meta-analysis involving ~12,000 patients from 50 studies suggested that at least five effective drugs were associated with better outcomes.[163] Thus, in addition to the core drugs already mentioned, additional drugs can be added depending on the resistance profile to create an optimal MDR-TB regimen.

The duration of treatment is also controversial, and the precise duration of therapy remains unclear.

The traditional duration of MDR-TB therapy has been 18–20 months. In 2016, the WHO recommended a shorter 9–11 month duration of treatment under certain conditions, the most important of which was that eligible patients should not likely be resistant to any component of the proposed regimen (except pyrazinamide).[164] This standardized regimen consists of an intensive phase of 4–6 months (depending on the time of sputum smear conversion) that includes amikacin,[165] moxifloxacin, clofazimine, prothionamide/ethionamide, high-dose isoniazid, ethambutol, and pyrazinamide. This is followed by a continuation phase of 5 months comprising moxifloxacin, clofazimine, ethambutol, and pyrazinamide.[164] The STREAM 1 study, a RCT (randomized-controlled trail) that evaluated the shorter course regimen in over 400 patients, demonstrated this regimen to be non-inferior to the longer regimen, though bacteriological outcomes were worse with the shorter regimen (higher rates of treatment failure and relapse), and lost to follow-up was higher with the longer regimen.[165] Interestingly, it did demonstrate that very good cure rates (~78%) could be achieved under research conditions with optimal patient adherence and psychosocial support even when bedaquiline and linezolid were not used. Thus, some programs were using the traditional 18–20-month duration of therapy, some the shorter course regimen, while others (like South Africa) were using both, depending on patient-specific characteristics. More recently, however, the South African National TB Programme took the bold but sensible step of including bedaquiline in 9–12 month regimen given the impact of bedaquiline in reducing mortality in MDR- and resistance beyond MDR-TB,[166–168] and the excellent culture conversion rate shown in several observational studies.[167–170] This regimen currently being used in South Africa (since approximately September 2018) is a 9–11-month regimen containing bedaquiline (instead of the SLID), a later-generation fluoroquinolone (levofloxacin), linezolid for 2–3 months, and other second-line drugs. Results of the performance outcomes of this regimen are awaited.

SLID, with appropriate monitoring, can still be considered in patients with fluoroquinolone-resistant MDR-TB, but where resources permit, a subcutaneous tunneled intravenous catheter should be inserted. Where this is unavailable, it is recommend that amikacin be given intramuscularly together with a local anesthetic, which seems feasible and does not affect the pharmacokinetics of the drug.[171] The use of kanamycin is no longer supported given its lack of association with better outcomes (low quality evidence); the same for capreomycin as it was associated with increased mortality. Hearing loss should be monitored, and it has become apparent that subclinical hearing loss is common in populations in TB-endemic countries because of poor access to health care during childhood years (thus access to regular testing is mandatory if injectables are to be used). SLIDs can be dosed at 3 times a week, where appropriate, to minimize toxicity.

The rate of adverse drug reactions in patients with MDR- and resistance beyond MDR-TB is high, and patients need to be carefully monitored (see later). When the adverse event is severe enough, the dose may need to be decreased or the drug may need to be stopped. Clofazimine is well tolerated but may often cause hyperpigmentation (poorly accepted by patients who may surreptitiously not take the drug) and prolong the QT interval. Bedaquiline is associated with QT prolongation, although this occurs in less than 10% of individuals and <1% stop the drug due to QT prolongation.[172] Thus, bedaquiline-associated QT prolongation is not a major problem in clinical practice.[172,173] When faced with an increased QT interval, it is first important to ensure that there are no other concomitant causative drugs (e.g., amitriptyline, citalopram, diphenhydramine, antipsychotics, etc.), electrolyte abnormalities (e.g., hypocalcemia and hypokalemia, often present in HIV-infected persons with diarrhea and malnutrition), or other factors (interactions or issues that increase bedaquiline concentration or duration of action, and genetic predisposition) causing QT prolongation. Occasionally, stopping other QT prolonging drugs such as clofazimine may be required. Linezolid is a particularly toxic drug and, in our experience, has to be discontinued in approximately one-third of patients.[174,175] The main adverse events include anemia, peripheral neuropathy, and optic neuritis. Most of the anemia-related toxicity occurs within the first 3 months. Neurotoxicity is evident at a median of 5–6 months.[174–176]

MEDICAL MANAGEMENT OF RESISTANCE BEYOND MDR-TB

The principles used to construct a regimen to manage resistance beyond MDR-TB are the same as those outlined in Table 16.3. In South Africa, the typical resistance beyond MDR-TB backbone used comprises bedaquiline, linezolid and PAS, with the addition of other drugs such as delamanid and the carbapenems, as appropriate, so that likely 4–5 effective drugs are used in the regimen. However, with bedaquiline and clofazimine now being used as frontline drugs in MDR-TB, constructing resistance beyond MDR-TB regimens will become more challenging. Treatment will have to rely on extended DST and individualized treatment. It is likely that such regimens will include delamanid and PAS as a backbone, with the addition of carbapenems, and other agents such as rifabutin where appropriate. Indeed, we recently showed that up to 22% of "XDR-TB" patients were susceptible to rifabutin despite being resistant to rifampicin.[118,177] Meropenem together with clavulanic acid (given as Augmentin® in endemic countries) has recently shown good EBA (early bactericidal activity) against *M. tuberculosis*. Delamanid may potentially be a useful drug for the treatment of DR-TB especially in settings where a regimen of at least 4–5 effective drugs cannot otherwise be constituted[178,179]; however, the preliminary results of the phase III trial showed that the primary outcome was not met (although significance was achieved when alternative methods for handling missing cultures were used[180]). Furthermore, the delamanid phase III trial also failed to meet its long-term (>20 month) efficacy outcomes. The reasons for the lack of delamanid efficacy in that trial remains unclear but may have been related to the dosing schedule used, i.e., once versus twice daily schedule.[180] In patients with high grade drug-specific resistance, who are often HIV-infected, management is complex and ideally such patients should be managed by multidisciplinary teams comprising social workers, occupational therapists, psychologists, pulmonologists or infectious disease physicians, adherence supporters, and cardiothoracic surgeons amongst others.

With the increasing use of bedaquiline and linezolid, programmatically incurable treatment failures (have failed bedaquiline-based regimens) are not infrequently encountered and pose a management problem. This is already a challenging problem in Cape Town and in other centers within South Africa. Managing such patients raises a number of ethical and logistical dilemmas including provision of long-term housing, right to work and live in the community, and access to facilities for palliative care. These have been discussed in detail elsewhere.[7] Although the majority of these patients succumb to their disease, some self-cures have

Table 16.5 Recommended principles for the surgical management of MDR and resistance beyond MDR-TB

- Patient selection for surgery and management should be interdisciplinary.
- Candidates include patients with unilateral disease (or apical bilateral disease in selected cases) with adequate lung function who have failed medical treatment.[309]
- In patients with rifampicin-resistant or MDR-TB, elective partial lung resection (lobectomy or wedge resection) was associated with improved treatment success.
- Surgical intervention may be appropriate in patients at high risk of relapse or failure despite response to therapy (e.g., resistance beyond MDR-TB or programmatically incurable TB).[309]
- Facilities for surgical lung resection are limited and often inaccessible.
- PET-CT may be useful for clarifying the significance of contralateral disease and may have prognostic significance but its role in this context requires validation.[310,311]
- It is critical that surgery be accompanied by an effective rescue regimen otherwise outcomes are suboptimal.
- The optimal duration of therapy post resection remains unclear.
- Surgery should be performed at a center with relevant experience.

Source: Adapted with permission from Dheda K. *Lancet,* 2016; Dheda K. *Lancet Resp Med,* 2017.
Abbreviations: MDR-TB, multidrug-resistant TB; XDR-TB, extensively drug-resistant TB (likely to be redefined soon).

been documented. Indeed, in the pre-chemotherapeutic era, about 15%–20% of patients self-cured their TB.[181]

The surgical management of MDR and resistance beyond MDR-TB is discussed later, however, when surgery is not an option (unfit for surgery or patient refusal) other experimental options may include the use of one-way valves for medical lung volume reduction.[182] There have been several case reports of the successful use of valves, though the valves are expensive, access is limited, and there are major infection control issues that need to be managed. A number of interesting research approaches are currently being pursued, including adjunct inhaled antibiotics, efflux pump inhibitors, therapeutic vaccines, host-directed therapies, and the use repurposed drugs including minocycline and ceftazidime-avibactam.[183,184]

SURGICAL MANAGEMENT OF DR-TB

The majority of patients with MDR-TB, as already outlined, can be cured with medical treatment alone, provided that medicines are available to design a DST-guided treatment regimen of at least five likely effective drugs. However, patients may benefit from additional surgical therapy depending on the physical status of a patient, the availability of drugs, and the extent of the disease (see Table 16.5).

The decision for a thoracosurgical intervention should be made by a multidisciplinary team of experts and the procedure should be performed in a center with experience in MDR-TB thoracic surgery.[185] Surgery should be considered in patients with localized pulmonary disease that cannot be cured by medical treatment alone (e.g., non-culture conversion after 6 months of adequate medical treatment, especially when there are large cavities) or when there are life-threatening complications, e.g., pulmonary hemorrhage, non-resolving pleural empyema, or extensive necrosis. The best treatment outcomes are achieved with partial unilateral lung resections though this likely reflects a selection bias.[186] Patients considered for pneumonectomy must be carefully selected. A recent meta-analysis on the role of surgery for patients with MDR-TB found no overall benefit of extensive surgical procedures though there were many confounders.[186]

Potential contraindications for surgical intervention include extensive fibrotic lung disease, bilateral cavitating disease, poor cardiopulmonary function, and endobronchial TB.[185] HIV coinfection should not be a contraindication for surgery, however, these patients should receive effective antiretroviral therapy (ideally, they should have undetectable viral replication). In addition to microbiological evaluation, preoperative assessment should ideally include spirometry, chest computed tomography imaging, a ventilation-perfusion scan, diffusion capacity testing, and an echocardiography (if indicated).

The optimal timing for surgery is after culture conversion so that the risk for bronchial stump breakdown is diminished. However, this is a theoretical concern and when culture conversion cannot be achieved by medical treatment, surgical treatment should not be delayed. Patients undergoing elective lung resection should improve their physical fitness prior to and post-surgery using physio- and respiratory therapy.

The WHO suggests that patients with MDR-TB who undergo pulmonary surgical therapy need postsurgical medical treatment.[185] It remains unclear if this is also the case in patients with very localized disease who undergo complete surgical resection of a lesion, though intuitively it should be the case. Recent data from the University of Cape Town suggests that surgical outcomes are poor unless accompanied by effective medical therapy (K Dheda; personal communication). The duration and intensity of post-surgery medical treatment to achieve relapse-free cure can be highly variable.[187,188] General recommendations can only be provided with a large degree of uncertainty.

MANAGEMENT IN SPECIAL SITUATIONS

MANAGEMENT OF DR-TB IN PATIENTS COINFECTED WITH HIV

Management of DR-TB in the setting of HIV-coinfection is challenging and associated with high mortality. This may be attributed to the potential for shared toxicity between TB and HIV treatment, the presence of HIV-related end-organ disease, pharmacokinetic drug-drug interactions, and immune reconstitution inflammatory syndrome (IRIS).[189]

Antiretroviral therapy (ART) should be initiated within 8 weeks of starting effective MDR-TB treatment irrespective of CD4+ count.[190] Patients with CD4+ counts <50 cells/mm³ should initiate antiretrovirals (ARVs) within 2 weeks of starting MDR-TB treatment as is the case for DS-TB treatment,[191–193] unless they are suspected to have TB meningitis, in which case the initiation of ARVs should be deferred by 6–8 weeks due to the risk of developing potentially fatal CNS IRIS (central nervous system immune reconstitution inflammatory syndrome).[194,195] The WHO has recently endorsed the use of dolutegravir as part of a first-line ART regimen.[196] This agent is not only more effective and better tolerated than previous ARVs but is also expected to be safe for coadministration with newer anti-TB agents such as bedaquiline and delamanid.[197,198]

New and repurposed drugs used in the treatment of MDR-TB and resistance beyond MDR-TB such as bedaquiline, linezolid, and delamanid have changed the face of MDR-TB treatment; however, significant adverse event profiles require that these agents be used with caution. This is particularly important in settings of high HIV coinfection where the potential for drug interactions is significant (Table 16.6[298] summarizes the shared toxicity between anti-TB therapy and ARVs).

MANAGEMENT OF DR-TB IN PREGNANCY

TB in pregnancy is associated with poor outcomes, including an increased risk of preterm birth, low birth weight, intrauterine growth restriction, and perinatal death.[199,200] Prevalence estimates for TB in pregnancy and in the postpartum period range from 0.06% to 7.2% and are as high as 11% in HIV coinfected patients.[201–203] This high prevalence may be attributed to the reduced ratio of T-helper 1 to T-helper 2 cells which predisposes pregnant women to acquire or reactivate TB.[204]

Some women may choose to terminate a pregnancy due to the potential teratogenic effects of anti-TB therapy.[205,206] All pregnant women should be started on treatment as soon as possible. However, the decision to initiate treatment for DR-TB and the construction of a DR-TB regimen must consider the gestational age of the fetus, and should weigh the risks of the teratogenicity

against potential benefit to the mother.[207] The teratogenic effects of anti-tuberculous treatment mainly occur during the first trimester. Therefore, treatment may be deferred until the second trimester in selected cases where the clinical condition of the mother is stable and where there is minimal radiological disease. This strategy, however, must be accompanied by close clinical follow-up as DR-TB in pregnancy, especially in the context of HIV coinfection, can have an accelerated course.[208,209] Mothers, especially if smear positive, should discontinue breastfeeding if possible, so as to limit proximity to the infant.

Aminoglycosides, specifically amikacin and kanamycin, are FDA class D agents. These should be excluded from TB treatment regimens during pregnancy because of the risk of ototoxicity and fetal malformation, especially within the first 20 weeks of gestation. Bedaquiline may be used instead of SLID as it is likely safer (FDA pregnancy risk category B) and animal reproduction studies have not demonstrated risk to the fetus.[210,211] Delamanid, however, should not be used in pregnancy until more safety data become available since animals studies have demonstrated potential teratogenic effects.[212] Both bedaquiline and delamanid are excreted in breast milk in animal studies and therefore, the decision to discontinue the drug or nursing should be taken within the clinical context. Ethionamide is generally avoided as it can increase the risk of nausea and vomiting associated with pregnancy. This drug may be reintroduced after delivery if needed to strengthen the regimen in the immediate postpartum period.

Last, it is critically important to offer individualized, long term, and effective contraception (e.g., medroxyprogesterone or an intrauterine contraceptive device) to all women of childbearing age who are receiving treatment for DR-TB considering the toxic effects of MDR-TB drugs to both the expectant mother and the fetus.

MANAGEMENT OF DR-TB IN PATIENTS WITH RENAL IMPAIRMENT

Factors contributing to the development of renal dysfunction, such as diarrhea and dehydration, should be addressed. Diuretic use and concomitant administration of other nephrotoxins should be rationalized.[213] The underlying cause of renal dysfunction may be due to a concomitant medical condition (e.g., hypertension, diabetes) or due to toxicity attributable to ARVs (e.g., tenofovir) and/or anti-tuberculous therapy (e.g., aminoglycoside). The risks of iatrogenic nephrotoxicity may be greater due to the background prevalence of HIV-associated nephropathy (HIVAN) in Africa.[213,214] The use of tenofovir and/or aminoglycoside should be avoided in such patients, especially if the patients have advanced HIV[215,216] with proteinuria.[215,217]

The WHO-recommended dosage (and dosing interval) for various anti-TB drugs is based according to the patient's creatinine clearance and the modality of dialysis.[207] In general, all nephrotoxic agents should be discontinued. Bedaquiline should be used in the setting of aminoglycoside-associated nephrotoxicity.

MANAGEMENT OF DR-TB IN PATIENTS WITH LIVER DYSFUNCTION

Patients with significant chronic liver disease should not receive pyrazinamide. Ethionamide, prothionamide, and PAS can also be

Table 16.6 Shared toxicity between antiretrovirals and anti-tuberculous therapy

Description of adverse event	Responsible antiretroviral agent/s	Responsible anti-tuberculous agent/s	Consideration
Renal toxicity	TDF	Aminoglycosides, Cm	• TDF causes renal failure with hypophosphatemia and proteinuria. Avoid in HIV-infected persons with renal impairment. • Avoid TDF in patients receiving aminoglycosides and Cm. • Serum creatinine should be checked before switching patients onto TDF after completion of aminoglycoside. • Caution is advised when administering TDF or aminoglycosides in patients with underlying comorbidities such as diabetes mellitus or in patients who are receiving concomitant nephrotoxic agents such as NSAIDS and amphotericin B. • If TDF is necessary monitoring of serum creatinine is required.
Electrolyte derangement	TDF	Aminoglycosides, Cm	• Minimize exacerbating factors such vomiting, diarrhea, dehydration, diuretics, etc.
Hepatitis/ hepatotoxicity	NVP, EFV, PI (especially RTV), NRTI	Z, Bdq,[299] PAS, FQ, Eto	• When severe (ALT≥ 3x ULN with symptoms or ALT>5x ULN) stop both ARVs and anti-TB agents, consider a non-hepatotoxic TB regimen. • Exclude other contributing or causative factors such as alcohol abuse, viral etiologies, and other drug toxicity. • The risk of NVP hepatotoxicity is highest in the first 3 months of starting therapy with higher risk in patients with CD4 >250[300]; the risk of NVP hepatotoxicity is lower if VL is suppressed.[301]
Myelosuppression	AZT	Lzd,[302] H	• Stop Lzd if myelosuppression occurs. Blood transfusion is indicated if hemoglobin falls below 8 g/dL.[285,286] • Avoid coadministration of AZT and Lzd. • Adverse events should be managed with a combination of temporary or permanent suspension of linezolid, dose reduction, and/or symptom management.[303] • Dose reduction to 300 mg daily may be associated with fewer neuropathic effects but may be associated with subtherapeutic levels.[304] • Consider stopping co-trimoxazole.
Peripheral neuropathy	ddI, d4T	Lzd,[290] Cs, H, Eto, E	• Avoid use of D4T or ddI in combination with Cs or Lzd. • Use pyridoxine as prophylaxis in patients receiving Cs, H, and Lzd.
QT prolongation		Bdq,[210] Mfx,[305] Cfz, Lfx[306]	• Close monitoring of QTc is recommended when using these agents in combination. • Lfx is associated with less QT prolongation compared to Mfx
Central Nervous system toxicity	EFV	Cs, H, Eto/Pto, FQ	• EFV toxicity generally occurs in first 2–3 weeks of treatment. • Concurrent use of EFV with CS needs close monitoring.
Headache	AZT, EFV	Cs, Bdq[299]	• Headaches may be self-limited in case of AZT, EFV and Cs. • Advise analgesia and hydration.
Nausea and vomiting	RTV, d4T, NVP	Eto, PAS, H, Bdq,[299] E, Z	• Many drugs will cause some degree of nausea. • If persistent, consider drug-induced pancreatitis or hepatitis.
Lactic acidosis	d4T, ddI, AZT, 3TC	Lzd[307]	• High index of suspicion needed to detect hyperlactatemia to prevent overt symptoms of lactic acidosis.
Pancreatitis	d4T, ddI	Lzd[302]	• Avoid coadministration where possible. • If pancreatitis occurs discontinue the relevant ARVs.
Diarrhea	PI, ddI	PAS, FQ, Eto	• For mild diarrhea, antimotility drugs can be used. • May be self-limited. Exclude opportunistic infections.
Optic neuritis	ddI	E, Lzd,[308] Eto	• Stop all suspected agents causing optic neuritis.
Hypothyroidism	d4T	Eto, PAS	• Monitor TSH for patients receiving these agents.
Joint pain		Z, Bdq, FQ	• Mild symptoms can be managed by simple analgesia.

Source: Reproduced with permission from Esmail A, Sabur NF, Okpechi I, and Dheda K. *J Thorac Dis.* 2018;10:3102–18.
Note: Abbreviations may be found in Table 16.4.

hepatotoxic while the fluoroquinolones are rarely implicated in hepatitis. Essentially, all second-line drugs may be used in chronic stable liver disease, but close monitoring of liver enzymes is mandatory and significant deterioration in liver function should trigger immediate withdrawal of the offending drug. The source of other causes of liver dysfunction, including viral hepatitis and alcohol consumption, should be addressed and treated to prevent further complications during treatment. A combination of four non-hepatotoxic drugs should ideally be used when formulating a regimen in patients with chronic liver dysfunction, including a fluoroquinolone, to ensure the efficacy of the regimen.[207]

Anti-TB treatment should be deferred until the hepatitis has stabilized in cases of acute hepatitis. Chronic hepatitis B infection is considered a risk factor for hepatotoxicity[218] in patients receiving TB treatment, especially if they are "e" antigen positive.[219] If treatment for hepatitis B infection is indicated, ART should be initiated with the combination of at least two agents active against hepatitis B, e.g., tenofovir and emtricitabine or lamivudine.[220,221] Entecavir may be used as a substitute to tenofovir in patients with renal dysfunction (dose adjustment may be required).[221] Drug interactions and overlapping toxicities with MDR-TB agents must be considered in HIV/HCV coinfection.[220]

MANAGEMENT OF DR-TB IN PATIENTS WITH DIABETES MELLITUS

Diabetes increases the risk of primary infection with MDR-TB and is associated with delayed sputum conversion.[222,223] Diabetes mellitus may also play a role in the development of DR-TB.[224,225] HbA1c may underestimate glycemic control (due to decreased red blood cell life span) in TB/HIV coinfected patients.[226]

Metformin may exaggerate gastrointestinal side effects when coadministered with anti-tuberculous agents such as ethionamide, PAS, and clofazimine, and can rarely cause lactic acidosis.[227] Caution is advised when using nephrotoxic agents and neurotoxic agents in patients with established diabetes. QTc monitoring is advised when using hypoglycemic agents such as sulphonylureas and glinides concurrently with bedaquiline and/or delamanid.[228] Furthermore, caution is also advised when using bedaquiline concurrently with potentially hepatotoxic antidiabetic agents such as thiazolidinediones.[229]

The management principles of DR-TB in patients with diabetes remain similar to nondiabetic patients. However, this may need reconsideration in view of the increased treatment failure rates seen in patients with uncontrolled diabetes.[230,231] Aggressive treatment is recommended for patients with uncontrolled diabetes[232] since these patients have increased rates of relapse and recurrence.[233–235] TB clinicians should leverage more frequent patient contact to counsel patients and optimize glycemic control.[236]

MANAGEMENT OF DR-TB IN THE INTENSIVE CARE UNIT

TB is frequently diagnosed in the intensive care unit (ICU) in patients presenting with or without a respiratory diagnosis.[237] The management of patients with DR-TB in ICU is complicated by pharmacokinetic concerns such as poor gastric absorption, high rates of organ dysfunction, and drug toxicity. Furthermore, concomitant renal failure is a common occurrence, which precludes

the use of aminoglycosides and impacts use of various anti-TB agents. Therapeutic drug monitoring (TDM) may be a valuable tool to advise on the timely adjustment of drug therapy.[238,239] However, TDM for second-line agents such as linezolid, fluoroquinolones, and injectable drugs is expensive and not widely available. Utilization of dried blood spots (DBS) for linezolid and fluoroquinolones are available and can overcome some of the logistical challenges of performing TDM.[240,241]

MANAGEMENT OF MDR-TB IN CHILDREN

This recently has been covered in detail by the same authors elsewhere,[6] and by others in Chapter 18.

RESPONSE TO THERAPY

The goal of anti-TB drug therapy is relapse-free cure by the eradication of *M. tuberculosis* in the human host. In routine clinical practice the effect of therapy is ascertained by sequential examination of sputum for the presence of acid-fast bacilli and viability of *M. tuberculosis* by mycobacterial cultures. When compared to patients with drug-susceptible TB, sputum smear microscopy and culture conversion is delayed in patients with MDR-TB on conventional regimens. Ongoing cigarette smoking further delays responses to anti-TB therapy; thus, smoking cessation is especially important for patients with MDR-TB. In a recent multicenter cohort of patients with non-MDR-TB and MDR-TB, the median (interquartile range) time to smear microscopy conversion was 19 days (10–32 days) and 32 days (17–67 days), and to culture conversion was 31 days (14–56 days) and 39 days (6–85 days), respectively. At 2 months of effective treatment, 90% and 78% of non-MDR-TB patients and MDR-TB patients achieved sputum microscopy conversion, and 67% and 61% of non-MDR-TB patients and MDR-TB patients achieved sputum culture conversion.[242] How long (from the initiation of treatment) should patients with MDR-TB observe infection control precautions (e.g., be isolated from the general public and the work place by remaining at home or in hospital if appropriate)? This remains unclear and contentious, and will depend on a number of factors including microbiological burden, presence of cavitation, disease extent and severity, HIV status, strain type, and most importantly the number and bactericidal activity of effective drugs used in the regimen. In situations where there are public health implications, and in patients likely to be more infectious, our policy is to confirm culture negativity before infection control precautions are rescinded (often this may occur 3–4 months into therapy when culture negative results become available). With modern regimens containing group A drugs, the time to culture negativity is likely to be shorter.

Ideally, sputum smear microscopy and cultures should be performed at least once every 2 weeks until culture conversion has been achieved (some centers perform weekly examinations) and thereafter on a monthly basis until the end of therapy (the reality in endemic countries is that only monthly sputum culture testing is performed). The kinetics of quantitative grading of the sputum bacillary load (Table 16.7) and the time to positivity of *M. tuberculosis* cultures are very good indicators of treatment responses.[243] A positive sputum culture status by the end of 6 months of therapy should be considered as failure of MDR-TB therapy.[244]

Table 16.7 Quantitative assessment of sputum specimens using microscopy[312]

Result	Number of acid-fast bacilli Bright light technique with 100-fold objective magnification
-	0 on smear (300 fields examined)
+/−	1–12 on smear (300 fields examined)
+	4–10 in 100 fields (100 fields examined)
++	1–10 in 10 fields (100 fields examined)
+++	1–10 per field of vision (50 fields examined)
++++	>10 per field of vision (20 fields examined)

While sputum microscopy and culture are suitable markers for the monitoring of the early phase of the treatment, other markers are needed for the later phase of the treatment, when bacteria cannot be detected from sputum specimens anymore.[245] Clinical and radiological scores have been proposed to monitor treatment responses in patients with MDR-TB, but these scores have not been validated as markers of cure or treatment failure thus far.[242] A biomarker from the blood, urine, or exhaled breath that can easily be measured, and that provides early indication of treatment failure or relapse-free cure, is currently not available. Such a marker would revolutionize the clinical management of drug-susceptible TB and DR-TB.[245]

There is an ongoing debate about how long patients should be considered infectious on DST-guided antimycobacterial therapy. While infectiousness declines rapidly in response to adequate therapy,[246] there is substantial concern for public health when discharging patients with MDR-TB from a hospital into the community when acid-fast bacilli are still detectable by sputum microscopy. In some countries, negative *M. tuberculosis* cultures are even required prior to hospital discharge of MDR-TB patients.[247]

PERSON-CENTERED CARE FOR DR-TB: HUMAN RIGHTS, TREATMENT SUPPORT, AND PALLIATIVE CARE

With the global goal of TB elimination, greater emphasis has been placed on providing services and care that focus on the unique and individual needs of those who are living with DR-TB. In fact, the first pillar of the WHO's "End TB" strategy is to provide "integrated, patient-centered care and prevention." Given that current TB services are structured in a way that prioritizes the needs of providers and programs, a truly person-centered model of care would be a radical shift in the field. In order to move from talking about such care to practicing some care, several actions need to be taken, including focusing on the rights of persons affected by TB, offering optimal treatment support, and working to alleviate suffering throughout the spectrum of care.

RIGHTS-BASED APPROACHES TO DR-TB

In the past, TB programs have focused on a "public health" approach to TB control, where the emphasis was placed on identifying the most infectious persons living with TB—those felt to be driving transmission—diagnosing them with simplified tools, and treating them with "universal"/standardized regimens.[248]

While it could be argued that this approach has resulted in tens of millions of people being diagnosed and successfully treated for TB, it is equally true that under this strategy, TB has once again become the leading infectious killer of adults, drug resistance has become global phenomenon, and little progress has been made in bending the pandemic curve.[249]

By contrast, a human rights-based approach focuses on preventing, diagnosing, and treating all persons with TB in a way that maximizes their chance of returning to a healthy and productive life.[250] This type of approach is essential for people affected by DR-TB who currently have almost no access to preventive treatment of infection, are misdiagnosed using conventional TB tools such as smear microscopy, and who are offered long and toxic treatment regimens that include drugs to which the mycobacteria may be resistant, and exclude effective drugs that could increase their chance of being cured. Continuing to offer minimal services violates the right to health clause in the United Nations Universal Declaration of Human Rights (article 25).[251] Person-centered care for DR-TB must also be built on the right to benefit from scientific progress, which would include universal and timely access to novel diagnostics and therapeutics, something which is clearly lacking in DR-TB today.[252]

COMPASSIONATE TREATMENT SUPPORT FOR DR-TB

Persons living with DR-TB face myriad challenges, and often their health issues are further complicated by pressing socioeconomic problems as well. These issues, including poverty, lack of transportation, and malnutrition have been well documented and are often compounded when DR-TB is diagnosed, since it causes catastrophic expenditures for individuals, families, and communities.[253] In spite of the compelling evidence about the myriad barriers to accessing diagnostic and treatment services,[254] current approaches to supporting adherence to DR-TB treatment focus largely on directly observed therapy, prolonged hospitalization, and minimalistic educational approaches. In fact, there seems to be a "blame-based" approach to adherence support[255] when it comes to DR-TB, even though a significant amount of DR-TB comes from primary transmission, inadequate drug dosing, and health systems errors.[256] For authentic person-centered care to be achieved, persons living with DR-TB should be offered treatment literacy, financial, nutritional, and transportation support, and flexible approaches to verifying adherence. Since the toxic nature of DR-TB treatment may be a key factor in nonadherence, persons should be offered regimens that minimize the risk of adverse events—including the use of injectable-free regimens.[257]

PALLIATIVE CARE TO ALLEVIATE SUFFERING

Discussions about palliative care in DR-TB often mistakenly focus on end-of-life issues. However, palliative services are aimed at relieving suffering—both physical and psychological—that can occur during the full spectrum of DR-TB care, including after completion of treatment. Because people with DR-TB face significant discrimination and stigma, it has been proposed that in addition to offering medical interventions to decrease pain, reduce air hunger, improve the work of breathing, and decrease adverse events, counseling and psychological support should also be offered.[258]

There will be some people living with DR-TB who are not able to achieve cure and will require end-of-life support. It is important that all efforts at cure—including the use of newer agents—are exhausted prior to declaring that a person has fatal DR-TB. It is also imperative that TB programs continue to engage with these individuals to ensure they can still meaningfully engage with others while minimizing the risk of transmission. Counseling support should also be provided as well as planning to help household and family members after the person succumbs to the disease.[259]

RESEARCH PRIORITIES AND CONCLUSION

There are a number of research priorities with regard to DR-TB, and these, together with timelines and barriers to achievement, have recently been covered in detail elsewhere.[7] However, four of the most important research priorities include: (i) development and evaluation of an effective TB vaccine; (ii) undertaking clinical trials to measure the effect of active case finding on individual treatment outcomes and transmission, (iii) improving knowledge about genetic predictors of resistance to the key first-line and second-line drugs, and develop DNA extraction and sequencing methodology suitable for routine use in a diagnostic laboratory, and (iv) clinical trials to evaluate the safety, optimal dosing, duration, efficacy and combinations of new and repurposed drugs. The elephant in the room remains the development of active case-finding strategies for the diagnosis of DR-TB. With current passive case-finding approaches, a DR-TB patient has already infected 10–15 other individuals and thus, diagnosis and treatment has limited impact on curtailing the burden of disease. Active case-finding strategies may include contact tracing, screening in congregate settings such as prisons, and mobile teams that go out into TB hot spots to find cases of DR-TB. We have recently shown that such an approach using a mobile van is feasible[139] and have extended this to a smaller scalable mini clinic concept using a low-cost vehicle manned by 2–3 health-care workers.

DR-TB still poses a major threat to TB control and has a high mortality (30%–60%), which is worse than most cancers and is associated with unsustainable costs. Recent news that the price of bedaquiline has been reduced to $400 per treatment course is welcomed.[260] However, how do we effectively tackle the complex problem of MDR- and resistance beyond MDR-TB? This will require a creative and committed multi-prong approach. Prevention is always better than cure and therefore, the first major step must be to prevent TB in the first place, and also to address its major drivers including poverty and overcrowding, malnutrition, and tobacco smoking.[6,7,116] An effective vaccine would go a long way to massively reducing TB burden over a relatively short period of time. Addressing such issues, including global economic transformation and reducing war and conflicts, together with developing an effective vaccine, will take many decades. In the meanwhile, we need to conserve existing drugs through robust and well-functioning health-care systems, well-trained health-care workers, correct dosing of drugs, ensuring that patients adhere to their therapy, practicing antibiotic stewardship, and by prioritizing and funding innovative research (e.g., optimal drug dosing, the use of adjunct inhaled antibiotics, the use of efflux pump inhibitors, the development of more accurate diagnostics that will allow the initiation of fully individualized regimens).

Other major priority areas include optimal treatment of DR-TB in children, the prioritization of optimal ART regimens, TDM, and management of DR-TB in special populations including pregnancy, HIV-infected persons, those with organ dysfunction, and in the critically ill. However, controlling MDR-TB, and TB as a whole, will only be possible with massive investment of resources, political will, and the eradication of poverty, overcrowding, wars and conflicts, developing universal access to health care, and a reorganized global economic system. There also needs to be a change in the current concept of leadership to one endorsing a global mindset of brotherhood and empathy, otherwise other challenges such as global warming, pollution, and destruction of the environment will wipe out mankind way before TB does.

REFERENCES

1. World Health Organization. *Global Tuberculosis Report*. Geneva, Switzerland, 2017.
2. Zager EM, and McNerney R. Multidrug-resistant tuberculosis. *BMC Infect Dis*. 2008;8:10.
3. *Global Tuberculosis Report*. World Health Organization; 2018 No. Licence: CC BY-NC-SA 3.0 IGO.
4. WHO. *Global Tuberculosis Report 2013*, 2013.
5. Resistance TROA. *Tackling Drug-Resistant Infections Globally: Final Report and Recommendations*, 2016.
6. Dheda K, Barry CE, 3rd, and Maartens G. Tuberculosis. *Lancet*. 2016;387:1211–26.
7. Dheda K et al. The epidemiology, pathogenesis, transmission, diagnosis, and management of multidrug-resistant, extensively drug-resistant, and incurable tuberculosis. *Lancet Respir Med*. 2017;5:291–360.
8. WHO. *Global Tuberculosis Report 2015*, 2015 [cited 2016 01/06/2016]. Available at: http://apps.who.int/iris/bitstream/10665/191102/1/9789241565059_eng.pdf
9. Pietersen E et al. Long-term outcomes of patients with extensively drug-resistant tuberculosis in South Africa: A cohort study. *Lancet*. 2014;383.
10. O'Donnell MR et al. High incidence of hospital admissions with multidrug-resistant and extensively drug-resistant tuberculosis among South African health care workers. *Ann Intern Med*. 2010;153:516–22.
11. Pooran A, Pieterson E, Davids M, Theron G, and Dheda K. What is the cost of diagnosis and management of drug resistant tuberculosis in South Africa? *PLOS ONE*. 2013;8:e54587.
12. KPMG. Global Economic Impact of Tuberculosis, 2016.
13. Lange C, van Leth F, Mitnick CD, Dheda K, and Gunther G. Time to revise WHO-recommended definitions of MDR-TB treatment outcomes. *Lancet Respir Med*. 2018;6:246–8.
14. Bifani PJ et al. Identification of a W variant outbreak of *Mycobacterium tuberculosis* via population-based molecular epidemiology. *JAMA*. 1999;282:2321–7.
15. Gandhi NR, Moll A, Sturm AW, Pawinski R, Govender T, Lalloo U, Zeller K, Andrews J, and Friedland G. Extensively drug resistant tuberculosis as a cause of death in patients co-infected with tuberculosis and HIV in a rural area of South Africa. *Lancet*. 2006;368:1575–80.

16. Van Rie A, Victor TC, Richardson M, Johnson R, van der Spuy GD, Murray EJ, Beyers N, Gey Van Pittius NC, van Helden PD, and Warren RM. Reinfection and mixed infection cause changing *Mycobacterium tuberculosis* drug-resistance patterns. *Am J Respir Crit Care Med.* 2005;172:636–42.

17. van Rie A, Warren RM, Beyers N, Gie RP, Classen CN, Richardson M, Sampson SL, Victor TC, and van Helden PD. Transmission of a multidrug-resistant *Mycobacterium tuberculosis* strain resembling "strain W" among noninstitutionalized, human immunodeficiency virus-seronegative patients. *J Infect Dis.* 1999;180:1608–15.

18. van Rie A, Warren R, Richardson M, Gie RP, Enarson DA, Beyers N, and van Helden PD. Classification of drug-resistant tuberculosis in an epidemic area. *Lancet.* 2000;356:22–5.

19. Niemann S, Rusch-Gerdes S, and Richter E. IS6110 fingerprinting of drug-resistant *Mycobacterium tuberculosis* strains isolated in Germany during 1995. *J Clin Microbiol.* 1997;35:3015–20.

20. Musser JM. Antimicrobial agent resistance in mycobacteria: Molecular genetic insights. *Clin Microbiol Rev.* 1995;8:496–514.

21. Sandgren A, Strong M, Muthukrishnan P, Weiner BK, Church GM, and Murray MB. Tuberculosis drug resistance mutation database. *PLoS Med.* 2009;6:e2.

22. Miotto P et al. A standardised method for interpreting the association between mutations and phenotypic drug resistance in *Mycobacterium tuberculosis. Eur Respir J.* 2017;50.

23. Coll F et al. Rapid determination of anti-tuberculosis drug resistance from whole-genome sequences. *Genome Med.* 2015;7:51.

24. Bifani PJ et al. Origin and interstate spread of a New York City multidrug-resistant *Mycobacterium tuberculosis* clone family. *JAMA.* 1996;275:452–7.

25. Casali N et al. Evolution and transmission of drug-resistant tuberculosis in a Russian population. *Nat Genet.* 2014;46:279–86.

26. Zhao Y et al. National survey of drug-resistant tuberculosis in China. *N Engl J Med.* 2012;366:2161–70.

27. Cohen KA et al. Evolution of extensively drug-resistant tuberculosis over four decades: Whole genome sequencing and dating analysis of *Mycobacterium tuberculosis* isolates from KwaZulu-Natal. *PLoS Med.* 2015;12:e1001880.

28. Merker M et al. Evolutionary history and global spread of the *Mycobacterium tuberculosis* Beijing lineage. *Nat Genet.* 2015;47:242–9.

29. Nsofor CA, Jiang Q, Wu J, Gan M, Liu Q, Zuo T, Zhu G, and Gao Q. Transmission is a noticeable cause of resistance among treated tuberculosis patients in Shanghai, China. *Sci Rep.* 2017;7:7691.

30. Yang C et al. Transmission of multidrug-resistant *Mycobacterium tuberculosis* in Shanghai, China: A retrospective observational study using whole-genome sequencing and epidemiological investigation. *Lancet Infect Dis.* 2017;17:275–84.

31. Muller B, Borrell S, Rose G, and Gagneux S. The heterogeneous evolution of multidrug-resistant *Mycobacterium tuberculosis. Trends Genet.* 2013;29:160–9.

32. WHO. Guidance for Surveillance of Drug Resistant Tuberculosis, 1997 [cited 2016 10/06/2016]. Available at: http://www.who.int/drugresistance/tb/en/TBguidelnes1.pdf

33. Shafer RW, Singh SP, Larkin C, and Small PM. Exogenous reinfection with multidrug-resistant *Mycobacterium tuberculosis* in an immunocompetent patient. *Tuber Lung Dis.* 1995;76:575–7.

34. Crofton J, and Mitchison D. Streptomycin resistance in pulmonary tuberculosis. *Br Med J.* 1948;2:1009–15.

35. Bloemberg GV et al. Acquired resistance to bedaquiline and delamanid in therapy for tuberculosis. *N Engl J Med.* 2015;373:1986–8.

36. Veziris N et al. MyRMA CNR, the tuberculosis consilium of the CNRM, MyRMA CNR, tuberculosis consilium of the CNRM. Rapid emergence of *Mycobacterium tuberculosis* bedaquiline resistance: Lessons to avoid repeating past errors. *Eur Respir J.* 2017;49.

37. Villellas C, Coeck N, Meehan CJ, Lounis N, de Jong B, Rigouts L, and Andries K. Unexpected high prevalence of resistance-associated Rv0678 variants in MDR-TB patients without documented prior use of clofazimine or bedaquiline. *J Antimicrob Chemother.* 2017;72:684–90.

38. Kendall EA, Fofana MO, and Dowdy DW. Burden of transmitted multidrug resistance in epidemics of tuberculosis: A transmission modelling analysis. *Lancet Respir Med.* 2015;3:963–72.

39. Cohen T, Sommers B, and Murray M. The effect of drug resistance on the fitness of *Mycobacterium tuberculosis. Lancet Infect Dis.* 2003;3:13–21.

40. Bottger EC, Springer B, Pletschette M, and Sander P. Fitness of antibiotic-resistant microorganisms and compensatory mutations. *Nat Med.* 1998;4:1343–4.

41. Comas I, Borrell S, Roetzer A, Rose G, Malla B, Kato-Maeda M, Galagan J, Niemann S, and Gagneux S. Whole-genome sequencing of rifampicin-resistant *Mycobacterium tuberculosis* strains identifies compensatory mutations in RNA polymerase genes. *Nat Genet* 2012;44:106–10.

42. Sherman DR, Mdluli K, Hickey MJ, Arain TM, Morris SL, Barry CE, III, and Stover CK. Compensatory ahpC gene expression in isoniazid-resistant *Mycobacterium tuberculosis. Science.* 1996;272:1641–3.

43. de Vos M, Muller B, Borrell S, Black PA, van Helden PD, Warren RM, Gagneux S, and Victor TC. Putative compensatory mutations in the rpoC gene of rifampin-resistant *Mycobacterium tuberculosis* are associated with ongoing transmission. *Antimicrob Agents Chemother.* 2013;57:827–32.

44. van Embden JD et al. Strain identification of *Mycobacterium tuberculosis* by DNA fingerprinting: Recommendations for a standardized methodology. *J Clin Microbiol.* 1993;31:406–9.

45. Kato-Maeda M, Metcalfe JZ, and Flores L. Genotyping of *Mycobacterium tuberculosis*: Application in epidemiologic studies. *Future Microbiol.* 2011;6:203–16.

46. Supply P et al. Proposal for standardization of optimized mycobacterial interspersed repetitive unit-variable-number tandem repeat typing of *Mycobacterium tuberculosis. J Clin Microbiol.* 2006;44:4498–510.

47. Kamerbeek J et al. Simultaneous detection and strain differentiation of *Mycobacterium tuberculosis* for diagnosis and epidemiology. *J Clin Microbiol.* 1997;35:907–14.

48. Roetzer A et al. Whole genome sequencing versus traditional genotyping for investigation of a *Mycobacterium tuberculosis* outbreak: A longitudinal molecular epidemiological study. *PLoS Med.* 2013;10:e1001387.

49. Walker TM et al. Whole-genome sequencing to delineate *Mycobacterium tuberculosis* outbreaks: A retrospective observational study. *Lancet Infect Dis.* 2013;13:137–46.

50. Walker TM et al. Assessment of *Mycobacterium tuberculosis* transmission in Oxfordshire, UK, 2007–12, with whole pathogen genome sequences: An observational study. *Lancet Respir Med.* 2014;2:285–92.

51. Gurjav U, Outhred AC, Jelfs P, McCallum N, Wang Q, Hill-Cawthorne GA, Marais BJ, and Sintchenko V. Whole genome sequencing demonstrates limited transmission within identified *Mycobacterium tuberculosis* clusters in New South Wales, Australia. *PLOS ONE.* 2016;11:e0163612.

52. Wyllie DH, Davidson JA, Grace Smith E, Rathod P, Crook DW, Peto TEA, Robinson E, Walker T, and Campbell C. A Quantitative evaluation of MIRU-VNTR typing against whole-genome sequencing for identifying *Mycobacterium tuberculosis* transmission: A Prospective Observational Cohort Study. *EBioMedicine.* 2018;34.

53. Niemann S, and Supply P. Diversity and evolution of *Mycobacterium tuberculosis*: Moving to whole-genome-based approaches. *CSH Perspect Med.* 2014;4:a021188.

54. Senghore M et al. Whole-genome sequencing illuminates the evolution and spread of multidrug-resistant tuberculosis in Southwest Nigeria. *PLOS ONE.* 2017;12:e0184510.

55. Zeng X, Kwok JS, Yang KY, Leung KS, Shi M, Yang Z, Yam WC, and Tsui SK. Whole genome sequencing data of 1110 *Mycobacterium tuberculosis* isolates identifies insertions and deletions associated with drug resistance. *BMC Genomics.* 2018;19:365.

56. Coscolla M, and Gagneux S. Consequences of genomic diversity in *Mycobacterium tuberculosis*. *Semin Immunol.* 2014;26:431–44.

57. Koser CU, Bryant JM, Becq J, Torok ME, Ellington MJ, Marti-Renom MA, Carmichael AJ, Parkhill J, Smith GP, and Peacock SJ. Whole-genome sequencing for rapid susceptibility testing of M. tuberculosis. *N Engl J Med.* 2013;369:290–2.

58. Klopper M et al. Emergence and spread of extensively and totally drug resistant tuberculosis in South Africa. *Emerg Infect Dis.* 2013;19:449–55.

59. Eldholm V, Monteserin J, Rieux A, Lopez B, Sobkowiak B, Ritacco V, and Balloux F. Four decades of transmission of a multidrug-resistant *Mycobacterium tuberculosis* outbreak strain. *Nat Commun.* 2015;6:7119.

60. Roycroft E et al. Molecular epidemiology of multi- and extensively drug-resistant *Mycobacterium tuberculosis* in Ireland, 2001–2014. *J Infect.* 2018;76:55–67.

61. Bainomugisa A et al. Multi-clonal evolution of multi-drug-resistant/extensively drug-resistant *Mycobacterium tuberculosis* in a high-prevalence setting of Papua New Guinea for over three decades. *Microb Genom.* 2018;4.

62. Trauner A et al. The within-host population dynamics of *Mycobacterium tuberculosis* vary with treatment efficacy. *Genome Biol.* 2017;18:71.

63. Wollenberg KR et al. Whole-genome sequencing of *Mycobacterium tuberculosis* provides insight into the evolution and genetic composition of drug-resistant tuberculosis in Belarus. *J Clin Microbiol.* 2017;55:457–69.

64. Mokrousov I. Molecular structure of *Mycobacterium tuberculosis* population in Russia and its interaction with neighboring countries. *Int J Mycobacteriol.* 2015;4(Suppl 1):56–7.

65. Perdigao J, Macedo R, Silva C, Pinto C, Furtado C, Brum L, and Portugal I. Tuberculosis drug-resistance in Lisbon, Portugal: A 6-year overview. *Clin Microbiol Infect.* 2011;17:1397–402.

66. Gandhi NR, Brust JC, Moodley P, Weissman D, Heo M, Ning Y, Moll AP, Friedland GH, Sturm AW, and Shah NS. Minimal diversity of drug-resistant *Mycobacterium tuberculosis* strains, South Africa. *Emerg Infect Dis.* 2014;20:426–33.

67. Cooke GS, Beaton RK, Lessells RJ, John L, Ashworth S, Kon OM, Williams OM, Supply P, Moodley P, and Pym AS. International spread of MDR TB from Tugela Ferry, South Africa. *Emerg Infect Dis.* 2011;17:2035–7.

68. WHO. World Heatlh Organization Treatment Guidelines for Drug-Resistant Tuberculosis, 2016;49.

69. Pym AS et al. Bedaquiline in the treatment of multidrug- and extensively drug-resistant tuberculosis. *Eur Respir J.* 2016;47:564–74.

70. MSF. *MSF Reports on Use of the New TB Drugs Bedaquiline and Delamanid*, 2016.

71. Pillay M, and Sturm AW. Evolution of the extensively drug-resistant F15/LAM4/KZN strain of *Mycobacterium tuberculosis* in KwaZulu-Natal, South Africa. *Clin Infect Dis.* 2007;45:1409–14.

72. Streicher EM et al. Emergence and treatment of multidrug resistant (MDR) and extensively drug-resistant (XDR) tuberculosis in South Africa. *Infect Genet Evol.* 2012;12:686–94.

73. Ho ZJM, Chee CBE, Ong RT, Sng LH, Peh WLJ, Cook AR, Hsu LY, Wang YT, Koh HF, and Lee VJM. Investigation of a cluster of multi-drug resistant tuberculosis in a high-rise apartment block in Singapore. *Int J Infect Dis.* 2018;67:46–51.

74. Outhred AC, Holmes N, Sadsad R, Martinez E, Jelfs P, Hill-Cawthorne GA, Gilbert GL, Marais BJ, and Sintchenko V. Identifying likely transmission pathways within a 10-year community outbreak of tuberculosis by high-depth whole genome sequencing. *PLOS ONE* 2016;11:e0150550.

75. Verver S et al. Transmission of tuberculosis in a high incidence urban community in South Africa. *Int J Epidemiol.* 2004;33:351–7.

76. Casali N, Broda A, Harris SR, Parkhill J, Brown T, and Drobniewski F. Whole genome sequence analysis of a large isoniazid-resistant tuberculosis outbreak in London: A Retrospective Observational Study. *PLoS Med.* 2016;13:e1002137.

77. Lalor MK et al. The use of whole-genome sequencing in cluster investigation of a multidrug-resistant tuberculosis outbreak. *Eur Respir J.* 2018;51.

78. Shah NS et al. Transmission of extensively drug-resistant tuberculosis in South Africa. *N Engl J Med.* 2017;376:243–53.

79. Dale KD, Globan M, Tay EL, Trauer JM, Trevan PG, and Denholm JT. Recurrence of tuberculosis in a low-incidence setting without directly observed treatment: Victoria, Australia, 2002–2014. *Int J Tuberc Lung Dis.* 2017;21:550–5.

80. Witney AA, Bateson AL, Jindani A, Phillips PP, Coleman D, Stoker NG, Butcher PD, McHugh TD, and Team RS. Use of whole-genome sequencing to distinguish relapse from reinfection in a completed tuberculosis clinical trial. *BMC Med.* 2017;15:71.

81. Korhonen V, Smit PW, Haanpera M, Casali N, Ruutu P, Vasankari T, and Soini H. Whole genome analysis of *Mycobacterium tuberculosis* isolates from recurrent episodes of tuberculosis, Finland, 1995–2013. *Clin Microbiol Infect* 2016;22:549–54.

82. Guerra-Assuncao JA et al. Recurrence due to relapse or reinfection with *Mycobacterium tuberculosis*: A whole-genome sequencing approach in a large, population-based cohort with a high HIV infection prevalence and active follow-up. *J Infect Dis.* 2015;211:1154–63.

83. Kuhnert D, Coscolla M, Brites D, Stucki D, Metcalfe J, Fenner L, Gagneux S, and Stadler T. Tuberculosis outbreak investigation using phylodynamic analysis. *Epidemics.* 2018;25.

84. Parvaresh L, Crighton T, Martinez E, Bustamante A, Chen S, and Sintchenko V. Recurrence of tuberculosis in a low-incidence setting: A retrospective cross-sectional study augmented by whole genome sequencing. *BMC Infect Dis.* 2018;18:265.

85. Chatterjee A, Nilgiriwala K, Saranath D, Rodrigues C, and Mistry N. Whole genome sequencing of clinical strains of *Mycobacterium tuberculosis* from Mumbai, India: A potential tool for determining drug-resistance and strain lineage. *Tuberculosis (Edinb).* 2017;107:63–72.

86. Williams OM et al. Fatal nosocomial MDR TB identified through routine genetic analysis and whole-genome sequencing. *Emerg Infect Dis.* 2015;21:1082–4;218.

87. Dalla Costa ER et al. Multidrug-resistant *Mycobacterium tuberculosis* of the Latin American Mediterranean Lineage, wrongly identified as *Mycobacterium pinnipedii* (Spoligotype International Type 863 [SIT863]), causing active tuberculosis in South Brazil. *J Clin Microbiol.* 2015;53:3805–11.

88. Nelson KN et al. Spatial patterns of extensively drug-resistant tuberculosis (XDR-tuberculosis) transmission in KwaZulu-Natal, South Africa. *J Infect Dis*. 2018;218.

89. Fiebig L et al. A joint cross-border investigation of a cluster of multidrug-resistant tuberculosis in Austria, Romania and Germany in 2014 using classic, genotyping and whole genome sequencing methods: Lessons learnt. *Euro Surveill*. 2017;22.

90. Hargreaves S, Lonnroth K, Nellums LB, Olaru ID, Nathavitharana RR, Norredam M, and Friedland JS. Multidrug-resistant tuberculosis and migration to Europe. *Clin Microbiol Infect*. 2017;23:141–6.

91. Gautam SS, Mac Aogain M, Cooley LA, Haug G, Fyfe JA, Globan M, and O'Toole RF. Molecular epidemiology of tuberculosis in Tasmania and genomic characterisation of its first known multidrug resistant case. *PLOS ONE*. 2018;13:e0192351.

92. Jensenius M et al. Multidrug-resistant tuberculosis in Norway: A nationwide study, 1995–2014. *Int J Tuberc Lung Dis*. 2016;20:786–92.

93. Hargreaves S, Lonnroth K, Nellums LB, Olaru ID, Nathavitharana RR, Norredam M, and Friedland JS. Response to Letter to the Editor by M. van der Werf, V. Hollo and C. Kodmon concerning "Multidrug-resistant tuberculosis and migration to Europe". *Clin Microbiol Infect*. 2017;23:580.

94. Coscolla M et al. Genomic epidemiology of multidrug-resistant *Mycobacterium tuberculosis* during transcontinental spread. *J Infect Dis* 2015;212:302–10.

95. Regmi SM, Chaiprasert A, Kulawonganunchai S, Tongsima S, Coker OO, Prammananan T, Viratyosin W, and Thaipisuttikul I. Whole genome sequence analysis of multidrug-resistant *Mycobacterium tuberculosis* Beijing isolates from an outbreak in Thailand. *Mol Genet Genomics*. 2015;290:1933–41.

96. Popovici O et al. Cross-border outbreak of extensively drug-resistant tuberculosis linked to a university in Romania. *Epidemiol Infect*. 2018;146:824–31.

97. Perez-Lago L, Martinez-Lirola M, Garcia S, Herranz M, Mokrousov I, Comas I, Martinez-Priego L, Bouza E, and Garcia-de-Viedma D. Urgent implementation in a hospital setting of a strategy to rule out secondary cases caused by imported extensively drug-resistant *Mycobacterium tuberculosis* strains at diagnosis. *J Clin Microbiol*. 2016;54:2969–74.

98. Smith CM, Lessells R, Grant AD, Herbst K, and Tanser F. Spatial clustering of drug-resistant tuberculosis in Hlabisa subdistrict, KwaZulu-Natal, 2011–2015. *Int J Tuberc Lung Dis*. 2018;22:287–93.

99. Kapwata T et al. Spatial distribution of extensively drug-resistant tuberculosis (XDR TB) patients in KwaZulu-Natal, South Africa. *PLOS ONE*. 2017;12:e0181797.

100. Doyle RM et al. Direct whole genome sequencing of sputum accurately identifies drug resistant *Mycobacterium tuberculosis* faster than MGIT culture sequencing. *J Clin Microbiol*. 2018.

101. McNerney R, Clark TG, Campino S, Rodrigues C, Dolinger D, Smith L, Cabibbe AM, Dheda K, and Schito M. Removing the bottleneck in whole genome sequencing of *Mycobacterium tuberculosis* for rapid drug resistance analysis: A call to action. *Int J Infect Dis*. 2017;56:130–5.

102. Mahomed S, Naidoo K, Dookie N, and Padayatchi N. Whole genome sequencing for the management of drug-resistant TB in low income high TB burden settings: Challenges and implications. *Tuberculosis (Edinb)*. 2017;107:137–43.

103. Votintseva AA et al. Same-day diagnostic and surveillance data for tuberculosis via whole-genome sequencing of direct respiratory samples. *J Clin Microbiol* 2017;55:1285–98.

104. Dookie N, Rambaran S, Padayatchi N, Mahomed S, and Naidoo K. Evolution of drug resistance in *Mycobacterium tuberculosis*: A review on the molecular determinants of resistance and

105. Shea J, Halse TA, Lapierre P, Shudt M, Kohlerschmidt D, Van Roey P, Limberger R, Taylor J, Escuyer V, and Musser KA. Comprehensive whole-genome sequencing and reporting of drug resistance profiles on clinical cases of *Mycobacterium tuberculosis* in New York State. *J Clin Microbiol* 2017;55:1871–82.

106. Brown TS, Narechania A, Walker JR, Planet PJ, Bifani PJ, Kolokotronis SO, Kreiswirth BN, and Mathema B. Genomic epidemiology of Lineage 4 *Mycobacterium tuberculosis* subpopulations in New York City and New Jersey, 1999–2009. *BMC Genomics*. 2016;17:947.

107. Aung HL et al. Whole-genome sequencing of multidrug-resistant *Mycobacterium tuberculosis* isolates from Myanmar. *J Glob Antimicrob Resist*. 2016;6:113–7.

108. Kidenya BR, Mshana SE, Fitzgerald DW, and Ocheretina O. Genotypic drug resistance using whole-genome sequencing of *Mycobacterium tuberculosis* clinical isolates from North-western Tanzania. *Tuberculosis (Edinb)*. 2018;109:97–101.

109. Black PA et al. Whole genome sequencing reveals genomic heterogeneity and antibiotic purification in *Mycobacterium tuberculosis* isolates. *BMC Genomics*. 2015;16:857.

110. Metcalfe JZ, Streicher E, Theron G, Colman RE, Penaloza R, Allender C, Lemmer D, Warren RM, and Engelthaler DM. *Mycobacterium tuberculosis* subculture results in loss of potentially clinically relevant heteroresistance. *Antimicrob Agents Chemother*. 2017;61.

111. Colman RE et al. Detection of low-level mixed-population drug resistance in *Mycobacterium tuberculosis* using high fidelity amplicon sequencing. *PLOS ONE*. 2015;10:e0126626.

112. Metcalfe JZ, Streicher E, Theron G, Colman RE, Allender C, Lemmer D, Warren R, and Engelthaler DM. Cryptic microheteroresistance explains *Mycobacterium tuberculosis* phenotypic resistance. *Am J Respir Crit Care Med*. 2017;196:1191–201.

113. Cox H, Hughes J, Daniels J, Azevedo V, McDermid C, Poolman M, Boulle A, Goemaere E, and van Cutsem G. Community-based treatment of drug-resistant tuberculosis in Khayelitsha, South Africa. *Int J Tuberc Lung Dis*. 2014;18:441–8.

114. Dave P et al. Has introduction of rapid drug susceptibility testing at diagnosis impacted treatment outcomes among previously treated tuberculosis patients in Gujarat, India? *PLOS ONE*. 2015;10:e0121996.

115. Loveday M, Wallengren K, Voce A, Margot B, Reddy T, Master I, Brust J, Chaiyachati K, and Padayatchi N. Comparing early treatment outcomes of MDR-TB in decentralised and centralised settings in KwaZulu-Natal, South Africa. *Int J Tuberc Lung Dis*. 2012;16:209–15.

116. Dheda K, Gumbo T, Gandhi NR, Murray M, Theron G, Udwadia Z, Migliori G, and Warren R. Global control of tuberculosis: From extensively drug-resistant to untreatable tuberculosis. *Lancet Resp Med*. 2014;2:321–38.

117. Parrish N, and Carrol K. Importance of improved TB diagnostics in addressing the extensively drug-resistant TB crisis. *Future Microbiol*. 2008;3:405–13.

118. Dheda K et al. Outcomes, infectiousness, and transmission dynamics of patients with extensively drug-resistant tuberculosis and home-discharged patients with programmatically incurable tuberculosis: A prospective cohort study. *Lancet Respir Med*. 2017;5:269–81.

119. Sharma A et al. and Global Preserving Effective TBTSI. Estimating the future burden of multidrug-resistant and extensively drug-resistant tuberculosis in India, the Philippines, Russia, and South Africa: A mathematical modelling study. *Lancet Infect Dis*. 2017;17:707–15.

120. Kim SJ. Drug-susceptibility testing in tuberculosis: Methods and reliability of results. *Eur Respir J.* 2005;25:564–9.

121. Van Deun A, Maug AK, Bola V, Lebeke R, Hossain MA, de Rijk WB, Rigouts L, Gumusboga A, Torrea G, and de Jong BC. Rifampicin drug resistance tests for tuberculosis: Challenging the gold standard. *J Clin Microbiol.* 2013.

122. Sanchez-Padilla E, Merker M, Beckert P, Jochims F, Dlamini T, Kahn P, Bonnet M, and Niemann S. Detection of drug-resistant tuberculosis by Xpert MTB/RIF in Swaziland. *N Engl J Med.* 2015;372:1181–2.

123. Martin A, and Portaels F. Methods for detection of drug resistance. In: Palomino J, Cardoso Leão S, Ritacco V (eds.). *Tuberculosis 2007; From Basic Science to Patient Care.* On Line: Amedeo, 2007. 640–54.

124. Brady MF, Coronel J, Gilman RH, and Moore DA. The MODS method for diagnosis of tuberculosis and multidrug resistant tuberculosis. *J Vis Exp.* 2008;18.

125. Huyen MN, Cobelens FG, Buu TN, Lan NT, Dung NH, Kremer K, Tiemersma EW, and van Soolingen D. Epidemiology of isoniazid resistance mutations and their effect on tuberculosis treatment outcomes. *Antimicrob Agents Chemother.* 2013;57:3620–7.

126. Chien JY, Chien ST, Chiu WY, Yu CJ, and Hsueh PR. Moxifloxacin improves treatment outcomes in patients with ofloxacin-resistant multidrug-resistant tuberculosis. *Antimicrob Agents Chemother.* 2016;60:4708–16.

127. Barrera L et al. *Policy Guidance on Drug-Susceptibility Testing (DST) of Second-Line Antituberculosis Drugs.* WHO. Geneva, 2008.

128. Ogwang S et al. Comparison of rapid tests for detection of rifampicin-resistant *Mycobacterium tuberculosis* in Kampala, Uganda. *BMC Infect Dis.* 2009;9:139.

129. Coll F, McNerney R, Preston M, Guerra-Assunção JA, Warry A, and Hill-Cawthorn G. Rapid determination of anti-tuberculosis drug resistance from whole-genome sequences. *Genome Med.* 2015;7.

130. Farhat MR et al. Genetic determinants of drug resistance in *Mycobacterium tuberculosis* and their diagnostic value. *Am J Respir Crit Care Med.* 2016;194.

131. Telenti A, Imboden P, Marchesi F, Lowrie D, Cole S, Colston MJ, Matter L, Schopfer K, and Bodmer T. Detection of rifampicin-resistance mutations in *Mycobacterium tuberculosis*. *Lancet.* 1993;341:647–50.

132. Steingart KR. Xpert MTB/RIF test for detection of pulmonary tuberculosis and rifampicin resistance. *J Evid Based Med.* 2013;6:58.

133. Theron G, Zijenah L, Chanda D, Clowes P, Rachow A, Lesosky M, Bara W, Mungofa S, Pai M, and Hoelscher M. Feasibility, accuracy, and clinical effect of point-of-care Xpert MTB/RIF testing for tuberculosis in primary-care settings in Africa: A multicentre, randomised, controlled trial. *Lancet.* 2013;383:424–35.

134. World Health Organization. Automated real-time nucleic acid amplification technology for rapid and simultaneous detection of tuberculosis and rifampicin resistance: Xpert MTB/RIF system for the diagnosis of pulmonary and extrapulmonary TB in adults and children. Publication number WHO/HTM/TB/2013.14. Geneva, Switzerland, 2013.

135. Press statement. FDA permits marketing of first U.S. test labeled for simultaneous detection of tuberculosis bacteria and resistance to the antibiotic rifampin. Available at; http://www.fda.gov/NewsEvents/Newsroom/PressAnnouncements/ucm362602.htm (last accessed January 13, 2014). Federal Drug Administration, 2013.

136. Steingart KR, Schiller I, Horne DJ, Pai M, Boehme CC, and Dendukuri N. Xpert(R) MTB/RIF assay for pulmonary tuberculosis and rifampicin resistance in adults. *Cochrane Database Syst Rev.* 2014:CD009593;1.

137. Dorman SE et al. and Denkinger CM, study t. Xpert MTB/RIF Ultra for detection of *Mycobacterium tuberculosis* and rifampicin resistance: A prospective multicentre diagnostic accuracy study. *Lancet Infect Dis.* 2018;18:76–84.

138. Bahr NC et al. Diagnostic accuracy of Xpert MTB/RIF Ultra for tuberculous meningitis in HIV-infected adults: A prospective cohort study. *Lancet Infect Dis.* 2018;18:68–75.

139. Calligaro GL et al. Effect of new tuberculosis diagnostic technologies on community-based intensified case finding: A multicentre randomised controlled trial. *Lancet Infect Dis.* 2017;17:441–50.

140. Baez-Saldana R et al. Isoniazid mono-resistant tuberculosis: Impact on treatment outcome and survival of pulmonary tuberculosis patients in Southern Mexico 1995–2010. *PLOS ONE.* 2016;11:e0168955.

141. Jenkins HE, Zignol M, and Cohen T. Quantifying the burden and trends of isoniazid resistant tuberculosis, 1994–2009. *PLOS ONE.* 2011;6:e22927.

142. Trajman A, Durovni B, Saraceni V, Cordeiro-Santos M, Cobelens F, and van den Hof S. High positive predictive value of Xpert in a low rifampicin resistance prevalence setting. *Eur Respir J.* 2014;44.

143. WHO. Molecular line probe assays for rapid screening of patients at risk of multi-drug resistant tuberculosis (MDR-TB) 2008 [Cited 2008 May]. Available at: http://www.who.int/tb/features_archive/expert_group_report_june08.pdf

144. Barnard M, van Pittius NCG, van Helden P, Bosman M, Coetzee G, and Warren R. Diagnostic performance of Genotype® MTBDRplus Version 2 line probe assay is equivalent to the Xpert® MTB/RIF assay. *J Clin Microbiol.* 2012;50.

145. Crudu V, Stratan E, Romancenco E, Allerheiligen V, Hillemann A, and Moraru N. First evaluation of an improved assay for molecular genetic detection of tuberculosis as well as RMP and INH resistances. *J Clin Microbiol.* 2012;50:1264–9.

146. Tomasicchio M, Theron G, Pietersen E, Streicher E, Stanley-Josephs D, van Helden P, Warren R, and Dheda K. The diagnostic accuracy of the MTBDRplus and MTBDRsl assays for drug-resistant TB detection when performed on sputum and culture isolates. *Sci Rep.* 2016;6:17850.

147. Meaza A et al. Evaluation of genotype MTBDRplus VER 2.0 line probe assay for the detection of MDR-TB in smear positive and negative sputum samples. *BMC Infect Dis* 2017;17:280.

148. Theron G, Peter J, Barnard M, Donegan S, Warren R, Steingart KR, and Dheda K. The GenoType® MTBDRsl test for resistance to second-line anti-tuberculosis drugs. *Cochrane Lib.* 2013;10:CD010705.

149. Theron G, Peter J, Richardson M, Warren R, Dheda K, and Steingart KR. GenoType((R)) MTBDRsl assay for resistance to second-line anti-tuberculosis drugs. *Cochrane Database Syst Rev.* 2016;9:CD010705.

150. World Health Organization. The use of molecular line probe assays for the detection of resistance to second-line anti-tuberculosis drugs. Policy guidance (WHO/HTM/TB/2016.07). Geneva, Switzerland, 2016.

151. Tagliani E et al. Diagnostic performance of the new version (v2.0) of GenoType MTBDRsl assay for detection of resistance to fluoroquinolones and second-line injectable drugs: A Multicenter Study. *J Clin Microbiol.* 2015;53:2961–9.

152. Orenstein E, Basu S, Shah N, Andrews J, Friedland G, Moll A, Gandhi N, and Galvani A. Treatment outcomes among patients with multidrug-resistant tuberculosis: Systematic review and meta-analysis. *Lancet Infect Dis.* 2009;9:153–61.

153. Votintseva AA et al. Mycobacterial DNA extraction for whole-genome sequencing from early positive liquid (MGIT) cultures. *J Clin Microbiol.* 2015;53:1137–43.

154. Theron G, Peter J, Richardson M, Barnard M, Donegan S, Warren R, Steingart KR, and Dheda K. The diagnostic accuracy of the GenoType((R)) MTBDRsl assay for the detection of resistance to second-line anti-tuberculosis drugs. *Cochrane Database Syst Rev.* 2014:Cd010705;10.

155. Steingart K, Sohn H, Schiller I, Kloda L, Boehme C, Pai M, and Dendukuri N. Xpert® MTB/RIF assay for pulmonary tuberculosis and rifampicin resistance in adults. *Cochrane Database Syst Rev.* 2013;1.

156. TB DOTS Strategy Coordination Directorate. *National Tuberculosis Control Guidelines.* Pretoria: Department of Health, Republic of South Africa, 2014.

157. Dlamini-Mvelase NR, Werner L, Phili R, Cele LP, and Mlisana KP. Effects of introducing Xpert MTB/RIF test on multi-drug resistant tuberculosis diagnosis in KwaZulu-Natal South Africa. *BMC Infect Dis.* 2014;14:442.

158. Saúde BMd. Secretaria de Vigilância em Saúde Programa Nacional de Controle da Tuberculose (2013) Programa Nacional de Controle da Tuberculose, 2013.

159. World Health Organization. Rapid Communication: Key changes to treatment of multidrug- and rifampicin-resistant tuberculosis (MDR/RR-TB), 2018. Licence: CC BY-NC-SA 3.0 IGO. Available at: http://www.who.int/tb/publications

160. Diseases NIo++C. *South African National Drug Resistant Tuberculosis Study,* 2014 [cited 2017, April 5, 2017]. Available at: http://www.nicd.ac.za/assets/files/K-12750%20NICD%20National%20Survey%20Report_Dev_V11-LR.pdf

161. Gunther G et al. Multidrug-resistant tuberculosis in Europe, 2010–2011. *Emerg Infect Dis* 2015;21:409–16.

162. Yuen CM et al. Association between regimen composition and treatment response in patients with multidrug-resistant tuberculosis: A prospective cohort study. *PLoS Med* 2015;12:e1001932.

163. The Collaborative Group for the Meta-Analysis of Individual Patient Data in MDR-TB treatment–2017: Nafees Ahmad, Shama D Ahuja OWA, Jan W C Alffenaar, Laura F Anderson, Parvaneh Baghaei, Didi Bang, Pennan M Barry, Mayara L Bastos,, Digamber Behera AB, Greg P Bisson, Martin Boeree, Maryline Bonnet, Sarah K Brode, James C M Brust, Ying Cai, Geisa F Carlessso,, Eric Caumes JPC, Rosella Centis, Pei-Chun Chan, Edward D Chan, Kwok-Chiu Chang, Macarthur Charles, Andra Cirule,, Margareth Pretti Dalcolmo LDA, Gerard de Vries, Keertan Dheda, Aliasgar Esmail, Jennifer Flood, Gregory Fox, Regina Gayoso,, Medea Gegia MTG, Sue Gu, Lorenzo Guglielmetti, Timothy H Holtz, Jennifer Hughes, Petros Isaakidis, Mathilde Frechet-Jachym,, Leah Jarlsberg RRK, Salmaan Keshavjee, Faiz Ahmad Khan, Maia Kipiani, Serena P Koenig, Won-Jung Koh, Afranio Kritski, Liga Kuksa, Charlotte L Kvasnovsky NK, Zhiyi Lan, Christoph Lange, Rafael Laniado-Laborín, Myungsun Lee, Vaira Leimane, Chi-Chiu Leung, Eric Chung-Ching Leung PZL, Phil Lowenthal, Ethel L Maciel, Suzanne M Marks, Sundari Mase, Lawrence Mbuagbaw, Giovanni B Migliori, Vladimir Milanov ACM, Carole Mitnick, Chawangwa Modongo, Erika Mohr, Ignacio Monedero, Payam Nahid, Norbert Ndjeka, Max R O'Donnell NP, Domingo Palmero, Jean William Pape, Laura J Podewils, Ian Reynolds, Vija Riekstina, Jérôme Robert, Maria Rodriguez BS, Kwonjune J Seung, Kathryn Schnippel, Tae Sun Shim, Rupak Singla, Sarah E Smith, Giovanni Sotgiu, Ganzaya Sukhbaatar PT, Simon Tiberi, Anete Trajman, Lisa Trieu, Zarir F Udwadia, Tjip S van der Werf, Nicolas Veziris, Piret Viiklepp, Stalz Charles Vilbrun KW, Janice Westenhouse, Wing-Wai Yew, Jae-Joon Yim, Nicola M Zetola, Matteo Zignol, Dick Menzies. Treatment correlates of successful outcomes in pulmonary multidrug-resistant tuberculosis: An individual patient data meta-analysis. *Lancet* 2018; THELANCET-D-18-00963R1, S0140-6736(18)31644–1.

164. WHO. *WHO Treatment Guidelines for Drug-Resistant Tuberculosis, 2016 Update.* Geneva, Switzerland: World Health Organisaion, 2016.

165. *WHO Treatment Guidelines for Multidrug- and Rifampicin-Resistant Tuberculosis 2018 Update (pre-final text) Annex 8.* World Health Organization, 2018.

166. Ndjeka N et al. Treatment of drug-resistant tuberculosis with bedaquiline in a high HIV prevalence setting: An interim cohort analysis. *Int J Tuberc Lung Dis.* 2015;19:979–85.

167. Olayanju O, Limberis J, Esmail A, Oelofse S, Gina P, Pietersen E, Fadul M, Warren R, and Dheda K. Long-term bedaquiline-related treatment outcomes in patients with extensively drug-resistant tuberculosis from South Africa. *Eur Respir J.* 2018;51.

168. Schnippel K et al. Effect of bedaquiline on mortality in South African patients with drug-resistant tuberculosis: A retrospective cohort study. *Lancet Respir Med.* 2018;6.

169. Diacon AH et al. Randomized pilot trial of eight weeks of bedaquiline (TMC207) treatment for multidrug-resistant tuberculosis: Long-term outcome, tolerability, and effect on emergence of drug resistance. *Antimicrob Agents Chemother* 2012;56:3271–6.

170. Diacon AH et al. The diarylquinoline TMC207 for multidrug-resistant tuberculosis. *N Engl J Med.* 2009;360:2397–405.

171. Court RG, Wiesner L, Chirehwa MT, Stewart A, de Vries N, Harding J, Gumbo T, McIlleron H, and Maartens G. Effect of lidocaine on kanamycin injection-site pain in patients with multidrug-resistant tuberculosis. *Int J Tuberc Lung Dis.* 2018;22:926–30.

172. Guglielmetti L, Tiberi S, Burman M, Kunst H, Wejse C, Togonidze T, Bothamley G, Lange C, and TBnet, of the TQs. QT prolongation and cardiac toxicity of new tuberculosis drugs in Europe: A Tuberculosis Network European Trials group (TBnet) study. *Eur Respir J.* 2018;52.

173. Shean K et al. Drug-associated adverse events and their relationship with outcomes in patients receiving treatment for extensively drug-resistant tuberculosis in South Africa. *PLOS ONE.* 2013;8:e63057.

174. Olayanju O, Esmail A, Limberis J, Gina P, and Dheda K. Linezolid interruption in patients with fluoroquinolone-resistant tuberculosis receiving a bedaquiline-based treatment regimen. *Int J Infect Dis,* 2019;85:74–9.

175. Zhang X, Falagas ME, Vardakas KZ, Wang R, Qin R, Wang J, and Liu Y. Systematic review and meta-analysis of the efficacy and safety of therapy with linezolid containing regimens in the treatment of multidrug-resistant and extensively drug-resistant tuberculosis. *J Thorac Dis.* 2015;7:603–15.

176. Fortún J, Martín-Dávila P, Navas E, Pérez-Elías MJ, Cobo J, Tato M, De la Pedrosa EG-G, Gómez-Mampaso E, and Moreno S. Linezolid for the treatment of multidrug-resistant tuberculosis. *J Antimicrob Chemother.* 2005;56:180–5.

177. Sirgel FA, Warren RM, Bottger EC, Klopper M, Victor TC, and van Helden PD. The rationale for using rifabutin in the treatment of MDR and XDR tuberculosis outbreaks. *PLOS ONE.* 2013;8:e59414.

178. Diacon AH, van der Merwe L, Barnard M, von Groote-Bidlingmaier F, Lange C, Garcia-Basteiro AL, Sevene E, Ballell L, and Barros-Aguirre D. beta-Lactams against tuberculosis—New trick for an old dog? *N Engl J Med.* 2016;375:393–4.

179. Payen MC, Muylle I, Vandenberg O, Mathys V, Delforge M, Van den Wijngaert S, Clumeck N, and De Wit S. Meropenem-clavulanate for drug-resistant tuberculosis: A follow-up of relapse-free cases. *Int J Tuberc Lung Dis.* 2018;22:34–9.

180. Organisation WH. WHO position statement on the use of delamanid for multidrug-resistant tuberculosis: Expedited review of the phase III clinical trial data of delamanid added to an optimised background MDR-TB regimen: WHO; 2018 No. CC BY-NC-SA 3.0 IGO.

181. Tiemersma EW, van der Werf MJ, Borgdorff MW, Williams BG, and Nagelkerke NJ. Natural history of tuberculosis: Duration and fatality of untreated pulmonary tuberculosis in HIV negative patients: A systematic review. *PLOS ONE*. 2011;6:e17601.

182. Giddings O, Kuhn J, and Akulian J. Endobronchial valve placement for the treatment of bronchopleural fistula: A review of the current literature. *Curr Opin Pulm Med*. 2014;20:347–51.

183. Deshpande D, Srivastava S, Chapagain M, Magombedze G, Martin KR, Cirrincione KN, Lee PS, Koeuth T, Dheda K, and Gumbo T. Ceftazidime-avibactam has potent sterilizing activity against highly drug-resistant tuberculosis. *Sci Adv*. 2017;3:e1701102.

184. Kawada H, Yamazato M, Shinozawa Y, Suzuki K, Otani S, Ouchi M, and Miyairi M. Achievement of sputum culture negative conversion by minocycline in a case with extensively drug-resistant pulmonary tuberculosis. *Kekkaku(Tuberculosis)*. 2008;83:725–8.

185. World Health Organization. *The Role of Surgery in the Treatment of Pulmonary TB and Multidrug- and Extensively Drug-Resistant TB*. Copenhagen, Denmark: World Health Organization European Region Office, 2014.

186. Fox GJ et al. Surgery as an adjunctive treatment for multidrug-resistant tuberculosis: An individual patient data meta-analysis. *Clin Infect Dis*. 2016;62:887–95.

187. Borisov SE et al. Outcomes of patients with drug-resistant-tuberculosis treated with bedaquiline-containing regimens and undergoing adjunctive surgery. *J Infect*. 2018;78.

188. Calligaro GL, Moodley L, Symons G, and Dheda K. The medical and surgical treatment of drug-resistant tuberculosis. *J Thorac Dis*. 2014;6:186–95.

189. Isaakidis P, Casas EC, Das M, Tseretopoulou X, Ntzani EE, and Ford N. Treatment outcomes for HIV and MDR-TB co-infected adults and children: Systematic review and meta-analysis. *Int J Tuberc Lung Dis*. 2015;19:969–78.

190. WHO. *Guidelines for the Programmatic Management of Drug-Resistant Tuberculosis*. Geneva: World Health Organization, 2011. No. WHO/HTM/TB/2009.420.

191. Abdool Karim SS et al. Integration of antiretroviral therapy with tuberculosis treatment. *N Engl J Med*. 2011;365:1492–501.

192. Blanc FX et al. Earlier versus later start of antiretroviral therapy in HIV-infected adults with tuberculosis. *N Engl J Med*. 2011;365:1471–81.

193. Havlir DV et al. and A ACTGS. Timing of antiretroviral therapy for HIV-1 infection and tuberculosis. *N Engl J Med*. 2011;365:1482–91.

194. Marais S, Pepper DJ, Marais BJ, and Torok ME. HIV-associated tuberculous meningitis—Diagnostic and therapeutic challenges. *Tuberculosis (Edinb)*. 2010;90:367–74.

195. Torok ME et al. Timing of initiation of antiretroviral therapy in human immunodeficiency virus (HIV)—Associated tuberculous meningitis. *Clin Infect Dis*. 2011;52:1374–83.

196. WHO. *Consolidated Guidelines on the Use of Antiretroviral Drugs for Treating and Preventing HIV Infection*. World Health Organization, 2016.

197. Sasabe H, Shimokawa Y, Shibata M, Hashizume K, Hamasako Y, Ohzone Y, Kashiyama E, and Umehara K. Antitubercular agent delamanid and metabolites as substrates and inhibitors of ABC and solute carrier transporters. *Antimicrob Agents Chemother*. 2016;60:3497–508.

198. UCSF. Database of Antiretroviral Drug Interactions. 2017. Available at: http://hivinsite.ucsf.edu/insite?pagear-00-02&param=235&post=4

199. Adhikari M. Tuberculosis and tuberculosis/HIV co-infection in pregnancy. *Semin Fetal Neonatal Med*. 2009;14:234–40.

200. Jana N, Vasishta K, Jindal SK, Khunnu B, and Ghosh K. Perinatal outcome in pregnancies complicated by pulmonary tuberculosis. *Int J Gynaecol Obstet*. 1994;44:119–24.

201. Mathad JS, and Gupta A. Tuberculosis in pregnant and postpartum women: Epidemiology, management, and research gaps. *Clin Infect Dis*. 2012;55:1532–49.

202. Nachega J, Coetzee J, Adendorff T, Msandiwa R, Gray GE, McIntyre JA, and Chaisson RE. Tuberculosis active case-finding in a mother-to-child HIV transmission prevention programme in Soweto, South Africa. *AIDS*. 2003;17:1398–400.

203. Sugarman J, Colvin C, Moran AC, Oxlade O. Tuberculosis in pregnancy: An estimate of the global burden of disease. *Lancet Glob Health*. 2014;2:e710–716.

204. Singh N, and Perfect JR. Immune reconstitution syndrome and exacerbation of infections after pregnancy. *Clin Infect Dis*. 2007;45:1192–9.

205. Palacios E et al. Drug-resistant tuberculosis and pregnancy: Treatment outcomes of 38 cases in Lima, Peru. *Clin Infect Dis*. 2009;48:1413–9.

206. Tabarsi P et al. Standardised second-line treatment of multidrug-resistant tuberculosis during pregnancy. *Int J Tuberc Lung Dis*. 2011;15:547–50.

207. WHO. *Companion Handbook to the WHO Guidelines for the Programmatic Management of Drug-Resistant Tuberculosis*. Geneva, Switzerland: World Health Organization, 2014.

208. Zvandasara P et al. Mortality and morbidity among postpartum HIV-positive and HIV-negative women in Zimbabwe: Risk factors, causes, and impact of single-dose postpartum vitamin A supplementation. *J Acquir Immune Defic Syndr*. 2006;43:107–16.

209. Gupta A et al. and Byramjee Jeejeebhoy Medical College-Johns Hopkins University Study G. Postpartum tuberculosis incidence and mortality among HIV-infected women and their infants in Pune, India, 2002–2005. *Clin Infect Dis*. 2007;45:241–9.

210. Centers for Disease Control and Prevention. Provisional CDC guidelines for the use and safety monitoring of bedaquiline fumarate (Sirturo) for the treatment of multidrug-resistant tuberculosis. *MMWR Recomm Rep*. 2013;62:1–12.

211. SIRTURO: Highlights of Prescribing Information: FDA Access Data, 2012.

212. *Best-Practice Statement on the Off-Label Use of Bedaquiline and Delamanid for the Treatment of Multidrug-Resistant Tuberculosis*. World Health Organization, 2017.

213. Reid A et al. and Development of Antiretroviral Therapy T. Severe renal dysfunction and risk factors associated with renal impairment in HIV-infected adults in Africa initiating antiretroviral therapy. *Clin Infect Dis*. 2008;46:1271–81.

214. Kasembeli AN, Duarte R, Ramsay M, and Naicker S. African origins and chronic kidney disease susceptibility in the human immunodeficiency virus era. *World J Nephrol*. 2015;4:295–306.

215. Bige N et al. Presentation of HIV-associated nephropathy and outcome in HAART-treated patients. *Nephrol Dial Transplant*. 2012;27:1114–21.

216. Williams DI, Williams DJ, Williams IG, Unwin RJ, Griffiths MH, and Miller RF. Presentation, pathology, and outcome of HIV associated renal disease in a specialist centre for HIV/AIDS. *Sex Transm Infect*. 1998;74:179–84.

217. Ramsuran D, Bhimma R, Ramdial PK, Naicker E, Adhikari M, Deonarain J, Sing Y, and Naicker T. The spectrum of HIV-related nephropathy in children. *Pediatr Nephrol*. 2012;27:821–7.

218. Wong WM, Wu PC, Yuen MF, Cheng CC, Yew WW, Wong PC, Tam CM, Leung CC, and Lai CL. Antituberculosis drug-related liver dysfunction in chronic hepatitis B infection. *Hepatology*. 2000;31:201–6.

219. Patel PA, and Voigt MD. Prevalence and interaction of hepatitis B and latent tuberculosis in Vietnamese immigrants to the United States. *Am J Gastroenterol*. 2002;97:1198–203.

220. *Guidelines for the Use of Antiretroviral Agents in HIV-1-Infected Adults and Adolescents*, AIDSInfo, 2016.

221. Prevention CfDCa. *Guidelines for Prevention and Treatment of Opportunistic Infections in HIV-Infected Adults and Adolescents*, AIDSInfo, 2016.

222. Restrepo BI, and Schlesinger LS. Impact of diabetes on the natural history of tuberculosis. *Diabetes Res Clin Pract*. 2014;106:191–9.

223. Salindri AD, Kipiani M, Kempker RR, Gandhi NR, Darchia L, Tukvadze N, Blumberg HM, and Magee MJ. Diabetes reduces the rate of sputum culture conversion in patients with newly diagnosed multi-drug-resistant tuberculosis. *Open Forum Infect Dis*. 2016;3:ofw126.

224. Baghaei P, Tabarsi P, Javanmard P, Farnia P, Marjani M, Moniri A, Masjedi MR, and Velayati AA. Impact of diabetes mellitus on tuberculosis drug resistance in new cases of tuberculosis. *J Glob Antimicrob Resist*. 2016;4:1–4.

225. Perez-Navarro LM, Fuentes-Dominguez FJ, and Zenteno-Cuevas R. Type 2 diabetes mellitus and its influence in the development of multidrug resistance tuberculosis in patients from southeastern Mexico. *J Diabetes Complications*. 2015;29:77–82.

226. Slama L, Palella FJ, Jr., Abraham AG, Li X, Vigouroux C, Pialoux G, Kingsley L, Lake JE, and Brown TT. Inaccuracy of haemoglobin A1c among HIV-infected men: Effects of CD4 cell count, antiretroviral therapies and haematological parameters. *J Antimicrob Chemother* 2014;69:3360–7.

227. Scheen AJ, and Paquot N. Metformin revisited: A critical review of the benefit-risk balance in at-risk patients with type 2 diabetes. *Diabetes Metab*. 2013;39:179–90.

228. Heller S et al. Considerations for assessing the potential effects of antidiabetes drugs on cardiac ventricular repolarization: A report from the Cardiac Safety Research Consortium. *Am Heart J*. 2015;170:23–35.

229. Tolman KG, and Chandramouli J. Hepatotoxicity of the thiazolidinediones. *Clin Liver Dis* 2003;7:369–79, vi.

230. Chiang CY et al. Glycemic control and radiographic manifestations of tuberculosis in diabetic patients. *PLOS ONE* 2014;9:e93397.

231. Ruslami R, Aarnoutse RE, Alisjahbana B, van der Ven AJ, and van Crevel R. Implications of the global increase of diabetes for tuberculosis control and patient care. *Trop Med Int Health*. 2010;15:1289–99.

232. Niazi AK, and Kalra S. Diabetes and tuberculosis: A review of the role of optimal glycemic control. *J Diabetes Metab Disord*. 2012;11:28.

233. Lee PH, Lin HC, Huang AS, Wei SH, Lai MS, and Lin HH. Diabetes and risk of tuberculosis relapse: Nationwide nested case-control study. *PLOS ONE*. 2014;9:e92623.

234. Wang JY, Lee MC, Shu CC, Lee CH, Lee LN, Chao KM, Chang FY. Optimal duration of anti-TB treatment in patients with diabetes: Nine or six months? *Chest*. 2015;147:520–8.

235. Hung CL, Chien JY, Ou CY. Associated factors for tuberculosis recurrence in Taiwan: A nationwide nested case-control study from 1998 to 2010. *PLOS ONE*. 2015;10:e0124822.

236. Riza AL et al. Clinical management of concurrent diabetes and tuberculosis and the implications for patient services. *Lancet Diabetes Endocrinol*. 2014;2:740–53.

237. Calligaro GL et al. Burden of tuberculosis in intensive care units in Cape Town, South Africa, and assessment of the accuracy and effect on patient outcomes of the Xpert MTB/RIF test on tracheal aspirate samples for diagnosis of pulmonary tuberculosis: A prospective burden of disease study with a nested randomised controlled trial. *Lancet Respir Med*. 2015;3:621–30.

238. Alsultan A, and Peloquin CA. Therapeutic drug monitoring in the treatment of tuberculosis: An update. *Drugs*. 2014;74:839–54.

239. Heysell SK, Moore JL, Peloquin CA, Ashkin D, and Houpt ER. Outcomes and use of therapeutic drug monitoring in multidrug-resistant tuberculosis patients treated in Virginia, 2009–2014. *Tuberc Respir Dis (Seoul)*. 2015;78:78–84.

240. Vu DH, Bolhuis MS, Koster RA, Greijdanus B, de Lange WC, van Altena R, Brouwers JR, Uges DR, and Alffenaar JW. Dried blood spot analysis for therapeutic drug monitoring of linezolid in patients with multidrug-resistant tuberculosis. *Antimicrob Agents Chemother*. 2012;56:5758–63.

241. Vu DH, Koster RA, Alffenaar JW, Brouwers JR, and Uges DR. Determination of moxifloxacin in dried blood spots using LC-MS/MS and the impact of the hematocrit and blood volume. *J Chromatogr B Analyt Technol Biomed Life Sci*. 2011;879:1063–70.

242. Heyckendorf J et al. Treatment responses in multidrug-resistant tuberculosis in Germany. *Int J Tuberc Lung Dis*. 2018;22:399–406.

243. Olaru ID, Heyckendorf J, Grossmann S, and Lange C. Time to culture positivity and sputum smear microscopy during tuberculosis therapy. *PLOS ONE*. 2014;9(8):e106075. doi: 10.1371/journal.pone.0106075.

244. Günther G et al. Treatment outcomes in multidrug-resistant tuberculosis. *N Engl J Med*. 2016;375:1103–5.

245. Heyckendorf J, Olaru ID, Ruhwald M, and Lange C. Getting personal perspectives on individualized treatment duration in multidrug-resistant and extensively drug-resistant tuberculosis. *Am J Respir Crit Care Med*. 2014;190:374–83.

246. van Cutsem G, Isaakidis P, Farley J, Nardell E, Volchenkov G, and Cox H. Infection control for drug-resistant tuberculosis: Early diagnosis and treatment is key. *Clin Infect Dis*. 2016;62(S3):S238–43.

247. Schaberg T et al. Tuberculosis guideline for adults—Guideline for diagnosis and treatment of tuberculosis including LTBI testing and treatment of the German Central Committee (DZK) and the German Respiratory Society (DGP). *Pneumologie*. 2017;71:325–97.

248. Dowdy DW, Azman AS, Kendall EA, and Mathema B. Transforming the fight against tuberculosis: Targeting catalysts of transmission. *Clin Infect Dis*. 2014;59:1123–9.

249. Keshavjee S, and Farmer PE. History of tuberculosis and drug resistance. *N Engl J Med* 2013;368:89–90.

250. Nicholson T, Admay C, Shakow A, and Keshavjee S. Double standards in global health: medicine, human rights law and multidrug-resistant TB treatment policy. *Health Hum Rights* 2016;18:85–102.

251. Amon JJ, . Limitations on human rights in the context of drug-resistant tuberculosis: A reply to Boggio et al. *HHR Journal*. 2009;11.

252. London L, Cox H, and Coomans F. Multidrug-resistant TB: Implementing the right to health through the right to enjoy the benefits of scientific progress. *Health Hum Rights*. 2016;18:25–41.

253. Kastor A, and Mohanty SK. Disease-specific out-of-pocket and catastrophic health expenditure on hospitalization in India: Do Indian households face distress health financing? *PLOS ONE*. 2018;13:e0196106.

254. Toczek A, Cox H, du Cros P, Cooke G, Ford N. Strategies for reducing treatment default in drug-resistant tuberculosis: Systematic review and meta-analysis. *Int J Tuberc Lung Dis*. 2013;17:299–307.

255. Benbaba S, Isaakidis P, Das M, Jadhav S, Reid T, and Furin J. Direct observation (DO) for drug-resistant tuberculosis: Do we really do? *PLOS ONE*. 2015;10:e0144936.

256. Keshavjee S, Dowdy D, and Swaminathan S. Stopping the body count: A comprehensive approach to move towards zero tuberculosis deaths. *Lancet*. 2015;386:e46–47.

257. Reuter A et al. The devil we know: Is the use of injectable agents for the treatment of MDR-TB justified? *Int J Tuberc Lung Dis*. 2017;21:1114–26.

258. Harding R, Foley KM, Connor SR, and Jaramillo E. Palliative and end-of-life care in the global response to multidrug-resistant tuberculosis. *Lancet Infect Dis*. 2012;12:643–6.

259. Hughes J, and Snyman L. Palliative care for drug-resistant tuberculosis: When new drugs are not enough. *Lancet Respir Med.* 2018;6:251–2.

260. Union T. *South Africa Announces Lower Price for TB Drug Bedaquiline.* International Union Against Tuberculosis and Lung Disease, 2018.

261. Jenkins HE et al. Assessing spatial heterogeneity of multidrug-resistant tuberculosis in a high-burden country. *Eur Respir J.* 2013;42:1291–301.

262. Farhat MR et al. Genetic determinants of drug resistance in *Mycobacterium tuberculosis* and their diagnostic value. *Am J Respir Crit Care Med.* 2016;194:621–30.

263. Daum LT, Rodriguez JD, Worthy SA, Ismail NA, Omar SV, Dreyer AW, Fourie PB, Hoosen AA, Chambers JP, and Fischer GW. Next-generation ion torrent sequencing of drug resistance mutations in *Mycobacterium tuberculosis* strains. *J Clin Microbiol.* 2012;50:3831–7.

264. Farhat MR et al. Genomic analysis identifies targets of convergent positive selection in drug-resistant *Mycobacterium tuberculosis.* *Nat Genet.* 2013;45:1183–9.

265. Zhang HT et al. Genome sequencing of 161 *Mycobacterium tuberculosis* isolates from China identifies genes and intergenic regions associated with drug resistance. *Nat Genet.* 2013;45:1255–U1217.

266. Stucki D et al. Tracking a tuberculosis outbreak over 21 years: Strain-specific single-nucleotide polymorphism typing combined with targeted whole-genome sequencing. *J Infect Dis.* 2015;211:1306–16.

267. Mokrousov I et al. Trends in molecular epidemiology of drug-resistant tuberculosis in Republic of Karelia, Russian Federation. *BMC Microbiol.* 2015;15:279.

268. Zanini F, Carugati M, Schiroli C, Lapadula G, Lombardi A, Codecasa L, Gori A, and Franzetti F. *Mycobacterium tuberculosis* Beijing family: Analysis of the epidemiological and clinical factors associated with an emerging lineage in the urban area of Milan. *Infect Genet Evol.* 2014;25:14–9.

269. Yen S, Bower JE, Freeman JT, Basu I, and O'Toole RF. Phylogenetic lineages of tuberculosis isolates in New Zealand and their association with patient demographics. *Int J Tuberc Lung Dis.* 2013;17:892–7.

270. Vasankari T, Soini H, Liippo K, and Ruutu P. MDR-TB in Finland—Still rare despite the situation in our neighbouring countries. *Clin Respir J.* 2012;6:35–9.

271. Rovina N, Karabela S, Constantoulakis P, Michou V, Konstantinou K, Sgountzos V, Roussos C, and Poulakis N. MIRU-VNTR typing of drug-resistant tuberculosis isolates in Greece. *Ther Adv Respir Dis.* 2011;5:229–36.

272. Bernard C, Brossier F, Sougakoff W, Veziris N, Frechet-Jachym M, Metivier N, Renvoise A, Robert J, Jarlier V, and NRC M-TMgot. A surge of MDR and XDR tuberculosis in France among patients born in the Former Soviet Union. *Euro Surveill.* 2013;18:20555.

273. Kubica T, Rusch-Gerdes S, and Niemann S. The Beijing genotype is emerging among multidrug-resistant *Mycobacterium tuberculosis* strains from Germany. *Int J Tuberc Lung Dis.* 2004;8:1107–13.

274. Jeon CY, Kang H, Kim M, Murray MB, Kim H, Cho EH, and Park YK. Clustering of *Mycobacterium tuberculosis* strains from foreign-born patients in Korea. *J Med Microbiol.* 2011;60:1835–40.

275. Gavin P et al. Multidrug-resistant *Mycobacterium tuberculosis* strain from Equatorial Guinea detected in Spain. *Emerg Infect Dis.* 2009;15:1858–60.

276. Farnia P et al. The recent-transmission of *Mycobacterium tuberculosis* strains among Iranian and Afghan relapse cases: A DNA-fingerprinting using RFLP and spoligotyping. *BMC Infect Dis.* 2008;8:109.

277. Stoffels K, Allix-Beguec C, Groenen G, Wanlin M, Berkvens D, Mathys V, Supply P, and Fauville-Dufaux M. From multidrug- to extensively drug-resistant tuberculosis: Upward trends as seen from a 15-year nationwide study. *PLOS ONE.* 2013;8:e63128.

278. Mor Z, Goldblatt D, Kaidar-Shwartz H, Cedar N, Rorman E, and Chemtob D. Drug-resistant tuberculosis in Israel: Risk factors and treatment outcomes. *Int J Tuberc Lung Dis.* 2014;18:1195–201.

279. Cain KP, Marano N, Kamene M, Sitienei J, Mukherjee S, Galev A, Burton J, Nasibov O, Kioko J, and De Cock KM. The movement of multidrug-resistant tuberculosis across borders in East Africa needs a regional and global solution. *PLoS Med.* 2015;12:e1001791.

280. Moniruzzaman A, Elwood RK, Schulzer M, and FitzGerald JM. Impact of country of origin on drug-resistant tuberculosis among foreign-born persons in British Columbia. *Int J Tuberc Lung Dis.* 2006;10:844–50.

281. Allix-Beguec C, Fauville-Dufaux M, and Supply P. Three-year population-based evaluation of standardized mycobacterial inter-spersed repetitive-unit-variable-number tandem-repeat typing of *Mycobacterium tuberculosis.* *J Clin Microbiol.* 2008;46:1398–406.

282. Mlambo CK, Warren RM, Poswa X, Victor TC, Duse AG, and Marais E. Genotypic diversity of extensively drug-resistant tuberculosis (XDR-TB) in South Africa. *Int J Tuberc Lung Dis.* 2008;12:99–104.

283. Gavin P, Iglesias MJ, Jimenez MS, Rodriguez-Valin E, Ibarz D, Lezcano MA, Revillo MJ, Martin C, Samper S, and Spanish Working Group on M-T. Long-term molecular surveillance of multidrug-resistant tuberculosis in Spain. *Infect Genet Evol.* 2012;12:701–10.

284. Svensson EM, Dooley KE, and Karlsson MO. Impact of lopinavir-ritonavir or nevirapine on bedaquiline exposures and potential implications for patients with tuberculosis-HIV coinfection. *Antimicrob Agents Chemother.* 2014;58:6406–12.

285. Senneville E, Legout L, Valette M, Yazdanpanah Y, Beltrand E, Caillaux M, Migaud H, and Mouton Y. Effectiveness and tolerability of prolonged linezolid treatment for chronic osteomyelitis: A retrospective study. *Clin Ther.* 2006;28:1155–63.

286. Gerson SL, Kaplan SL, Bruss JB, Le V, Arellano FM, Hafkin B, and Kuter DJ. Hematologic effects of linezolid: Summary of clinical experience. *Antimicrob Agents Chemother* 2002;46:2723–6.

287. Xavier AS, and Lakshmanan M. Delamanid: A new armor in combating drug-resistant tuberculosis. *J Pharmacol Pharmacother.* 2014;5:222–4.

288. WHO. *WHO Updated References on Management of Drug-Resistant Tuberculosis: Guidelines for the Programmatic Management of Drug-Resistant Tuberculosis—2011 update.* Geneva: World Health Organization, 2011.

289. Lange C et al. *Management of Patients with Multidrug-resistant/Extensively Drug-Resistant Tuberculosis in Europe: A TBNET Consensus Statement.* ERS Publications, 2014.

290. Sotgiu G et al. Efficacy, safety and tolerability of linezolid containing regimens in treating MDR-TB and XDR-TB: Systematic review and meta-analysis. *Eur Respir J.* 2012;40:1430–42.

291. Chang KC, Yew WW, Tam CM, and Leung CC. WHO group 5 drugs and difficult multidrug-resistant tuberculosis: A systematic review with cohort analysis and meta-analysis. *Antimicrob Agents Chemother.* 2013;57:4097–104.

292. World Health Organization. *WHO Treatment Guidelines for Drug-Resistant Tuberculosis,* 2016 update. WHO/HTM/TB/201604, 2016.

293. WHO. *The Use of Bedaquiline in the Treatment of Multidrug-Resistant Tuberculosis: Interim Policy Guidance.* Geneva: World Health Organisation, 2013.

294. WHO. *The Use of Delaminid in the Treatment of Mutlidrug-Resistant Tuberculosis: Interim Policy Guidance.* Geneva: World Health Organisation, 2014.

295. Garcia-Prats AJ, Rose PC, Draper HR, Seddon JA, Norman J, McIlleron HM, Hesseling AC, and Schaaf HS. Effect of coadministration of lidocaine on the pain and pharmacokinetics of intramuscular amikacin in children with multidrug-resistant tuberculosis: A randomized crossover trial. *Pediatr Infect Dis J*. 2018;37:1199–203.

296. Muller B, Borrell S, Rose G, and Gagneux S. The heterogeneous evolution of multidrug-resistant *Mycobacterium tuberculosis*. *Trends Genet*. 2013;29:160–9.

297. Taneja R, Garcia-Prats AJ, Furin J, and Maheshwari HK. Paediatric formulations of second-line anti-tuberculosis medications: Challenges and considerations. *Int J Tuberc Lung Dis*. 2015;19(Suppl 1):61–8.

298. Esmail A, Sabur NF, Okpechi I, and Dheda K. Management of drug-resistant tuberculosis in special sub-populations including those with HIV co-infection, pregnancy, diabetes, organ-specific dysfunction, and in the critically ill. *J Thorac Dis*. 2018;10:3102–18.

299. Worley MV, and Estrada SJ. Bedaquiline: A novel antitubercular agent for the treatment of multidrug-resistant tuberculosis. *Pharmacotherapy*. 2014;34:1187–97.

300. Zhang C et al. The interaction of CD4 T-cell count and nevirapine hepatotoxicity in China: A change in national treatment guidelines may be warranted. *J Acquir Immune Defic Syndr* 2013;62:540–5.

301. De Lazzari E et al. Hepatotoxicity of nevirapine in virologically suppressed patients according to gender and CD4 cell counts. *HIV Med* 2008;9:221–6.

302. Fortun J, Martin-Davila P, Navas E, Perez-Elias MJ, Cobo J, Tato M, De la Pedrosa EG, Gomez-Mampaso E, and Moreno S. Linezolid for the treatment of multidrug-resistant tuberculosis. *J Antimicrob Chemother*. 2005;56:180–5.

303. Anger HA, Dworkin F, Sharma S, Munsiff SS, Nilsen DM, and Ahuja SD. Linezolid use for treatment of multidrug-resistant and extensively drug-resistant tuberculosis, New York City, 2000–06. *J Antimicrob Chemother*. 2010;65:775–83.

304. Koh WJ, Kang YR, Jeon K, Kwon OJ, Lyu J, Kim WS, and Shim TS. Daily 300 mg dose of linezolid for multidrug-resistant and extensively drug-resistant tuberculosis: Updated analysis of 51 patients. *J Antimicrob Chemother*. 2012;67:1503–7.

305. Mehrzad R, and Barza M. Weighing the adverse cardiac effects of fluoroquinolones: A risk perspective. *J Clin Pharmacol*. 2015;55.

306. Stancampiano FF et al. Rare incidence of ventricular Tachycardia and Torsades de pointes in hospitalized patients with prolonged QT who later received levofloxacin: A retrospective study. *Mayo Clin Proc*. 2015;90:606–12.

307. Im JH, Baek JH, Kwon HY, and Lee JS. Incidence and risk factors of linezolid-induced lactic acidosis. *Int J Infect Dis*. 2015;31:47–52.

308. Roongruangpitayakul C, and Chuchottaworn C. Outcomes of MDR/XDR-TB patients treated with linezolid: Experience in Thailand. *J Med Assoc Thai*. 2013;96:1273–82.

309. WHO. *The Role of Surgery in the Treatment of Pulmonary TB and Multidrug- and Extensively Drug-Resistant TB. Regional Office for Europe*. Copenhagen: World Health Organization, 2014.

310. Chen RY 3rd et al.. PET/CT imaging correlates with treatment outcome in patients with multidrug-resistant tuberculosis. *Sci Transl Med* 2014;6:265ra166.

311. Vorster M, Sathekge MM, and Bomanji J. Advances in imaging of tuberculosis: The role of (1)(8)F-FDG PET and PET/CT. *Curr Opin Pulm Med*. 2014;20:287–93.

312. Diagnosis of Tuberculosis. *Part 32: Detection of Mycobacteria by Microscopic Methods*. Berlin, Germany: Medical Microbiology: German Institute for Standardisation (Deutsches Institut für Normung), Beuth Verlag, 1995.

17

The Surgical Management of Tuberculosis and Its Complications

RICHARD S. STEYN

INTRODUCTION

Pulmonary tuberculosis led to the birth of thoracic surgery. The techniques of pulmonary resection in use today were developed to deal with the persisting problem of tuberculosis (TB) in the 1930s, 1940s, and 1950s. In addition, collapse therapy led to the development of thoracoplasty, still of value in rare circumstances today,[1] now refined by the development of video-assisted technology. Plombage has evolved into techniques of space reduction, such as myoplasty and omentoplasty. As the incidence of TB declined in developed countries, these techniques were left as a valuable legacy and were available to deal with the next epidemic—lung cancer and the chronic infective complications that resulted from this surgery.

Today, however, the management of TB and its sequelae is benefiting from the subsequent development of techniques such as mediastinoscopy, video-assisted thoracic surgery (VATS) and myoplasty. This cross-pollination has provided the modern thoracic surgeon with a broad range of procedures to deal with the continued threat of TB in Western countries, the rising incidence of multidrug-resistant organisms and the continued epidemic of TB in underdeveloped countries. The thoracic surgeon still has an important role, supporting the respiratory physician, in the diagnosis and management of difficult cases.

DIAGNOSIS

The sputum-negative patient may present with mediastinal lymphadenopathy, a pleural effusion or a pulmonary nodule, requiring biopsy to exclude other conditions, especially sarcoidosis, carcinoma and lymphoma, and to obtain tissue for culture and sensitivity. Although the chest radiograph may clearly demonstrate lymphadenopathy, a computed tomographic (CT) scan will often be requested to confirm that lymph nodes within reach of biopsy techniques are enlarged, to help in the choice of the appropriate technique (Figure 17.1), to identify any pulmonary focus and to clarify the relationship of vital structures that present a hazard at surgery. The surgeon has several biopsy techniques from which to choose the one that will most reliably establish the diagnosis, and if more than one is possible will choose on the basis of familiarity, the equipment available and cosmetic considerations (Figure 17.2).

CERVICAL MEDIASTINOSCOPY

Cervical mediastinoscopy is undertaken under general anesthesia using a 2–3 cm incision midway between the suprasternal notch and the thyroid cartilage. Although a safe and relatively minor procedure, considerable experience is needed to avoid damage to the recurrent laryngeal nerves and major blood vessels in this crowded anatomical region.[2] The development of video-assisted mediastinoscopy has been of considerable benefit in training surgeons to navigate safely through this region.[3] The view of the surgeon is enhanced, the assistant can take part in the procedure and each case is a teaching experience (Figure 17.3).

Mediastinoscopy allows access to, and biopsy from, the nodes in the superior mediastinum that lie on either side of the trachea, in the pretracheal position and at the main carina (Figure 17.4). Nodes in the upper pole of the right hilum may be reached, but caution is necessary to avoid damage to the azygos vein and the branch of the pulmonary artery to the upper lobe.

Biopsy material, as in all these techniques, will be sent for culture in addition to histological examination, and because sarcoidosis is an ever-present possibility, biopsies should be taken from several nodal stations to avoid the pitfall of detecting only the granulomatous response in a lymph node adjacent to malignancy. Increasingly mediastinoscopy is undertaken as a day case.[4]

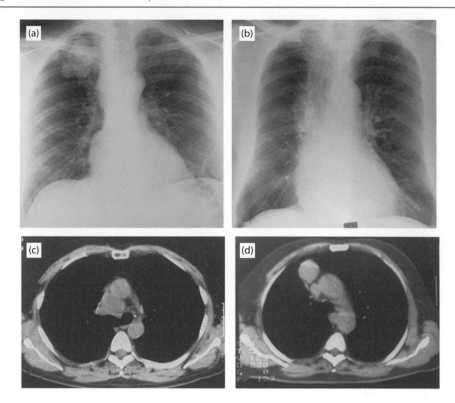

Figure 17.1 Although postero-anterior chest x-rays can show that there is a mediastinal abnormality, a CT scan is necessary to show the precise site and route for biopsy. The chest film in (a) shows mediastinal widening in a patient with lung cancer, similar in appearance to the mediastinum in (b) of a patient subsequently shown to have a thymoma. The CT films in (c) and (d) clearly show that the abnormality in (a) would be accessible to cervical mediastinoscopy, while that in (b) could not be reached by this route and requires right anterior mediastinotomy.

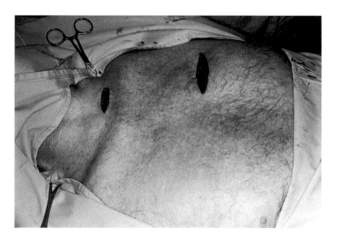

Figure 17.2 The incisions used to explore the mediastinum surgically. The patient's chin is to the left, the clavicles are visible, as is the right nipple. The upper incision at the root of the neck provides access for cervical mediastinoscopy, the longer incision on the left chest wall is for anterior mediastinotomy. The cosmetic result of the former is very satisfactory as the scar is in the skin crease. The latter results in a visible scar that is less satisfactory.

ANTERIOR MEDIASTINOTOMY

Anterior mediastinotomy is undertaken under general anesthesia utilizing a 3–5 cm incision through the intercostal interspace over the area to be biopsied,[2] most commonly the second intercostal space on the left or right (Figure 17.2). Resection of the costal cartilage is unnecessary and results in an ugly sulcus beneath the scar

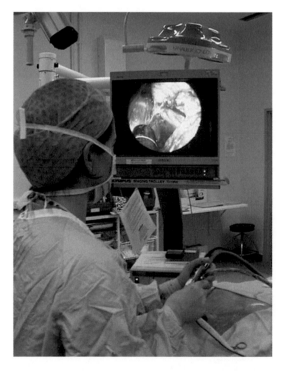

Figure 17.3 A patient undergoing cervical video mediastinoscopy. The instrument is inserted beneath the pretracheal fascia, and dissection proceeds to the main carina. The surgeon and assistant view the field on the monitor allowing both to participate in the operation. The view is magnified and structures are more clearly seen than with conventional mediastinoscopy.

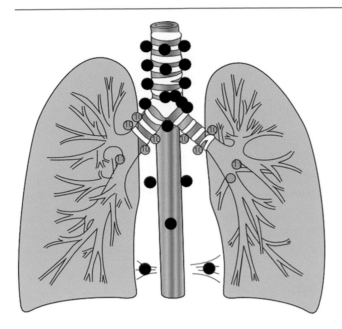

Figure 17.4 A nodal chart used to describe node positions. Those nodes in stations 1–4 in the paratracheal areas, stations 1 and 3 in the pretracheal area and station 7 at the main carina are accessible to cervical mediastinoscopy. Stations 5 and 6 lying beneath the aortic arch and over the ascending aorta are only accessible by anterior mediastinotomy.

that is prone to hematoma and infection. In any event, the scar is cosmetically less acceptable, particularly for younger women and those who are heavy breasted. This approach provides safe access to nodes in the anterior mediastinum and those outside the aortic arch (Figure 17.4).

Digital examination through the interspace will identify a safe target that can be incised to provide a large biopsy. The procedure can be enhanced by using the video mediastinoscope (as used for cervical mediastinoscopy). The use of the diathermy should be reserved for hemostasis after a representative biopsy has been secured; one should avoid the temptation to biopsy vascular nodes using the diathermy ventilation, and this is mandatory if more complex procedures are contemplated involving several access

ports. Although VATS can be used to access mediastinal lymph nodes that lie in a suitable location, these are usually accessible with greater ease and less equipment using one of the previous techniques. VATS is of value when biopsy of the pleura (Figure 17.5) or lung is needed.

THORACOTOMY AND PULMONARY RESECTION

Thoracotomy and pulmonary resection will on occasions prove the only technique that will allow a firm diagnosis and exclude covert malignancy.[6] VATS surgery is becoming the preferred approach for excision of lung lesions less that 3 cm in size (although increasingly some units are utilizing a VATS approach for even larger lesions). Where the lung abnormalities are larger or confluent or dense adhesions are present, thoracotomy may be necessary to fully explore the chest (Figure 17.6). The surgeon will wish to avoid taking biopsies from the periphery of such consolidated areas because this may miss an underlying neoplasm, and the procedure must ensure for the patient a full and reliable assessment.

Progressive dissection, with frequent frozen-section biopsies, is necessary to encircle the abnormality. Often during such a dissection, the true pathology becomes apparent because this will result in material of little value to the histopathologist. The pleura is often entered when undertaking biopsy through the right side, but this is of little consequence if the breach is recognized and air evacuated before closing the wound using a temporary drain through the incision. A post-operative chest radiograph is mandatory. Most patients will wish to stay overnight before discharge.

ENDOBRONCHIAL ULTRASOUND AND BIOPSY

Endobronchial ultrasound (EBUS)-guided fine-needle aspiration biopsy of mediastinal nodes offers a less invasive alternative for sampling of the mediastinal nodes (http://guidance. nice.org. uk/IPG254). The procedure is being widely adopted by respiratory physicians and is reducing the practice of mediastinoscopy.[5] This procedure is very similar to flexible bronchoscopy and can be undertaken with conscious sedation or under general anesthesia.

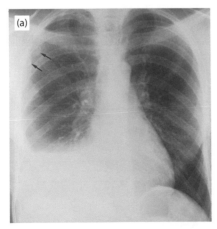
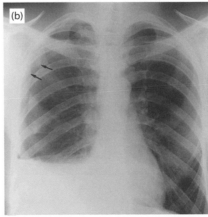

Figure 17.5 (a) The chest x-ray of a patient presenting with a right pleural effusion. The underlying pleural nodules (arrowed) are easier to see on (b) a second radiograph taken after aspiration had resulted in an inadvertent pneumothorax. Biopsy by video-assisted thoracoscopy showed the presence of necrotizing granulomata and acid-fast bacilli.

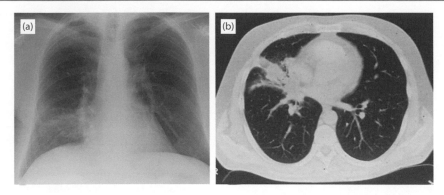

Figure 17.6 (a) The postero-anterior chest x-ray and (b) computed tomographic film of a middle-aged smoker with hemoptysis. The extensive consolidation required exploratory thoracotomy and middle lobectomy to establish a diagnosis of TB and to exclude an underlying neoplasm.

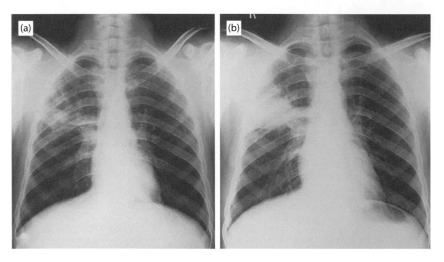

Figure 17.7 (a) The chest x-ray of a patient sputum-positive for TB. During treatment with appropriate antibiotics, (b) a second x-ray showed the opacity to have progressed. At thoracotomy, a carcinoma was confirmed and resected.

The EBUS bronchoscope is similar in dimensions to a standard adult fiber-optic bronchoscope but has an ultrasound probe at its distal end. Proximal to the ultrasound probe, and at 30 degrees to the long axis of the bronchoscope, are a fiber-optic lens and a biopsy channel, through which a 22-G biopsy needle can be passed.

VIDEO-ASSISTED THORACOSCOPY

VATS can be undertaken with a single 2-cm access port under local anesthesia with the patient breathing spontaneously. However, better access is afforded with greater comfort for the patient and surgeon if general anesthesia and single-lung diagnosis of malignancy or clear proof of TB is found, but if the biopsy reports are of non-specific inflammation, the surgeon will feel that lobectomy is necessary. It is uncertain whether resection in these circumstances speeds resolution of the infective process, but it is certainly preferable to failing to resect a potentially curable cancer. Of course, if TB is established subsequently or seems probable on macroscopic examination of the resection specimen, conventional drug treatment should be started immediately, ahead of culture results.

Lung cancer can occur in conjunction with active TB, or follow years after exposure or effective therapy (Figure 17.7). The supervising clinician needs to be aware of this possibility if radiological progression is observed despite "adequate" therapy or if "reactivation" is suggested by the development of a new opacity. Many such patients are too frail or have insufficient pulmonary reserve to tolerate resection, but needle biopsy is warranted and effective non-surgical therapy should not be withheld. The fear of reactivation of dormant tuberculous infection by chemotherapy or radiotherapy makes the use of prophylactic anti-tuberculous therapy justified in such circumstances.

MANAGEMENT

RESISTANT TB

Occasionally, organisms that are sensitive to drug therapy, if sequestered within lung cavities, may not be eradicated by "adequate" drug therapy (Figure 17.8). The surgeon may complete sterilization in such cases by resecting the cavity. For such major surgery, the patient should be in a good nutritional state with adequate lung function to withstand resection and should have had a course of appropriate anti-tuberculous chemotherapy for at least

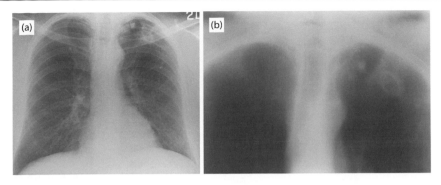

Figure 17.8 (a) The postero-anterior chest x-ray and (b) tomograms of a patient with "resistant" TB. Bacteriological clearance was obtained by excision of the upper division of the left upper lobe.

three months. In practice, in the undernourished subjects who are likely to require such surgery, a considerable period of in-patient preparation will be required to optimize their condition with nutritional support and intensive physiotherapy.[7,8]

The surgeon will wish to document the full extent of the lung disease before surgery, to see the size and extent of the cavity, to visualize any additional cavities, to anticipate the probable extent of resection and to assess the degree to which fibrosis involves adjacent lung segments. In the past, bronchography was extremely useful in this respect but has now been superseded by CT scanning.

Resection in these circumstances is often technically demanding.[8–10] The pleural space and fissural planes are usually obliterated by chronic inflammation, and hard, adherent nodes surround the hilar structures. The surgeon's attempts to be conservative will be made difficult by such problems and by the surrounding fibrosis that usually extends into lung parenchyma beyond the area of the cavity. Careful and technically taxing dissection is necessary. Despite meticulous hemostasis, blood transfusion is frequently required.[11]

The surgeon must make every attempt to preserve lung tissue that is judged to be recoverable. This will on occasion present the clinician with the additional problem posed by a small lung remnant failing to fill the hemithorax. The combination of a small residual lung, fibrotic or emphysematous lung parenchyma with a persistent air-leak and the consequent need for prolonged drainage is a recipe for the development of a chronic space infection. The surgeon will wish to avoid this and, if this scenario seems probable, will add a space reduction procedure to the operation, either immediately or after a period of drainage has established the maximal expansion to which the residual lung is capable and defined the extent of chest cavity reduction that is required.[5,12]

There are a number of such techniques available to the surgeon. A "trimming" thoracoplasty is an old and welltried operation.[13] This involves the subperiosteal resection of the upper ribs sufficient to reduce the chest cavity to the size that will accommodate the residual lung. The first rib is removed from the sternum to the neck, protecting the neurovascular structures at the apex and usually two to four other ribs, from the head of the rib forward over a sufficient arc of the rib. The anterior extent of the resection of these ribs is progressively tailored to leave the new apex of the chest cavity configured to the shape of the remaining lung segments (Figure 17.9). In this context, it is not usually necessary to

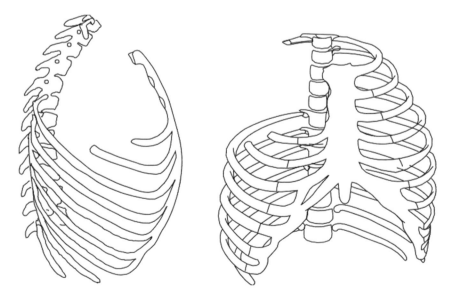

Figure 17.9 A diagram to illustrate the skeletal resection associated with a five-rib thoracoplasty. In this case, the majority of the first rib has been resected, the whole of ribs 2 and 3, with the transverse processes, and tailored resection of ribs 4 and 5 with the transverse processes.

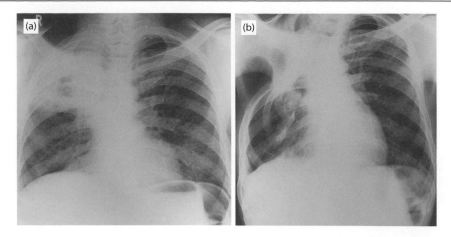

Figure 17.10 (a) The chest x-ray of a patient with extensive cavitation due to TB presenting with life-threatening hemoptysis. (b) Emergency surgery was successful but entailed resection of the right upper lobe, the apical segment of the lower lobe and a trimming, five-rib thoracoplasty (note the first rib was left on this occasion).

resect the transverse processes of the vertebrae. The removal of up to three ribs has little cosmetic impact, although physiotherapy is necessary to preserve posture and good shoulder movement, but more than this is probably now unacceptable (Figure 17.10) because other techniques are available.

A pleural tent can be fashioned by extrapleural mobilization over the apex. This produces a hematoma above the tent and will reduce intrapleural volume without irreversibly compressing the lung parenchyma. Unfortunately, in this context, the pleura is usually damaged during dissection and is not available for this technique. The diaphragm may be temporarily paralyzed by cryoablation of the phrenic nerve immediately above its insertion, allowing the diaphragm to rise to obliterate any residual space. Unfortunately, this development of the phrenic crush procedure may not prove adequate if the diaphragmatic position is fixed by chronic inflammation and fibrosis. A myoplastic rotation flap provides healthy tissue to help fill the hemithorax. If the services of an expert reconstructive surgeon are on hand, the ipsilateral latissimus dorsi, the pectoralis major and the serratus anterior, separately or in combination, can be mobilized on their vascular pedicle and transposed into the chest cavity through a short rib resection at an appropriate level.

Although such techniques are technically demanding and require some anticipation on the part of the thoracic surgeon, they provide a good cosmetic result with rapid recovery.[14] In practice, a limited "trimming" thoracoplasty combined with a myoplastic flap provides good space reduction with a satisfactory cosmetic result, even if only the basal segments of the lower lobe can be preserved.

Sadly, pneumonectomy will still prove necessary on occasions when all function has been lost on one side and the other lung is normal or the site of minimal disease (Figure 17.11). In such circumstances, it is may be appropriate to undertake pleuropneumonectomy because this facilitates dissection and ensures the clearance of any infected collections within the pleural space. Although the mortality of this formidable operation is now less than 10%,[7,9,15] the morbidity remains high, around 30%, chiefly through the development of infective problems often linked with

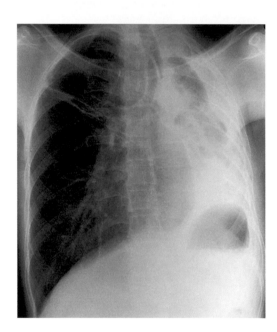

Figure 17.11 The chest x-ray of a patient with "resistant" TB with extensive destruction of the left lung and minimal disease on the right. Pleuropneumonectomy was performed after three months of drug therapy and resulted in sputum conversion.

bronchopleural fistula (BPF). This complication can be reduced by meticulous surgical technique and the use of pedicled muscle flaps.[16] Anti-tuberculous chemotherapy should be continued postoperatively, modified by bacteriological information from the resection specimen. Most authors suggest at least a further six months of drug therapy, although others recommend 12 months.[6]

MULTIDRUG-RESISTANT TB

Mycobacteria resistant to one or more first-line drugs are now increasingly being encountered in developed countries. Although multidrug-resistant TB (MDR-TB) is relatively uncommon in Northern Europe,[17] it presents the most common indication for surgery in TB in North America.[12,18] The World Health

Organization (WHO) has issued recommendations for treating (https://www.who.int/tb/publications/2019/consolidated-guidelines-drug-resistant-TB-treatment/en/); however, most of the evidence is based on case series and expert consensus rather than randomized-controlled studies.[19] Surgery is recommended in patients with a high risk of relapse based on drug-resistance profile and persistently positive sputum despite aggressive drug therapy but with localized disease amenable to resection. Prolonged medical therapy is important in the selection and preparation of patients for surgery, and, ideally, sputum conversion should be obtained before an operation.[12,18] Patients who do not become sputum-negative and those with residual cavities or destroyed lung parenchyma should undergo surgery, as long as the areas of the lung acting as reservoirs of infection can be encompassed by resection (Figure 17.11).

Those who have widespread, bilateral parenchymal disease are not suitable (Figure 17.12). The risks of BPF make the addition of a myoplastic flap to cover the bronchial stump justified, at least in those undergoing pneumonectomy,[12] and some authors would add this routinely to any patient undergoing pulmonary resection for MDR-TB.[18] Drugs are continued post-operatively for a prolonged period, but many patients will default despite careful supervision. Prolonged disease control will be achieved with surgery and drug therapy in up to 90% of this difficult population,[12,20] an improvement on the high relapse rate seen with medical therapy alone.[21]

SURGERY FOR THE COMPLICATIONS OF TB

A tuberculous effusion will resolve with drug therapy unless complicated by pyogenic infection, or the development of a BPF, resulting in an empyema. Such septic complications usually occur during the acute illness, but if resolution is incomplete, the presence of a persisting loculus may lead to empyema many years after successful eradication of the tuberculous infection. The treatment of such a complication, whatever the time course, follows the general principles of any empyema: drainage followed by definitive therapy and identify the organism. Occasionally, mycobacteria will be found if the original infection was not treated adequately, but usually pyogenic bacteria are responsible. An intercostal drain may be necessary if the patient is toxic and unwell, but in most cases, drainage will be surgical, by rib resection at the most dependent point of the empyema. If this site is not obvious on either CT scan or erect ultrasound scan, a small volume of heavy radio-opaque contrast material will demonstrate the optimal point for drainage on subsequent erect, lateral and postero-anterior chest x-rays.

At the time of drainage, the surgeon will evacuate all fibrin debris and, if there is no clinical or radiographic evidence to suggest a BPF, will irrigate the cavity to clean the space. Such debridement can be facilitated by VATS,[22] and at times this may amount to video-assisted decortication.[23] Adequate open drainage, given time, will lead to the slow reexpansion of the underlying lung, as long as the lung has fully recovered from the tuberculous infection (Figure 17.13). In frail, debilitated individuals, the clinician may persist with drainage in the hope that resolution occurs or their condition improves sufficiently to allow other options to be considered. Fenestration, the creation of a skin-lined window or Eloesser flap,[24] facilitates prolonged drainage without the logistical problems associated with tube drainage.

Definitive surgical treatment will speed re-expansion and resolution of the chronic infection but is dependent upon the fitness of the patient and the state of the lung as assessed by CT scanning. Decortication can be difficult if the visceral cortex is calcified, as may be the case in empyemata that occur many years after the tuberculous infection, and this situation is akin to the problems associated with collapse therapy. If the cortex can be removed, the lung will re-expand if the parenchyma is healthy. If bronchiectasis is present in a segment, lobe or the whole lung, pulmonary resection should be combined with decortication. If the residual lung is too small to fill the hemithorax, due to extensive resection or parenchymal fibrosis, one of the space-filling techniques described earlier will be added to decortication, unless pneumonectomy has proven necessary. Given the bilateral nature of the lung damage that is often present, the surgeon will strive to preserve any functioning lung tissue on the side of the empyema.

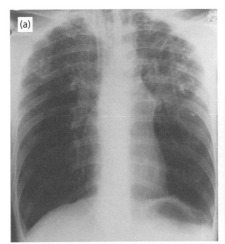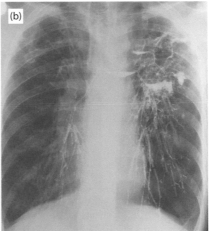

Figure 17.12 (a) The postero-anterior x-ray of a patient with "resistant" TB referred for surgery. (b) The bronchogram shows that the extent of cavitation would have required bilateral resections, involving upper lobectomy on the right, upper lobectomy and apical sementectomy with trimming thoracoplasty on the left, which was judged too extensive for this patient's fitness.

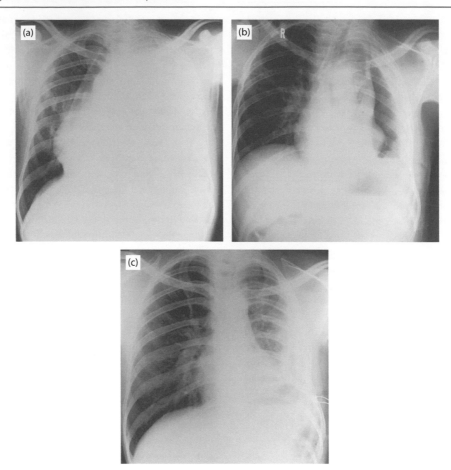

Figure 17.13 (a) The presentation x-ray of a patient with a large, post-tuberculous left empyema. (b) After rib resection and drainage, the mediastinum has moved centrally, but a large space remains on the left. (c) After three months, the space has all but resolved with re-expansion of the left lung. Such recovery suggests that the lung has not suffered severe damage from the tuberculous infection. After a further six weeks, a sinogram showed no residual space and the drain was removed.

The severity of symptoms may make surgery necessary for some of the other complications of TB.[8] A persistent cough, productive of large quantities of purulent sputum, may result from bronchiectasis, destroyed lung parenchyma or may be due to a persistent cavity. Post-tuberculous bronchiectasis usually results in progressive loss of the lung parenchyma subserved by the affected bronchi and associated atelectasis (Figure 17.14). Resection of such grossly diseased and functionless lung tissue has little impact on residual lung function. Therefore, if the bronchiectatic segments can be encompassed by pulmonary resection, even if this entails

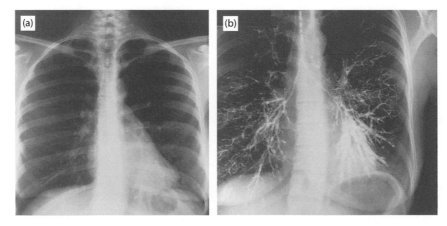

Figure 17.14 (a) The chest x-ray of a patient with collapse of the left lower lobe following TB. (b) Persistent sputum production was resolved after a bronchogram showed complete bronchiectasis of the left lower lobe, sparing of any other segments, and left lower lobectomy successfully relieved the symptoms.

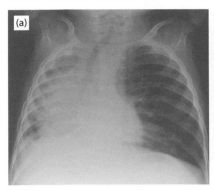
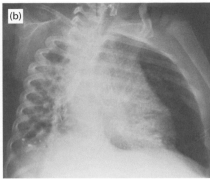

Figure 17.15 (a) The chest x-ray of a three-year-old child following TB left with severe cough with sputum production and failure to thrive. (b) The bronchogram shows total destruction of the right lung and left lower lobe bronchiectasis. He successfully underwent right pneumonectomy and left lower lobectomy, with relief of symptoms and no change in exercise capacity.

bilateral thoracotomies, surgery offers good symptomatic relief (Figure 17.15). The severity of such disease in each lobe or segment correlates well with the contribution it is making to the patient's symptoms. On occasion, therefore, it may be justified to remove a grossly diseased lobe, even if areas of minor damage are left in the ipsilateral or contralateral lung. This can be a difficult decision for the surgeon, but in properly selected cases, significant, if incomplete, relief of symptoms can be expected.

Hemoptysis may be small and repeated or dramatic and life-threatening, and may result from an area of bronchiectasis or destroyed lung, or an uncomplicated cavity. Hemoptysis is much more common and far more problematical when the cavity has been colonized by a fungal ball. Although CT scanning is valuable to demonstrate the presence of fungal colonization of a small cavity (Figure 17.16),[25] this is usually obvious on the chest radiograph with large cavities (Figure 17.17). Cough is then also more persistent and especially debilitating when the patient is supine at night.

The technical problems associated with resection for TB, described previously, are even greater in these circumstances, and surgery is only indicated if symptoms are severe. In many patients, the extent of the disease and their poor health will make such surgery excessively hazardous. Certainly a much greater level of fitness is required than would be needed if undertaking

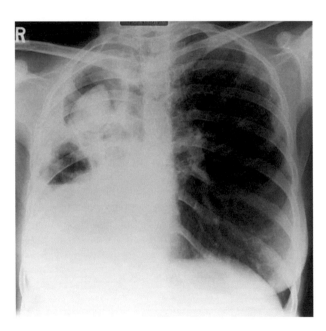

Figure 17.17 The chest x-ray of a patient with total destruction of the right lung following TB. The largest cavity has been colonized by a large fungal ball. Repeated hemoptysis required pleuropneumonectomy.

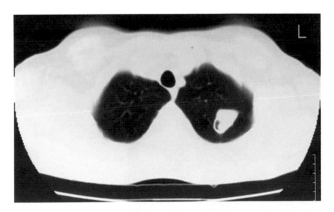

Figure 17.16 The CT scan of an apical mass showing the typical appearances of a fungal ball, allaying suspicions of a neoplasm.[25] (From Roberts CM et al. *Radiology* 165, 123–8, 1987. With permission.)

the relatively straightforward resection of a cancer. The surgeon should strive to be conservative, using space reduction techniques where appropriate. The mortality rate remains high, usually in the region of 10%[6,26] although others have found it as high as 30%.[27]

In the emergency setting, preparation is denied and the risks are even greater. It is not surprising therefore that bronchial embolization is appealing to patient and doctor alike. Even though some radiologists, with diligence and persistence, have managed good results,[28] these are often short-lived, although still of value in permitting surgery to be delayed for more thorough assessment. Surgery, however, is justified in this taxing situation because the risk of further fatal bleeding with medical therapy offsets the appeal of conservative management.[29,30]

If fungal balls are present bilaterally, the associated widespread parenchymal disease will leave few patients with sufficient respiratory reserve to tolerate complex, bilateral resections. If the radiologist can identify the bronchial vessel responsible for the hemorrhage, this should be embolized. If not, then all large bronchial vessels will have to be embolized on both sides, taking care to avoid any important spinal branches. Success in such circumstances is lower, but one has little option in such dire situations. The risk of bleeding seems related to the size of the cavity not the fungal ball.[29] Therefore, if the cavity on one side is considerably larger than on the other side, and if the patient is fit for unilateral surgery, then the clinician may be forced to undertake the speculative resection of the dominant lesion in the hope of salvaging the patient.

For patients in whom embolization has failed repeatedly, and who are unfit for conventional surgery, the surgeon may have to resort to unconventional techniques. Injecting antifungal agents such as brilliant green, natamycin and "Polish paste" into the cavity, bronchoscopically or percutaneously, has been advocated,[31] but the results are unconvincing. Cavernostomy has been tried in the emergency setting with limited success.[32] Cavernostomy in the elective situation is successful at relieving cough and less dramatic bleeding, and the cavity may remain radiologically free of colonization. Transposing a myoplastic flap into the cavity seems to be beneficial even if the flap fails to fill all the interstices of the cavity. Perhaps the muscle with its blood supply exudes cytokines that prevent further colonization. Simultaneous thoracoplasty to collapse the cavity should also be considered.[33]

Endobronchial TB can result in bronchial stenosis and subsequent destruction of the subserved lung parenchyma. If medical therapy with the addition of steroids does not lead to resolution, early recourse to surgery is necessary to preserve lung function.[34,35] Conservative surgery is often possible, and bronchoplastic repair will conserve some or all of the lung parenchyma (Figure 17.18).

SURGERY FOR THE LATE SEQUELAE OF COLLAPSE THERAPY

We are often haunted by our successes. Patients who had cavitating TB in the 1940s and early 1950s and were salvaged from this dismal situation by "novel" collapse procedures may return in their twilight years with the late, infective complications of induced pneumothorax, extrapleural pneumothorax, plombage (Figure 17.19) or

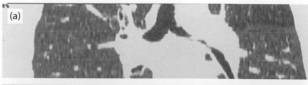
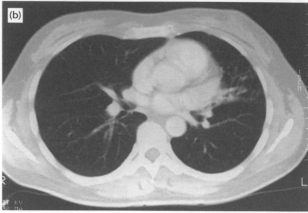

Figure 17.18 (a) A spiral CT reconstruction of a patient who suffered tuberculous endobronchial infection showing stenosis of the termination of the left main bronchus. (b) The scan also confirmed damage to the left upper lobe by obstruction with subsequent bronchiectasis. Bronchoplastic resection of the main bronchus with upper lobectomy restored function to the lower lobe and prevented progressive loss of the whole lung.

an inadequate thoracoplasty. The responsible clinician, and even the patient themselves, may overlook the distant history. Indeed, many of the doctors treating such patients would not have been born at the time of the initial treatment. As a consequence, it is not unusual for such problems to be undiagnosed for many months or dismissed as chest infections or simple empyema.

Once considered, the diagnosis is not difficult and CT scanning will confirm the situation (Figure 17.20). The intrathoracic space will be seen on serial chest x-rays to have enlarged (Figure 17.21) or to have developed a fluid level (Figure 17.22). The infective agent is usually a pyogenic organism, such as *Staphylococcus aureus*, but myobacterium TB may be present and may require additional drug therapy. Surgical management is complex and further complicated by the age and frailty of many patients. Initial

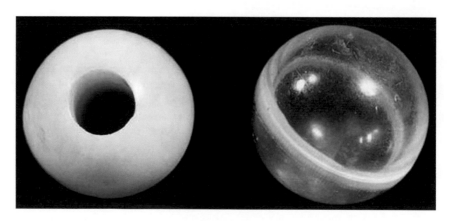

Figure 17.19 Plombage was previously undertaken to facilitate "collapse therapy", using materials such as "polystan balls" (left) and "lucite balls" (right).

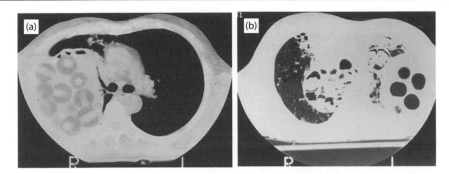

Figure 17.20 CT cuts showing the characteristic appearances of (a) "polystan balls" and (b) "lucite balls". In addition, this patient also had extensive cavitation and fungal colonization.

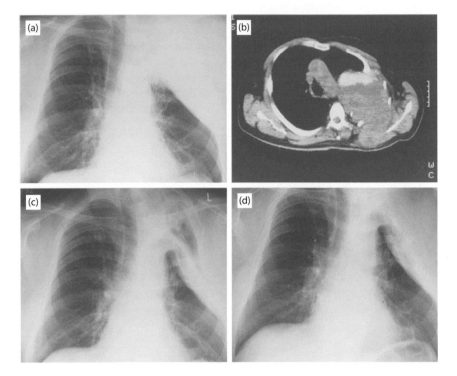

Figure 17.21 (a) The chest x-ray of a patient presenting with chest wall pain and a mass 40 years after plombage for TB. A sarcoma was suspected, but (b) the CT scan shows the underlying plombage expanding through the chest wall. (c) After the evacuation of the shredded plastic plombage material, drainage shows the size of the residual cavity. (d) Six months later, the patient accepted surgery to obliterate the space by trimming thoracoplasty and omental transfer, with complete resolution.

drainage should be performed surgically. Any foreign material is removed from the pleural cavity, which is not difficult if polystan or lucite balls had been used but can be more troublesome if shredded plastic had been inserted without an envelope (Figure 17.21). Subsequent management, and its timing, will depend upon the level of fitness achieved following drainage and the patient's attitude to long-term drainage. If they are sufficiently fit to be offered a permanent solution, most will opt for surgery, despite the obvious risks. If the underlying lung is of reasonable volume and CT suggests it has recovered well from the initial infection and years of collapse, decortication may be attempted. Usually, however, this alone will prove inadequate. The lung may fail to fill the hemithorax, or surgical trauma will leave an excessive air-leak. Space obliteration by myoplasty and/or omentoplasty is often necessary, often combined with a "trimming" thoracoplasty that

reduces the cavity to be filled and allows access for the muscle flap. The omentum is particularly well suited to this situation because of its ability to "mop up" infection and adhere to the underlying lung. A pedicled, rotation flap of omentum may not reach the apex of the chest cavity (Figure 17.23). The addition of a myoplastic flap, based on pectoralis major or serratus anterior, may serve to fill this part of the cavity or the technically more demanding technique of a free graft of omentum may be necessary, using microsurgical re-anastamosis of the vascular pedicle of the omentum to a suitable artery and vein in the thorax, usually the internal mammary vessels.[14]

A shallow, infected pneumothorax cavity may be treated by a localized, Schede type of thoracoplasty[13] with little impact on functional or cosmetic result (Figure 17.24). More extensive thoracoplasty operations of this type are complicated by the subsequent

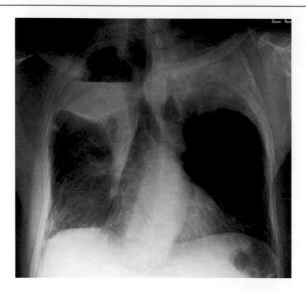

Figure 17.22 The chest x-ray of a patient presenting with fever, cough and hemoptysis 35 years after right extrapleural pneumothorax and right-sided plombage. The fluid level indicates the infection is within the right space.

onset of respiratory failure as a consequence of denervation of the accessory, abdominal muscles of respiration. Revision of the original thoracoplasty may eradicate the residual space (Figure 17.25). If the patient is unfit for definitive surgery, then the options are limited. Long-term drainage requires domiciliary nursing care, and the patient may prefer a fenestrum or Eloesser flap procedure.[24] The best quality of life may be afforded by leaving nature alone and the patient with an intermittent discharging sinus.

Diagnostic procedures for TB, such as mediastinoscopy and VATS, can be performed virtually without risk if the patient is reasonably fit and the surgeon experienced with such techniques,[2] but the risks increase as the procedure becomes more invasive and resection becomes necessary. In such circumstances, considerable experience is necessary to select and prepare the patient and to choose the appropriate technique from the wide range of options available. Although lesser resections can be performed with an operative mortality less than 5%,[6,8] if operating for the severe complications, such as fungal infection especially with massive hemoptysis, or if pneumonectomy proves necessary, expert surgery is needed to keep the mortality around 10%.[6,9,26] Such surgery is technically challenging but worthwhile in the desperate situation faced by such patients.

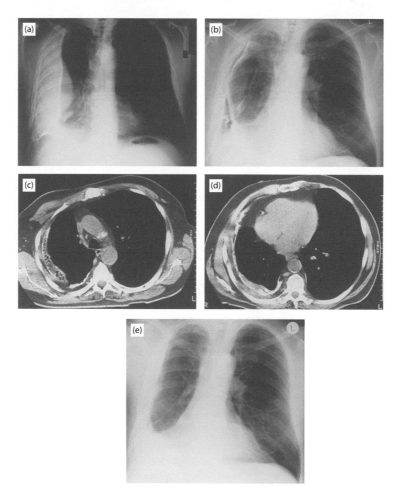

Figure 17.23 (a) The chest x-ray of a patient with right chest pain many years after "collapse therapy" for TB. The presence of the wound and the extensive pleural calcification should have alerted the physician to the underlying cause. The patient neglected to mention the history, and malignancy was suspected. (b) Eventually, rather inadequate drainage was performed by a surgeon who attempted pleurodesis. (c, d) The CT cuts, clearly show the residual space and heavily calcified visceral and parietal cortex. The patient was reluctant to accept surgery and persisted with drainage for one year. (e) The chest x-ray after corrective surgery shows the space obliterated by decortication, omental transfer and a myoplastic flap to the apex of the space.

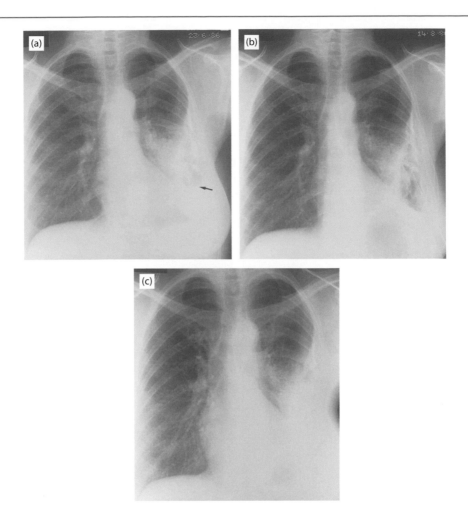

Figure 17.24 (a) The chest x-ray of a female with persistent fever and cough many years after an artificial pneumothorax for TB, showing a fluid level (arrow) in the space. (b) After drainage, acid-fast bacilli were recovered, and the symptoms were relieved. (c) After appropriate drug therapy for three months, the space was obliterated by a localized, "Schede-type" thoracoplasty with acceptable cosmetic results and long-term relief.

OUR APPROACH TO INFECTION CONTROL AND SURGERY FOR MDR-TB

When performing surgery on patients with MDR-TB, in addition to achieving the desired outcome for the patient, the surgical and anesthetic teams must minimize the risk of infection for the staff and other patients. This can only be achieved by ensuring there is good prior preparation, involvement of the infection control team and co-ordinated teamwork. All staff present in the operating room will have fit testing performed with retraining as necessary to ensure correct wearing of filtering facepiece (FFP) masks. Traditionally, operating rooms are positive pressure ventilated with air being pushed out of the room into the surrounding corridors. In MDR-TB cases, it would be ideal to have a negative pressure operating room to allow potentially contaminated air to be removed safely and further reduce risk to staff.[36]

Our patients usually come to the operating theater wearing an FFP2 or FFP3 mask. All staff present in the theater will also don FFP2 or FFP3 masks prior to the patient removing their mask. During the procedure, we minimize staff leaving and re-entering the operating room by ensuring that whenever possible all equipment is available either in the theater or in the adjacent anteroom/ preparation room. We have found however that if the surgery is prolonged, staff wearing FFP masks for sustained periods find this tiring and many have reported developing headaches or feeling uncomfortable. Non-scrub staff may leave the theater for a comfort break; however, the scrub team normally does not; therefore, we normally wear FFP 2/3 masks with an exhale valve to reduce this effect.

After removal of the patient's FFP mask, the patient will breathe oxygen/air mix as appropriate using a face mask connected to the anesthetic machine circuit with waste gas being extracted via a scavenging system. Following induction of anesthesia, our patients always have a bronchoscopy performed. Our preference is to perform a rigid bronchoscopy followed by passage of a flexible fiber-optic bronchoscope via the rigid bronchoscope. Video bronchoscopes allow the surgeon to avoid placing their face near to the patient's face. The combination of rigid and flexible bronchoscopy allows very good rapid clearance of any retained secretions and thorough inspection of the bronchial tree to identify the anatomy

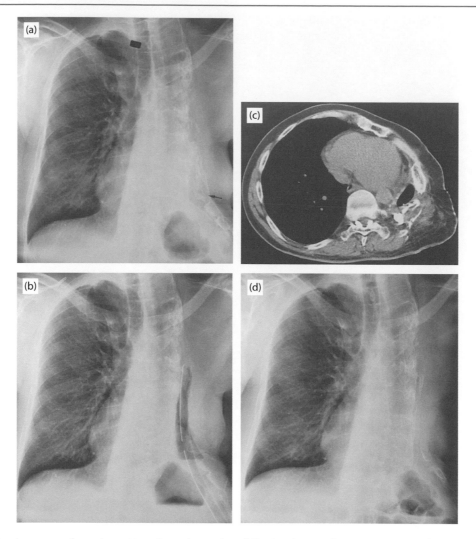

Figure 17.25 (a) The chest x-ray of a patient with an intermittent sinus following thoracoplasty many years earlier, a space is seen (arrow) at the left base beneath the thoracoplasty. (b) After drainage, the extent of the cavity is seen, better demonstrated on CT scan. (d) Revision of the thoracoplasty dealt with the problem with no additional deformity.

and any abnormalities (e.g., bronchial stenosis) that may be present. Normally, for rigid bronchoscopy, patients are ventilated during the procedure using venturi jet insufflation. This is not done in MDR-TB cases; instead patients are kept apnoeic and the procedure is kept short with early return to facemask with waste gas scavenging. Bronchoscopy can be repeated if needed or alternatively the patients can be intubated using a single-lumen endotracheal tube, and the fiber-optic bronchoscopy can be passed via a catheter mount. Once again waste gases are removed using the anesthetic scavenging circuit.

After completion of the bronchoscopic procedures, the patient is intubated with a double-lumen endotracheal tube or, in challenging cases, with a single-lumen tube with bronchial blocker to allow single-lung ventilation. The operative side is now collapsed. Traditionally, in pulmonary surgery, many surgeons would often partially inflate the lung to facilitate dissection of the fissure or lung. However, in MDR-TB, the lung is kept collapsed ideally throughout the procedure until the final stages when the lung is re-inflated under water to check for air leaks prior to closure. This is done immediately prior to closing the

chest. The dissection of fissures or lung itself is performed on the deflated lung to avoid aerosolization and to minimize potential contamination of the surgical team. If, during the procedure, the operative side lung does need to be re-inflated to maintain adequate gas exchange, then this is co-ordinated with the surgeon and the incision is temporally covered while the lung is re-inflated and then deflated.

As mentioned earlier, surgical dissection for TB can be particularly challenging and significant blood loss can occur. Our preference to avoid this is by very meticulous dissection predominantly using diathermy to divide adhesions and tissue rather than sharp dissection. We have also found that hemostatic agents—for example, chitosan (Celox⁻) and gelatin–thrombin matrix (Floseal⁻)—are useful adjuncts for control of bleeding. Attention to detail is essential combined with a thorough understanding of the anatomy and particularly constantly maintaining awareness of the anatomical relations at all times. This is especially important when the inter-lobar fissures have been obliterated by the disease process, and successful surgery may be dependent on being able to create a "new fissure" by dividing the lung parenchyma and individually ligating vessels and bronchi until the pulmonary artery at the base of the fissure is identified. Special attention is paid to identifying and ligating the small bronchi to reduce any air leak and to prevent prolonged post-operative drainage.

REFERENCES

1. Peppas G, Molnar TF, Jeyasingham K, and Kirk AB. Thoracoplasty in the context of current surgical practice. *Ann Thorac Surg.* 1993;56:903–9.

2. Goldstraw P. Mediastinal exploration by mediastinoscopy and mediastinotomy. *Br J Dis Chest.* 1988;82:111–20.

3. Mouroux J, Venissac N, and Alifano M. Combined video-assisted mediastinoscopy and video-assisted thoracoscopy in the management of lung cancer. *Ann Thorac Surg.* 2001;72:1698–704.

4. Cybulsky IJ, and Bennett WF. Mediastinoscopy as a routine outpatient procedure. *Ann Thorac Surg.* 1994;58:176–8.

5. Navani N et al. EBUS-TBNA prevents mediastinocopies in the diagnosis of isolated mediastinal lymphadenopathy: A prospective trial. *Am J Respir Crit Care Med.* 2012;186:255–60.

6. Mouroux J et al. Surgical management of pleuropulmonary tuberculosis. *J Thorac Cardiovasc Surg.* 1996;111:662–70.

7. Conlan AA, Lukanich JM, Shutz J, and Hurwitz SS. Elective pneumonectomy for benign lung disease: Modern day mortality and morbidity. *J Thorac Cardiovasc Surg.* 1995;110:1118–24.

8. Rizzi A et al. Results of surgical management of tuberculosis: Experience in 206 patients undergoing operation. *Ann Thorac Surg.* 1995;59:896–900.

9. Reed CE. Pneumonectomy for chronic infection: Fraught with danger? *Ann Thorac Surg.* 1995;59:408–11.

10. Goldstraw P. Surgery for pulmonary tuberculosis. *Surgery.* 1987;145:1071–82.

11. Griffiths EM, Kaplan DK, Goldstraw P, and Burman JF. Review of blood transfusion practices in thoracic surgery. *Ann Thorac Surg.* 1994;57:736–9.

12. Treasure RL, and Seaworth BJ. Current role of surgery in *Mycobacterium tuberculosis. Ann Thorac Surg.* 1995;59:1405–7.

13. Langston HT. Thoracoplasty: The how and the why. *Ann Thorac Surg.* 1991;52:1351–3.

14. al-Kattan KM, Breach NM, Kaplan DK, and Goldstraw P. Soft-tissue reconstruction in thoracic surgery. *Ann Thorac Surg.* 1995;60:1372–5.

15. al-Kattan KM, and Goldstraw P. Completion pneumonectomy: Indications and outcome. *J Thorac Cardiovasc Surg.* 1995;110:1125–9.

16. Cerfolio RJ. The incidence, etiology, and prevention of postresectional bronchopleural fistula. *Semin Thorac Cardiovasc Surg.* 2001;13(1):3–7.

17. Medical Research Council Cardiothoracic Epidemiology Group. National survey of notifications of tuberculosis in England and Wales in 1988. *Thorax.* 1992;47:770–5.

18. Pomerantz M, Madsen L, Goble M, and Iseman M. Surgical management of resistant *Mycobacterial tuberculosis* and other mycobacterial pulmonary infections. *Ann Thorac Surg.* 1991;52:1108–12.

19. Marrone MT, Venkataramanan V, Goodman M, Hill AC, Jereb JA, and Mase SR. Surgical interventions for drug-resistant tuberculosis: A systematic review and meta-analysis. *Int J Tuberc Lung Dis.* 2013;17:6–16.

20. Yu JA, Weyant MJ, and Mitchell JD. Surgical treatment of atypical mycobacterial infections. *Thorac Surg Clin.* 2012;22(3):277–85.

21. Goble M et al. Treatment of 171 patients with pulmonary tuberculosis resistant to isoniazid and rifampin. *N Engl J Med.* 1993;328:527–32.

22. Lawrence DR, Ohri SK, Moxon RE, and Fountain SW. Thoracoscopic debridement of empyema thoracis. *Ann Thorac Surg.* 1997;64:1448–50.

23. Ferguson MK. Thoracoscopy for empyema, bronchopleural fistula, and chylothorax. *Ann Thorac Surg.* 1993;56:644–5.

24. Eloesser L. An operation for tuberculous empyema. *Surg Gynaecol Obstet.* 1935;60:1096.

25. Roberts CM, Citron KM, and Strickland BS. Intrathoracic aspergilloma: Role of CT in diagnosis and treatment. *Radiology.* 1987;165:123–8.

26. Massard G et al. Pleuropulmonary aspergilloma: Clinical spectrum and results of surgical treatment. *Ann Thorac Surg.* 1992;54:1159–64.

27. Daly RC et al. Pulmonary aspergillomas. Results of surgical treatment. *J Thorac Cardiovasc Surg.* 1986;92:981–8.

28. Remy J et al. Treatment of hemoptysis by embolization of bronchial arteries. *Radiology.* 1977;122:33–7.

29. Jewkes J, Kay PH, Paneth M, and Citron KM. Pulmonary aspergilloma: Analysis of prognosis in relation to haemoptysis and survey of treatment. *Thorax.* 1983;38:572–8.

30. Knott-Craig CJ et al. Management and prognosis of massive hemoptysis: Recent experience with 120 patients. *J Thorac Cardiovasc Surg.* 1993;105:394–7.

31. Henderson AH, and Pearson JEG. Treatment of bronchopulmonary aspergillosis with observations on the use of natamycin. *Thorax.* 1968;23:519–23.

32. Rergkliang C et al. Surgical management of pulmonary cavity associated with fungus ball. *Asian Cardiovasc Thorac Ann.* 2004; 12(3):246–9.

33. Massard G, Olland A, Santelmo N, and Falcoz PE. Surgery for the sequelae of postprimary tuberculosis. *Thorac Surg Clin.* 2012;22:287–300.

34. Watanabe Y et al. Results in 104 patients undergoing bronchoplastic procedures for bronchial lesions. *Ann Thorac Surg.* 1990;50:607–14.

35. Frist WH, Mathisen DJ, Hilgenberg AD, and Grillo HC. Bronchial sleeve resection with and without pulmonary resection. *J Thorac Cardiovasc Surg.* 1987;93:350–7.

36. Chow TT, Kwan A, Lin Z, and Bai W. Conversion of operating theatre from positive to negative pressure environment. *J Hosp Infect.* 2006;64:371–8.

18

Tuberculosis in Childhood and Pregnancy

LINDSAY H. CAMERON AND JEFFREY R. STARKE

TUBERCULOSIS IN CHILDREN

INTRODUCTION

Childhood tuberculosis differs from adult tuberculosis in epidemiology, clinical and radiographic presentation, and treatment. The risk of a child developing tuberculosis is influenced by age, immune status, and the intensity of exposure to a source case with tuberculosis disease.[1,2]

Much of adult pulmonary tuberculosis is caused by a reactivation of *Mycobacterium tuberculosis* bacilli contained in the apices of the lungs following hematogenous dissemination at the time of infection. Childhood tuberculosis is most often a complication of the pathophysiologic events following the initial infection. The interval between infection and disease is often years in immunocompetent adults but is often only weeks to months in young children.[1] Young children rarely develop contagious pulmonary disease and are more likely than adults to develop extrapulmonary manifestations of tuberculosis. Based on the differences in the pathophysiology of tuberculosis and the clinical manifestations between adults and children, the approaches to the diagnosis, treatment, and prevention of tuberculosis infection and disease in children are different.[3]

TERMINOLOGY

The terminology used to describe the various stages and clinical presentations of childhood tuberculosis follow the pathophysiology from the initial transmission of *M. tuberculosis* through infection and disease. The stages may not be completely distinct in young children.

Exposure occurs when a child has had significant contact with an adult or adolescent source case with potentially contagious pulmonary tuberculosis. The likelihood of an exposure leading to infection in a child is associated with the contagiousness of the source case and the child's proximity and duration of exposure. The most frequent location for exposure of a child is her household, but it can occur at school, a day care center, or other closed setting. In this stage, the initial test of infection (either a tuberculin skin test [TST] or interferon gamma release assay [IGRA]) is negative, the child lacks signs and symptoms of disease and the chest radiograph is normal. Some children may have inhaled droplet nuclei containing *M. tuberculosis* and have early infection, which is unapparent to a clinician as it takes 2–3 months for a TST or IGRA to become positive. A contact investigation—evaluating those close to the suspected source case with tuberculosis—is the most important activity in a community to prevent cases of tuberculosis in children.[4,5] The US Centers for Disease Control and Prevention (CDC) and the American Academy of Pediatrics (AAP) recommend that children younger than 4 years of age and HIV (human immunodeficiency virus)-infected children at any age who are exposed to a source case with tuberculosis be evaluated for tuberculosis infection and be started on treatment to prevent rapid development of disseminated or meningeal tuberculosis, which can occur before the TST or IGRA become reactive.[6,7]

Infection occurs when a child inhales droplet nuclei containing *M. tuberculosis*, which are deposited in the lung and are established intracellularly within the lung parenchyma and/or the draining lymph system. The hallmark of this stage is a reactive TST or IGRA in an asymptomatic child. The child's chest radiograph is either normal or reveals only granuloma or calcification in the lung parenchyma and/or regional lymph nodes. In developed countries, all children infected with *M. tuberculosis* are treated to prevent the development of disease in the near or distant future.

Disease occurs when a child develops signs and symptoms or radiographic manifestations caused by *M. tuberculosis*. Not all infected individuals will develop disease. An immunocompetent adult with untreated tuberculosis infection has a 5%–10% chance of tuberculosis infection progressing to disease; one-half of this risk occurs within 2–3 years of infection. In contrast, up to 50% of immunocompetent infants with untreated tuberculosis infection will develop disease which is often serious and life threatening, most often 6-9 months after the initial exposure.[1] Children typically have closed caseous lesions with relatively few mycobacteria (termed paucibacillary disease) and, until adolescence, lack the tussive force to transmit bacteria in their environment.

This contributes to the complexity in confirming a diagnosis of childhood tuberculosis; compared to adults, most children have both acid-fast sputum smear and culture negative tuberculosis. Therefore, most children are diagnosed with tuberculosis disease based on a known exposure to tuberculosis, a positive test of infection, clinical symptoms, and supportive radiographic studies. In contrast, adolescents may develop adult-type or reactivation disease with a high burden of bacilli that can be easily transmitted into the environment.

Infection and the onset of tuberculosis disease are often distinct events in adolescents and adults, separated in time. In young children, tuberculosis disease often complicates the initial infection, suggesting that the two stages occur on a continuum.[8] This can cause confusion regarding the optimal treatment regimen for young children with tuberculosis. The current consensus in the United States is to consider disease to be present if thoracic adenopathy or other concerning chest radiographic findings caused by *M. tuberculosis* are identified, even if the child is asymptomatic.

EPIDEMIOLOGY

As most children with tuberculosis infection and disease acquire *M. tuberculosis* from an adult in their environment, the epidemiology of childhood tuberculosis tends to follow that in adults. The risk of a child acquiring tuberculosis infection is environmental, determined by the likelihood that she will be in contact with an adult with contagious disease. In contrast, the risk of a child infected with *M. tuberculosis* progressing to disease depends mainly on host immunologic and genetic factors.

CHILDHOOD TUBERCULOSIS WORLDWIDE

Tuberculosis has surpassed HIV/AIDS as the most frequent infectious disease cause of death worldwide.[9] Approximately 95% of tuberculosis cases occur in the developing world. The global burden of tuberculosis is influenced by several factors including: the HIV pandemic, the development of multidrug-resistant tuberculosis (MDR-TB), and the disproportionately low access of populations in low-resource settings worldwide to both diagnostic tests and effective medical therapy. Due to a lack of laboratory infrastructure in low-resource settings, few children have culture-confirmed tuberculosis, which leads to variation in country-specific childhood tuberculosis case reporting.

The first estimate of the global burden of childhood tuberculosis was published by the WHO in 2012. More recently, mathematical models have been used to estimate the global burden of childhood tuberculosis infection and disease.[9–11] At least 1 million children develop tuberculosis disease each year, and 233,000 die from complications of tuberculosis.[9,10,12] The youngest and most vulnerable children are at highest risk of death from tuberculosis. According to more recent reports from the WHO, nearly 650 children die each day, 80% of whom are less than 5 years of age.[13] The highest overall numbers of childhood tuberculosis cases occur in Southeast Asia followed by Africa. The proportion of pediatric cases is higher in Sub-Saharan Africa than in any other area of the world.[14] India has the largest number of newly diagnosed childhood tuberculosis cases worldwide, followed by the People's Republic of China. Vietnam has had the greatest recent increase in reported rates.

The incidence of drug-resistant tuberculosis has increased in some areas of the world in both adults and children. MDR-TB is defined as resistance to at least isoniazid and rifampin; extensively drug-resistant tuberculosis (XDR-TB) includes MDR-TB plus resistance to any fluoroquinolone and at least one of the three injectable drugs (kanamycin, capreomycin, or amikacin). In 2014, the worldwide estimate for MDR-TB in children was 2.9% of all cases, and for XDR-TB it was 0.1%. The highest incidence of MDR-TB in children occur in the Southeast Asian, African, and Western Pacific Regions; however, the proportion of drug-resistant cases is highest in countries belonging to the Russian Federation, where over 30% of children with tuberculosis have a drug-resistant organism.[11]

CHILDHOOD TUBERCULOSIS IN THE UNITED STATES

Tuberculosis case rates in the United States decreased during the first half of the twentieth century, long before the advent of antituberculosis drugs, as a result of improved living conditions and, likely, genetic selection favoring persons resistant to developing disease. A resurgence of tuberculosis in the late 1980s was associated primarily with: the HIV epidemic; transmission of the organism in congregate settings including health-care institutions; disease occurring in recent immigrants; and poor conduct of community tuberculosis management, specifically contact tracing. Since 1992, the tuberculosis incidence in the United States has decreased, however, the case rate has remained stable at approximately 3 cases per 100,000 persons.[15] From 2007 to 2017, 121,209 tuberculosis cases had complete data reported to the National Tuberculosis Surveillance System, of whom 9,276 (8%) were children and adolescents less than 18 years of age.[16] The incidence rate of tuberculosis among children and adolescents was 1 case per 100,000 person-years and declined by 47.8% from 2007 to 2017. The tuberculosis incidence rates were highest in children less than 12 months of age (1.9 per 100,000 person-years), followed by adolescents aged 15–17 years (1.4 per 100,000 years), and were lowest among children aged 7–12 years (0.5 per 100,000 person-years).

From 2010 to 2017, non-US born children, children born to non-US-born parents, and children of racial or ethnic minority status were disproportionately affected by tuberculosis.[16] The age-specific incidence rate of non-US-born children was 13 times that of US-born children. Non-US-born children accounted for approximately 32% of the total number of childhood tuberculosis cases, the majority being from Mexico followed by Ethiopia, the Philippines, Myanmar, and Haiti. In US-born children, the incidence rates of tuberculosis if both parents were non-US-born and if one parent was non-US-born were 8 and 3 times as high, respectively, compared to US-born children with both parents being US-born. This is supported by prior research that found among the US-born children with tuberculosis that 75% had some international connection through a family member or previous travel or residence in a tuberculosis endemic country.[17,18] Similar to adults in the United States, tuberculosis occurs disproportionately among children of racial-ethnic minority status. The incidence rates of tuberculosis among children of Native Hawaiian or Pacific Islander, Asian, Native American or Native Alaskan, black, and Hispanic children were 144, 44, 22, 19, and 18 times as high, respectively, as among non-Hispanic white children.[16]

The rates of drug-resistant tuberculosis in children in the United States remain low.[18,19] A total of 89 childhood cases of MDR tuberculosis were reported in the United States in 2015; of those, 70.8% were non-US-born. Among children with culture-confirmed tuberculosis in the United States in 2015, 15.2% had organisms with resistance to at least one first-line drug and 0.9% had MDR organisms.

CHILDHOOD TUBERCULOSIS INFECTION

Modeling studies estimate that 75,000,000 children under the age of 15 years worldwide are infected with *M. tuberculosis*.[10,11,13] In high-prevalence countries, rates of tuberculosis infection among the young population average 20%–50%. However, reliable estimates in these countries are difficult to obtain due to lack of diagnostic resources, which has led to an underdiagnosis and underreporting of infected children.

In the United States, only a few states consider tuberculosis infection to be a reportable condition. Most children are infected in the home; however, outbreaks of childhood and adolescent tuberculosis infection and disease continue to occur in schools, day care centers, and other congregate settings. The most efficient method of identifying children with recent tuberculosis infection is through contact tracing of adults with contagious pulmonary tuberculosis.[3,5,6] On average, 30%–50% of household contacts of an index case will have a positive test of infection.

TUBERCULOSIS IN HIV-INFECTED CHILDREN

Most cases of tuberculosis in HIV-infected children occur in developing countries. A study conducted in South Africa demonstrated that the incidence of tuberculosis disease in HIV-infected children is 42 times higher than that in HIV-uninfected children.[20] Establishing the diagnosis of tuberculosis in an HIV-infected child may be difficult because the immune based tests (TST or IGRA) may be negative and many other HIV-related opportunistic infections and conditions have overlapping clinical features with tuberculosis.[21,22] HIV-infected children suffer from more severe and progressive forms of tuberculosis, and more often have disease in extrapulmonary sites, including meningitis and abdominal disease.[23–26] Radiographic findings are similar to those in children with normal immune systems, but lobar disease and lung cavitation are more common. The most common symptoms include fatigue, malaise, weight loss, nonspecific respiratory symptoms, and fever. Tuberculosis is often suspected when a HIV-infected child has symptom persistence after treatment for a community-acquired pneumonia. Recurrent tuberculosis disease and relapse occur more frequently in HIV-infected children, and they are also at increased risk to have primary or secondary drug resistance.

The mortality rate of HIV-infected children with untreated *M. tuberculosis* is high and correlates with their CD4 counts. The host immune response to tuberculosis infection appears to enhance HIV replication and accelerate the immune suppression caused by HIV.[27,28] Increased mortality rates are often attributable to progressive HIV infection rather than tuberculosis. Therefore, HIV-infected children with potential tuberculosis exposures or recent documented infection should be promptly evaluated and treatment for tuberculosis infection should be started. Conversely, all children with suspected tuberculosis should be tested for HIV.[10] In general, HIV-infected children with tuberculosis have a favorable prognosis as long as they do not have severe or progressive tuberculosis and appropriate antituberculosis drugs and antiretroviral therapy are available.[18]

CHILDHOOD TUBERCULOSIS TRANSMISSION

The diagnosis of a case of childhood tuberculosis is a sentinel event in a community. Children are most often infected with *M. tuberculosis* by an adult or adolescent in their immediate household with contagious tuberculosis disease, most often a parent, grandparent, older sibling, or aunt/uncle. Transmission from an extrafamilial source case occurs but is much less common and has been reported by babysitters, school teachers, music teachers, school bus drivers, church attendees, classmates, gardeners, and candy store keepers leading to hundreds of mini epidemics within population groups.[29] A study from Texas Children's Hospital in Houston, Texas reported that when chest radiographs were obtained of adult care takers of children admitted with suspected tuberculosis, 15% had previously undetected pulmonary tuberculosis.[30] In the household of an adult with smear positive, cavitary tuberculosis, infants and toddlers are frequently infected. Adolescents are also at increased risk of becoming infected, while school-aged children are less often affected.[1,31] Once an adult has been started on antituberculosis therapy, their risk of transmitting *M. tuberculosis* to children in their environment is low. Adults with smear and culture positive tuberculosis are assumed to be infectious for at least 2 weeks after the start of effective chemotherapy. Those with chronic tuberculosis who go undetected, or those who are inadequately treated, pose the highest risk of transmitting *M. tuberculosis,* including the transmission of drug-resistant bacteria.

Early observational studies of young children in orphanages with pulmonary tuberculosis revealed that children rarely, if ever, infect other children.[32] Young children often lack the tussive force to expectorate bacilli into their environment. Children who were more likely to transmit *M. tuberculosis* were found to have imaging findings most consistent with adult-type tuberculosis.[33] Siblings, parents, or nurses who care for children with pulmonary tuberculosis often remain TST or IGRA negative.[34] When *M. tuberculosis* has been documented in children's hospitals, it is invariably due to transmission from an adult caregiver of a child with undiagnosed pulmonary tuberculosis.[35–37] Guidelines issued by the CDC state that most children with typical tuberculosis do not require isolation in the hospital unless they have uncontrolled productive cough, a cavitary lesion, or acid-fast smear positive sputa.[38] Tuberculosis in childhood must be considered in the transmission of tuberculosis in a community, not due to the likelihood of their transmitting infectious droplets into their immediate environment, but rather because, if untreated, they can harbor a partially healed infection that lies dormant, which remains at risk of reactivating as contagious pulmonary tuberculosis many years later. This most often occurs during times of emotional or physiologic stress including: adolescence, pregnancy, immunosuppression, or old age. Children with tuberculosis infection constitute a long-lasting reservoir of tuberculosis in a community. Programs targeting children for prevention and treatment of tuberculosis will have a limited impact on immediate disease rates in a community, but a profound impact on the long-term control of the disease.[3]

CHILDHOOD TUBERCULOSIS PATHOGENESIS AND IMMUNOLOGY

In over 95% of cases of childhood tuberculosis, the portal of entry for *M. tuberculosis* is the lung.[39] Respiratory particles larger than 10 μm containing tubercle bacilli are often caught by the muco-ciliary clearance mechanisms of the bronchial tree and are expectorated with cough. Small particles are easily inhaled beyond the bronchial tree into the alveoli of the lung parenchyma. The primary complex of tuberculosis consists of local disease at the portal of entry and the regional lymph nodes. While primary infection most often occurs in the lung, it can occur in any location in the body.[40] Ingestion of infected milk with bovine tuberculosis can lead to a gastrointestinal primary lesion. Infection of the skin or mucous membrane can occur through a skin abrasion, laceration, or an insect bite. The number of bacilli necessary to establish an infection in children is unknown, but is thought to be only a few organisms.

The time period from entrance of the tubercle bacilli to a person's development of cutaneous hypersensitivity is usually 2–12 weeks, most often 4–8 weeks. The onset of hypersensitivity in children may be accompanied by upper respiratory congestion, cough, and fever that can last 1–3 weeks. During this phase, there is an intensified tissue reaction, and the primary complex may be evident on chest radiograph. The primary focus increases in size during this time, but is not encapsulated. As hypersensitivity evolves, the inflammatory response becomes more intense and the regional lymph nodes often enlarge. The parenchymal portion of the primary complex undergoes caseous necrosis and encapsulation, and can either continue to enlarge or heal completely by fibrosis or calcification. If the parenchymal lesion continues to enlarge, it may result in focal pneumonitis and thickening of the underlying pleura or intense caseation may occur in the center of the lesion with liquefaction and extension into the adjacent bronchus, leaving a residual primary tuberculosis cavity.[39,40]

During the development of the primary parenchymal lesion and accelerated caseation brought on by the development of hypersensitivity, tubercle bacilli from the primary complex spread via the bloodstream and lymphatics throughout the body. The areas most commonly seeded are the apices of the lungs, liver, spleen, meninges, peritoneum, lymph nodes, pleura, and bone. If large numbers of bacilli are disseminated, a child is at risk of developing miliary (disseminated) tuberculosis. When small numbers of bacilli are disseminated, microscopic foci are scattered to various tissues. These areas are the most common extrapulmonary sites for childhood or adult onset tuberculosis disease (months to years later).[40]

The tubercle foci in the regional lymph nodes develop some fibrosis and encapsulation, but the healing in this location is often less complete than in parenchymal lesions. Viable *M. tuberculosis* bacilli may persist for decades after calcification of these nodes.

The size of these lymph nodes remains normal in most cases of primary tuberculosis infection. If these lymph nodes enlarge during the host inflammatory reaction, due to their location, hilar and paratracheal lymph nodes may exert external pressure on a regional bronchus. Partial obstruction caused by external compression leads to hyperinflation of the distal lung segment. Complete obstruction may result in atelectasis of the entire lung segment.[2,41,42] These children often present with respiratory distress or failure and can have audible wheeze or diminished breath sounds on pulmonary examination. More often, caseous lymph nodes attach to and erode through the bronchial wall and can transmit infection to the lung parenchyma leading to bronchial obstruction and atelectasis. The resultant radiographic finding is referred to as "epituberculosis," "collapse-consolidation," and "segmental" tuberculosis. Rarely, intrathoracic tuberculous nodes invade adjacent structures, such as the pericardium or esophagus.

The timeline for primary tuberculosis and its complications in infants and children is well documented.[40] Widespread lympho-hematogenous dissemination leading to miliary (disseminated) tuberculosis, including tuberculous meningitis, occurs in 0.5%–2% of infected children usually 2–6 months after initial infection. Intrathoracic manifestations generally occur within the first year. Clinically apparent lymph node or endobronchial tuberculosis usually appears within the first 3–9 months. Musculoskeletal lesions often take 12 months to develop; renal lesions may not present clinically for 5–25 years after initial infection.

Tuberculosis disease that occurs more than a year after the primary infection is thought to be secondary to endogenous regrowth of persistent bacilli from the primary infection and subclinical dissemination. Exogenous reinfection rarely results in tuberculosis disease; most cases of postprimary or reactivation tuberculosis in adolescents are believed to be secondary to endogenous organisms. Reactivation tuberculosis affects female adolescents twice as often as males; the reason for their increased risk is unknown but likely related to physiologic and hormonal changes during this time period. The most common disease manifestation of tuberculosis disease is a pulmonary infiltrate or cavitary lesion in the lung apices, where oxygen tension is high. Dissemination of bacilli during reactivation is uncommon in immunocompetent adolescents.

The age of the child at the time of acquisition of tuberculosis infection is the most influential factor on their development of both primary and reactivation tuberculosis. Disseminated (miliary and tuberculous meningitis), lymph node and subsequent segmental disease complicating primary infection occur most often in young children. Approximately 50% of untreated children less than 12 months of age develop radiographically significant tuberculosis disease, compared with 24% of children 1–10 years of age and 16% of children aged 11–15 years.[43,44] If young children do not suffer from early complications following primary infection, their risk of developing reactivation tuberculosis later in life is low. Conversely, older children and adolescents rarely experience complications following primary infection but have a greater risk of developing reactivation pulmonary tuberculosis in adolescence or adulthood.

There is increasing knowledge on the primary immune response to tuberculosis. As shown in children with underlying immunodeficiency, immune control of mycobacteria is dependent on cell-mediated immunity (*M. tuberculosis* specific T-lymphocytes, macrophages, monocytes, neutrophils, dendritic cells, Toll-like receptors, INF-γ, TNF [tumor necrosis factor]-α, and interleukin-2).[45,46] The increased risk of progression from infection to disease that exists among young children and adolescents compared to school-age children is thought to be due to an insufficient production and function of Toll-like receptors, dendritic cells, macrophages in addition to a deficient ability for CD4+ cells to express Th1 effector function. This immune dysfunction is highest among neonates, young infants, and immunosuppressed children. As the immune system matures or becomes functional (with immune reconstitution), the risk of progression to disease decreases.

CLINICAL MANIFESTATIONS AND DIAGNOSIS OF CHILDHOOD TUBERCULOSIS

The timing of the diagnosis of tuberculosis in children differs between high- and low-burden settings.[47] In high-burden countries, most children are passively diagnosed when they present for medical care with symptomatic tuberculosis disease.[48] Tuberculosis is suspected in a symptomatic child when a household or adult contact also has tuberculosis. In these settings, most children are diagnosed based on clinical symptoms, without radiologic data or microbiologic confirmation. To aid in the diagnosis of tuberculosis in children in resource limited settings, a variety of scoring systems have been devised based on clinical signs and symptoms, known epidemiologic exposure, and the available tests.[49] However, the sensitivity and specificity of these systems varies by location, leading to both over- and underdiagnosis of childhood tuberculosis. No clinical scoring system has been adequately validated in a clinical trial.

Since 2013, the WHO has published guidelines for intensive case-finding strategies (active case-finding) in high-burden countries, which improves the identification of both adults and children with tuberculosis.[50] Several countries have implemented this practice, which includes screening close contacts of those with symptomatic tuberculosis, those who are HIV infected, and those with poor access to health-care services. There are published screening algorithms for children, although the most common practice is an interview to identify those at risk (including symptoms screen and HIV testing).[50] Active case-finding strategies improve rates of diagnosis of tuberculosis in a community, allows for earlier diagnosis and is cost-effective.[51-53]

In low-burden countries, children with tuberculosis are discovered one of three ways: they present for medical care with symptomatic tuberculosis, they are diagnosed during contact tracing, or are diagnosed through a community- or school-based testing program. The most cost-effective method to identify children at risk for tuberculosis is through contact tracing for an adult case. In the United States, up to 50% of children with pulmonary tuberculosis are diagnosed during contact tracing. The affected child typically has few or no symptoms, but the investigation reveals a positive test of infection (TST or IGRA) and an abnormal chest radiograph.

CHILDHOOD TUBERCULOSIS DISEASE: CLINICAL MANIFESTATIONS

Pulmonary

The primary pulmonary complex includes the parenchymal pulmonary focus and the regional lymph nodes.[38] Approximately 70% of lung foci are subpleural, and localized pleurisy is common. The initial parenchymal inflammation is not usually visible on chest radiograph, but a localized, nonspecific infiltrate may be seen before the development of tissue hypersensitivity. During the initial infection, all lobar segments of the lung are at equal risk of being involved, and 25% of cases have multiple primary lung foci.[54] The hallmark of primary tuberculosis in the lung is the relatively large size of the regional lymphadenitis compared with the relatively small size of the initial lung focus. As delayed-type hypersensitivity develops, the hilar lymph nodes continue to enlarge in some children, especially infants, compressing the regional bronchus and causing obstruction. The usual sequence is hilar lymphadenopathy, focal hyperinflation, and then atelectasis. The resulting radiographic shadows have been called collapse-consolidation or segmental tuberculosis (Figure 18.1). Inflamed caseous nodes may attach to the endobronchial wall and erode through it, causing endobronchial tuberculosis or a fistulous tract.[55] The caseum causes complete obstruction of the bronchus, resulting in extensive infiltrate and collapse.[56,57] The radiographic picture is similar to that caused by the aspiration of a foreign body but is usually quite different from bacterial or viral pneumonia. In pulmonary tuberculosis, the lymph nodes act as the "foreign body." Enlargement of the subcarinal lymph nodes can cause compression of the esophagus and, rarely, a bronchoesophageal fistula.[58]

Most cases of tuberculous bronchial obstruction in children resolve fully with appropriate treatment.[59] There is occasionally a residual calcification of the primary focus or regional lymph nodes. The appearance of calcification implies that the lesion has been present for at least 6–12 months. Healing of the segment can be complicated by scarring or contraction associated with cylindrical bronchiectasis, but this is rare.

Children can have lobar pneumonia without impressive hilar lymphadenopathy. If the primary infection is progressively

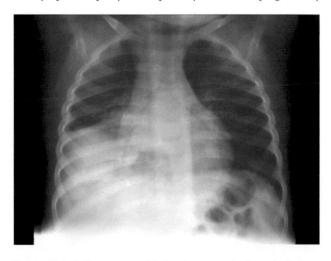

Figure 18.1 Collapse-consolidation/segmental tuberculosis.

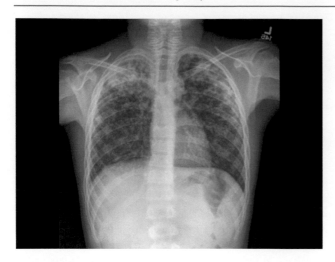

Figure 18.2 Miliary tuberculosis.

destructive, liquefaction of the lung parenchyma can lead to the formation of a thin-walled primary tuberculosis cavity. Bullous tuberculous lesions rarely occur in the lungs and, if they rupture, can lead to pneumothorax. Erosion of a parenchymal focus of tuberculosis into a blood or lymphatic vessel can result in dissemination of the bacilli and a miliary pattern, with small nodules evenly distributed on the chest radiograph (Figure 18.2).

The symptoms and physical signs of primary pulmonary tuberculosis in children are surprisingly meager considering the degree of radiographic changes often present. The physical manifestations of disease and associated symptoms differ by age of onset (Table 18.1). Young infants and adolescents are more likely to experience signs and symptoms of tuberculosis, while school-age children are more likely to have clinically silent disease. When active case finding is performed, up to 50% of infants and children with radiographically moderate to severe pulmonary tuberculosis have no physical findings. Nonproductive cough and mild dyspnea are the most common symptoms in infants, which is probably due to their smaller airway diameters relative to the parenchymal and lymph node changes in pulmonary tuberculosis. Systemic symptoms such as fever, night sweats, anorexia, and decreased activity are less

Table 18.1 Symptoms and signs of pulmonary tuberculosis in childhood

Symptom or sign	Infants and young children	Older children and adolescents
Fever	Common	Uncommon
Night sweats	Rare	Uncommon
Cough	Common	Common
Productive cough	Rare	Common
Hemoptysis	Never	Rare
Dyspnea	Common	Rare
Rales	Common	Uncommon
Wheezing	Common	Uncommon
Dullness to percussion	Rare	Uncommon
Diminished breath sounds	Common	Uncommon

Table 18.2 Comparison of chest radiographs of pulmonary tuberculosis in adults and children

Characteristic(s)	Adults	Children
Location	Apical	Anywhere (25% multilobar)
Adenopathy	Rare	Usual
Cavitation	Common	Rare (except in adolescence)
Signs and symptoms	Consistent	Relative paucity

common. Some infants present with poor weight gain or develop failure to thrive, which may not improve until several months into their treatment course. Pulmonary signs are even less common. Some infants and young children with bronchial obstruction have signs from air trapping such as localized wheezing or decreased breath sounds that may be accompanied by tachypnea or, rarely, respiratory distress. The pulmonary symptoms and signs occasionally are alleviated by antibiotics, suggesting a bacterial superinfection distal to the focus of tuberculous bronchial obstruction, which contributes to the clinical presentation of disease.

As expected, the radiographic findings in childhood tuberculosis reflect the pathophysiology and are different from the findings in adults (Table 18.2).[60] The majority of cases of pulmonary tuberculosis in children resolve radiographically with or without antituberculosis chemotherapy; however, in the pretreatment era, up to 60% of children had residual anatomic sequelae not apparent on radiographs. With delayed or no treatment, calcification of the caseous lesions is common. Healing of the pulmonary segment can be complicated by scarring or contraction associated with cylindrical bronchiectasis or bronchostenosis. When these complications occur in the upper lobes they are usually clinically silent. They are rare in children who have successfully completed current regimens of chemotherapy.[61]

A rare but serious complication of tuberculosis in a child occurs when the primary focus enlarges steadily and develops a large caseous center.[62] Liquefaction can cause formation of a primary cavity associated with a high burden of tubercle bacilli. The radiographic and clinical picture of progressive primary tuberculosis is closest to that of bronchial pneumonia. The child commonly presents with high fever, moderate to severe cough with sputum production, weight loss, and night sweats. Physical signs include diminished breath sounds, rales, and dullness to percussion over the cavity. The enlarging focus can slough necrotic debris into the adjacent bronchus, leading to further intrapulmonary dissemination. Rupture of this cavity into the pleural space causes a bronchopleural fistula or pyopneumothorax. Rupture into the pericardium can cause acute pericarditis with constriction. Prior to the advent of antituberculosis chemotherapy, the mortality of progressive pulmonary tuberculosis in children was 30%–50%; with current treatment, the prognosis is excellent for full recovery.

Pulmonary tuberculosis in adults usually represents endogenous reactivation of a site of tuberculosis infection previously established in the body. This form of tuberculosis is rare in childhood but can occur in adolescence.[40] Children with a healed tuberculosis infection acquired when they were younger than 2 years of age rarely develop reactivation pulmonary disease, which is more common in those who acquire the initial infection when they are older than 7 years of age.[62] The most common pulmonary sites are the original parenchymal focus, lymph nodes, or the apical seedings (Simon foci) established during the hematogenous phase of the early infection.[63] This form of tuberculosis disease usually remains localized in the lungs, as the established immune response prevents further extrapulmonary spread. The most common radiographic findings are extensive infiltrates or thick-walled cavities in the upper lobes.

Older children and adolescents with reactivation tuberculosis are more likely to experience fever, anorexia, malaise, weight loss, night sweats, productive cough, hemoptysis, and chest pain compared to children with primary pulmonary tuberculosis. However, physical examination findings often are minor or absent, even when cavities or large infiltrates are present. Most symptoms improve within several weeks of starting effective treatment, although cough may last for several months. This form of tuberculosis usually remains localized to the lungs, however, the child may be highly contagious if there is significant sputum production and cough. The prognosis for full recovery is excellent with appropriate therapy.

Pleural

Tuberculous pleural effusions are caused by the hypersensitivity response to the discharge of bacilli into the pleural space from a subpleural pulmonary focus or from subpleural caseous lymph node.[62] The discharge is usually small and the subsequent pleuritis is localized and asymptomatic. Larger and clinically significant effusions occur months to years after the primary infection. Often the radiographic abnormality is more extensive than would be suggested by physical findings or symptoms (Figure 18.3). A clinically significant pleural effusion occurs in 10%–30% of tuberculosis cases in young adults, is infrequent in children younger than 6 years of age, and rare in children younger than 2 years of age.[63] Tuberculous pleural effusions are usually unilateral in children. They are rarely associated with a segmental pulmonary lesion and are uncommon in disseminated tuberculosis.

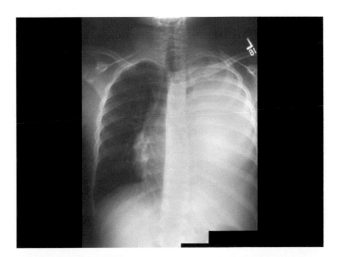

Figure 18.3 Pleural effusion.

The onset of symptoms and signs usually is abrupt with fever, chest pain, shortness of breath, dullness to percussion, and diminished breath sounds on the affected side. The fever can be high and may last for several weeks after the initiation of antituberculosis chemotherapy. The diagnosis may be difficult to make as the acid-fast stain of the pleural fluid is nearly always negative and the culture is positive in only 30%–50% of cases. The best material for the diagnosis is a pleural biopsy, which will reveal caseating granulomas on pathologic examination in up to 90% of cases, and up to 70% are culture positive. The prognosis is excellent, but radiographic resolution often takes months.

Lymphohematogenous (disseminated) disease

Tubercle bacilli are disseminated to distant anatomic sites in virtually all cases of asymptomatic tuberculosis infection.[39,44,62] Autopsy evaluation of persons who died of other causes within days to weeks after an initial tuberculosis infection demonstrated organisms in many organs and tissues, most commonly the liver, spleen, skin, and lung apices. The clinical manifestations produced by lymphohematogenous tuberculosis depends on the quantity of organisms released from the primary focus and the host immune response. Children with an impaired immune response, including infants or those who are HIV infected, are more likely to develop severe forms of disseminated disease.

The occult dissemination of tubercle bacilli during the initial infection usually produces no symptoms, but it is the event that results in extrapulmonary foci that can become the site of disease month to years after the initial infection. Children rarely experience protracted hematogenous tuberculosis caused by the intermittent release of tubercle bacilli as a caseous focus erodes through the wall of a blood vessel in the lung. The clinical picture may be acute, but more often it is indolent and prolonged, with spiking fever accompanying the release of organisms into the bloodstream. Multiple organ involvement is common, leading to hepatomegaly, splenomegaly, lymphadenitis in superficial or deep nodes, and papulonecrotic tuberculids appearing on the skin. Bones and joints or kidneys also can be involved. Meningitis occurs only late in the course and was the main cause of death in the prechemotherapy era. Pulmonary involvement is surprisingly mild early in the course, but diffuse involvement becomes apparent if treatment is not initiated early. Culture confirmation of this complication can be difficult; bone marrow or liver aspirate stains and cultures may be necessary and should be performed if the diagnosis is considered and other diagnostic testing is unrevealing.

The most common clinically significant form of disseminated tuberculosis is miliary disease, which occurs when massive numbers of tubercle bacilli are released into the bloodstream, leading to disease in two or more organs.[44,63,64] Miliary tuberculosis is most often a complication of primary infection, occurring within 2–6 months of the primary inoculation. While this form of disease is most common in those who are immunosuppressed or in infants and young children, it also occurs in adolescents and older adults, resulting from the breakdown of a previously healed or calcified primary pulmonary lesion.

The clinical manifestations of miliary tuberculosis are protean and depend on the load and final location of disseminated organisms. Lesions are often larger and more numerous in the lungs, spleen, liver, and bone marrow than other tissues.[65] The distribution may correlate with both the blood supply and the number of reticuloendothelial cells and tissue phagocytes.

The onset of miliary tuberculosis can be explosive when the patient becomes gravely ill in several days.[66] More often, the onset is insidious and the patient may not be able to accurately pinpoint the time of initial symptoms. Early systemic signs include malaise, anorexia, weight loss, and low-grade fever. At this time, abnormal physical signs are usually absent. Within weeks, generalized lymphadenopathy and hepatosplenomegaly develop in approximately 50% of cases. The fever can become higher and more sustained although the chest radiograph at this stage is usually normal and respiratory symptoms are few. Within several more weeks, the lungs can become filled with tubercles, accompanied by dyspnea, cough, rales, or wheezing. As the pulmonary disease progresses, an alveolar-air block syndrome can result in frank respiratory distress, hypoxia, and pneumothorax, or pneumomediastinum. Signs or symptoms of meningitis or peritonitis are found in 20%–40% of patients with advanced disease.[65,66] Chronic or recurrent headache in a child with miliary tuberculosis usually indicates the presence of central nervous system (CNS) involvement, whereas the onset of abdominal pain or tenderness is a sign of tuberculous peritonitis. Cutaneous lesions include papulonecrotic tuberculids, nodules, or purpura; which often occur in crops. Choroid tubercles occur in 13%–87% of patients and are highly specific for the diagnosis of miliary tuberculosis.

The early diagnosis of disseminated tuberculosis can be difficult, requiring a high index of suspicion by the clinician. Often the patient presents with fever of unknown origin. Mycobacterial blood cultures are rarely, if ever, positive. Early sputum or gastric aspirate cultures have a low sensitivity. Biopsy of the liver or bone marrow are the best methods to attempt to establish an early diagnosis.

With proper treatment, the prognosis of miliary tuberculosis in children is excellent. However, resolution of signs and symptoms may be slow with fever declining in 2–3 weeks of starting chemotherapy, and chest radiographic abnormalities persisting for several months.

Lymphatic

Tuberculosis of the superficial lymph nodes, historically referred to as scrofula, is the most common form of extrapulmonary tuberculosis in children, accounting for approximately 67% of cases.[63,67] Historically, scrofula was usually caused by drinking unpasteurized cow's milk laden with *Mycobacterium bovis*. However, through effective veterinary control, *M. bovis* has been nearly eliminated from North America. Most current cases of tuberculous lymphadenitis occur within 6–9 months of the initial infection, although some cases arise years later. The tonsillar, anterior cervical, submandibular, and supraclavicular nodes become involved secondary to extension of a primary lesion of the upper lung fields or abdomen. Infected lymph nodes in the inguinal, epitrochlear, or axillary regions result from regional adenitis associated with tuberculosis of the skin or skeletal system.

In the early stages of infection, the lymph nodes enlarge gradually. The nodes are discrete, nontender, and firm but not hard. The nodes often feel fixed to underlying or overlying tissue. Disease is most often unilateral, but because of the crossover drainage patterns of lymphatic vessels in the chest and lower neck, can present bilaterally. As infection progresses, multiple nodes can become infected, resulting in a mass of matted nodes. Other than low-grade fever, systemic signs and symptoms are usually absent. The TST or IGRA is often positive but the chest radiograph is normal in up to 70% of cases. The onset of illness occasionally is more acute, with rapid enlargement of lymph nodes associated with high fever, tenderness, and fluctuance. Rarely children will present with a tender fluctuant mass with overlying cellulitis or skin discoloration.

If left untreated, lymph node tuberculosis can resolve spontaneously, but more often progresses to caseation and lymph node necrosis.[68] The capsule of the node breaks down, resulting in the spread of infection to adjacent nodes. The skin overlying the mass of nodes becomes thin, shiny, and erythematous. Rupture through the skin results in a draining sinus tract that may require surgical removal.

The most difficult diagnostic dilemma in the differential diagnosis of tuberculous adenitis is distinguishing this condition from lymphadenitis caused by nontuberculous mycobacteria. Both conditions can cause chronic, nontender adenopathy with overlying skin changes, and the eventual creation of tissue breakdown and sinus tracts.[7] The chest radiograph is usually normal in both conditions and the TST reaction may be positive with either infection. The most important diagnostic clue for the diagnosis of tuberculous adenitis in a child is finding an adult source case in the child's environment. Fine needle aspiration or excisional biopsy and culture of the lymph nodes are often required to definitively establish the etiology. However, the cultures can be negative in up to 50% of reported cases of both tuberculous and nontuberculous mycobacterial lymphadenitis.

Central nervous system

Meningitis

CNS tuberculosis is the most serious complication in children and is universally fatal without effective treatment. It usually arises from the formation of a metastatic caseous lesion in the cerebral cortex or meninges that develops during the lymphohematogenous dissemination of the primary infection.[69] This lesion, often called a Rich focus, increases in size and discharges small numbers of tubercle bacilli into the subarachnoid space. The resulting gelatinous exudate can infiltrate the cortical or meningeal blood vessels, producing inflammation, obstruction, and subsequent infarction of the cerebral cortex. The brainstem is the area most commonly affected, accounting for the frequent involvement of cranial nerves III, VI, and VII. The exudate interferes with the normal flow of cerebrospinal fluid (CSF) in and out of the ventricular system at the level of the basilar cisterns, leading to a communicating hydrocephalus. This combination of vasculitis, infarction, cerebral edema, and hydrocephalus results in severe damage that can occur gradually or rapidly with this disease. Profound abnormalities in electrolyte metabolism, especially hyponatremia secondary to inappropriate secretion of antidiuretic hormone or salt wasting, are common and may contribute to the pathophysiology.

Salt wasting may make correction of the electrolyte disturbances difficult.[70]

Tuberculous meningitis complicates approximately 0.5% of untreated primary infections in children of all ages, but up to 10% of children less than 1 year of age. It is most common in children between 6 months and 4 years of age.[71,72] It is extremely rare in infants less than 4 months of age because, in general, it takes that long for the pathologic events to take place. Since it is an early manifestation of the primary infection, the initial exposure history is negative but the adult source case can be identified soon after the diagnosis of tuberculosis meningitis in the child is suspected.[73]

The clinical progression of tuberculous meningitis may be rapid or gradual. Rapid progression tends to occur more often in infants and young children, who can experience symptoms for only several days before the onset of acute hydrocephalus, seizure activity, and cerebral edema.[74] More often, the signs and symptoms progress slowly over weeks and are divided into three clinical stages. The first stage typically lasts 1–2 weeks and is characterized by non-specific symptoms such as fever, headache, irritability, drowsiness, and malaise. Focal neurologic signs are absent, but infants can experience a stagnation or loss of developmental milestones. The second stage usually begins more abruptly with lethargy, nuchal rigidity, seizures, positive Kernig and Brudzinski signs, hyperto-nia, vomiting, cranial nerve palsies, and other focal neurologic signs. The accelerating clinical illness usually correlates with the development of hydrocephalus with subsequent increased intra-cranial pressure and vasculitis. Some children do not have evidence of meningeal irritation but have signs of encephalitis such as disorientation, abnormal movement, or speech impairment.[75] The third stage is marked by coma, hemiplegia or paraplegia, hyperten-sion, decerebrate posturing, deterioration of vital signs, and even-tually death. The prognosis of tuberculous meningitis correlates most closely with the clinical stage of illness at the time treatment is initiated. The majority of patients in the first stage have an excel-lent outcome, whereas most patients in the third stage who survive have permanent disabilities which include blindness, deafness, paraplegia, diabetes insipidus, or mental retardation. It is impera-tive that antituberculosis treatment be considered strongly for any child with meningitis and no other established etiology who devel-ops basilar meningitis and hydrocephalus, cranial nerve palsy, or stroke. The key to the diagnosis of tuberculous meningitis in chil-dren is often identifying the adult source case.

Confirming a diagnosis of tuberculous meningitis can be extremely difficult. The TST and IGRAs are negative in up to 50% of cases, and 20%–50% of children have a normal chest radio-graph.[76] The most important laboratory test for the diagnosis of tuberculous meningitis is examination and culture of the lumbar cerebrospinal fluid (CSF). The CSF leukocyte count usually ranges from 10 to 500 cells/μL. Polymorphonuclear leukocytes may be present initially and may portend a poorer prognosis, but a lym-phocyte predominance is more typical. The CSF glucose is usually between 20 and 40 mg/dL, whereas the CSF protein level is ele-vated and may be markedly high (400–5,000 mg/dL). The success of the microscopic examination of stained CSF and mycobacterial cultures correlates with the volume of the CSF sample. When a minimum of 10 mL of lumbar CSF is available, the acid-fast stain of the CSF sediment is positive in up to 30% of cases and the cul-ture is positive in up to 70% of cases. Unfortunately, a volume of 1–2 mL is usually all that can be obtained from a young child. Polymerase chain reaction (PCR) testing of the CSF can improve diagnosis. Cultures of other body fluids can help confirm the diagnosis.

Computed tomography or magnetic resonance scans often help establish the diagnosis of tuberculous meningitis and can aid in evaluating the success of therapy. The classic imag-ing finding of tuberculous meningitis is abnormal enhance-ment in the posterior fossa (basal enhancement), which may involve the meninges or cisterns.[77] Both computed tomography and magnetic resonance imaging are capable of demonstrating hydrocephalus, the most common complication of tuberculous meningitis. Computed tomography is capable of identifying abnormal enhancement in the basal cisterns but cannot distin-guish between vessels and cistern enhancement as with magnetic resonance imaging. Contrasted magnetic resonance imaging is more sensitive for the identification of miliary foci/nodules in the leptomeninges and inflammatory pan-arteritis (and associ-ated cerebral infarction) which are rarely identified on computed tomography imaging.[78–80] Any child with a triad of imaging find-ings including basal enhancement, hydrocephalus, and cerebral infarction has tuberculous meningitis until proven otherwise.

Tuberculoma

Another manifestation of CNS tuberculosis is the tuber-culoma which usually presents clinically as a brain tumor. Tuberculomas account for up to 30% of brain tumors in some areas of the world. They occur most often in children less than 10 years of age and most often present as a solitary lesion. While tuberculoma lesions in adults are most often supratentorial, in children, they are often infratentorial, located at the base of the brain near the cerebellum (Figure 18.4). The most common

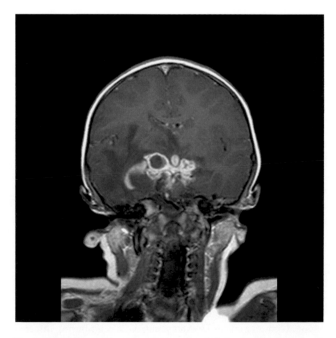

Figure 18.4 Magnetic resonance imaging: infratentorial tuberculosis.

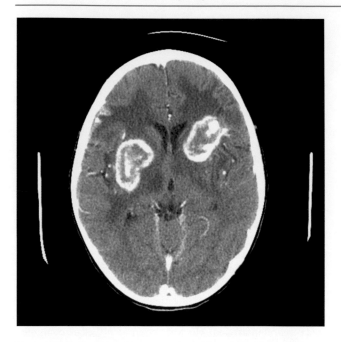

Figure 18.5 Computed tomography: tuberculoma.

symptoms in children include headache, fever, focal neurologic findings, and seizures. The TST or IGRA is usually positive, but the chest radiograph is often normal. Advanced imaging of the brain reveals tuberculomas as discrete lesions with a significant amount of surrounding edema. Contrast enhancement is often impressive and can reveal a ring-like lesion (Figure 18.5). Surgical excision of tuberculomas may be necessary to distinguish tuberculoma from other causes of brain tumor or other ring enhancing lesions. However, if the clinical suspicion for tuberculoma is high, surgical removal is not necessary as most tuberculomas resolve with medical management alone. These lesions can persist for months or years.

Since the advent of contrast-enhanced brain imaging, the paradoxical development of tuberculomas has been recognized in children with and without HIV infection who have an initial diagnosis of tuberculous meningitis while they are receiving effective chemotherapy.[81,82] The cause and nature of these tuberculomas are poorly understood but they likely represent a form of immune reconstitution inflammatory syndrome (IRIS). Their development is not thought to be a failure of drug treatment and does not necessitate a change in therapeutic regimen. This phenomenon should be considered whenever a child with tuberculous meningitis deteriorates or develops focal neurologic findings while on treatment. Corticosteroids can alleviate the occasionally severe clinical signs and symptoms that occur. Thalidomide, a potent TNF-α inhibitor, is now also being used by experts in the treatment of refractory tuberculomas.[83]

Skeletal tuberculosis

Skeletal tuberculosis usually results from lymphohematogenous seeding of tubercle bacilli at the time of a primary infection. Bone infection may also originate by direct extension from a caseous regional lymph node or by extension from a neighboring infected tissue. The time interval between infection and disease can be as

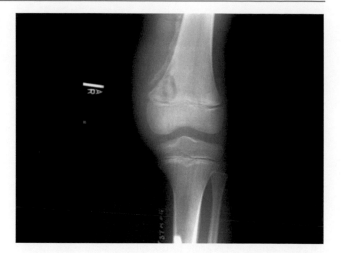

Figure 18.6 Tuberculous lesion in metaphysis of femur.

short as 1 month in cases of tuberculous dactylitis or years for tuberculosis of the hip. Joints of weight bearing bones are most commonly affected. The infection usually begins in the metaphysis (Figure 18.6). Granulation tissue and caseation develop, which can destroy bone both by direct infection and pressure necrosis. Soft tissue abscess and extension of the infection through the epiphysis into the nearby joint often complicate the bone lesion. The infection frequently becomes clinically apparent when the joint involvement progresses.

Most cases of bone tuberculosis occur in the vertebrae causing tuberculosis of the spine, known as Pott's disease.[84] Although any vertebral body can be involved, there is a predilection for the lower thoracic and upper lumbar vertebrae. Involvement of two or more vertebrae is common; they usually are continuous but there may be skip areas between lesions. The infection is in the body of the vertebra leading to bony destruction and collapse. The usual progression of tuberculous spondylitis is from initial narrowing of one or several disc spaces to collapse and wedging of the vertebral body with subsequent angulation of the spine (gibbus) or kyphosis. The infection may extend out from the bone causing paraspinal (Pott's), psoas, or retropharyngeal abscess. The most frequent clinical signs and symptoms of tuberculous spondylitis in children are low-grade fever, irritability and restlessness (especially at night), back pain usually without significant tenderness, and abnormal positioning and gait or refusal to walk. Rigidity of the spine may be caused by profound muscle spasm resulting from the child's involuntary effort to immobilize the spine.

Other sites of skeletal tuberculosis, in approximate order of frequency, are the knee, elbow, and ankle.[85] The degree of involvement ranges from joint effusion without bone destruction to frank destruction of bone and restriction of the joint caused by chronic fibrosis of the synovial membrane. The process usually evolves over months to years, most commonly causing mild pain, stiffness, limping, and restricted movement. The TST or IGRA is positive in 80%–90% of cases. In most cases, culture of the joint fluid or bone biopsy yields the organism. Tuberculosis should be considered in any child with risk factors and a persistent bone or joint lesion.

One form of bony tuberculosis peculiar to infants is tuberculous dactylitis. Affected children develop distal endarteritis followed by painless swelling and cystic bone lesions. Abscesses are rare.

Abdominal tuberculosis

Abdominal tuberculosis can result from ingestion of mycobacterium, hematogenous dissemination or lymphatic spread from a pulmonary focus. Abdominal tuberculosis is one of the most common sites for extrapulmonary infection; and it may be underdiagnosed in children. A retrospective study from a high-tuberculosis burden country found that among 47 children with culture positive pulmonary tuberculosis (20 of whom were HIV infected), 23% of children had ultrasound findings consistent with abdominal infection.[86] The most common manifestation was lymphadenopathy followed by hepatosplenomegaly, hepatic and splenic lesions, and ascites. The presence of abdominal adenopathy correlated with thoracic adenopathy. Children with gastrointestinal tuberculosis can present with intestinal inflammation with or without peritonitis.[87] A primary intestinal infection rarely will occur after ingestion of a bacilli laden sputum, which is more common in adolescents with cavitary tuberculosis. *M. bovis* also causes a primary intestinal infection following the ingestion of contaminated milk products.

The most common manifestations of abdominal tuberculosis include abdominal pain, abdominal distension, malnutrition, and prolonged fever.[85–88] It is uncommon for a child to have a palpable abdominal mass. The TST or IGRA is likely to be negative if a child is severely malnourished. If present, ascitic fluid should be collected and analyzed for infection. The fluid is exudative with a high albumin level and lymphocytic predominance.[89] Microbiologic studies, including acid-fast smear, culture, PCR, and drug-susceptibility testing (DST) should be obtained. Laparoscopic examination allows for direct visualization of the peritoneal space, which often reveals ascites, fibrous bands, mesenteric adhesions, nodules throughout the peritoneum, lymphadenopathy, and edematous loops of bowel. Tissue samples can be sent for histologic and bacteriologic examination. Colonoscopy may be helpful in the evaluation of intestinal tuberculosis, which most often reveals mucosal ulceration in the ileocecal region. These ulcers should be biopsied for histopathologic examination and culture. Intestinal tuberculosis remains on the differential diagnosis for inflammatory bowel disease in children.[90]

Female genitourinary

Tuberculosis of the female genital tract is uncommon in prepubescent girls. This condition usually originates from lymphohematogenous spread, although it can be caused by direct spread from the intestinal tract or bone.[91] Adolescent girls can develop genital tract tuberculosis during a primary infection. The fallopian tubes are most often involved (90%–100% of cases), followed by the endometrium (50%), ovaries (25%), and cervix (5%). Tuberculous involvement of the fallopian tubes may lead to distension and obstruction; progression may lead to the development of a tubo-ovarian abscess. With uterine involvement, fluid accumulation will occur and may cause cervical obstruction. Extra-pelvic spread can lead to inflammation of the peritoneum, omentum, mesentery, and bowel. The most common symptoms are lower abdominal pain, dysmenorrhea or amenorrhea, or infertility. Systemic manifestations are usually absent, and most patients have a normal chest radiograph. The TST or IGRA is usually positive. Imaging findings are nonspecific as the differential diagnosis includes sexually transmitted infections and malignant conditions. Clinicians should consider genital tuberculosis in asexual adolescent females at risk for tuberculosis who have a negative infectious or pathologic work-up for alternative diagnoses and have a positive TST or IGRA.

DIAGNOSTIC EVALUATION

Many children with tuberculosis in low-burden areas are discovered through contact tracing of adults with infectious pulmonary tuberculosis. Most of these children have tuberculosis infection or asymptomatic disease that would have progressed or escaped detection if the contact tracing had not occurred. In most high-tuberculosis burden areas, children with pulmonary tuberculosis are discovered only after a symptomatic illness begins. A strong index of suspicion for tuberculosis is required to correctly identify the cause of illness in children since the signs and symptoms of most forms of tuberculosis are similar to those of other infections and conditions. The importance of the epidemiologic setting of the child in establishing the diagnosis of tuberculosis cannot be overemphasized.

Routine laboratory tests such as complete blood count and differential, C-reactive protein (CRP), erythrocyte sedimentation rate (ESR), urinalysis, and blood chemistries are usually normal in children with early manifestations of tuberculosis disease. Anemia, hypoalbuminemia, and abnormalities in liver serum enzyme tests may indicate more severe forms of or disseminated tuberculosis.

IMMUNE-BASED TESTING "TESTS OF TUBERCULOSIS INFECTION"

Tuberculin skin test

The principles for tuberculin skin testing of children are the same as those for adults.[92] The tuberculin skin test (TST) measures a delayed-type hypersensitivity reaction to tuberculous antigens. T-lymphocytes sensitized by prior tuberculosis infection are recruited to the skin, where they release lymphokines that induce induration through local vasodilation, edema, fibrin deposition, and recruitment of other inflammatory cells to the area. The amount of induration in response to the test should be measured by a trained person 48–72 hours after administration. In some children the onset of induration is longer than 72 hours after placement; this is also a positive result. Immediate hypersensitivity reactions to tuberculin or other constituents of the preparation are short-lived (<24 hours) and not considered a positive result. Tuberculin sensitivity develops between 3 weeks and 3 months (most often in 4–8 weeks) after the inhalation of organisms. Approximately 10% of immunocompetent children with culture-documented tuberculosis do not react initially to tuberculin, although most become reactive after several months of therapy.[93,94] The tuberculin reaction persists for many years, even after successful completion of chemotherapy.[94]

Young infants generally produce less induration and response to tuberculin than older children. Additional host-related factors, including malnutrition, immunosuppression by disease or drugs, viral infections (measles, mumps, varicella, or influenza), vaccination with live-virus vaccines, and overwhelming tuberculosis, can depress the TST reaction in an infected child. Corticosteroid therapy can decrease the reaction to the tuberculin proteins, but the effect is variable; in general, TST placement at the time of initiating corticosteroid therapy is reliable. False-positive reactions to tuberculin can be caused by cross-sensitization to antigens of nontuberculous mycobacteria. These cross-reactions are usually transient over months to years and produce <10–12 mm of induration, but larger areas of induration can occur. Previous vaccination with bacille Calmette-Guérin (BCG) also can cause a reaction to a TST, which is partly related to the strain of BCG used.[95–97] This reaction is most prominent if a person has received two or more BCG vaccinations (at birth and then later in childhood). At least 50% of the infants who receive a BCG vaccine do not develop a positive TST and 80%–90% of those who have a positive reaction initially have a negative TST within 2–5 years. When BCG-induced TST reactivity is present, it usually causes <15 mm of induration, although larger reactions occur in some persons.

Routine testing of all children for tuberculosis infection in low-burden settings is no longer recommended; this practice has been replaced by targeted testing of children with specific risk tuberculosis factors.[7,98] In children with no tuberculosis risk factors, the vast majority of "positive" TST results will be false-positive results. The appropriate size of induration indicating a positive TST result varies with related epidemiologic risk factors (Table 18.3).[7] For children at the highest risk of progression to tuberculosis disease, TST sensitivity is most important whereas specificity is more important for children at low risk of progression.

Table 18.3 Definitions of positive TST results in infants, children, and adolescents[7]

Induration ≥5 mm

Children in close contact with a known or suspected source case with tuberculosis disease

Children suspected to have tuberculosis disease:

- Chest radiograph findings consistent with active tuberculosis disease
- Clinical signs or symptoms of tuberculosis disease

Children receiving immunosuppressive therapy (including high-dose corticosteroids or TNF-α antagonists), or immunosuppressive conditions, including HIV

Induration ≥10 mm

Children at increased risk of disseminated tuberculosis disease:

- Children younger than 4 years
- Children with a chronic medical condition, including lymphoma (including Hodgkin's disease), diabetes mellitus, chronic renal failure, or malnutrition
- Children born in high-prevalence regions of the world
- Children frequently exposed to adults who are HIV infected, homeless, users of illicit drugs, or incarcerated

Induration ≥15 mm

Children aged 4 years or older without any risk factors

Interferon-γ release assays

There are two interferon-γ release assays (IGRAs) available for commercial use in the United States: (T-SPOT.*TB* [Oxford Immunotec; Marlborough, MA] and QuantiFERON-TB [QFT] [QIAGEN; Germantown, MD]). They have clear advantages for the diagnosis of tuberculosis infection over the TST. Both IGRAs detect IFN-γ production by T-lymphocytes in response to specific tuberculosis antigens. The QFT test measures whole blood concentrations of IFN-γ to three specific antigens (ESAT-6, CFP-10, and TB7.7) while the T-SPOT.*TB* test measures the number of T-lymphocytes/monocytes producing IFN-γ in response to two antigens (ESAT-6 and CFP-10). The test antigens are not present on *M. bovis*-BCG and most species of environmental mycobacteria (including *Mycobacterium avium* complex). This improves the IGRA specificity compared with the TST, leading to fewer false-positive results. Both IGRAs have internal positive and negative controls. Indeterminate (QuantiFERON-TB)/invalid (T-SPOT.*TB*) responses occur when the test sample is negative but the positive control has insufficient activity, or if the negative control has high background activity. Indeterminate/invalid results may be caused by technical factors (such as insufficient shaking of QFT tubes or delayed processing time).[99–101] Most studies report indeterminate/invalid rates in children from 0%-10%, which is influenced by a child's age and immune status. In children <2 years of age, indeterminate rates can be as high as 8.1%, compared to 2.7% in older children, although more recent studies generally report much lower rates.[102–106] An indeterminate or invalid IGRA result is neither negative nor positive and should not guide treatment decisions. Neither IGRA test has proven to be superior to the other in children.

Similar to the TST, IGRAs cannot differentiate between tuberculosis infection and disease. Studies comparing IGRA and TST performance in children have shown comparable sensitivity (85% in culture-confirmed children) but superior IGRA specificity (95% vs. 49%) in BCG-immunized, low-risk children. Neither the TST nor the IGRAs perform well in infants and young children who are malnourished, severely immunocompromised, or have disseminated tuberculosis disease. Most experts use an IGRA in the evaluation of healthy young children down to 2 years of age who are at low risk of tuberculosis infection, especially in those who have received a BCG vaccine.[7,107] Both TST and IGRA testing should be considered in children whose initial TST or IGRA result is negative for whom the risk of tuberculosis is high (to enhance the sensitivity of the combination of the two tests).

Technical advantages of the IGRAs over the TST include: the need for a single patient encounter (vs. 2 spaced in time with the TST) and the lack of cross-reaction with BCG vaccination and most environmental mycobacteria. IGRAs are also useful for those: who are unlikely to return for TST interpretation; whose family is reluctant to treat a child with tuberculosis infection based on a TST result alone; and, with a positive TST result in whom nontuberculous mycobacterial disease is suspected.[104]

MICROBIOLOGIC TESTING

Acid-fast stain, culture, and drug susceptibility testing

The isolation of *M. tuberculosis* from a clinical sample remains the gold standard for the diagnosis of tuberculosis disease. The collection of a respiratory specimen from a child with suspected pulmonary tuberculosis provides samples for acid-fast bacilli staining, PCR, culture, and DST. Sputum specimens for culture should be collected from adolescents and older children who are able to expectorate spontaneously. Induced sputum with a jet nebulizer, inhaled saline, and chest percussion followed by nasopharyngeal suctioning are effective methods to obtain a respiratory specimen from children as young as 12 months of age.[107,108] The most commonly obtained culture specimen for young children with suspected pulmonary tuberculosis is the early morning gastric aspirate obtained before the child has arisen and peristalsis has emptied the stomach of the pooled, swallowed overnight respiratory secretions.[108] Unfortunately, even under optimal conditions, three consecutive induced sputum samples or gastric aspirates yield the organism in fewer than 50% of clinically diagnosed cases; negative cultures never exclude the diagnosis of tuberculosis in a child.[109] The yield from culture obtained via flexible bronchoscopy is significantly less than that from properly obtained gastric aspirates.[110] However, bronchoscopy can be useful to examine the anatomy of the bronchial tree when the diagnosis is uncertain.

Fortunately, there is often little need for culture confirmation for many children with suspected pulmonary tuberculosis, especially in low-burden settings. If the child has a positive TST or IGRA, clinical or radiographic findings suggestive of tuberculosis and known recent contact with an adult case with infectious tuberculosis, the child should be treated for tuberculosis disease. The drug-susceptibility test results from the source case's isolate can be used to determine the best treatment regimen for the child. However, PCR, cultures, and DST should always be performed on specimens from the child under four conditions: (1) the source case is unknown, (2) the source case has a drug-resistant organism, (3) the child has rapidly progressive disease or severe disseminated disease, (4) the child has extrapulmonary tuberculosis (which has a broader differential diagnosis than is usual for pulmonary tuberculosis). Unfortunately, while acid-fast stains of gastric contents may have a specificity for tuberculosis greater than 90%, the sensitivity is usually less than 10%.

Molecular techniques

Molecular techniques to identify *M. tuberculosis* specific DNA and RNA genomic targets have clear advantages over the traditional microbiologic methods including: increased sensitivity compared to smear microscopy in respiratory specimens, decreased turnaround time compared to traditional culture, and more rapid drug-susceptibility information. These techniques are increasingly popular to confirm or support the diagnosis of tuberculosis in adults and children in both high-burden and low-burden settings.[111–114] The application of molecular testing of clinical samples from children to confirm tuberculosis disease has the potential to improve estimates of childhood tuberculosis in high-burden settings.

The first form of nucleic amplification studied in children with tuberculosis was the traditional PCR technique, which identifies *M. tuberculosis* specific DNA sequences as markers for microorganisms in clinical specimens. Epidemiologic studies have revealed that most strains of *M. tuberculosis* carry 10–15 randomly distributed repetitive DNA sequences of IS6110 restriction fragment length polymorphism (RFLP) along the chromosome. Most PCR techniques identify insertion element IS6110 as the DNA marker for *M. tuberculosis* complex organisms and have a sensitivity of more than 90% compared with sputum culture for detecting pulmonary tuberculosis in adults. Unfortunately, this test is expensive, requires sophisticated equipment and technical competence to avoid cross-contamination of specimens, and is, therefore, restricted to reference laboratories and clinical studies.

Compared with a clinical diagnosis of pulmonary tuberculosis in children, the sensitivity of DNA PCR has varied from 25% to 83%, and specificity has varied from 80% to 100%.[111–114] The DNA PCR of gastric aspirates may be positive in a recently infected child even when the child is asymptomatic and the chest radiograph is normal, demonstrating the occasional difficulty in distinguishing between tuberculosis infection and disease in children. A negative PCR result never eliminates the diagnosis of tuberculosis, and a positive PCR result supports, but never confirms, the diagnosis.

GeneXpert MTB/RIF (Xpert) (Cepheid; Sunnyvale, CA) is a cartridge-based nucleic acid amplification test that simultaneously identifies *M. tuberculosis* DNA and rifampin resistance. GeneXpert is often used as a proxy for identifying multidrug-resistant tuberculosis. This assay uses a self-contained cartridge system, which yields results from direct specimens in 2 hours and is less operator-dependent than traditional PCR detection methods. Multiple meta-analyses of studies involving children with a confirmed or suspected diagnosis of pulmonary tuberculosis have demonstrated improved sensitivity (62%–98%) and specificity (66%–98%) of Xpert on induced or expectorated sputa compared to smear microscopy for the diagnosis of pulmonary tuberculosis.[115–117] The sensitivity of Xpert is similar on acid-fast smear gastric aspirate samples from children with suspected pulmonary tuberculosis and smear positive-induced sputum samples (77% vs. 86%). However, the combination of the two methods on smear positive samples improves sensitivity (96% for smear and culture positive samples and 63% for smear negative-culture positive samples). Although cartridges for the Xpert system are expensive, it offers advantages in rapid detection of MDR tuberculosis and is especially useful in settings lacking more sophisticated laboratory infrastructure. In low-resource settings, Xpert may replace smear microscopy; however, it should never replace mycobacterial culture and drug-susceptibility testing.

An additional application of molecular testing is a genome-wide analysis of RNA expression of *M. tuberculosis* genomic targets in host blood. This has potential to distinguish tuberculosis from other diseases in high-burden settings, which is especially promising in areas with a high prevalence of HIV infection. A multicenter study enrolled 346 children from three high-tuberculosis burden countries to evaluate the performance of genome-wide RNA expression.[118] Among the children enrolled, 114 had culture-confirmed tuberculosis disease (32%). Fifty-one RNA transcripts were identified that distinguished tuberculosis from other diseases and 42 transcripts distinguished between tuberculosis disease and infection. In a validation cohort of Kenyan children with culture-confirmed disease, the transcript signature was 82.9% sensitive [CI: 69%–94%], and 84% specific [CI: 75%–93%].

An additional application of whole-genome sequencing is to identify molecular drug resistance gene targets and offers more timely information (days compared to weeks) on drug susceptibility compared with traditional phenotypic DST.[119] This technology is especially useful in providing treatment recommendations for children who are contacts of adult source cases who have been treated previously for tuberculosis or who have failed to improve on their tuberculosis treatment regimen. The availability of this technology is currently limited to reference laboratories.

TREATMENT

The general principles that have governed the development of treatment regimens for adults with tuberculosis apply to children. Most childhood tuberculosis experts believe that if a regimen is efficacious for treating adults with tuberculosis, it will be effective for childhood tuberculosis. However, there are several special considerations for children with tuberculosis based on the natural history of the disease, the lower bacillary burden in young children, drug pharmacokinetics and dynamics, safety and tolerability, and the formulations of the available drugs. First, children usually develop tuberculosis disease as an immediate complication of a primary infection. Children typically have low numbers of bacteria enclosed in caseous lesions with relatively few mycobacteria (termed paucibacillary disease). The large bacterial populations found within cavities or infiltrates that are characteristic of adult pulmonary tuberculosis can be seen in adolescents, but are usually absent in young children. Since the likelihood of *M. tuberculosis* developing resistance to any antimycobacterial drug is proportional to the mycobacterial population size, in general, children are less likely than adults to develop secondary drug resistance while receiving therapy.[120]

A related problem concerns the natural history of primary tuberculosis in children. While asymptomatic infection and pulmonary disease are easily distinguishable events in adults, the range of microbiologic and host response events exists on a continuum in children. In asymptomatic children, with a positive TST or IGRA, who are identified at the time of a contact investigation with a known exposure to a symptomatic adult, it may be difficult for clinicians to distinguish between infection and disease. Furthermore, pediatric radiographs can be difficult to interpret and there are no standards for what constitutes hilar or mediastinal adenopathy in a child. In general, a clinician should consider a child to have tuberculosis disease if adenopathy is readily visible on chest radiograph, even if the child has no signs or symptoms of tuberculosis. When determining the best treatment regimen for a child (which in most cases is very well tolerated), in general, it is safer to overestimate rather than underestimate the extent of disease, particularly in a child known to be at high risk for recent acquisition of tuberculosis infection.

Third, young children have a higher propensity than adults to develop extrapulmonary forms of tuberculosis, especially disseminated tuberculosis and meningitis. It is important that antituberculosis drugs penetrate into a variety of tissues and fluids, especially across the blood brain barrier into the meninges. Isoniazid, rifampin, pyrazinamide, ethionamide, fluoroquinolones, and linezolid cross both inflamed an uninflamed

meninges adequately to kill virtually all strains of drug-susceptible *M. tuberculosis.*

Fourth, the pharmacokinetics and dynamics and safety and tolerability of antituberculosis drugs differ between children and adults.[121] In general, children tolerate larger doses per kilogram of body weight and have fewer adverse events than adults.[122,123] It is unclear whether the higher serum concentration of drugs achieved in children has any therapeutic advantage.[124] The lower rates of toxicity in children usually correlate with fewer interruptions of treatment.

Finally, the most important difference between children and adults concerns the formulations, and, therefore, the administration of antituberculosis medications. Most available dosage formulations worldwide are in pill or tablet form, and were designed for use in adults. The administration of these preparations to children often involves crushing pills or constituting suspensions, which may lead to inadequate absorption of oral medications.[125] More recent pharmacokinetic studies using increased doses of commonly used drugs have demonstrated higher blood levels of antituberculosis drugs than in previous studies without increased toxicity, which has guided new dosing recommendations by the WHO for the management of childhood tuberculosis.[126–128] The "pill burden" may be difficult for young children at the start of therapy. If these problems are not anticipated or discussed with families, they may cause significant delays and interruptions of treatment. To overcome some of these barriers, fixed-dose multidrug combinations (FDCs) tablets have been developed recently which easily dissolve in water and have improved palatability. These FDCs have improved childhood tuberculosis disease treatment completion rates.[125] In the United States, FDCs are not readily available for the treatment of childhood tuberculosis. The most effective intervention in the United States that has been shown to improve childhood tuberculosis treatment completion rates is the administration of treatment via directly observed therapy (DOT) with trained health-care workers who are educated and trained in techniques to assist parents in the administration of the treatment.[129–131]

ANTITUBERCULOSIS DRUGS FOR CHILDREN

Several antituberculosis drugs are used to achieve a relatively rapid cure and prevent the emergence of secondary drug resistance during therapy (Table 18.4).[7] The choice of regimen depends on the extent of tuberculosis disease, the host, and the likelihood of drug resistance. Isoniazid is familiar to pediatricians, as it is effective and well tolerated by children. It is metabolized by acetylation in the liver, however, there is no correlation in children between the acetylation rate and either drug efficacy or adverse reactions.[132] The major toxic effects of isoniazid in adults are very rare in children. Hepatotoxicity among children taking isoniazid is exceedingly rare.[122,133] Only 3%–10% of children taking isoniazid experience a transient elevation in liver enzyme levels; clinically significant hepatitis occurs in far less than 1% of children.[122] Adolescents are more likely than younger children to experience hepatotoxicity.[134] For most children and adolescents, toxicity can be monitored using only clinical signs and symptoms of hepatitis; routine biochemical monitoring is not necessary. Pyridoxine levels are decreased in children taking isoniazid, but symptomatic

Table 18.4 First-line drugs for the treatment of childhood tuberculosis infection and disease

Drug	Dosage forms	Daily dosage (mg/kg/day)	Twice weekly dosage (mg/kg/dose)	Weekly dosage (mg/kg/dose)	Maximum dose
Ethambutol	Tablets 100 mg 400 mg	20–25	50		2.5 g
Isoniazid	Scored tablets 100 mg 300 mg	10–15	20–30	Age 2–11 years, ≥10 kg: 25 Age ≥12 years: 15	Daily, 300 mg Once weekly or twice weekly, 900 mg
Pyrazinamide	Scored tablets 500 mg	30–40	50		2 g
Rifampin	Capsules 150 mg 300 mg	15–20	15–20[a]		Daily, 600 mg Twice weekly, 600 mg
Rifapentine	Tablets 150 mg			Wt 10–14.0 kg: 300 mg/dose Wt 14.1–25.0 kg: 450 mg/dose Wt 25.1–32.0 kg: 600 mg/dose Wt 32.1–49.9 kg: 750 mg/dose ≥50.0 kg: 900 mg maximum	Weekly: 900 mg

[a] For infants and toddlers, and children of any age with tuberculous meningitis, higher oral doses (20–30 mg/kg/day) of rifampin should be considered.

peripheral neuritis is exceedingly rare.[133] However, certain children—especially adolescents with poor nutritional habits, children with diets low in meat and milk intake, HIV-infected children, and breastfeeding infants—should receive pyridoxine supplementation.[7]

Rifampin and rifapentine are rifamycins that are also well tolerated by children. Hepatotoxicity is infrequent and other adverse reactions that occur in adults, including leukopenia, thrombocytopenia and immunologically mediated flu-like syndrome, are rare. Clinicians should consider the risk of drug-drug interactions as rifamycins may influence the metabolism of various classes of medications (including antiretroviral medications, antiepileptic medications, and antihypertensive medications). In addition, the effectiveness of most oral contraceptives will be decreased, and alternative birth control methods should be used.

Pyrazinamide has been used extensively in children; hepatitis and complications of hyperuricemia are exceedingly rare events. Ethambutol is also safe in children and is widely used in the first-line regimen for the treatment of childhood tuberculosis. Optic toxicity is rare in children, and formal ophthalmologic evaluation of asymptomatic children is not necessary. Ethionamide is well tolerated in children and is considered a first-line therapy for tuberculous meningitis. Children may experience nausea and vomiting, but less frequently than adults. Baseline thyroid function testing followed by monitoring 6-month intervals is recommended for children receiving long-term ethionamide therapy.

Fluoroquinolones are the major class of medications used in children with known or suspected drug resistance.[135] Tendon rupture, which has been observed in adults and rarely in adolescents, has not been observed in children. Fluoroquinolones are well tolerated by children and are safe.[136–138] Hepatoxicity is exceedingly rare, including with long-term administration.[135,138]

SPECIFIC TREATMENT

Thoracic disease

The standard therapy of intrathoracic, drug-susceptible tuberculosis (non-cavitary pulmonary disease and/or hilar lymphadenopathy) in children, as recommended by the AAP and the CDC, is a minimum of 6 months which includes isoniazid and rifampin supplemented in the first 2 months by pyrazinamide and ethambutol. Several clinical trials have shown that this regimen yields a success rate approaching 100%, with an incidence of clinically significant adverse reactions of <2%. Nine-month regimens of only isoniazid and rifampin are also effective for drug-susceptible tuberculosis, but the necessary length of treatment, the need for good adherence by the patient, and the relative lack of protection against possible initial drug resistance have led to the favoring of treatment regimens with additional drugs for a short time period. Most experts recommend that children receive their antituberculosis drugs via DOT, when a health-care worker is present during medication administration (often by a parent or adult caregiver). When DOT is used, intermittent (twice or thrice weekly) administration of drugs after an initial period as short as 2 weeks of daily therapy has been shown to be as effective as daily therapy for the treatment of drug-susceptible tuberculosis in children.[139–141] Children or adolescents with disseminated (miliary) tuberculosis or adult-type cavitary tuberculosis are treated for a minimum of 6 months from culture conversion, and the medications are given daily.[140]

Extrathoracic disease

In general, extrathoracic tuberculosis in children is caused by small numbers of mycobacteria. Therefore, the treatment of most manifestations of extrathoracic tuberculosis in children, including cervical lymphadenopathy, intra-abdominal tuberculosis and tuberculosis of the genital tract, is the same as for pulmonary tuberculosis. Exceptions are bone and joint, disseminated, and tuberculous meningitis/tuberculomas, for which there are inadequate data to recommend a 6-month duration of therapy. These conditions are treated for a minimum of 9–12 months. Surgical debridement of bone and joint disease may be necessary in addition to medical therapy.[142]

Children with tuberculous meningitis are treated initially with four-drug therapy (isoniazid, rifampin, pyrazinamide, and ethionamide or an injectable aminoglycoside). In most cases, the pyrazinamide and fourth medication are discontinued after 2 months, and isoniazid and rifampin are continued for an additional 7–10 months.[143,144] In adults, the use of linezolid or a fluoroquinolone has shown clinical benefit, especially when drug resistance is expected or if other medications are poorly tolerated.[145,146] Corticosteroids are administered in conjunction with antituberculosis treatment for tuberculous meningitis, and reduce the associated morbidity and mortality.[147] In children who have refractory inflammation, thalidomide has been used successfully, on a case-by-case basis.[83,148] Neurosurgical ventriculoperitoneal shunting is frequently required when significant hydrocephalus is present. When surgical shunting cannot be performed safely or urgently, acetazolamide with or without a diuretic medication has been used to decrease CSF production, as a medical adjunct to decrease intracranial pressure.

Tuberculous lymphadenitis responds well to antituberculosis chemotherapy alone.[149] Surgical resection of involved lymph nodes usually is not necessary and may lead to the formation of cutaneous fistula tracts or severe scarring. If performed, excisional biopsy is preferred over incisional biopsy. However, surgical biopsy and mycobacterial culture may be necessary to distinguish tuberculous adenitis from other entities, most notably infection due to *Bartonella henselae* or nontuberculous mycobacteria.

Tuberculosis treatment in HIV-infected children

Treatment of tuberculosis in HIV-infected children is often empiric based on epidemiologic and radiographic information, because the radiographic appearance of other pulmonary complications of HIV in children, such as bacterial pneumonia, lymphoid interstitial pneumonitis, and nontuberculous mycobacterial infection, may be similar to that of tuberculosis. In HIV-infected children who do not respond to treatment for community-acquired pneumonia and tuberculosis cannot be excluded, antituberculosis therapy should be considered.

Children with suspected or confirmed tuberculosis and newly diagnosed or previously untreated HIV infection should be evaluated for starting early combined antiretroviral therapy (cART), preferably within 2–8 weeks of starting tuberculosis treatment, irrespective of their immune status.[150,151] HIV-infected children who are severely immunocompromised (CD4+ count <50 cells/mL), should be monitored closely for a paradoxical worsening of their tuberculosis disease, which supports a diagnosis of IRIS.[149–152] IRIS occurs when the initial cART therapy causes a rapid decrease in the HIV load and an increase in CD4+ cell counts, resulting in an exaggerated inflammatory reaction to *M. tuberculosis*. IRIS manifests in two forms: "unmasking IRIS" occurs when a child

develops symptoms from an undiagnosed tuberculosis infection soon after cART is started and "paradoxical IRIS" occurs when a child who is receiving cART and antituberculosis therapy develops a worsening of tuberculosis symptoms despite previous clinical improvement and evidence of HIV control (improving CD4+ count and reduced HIV viral load).[150] HIV-infected children who develop tuberculosis-related IRIS most commonly present with fever, cough, new skin lesions, enlarging cervical or thoracic lymph nodes, and new or enlarging brain tuberculomas, with or without associated meningitis.[150–155] Treatment of tuberculosis-related IRIS in HIV-infected children should occur in consultation with a physician who has expertise in the management of both diseases.

Following receipt of the *M. bovis* vaccine (BCG vaccine), HIV-infected infants are at increased risk of developing disseminated *M. bovis*-BCG disease. Studies have revealed that HIV-infected infants have more than a 100-fold increased risk of developing disseminated *M. bovis* disease following their receipt of the vaccine compared to HIV-uninfected children.[156,157] This has led to the recommendation that the BCG vaccine should not be administered to infants born to women with HIV or to infants and children with a confirmed HIV diagnosis.[150,158]

HIV-infected children are usually started on standard antituberculosis regimens that include isoniazid, rifampin, pyrazinamide, and ethambutol. All treatment should be administered daily, not intermittently. Most experts believe that HIV-infected children with drug-susceptible tuberculosis should receive the standard four-drug regimen for the first 2 months followed by isoniazid and rifampin for a total duration of at least 9 months.[147] A major consideration prior to choosing a cART regimen is that the coadministration of rifampin and some antiretroviral agents results in subtherapeutic blood levels of protease inhibitors and nonnucleoside reverse transcriptase inhibitors. Concomitant administration of these drugs should be avoided. Based on the child's age, HIV drug resistance profile and previous cART exposure, an efavirenz-based regimen is preferred. If nevirapine is used, the dose must be adjusted for concomitant rifampin administration. If a protease inhibitor combination is used, a higher dose of ritonavir (termed "superboosting") equal to that of the lopinavir dose, for the full duration of the rifampin treatment plus an additional 2 weeks is recommended. Pyridoxine supplementation (1–2 mg/kg/day, maximum dose 50 mg/day) should be provided to all HIV-infected children who are receiving isoniazid.[7,147] HIV-infected children with extrapulmonary disease, including tuberculous meningitis, miliary/disseminated tuberculosis, or musculoskeletal disease, should be treated for a minimum of 12 months. For children with tuberculous meningitis, ethambutol is replaced with ethionamide or an injectable aminoglycoside due to their superior CNS penetration. The addition of corticosteroids is indicated for HIV-infected children with tuberculous meningitis, pleural effusion, airway compromise, or severe IRIS. HIV-infected children appear to have more frequent adverse reactions to antituberculosis drugs and must be monitored closely during therapy.[159] Liver enzyme testing should be obtained after 2, 4, and 8 weeks of treatment for tuberculosis. After 2 months, routine testing can be spaced to every 2–3 months in asymptomatic children, or more frequently as clinically indicated.[150]

Drug-resistant tuberculosis

There are two major types of drug resistance: primary resistance and secondary resistance. Primary resistance occurs when a child is infected with *M. tuberculosis* that is already resistant to a particular drug. Secondary resistance occurs when drug-resistant organisms emerge as the dominant population during a treatment course. The major causes of secondary drug resistance are poor adherence to the medication by the patient or inadequate treatment regimens prescribed by the physician. Nonadherence to one drug is more likely to lead to secondary resistance than is failure to take all drugs. Secondary resistance is rare in young children because of the small size of the mycobacterial population. Consequently, most drug resistance in children is primary, and patterns of drug resistance among children tend to mirror those found among adults in the same population.[160,161] The main predictors of drug-resistant tuberculosis among adults are history of previous antituberculosis treatment, coinfection with HIV, and exposure to another adult with infectious drug-resistant tuberculosis.

Treatment of drug-resistant tuberculosis is successful only when at least two bactericidal drugs to which the infecting strain of *M. tuberculosis* is susceptible are given.[162,163] When a child has suspected drug-resistant tuberculosis, usually at least four or five drugs should be administered initially until the susceptibility pattern is determined and a more specific regimen can be designed (Table 18.5).[164–166] The specific treatment plan must be individualized for each patient according to the results of susceptibility testing on the isolates from the child or her adult source case. When isoniazid mono-resistance is present, a total treatment duration of 9 months with rifampin, pyrazinamide, and ethambutol is usually adequate. When resistance to both isoniazid and rifampin is present, the total duration of therapy is often extended to 12–24 months. Daily therapy should be administered to any child with drug-resistant tuberculosis. In 2016, the WHO endorsed a 9–12 month treatment regimen for adults and children with MDR-TB who were not previously treated with second-line drugs or who were unlikely to have a strain with resistance to second-line injectable agents or fluoroquinolones.[163] This recommendation was based on the results of adult observational studies and extrapolated for use in children. Furthermore, as second-line treatment options for MDR-TB in children, there is increasing use of new antituberculosis medications (bedaquiline and delamanid) and repurposed drugs (linezolid and clofazimine).[167,168] Delamanid is a nitroimidazole that has been studied for the treatment of MDR-TB in children since 2013. This includes two pharmacokinetic studies in HIV-uninfected children down to age 6 years.[168,169] Based on these studies, delamanid is endorsed for use in children ≥6 years and ≥20 kg in whom a four-drug regimen cannot be constructed due to drug resistance, the child experiences significant drug intolerance, or is at high risk of treatment failure. Further studies are ongoing to evaluate the safety and efficacy of delamanid in children with MDR-TB who are HIV-infected and those who are 3–5 years of age. Bedaquiline is considered acceptable for treatment of children ≥12 years of age and >33 kg with the same tuberculosis treatment indications specified for delamanid. Bedaquiline should not be given with efavirenz due to reduced bedaquiline levels with coadministration. For HIV-infected children, efavirenz should be replaced with nevirapine or raltegravir while they are receiving bedaquiline. A baseline EKG and monitoring of QTc is recommended in patients receiving bedaquiline and/or delamanid. Children with a baseline QTc interval ≥500 ms should not be started on bedaquiline or delamanid until the QTc interval is corrected.[169,170] In addition, a child's baseline albumin should be ≥2.8 g/dL prior to starting delamanid. Trials evaluating the clinical efficacy of the use of combined treatment with bedaquiline and delamanid for the treatment of MDR-TB in children are lacking. Both linezolid and clofazimine are now included as core second-line agents in treatment regimens for children with MDR-TB. Both drugs require close monitoring for adverse effects and toxicity.[167]

The prognosis of single drug or MDR tuberculosis in children is usually good if the drug resistance is identified early in the treatment, appropriate drugs are administered under DOT, adverse reactions from the drugs are minor, and the child and family are in a supportive environment. The treatment of drug-resistant tuberculosis in children should always be undertaken by a clinician with specific expertise in the treatment of tuberculosis. Clinical trials to evaluate the efficacy, safety, pharmacokinetics, and pharmacodynamics of the administration of combinations and shorter regimens of new and repurposed antituberculosis medications for the treatment of childhood tuberculosis are needed.[171]

Table 18.5 Drugs used for treatment of MDR tuberculosis in children

Fluoroquinolones	Levofloxacin
	Moxifloxacin
	Gatifloxacin
Second-line injectable agents	Amikacin
	Capreomycin
	Kanamycin
	Streptomycin
Other core second-line agents	Ethionamide/prothionamide
	Cycloserine/terizidone
	Linezolid
	Clofazimine
Add-on agents	Pyrazinamide[a]
	Ethambutol[a]
	High-dose isoniazid[a]
	Bedaquiline[b]
	Delamanid[b]
	p-aminosalicylic acid[c]
	Imipenem-cilastain[c]
	Meropenem[c,d]
	Amoxicillin-clavulanate[c,d]
	(Thioacetazone)[c,e]

Source: World Health Organization: WHO treatment guidelines for drug-resistant tuberculosis, 2016 update. Geneva, Switzerland. http://apps.who.int/iris/bitstream/10665/250125/1/9789241549639-eng.pdf
[a] Considered first-line add-on agent.
[b] Considered second-line add-on agent.
[c] Considered third-line add-on agent.
[d] Carbapenems and amoxicillin-clavulanate are given together.
[e] Confirm patient is HIV negative prior to starting thioacetazone.

Anti-inflammatory therapy

Corticosteroids are useful in treating some children with tuberculosis disease but only when used in combination with effective antituberculosis drugs. They are beneficial for tuberculosis in children where the host inflammatory reaction contributes significantly to tissue damage or impairment of organ function (Table 18.6). There is convincing evidence that corticosteroids decrease mortality rates and long-term neurologic sequelae in some patients with tuberculous meningitis by reducing vasculitis, inflammation, and, ultimately, intracranial pressure.[172] Lowering the intracranial pressure limits tissue damage and favors circulation of antituberculosis drugs through the brain and meninges. Short courses of corticosteroids also may be effective for children with enlarged hilar lymph nodes that compress the tracheobronchial tree causing respiratory distress, localized emphysema, or segmental pulmonary lesions.[173,174] Several randomized clinical trials have shown that corticosteroids can help relieve symptoms and constriction associated with acute tuberculous pericardial effusion.[175] In patients with tuberculous pleural effusion in whom there is a shift of the mediastinum and acute respiratory compromise, corticosteroids may cause dramatic improvement in symptoms, although the long-term course is probably unaffected.[176] Some children with severe miliary tuberculosis have dramatic improvement with corticosteroids if the inflammatory reaction is so severe that alveolocapillary block is present. There is no convincing evidence that one corticosteroid is superior over the other. The most commonly used regimen is prednisone, 1–2 mg/kg/day divided in one or two doses orally for 4–6 weeks, followed by a gradual taper. Thalidomide (3–5 mg/kg/day), a potent TNF-α inhibitor of monocytes and macrophages, has been used as a successful adjuvant therapy for the treatment of children with tuberculous arachnoiditis of the optic chiasm leading to visual loss, and large tuberculous pseudo-abscesses in the brain and spinal cord.[83,148]

Treatment of tuberculosis infection

The goal of treatment of children with asymptomatic tuberculosis infection is to prevent progression to disease. This treatment is an established practice. The effectiveness of isoniazid therapy in children infected by a source case with an isoniazid-susceptible isolate has approached 100%.[177]

The following aspects of the natural history and treatment of tuberculosis infection in children must be considered in the formulation of recommendations about therapy: (1) recently infected immunocompromised children and children younger than 5 years have a high risk of progression to disease with untreated infants having up to a 40% chance of developing tuberculosis disease; (2)

Table 18.6 Manifestations of tuberculosis that may benefit from corticosteroid therapy

- Tuberculous meningitis
- Tuberculoma with edema or mass effect
- Miliary disease with alveolar-capillary block
- Constrictive pericarditis
- Massive pleural effusion
- Pott's disease (vertebral tuberculosis) with nerve compression

infants and young children are more likely to have life-threatening forms of tuberculosis, including meningitis and disseminated disease; (3) the risk for progression from tuberculosis infection to disease decreases gradually through childhood, until adolescence when the risk increases; and (4) children with tuberculosis infection have more years at risk for the development of disease than adults. Because of these factors, and the excellent safety profile of antituberculosis drugs in children, children and adolescents with tuberculosis infection should always be treated.

The standard treatment regimens for the treatment of tuberculosis infection in children include: 6–9 months of isoniazid (daily, or twice weekly via DOT); 3 months of daily rifampin and isoniazid; 4 months of daily rifampin; and once weekly isoniazid and rifapentine for 12 weeks.[7,178]

Isoniazid therapy for tuberculosis infection appears to be more effective for children than adults, with several large clinical trials demonstrating risk reduction of 70%–90%. Analysis of data from several studies has demonstrated a 20%–30% decreased efficacy of isoniazid treatment if it was taken for 6 months rather than 9 months. However, due to resource constraints on the international scale, the WHO-recommended duration of isoniazid therapy for tuberculosis infection is 6 months.[179] Isoniazid given twice weekly for 9 months via DOT has been used extensively and is as effective as daily therapy. For healthy children taking isoniazid but no other potentially hepatotoxic drugs, routine biochemical monitoring and supplementation with pyridoxine are not necessary. Three months of daily rifampin and isoniazid has been used throughout Europe, with programmatic data suggesting that the regimen is effective, but this regimen is not recommended in the United States.[180] Rifampin alone is a safe, well tolerated, acceptable alternative to daily or twice weekly isoniazid for 9 months. A multicenter, open-label trial randomized 844 children (<18 years of age) to receive either 4 months of daily rifampin or 9 months of isoniazid; 13% more children completed 4 months of rifampin compared to isoniazid, and no children in either group discontinued the drug due to a serious adverse event.[181] Due to superior treatment completion rates compared to 9 months of isoniazid, 4 months of rifampin is now considered by many experts to be a better treatment option.[178,181–184] Rifapentine is a rifamycin with a very long half-life, allowing for weekly administration in conjunction with high-dose isoniazid. Twelve doses of once weekly high-dose isoniazid and rifapentine are as safe and effective for treating tuberculosis infection as 9 months of daily isoniazid for children down to 2 years of age.[129,183,185] Traditionally, this regimen has been given via DOT. In areas of the United States where DOT and funding are available, this is becoming the preferred regimen for the treatment of tuberculosis infection in age-eligible children who are exposed to a contact with a pansusceptible isolate of *M. tuberculosis*.

For children who develop tuberculosis infection after being in contact with a source case with a MDR strain of *M. tuberculosis*, the treatment regimen depends on the drug-susceptibility profile of the source case's organism. The most commonly used regimen includes a fluoroquinolone—often levofloxacin—with or without other oral drugs.[186] In most cases, an expert in tuberculosis should be consulted.

Few controlled studies have been published regarding the efficacy of treatment regimens other than isoniazid for tuberculosis infection in HIV-infected children. The most commonly used regimen is a 6–9-month course of daily isoniazid. Most experts recommend that routine monitoring of serum hepatic enzyme concentrations be performed and pyridoxine be given when HIV-infected children are treated with isoniazid. In children who are not receiving protease inhibitor or nonnucleoside reverse transcriptase inhibitors, the optimal duration of rifampin therapy is not known, but most experts recommend at least a 6-month course if isoniazid cannot be used.

Postexposure treatment "window prophylaxis"

Serious tuberculosis disease can develop rapidly in a young child, even before a test of infection becomes positive. Therefore, children younger than 5 years of age who are initially TST or IGRA negative but have been in contact with a potentially contagious adult should receive isoniazid therapy until 8–10 weeks after contact has been broken by either physical separation from the source case or chemotherapy.[187] This practice is often referred to as "window prophylaxis." For these children, TST or IGRA testing is repeated after 8–10 weeks; if the second test result is positive, isoniazid therapy is continued for 9 months, but if the result is negative, treatment can be stopped.

Supportive and follow-up care

Children receiving treatment should be followed carefully to promote adherence to therapy, to monitor for adverse reactions to medications, and to ensure that the tuberculosis is being adequately treated. The clinician must report all clinically suspected and microbiologically confirmed childhood tuberculosis cases to the local health authority. This is to ensure that the child and the family receive appropriate care and evaluation. Adequate nutrition is important during the treatment of tuberculosis. Activity restriction is not necessary unless the child develops respiratory embarrassment or immobilization is necessary (in some cases of vertebral tuberculosis). Patients should be clinically evaluated every 4–6 weeks while receiving therapy. Anticipatory guidance with regard to the administration of medications to children is crucial. The clinician should foresee difficulties that the family might have in introducing several new medications in inconvenient dosage formulations to a young child. Pill forms of isoniazid, rifampin, pyrazinamide, and ethambutol can be crushed and given with small amounts of food.

Nonadherence to treatment is a major problem due to the long-term nature of treatment and sometimes difficult social circumstances of the patients. The child or adolescent and family must know what is expected of them through verbal and written instructions in their primary language. Approximately 30%–50% of children taking long-term treatment are nonadherent with self-administered medications, and clinicians are usually not able to determine in advance which children or adolescents will be nonadherent. Preferably, DOT should be instituted by the local health authority.[130]

The rates of adverse reactions to antituberculosis medications are low enough in children and adolescents that routine baseline and monitoring of hepatic function tests is not necessary. If there is a previous history of hepatitis, obesity (fatty liver) or other chronic illness, it is advisable to obtain a baseline hepatic function

panel. If the patient or family reports any symptoms that could be adverse reactions to antituberculosis medications, the child should have a complete physical examination and a hepatic function panel (including bilirubin level determination). Serum liver enzyme elevations of 2 times normal are fairly common and do not necessitate discontinuation of medications if all other findings are normal. Pyrazinamide may cause mild arthralgia or arthritis that is usually transient. Rash and severe pruritus are less common in children. Children receiving ethionamide should have baseline thyroid function testing and monitoring every 6 months to evaluate for hypothyroidism. Rifapentine can cause muscle aches that are generally self-limited and require no intervention. Adverse reactions with fluoroquinolones are uncommon.

Radiographic improvement of intrathoracic disease in children occurs very slowly. A common practice is to obtain a chest radiograph at diagnosis and 4–8 weeks into therapy to be sure that no progression or unusual changes have occurred. If these radiographs are satisfactory, interim chest radiographs are not necessary, and an end of treatment radiograph is recommended. A significant proportion of children with intrathoracic adenopathy have abnormal radiographic findings for 1–3 years, after effective antituberculosis treatment has been completed. If clinical and radiographic improvement has occurred after 6 months of therapy, medications can be discontinued, and the child can be followed at intervals of 6–12 months with appropriate chest radiographs to determine continued improvement in radiographic appearance.

TUBERCULOSIS IN PREGNANT WOMEN AND THE NEWBORN

INTRODUCTION

The influence of pregnancy on the incidence and prognosis of tuberculosis has been debated since antiquity.[188] At various times, pregnancy has been thought to improve, worsen, or have no effect on the prognosis of tuberculosis. This controversy has lost some of its importance since the advent of effective antituberculosis therapy. With adequate treatment, a pregnant woman with tuberculosis has a prognosis equivalent to that of a comparable nonpregnant woman. If untreated, tuberculosis disease during pregnancy may result in unfavorable outcomes for both the pregnant woman and the fetus. Tuberculosis during pregnancy increases the risk of premature birth, low birth weight, intrauterine growth retardation, and perinatal death. Infants born to mothers with tuberculosis disease should be evaluated and treated to prevent the development of serious tuberculosis.[189]

PATHOGENESIS

The pathogenesis of pulmonary tuberculosis during pregnancy is similar to that for nonpregnant women. Shortly after the initiation of infection, some organisms enter the lymphatic and blood vessels and disseminate throughout the body. During this phase of infection, the genitalia, endometrium, or placenta may become involved. Genital tuberculosis is most likely to occur at the time of menarche and can have a very long and relatively asymptomatic course. The fallopian tubes are most often involved (90%–100%), followed by the uterus (50%–60%), ovaries (20%–30%), and cervix (5%–15%).[190] Sterility is often the presenting complaint of tuberculous endometritis, which diminishes the likelihood of congenital tuberculosis occurring.[191] Worldwide estimates are that tuberculosis is the cause of infertility in 1%–13% of women. An Egyptian study of 420 infertile women who were admitted for diagnostic laparoscopy, endometrial biopsy, and *M. tuberculosis* PCR testing[192] identified tuberculosis as the cause in 24 women (5.7%); 17 of these women (71%) were found to have fallopian tube involvement (beading, sacculation or rigid appearance), 7 (29%) had ovarian disease, and 6 (25%) had peritoneal seeding. Tuberculous endometritis can lead to congenital infection in the newborn, but it results more frequently from disseminated tuberculosis in the mother than from direct extension from endometritis.[193,194]

The potential modes of inoculation of the newborn infant with tuberculosis from the mother are listed in Table 18.7. Infection of the neonate through the umbilical cord is a rare event. These infants' mothers frequently suffer from pleural effusion, meningitis, or disseminated disease during pregnancy or soon afterwards.[195–199] In many of these cases, a diagnosis of tuberculosis in the child leads to the discovery of the mother's tuberculosis. The intensity of lymphohematogenous spread during pregnancy is one of the factors that determines if congenital tuberculosis will occur. Hematogenous dissemination in the mother leads to the infection of the placenta with subsequent transmission to the fetus. Tubercle bacilli have been demonstrated in the decidua, amnion, and chorionic villi of the placenta.[191] However, even massive involvement of the placenta with tuberculosis does not always give rise to congenital infection. It is not clear whether the fetus can be directly infected from the mother's bloodstream without a caseous lesion first forming in the placenta.

In hematogenous congenital tuberculosis, *M. tuberculosis* reaches the fetus via the umbilical vein. If some bacilli infect the liver, a primary focus develops with involvement of the periportal lymph nodes. However, the bacilli can pass through the liver into the main circulation leading to a primary focus in the fetus' lung. The tubercle bacilli in the lung often remain dormant until after birth when oxygenation and circulation increase significantly, leading to pulmonary tuberculosis in the young infant.

Congenital infection of the infant may also occur via aspiration or ingestion of amniotic fluid.[199] The fetus may inhale or ingest the tubercle bacilli when the caseous lesion in the placenta ruptures directly into the amniotic cavity. Inhalation or ingestion of infected amniotic fluid is the most likely cause of tuberculosis

if the infant presents with multiple primary foci in the lung, liver, gastrointestinal tract, or middle ear.[200]

The pathology of tuberculosis in the fetus and newborn usually demonstrates the predisposition to dissemination and fatal disease.[201] The liver and lungs are primarily involved followed by the bone marrow, bone, gastrointestinal tract, adrenal glands, spleen, kidney, abdominal lymph nodes, and skin. The histologic patterns of involvement are similar to those in adults; tubercles and granulomas are common.[202] CNS involvement occurs in fewer than 50% of cases. The mortality of congenital tuberculosis reaches 50% due primarily to the failure to suspect the correct diagnosis. Most fatal cases are diagnosed at autopsy.[197,198]

Postnatal acquisition of tuberculosis via airborne inoculation is the most common route of infection for the neonate. It may be impossible to differentiate postnatal infection from prenatal acquisition on clinical grounds alone. It is important to remember that any adult in the neonate's environment can be a source of airborne tuberculosis. Since newborns infected with tuberculosis are at extremely high risk of developing severe forms of disease, investigation of an adult with tuberculosis whose household contains a pregnant woman should be considered a public health emergency. In addition, all adults in contact with an infant suspected of having infection or disease should undergo a thorough investigation for tuberculosis.

EPIDEMIOLOGY: INTERACTION OF TUBERCULOSIS AND PREGNANCY

The true burden of tuberculosis disease among pregnant women is unknown. An estimate of the global burden of tuberculosis disease during pregnancy that was extrapolated from the WHO tuberculosis case incidence data in 2011 from 217 countries estimated that 216,500 (range 192,100–247,000) tuberculosis cases occurred among pregnant women worldwide.[203] The greatest burdens of disease were found in the WHO African region (89,400 cases) followed by the South East Asian region (67,500 cases). The lowest burden of disease occurred in the WHO region of the America with 4800 cases. Due to nonspecific signs and symptoms that occur in pregnant women with tuberculosis, this is thought to be an underestimate of the true burden of disease.

From ancient times, medical opinions regarding the interaction of pregnancy and tuberculosis have varied considerably. Hippocrates thought that pregnancy had a beneficial effect on tuberculosis, a view that persisted virtually unchallenged into the nineteenth century, when an opposite view emerged. In 1850, Grisolle reported 24 cases of tuberculosis that developed during pregnancy.[204] In all patients, the progression of tuberculosis was more severe than usually seen in nonpregnant women of the same age. Shortly thereafter, further reports were published that implied pregnancy had a deleterious effect on tuberculosis. This view gained so much support that by the early twentieth century, the concept of induced abortion as a solution to avoid the consequences of tuberculosis during pregnancy became accepted practice.

The opinion that pregnancy had a deleterious effect on tuberculosis predominated until the late 1940s. In 1943, Cohen detected no increase rate of progression of tuberculosis among 100 pregnant

Table 18.7 Potential modes of inoculation of a neonate or infant with *M. tuberculosis*

Maternal focus	Mode of spread
Pneumonia or pneumonitis	Airborne
Placentitis	Hematogenous (umbilical vessel)
Amniotic	Aspiration of infected fluid
Cervicitis, Endometritis	Direct contact, aspiration

women with abnormal chest radiographs.[205] In 1953, Hedvall presented a comprehensive review of the published studies concerning tuberculosis in pregnancy in the prechemotherapy era.[206] He cited studies totaling over 1000 cases that reported negative effects of pregnancy on tuberculosis. However, he discovered a nearly equal number of reported cases in which a neutral or favorable relationship between pregnancy and tuberculosis was observed. In his own study involving 250 pregnant women with abnormal chest radiographs consistent with tuberculosis, he noted that 9% improved, 7% worsened, and 84% remained unchanged during pregnancy. In follow-up, during the first postpartum year, 9% improved, 15% worsened, and 76% were stable. Crombie noted that 31 of 101 pregnant women with quiescent tuberculosis experienced a relapse after delivery; 20 of the 31 relapses occurred in the first postpartum year.[207] Several other investigators observed a higher risk of relapse during the puerperium. However, other studies failed to support an increased risk of progression of tuberculosis in the postpartum period. Cohen's study failed to show a major increase in activity of tuberculosis during pregnancy or any postpartum interval.[208] Other studies had similar results and, although they did not have controlled populations, it was estimated that the rates of progression would be comparable to nonpregnant age-matched control subjects.[208,209] From these and other studies it became clear that the anatomic extent of disease, the radiographic pattern, and the susceptibility of the individual patient to tuberculosis are more important than pregnancy itself in determining the course and prognosis of the pregnant woman with tuberculosis.

The controversy concerning the effect of pregnancy or the postpartum period on tuberculosis has lost most of its importance since the advent of effective chemotherapy. With adequate treatment, pregnant women with tuberculosis have the same excellent prognosis as nonpregnant women. Several studies could document no adverse effects of pregnancy, birth, the postpartum period, or lactation on the course of tuberculosis in women receiving chemotherapy.[189,210]

In the prechemotherapy era, active tuberculosis at an advanced stage carried a poor prognosis for both the mother and the child. Shaefer et al. reported that the infant and maternal mortality from untreated tuberculosis was between 30% and 40%.[189] In the chemotherapy era, the outcome of pregnancy rarely is altered by the presence of tuberculosis in the mother, except in rare cases of congenital tuberculosis. One study from Norway revealed a higher incidence of toxemia, postpartum hemorrhage, and difficult labor in mothers with tuberculosis compared to controls.[211] The incidence of miscarriage was almost 10 times higher in mothers with tuberculosis, but there was no significant difference in the rate of congenital malformations between children born to mothers with and without tuberculosis. One study reported an incidence of prematurity among infants born to untreated mothers in a tuberculosis sanatorium ranging from 23%–64%, depending on the severity of tuberculosis in the mother.[212] However, most experts now believe that with adequate treatment of the pregnant woman with tuberculosis, the prognosis of pregnancy should not be affected adversely by the presence of tuberculosis. Because of the excellent prognosis for both mother and child, the recommendation for the therapeutic abortion has been abandoned.

CLINICAL MANIFESTATIONS, DIAGNOSIS, AND MANAGEMENT

PREGNANT WOMAN

The clinical manifestations of tuberculosis in pregnant women can overlap with those related to pregnancy (including tiredness, fatigue, shortness of breath, sweating, and low-grade fevers) which may lead to a delay in a diagnosis of tuberculosis.[213,214] In one series of 27 pregnant and postpartum women with pulmonary tuberculosis, the most common clinical findings were cough, fever, weight loss, malaise, and fatigue.[215] However, almost 20% of pregnant women lacked significant symptoms. The TST was positive in 26 of 27 patients. Diagnosis was established in all cases by culture of sputum for *M. tuberculosis*. Sixteen of these patients had drug-resistant tuberculosis and their clinical course was marked by more extensive pulmonary involvement, higher incidence of pulmonary complications, longer sputum conversions times, and a higher incidence of death. In another series, approximately 5%–10% of pregnant women with tuberculosis had extrapulmonary disease, a rate comparable to the nonpregnant population.[216]

The indications for treatment and the basic principles for management of tuberculosis disease in the pregnant women are not much different from those in the nonpregnant patient. However, the recommended drug regimens and drugs used are slightly different, mostly due to possible toxic effects of several drugs on the developing fetus. There is no doubt that untreated tuberculosis disease represents a far greater risk to the pregnant woman and her fetus than dose appropriate treatment of the disease.[217] However, if there is a delay in diagnosis, there is great risk of morbidity and mortality in both the woman (including a higher risk of abortion, postpartum hemorrhage, labor difficulties, and preeclampsia) and her developing fetus (including low birth weight, prematurity, and neonatal mortality).[213] The currently recommended treatment for drug-susceptible tuberculosis in pregnancy is 6 months of isoniazid and rifampin daily, supplemented by ethambutol and pyrazinamide for the first 2 months.[218,219] The drugs are usually given daily for the first 2 weeks to 2 months; then they can be given daily or intermittently for the remainder of therapy with equal effectiveness. Pyridoxine should also be given because of increased requirements for this vitamin in pregnancy.[220] Extensive experience with isoniazid, rifampin, and ethambutol has shown that they are safe in both the mother and the fetus.[218–220] Several antituberculosis drugs are not used in pregnancy because of possible toxicity to the fetus.[221] Streptomycin should be avoided during pregnancy, if possible, since almost 20% of infants will have eighth nerve damage if the drug is given to their mothers during pregnancy.[219,222] Other injectable drugs with antituberculosis activity, including capreomycin, kanamycin, and amikacin, could have the same toxic potential as streptomycin.

In women with multidrug-resistant tuberculosis, second-line agents (cycloserine, ethionamide, fluoroquinolones, para-aminosalicylic acid, and aminoglycosides) have been used successfully for treatment, and short term follow-up analyses found no evidence of teratogenicity, toxicity, or transmission of tuberculosis to the infant.[223,224] The treatment of any form of drug-resistant tuberculosis during pregnancy is extraordinarily difficult and should be handled by an expert with great experience with the disease.

NEWBORN

The clinical manifestations of tuberculosis in the fetus or newborn are listed in Table 18.8. Most newborns with tuberculosis have an abnormal chest radiograph and approximately 50% have a miliary pattern of disease. Some infants with a normal chest radiograph early in the course develop profound radiographic abnormalities as the disease progresses. The most common findings are adenopathy and parenchymal infiltrates. Occasionally, the pulmonary involvement progresses very rapidly, leading to the development of a thin-walled cavity.

The clinical presentation of tuberculosis in the newborn is similar to that caused by bacterial sepsis and other congenital infections such as syphilis and cytomegalovirus. The diagnosis of congenital tuberculosis should be suspected in any infant with appropriate signs and symptoms who does not respond to vigorous antibiotic therapy and whose evaluation for other congenital infections is unrevealing. Of course, clinical suspicion should be high if the mother has or has had tuberculosis or if she has tuberculosis risk factors. If possible, an examination of the placenta for granulomatous inflammation, acid-fast bacilli, and by PCR and culture should be performed.[225]

The timely diagnosis of congenital or neonatal tuberculosis is often difficult. The TST is always negative initially, although it may become positive after 1–3 months. Occasionally, an IGRA is positive. The diagnosis must be established by finding acid-fast bacilli in body fluids or tissue and by culturing *M. tuberculosis*. A positive acid-fast smear of an early morning gastric aspirate in a newborn should be considered indicative of tuberculosis, although false-positive smears occur. Direct acid-fast smears, PCR, and culture from middle ear fluid, bone marrow, tracheal aspirate, or tissue biopsy can be useful and should be attempted. One study found positive cultures for *M. tuberculosis* in 10 of 12 gastric aspirates, 3 of 4 liver biopsies, 3 of 3 lymph node biopsies, and 2 of 4 bone marrow biopsies from children with congenital tuberculosis.[226] Open lung biopsy has also been used to establish a diagnosis. The CSF should be examined, sent for routine studies, cultured for mycobacteria, and sent for molecular testing; however, the yield for isolation of *M. tuberculosis* is low.[226,227]

The most important clue to rapidly establish the diagnosis of congenital or neonatal tuberculosis is the maternal and family history. Suspicion should increase if the mother of other family members suffer from unexplained pneumonia, bronchitis, pleural effusion, meningitis, or endometritis shortly before, during, or after pregnancy. Testing of both parents and other family members can yield important clues about the presence of tuberculosis in the family. The importance of this epidemiologic information cannot be overemphasized. The need for thorough investigation of the mother was emphasized by Hageman et al. who found that only 10 of 26 mothers who gave birth to neonates with congenital tuberculosis were diagnosed prior to their infants; the other 16 were discovered as part of the investigation of the infant.[226]

The optimal treatment of congenital tuberculosis has not been established since the rarity of the condition precludes formal treatment trials. The basic principles for treatment of older children also apply to the treatment of congenital tuberculosis. All neonates with suspected congenital tuberculosis should be started on four antituberculosis medications (isoniazid, rifampin, pyrazinamide plus either ethambutol or an aminoglycoside) until the diagnostic evaluation and susceptibility testing of isolated organisms are concluded.[227] Although the optimal duration of therapy has not been established, many experts treat infants with congenital tuberculosis for a total duration of 9–12 months. Young infants receiving multidrug therapy should have serum liver enzymes and uric acid (for pyrazinamide) monitored. Hearing screens and renal function testing should be obtained for infants receiving long-term aminoglycoside therapy. All neonates and infants should receive tuberculosis treatment under DOT.

SCREENING AND TESTING FOR TUBERCULOSIS DURING PREGNANCY

For all pregnant women, the history obtained in an early visit should include questions about tuberculosis risk factors (including birth in or regular travel to a country with a high burden of tuberculosis or known exposure to an adult with known tuberculosis disease), previous positive test for tuberculosis infection (either TST or IGRA), previous treatment for tuberculosis, and current symptoms compatible with tuberculosis. The WHO recommends systematic tuberculosis screening of pregnant women who live in settings where the tuberculosis prevalence is 100 cases per 100,000 population or higher.[228] In the United States, the CDC and the American College of Obstetrics and Gynecology (ACOG) recommend screening for tuberculosis in women at high risk at the time of prenatal care visits.[229] Any pregnant woman with risk factors for tuberculosis and all HIV-infected women should be tested with either a TST or IGRA. An IGRA is the preferred method for testing women who have received a BCG vaccination and in those who are less likely to return for a TST reading. It must be emphasized that HIV-infected women and *M. tuberculosis* may have a falsely negative TST or IGRA, especially if her HIV infection is poorly controlled; these women should be screened for symptoms of tuberculosis with a low threshold for chest imaging to evaluate for pulmonary tuberculosis. For many high-risk women, prenatal or peripartum care represents their only contact with the health-care system and the opportunity to test them for tuberculosis infection or disease should not be lost. Any pregnant

Table 18.8 Most frequent signs and symptoms of congenital tuberculosis

Sign or symptom	Frequency (in percentage)
Respiratory distress	77
Fever	62
Hepatic and/or splenic enlargement	62
Poor feeding	46
Lethargy or irritability	42
Lymphadenopathy	35
Abdominal distension	27
Failure to thrive	19
Ear discharge	15
Skin lesions	12

Source: Adapted from Hageman J et al. *Pediatrics.* 1980;66:980.

woman with a positive TST or IGRA result should receive a chest radiograph with appropriate abdominal shielding. In addition, a thorough review of systems and physical examination should be carried out to exclude extrapulmonary tuberculosis.

The principles of treatment of asymptomatic tuberculosis infection are similar for pregnant women and other adults of comparable age. Although treatment of tuberculosis disease during pregnancy is unquestioned, the treatment of the pregnant woman who has an asymptomatic tuberculosis infection is more controversial. As pregnancy does not seem to increase the risk of a woman progressing from infection to disease, some clinicians prefer to delay treatment of tuberculosis infection until after delivery. Others believe that because recent infection can be accompanied by hematogenous spread to the placenta, it is preferable to treat without delay or defer initiating treatment until the second trimester.[230] The benefits of immediate treatment may be greater in high-risk patients such as HIV-infected women or close contacts to a person with tuberculosis. There appears to be an increased risk of isoniazid-associated hepatoxicity during the postpartum period.[231-233] This was highlighted in multicenter, randomized, non-inferiority trial including HIV-infected pregnant women. The women were randomized to receive isoniazid during pregnancy (immediate group) or in the postpartum period (deferred group). Approximately 6% of women developed hepatotoxicity of grade 3 or higher, including four who were symptomatic and two (0.2%) died of hepatotoxicity. More women in the immediate group experienced hepatotoxicity than those in the deferred group. All of the events occurred during the postpartum period in participants receiving efavirenz-based antiretroviral treatment (ART) regimens.[233] If isoniazid treatment is started or continued during pregnancy or the postpartum period, women should be followed closely for signs, symptoms, and abnormalities in liver enzymes. The possible increased risk of isoniazid-associated hepatotoxicity must be weighed against the risk of developing tuberculosis disease as well as the subsequent consequences to both the mother and the baby.

In mothers who are continued on tuberculosis treatment following the delivery of the infant, questions arise regarding the safety of breastfeeding while the mother is receiving antituberculosis drugs. Snider and Powell showed that a breastfeeding infant would receive no more than 20% of the usual therapeutic dosage of isoniazid and less than 11% for other antituberculosis drugs.[234] Potential toxic effects of drugs delivered via breast milk have not been reported. However, because pyridoxine deficiency in the neonate can cause seizures, and breast milk contains relatively low levels of pyridoxine, the infant whose breastfeeding mother is taking isoniazid should receive supplemental pyridoxine. This is often administered in the form of an infant multi-vitamin.[235]

MANAGEMENT OF A MOTHER WITH A POSITIVE TEST FOR TUBERCULOSIS INFECTION

NEGATIVE CHEST RADIOGRAPH AND ASYMPTOMATIC

If the mother has a positive TST or IGRA, a negative chest radiograph, and is clinically well, no separation of the infant and the mother is needed after delivery. The child needs no special evaluation or treatment if the child remains asymptomatic. Because the mother's test of infection may be a signal that there is infectious tuberculosis within the household, all other household members and close contacts should undergo testing for tuberculosis infection and further evaluation as indicated. The mother is usually a candidate for therapy for tuberculosis infection.

ABNORMAL CHEST RADIOGRAPH

If the mother has suspected tuberculosis at the time of delivery (based on her tuberculosis risk factors, symptoms with or without a positive TST or IGRA), the newborn should be separated from the mother until the chest radiograph is obtained. If the mother's chest radiograph is abnormal, separation should be maintained until the mother has been evaluated thoroughly, including examination of her sputum. If possible, the placenta should be examined for evidence of granulomoatous inflammation and tissue specimens should be sent for acid fast smear and mycobacterial culture. If the mother's chest radiograph is abnormal but the history, physical examination, sputum examination, and evaluation of the radiograph show no evidence of current active tuberculosis, it is reasonable to assume that the infant is at low risk for infection. The radiographic abnormality may be due to another cause or a quiescent focus of past tuberculosis. If the mother remains untreated, she may develop active tuberculosis and expose her infant (who is at very high risk of a tuberculosis infection progressing to disease).[236] The untreated mother should receive appropriate treatment, and she and her infant should receive careful follow-up care. In addition, all other household members and close contacts should undergo testing for tuberculosis infection and further evaluation as indicated.

If the mother's chest radiograph, acid-fast sputum smear, or rapid molecular testing shows evidence of current tuberculosis disease, additional steps are necessary to protect the infant. Isoniazid therapy for newborns has been so effective that separation of the mother and the infant is no longer considered mandatory.[237,238] Separation should occur only if the mother is ill enough to require hospitalization, she has been or is expected to become nonadherent to treatment, or she has confirmed or suspected drug-resistant tuberculosis. As isoniazid resistance is increasing, it is not always clear if isoniazid therapy will be effective. If, due to epidemiologic factors, isoniazid resistance is suspected or the mother's adherence with medication is in question, rigorous separation of the infant from the mother must be considered. The duration of the separation will vary but must be as long as it takes to render the mother noninfectious. An expert in tuberculosis should be consulted if the young infant has potential exposure to the mother or another adult with tuberculosis disease caused by an isoniazid-resistant strain of *M. tuberculosis*. A conservative suggestion for the duration of separation would be 6–12 weeks of culture negativity for the mother. In cases when the organism is drug-susceptible, isoniazid should be continued in the infant at least until the mother is sputum culture negative for 3 months. At that time, a TST should be performed; if the test is positive, the infant should be evaluated for the presence of tuberculosis disease with a physical examination and chest radiograph and further evaluation for extrapulmonary sites of disease. If disease is absent, the infant should continue isoniazid for a total duration of 6–9 months. If the TST is negative, and the mother has good adherence and response to treatment, isoniazid can be discontinued.

REFERENCES

1. Marias BJ, Gie RP, Schaaf HS, Beyers N, Donald PR, and Starke JR. Childhood pulmonary tuberculosis: Old wisdom and new challenges. *Am J Respir Crit Care Med*. 2006;173:1078.

2. Perez-Velez CM, and Marais BJ. Tuberculosis in children. *N Engl J Med*. 2012;367:348.

3. Starke JR. New concepts in childhood tuberculosis. *Curr Opin Pediatr*. 2007;19:306.

4. Jaganath D et al. Contact investigations for active tuberculosis among child contacts in Uganda. *Clin Infect Dis*. 2013;57:1685.

5. Kimerling ME, Barker JT, Bruce F, Brook NL, and Dunlap NE. Preventable childhood tuberculosis in Alabama: Implications and opportunities. *Pediatrics*. 2000;105:E53.

6. Centers for Disease Control and Prevention. Guidelines for the investigation of contacts of persons with infectious tuberculosis. *Morb Mortal Wkly Rep (MMWR)*. 2005;55(RR15).

7. American Academy of Pediatrics. Tuberculosis. In: Kimberlin DW (ed.). Brady MT, Jackson MA, and Long SA (associate editors). *Red Book, 2018 Report of Committee on Infectious Diseases*. 31st ed. Elk Grove Village, IL: American Academy of Pediatrics, 2018.

8. Khan EA, and Starke JR. Diagnosis of tuberculosis in children: Increased need for better methods. *Emerging Infect Dis*. 1995;1.

9. World Health Organization. *Global Tuberculosis Report*. Geneva, Switzerland: World Health Organization, 2019.

10. Dodd PJ, Gardiner E, Coghlan R, and Seddon JA. Burden of childhood tuberculosis in 22 high-burden countries: A mathematical modeling study. *Lancet Glob Health*. 2014;2:e453.

11. Dodd PJ, Sismanidis C, and Seddon JA. Global burden of drug resistant tuberculosis in children: A mathematical modeling study. *Lancet Infect Dis*. 2016;16.

12. Murray CJ et al. Global, regional, and national incidence and mortality for HIV, tuberculosis and malaria during 1990–2013: A systematic analysis for the Global Burden of Disease Study. *Lancet*. 2013;384.

13. World Health Organization. *Roadmap towards Ending TB in Children and Adolescents*. Geneva, Switzerland: World Health Organization, 2019.

14. Seddon JA, and Shingadia D. Epidemiology and disease burden of tuberculosis in children: A global perspective. *Infect Drug Resist*. 2014;7.

15. Centers for Disease Control and Prevention. Tuberculosis—United States, 2018. *Morb Mortal Wkly Rep (MMWR)*. 2018;68(11):257.

16. Cowager TL, Wortham JM, and Burton DC. Epidemiology of tuberculosis among children and adolescents in the USA, 2007–17: An analysis of national surveillance data. *Lancet Public Health*. 2019;4:e5006–16.

17. Winston CA, and Menzies HJ. Pediatric and adolescent tuberculosis in the United States, 2008–2010. *Pediatrics*. 2012;130:6.

18. Centers for Disease Control and Prevention. Slide sets—Epidemiology of pediatric tuberculosis in the United States. 2017. Available at: https://www.cdc.gov/tb/publications/slidesets/pediatrictb/default.htm

19. Smith SE, Pratt R, Trieu L, Barry PM, Thai DT, Desai Ahuja S, and Shah S. Epidemiology of pediatric multidrug-resistant tuberculosis in the United States, 1993–2014. *Clin Infect Dis*. 2017;65.

20. Dangour Z, Izu A, Hillier K, Solomon F, Beylis N, Moore DP, Nunes MC, and Madhi SA. Impact of the antiretroviral treatment program on the burden of hospitalization for culture-confirmed tuberculosis in South African children: A time-series analysis. *Pediatr Infect Dis J*. 2013;32:972.

21. Venturini E, Turkova A, Chiappini E, Galli L, de Martino M, and Thorne N. Tuberculosis in HIV co-infection in children. *BMC Infect Dis J*. 2013;32:972.

22. Elenga N, Kouakoussui KA, Bonard D, Fassinou P, Anaky MF, Wemin ML, Dick-Amon-Tanoh F, Rouet F, Vincent V, and Msellati P. Diagnosed tuberculosis during the follow-up of a cohort of human-immunodeficiency virus-infected children in Abidjan, Côte d'Ivoire: ANRS 1278 study. *Pediatr Infect Dis J*. 2005;24:1077.

23. Braitstein P, Nyandiko W, Vreeman R, Wools-Kaloustian K, Sang E, Musick B, Sidle J, Yiannoutsos C, Ayaya S, and Carter EJ. The clinical burden of tuberculosis among human immunodeficiency virus-infected children in Western Kenya and the impact of combination antiretroviral treatment. *Pediatr Infect Dis J*. 2009;28:626.

24. Stop TB. Partnership Childhood TB Subgroup. Chapter 3: Management of TB in the HIV-infected child. *Int J Tuberc Lung Dis*. 2006;9:477.

25. Chintu C, Bhat G, Luo C, Raviglione M, Diwan V, Dupont HL, and Zumla A. Seroprevalence of human immunodeficiency virus type 1 infection in Zambian children with tuberculosis. *Pediatr Infect Dis J*. 1993;12:499.

26. Blussé van Oud-Alblas HJ, van Vliet ME, Kimpen JL, de Villiers GS, Schaaf HS, and Donald PR. Human immunodeficiency virus infection in children hospitalized with tuberculosis. *Ann Trop Paediatr*. 2002;22:115.

27. Pawlowski A, Jansson M, Sköld M, Rottenberg ME, and Källenius G. Tuberculosis and HIV Co-Infection. *PLoS Pathog*. 2012;8:2.

28. Geldmacher C, Zumla A, and Hoelscher M. Interaction between HIV and *Mycobacterium tuberculosis*: HIV-1 induced CD4 T-cell depletion and the development of active tuberculosis. *Curr Opin HIV AIDS*. 2012;73:3.

29. Lincoln EM. Epidemics of tuberculosis. *Bibliogr Tuberc*. 1965;21.

30. Muñoz FM, Ong LT, Seavy D, Medina D, Correa A, and Starke JR. Tuberculosis among adult visitors of children with suspected tuberculosis and employees at a children's hospital. *Infect Control Hosp Epidemiol*. 2002;32.

31. Marais BJ, Gie RP, Schaaf HS, Hesseling AC, Obihara CC, Starke JR, Enarson DA, Donald PR, and Beyers N. The natural history of childhood intra-thoracic tuberculosis—A critical review of the pre-chemotherapy literature. *Int J Tuberc Lung Dis*. 2004;8:392.

32. Wallgren A. On contagiousness of childhood tuberculosis. *Acta Paediatr*. 1937;22.

33. Curtis AB, Ridzon R, Vogel R, McDonough S, Hargreaves J, Ferry J, Valway S, and Onorato IM. Extensive transmission of *Mycobacterium tuberculosis* from a child. *N Engl J Med*. 1999;314.

34. Cruz AT, Medina D, Whaley EM, Ware KM, Koy TH, and Starke JR. Tuberculosis among families of children with suspected tuberculosis and employees at a children's hospital. *Infect Control Hosp Epidemiol*. 2002;23.

35. Ahn JG, Kim DS, and Kim KH. Nosocomial exposure to active pulmonary tuberculosis in a neonatal intensive care unit. *Am J Infect Control*. 2015;43.

36. Millership SE, Anderson C, Cummins AJ, Braecebridge S, and Abubakar I. The risk of infants from nosocomial exposure to tuberculosis. *Pediatr Infect Dis J*. 2009;28.

37. Weinstein JW, Barrett CR, Baltimore RS, and Hierholzer WJ Jr. Nosocomial transmission of tuberculosis from a hospital visitor on a pediatrics ward. *Pediatr Infect Dis J*. 1995;14.

38. Centers for Disease Control and Prevention. Guidelines for preventing the transmission of *Mycobacterium tuberculosis* in healthcare facilities. *Morb Mortal Wkly Rep (MMWR)*. 1994;43(RR-17).

39. Wallgren A. Primary pulmonary tuberculosis in childhood. *Am J Dis Child*. 1935;49:1105.

40. Wallgren A. Primary tuberculosis—Relation of childhood infection to disease in adults. *Lancet*. 1938;1:5973.

41. Wallgren A. The time-table of tuberculosis. *Tubercle*. 1948;29:245.

42. Marais BJ, Donald PR, Gie RP, Schaaf HS, and Beyers N. Diversity of disease manifestations in childhood pulmonary tuberculosis. *Ann Trop Paediatr*. 2005;25:79.

43. Marias BJ, and Schaaf HS. Tuberculosis in children. *Cold Spring Harb Perspect Med*. 4:a017855, 2014.

44. Miller FJW, Seal RME, and Taylor MD. *Tuberculosis in Children*. London: J. and A. Churchill, Ltd., 1963, 163, 466.

45. Jones C, Whittaker E, Bamford A, and Kampmann B. Immunology and pathogenesis of childhood TB. *Pediatr Respir Rev*. 2011;12.

46. Imperiali FG, Zaninoni A, La Maestra L, Tarsia P, Blasi F, and Barcellini W. Increased *Mycobacterium tuberculosis* growth in HIV-1-infected human macrophages: Role of tumour necrosis factor-α. *Clin Exp Immunol*. 2001;123:3.

47. Newton SM, Brent AJ, Anderson S, Whittaker E, and Kampmann B. Paediatric tuberculosis. *Lancet Infect Dis*. 2008;8.

48. Salazar GE et al. Working Group on TB in Peru. Pulmonary tuberculosis in children in a developing country. *Pediatrics*. 2001;108.

49. Hesseling AC, Schaaf HS, Gie RP, Starke JR, and Beyers NA. Critical review of diagnostic approaches used in the diagnosis of childhood tuberculosis. *Int J Tuberc Lung Dis*. 2002;6.

50. World Health Organization. *Systematic Screening for Active Tuberculosis. Principles and Recommendations*. Geneva, Switzerland: World Health Organization, 2013.

51. Marias BJ. Strategies to improve tuberculosis case finding in children. *Public Health Action*. 2015;5.

52. Eang MT, Satha P, Yadav RP, Morishita F, Nishikiori N, van-Maaren P, and Weezenbeek CL. Early detection of tuberculosis through community-based active case finding in Cambodia. *BCM Public Health*. 2012;12.

53. Joshi B, Chinnakali P, Shrestha A, Das M, Kumar AMV, Pant R, Lama R, Sarraf RR, Dumre SP, and Harries AD. Impact of intensified case finding strategies on childhood TB case registration in Nepal. *Public Health Action*. 2015;5.

54. Starke JR, and Taylor-Watts KT. Tuberculosis in the pediatric population of Houston, Texas. *Pediatrics*. 1989;84:28.

55. Daly JF, Brown DS, Lincoln EM, and Wilkins VN. Endobronchial tuberculosis in children. *Dis Chest*. 1952;22:380

56. Lorriman G, and Bentley FJ. The incidence of segmental lesions in primary tuberculosis of childhood. *Am Rev Tuberc*. 1959;79:756.

57. Morrison JB. Natural history of segmental lesions in primary pulmonary tuberculosis. *Arch Dis Child*. 1973;48:90.

58. Stansberry SD. Tuberculosis in infants and children. *J Thorac Imaging*. 1990;5:17.

59. Giammona ST, Poole CA, Zelowitz P, and Skrovan C. Massive lymphadenopathy in primary pulmonary tuberculosis in children. *Am Rev Resp Dis*. 1969;100:480.

60. Marias BJ, Gie RP, Schaaf HS, Starke JR, Hesseling AC, Donald PR, and Beyers N. A proposed radiological classification of childhood intrathoracic tuberculosis. *Pediatr Radiol*. 2004;34:886.

61. Lincoln EM, Gilbert L, and Morales SM. Chronic pulmonary tuberculosis in individuals with known previous primary tuberculosis. *Dis Chest*. 1960;38:473.

62. Lincoln EM, and Sewell EM. *Tuberculosis in Children*. New York: McGraw-Hill Book Company, 1963, 1.

63. Reider HL, Snider DE Jr, and Cauthen GM. Extrapulmonary tuberculosis in the United States. *Am Rev Resp Dis*. 1990;141:347.

64. Boyd GL. Tuberculous pericarditis in children. *Am J Dis Child*. 1953;86:293.

65. Schuitt KE. Miliary tuberculosis in children. Clinical and laboratory manifestations in 19 patients. *Am J Dis Child*. 133:583, 1979.

66. Hussey G, Chilsholm T, and Kibel M. Miliary tuberculosis in children: A review of 94 cases. *Pediatr Infect Dis J*. 1991;10:832.

67. Margileth AM, Chandra R, and Altman RP. Chronic lymphadenopathy due to mycobacterial infection. Clinical features, diagnosis, histopathology and management. *Am J Dis Child*. 1984;138:917.

68. Appling D, and Miller RH. Mycobacterial cervical lymphadenopathy: 1981 update. *Laryngoscope*. 1981;91:1259.

69. Rich AR, and McCordock HA. The pathogenesis of tuberculous meningitis. *Bull Johns Hopkins Hosp*. 1933;52:5.

70. Cotton MF, Donald PR, Schoeman JF, Aalbers C, VanZyl LE, and Lombard C. Plasma arginine vasopressin and the syndrome of inappropriate antidiuretic hormone secretion in tuberculous meningitis. *Pediatr Infect Dis J*. 1991;10:837.

71. Jaffe IP. Tuberculous meningitis in childhood. *Lancet*. 1982;1:738.

72. Waecker NJ Jr, and Conners JD. Central nervous system tuberculosis in children: A review of 30 cases. *Pediatr Infect Dis J*. 1990;9:539.

73. Doerr CA, Starke JR, and Ong LT. Clinical and public aspects of tuberculous meningitis in children. *J Pedaitr*. 1995;172(1).

74. Idriss ZH, Sinno A, and Kronfol NM. Tuberculous meningitis in childhood: 43 cases. *Am J Dis Child*. 1976;130:364.

75. Udani PM, Parkeh UC, and Dastur DK. Neurologic and related syndromes in CNS tuberculosis: Clinical features and pathogenesis. *J Neurol Sci*. 1971;14:341.

76. Zarabi M, Sane S, and Girdany BR. Chest roentgenogram in the early diagnosis of tuberculous meningitis in children. *Am J Dis Child*. 1971;121:389.

77. Andronikou S, Smith B, Hatherhill M, Douis H, and Wilmshurst J. Definitive neuroradiological diagnostic features of tuberculous meningitis in children. *Pediatr Radiol*. 2004;34.

78. Pienaar M, Andronikou S, and van Toorn R. MRI to demonstrate diagnostic features and complications of TBM not seen with CT. *ChNS*. 2009;25.

79. Janse van Rensburg P, Andronikou S, van Toorn R, and Pienaar M. Magnetic resonance imaging of miliary tuberculosis of the central nervous system in children with tuberculous meningitis. *Pediatr Radiol*. 2008;38.

80. van der Merwe DJ, Andronikou S, van Toorn R, and Pienaar M. Brainstem ischemic lesions on MRI in children with tuberculous meningitis: With diffusion weighted confirmation. *ChNS*. 2009;25.

81. Chambers ST, Hendrickse WA, Record C, Rudge P, and Smith H. Paradoxical expansion of intracranial tuberculomas during chemotherapy. *Lancet*. 1984;2:181.

82. Teoh R, Humphries MJ, and O'Mahony SG. Symptomatic intracranial tuberculoma developing during treatment of tuberculosis: A report of 10 patients and review of the literature. *Q J Med*. 1987;63:449.

83. van Toorn R, du Plessis AM, Schaaf HS, Buys H, Hewlett RH, and Schoeman JF. Clinicoradiologic response of neurologic tuberculous mass lesions in children treated with thalidomide. *Pediatr Infect Dis J*. 2015;34(2):214.

84. Janssens JP, and deHaller R. Spinal tuberculosis in a developed country. *Clin Ortho Rel Res*. 1990;257:67.

85. Bavadekar A. Osteoarticular tuberculosis in children. *Prog Pediatr Surg*. 1982;15:131.

86. Scheepers S, Andronikou S, and Mapukata A. Abdominal lymphadenopathy in children with tuberculosis presenting with respiratory symptoms. *Ultrasound*. 2011;19.

87. Shah I, and Uppuluri R. Clinical profile of abdominal tuberculosis in children. *Indian J Med Sci*. 2010;64.

88. Basu S, Ganguly S, Chandra PK, and Basu S. Clinical profile and outcome of abdominal tuberculosis in Indian children. *Singapore Med J*. 2007;48.

89. Dinler G, Şensory G, Helek D, and Kalayci AG. Tuberculous peritonitis in children: Report of nine patients and review of the literature. *World J Gastroenterol*. 2008;14.

90. Makharia GK et al. Clinical, endoscopic, and histological differentiations between Chron's disease and intestinal tuberculosis. *Am J Gastroenterol*. 2010;105:3.

91. De Backer AI, Mortelé KJ, Bomans P, De Keulenaer BL, Bourgeois SA, Kockx MM. Female genital tract tuberculosis with peritoneal involvement: CT and MR imaging features. *Eur J Radiol Extra*. 2005;53:71.

92. American Thoracic Society. Diagnostic standards and classification of tuberculosis. *Am Rev Resp Dis*. 1990;142:725.

93. Hsu KH. Tuberculin reaction in children treated with isoniazid. *Am J Dis Child*. 1983;137:1090.

94. Steiner P, Rao M, Victoria MS, Jabbar H, and Steiner M. Persistently negative tuberculin reactions: Their presence among children culture positive for *Mycobacterium tuberculosis*. *Am J Dis Child*. 1980;134:747.

95. Karalliedde S, Katugaha LP, and Uragoda CG. Tuberculin response of Sri Lankan children after BCG vaccination at birth. *Tubercle*. 1987;68(1):33.

96. Menzies R, and Viassandjee B. Effect of bacille Calmette-Guérin vaccination on tuberculin reactivity. *Am Rev Respir Dis*. 1992;145(3):621.

97. Menzies R, Vissandjee B, and Amyot D. Factors associated with tuberculin reactivity among the foreign-born in Montreal. *Am Rev Repir Dis*. 1992;146(3):752.

98. Mandalakas AM, Kirchner HL, Lombard C, Walzl G, Grewal HMS, Gie RP, and Hesseling AC. Well-quantified tuberculosis exposure is a reliable surrogate measure of tuberculosis infection. *Int J Tuberc Lung Dis*. 2012;16:1033.

99. Bianchi L, Galli L, Moriondo M, Veneruso G, Becciolini L, Azzari C, Chiappini E, and de Martino M. Interferon-gamma release assay improves the diagnosis of tuberculosis in children. *Pediatr Infect Dis J*. 2009;28:510.

100. Mazurek GH, Jereb J, Vernon A, LoBue P, Goldberg S, Gastro K, and IGRA Expert Committee. Centers for Disease Control and Prevention. Updated guidelines for using interferon gamma release assays to detect *Mycobacterium tuberculosis* infection in the United States—2010. *Morb Mortal Wkly Rep (MMWR)*. 2010;59:RR-5.

101. Detjen AK, Keil T, Roll S, Hauer B, Mauch H, Wahn U, and Magdorf K. Interferon-gamma release assays improve the diagnosis of tuberculosis and nontuberculous mycobacterial disease in children in a country with a low incidence of tuberculosis. *Clin Infect Dis*. 2007;45:322.

102. Machingaidze S, Wiysonge CS, Gonzales-Angulo Y, Hatherill M, Moyo S, Hanekom W, and Mahomed H. The utility of interferon gamma release assay for diagnosis of latent tuberculosis infection and disease in children: As systematic review and meta-analysis. *Pediatr Infect Dis J*. 2011;30:694.

103. Mandalakas AM, Detjen AK, Hesseling AC, Benedetti A, and Menzies D. Interferon-gamma release assays and childhood tuberculosis: Systematic review and meta-analysis. *Int J Tuberc Lung Dis*. 2011;15:1018.

104. Sun L et al. Interferon gamma release assay in diagnosis of pediatric tuberculosis: A meta-analysis. *FEMS Immunol Med Microbiol*. 2011;63:165.

105. Starke JR. Interferon-γ release assays for diagnosis of tuberculosis infection and disease in children. *Pediatrics*. 2014;134:e1763.

106. Kay AW, Islam SM, Wendorf K, Westenhouse J, and Barry PM. Interferon-γ release assay performance for tuberculosis in childhood. *Pediatrics*. 2018;141.

107. Grant LR, Hammitt LL, Murdoch DR, O'Brien KL, and Scott JA. Procedures for collection of induced sputum specimens from children. *Clin Infect Dis*. 2012;54(Suppl 2):S140.

108. Ruiz-Jiménez M, Guillén Martín S, Prieto Tato LM, Cacho Clavo JB, Álvarez García A, Soto Sánchez B, and Ramos Amador JT. Induced sputum versus gastric lavage for the diagnosis of pulmonary tuberculosis in children. *BMC Infect Dis*. 2013;13:222.

109. Cruz AT, Revell PA, and Starke JR. Gastric aspirate yield for children with suspected pulmonary tuberculosis. *J Pediatr Infect Dis Soc*. 2013;2:171.

110. Abadco DL, and Steiner P. Gastric lavage is better than bronchoalveolar lavage for isolation of *Mycobacterium tuberculosis* in childhood pulmonary tuberculosis. *Pediatr Infect Dis J*. 1992;11:735.

111. Delacourt C, Poveda JD, Chureau C, Beydon N, Mahut B, de Blic J, Scheinmann P, and Garrigue G. Use of polymerase chain reaction for improved diagnosis of tuberculosis in children. *J Pediatr*. 1995;126:703.

112. Gomez-Pastrana D, Torronteras R, Caro P, Anguita ML, López-Barrio AM, Andres A, and Navarro J. Comparison of amplicor, in-house polymerase chain reaction, and conventional culture for the diagnosis of tuberculosis in children. *Clin Infect Dis*. 2001;32:17.

113. Pierre C, Olivier C, Lecossier D, Boussougant Y, Yeni P, and Hance AJ. Diagnosis of primary tuberculosis in children by amplification and detection of mycobacterial DNA. *Am Rev Respir Dis*. 1993;147:420.

114. Smith KC, Starke JR, Eisenach K, Ong LT, and Denby M. Detection of *Mycobacterium tuberculosis* in clinical specimens from children using polymerase chain reaction. *Pediatrics*. 1996;97:155.

115. Detjen AK, DiNardo AR, Leyden J, Steingart KR, Menzies D, Schiller I, Dendukuri N, and Mnadalakas AM. Xpert MTB/RIF assay for the diagnosis of pulmonary tuberculosis in children: A systematic review and meta-analysis. *Lancet Respir Med*. 2015;3:415.

116. Zar HJ, Workman LJ, Prins M, Bateman LJ, Mbhele SP, Whitman CB, Denkinger CM, and Nicol MP. Tuberculosis diagnosis in children using Xpert Ultra on different respiratory specimens. *Am J Respir Crit Care Med*. 2019;200(12):1531.

117. Denkinger CM, Schumacher SG, Boehme CC, Dendukuri N, Pai M, and Steingart KR. Xpert MTB/RIF assay for the diagnosis of extrapulmonary tuberculosis: A systematic review and meta-analysis. *Eur Respir J*. 2014;44:435.

118. Anderson ST et al. Diagnosis of childhood tuberculosis and host RNA expression in Africa. *N Engl J Med*. 2014;370:1712–1723.

119. Brown AC et al. Rapid whole-genome sequencing of *Mycobacterium tuberculosis* isolates directly from clinical samples. *J Clin Microboiol*. 2015;53(7):2230.

120. Starke JR. Multidrug therapy for tuberculosis in children. *Pediatr Infect Dis J*. 1990;9:785.

121. Reed MD, and Blumber JL. Clinical pharmacology of antitubercular drugs. *Pediatr Clin North Am*. 1983;30:177.

122. Stein MT, and Liang D. Clinical hepatotoxicity of isoniazid in children. *Pediatrics*. 1979;64:499.

123. O'Brien RJ, Long MW, Cross FS, Lyle MA, and Snider DE Jr. Hepatotoxicity from isoniazid and rifampin among children treated for tuberculosis. *Pediatrics*. 1983;72:491.

124. Olson WA, Pruitt AW, and Dayton PG. Plasma concentrations of isoniazid in children with tuberculosis infections. *Pediatrics*. 1981;67:876.

125. Notterman DA, Nardi M, and Saslow JG. Effect of dose formulation on isoniazid absorption in two young children. *Pediatrics.* 1986;77:850.

126. McIllleron H, Willemse M, Werely CJ, Hussey GD, Schaaf HS, Smith PJ, and Donald PR. Isoniazid plasma concentrations in a cohort of South African children with tuberculosis: Implications for international dosing guidelines. *Clin Infect Dis.* 2009;48:1547.

127. Thee S, Seddon JA, Donald PR, Seifart HI, Werely CJ, Hesseling AC, Rosenkranz B, Roll S, Magdorf K, and Schaaf HS. Pharmacokinetics of isoniazid, rifampin, and pyrazinamide in children younger than two years of age with tuberculosis: Evidence for implementation of revised World Health Organization recommendations. *Antimicrob Agents Chemother.* 2011;55:5560.

128. World Health Organization. *New Fixed-Dose Combinations for the Treatment of TB in Children.* Geneva, Switzerland. 2016. Available at: http://www.who.int/tb/FDC_Factsheet.pdf

129. Cruz AT, Ahmed A, Mandalakas AM, and Starke JR. Treatment of latent tuberculosis infection in children. *J Pediatr Infect Dis Soc.* 2013;2:2248.

130. Cruz AT, and Starke JR. Safety and adherence for 12 weekly doses of isoniazid and rifapentine for pediatric tuberculosis infection. *Pediatr Infect Dis J.* 2016;35:811.

131. Cruz AT, and Starke JR. Increasing adherence for latent tuberculosis infection therapy with health department-administered therapy. *Pediatr Infect Dis J.* 2012;31:193.

132. Martinez-Roig A, Roig A, Cami J, Llorens-Terol. J, de la Torre R, and Perich F. Acetylation phenotype and hepatotoxicity in the treatment of tuberculosis in children. *Pediatrics.* 1986;77:912.

133. Pellock JM, Howell J, Kendig EL Jr, and Baker H. Pyridoxine deficiency in children treated with isoniazid. *Chest.* 1985;87:658.

134. Litt IF, Cohen MI, and McNamara H. Isoniazid hepatitis in adolescents. *J Pediatr.* 1976;89:133.

135. Seddon JA et al. High treatment success in children treated for multi-drug resistant tuberculosis: An observational cohort study. *Thorax.* 2003;69:5.

136. Forsythe CT, and Ernst ME. Do fluoroquinolones commonly cause arthropathy in children? *CJEM.* 2007;9(6):459–62.

137. Burkhardt JE, Walterspiel JN, and Schaad UB. Quinolone arthropathy in animals versus children. *Clin Infect Dis.* 1997;25:5.

138. Yee CL, Diffy C, Gerbino PG, Stryker S, and Noel GJ. Tendon or joint disorders in children after treatment with fluoroquinolones or azithromycin. *Pediatr Infect Dis J.* 2002;21:6.

139. Kumar L, Dhand R, Singhi PD, Rao KL, and Katariaya S. A randomized trial of fully intermittent vs. daily followed by intermittent short course chemotherapy for childhood tuberculosis. *Pedaitr Infect Dis J.* 1990;9:802.

140. Te Water Naude JM, Donald PR, Hussey GD, Kibel MA, Louw A, Perkins DR, and Schaaf HS. Twice weekly vs. daily chemotherapy for childhood tuberculosis. *Pediatr Infect Dis J.* 2000;19:405.

141. Donald PR, Maher D, Martiz JS, and Qazi S. Ethambutol dosage for the treatment of children: Literature review and recommendations. *Int J Tuberc Lung Dis.* 2006;10:1381.

142. Agarwal A, Khan SA, and Qureshi NA. Multifocal osteoarticular tuberculosis in children. *J Orthop Surg, (Hong Kong).* 2011;19:336.

143. Visudhiphan P, and Chiemchanya S. Tuberculous meningitis in children: Treatment with isoniazid and rifampicin for twelve months. *J Pediatr.* 1989;114:875.

144. van Well GTJ, Paes BF, Terwee CB, Springer P, Rood JJ, Donald PR, van Furth AM, Schoeman JF. Twenty years of pediatric tuberculosis meningitis: A retrospective cohort study in the western cape of South Africa. *Pediatrics.* 2009;123.

145. Li H, Lu J, Liu J, Zhao Y, Ni X, and Zhao S. Linezolid is associated with improved early outcomes of childhood tuberculous meningitis. *Pediatr Infect Dis J.* 2016;35.

146. Twaites GE, van Toorn R, and Schoeman J. Tuberculous meningitis: More questions, still too few answers. *Lancet Neurol.* 2013;12.

147. Schoeman JF, Van Zyl LE, Laubscher JA, and Donald PR. Effect of corticosteroids on intracranial pressure, computed tomographic findings, and clinical outcome in young children with tuberculous meningitis. *Pediatrics.* 1997;99.

148. Schoeman JF, Andronikou S, and Sefan DC. Tuberculous meningitis-related optic neuritis recovery of vision with thalidomide in 4 consecutive cases. *J Child Neurol.* 2010;25:822.

149. Jawahar MS, Sivasubramanian S, Vijayan VK, Ramakrishnan CV, Paramasivan CN, Selvakumar V, Paul S, Tripathy SP, and Prabhakar R. Short-course chemotherapy for tuberculous lymphadenitis in children. *Br Med J.* 1990;201:359.

150. United States Department of Health and Human Services. AIDSinfo. Guidelines for the prevention and treatment of opportunistic infections in HIV-exposed and HIV-infected children. 2019. Available at: https://aidsinfo.nih.gov/guidelines/html/5/pediatric-opportunistic-infection/414/mycobacterium-tuberculosis

151. Martinson NA et al. HAART and risk of tuberculosis in HIV-infected South African children: A multi-site retrospective cohort. *Int J Tuberc Lung Dis.* 2009;13:862–7.

152. Zampoli M, Kilborn T, and Eley B. Tuberculosis during early antiretroviral-induced immune reconstitution in HIV-infected children. *Int J Tuberc Lung Dis.* Apr 2007;11(4):417–23. Available at: http://www.ncbi.nlm.nih.gov/pubmed/17394688.

153. Lawn SD, Wilkinson RJ, Lipman MC, and Wood R. Immune reconstitution and "unmasking" of tuberculosis during antiretroviral therapy. *Am J Respir Crit Care Med.* Apr 1 2008;177(7):680–5. Available at: http://www.ncbi.nlm.nih.gov/pubmed/18202347.

154. Meintjes G et al. Tuberculosis-associated immune reconstitution inflammatory syndrome: Case definitions for use in resource-limited settings. *Lancet Infect Dis.* 2008;8:8.

155. Puthanakit T, Oberdorfer P, Akarathum N, Wannarit P, Sirisanthana T, and Sirisanthana V. Immune reconstitution syndrome after highly active antiretroviral therapy in human immunodeficiency virus-infected Thai children. *Pediatr Infect Dis J.* 2006;25:53.

156. Hesseling AC et al. Bacille Calmette-Guérin vaccine-induced disease in HIV-infected and HIV-uninfected children. *Clin Infect Dis.* 2006;42:548.

157. Puthanakit T, Oberdorfer P, Punjaisee S, Wannarit P, Sirisanthana T, and Sirisanthana V. Immune reconstitution syndrome due to bacillus Calmette-Guerin after initiation of antiretroviral therapy in children with HIV infection. *Clin Infect Dis.* Oct 1 2005;41(7):1049–52. Available at: http://www.ncbi.nlm.nih.gov/pubmed/16142674.

158. Hesseling AC, Cotton MF, Fordham von Reyn C, Graham SM, Gie RP, and Hussey GD. Consensus statement on the revised World Health Organization recommendations for BCG vaccination in HIV-infected infants. *Int J Tuberc Lung Dis.* 2008;12:1376.

159. Barnes PF, Bloch AB, Davidson PT, Snider DE Jr. Tuberculosis in patients with human immunodeficiency virus infection. *N Engl J Med.* 1991;324:1644.

160. Steiner P, Rao M, Victoria MS, Hunt J, and Steiner M. A continuing study of primary drug-resistant tuberculosis among children observed at Kings County Hospital Medical Center between the years 1961–1980. *Am Rev Resp Dis.* 1983;128:425.

161. Steiner P, Rao M, Mitchell M, and Steiner M. Primary drug-resistant tuberculosis in children. Correlation of drug-susceptibility patterns in matched patient and source case strains of *Mycobacterium tuberculosis*. *Am J Dis Child*. 1985;139:780.

162. Steiner P, and Rao M. Drug-resistant tuberculosis in children. *Semin Pediatr Infect Dis*. 1993;4:275.

163. Swanson DS, and Starke JR. Drug-resistant tuberculosis in pediatrics. *Pediatr Clin North Am*. 1995;42:553.

164. Partners in Health. *The PIH Guide to the Medical Management of Multidrug-Resistant Tuberculosis*. 2nd ed. *Partners in Health*. Boston, USA: USAID TB Care II, 2013. Available at: https://www.pih.org/sites/default/files/2017-07/PIH%2520Guide%2520Medical%2520Management%2520of%2520MDR-TB%25202013.pdf.

165. *Management of Drug-Resistant Tuberculosis in Children: A Field Guide*. 2nd ed. Boston, USA: The Sentinel Project for Pediatric Drug-Resistant Tuberculosis, 2015. Available at: http://sentinel-project.org/wp-content/uploads/2015/03/Field_Handbook_2nd_Ed_revised-no-logos_03022015.pdf

166. World Health Organization. *WHO Treatment Guidelines for Drug-Resistant Tuberculosis, 2016 update*. Geneva, Switzerland. Available at: http://apps.who.int/iris/bitstream/10665/250125/1/9789241549639-eng.pdf

167. D'Ambrosio L, Centis R, Sotgiu G, Pontali E, Spanevello A, and Migliori GB. New anti-tuberculosis drugs and regimens: 2015 update. *ERJ Open Res*. 2015;1:00010.

168. Harausz EP et al. Sentinel Project on Pediatric Drug-Resistant Tuberculosis. New and repurposed drugs for pediatric multi-drug resistant tuberculosis, practice-based recommendations. *Am J Respir Crit Care Med*. 2017;195:10.

169. The Sentinel Project on Pediatric Drug-Resistant Tuberculosis. *Rapid Clinical Advice: The Use of Delamanid and Bedaquiline for Children with Drug Resistant Tuberculosis*. Boston, USA: The Sentinel Project on Pediatric Drug-Resistant Tuberculosis. Available at: http://sentinel-project.org/wp-content/uploads/2016/05/Rapid-Clinical-Advice_May-16-2016.pdf.

170. Tadolini M et al. Compassionate use of new drugs in children and adolescents with multidrug-resistant tuberculosis; early experiences and challenges. *Eur Respir J*. 2016;48:938.

171. Garcia-Prats AJ, Svensson EM, Weld ED, Schaaf HS, and Hesseling AC. Current status of pharmacokinetic and safety studies of multidrug resistant tuberculosis treatment in children. *Int J Tuberc Lung Dis*. 2018;22(5).

172. Girgis NI, Farid Z, Kilpatrick ME, Sulatn Y, and Mikahail IA. Dexamethasone adjunctive treatment for tuberculous meningitis. *Pediatr Infect Dis*. 1991;10:179.

173. Nemir RL, Cordova J, Vaziri F, and Toledo F. Prednisone as an adjunct in the chemotherapy of lymph node-bronchial tuberculosis in childhood: A double-blinded study. II. Further term observation. *Am Rev Resp Dis*. 1967;95:402.

174. Toppet M, Malfroot A, Derde MP, Toppet V, Spehl M, and Dab I. Corticosteroids in primary tuberculosis with bronchial obstruction. *Arch Dis Child*. 1990;65:1222.

175. Strang JIG, Kakaza HHS, Gibson DG, Allen BW, Mitchinson DA, Evans DJ, Girling DJ, Nunn AJ, and Fox W. Controlled clinical trial of complete open surgical drainage and prednisolone in treatment of tuberculous pericardial effusion in Transkei. *Lancet*. 1988;2:759.

176. Smith MHD, and Matasaniotis N. Treatment of tuberculous pleural effusions with particular reference to adrenal corticosteroids. *Pediatrics*. 1958;22:1074.

177. Hsu KHK. Thirty years after isoniazid. Its impact on tuberculosis in children and adolescents. *J Am Med Assoc*. 1984;251:1283.

178. Cruz AT, Ahmed A, Mandalakas AM, and Starke JR. Treatment of latent tuberculosis infection in children. *J Pediatr Infect Dis Soc*. 2013;2:2248.

179. Pediatric Tuberculosis Collaborative Group. Diagnosis and treatment of latent tuberculosis infection in children and adolescents. *Pediatrics*. 2004;114:1175.

180. Spyridis NP, Spyridis PG, Gelemse A, Sypsa V, Valianatou M, Metsou F, Gourgiotis D, and Tsolia MN. The effectiveness of a 9-month regimen of isoniazid alone versus 3- and 4-month regimens of isoniazid plus rifampin for treatment of latent tuberculosis infection in children: Results of an 11-year randomized study. *Clin Infect Dis*. 2007;45:715.

181. Diallo T et al. Safety and side effects of rifampin versus isoniazid in children. *New Engl J Med*. 2018;379(5):454.

182. Cruz AT, and Starke JR. Safety and completion of a 4-month course of rifampicin for latent tuberculosis infection in children. *Int J Tuberc Lung Dis*. 2014;18(9):1057–61.

183. Cruz AT, and Starke JR. Completion rate and safety of tuberculosis infection treatment with shorter regimens. *Pediatrics*. 2018;141(2):e20172838.

184. Villarino ME, Rizdon R, Weismuller PC, Elcock M, Maxwell RM, Meador J, Smith PJ, Carson MJ, and Geiter LJ. Rifampin preventive therapy for tuberculosis infection: Experience with 157 adolescents. *Am J Respir Crit Care Med*. 1997;155:1735–8.

185. Villarino ME et al. Treatment for preventing tuberculosis in children and adolescents: A randomized clinical trial of a 3-month, 12-dose regimen of a combination of rifapentine and isoniazid. *JAMA Pedaitr*. 2015;169:247.

186. Starke JR, and Donald PR. (eds).*Handbook of Child & Adolescent Tuberculosis*. Oxford University Press, New York, NY, 2016.

187. Lanciella L et al. How to manage children who have come into contact with patients affected by tuberculosis. *J Clin Tuberc Other Mycobact Dis*. 2015;1:1.

188. Snider DE Jr. Pregnancy and pulmonary tuberculosis. *Chest*. 1984;86:11.

189. Starke JR. Pediatric tuberculosis: A time for a new approach. *Tuberculosis*. 2002;82:208.

190. Schaefer G, Zervoudakis IA, and Fuchs FF. Pregnancy and pulmonary tuberculosis. *Obstet Gynecol*. 1975;46:706.

191. Bazaz-Malik G, Maheshwari B, and Lal N. Tuberculous endometritis: A clinicopathologic study of 1000 cases. *Br J Obstet Gynaecol*. 1983;90:84.

192. Nezar M, Goda H, and El-Negery M. Genital tract tuberculosis among infertile women: An old problem revisited. *Arch Gynecol Obstet*. 2009;280.

193. Hallum JL, and Thomas HE. Full term pregnancy after proved endometrial tuberculosis. *J Obstet Gynaecol Br Emp*. 1955; 62:548.

194. Kaplan C, Benirschke K, and Tarzy B. Placental tuberculosis in early and late pregnancy. *Am J Obstet Gynecol*. 1980;137:858.

195. Ceneno RS, Winter J, and Bentson JR. Central nervous system tuberculosis related to pregnancy. *J Comput Tomogr*. 1982;6:141.

196. Grenville-Mathers R, Harris WC, and Trenchard HJ. Tuberculous primary infection in pregnancy and its relation to congenital tuberculosis. *Tubercle*. 1960;41:181.

197. Hageman J, Shulman S, and Schreiber M. Congenital tuberculosis: Critical reappraisal of clinical findings and diagnostic procedures. *Pediatrics*. 1980;66:980.

198. Nemir RL, and O'Hare D. Congenital tuberculosis. *Am J Dis Child*. 1985;139:284.

199. Hertzog AJ, Chapman S, and Herring J. Congenital primary aspiration-tuberculosis. *Am J Clin Pathol*. 1940;19:1139.

200. Hughesdon MR. Congenital tuberculosis. *Arch Dis Child.* 1946;21:131.

201. Jacobs RF, and Abernathy RS. Management of tuberculosis in pregnancy and the newborn. *Clin Perinatol.* 1988;15:305.

202. Siegel M. Pathologic findings and pathogenesis of congenital tuberculosis. *Am Rev Tuberc.* 1934;29:297.

203. Sugarman J, Colvin C, Moran AC, and Oxalde O. Tuberculosis in pregnancy: An estimate of the global burden of disease. *Lancet Glob Health.* 2014;2:e710.

204. Grisolle A. De l'influence que la grossesse et la phthisie pulmonary excercetn reciproquement l'une sur l'autre. *Arch Gener Med.* 1850;22:41.

205. Cohen RC. Effects of pregnancy on partuition on pulmonary tuberculosis. *Br Med J.* 1943;2:775.

206. Hedvall E. Pregnancy in tuberculosis. *Acta Med Scand.* 1953;147(Suppl. 286).

207. Crombie RC. Pregnancy and pulmonary tuberculosis. *Br J Tuberc.* 1954;48:97.

208. Cohen JD, Patton EA, and Badger TL. The tuberculous mother. *Am Rev Resp Dis.* 1952;65:1.

209. Edge JR. Pulmonary tuberculosis and pregnancy. *Br Med J.* 1952;2:845.

210. De March P. Tuberculosis and pregnancy. *Chest.* 1975;68:800.

211. Bjerkedal T, Bahna SL, and Lehmann EH. Course and outcome of pregnancy in women with pulmonary tuberculosis. *Scand J Resp Dis.* 1975;56:245.

212. Ratner B, Rostler AE, and Salgado PS. Care, feeding and fate of premature and full term infants born of tuberculous mothers. *Am J Dis Child.* 1951;81:471.

213. Knight M, Kurinczuk JJ, Nelson-Piercy C, Spark P, Brocklehurst P, and on behalf of UKOSS. Tuberculosis in pregnancy in the U.K. *BJOC.* 2009;116.

214. Llewelyn M, Cropley I, Wilkinson RJ, and Davidson RN. Tuberculosis diagnosed during pregnancy: A prospective study from London. *Thorax.* 2000;55:2.

215. Good JT Jr, Iseman MD, and Davidson PT. Tuberculosis in association with pregnancy. *Am J Obstet Gynecol.* 1981;140:492.

216. Wilson EA, Thelin TJ, and Dilts PV. Tuberculosis complicated by pregnancy. *Am J Obstet Gynecol.* 1972;115:526.

217. Lowe CR. Congenital defects among children born to women under supervision or treatment for tuberculosis. *Br J Prev Soc Med.* 1964;18:14.

218. Cziezel AE, Rockenbauer M, Olsen J, and Sørensen HT. A population-based case-control study of the safety of oral anti-tuberculosis drug treatment during pregnancy. *Int J Tuberc Lung Dis.* 2001;5:564.

219. Snider DE Jr, Layde PM, Johnson MW, and Lyle MA. Treatment of tuberculosis during pregnancy. *Am Rev Respir Dis.* 1980;122(1):65.

220. Atkins JN. Maternal plasma concentrations of pyridoxal phosphate during pregnancy; adequacy of vitamin B_6 supplementation during isoniazid therapy. *Am Rev Resp Dis.* 1982;126:714.

221. Lewit T, Nebel L, and Terrancina S. Ethambutol in pregnancy: Observations on embryogenesis. *Chest.* 1974;68:25.

222. Robinson GC, and Cambon KG. Hearing loss in infants of tuberculous mothers treated with streptomycin during pregnancy. *N Engl J Med.* 1964;271:949.

223. Shin S et al. Treatment of multidrug-resistant tuberculosis during pregnancy: A report of 7 cases. *Clin Infect Dis.* 2003;36:996.

224. Drobac PC, del Castillo H, Sweetland A, Anca G, Joseph JK, Furin J, and Shin S. Treatment of multidrug-resistant tuberculosis during pregnancy: Long-term follow-up of 6 children with intrauterine exposure to second-line agents. *Clin Infect Dis.* 2005;40(11):1689.

225. Nhan-Chang CL, and Jones TB. Tuberculosis in pregnancy. *Clin Obst Gyn.* 2010;53:2.

226. Hageman J, Shulman S, and Schreiber M. Congenital tuberculosis: Critical reappraisal of clinical findings and diagnostic procedures. *Pedaitrics.* 1980;66:980.

227. Nemir RL, and O'Hare D. Congenital tuberculosis. *Am J Dis Child.* 1985;139:284.

228. World Health Organization. *WHO recommendation on tuberculosis testing in pregnancy.* Geneva, Switzerland. 2018. Available at: http://apps.who.int/iris/bitstream/handle/10665/259947/WHO-RHR-18.02-eng.pdf?sequence=1

229. Centers for Disease Control and Prevention. *Targeted testing and treatment of women at high risk for tuberculosis.* Atlanta, GA. 2018. Available at: https://www.cdc.gov/nchhstp/pregnancy/screening/tb-testing.html

230. Vallejo JG, and Starke JR. Tuberculosis and pregnancy. *Clin Chest Med.* 1992;13:693.

231. Franks AL, Binkin NJ, and Snider DE Jr. Isoniazid hepatitis among pregnant and postpartum Hispanic patients. *Public Health Rep.* 1989;104:151.

232. Snider DE Jr, and Caras GJ. Isoniazid associated hepatitis deaths: A review of available information. *Am Rev Resp Dis.* 1992;145:494.

233. Gupta A et al. Isoniazid preventive therapy in HIV-infected pregnant and postpartum women. *New Engl J Med.* 2019;381:14.

234. Snider DE Jr, and Powel KE. Should mothers taking antituberculosis drugs breast-feed? *Arch Intern Med.* 1984;144:589.

235. McKenzie SA, Macnab AJ, and Katz G. Neonatal pyridoxine responsive convulsions due to isoniazid therapy. *Arch Dis Child.* 1976;51:567.

236. Kendig EL, and Rogers WL. Tuberculosis in the neonatal period. *Am Reve Tuberc.* 1958;77:418.

237. Dormer BA, Swarit JA, and Harrison I. Prophylactic isoniazid protection of infants in a tuberculosis hospital. *Lancet.* 1959;2:902.

238. Light IJ, Saidelman M, and Sutherland JM. Management of newborns after nursery exposure to tuberculosis. *Am Rev Resp Dis.* 1974;109:415.

Treatment of Latent Tuberculosis Infection Including Risk Factors for the Development of Tuberculosis

MARTIN DEDICOAT

SCREENING

A quarter of the world's population may be infected with tuberculosis (TB).[1] In the majority of these people the infection will remain dormant. A variety of risk factors may lead to this latent TB infection (LTBI) becoming active. Treatment of LTBI has been shown to reduce the risk of developing active TB.[2]

One of the pillars of the "WHO End TB Strategy" includes the identification of people who have LTBI and who would benefit from preventive therapy.[3] In order to achieve global TB eradication the vast pool of individuals with LTBI need to be identified and offered effective treatment to prevent progression to active infectious TB.

It is not possible to test and treat everyone for LTBI and the risk of infection is low in many groups of people, as is the risk of progression of LTBI to active TB in many cases, so targeted testing is recommended by the National Institute of Clinical Excellence (NICE),[4] Centers for Disease Control and Prevention (CDC),[5] and the World Health Organization (WHO).[3-5] Individuals at increased risk of LTBI and increased risk of progression to active TB are detailed in this chapter. In all cases, when treatment for LTBI is being considered, a careful clinical evaluation including a chest radiograph should be undertaken to exclude active TB. Rules have been developed for HIV infected and uninfected patients to exclude active TB. The absence of TB symptoms such as cough, fever, night sweats, hemoptysis, weight loss, chest pain, shortness of breath, or fatigue, as well as lack of chest radiograph abnormalities, had the highest sensitivity and best negative predictive value to exclude TB. Presence of any TB symptom followed by chest radiograph had 99.8% negative predictive value to exclude active TB.[6-8]

INTERPRETATION

Both the tuberculin skin test (TST) and interferon gamma release assays (IGRA) can indicate infection with *Mycobacterium tuberculosis* (MTB). Both tests, when positive, have been shown to be associated with an increased risk of developing active TB.[9,10] For the purpose of this chapter, a TST>5 mm or a positive TB IGRA test will be considered to indicate infection with MTB. The rest of this chapter focuses on who to screen for LTBI, who is most at risk of progression to active TB, and how to treat LTBI.

TREATMENT OF LATENT TB

Good evidence exists for the efficacy of treating LTBI in preventing individuals from progressing to active disease. The number of bacteria present in a person with TB in the latent state is several orders of magnitude lower than in people with active TB, therefore the use of single agents and shorter than 6-month courses of treatment have been shown to be effective. WHO recommends four possible regimens for LTBI treatment—6–9 months of daily isoniazid (INH) monotherapy, 4 months of daily rifampicin (RIF) monotherapy, 3 months of daily RIF and INH, and 12 weekly doses of rifapentine (RPT) with INH. The evidence for each regimen, which is variable, is summarized in the following sections and in Tables 19.1 and 19.2.

Table 19.1 Recommended groups for latent TB screening

Risk factor	WHO	CDC	NICE
Close contacts	Yes	Yes	Yes
HIV infection	Yes	Yes	Yes
Dialysis	Yes	Yes	Yes
Chronic renal disease	No	Yes	Yes
Anti-TNF drugs	Yes	Yes	Yes
Silicosis	Yes	Yes	Yes
Fibrosis/old TB on chest x-ray	No	Yes	No
Pre-organ transplant	Yes	Yes	Yes
Haematological malignancy	No	No	Yes
Head and neck cancer	No	Yes	No
Patients receiving chemotherapy	No	No	Yes
Jejunal bypass or gastrectomy	No	Yes	Yes
New entrants from high TB incidence countries	Yes	Yes	Yes
Health-care workers	Yes	Yes	Yes
Underserved population[a]	Yes	Yes	Yes
Diabetes	No	Yes	Yes
Smoking	No	No	No
Excessive alcohol	No	No	Yes
Steroids	No	Yes	No
Underweight	No	Yes	No

[a] IVDU, prisoners, homeless, and nursing home residents.

MEDICATION

Medications used to treat latent TB and doses are presented in Table 19.1. Details of the mechanism of action of these drugs and their common adverse effects are covered in Chapter 10. Regimens recommended by WHO, CDC, and NICE[4–6] will be discussed in the following section, specifically INH monotherapy, RIF monotherapy, RIF and INH in combination, and RPT and INH in combination. RIF and pyrazinamide (PZA) in combination is also discussed but is no longer recommended.

INH MONOTHERAPY

INH was the first agent to be shown to be effective in preventing LTBI from progressing to active TB in a number of large studies.[11] Details of some of the studies for specific risk groups such as patients with fibrotic lesions and HIV infection are outlined here.

WHO and NICE recommend 6 months of daily INH for LTBI. The WHO and CDC also recommend 9 months of daily INH with 6 months as an alternative, including twice weekly directly observed options. WHO recommendations are based on evidence from recent systematic reviews among HIV infected patients showing reduced TB incidence with INH monotherapy in patients with a positive TST.[12] The odds ratio for the prevention of active TB by INH compared to placebo was: for 6 months of INH, OR 0.65 (95% CI 0.5–0.83); for 9 months of INH, OR 0.75 (95% CI 0.35–1.62); and for 12–72 months of INH, OR 0.5 (95% CI 0.41–0.62).[13] A 9-month INH regimen is recommended based on reanalysis of data from trials of 6–24 months of INH treatment; the ideal treatment duration beyond which the protective effect did not increase much but cost and toxicity became less favorable was 9 months.[14]

Table 19.2 WHO recommended regimens for treating latent TB infection in adults

Regimen	Dose, frequency, and duration	Notes	Evidence
Isoniazid	Adults 5 mg/kg (max 300 mg) daily for 6–9 months—with pyridoxine Children 10 mg/kg	CDC and NICE recommended 9 months of daily CDC preferred regimen for 　1. HIV infected 　2. Children 2–11 　3. Pregnancy	
Isoniazid		Twice weekly for 9 months recommended for pregnancy—directly observed	
RIF	Adults and children 10 mg/kg (max 600 mg) daily for 4 months	CDC and NICE recommended	
RIF and INH	Adults and children—RIF 10 mg/kg (600 mg max) Adults INH5 mg/kg (300 mg max) Children 10 mg/kg With pyridoxine	Usually given as a combination preparation, e.g., Rifinah 300/150 NICE recommended	
RPT and INH	Weekly directly observed dose—for 3 months (12 doses) RPT Weight 10–14 kg 300 mg weekly 14.1–25 kg 450 mg weekly 25.1–32 kg 600 mg weekly 32.1–50 kg 750 mg weeky >50 kg 900 mg weekly INH15 mg/kg max 900 mg weekly—with pyridoxine 50 mg	CDC recommended for children aged over 2 years Not recommended for 1. Pregnancy 2. If RIF/INH resistance suspected	

The duration of protection after taking INH chemoprophylaxis is variable and probably depends on a number of factors including the background TB prevalence of the setting being studied and the vulnerability of the people exposed. Comstock reported that the protective effect of INH exceeded 19 years among the Inuit in Alaska.[15] In contrast, a study of South African miners found protection only lasted a couple of years, possibly due to the high TB incidence in this setting.[16]

INH prophylaxis has been shown to be efficacious in preventing TB in children. Meta-analyses of eight studies including 10,320 children aged under 15 years found a pooled risk ratio (RR) of 0.65 (95% CI 0.47–0.98). In this review, primary prophylaxis was not found to be protective, RR 0.93 (95% CI 0.71–1.21).[17]

The main adverse effects of INH are hepatotoxicity and peripheral neuropathy. An open label study comparing 4 months of RIF to 9 months of INH found 14% had to discontinue therapy in the INH group compared to 3% in the RIF group; drug-induced hepatitis was only seen in the INH group.[18] An analysis of studies comparing 6, 9, and 12 months of INH compared to 4 months of RIF or 3 months of RIF/INH found higher hepatotoxicity in the INH-only regimens compared to the others.[13] Patients with pre-existing liver disease or at high risk of hepatoxicity such as heavy alcohol drinkers should be carefully monitored when taking INH or should be offered a less hepatotoxic regimen. NICE guidelines recommend pyridoxine be given with INH to help reduce the incidence of peripheral neuropathy.[4] Patients should be advised to stop treatment and inform their key worker if they develop adverse effects such as nausea, vomiting, reduced appetite, jaundice, or signs of peripheral neuropathy.

RIF MONOTHERAPY

RIF monotherapy has been shown to reduce the incidence of TB compared to placebo by approximately 50% in an initial study in Hong Kong.[19] A network meta-analysis found that compared to placebo the odds ratio of developing TB after taking RIF monotherapy was 0.41 (95% CI 0.19–0.85).[13]

A Cochrane review looked at the evidence for using RIF monotherapy compared to INH monotherapy for preventing TB; the incidence of TB after 5 years of follow-up was the outcome measure. Only one study was used in this part of the analysis. RIF for 4 months appeared to be as effective as 6–9 months of INH in the study, relative risk 0.81 (95% CI 0.47–1.4) but the overall quality of the study was rated as low.[20–22] No difference in adherence or treatment limiting effects was seen but there was a lower risk of grade 3 or 4 hepatotoxicity with RIF compared to INH, RR 0.15 (95% CI 0.07–0.4); this part of the review looked at five studies with a total of 1774 patients. There does not appear to be an excess of RIF resistance in patients treated with RIF for LTBI. A review of six randomized controlled trials found relative risk of RIF resistance in subsequent active TB cases was 3.45 (95% CI 0.72–16.56) compared to non-RIF-containing regimens, but this was not statistically significantly different.[23] Rifamycin-containing regimens are associated with higher rates of completion compared to other regimens.[24] Two recent open label trials have compared 4 months of RIF monotherapy to 9 months of INH monotherapy in adults and children, respectively. The trial, involving over 6800 adults,

was conducted in nine countries. RIF monotherapy for 4 months was found to be non-inferior to 9 months of INH in preventing active TB during 28 months following randomization. The completion rate was higher in the RIF group at 78.8% versus 63.2%, a 15.1% difference (95% CI 12.7–17.4). There was a lower rate of adverse events, especially hepatotoxicity, in the RIF group.[18] A similar trial in children aged <18 years involving 829 children found similar safety and efficacy between 4 months of RIF compared to 9 months of INH but with better treatment completion in the RIF group at 85.3% versus 76.4%, a 13.4% difference (95% CI 7.5–19.3).[25]

RIF monotherapy is recommended for patients who cannot take INH, such as patients with peripheral neuropathy or those with exposure to INH-resistant TB. Patients with liver disease may tolerate RIF better than INH but would still require frequent clinical and biochemical monitoring. The recent trials mentioned previously are likely to result in changes to guidelines in the near future.

RIF AND INH FOR 3 MONTHS

Daily RIF with INH for 3 months was shown to be as effective in preventing TB as 6 months of daily INH in a trial in Hong Kong in patients with silicosis.[21] There have not been as many subsequent trials as there have been with INH but the convenience of 3 months as opposed to 6–9 months of treatment has led to widespread adoption of this regimen in some countries, such as the UK.[4] Meta-analyses of five studies comprising 1926 patients found that with regard to development of active TB, 3 months of RIF and INH was equivalent to 6–12 months of INH monotherapy; severe adverse events were equal between the two therapies.[26] A retrospective review of patients in South Korea taking latent TB treatment prior to antitumor necrosis factor (aTNF)-alpha therapy found completion rates of 94.2% for patients taking 3 months of RIF and INH compared to 73.8% for those receiving 9 months of INH.[27] A network meta-analysis for the prevention of active TB found an odds ratio of 0.53 (95% CI 0.36–0.78) for the prevention of active TB compared to placebo with 3–4 months of daily RIF and INH.[13] The most recent WHO LTBI treatment guidelines recommend 3 months of RIF with INH as an alternative to 6 months of INH for children aged <15 years.[28] The guideline group conducted a further evidence review of trials and observation studies focusing on children and found that fewer participants given RIF and INH for 3 months developed radiographic evidence of TB than those given 9 months of INH, relative risk 0.49 (95% CI 0.2–0.56). There was also higher adherence among children, RR 1.07 (95% CI 1.01–1.14).[6,29,30,31] It is not clear if this regimen is more hepatotoxic than 4 months of RIF monotherapy.

INH AND RPT

RPT is a rifamycin with a long half-life. It was shown many years ago that RPT was more bactericidal than RIF in a mouse TB model and, due to its long half-life, could be administered less frequently.[32] A large multicountry trial of 3986 patients comparing weekly RPT with INH for 3 months (12 doses) to 9 months of daily INH found a cumulative rate of TB of 0.19% in the RPT/INH group compared to 0.43% in the INH-only group. Rates of treatment completion were 82.1% in the RPT/INH group compared to 69% in the INH-only group (P<0.001), hepatotoxicity occurred in 0.4% of the RPT/INH group and 2.7% of the INH group (P=0.009).[33] Further study of hepatoxicity found that of 6862 patients evaluated, 1.8% of patients receiving 9 months of INH developed hepatotoxicity compared to 0.4% of patients receiving 12 doses of RPT/INH (p<0.001).[34,35] Based on the data from the study, RPT/INH was adopted as a recommended regimen by the CDC and later by WHO.[5,6] One hundred and twenty-six pregnancies occurred among trial participants and no unexpected fetal loss or congenital abnormalities were detected.[36]

An open label trial of 12 doses of RPT/INH versus 9 months of INH in HIV infected patients with median CD4 counts of around 500 cells/μL found cumulative TB incidence rates of 1.1% in the RPT/INH group and 3.5% in the 9-month INH group, treatment completion rate was 89% in the RPT/INH group and 64% in the INH group (P<0.001).[37]

A randomized controlled trial conducted across several countries compared daily RPT/INH for 1 month to daily INH for 9 months in HIV infected persons. RPT was dosed according to weight 300–600 mg daily, INH was given at a dose of 300 mg daily in both arms. The trial was open label with a non-inferiority design. Three thousand patients were enrolled in the study. The primary end point of TB or death from TB was seen in 2% of both treatment arms indicating non-inferiority of the short regimen compared to 9 months of INH. Also, treatment completion at 97% versus 90% was higher in the 1-month regimen group. Adverse effects were not different between the two arms of the trial.[38]

Flu-like reactions can occur with this regimen as have been seen with intermittent RIF dosage regimens.[39]

3 months of weekly RPT/INH has been modeled to be cheaper and result in fewer cases of active TB compared to 9 months of daily INH.[40] The regimen has favorable pharmacokinetics and can be used in children aged 2–17 years; higher treatment completion rates were seen in children compared to 9 months of INH monotherapy.[41,42] Dose regimens are shown in Table 19.2. A twelve-dose cycle of RPT/INH is recommended by the CDC and WHO for adults and children aged over 2 years. RPT should be used with caution in patients with HIV infection taking antiretroviral therapy (ART) due to potential interactions. The CDC recently conducted a systematic meta-analysis of RPT/INH studies and extended their recommendations for use in children, HIV infected patients, and for self-administered therapy.[43,44]

RIF AND PZA FOR 8 WEEKS

RIF in combination with PZA for 8 weeks given as a daily dose or twice weekly for 8–12 weeks has been shown to be effective in treating latent TB. A multicenter study of 1583 HIV infected patients with positive TSTs comparing 2 months of daily RIF and PZA with 12 months of daily INH found 80% of patients in the RIF/PZA group completed treatment compared to 69% in the INH group. After a mean of 37 months of follow-up rates of TB in the RIF/PZA group were 0.8 per 100 person years compared to 1.1 per 100 person years in the INH group. This regimen was endorsed initially by the CDC for use in HIV infected patients as well as HIV uninfected patients.[44]

Shortly after this regimen was recommended reports emerged on high rates of liver toxicity and, in some cases, death. The CDC carried out a retrospective survey of 7737 patients who had received either daily or intermittent RIF/PZA for LTBI, 204 (26.4 per 1000 treatments, 95% CI 22.8–30) patients discontinued treatment due to a rise in aspartate transaminase (AST) to greater than 5 times the normal upper limit, and an additional 146 patients stopped therapy due to hepatitis (18.9 per 1000 treatments, 95% CI 17.4–20.4). In comparison the mortality rate in patients being treated with INH was 0–0.3 per 1000.[45–47]

These findings were confirmed in a meta-analysis looking at six studies involving patients from seven countries including HIV and non-HIV infected patients comparing 2–3 months of RIF/PZA to 12 months of INH treatment. Both regimens showed similar efficacy in preventing TB developing but the RIF/PZA regimen was associated with a much higher risk of severe adverse effects compared to 12 months of INH (risk difference 29%, 95% CI 13–46 vs. risk difference 7%, 95% CI 4–10).[48–50] In view of these findings, RIF/PZA is not recommended for the treatment of LTBI.

RISK FACTORS

Risk factors for people with LTBI developing active TB are many and often there is complex interplay between different risks. Apart from well-known comorbidities such as HIV infection, which increase the risk of developing active TB manyfold, there is increasing recognition of more common comorbidities such as diabetes, which—although having a much smaller effect on the risk of developing active TB—may have a large impact at a population level because of its prevalence, especially in countries with a high incidence of both conditions.[51] Another important and emerging risk factor for developing active TB is the use of novel immunomodulatory agents such as TNF-alpha agents. These agents were first noted to increase the risk of developing active TB several years after their introduction to treat conditions such as inflammatory bowel disease.[52] This increased risk was not predicted from animal models or noted in prelicensing studies. Many new immunomodulators that only recently entered clinical practice have a relatively unknown TB reactivation risk.

All of these risks are discussed individually in the following sections.

CLOSE CONTACTS AND RECENT CONVERTORS

People who are in close contact with a case of infectious TB are at increased risk of progressing to active TB if they become latently infected. The rate of progression to active TB after exposure is around 0.6%–7.5% in the first year; it is lower in the second year but adds up to around 10% in total over 2 years. This can be reduced with chemoprophylaxis as described previously.[53] Close contacts of infectious TB cases should be screened, assessed for active TB, and offered an appropriate test for latent TB. The test offered will depend on local guidelines and circumstances, e.g., if people from a large congregate setting need to be screened, a single IGRA test after an appropriate interval may be the most efficient and cost effective strategy. If positive they should be offered treatment for LTBI.

Close contacts with HIV infection are more likely to progress to active disease and after exclusion of active disease those with advanced immunosuppression (CD4<200 cells/mm^3) should be offered chemoprophylaxis.[4]

Children aged under 5 years are at the highest risk of progression to active TB. WHO recommends that HIV-uninfected children under the age of 5 years in high TB incidence countries who are exposed to infectious TB be screened for active disease and, if excluded, be given treatment for LTBI. In low-incidence countries, latent TB treatment is recommended after appropriate testing with TST or IGRA. For HIV infected infants <12 months old who are in contact with infectious TB, treatment with INH prophylaxis should ensue once active disease has been excluded.[3] NICE guidelines recommend neonates (<4 weeks old) in contact with smear positive respiratory TB should be assessed for active TB and, if it is excluded, started on INH; a tuberculin skin test is carried out at 6 weeks. If it is positive, reassess for active TB and if excluded continue INH for 6 months. If the TST is negative, reassess for active disease and consider an IGRA test; if negative, give bacillus Calmette-Gùerin (BCG) vaccine and if positive continue INH treatment for 6 months. A similar strategy is recommended for children aged 4 weeks to 2 years.[4] Older children are assessed in a similar fashion to adults: first exclude active disease then carry out a screening test or combination of tests and give chemoprophylaxis if the test or tests are positive, and offer BCG vaccine if the tests are negative.

FIBROTIC LESIONS

Fibrotic lung lesions mainly in the upper lobes increase the risk of a person with latent TB developing active TB 6–19-fold.[54,55] Before treating a patient with a fibrotic lung lesion for latent TB, a full evaluation should be carried out to ensure the patient does not have active disease. Sputum samples should be taken and further imaging, including cross-sectional imaging, may be appropriate, possibly followed by bronchoscopy. Often patients with fibrotic lung lesions may have been evaluated for lung cancer and have had a CT–PET (computerized tomography–positron emission tomography) scan.[56] Treatment for active TB may be appropriate in these cases where the PET scan reveals a metabolically active lesion confirmed to be TB by histology.

If a thorough evaluation does not reveal active TB, treatment of these patients for latent TB is appropriate.

Treatment of these individuals has been shown to be very effective in preventing active TB. A large study conducted in 115 dispensaries in seven European countries by the International Union against Tuberculosis recruited 28,000 patients with stable (for 1 year) fibrotic lung lesions and reactive tuberculin skin tests of at least 6 mm (mean 15 mm). Patients were given 12, 24, or 52 weeks of INH treatment or placebo. The rate of development of active TB in the placebo group, defined as culture positive cases during the first 12 months, was 0.4%, and during the first 5 years, 1.4%. People receiving 12 weeks of INH showed a 21% reduction in cases; those who received 24 weeks of INH showed a 65% reduction and those who received 52 weeks of INH showed a 75% reduction. When the analysis was confined only to patients who had completed therapy as opposed to those who had started

therapy but may not have finished, reduction in cases were 69% for those completing 24 weeks of treatment and 93% for those completing 52 weeks of therapy. Larger fibrotic lesions >2 cm^2 were more likely to reactivate and appeared to benefit more from 52 weeks of treatment.[57] Another study also showed the benefit of treating LTBI in patients with fibrotic lesions but no benefit in treating patients who had previously received treatment for active TB.[58]

The data presented previously is based on INH treatment. There are no specific trials to support the use of RIF-based treatment of LTBI in patients with fibrotic lung lesions but it is probably reasonable to extrapolate the findings of LTBI in patients with silicosis treated by the Hong Kong Chest Service.[21]

Interestingly, despite strong evidence showing the benefit of treating LTBI in patients with fibrotic lesions, only CDC guidelines specifically recommend treatment of this group.[5]

HIV INFECTION

Around a quarter of all deaths in HIV infected individuals are due to TB.[59] The relative risk of TB reactivating in HIV infected individuals compared to the general population has been estimated to be over 100 times.[60] In HIV infected people not receiving ART, the rate of progression for latent to active TB is 5%–10% per year.[61] Chemoprophylaxis for LTBI in HIV infected individuals has been shown to be effective. There are two strategies with regard to selecting whom to treat. In resource-limited settings with high TB incidence, INH has been shown to reduce the incidence of TB in HIV infected people regardless of their TST result. There, people with HIV can be treated without needing a test for LTBI. The current recommended duration of treatment is 36 months; this is a proxy for lifelong treatment.[3,62–64] Despite WHO recommending INH therapy for HIV infected people in 1990, there has been relatively poor uptake in the highest incidence countries. A recent study in Malawi found that around a quarter of patients enrolled in INH preventive therapy programs in a well-managed cohort did not complete treatment. In Uganda, in an operational setting, 60% of patients were lost from the program.[65,66] Integration with ART programs can help.

In low-incidence, high income countries, targeted LTBI testing among HIV infected people is recommended. In the UK, the British HIV association (BHIVA) recommends testing of all HIV infected patients from medium and high incidence TB countries (>40/100,000 per year), regardless of CD4 count or concurrent ART;[67] the CDC recommends offering treatment to HIV infected people with a TST >5 mm or positive IGRA test. BHIVA recommends using an IGRA test for screening for LTBI in HIV infected people; clinical judgment should be used if the test is indeterminate. The incidence of hepatotoxicity has been found to be low but increased when other risk factors such as excess alcohol are also present; clinical monitoring for adverse effects is recommended.[68]

INH monotherapy and INH with RIF are both recommended for the treatment of LTBI in HIV infected people, and more recently, weekly RPT/INH. Care should be taken when using RIF due to possible interactions with ART.

OTHER IMMUNOSUPPRESSED INDIVIDUALS INCLUDING ANTI-TNF THERAPY

Various agents have been associated with reactivation of latent TB. Corticosteroids have been shown in mouse and rabbit models to reactivate latent TB.[69,70] The risk in humans is less clear. There are multiple case reports of TB in patients receiving steroids, but there are no high quality studies. A retrospective review of over 1000 patients did not show an excessive risk over background.[71] A study in Taiwan of patients with rheumatoid arthritis receiving a corticosteroid dose of more than 5 mg a day found an excess risk of active TB of 5 times (95% CI 1.47–17.16) compared to the background risk.[72]

The use of aTNF-alpha inhibitors has revolutionized the management of inflammatory bowel disease as well as many rheumatological and dermatological conditions. Wider off-license use of these drugs is continuing. An increased risk of TB in patients being treated with aTNF drugs was noted soon after their introduction into routine clinical practice.[51] TB developing in patients receiving aTNF therapy may be difficult to diagnose and may be disseminated.[73–75] It appears that aTNF drugs interfere with the immune system's ability to control TB infection at a number of places in both the innate and adaptive parts of the system, as reviewed by Harris and Keane.[76] There are currently five licensed aTNF agents, infliximab, adalimumab, etanercept, golimumab, and certolizumab pegol, the risk of TB reactivation is different with each agent (Table 19.3); the highest risk of TB activation is increased up to 25 times that of background. The use of any of the agents should be preceded by screening for active and LTBI in line with national and specialist society guidelines.[77] Treatment of LTBI prior to aTNF therapy has been shown to be effective and to reduce the rate of active TB by around two-thirds.[78] There are no clear data on the optimal timing to start aTNF agents in patients being treated for LTBI; ideally LTBI treatment should be completed but if aTNF therapy is urgently needed, a minimum of a month of antituberculosis therapy prior to starting has been suggested.[79] There have been a plethora of biologic agents other than aTNF introduced over the past few years that target parts of the immune system. The risk of TB reactivation with these agents is not as yet clearly defined, but to date there appears to be little if any risk with the anti-interleukin 1 agent anakinra, anti-CD20 agent rituximab, and anti-CD80/CD86 abatacept. The risk with tocilizumab, a humanized monoclonal antibody against interleukin 6 receptor, is not clear, although probably not increased, but post-marketing surveillance of this and other new biological agents needs to continue.[80–82]

INTRAVENOUS DRUG USERS (NON-HIV INFECTED)

Intravenous drug users (IVDU) have been shown to have a higher risk of developing active TB compared to the background population. One of the first studies to report the increased incidence in New York found a city-wide prevalence of TB of 1,372/100,000 among IVDU compared to a prevalence of 64.7/100,000 in the city as a whole.[82] This increased prevalence may have been due partially to the early HIV epidemic. In later studies, the effect of HIV infection on TB reactivation and transmission was shown to be more marked than the risk posed by intravenous drug use alone, but this group of patients are liable to present late with advanced active TB and thus cause microepidemics of TB transmission in their communities. In cities such as Barcelona, where the early HIV epidemic was concentrated among IVDU, large rises in TB incidence were seen.[83]

WHO, NICE, and CDC guidelines recommend testing and treating latent TB in IVDU. IVDU may be difficult to access and screen, but once they have entered a methadone treatment program there is an opportunity for testing and treating LTBI. A study of IVDU taking methadone and given directly observed INH along with their methadone had completion rates of 77% compared to 13% for those patients referred to a TB clinic for standard care.[84] Joint cooperation should be encouraged and include blood-borne virus screening.

HEALTH-CARE WORKERS

Prior to effective treatment for TB, i.e., before 1950, there was a very high risk of TB in health-care workers. This risk fell until the resurgence of TB in the mid-1980s to mid-1990s. Risks in hospitals apply to health-care workers involved in direct patient care as well as laboratory technicians and mortuary staff. Improvements in infection control such as improved ventilation, both high and low tech ultraviolet light, and the appropriate isolation of infectious patients have resulted in reduced transmission in health-care settings. The use of correctly fitting masks by health-care workers also contributes to reduced risk.[85] Multiple preventive methods need to be employed to protect patients and staff in health-care institutions.[86]

In high incidence TB countries, rates of TB infection among health-care workers have been found to be very high; a recent review found a pooled prevalence of 47% (95% CI 34%–60%) of LTBI and was as high as 63% in South Africa.[87] There are few studies looking at TB incidence among health-care workers in high incidence countries; a study of nursing students in Zimbabwe found 19.3 TST conversions per 100 person-years (95% CI 14.2–26.2), compared to 6.0 (3.5–10.4) conversions per 100 person-years among polytechnic students, showing a substantial risk of nurses acquiring TB in the workplace, not surprising in view of the high volume of patients with TB managed by these nurses.[88] A recent systematic review found the overall prevalence of LTBI

Table 19.3 Risk of TB with aTNF agents

Agent	Risk	Reference
Adalimumab	IR 176–215/100,000	173,174
Certolizumab pegol	Rate 0.42/100 person years (0.31–0.57)	175
Etanercept	IR 9.3–144/100,000	173,174,176,177
Golimumab	Rate 0.55/100 person years (0.07–1.98)[a]	178
Infliximab	IR 54–383/100,000	173,174,176,177

[a] Patients also taking methotrexate. Abbreviation: IR, incidence ratio.

among health-care workers was 37%, with a cumulative incidence of 97/100,000 per year. The risk of LTBI was at least twice that of the general population.[89]

The risk of transmission of TB from health-care workers to their clients can be difficult to determine. Whole-genome sequencing may shed more light on this in the future. A systematic review and meta-analyses of reported cases of TB transmitted by health-care workers to patients found that the rate of transmission was 0.09% (95% CI 0.02–0.22) for adult patients and 2.6% (95% CI 1–4.9) for other health-care workers indicating the risk to patients from health-care workers with TB is present but several orders of magnitude less than the risk of health-care workers transmitting TB to their colleagues. It is important that appropriate screening is carried out when a case of active infectious TB is discovered in a health-care worker.[90]

OTHER GROUPS WITH HIGH RISK OF EXPOSURE

There are other groups at increased risk of developing active TB due to their social circumstances, specifically recent immigrants, prisoners, and homeless individuals. Often individuals in these groups may have multiple risk factors, including HIV infection and IVDU, putting them at even higher risk of developing active disease making this a high priority group to screen and treat, but social risk factors can make these individuals difficult to find and engage in treatment programs.

Numbers of international migrants are growing; in 2017 the United Nations estimated there were 258 million migrants, the majority of migration is from lower to higher income countries and also from higher to low incidence TB areas.[91] People migrating from high incidence to low-incidence TB prevalence countries are at increased risk of developing active TB for a variety of reasons. In some low incidence countries the vast majority of active cases of TB are seen in recently arrived and settled migrants. In England around 75% of annual active TB cases are seen in people born overseas in high TB incidence countries.[92] There are several ways to address this issue, one of which is pre-entry screening for active TB, which has been shown to be useful but will not address the large numbers of people arriving with LTBI.[93] Screening for active TB in migrants once they arrive in their destination country is fairly widely undertaken. Screening for LTBI is less widely practiced although recommended by WHO, NICE, and CDC. The definition of whom to screen also varies in the UK. People arriving from countries with a TB incidence >150/100,000 are offered screening if aged between 16 and 35 years. In Canada, those arriving from countries with a TB incidence >30/100,000 are screened. Asylum seekers are in some cases screened even if their country of origin is low incidence due to the possibility of TB contact during their migration.[94,95] Data on the outcome of treating migrant groups for LTBI at a country level is lacking but should be available in the next few years from PHE (Public Health England), following evaluation of the national LTBI screening program. Reducing barriers to screening and providing information in culturally appropriate language is important.[96] Also, offering screening in convenient locations such as at language classes may improve uptake.[97]

Homeless people have benefited from screening for active TB where this has been undertaken.[98] Screening and treating homeless people for LTBI is more complex but possible. LTBI prevalence has been found to be as high as 50% in a recent review; also the presence of blood-borne virus infections is common in this group, making treatment potentially more complex. A major risk factor for LTBI among homeless people in England was previous incarceration, confirming the interplay of risk factors but also strengthening the case for joining health-care services and screening to identify and treat people with social risk factors at multiple sites.[99]

Prisoners are at high risk of developing active TB and, due to the nature of incarceration, spread to others is likely and often extensive. Screening of prisoners is recommended by WHO, NICE, and the CDC but, whereas screening for active disease is often undertaken, LTBI screening is not. There are a number of barriers to effective LTBI screening in prisons such as poor health care, lack of facilities for TB screening, and poor access to necessary medication; prison health services are often not priorities for investment.[100]

Mathematical modeling carried out by the European Centre for Disease Control has calculated that current screening for LTBI in low incidence countries will not allow the WHO target for TB elimination by 2050 to be met. But if homeless people, IVDU, prisoners, and recently arrived migrants from high incidence TB countries are screened and treated for LTBI then significant decreases in active TB would be seen.[101]

MEDICAL RISK FACTORS

Certain medical conditions increase the risk of people with LTBI developing active TB. The magnitude of increase varies between studies and between high and low prevalence countries. Certain risk factors such as diabetes are emerging as increasingly important due to the changing prevalence of the condition across the world, especially in developing settings with high rates of LTBI. Data on the benefit of chemoprophylaxis for all the risk factors mentioned in the following sections is lacking in some cases, but individuals often have more than one risk factor for developing active TB and the benefit of chemoprophylaxis usually outweighs the risk of not treating individuals. The conditions to be discussed are silicosis, diabetes, renal disease, malignancy, weight loss, chronic peptic ulcer disease, gastrectomy, weight loss surgery, and smoking.

SILICOSIS

Silicosis has long been recognized as a risk factor for developing pulmonary TB. Also, it has been observed that patients with silicosis who develop pulmonary TB have worse outcomes and may need extended therapy.[19,21] This may be because of impaired alveolar macrophage function due to silica. The increased risk is related to the amount of silica and other dust exposure, with the risk being increased even in people who have not developed overt silicosis.[102] The increased risk of TB in people with silica exposure compared to others may be difficult to determine, as other risk factors such as HIV infection, smoking, and other dust exposure are often present, but it is in the order of magnitude of an increased risk of 3 times[102,103]; there have been much higher estimates. A 10-year retrospective study of copper miners from what is now Zambia found that there was a 26-fold increase in silicotic miners (2.89%/year) compared to nonsilicotic miners (0.11%/year); this is on the background of a very high TB incidence setting.[104] The increased risk remains after the cessation of dust exposure. A study of former miners in Oklahoma aged over 50 years of whom a third had silicosis observed 8 (1.1%/year) of 367 people developed culture positive TB over a 2-year period.[105] Despite improved working practices in many settings, there has not been a significant decrease in the number of miners with silicosis over the last 30 years, so silicosis as a risk for TB seems unlikely to disappear soon.[106]

Chemoprophylaxis has been shown to be effective in patients with LTBI and silicosis, but there are few high quality studies and the evidence base is weaker than that for many other risk groups such as HIV infected patients. A study using INH monotherapy showed a 93% reduction in active TB cases compared to placebo, but the study included people with other risk factors such as recent skin test convertors, close contacts of TB patients, and people with fibrotic lung lesions all of which have previously been shown to independently benefit from chemoprophylaxis.[107] Another study from Hong Kong where many people are exposed to silica via the construction industry randomized a group of 625 patients with LTBI. Patients received 24 weeks of 300 mg INH daily, 12 weeks of 300 mg INH with 600 mg RIF daily, 600 mg RIF daily, or placebo daily for 24 weeks of therapy, all self-directed. After 5 years of follow-up, a 50% reduction in TB was seen; TB occurred in 13% of the chemoprophylaxis groups compared to 27% of the placebo group. There was no difference in efficacy between the different chemoprophylaxis groups.[108]

Diabetes mellitus

Diabetes mellitus (DM) is becoming more prevalent across the world. The 2017 International Diabetes Federation Atlas reports that there are 425 million people worldwide with DM, half of whom are undiagnosed; a further 325 million people are at risk of developing type 2 DM. Eighty percent of people with DM live in low or middle income countries; the same countries that have the highest incidence of TB. Although the prevalence of DM is predicted to rise across the world, the biggest increases over the next 3 decades are likely to be in the poorest and most populous regions, e.g., Africa, 156% predicted increase, and South East Asia, 84% predicted increase. In view of this, any interaction between the two epidemics of DM and TB could have important adverse consequences.[109] The overall prevalence of diabetes among incident TB patients varies across countries but has been estimated to be between 1.9% and 45% with a median prevalence of 16%.[110]

DM has been associated with an increased risk of active TB in a number of studies. This risk varies between studies. A recent systematic review and meta-analyses that included studies with a total of over 58 million subjects including over 89,000 TB cases and involving 16 countries found that the measure of association between DM and TB varied from a relative risk or hazard ratio of 3.59 (95% CI 2.25–5.73) for prospective studies to a relative

risk (RR) or hazard ratio of 1.55 (95% CI 1.39–1.72) for retrospective studies. Overall when all the studies were combined, despite varying methodology, the measure of association was 2 (95% CI 1.78–2.24).[111]

The biological mechanism that predisposes people with DM to develop active TB is not well defined. There does appear to be an association with poorly controlled DM as well as competing factors such as excessive use of alcohol and smoking. It has been shown that people with poorly controlled DM and hyperglycemia have reduced intracellular killing of bacteria by leucocytes.[112] Also, type 2 DM patients have been shown to have reduced interferon gamma production in response to stimuli; this could affect a person's ability to control early TB infection, predisposing them to developing active disease.[113] The association between hyperglycemia and TB has been observed in a cohort of African people, but the overall additional contribution of hyperglycemia to TB prevalence was felt to be small, and it is likely that the effect of DM will be less significant when other competing risk factors such as HIV infection are dominant in the population under study.[114,115]

One of the biggest risk factors for type 2 DM is obesity. Obesity has been shown to have a protective effect with regard to developing active TB. There is a complex interplay of risks between DM, obesity, and TB that may not cancel each other out. A large cohort study based in Taiwan involving 167,392 patients followed for a median of 7 years found individuals with a body mass index (BMI) >30 kg/m^2 had a 67% (95% CI −3% to −90%) and 64% (95% CI 31%–81%) reduction in risk of developing TB in two cohorts. Overall, obesity appeared to have a protective effect with regard to developing TB that was canceled out in people who were both obese and had DM, compared to people who were neither obese nor had DM.[116]

Although the risk of active TB is clearly increased by DM, the relationship between TB infection and DM is less clear. A recent systematic review that included over 38,000 individuals found inconsistent associations between different study methodologies and designs. Overall there was a small but statistically significant association between DM and an increased risk of LTBI with a pooled odds ratio of 1.18 (95% CI 1.06–1.3).[117] Screening patients with DM for LTBI in low TB incidence countries is not currently recommended in WHO guidelines unless other risk factors are present, but this may change as more evidence becomes available and prevalence of other risk factors changes.[6,8]

Chronic renal failure, dialysis

Chronic renal disease was recognized as a risk factor for the development of active TB over 40 years ago. The risk varies between studies and depends to some extent on the background of patients and coexisting conditions.[118–121] A large study from Australia found the incidence of TB in dialysis patients was 66.8/100,000 per year compared to 5.7/100,000 per year in the population as a whole. This gave an adjusted RR for people on dialysis of 7.8 (95% CI 3.3–18.7).[122] A study from London, UK, showed a much higher TB prevalence; the cumulative TB incidence was 1,267/100,000 (95% CI 630–1904) in hemodialysis patients, 398/100,000 (95% CI, 80–1160) in peritoneal dialysis patients and 522/100,000 (95% CI 137–909) in renal transplant patients. These rates are 85, 26, and 35 times greater than the background rate of TB in the UK.[123] Active TB can be difficult to diagnose in patients with renal disease and may be more likely to be extrapulmonary and often peritoneal, especially in peritoneal dialysis patients. In view of being difficult to diagnose, screening and treatment of latent TB in this patient group is of particular importance.[124]

The choice of screening test for latent TB in patients with renal disease is important, TSTs are not sensitive due to energy with advanced renal disease, therefore IGRA tests are preferred.[125,126]

Chemoprophylaxis is recommended for patients with chronic kidney disease by NICE and CDC guidelines, also for patients receiving dialysis. WHO, NICE, and CDC recommend screening and treatment of LTBI.[4-6] INH is removed to some extent by dialysis so should be given after completion of a hemodialysis session. Patients with renal failure are more liable to develop peripheral neuropathy so pyridoxine should be given with INH. RIF may reduce the level of immunosuppressant drugs given to patients with renal transplants, such as tacrolimus, so these drug levels should be carefully monitored if RIF is coadministered.[127]

MALIGNANCY

Malignancy, especially head and neck cancer and hematological malignancy, are associated with reactivation of LTBI. A strong association with head and neck cancer compared to other malignancies was noted many years ago; the reason for this is multifactorial and may be related to weight loss, immunosuppression, chemotherapy, and radiotherapy.[128]

The largest recent study of the additional risk of TB reactivation posed by malignancy was based on a study of the Danish national medical databases. The study looked at 290,944 patients with cancer. The overall adjusted hazard ratio for TB among cancer patients was 2.48 (95% CI 1.99–3.1). The cancers with the three highest risks of TB reactivation were those of the aerodigestive tract, tobacco-related cancer, and hematological malignancies. High risk was also noted to occur in the first year after cancer diagnosis, but remained elevated 5 years after diagnosis. Patients receiving chemotherapy or radiotherapy had an adjusted hazard ratio of 6.78 compared to the background rate.[129] It therefore seems sensible to offer latent TB testing and treatment for patients with these types of malignancies and those due to undergo cytotoxic or radiotherapy.

Guidelines for testing and treating patients with malignancy for LTBI vary. In the UK, NICE 2016 recommends testing for LTBI and treating patients with hematological malignancies and patients receiving chemotherapy for other malignancies.[4] In the United States, CDC guidelines recommend treatment for patients with head and neck cancer. Toxicity of LTBI treatment and interactions with chemotherapy agents should be taken into account, e.g., peripheral neuropathy caused by both INH and some cytotoxic drugs may be alleviated by pyridoxine. RIF may render some agents less effective by increasing their metabolism, such as corticosteroids.

RAPID WEIGHT LOSS AND MALNUTRITION

Active TB is associated with weight loss which, if treatment is delayed, can be marked. Rapid significant weight loss as a risk factor for developing active TB has been described.[130,131] Weight loss of more than 10% of ideal weight is probably an independent risk factor for developing active TB and is an indication for treatment of LTBI. In these cases the cause of weight loss may also be an additional risk factor such as malnutrition, malabsorption, gastrectomy, malignancy, intestinal bypass surgery, or starvation. Low BMI has also been recognized as a risk factor for developing TB disease, a relationship between BMI and the risk of developing TB has been shown in several cohorts.[132]

Being underweight and having a low BMI does not appear to be linked to a higher likelihood of having LTBI, as recent careful systematic review has shown.[133]

The effect of malnutrition on the success of LTBI treatment is not well defined but may be lowered due to a less effective immune system; medication used to treat LTBI has been reported to be more toxic in malnourished patients.[134,135]

CHRONIC PEPTIC ULCER DISEASE, POSTGASTRECTOMY

Reactivation of latent TB and increased susceptibility to TB following subtotal gastrectomy has long been recognized.[136] Gastrectomy for the treatment of gastric cancer has been associated with an increased risk of TB compared to the general population in the Republic of Korea, which has a current TB incidence of 39/100,000.[137] A retrospective study of 1776 individuals who had undergone gastrectomy found 0.9% (16/1776) patients developed active TB, which equates to an annual incidence of 223.7 cases per 100,000. Other risk factors identified included previous TB and low BMI, possibly demonstrating the interplay between different risk factors.[137] Interestingly, treatment of active TB in postgastrectomy patients has been associated with higher treatment failure rates; in one small case–control study 26% of patients had clinical treatment failure at 4 months.[138,139]

INTESTINAL BYPASS SURGERY

Surgery for morbid obesity, especially jejunoileal bypass surgery, has been shown to be very effective, leading to significant weight loss. It has also been associated with an increased risk of TB. The increased risk has been reported to be between 27 and 63 that of the general population.[140,141] Laparoscopic weight loss techniques such as gastric banding do not seem to confer the same risk of TB compared to older surgical techniques, although there are case reports of TB after these procedures.[142] This reduced risk may be because laparoscopic techniques cause less profound weight loss.

SMOKING

A link between cigarette smoke and TB was first postulated as early as 1918 by G. B. Webb based on observations of TB rates in American soldiers who smoked.[143] There have been many observational studies looking at the additional risk that smoking adds to the chance of a person becoming infected with TB and going on to develop active TB. Many of these studies have been confounded by other risk factors and behaviors that may put people at higher risk of TB such as homelessness, alcohol misuse, intravenous drug use, poverty, malnutrition, and other lung diseases. This makes it difficult to clearly define the additional risk for TB due to smoking alone. Some of these factors may also affect the results of TB IGRA tests, making the situation even more complicated. A systematic review and meta-analyses by Jayes et al. summarized four cohort studies published since 2000 looking at the increased risk of active TB; three of the studies were graded as high quality. The summary estimate for the relative RR attributed to active smoking was 1.57 (95% CI 1.18–2.10); increasing risk was seen with increased number of cigarettes smoked. Other reviews have broken the risk down between three outcomes, TB infection, TB disease, and TB mortality. The evidence is strongest for TB disease with a relative risk of around 2.2. For TB infection, the evidence is less strong but the relative risk is around 1.5. For TB mortality, the relative risk is around 2.0.[144–149] Generally, smoking is not identified in guidelines as a risk factor justifying treatment of LTBI unless associated with other risks.

The risk of TB in relation to secondhand or passive tobacco smoke is less clear cut. In a recent systematic review that assessed 12 studies there did not appear to be an increased risk of acquiring TB infection related to secondhand smoke exposure (RR 1.19, 95% CI 0.9–1.57), but there did appear to be an increased risk of developing TB disease (RR 1.59, 95% CI 1.11–2.27). The authors noted that the studies reviewed had quite marked heterogeneity so the overall risk in different setting remains unclear and more evidence is required.[150]

LOW-RISK INDIVIDUALS

Individuals at low risk of having latent TB and at low risk of developing active TB are not usually screened for LTBI unless they are entering a high risk setting for acquiring disease, or are vulnerable to active TB, such as patients starting aTNF treatment. Another low risk group of people who may be screened for LTBI are those entering occupations where the development of active TB would be potentially deleterious to those around them, such as health-care workers. In these cases, the benefit of treatment probably outweighs the risk of toxicity secondary to treatment. For other low risk individuals, the decision is more finely balanced, but online evidence-based decision tools exist that can help clinicians and individuals make decisions around treatment benefits and risks. One such calculator is the online TST/IGRA interpreter maintained by McGill University, Canada.[151,152] Using this calculator, for example, an 18-year-old white person from the United States found to have a positive IGRA and TST>15 mm but with no recent TB contact and no other risk factors may have a lifetime risk of active TB of around 6% but a risk of hepatotoxicity secondary to INH close to 0. In contrast, a 65-year-old white person from the United States with no recent TB contact and no risk factors, with the same screening results, has a risk of 1.5% of developing active TB before the age of 80, but a risk of hepatotoxicity secondary to INH is around 5%. In general, young low risk individuals probably will benefit from chemoprophylaxis, but screening should follow local and national guidelines.[153]

MONITORING CHEMOPROPHYLAXIS

Individuals being treated for LTBI, as they do not have active disease, must be carefully monitored for adverse effects of medication to minimize risks of harm. All patients should be counseled in terms and language that they can understand about what side effects to look out for and what action to take if they develop them, namely nausea, vomiting, itching rash, jaundice, and painful feet. Clinical evaluation on a monthly basis enquiring about gastrointestinal disturbance, rash, peripheral neuropathy, and jaundice should be undertaken.

Baseline liver enzymes are usually measured prior to starting LTBI treatment, even though there is not a strong evidence base to support this. Some authorities do not recommend measuring liver enzymes in all patients but just those at higher risk of hepatotoxicity such as patients with hepatitis B and C, HIV infection, heavy alcohol users, patients on hepatoxic medication, over 35 years of age, pregnant patients, and those in the postpartum period up to 90 days. A careful risk–benefit analysis should be undertaken before treating patients for latent TB with advanced liver disease, such as Child Pugh grade 3 and above, as the risks of life-threatening hepatotoxicity are high. Patients with raised baseline alanine transaminase (ALT) or AST should be closely monitored with repeat liver enzyme tests after 2 weeks, then monthly. With this in mind it is good practice to measure liver enzymes on all patients prior to starting LTBI treatment and, where possible, blood-borne virus screening should be done.[154]

Hepatotoxicity secondary to LTBI treatment defined as a rise in ALT of greater than 3 times the upper limit of normal with symptoms or greater than 5 times the upper limit of normal without symptoms necessitates stopping treatment. The frequency of occurrence varies between regimens and individuals based on preexisting risk. RIF monotherapy is rarely associated with drug-induced hepatitis but may cause a rise in bilirubin.[154] INH has been associated with fatal hepatotoxicity.[11,14,15] A study from a public health clinic in the United States, which looked at 3377 patients treated with INH for latent TB found hepatotoxicity, defined as a rise in AST to greater than 5 times the upper limit of normal, occurred at a rate of 5.6 per 1000 patients; the number of hepatotoxic events per 1000 patients after 1, 3, and 6 months were 2.5, 7.2, and 4.1, respectively. There was also a strong association between hepatotoxicity and age with events occurring at a rate of 4.4 per 1000 patients in those aged 25–34 years compared to 20.8 per 1000 patients in those aged over 50 years.[155,156] RPT/INH weekly treatment has been shown to be associated with a lower rate of hepatotoxicity compared to daily INH for 9 months. A study of 6862 participants found hepatotoxicity developed in 1.8% of patients receiving 9 months of INH compared to 0.4% of those receiving 3 months of RPT/INH. One of the risk factors identified for hepatotoxicity was hepatitis C infection, strengthening the argument for screening all latent TB patients for hepatitis prior to starting treatment, as well as closely monitoring these patients.[34]

COMPLETION OF TREATMENT

Completion of LTBI treatment is based not only on the duration of therapy but also on the total number of drug doses taken. For the 9-month INH monotherapy, the patient should receive at least 240 of the prescribed 270 doses of treatment within a year of starting therapy. For the 6-month INH regimen, 180 doses should be taken within 9 months of starting therapy. For the 3-month regimen of INH and RIF, 90 doses should be taken within 4 months and for the 4-month regimen of RIF monotherapy, 120 doses should be taken within 3 months. These regimens are usually self-directed so are more difficult to monitor other than by pill count. The weekly regimen of RPT/INH consists of 12 doses and successful therapy is defined as at least 11 doses of medication taken within 16 weeks of starting therapy.[34,37] If longer gaps in therapy than those given previously occur or if less than 75% of the prescribed doses are taken then retreatment should be considered after excluding the possibility of active TB. Supportive interventions such as dosette boxes, weekly key worker contacts, directly observed therapy, or video observed therapy should be considered for high risk individuals.[157] A review into completion of latent TB treatment looking at 54 studies found one of the main barriers to completing treatment was length of treatment, which would favor the use of shorter, especially intermittent, regimens such as RPT/INH, Also culturally specific case management was found to improve adherence, which is important to consider in services covering a diverse population group.[158] It should also be remembered that there is a high rate of drop out all the way through the care pathway of patients being screened and treated for LTBI, with a large proportion of patients not completing screening or starting treatment.[24]

RETREATMENT AND EXOGENOUS REINFECTION

There is not a body of evidence to support the retreatment of people who have been treated for LTBI or active TB who go on to develop a medical condition that puts them at risk of TB reactivation. Several scenarios bear consideration though. Firstly, if a person has previously been treated for active TB prior to the introduction of RIF or if the person's treatment for active TB was not completed, then LTBI treatment may be considered. Secondly, a person who has been reexposed to TB via, for example, a household contact, may benefit from repeat LTBI treatment. The contribution of exogenous reinfection with TB versus reactivation of latent disease even after previous treatment has become more clear with the widespread advent of typing. In the low TB incidence countries like United States and Italy, about 15%–23% of late recurrent TB cases are due to exogenous reinfection, respectively. This figure rises to 60% in certain groups such as recent immigrants who may be frequently reexposed to TB. In China, a high burden TB country, over 60% of recurrent TB cases have been shown to be due to exogenous reinfection.[159–161]

Lastly, people with fibrotic chest radiograph changes who have been previously treated for active or LTBI should be monitored closely if they undergo immunosuppressive treatment.

CONTACTS OF DRUG-RESISTANT TB CASES

There is sparse evidence on the correct approach to take with regard to chemoprophylaxis of LTBI in people exposed to drug-resistant TB (DRTB). Often the drug sensitivity of the index case

is not known in which case use of standard chemoprophylaxis is indicated even for patients with LTBI from high DRTB incidence countries. For mono-resistant TB it seems logical to use the agent that the index case is sensitive to, so 4 months of daily RIF can be used for contacts of an INH mono-resistant index case and 6–9 months of INH monotherapy can be used for contact with RIF mono-resistant index cases. The situation is more difficult for contacts of multidrug-resistant index cases.

There are estimated to be around 490,000 cases of multidrug-resistant TB (MDRTB) in the world in 2016, with around 190,000 deaths.[59] These MDRTB cases may generate upwards of 3 million cases of latent MDRTB.[162] The need for effective chemoprophylaxis is great as MDRTB is much more difficult to treat, needs longer treatment, and uses more toxic, less well-tolerated agents than drug-sensitive TB. Outcomes are also poor compared to drug-sensitive TB, so the potential gain from preventing MDRTB on an individual as well as population level is potentially greater than that of drug-sensitive TB.

There is lack of consensus on how to manage people with latent MDRTB infection. Some guidelines recommend close monitoring for 24 months, others advise individualized chemoprophylaxis.[163,164] Both approaches will be discussed in the following section. Currently, there is a lack of good quality randomized trials on the effectiveness of chemoprophylaxis in these cases, but three trials are underway that may provide a useful guide. The three trials started recruiting in 2015 and will report hopefully by 2020. TB CHAMP (child multidrug-resistant preventive therapy) is being conducted in South Africa on children under 5 years. It is looking at levofloxacin versus placebo for 6 months and will follow patients for 18 months. PHOENix (Protecting Households On Exposure to Newly Diagnosed Index) is a multicenter trial recruiting adults and children looking at delamanid versus INH for 6 months with 22 months of follow-up and Levofloxacin versus placebo for the treatment of latent tuberculosis among contacts of patients with multidrug-resistant tuberculosis (V-QUIN MDRTB). The trial is recruiting adults and children in Vietnam, looking at 6 months of levofloxacin versus placebo with 30 months of follow-up.

Until these trials report there are two possible strategies for patients with possible latent MDRTB. Firstly, close observation for 24 months as recommended by WHO.[6] This strategy involves identifying and registering contacts of MDRTB cases and performing clinical follow-up for at least 2 years, the period of highest risk of developing active TB. This strategy is far from passive and involves much effort to keep the patients involved, engaged, and not lost to follow-up. Early detection of active TB in these patients should allow the institution of appropriate therapy at an early stage of disease before significant lung damage has occurred, and could reduce the risk to others by allowing the patient to be isolated and rendered noninfectious.[165]

The second strategy involves giving targeted chemoprophylaxis based on the sensitivity of the index case isolate or based on the epidemiology of isolates in the area concerned. A study from the Federated States of Micronesia looked at 119 contacts of MDRTB patients. All were offered chemoprophylaxis. One hundred and four patients initiated chemoprophylaxis with daily fluoroquinolone-based regimens for 12 months either alone or with ethambutol or ethionamide depending on the index case sensitivity; 15 participants refused to take treatment. No cases of MDRTB were detected in the 104 patients given treatment compared to 3/15 cases in those who refused treatment. No serious adverse effects were reported.[166] In a South African study of children who were contacts of ofloxacin-sensitive MDRTB patients, ofloxacin, ethambutol, and high dose INH for 6 months were given to 186 children regardless of skin test results, including HIV infected children. 3.2% of children developed TB, which is lower than the rates in historical controls. 3.7% of children developed a serious adverse effect and one child died.[167] This compares to the observation from the same setting of 29/125 (29%) of MDRTB exposed but untreated children who went on to develop active MDRTB during a 30-month follow-up period.[168]

The overall quality of evidence in favor of treating contacts of MDRTB patients with chemoprophylaxis remains poor but a fluoroquinolone and ethambutol combination appears promising if the index case is sensitive. Current guidelines are therefore mainly based on expert opinion. A recent systematic review and meta-analyses reported that of the studies assessed, there was a 90% (9%–99%) reduction in MDRTB incidence among those receiving chemoprophylaxis; fluoroquinolone/ethambutol regimens had the greatest cost-effectiveness.[169] Until clinical trial evidence is available, decisions around chemoprophylaxis should be based on local guidelines and conducted by centers experienced in the management of MDRTB.

PREGNANCY AND LACTATION

INH and RIF are safe for women to take during pregnancy, but women diagnosed with LTBI while pregnant can be treated after delivery. In some high risk cases such as women with advanced HIV infection, treatment of LTBI during pregnancy may be considered, but with the advent of highly effective ART, which is usually given during pregnancy, the risk of these women developing TB has been reduced, allowing LTBI treatment to be deferred.

An evaluation of pregnancies that occurred during two large trials of 12 weekly doses of INH/RPT and 9 months of INH alone for the treatment of latent TB found no excess of fetal abnormalities or fetal loss in either treatment group among 126 pregnancies that occurred during treatment or follow-up, including 87 pregnancies where the mother was exposed to the study drugs, compared to the background rate for the United States.[170]

There is some evidence that women are more likely to develop active TB during the first 180 days postpartum period, so starting LTBI treatment postpartum maybe particularly effective. There is some suggestion that hepatotoxicity due to INH is more likely in the puerperal period, so liver enzyme monitoring is suggested.[171,172]

Breastfeeding is safe while taking LTBI treatment. INH is found in breast milk at concentrations 20% of that in plasma. This probably does not pose a risk to a breastfeeding infant, although some authorities recommend giving pyridoxine to premature or low weight breastfed infants in these cases.

REFERENCES

1. Houben RMGJ, and Dodd PJ. The global burden of latent tuberculosis infection: A re-estimation using mathematical modelling. *PLoS Med.* 2016;13:e1002152.
2. LoBue P, and Menzies D. Treatment of latent tuberculosis infection an update. *Respirology.* 2010;15(4): 603–22.
3. WHO. *End TB Strategy.* Geneva: WHO. Available at: http://www.who.int/tb/strategy/End_TB_Strategy.pdf?ua=1 (accessed March 6, 2017).
4. National Institute for Health and Clinical Excellence (NICE). Tuberculosis (NG33), London. Available at: https://www.nice.org.uk/guidance/ng33.
5. Centers for Disease Control and Prevention. Latent tuberculosis infection a guide for primary health care providers. Atlanta. Available at: https://www.cdc.gov/tb/publications/ltbi/treatment.htm.
6. Getahun H et al. Management of latent *Mycobacterium tuberculosis* infection: WHO guidelines for low tuberculosis burden countries. *Eur Respir J.* 2015;46(6):1563–76.
7. van't Hoog AH, Meme HK, Laserson KF, Agaya JA, Muchiri BG, Githui WA, Odeny LO, Marston BJ, and Borgdorff MW. Screening strategies for tuberculosis prevalence surveys: The value of chest radiography and symptoms. *PLOS ONE.* 2012;7(7):e38691.
8. Getahun H et al. Development of a standardized screening rule for tuberculosis in people living with HIV in resource-constrained settings: Individual participant data meta-analysis of observational studies. *PLoS Med.* 2011 Jan 18;8(1):e1000391.
9. Watkins RE, Brennan R, and Plant AJ. Tuberculin reactivity and the risk of tuberculosis: A review. *Int J Tuberc Lung Dis.* 2000;4(10):895–903.
10. Kahwati LC, Feltner C, Halpern M, Woodell CL, Boland E, Amick HR, Weber RP, and Jonas DE. *Screening for Latent Tuberculosis Infection in Adults: An Evidence Review for the U.S. Preventive Services Task Force [Internet].* Rockville, MD: Agency for Healthcare Research and Quality (US), 2016 Sep. Available at: http://www.ncbi.nlm.nih.gov/books/NBK385122/
11. Comstock GW, Baum C, and Snider DE Jr. Isoniazid prophylaxis among Alaskan Eskimos: A final report of the bethel isoniazid studies. *Am Rev Respir Dis.* 1979;119(5):827–30.
12. Akolo C, Adetifa I, Shepperd S, and Volmink J. Treatment of latent tuberculosis infection in HIV infected persons. *Cochrane Database Syst Rev.* 2010;(1):CD000171.
13. Zenner D, Beer N, Harris RJ, Lipman MC, Stagg HR, and van der Werf MJ. Treatment of latent tuberculosis infection: An updated network meta-analysis. *Ann Intern Med.* 2017;167(4):248–55.
14. Comstock GW. How much isoniazid is needed for prevention of tuberculosis among immunocompetent adults? *Int J Tuberc Lung Dis.* 1999;3(10):847–50.
15. Comstock GW. Prevention of tuberculosis among tuberculin reactors: Maximizing benefits, minimizing risks. *JAMA.* 1986;256(19):2729–30.
16. Churchyard GJ, Fielding KL, Lewis JJ, Coetzee L, Corbett EL, Godfrey-Faussett P, Hayes RJ, Chaisson RE, Grant AD, and Thibela TB Study Team. A trial of mass isoniazid preventive therapy for tuberculosis control. *N Engl J Med.* 2014;370(4):301–10.
17. Ayieko J, Abuogi L, Simchowitz B, Bukusi EA, Smith AH, and Reingold A. Efficacy of isoniazid prophylactic therapy in prevention of tuberculosis in children: A meta-analysis. *BMC Infect Dis.* 2014;14:91.
18. Menzies D et al. Four months of rifampin or nine months of isoniazid for latent tuberculosis in adults. *N Engl J Med.* 2018 Aug 2;379(5):440–53.

19. Hong Kong Chest Service. A controlled clinical comparison of 6 and 8 months of antituberculosis chemotherapy in the treatment of patients with silicotuberculosis in Hong Kong. Hong Kong Chest Service/tuberculosis Research Centre, Madras/British Medical Research Council. *Am Rev Respir Dis*. 1991;143(2):262–7.

20. Sharma SK, Sharma A, Kadhiravan T, and Tharyan P. Rifamycins (rifampicin, rifabutin and rifapentine) compared to isoniazid for preventing tuberculosis in HIV-negative people at risk of active TB. *Cochrane Database Syst Rev*. 2013;(7):CD007545.

21. Hong Kong Chest Service/Tuberculosis Research Centre, Madras/British Medical Research Council. A double-blind placebo-controlled clinical trial of three antituberculosis chemoprophylaxis regimens in patients with silicosis in Hong Kong. *The American Review of Respiratory Disease*. 1992;145(1):36–41.

22. Menzies D, Dion MJ, Rabinovitch B, Mannix S, Brassard P, and Schwartzman K. Treatment completion and costs of a randomized trial of rifampin for 4 months versus isoniazid for 9 months. *Am J Respir Crit Care Med*. 2004;170(4):445–9.

23. den Boon S, Matteelli A, and Getahun H. Rifampicin resistance after treatment for latent tuberculous infection: A systematic review and meta-analysis. *Int J Tuberc Lung Dis*. 2016;20(8):1065–71.

24. Alsdurf H, Hill PC, Matteelli A, Getahun H, and Menzies D. The cascade of care in diagnosis and treatment of latent tuberculosis infection: A systematic review and meta-analysis. *Lancet Infect Dis*. 2016;16(11):1269–78.

25. Diallo T et al. Safety and side effects of rifampin versus isoniazid in children. *N Engl J Med*. 2018 Aug 2;379(5):454–63.

26. Ena J, and Valls V. Short-course therapy with rifampin plus isoniazid, compared with standard therapy with isoniazid, for latent tuberculosis infection: A meta-analysis. *Clin Infect Dis*. 2005;40(5):670–6.

27. Park SJ et al. Comparison of LTBI treatment regimens for patients receiving anti-tumour necrosis factor therapy. *Int J Tuberc Lung Dis*. 2015;19(3):342–8.

28. Spyridis NP et al. The effectiveness of a 9-month regimen of isoniazid alone versus 3- and 4-month regimens of isoniazid plus rifampin for treatment of latent tuberculosis infection in children: Results of an 11-year randomized study. *Clin Infect Dis*. 2007;45(6):715–22.

29. Galli L et al. Pediatric tuberculosis in Italian children: Epidemiological and clinical data from the Italian register of pediatric tuberculosis. *Int J Mol Sci*. 2016;17(6):pii: E960.

30. van Zyl S, Marais BJ, Hesseling AC, Gie RP, Beyers N, and Schaaf HS. Adherence to anti-tuberculosis chemoprophylaxis and treatment in children. *Int J Tuberc Lung Dis*. 2006;10(1):13–8.

31. Blake MJ, Abdel-Rahman SM, Jacobs RF, Lowery NK, Sterling TR, and Kearns GL. Pharmacokinetics of rifapentine in children. *Pediatr Infect Dis J*. 2006;25(5):405–9.

32. Ji B, Truffot-Pernot C, Lacroix C, Raviglione MC, O'Brien RJ, Olliaro P, Roscigno G, and Grosset J. Effectiveness of rifampin, rifabutin, and rifapentine for preventive therapy of tuberculosis in mice. *Am Rev Respir Dis*. 1993;148(6 Pt 1):1541–6.

33. Weiner M et al. Pharmacokinetics of rifapentine at 600, 900, and 1,200 mg during once-weekly tuberculosis therapy. *Am J Respir Crit Care Med*. 2004;169(11):1191–7.

34. Sterling TR et al. Three months of rifapentine and isoniazid for latent tuberculosis infection. *N Engl J Med*. 2011;365(23):2155–66.

35. Bliven-Sizemore EE, Sterling TR, Shang N, Benator D, Schwartzman K, Reves R, Drobeniuc J, Bock N, Villarino ME, and TB Trials Consortium. Three months of weekly rifapentine plus isoniazid is less hepatotoxic than nine months of daily isoniazid for LTBI. *Int J Tuberc Lung Dis*. 2015;19(9):1039–44.

36. Moro RN et al. Exposure to latent tuberculosis treatment during pregnancy: The PREVENT TB and the iAdhere Trials. *Ann Am Thorac Soc*. 2018;15(5):570–80. doi: 10.1513/AnnalsATS.201704-326OC.

37. Sterling TR et al. Three months of weekly rifapentine and isoniazid for treatment of *Mycobacterium tuberculosis* infection in HIV-coinfected persons. *AIDS*. 2016;30(10):1607–15

38. Swindells S et al. One month of rifapentine plus isoniazid to prevent HIV-related tuberculosis. *N Engl J Med*. 2019;380:1001–11.

39. Sterling TR, Moro RN, Borisov AS, Phillips E, Shepherd G, Adkinson NF, Weis S, Ho C, and Villrino ME, Tuberculosis Trials Consortium. Flu-like and other systemic drug reactions among persons receiving weekly rifapentine plus isoniazid or daily isoniazid for treatment of latent tuberculosis infection in the PREVENT tuberculosis study. *Clin Infect Dis*. 2015;61(4):527–35.

40. Shepardson D et al. Cost-effectiveness of a 12-dose regimen for treating latent tuberculous infection in the United States. *Int J Tuberc Lung Dis*. 2013;17(12):1531–7.

41. Weiner M et al. Rifapentine pharmacokinetics and tolerability in children and adults treated once weekly with rifapentine and isoniazid for latent tuberculosis infection. *J Pediatric Infect Dis Soc*. 2014;3(2):132–45.

42. Borisov AS et al. Update of recommendations for use of once-weekly isoniazid-rifapentine regimen to treat latent *Mycobacterium tuberculosis* infection. *MMWR Morb Mortal Wkly Rep*. 2018 Jun 29;67(25):723–6.

43. Diallo T et al. Safety and side effects of rifampin versus isoniazid in children. *N Engl J Med*. 2018 Aug 2;379(5):454–63.

44. Njie GJ, Morris SB, Woodruff RY, Moro RN, Vernon AA, and Borisov AS. Isoniazid-rifapentine for latent tuberculosis infection: A systematic review and meta-analysis. 2018;55(2):244–52.

45. Villarino ME et al. Treatment for preventing tuberculosis in children and adolescents: A randomized clinical trial of a 3-month, 12-dose regimen of a combination of rifapentine and isoniazid. *JAMA Pediatr*. 2015;169(3):247–55.

46. Gordin F et al. Rifampin and pyrazinamide vs isoniazid for prevention of tuberculosis in HIV-infected persons: An international randomized trial. Terry Beirn Community Programs for Clinical Research on AIDS, the Adult AIDS Clinical Trials Group, the Pan American Health Organization, and the Centers for Disease Control and Prevention Study Group. *JAMA*. 2000; 283:1445–50.

47. Nolan CM, Goldberg SV, and Buskin SE. Hepatotoxicity associated with isoniazid preventive therapy: A 7-year survey from a public health tuberculosis clinic. *JAMA*. 1999;281:1014–8.

48. Lee AM et al. Risk factors for hepatotoxicity associated with rifampin and pyrazinamide for the treatment of latent tuberculosis infection: Experience from three public health tuberculosis clinics. *Int J Tuberc Lung Dis*. 2002;6:995–1000.

49. Gao XF, Wang L, Liu GJ, Wen J, Sun X, Xie Y, and Li YP. Rifampicin plus pyrazinamide versus isoniazid for treating latent tuberculosis infection: A meta-analysis. *Int J Tuberc Lung Dis*. 2006 Oct;10(10):1080–90.

50. McNeill L et al. Pyrazinamide and rifampin vs isoniazid for the treatment of latent tuberculosis: Improved completion rates but more hepatotoxicity. *Chest*. 2003;123:102–6.

51. Horsburgh CR Jr, and Rubin EJ. Clinical practice. Latent tuberculosis infection in the United States. *NEJM*. 2011;364(15):1441–8.

52. Keane J, Gershon S, Wise RP, Mirabile-Levens E, Kasznica J, Schwieterman WD, Siegel JN, and Braun MM. Tuberculosis associated with infliximab, a tumor necrosis factor alpha-neutralizing agent. *N Engl J Med*. 2001 Oct 11;345(15):1098–104.

53. Ferebee SH. Controlled chemoprophylaxis trials in tuberculosis. A general review. *Bibl Tuberc.* 1970;26:28–106.

54. Nolan CM, Aitken ML, Elarth AM, Anderson KM, and Miller WT. Active tuberculosis after isoniazid chemoprophylaxis of Southeast Asian refugees. *Am Rev Respir Dis.* 1986;133(3):431–6.

55. Grzybowski S, Fishaut H, Rowe J, and Brown A. Tuberculosis among patients with various radiologic abnormalities, followed by the chest clinic service. *Am Rev Respir Dis.* 1971;104(4):605–8.

56. Feng M, Yang X, Ma Q, and He Y. Retrospective analysis for the false positive diagnosis of PET-CT scan in lung cancer patients. *Medicine (Baltim).* 2017;96(42):e7415.

57. International Union Against Tuberculosis Committee on Prophylaxis. Efficacy of various durations of isoniazid preventive therapy for tuberculosis: Five years of follow-up in the IUAT trial. *Bull World Health Organ.* 1982;60(4):555–67.

58. Falk A, and Fuchs GF. Prophylaxis with isoniazid in inactive tuberculosis. A Veterans Administration Cooperative Study XII. *Chest.* 1978;73(1):44–8.

59. World Health Organisation. *Global Tuberculosis Report 2017*, 2017.

60. Selwyn PA, Hartel D, Lewis VA, Schoenbaum EE, Vermund SH, Klein RS, Walker AT, and Friedland GH. A prospective study of the risk of tuberculosis among intravenous drug users with human immunodeficiency virus infection. *N Engl J Med.* 1989;320(9):545–50.

61. Markowitz N et al. Tuberculin and anergy testing in HIV-seropositive and HIV-seronegative persons. Pulmonary Complications of HIV Infection Study Group. *Ann Intern Med.* 1993 Aug 1;119(3):185–93.

62. Kufa T, Chihota VN, Charalambous S, and Churchyard GJ. Isoniazid preventive therapy use among patients on antiretroviral therapy: A missed opportunity. *Int J Tuberc Lung Dis.* 2014;18(3):312–4.

63. Rangaka MX et al. Isoniazid plus antiretroviral therapy to prevent tuberculosis: A randomised double-blind, placebo-controlled trial. *Lancet.* 2014 Aug;384(9944):682–90.

64. *Recommendation on 36 Months Isoniazid Preventive Therapy to Adults and Adolescents Living with HIV in Resource-Constrained and High TB- and HIV-Prevalence Settings: 2015 Update.* Geneva: World Health Organization, 2015.

65. Thindwa D, MacPherson P, Choko AT, Khundi M, Sambakunsi R, Ngwira LG, Kalua T, Webb EL, and Corbett EL. Completion of isoniazid preventive therapy among human immunodeficiency virus positive adults in urban Malawi. *Int J Tuberc Lung Dis.* 2018;22(3):273–9.

66. Namuwenge PM, Mukonzo JK, Kiwanuka N, Wanyenze R, Byaruhanga R, Bissell K, and Zachariah R. Loss to follow up from isoniazid preventive therapy among adults attending HIV voluntary counseling and testing sites in Uganda. *Trans R Soc Trop Med Hyg.* 2012;106(2):84–9.

67. *British HIV Association guidelines for the management of HIV/TB co-infection in adults 2017.* London: BHIVA. Available at: http://www.bhiva.org/documents/Guidelines/TB/BHIVA-TB-HIV-co-infection-guidelines-consultation.pdf (accessed April 2, 2018).

68. Grant AD, Mngadi KT, van Halsema CL, Luttig MM, Fielding KL, and Churchyard GJ. Adverse events with isoniazid preventive therapy: Experience from a large trial. *AIDS.* 2010;24(Suppl 5):S29–36.

69. Manabe YC et al. The aerosol rabbit model of TB latency, reactivation and immune reconstitution inflammatory syndrome. *Tuberculosis (Edinb).* 2008;88(3):187–96.

70. Scanga CA, Mohan VP, Joseph H, Yu K, Chan J, and Flynn JL. Reactivation of latent tuberculosis: Variations on the Cornell murine model. *Infect Immun.* 1999;67(9):4531–8.

71. Haanaes OC, and Bergmann A. Tuberculosis emerging in patients treated with corticosteroids. *Eur J Respir Dis.* 1983;64(4):294–7.

72. Lim CH et al. The risk of tuberculosis disease in rheumatoid arthritis patients on biologics and targeted therapy: A 15-year real world experience in Taiwan. *PLOS ONE.* 2017 Jun 1;12(6):e0178035.

73. Bourikas LA, Kourbeti IS, Koutsopoulos AV, and Koutroubakis IE. Disseminated tuberculosis in a Crohn's disease patient on anti-TNF alpha therapy despite chemoprophylaxis. *Gut.* 2008;57:425.

74. Cantini F, Niccoli L, and Goletti D. Adalimumab, etanercept, infliximab, and the risk of tuberculosis: Data from clinical trials, national registries, and postmarketing surveillance. *J Rheumatol Suppl.* 2014;91:47–55.

75. Unlu M, Cimen P, Ayranci A, Akarca T, Karaman O, and Dereli MS. Disseminated tuberculosis infection and paradoxical reaction during antimycobacterial treatment related to TNF-alpha blocker agent Infliximab. *Respir Med Case Rep.* 2014;13:43–7.

76. Harris J, and Keane J. How tumour necrosis factor blockers interfere with tuberculosis immunity. *Clin Exp Immunol.* 2010;161(1):1–9.

77. Solovic I et al. The risk of tuberculosis related to tumour necrosis factor antagonist therapies: A TBNET consensus statement. *Eur Respir J.* 2010;36(5):1185–206

78. Ai JW, Zhang S, Ruan QL, Yu YQ, Zhang BY, Liu QH, and Zhang WH. The risk of tuberculosis in patients with rheumatoid arthritis treated with tumor necrosis factor-α antagonist: A meta-analysis of both randomized controlled trials and registry/cohort studies. *J Rheumatol.* 2015;42(12):2229–37.

79. Shim TS. Diagnosis and treatment of latent tuberculosis infection due to initiation of anti-TNF therapy. *Tuberc Respir Dis (Seoul).* 2014;76(6):261–8.

80. Cantini F, Niccoli L, and Goletti D. Tuberculosis risk in patients treated with non-anti-tumor necrosis factor-α (TNF-α) targeted biologics and recently licensed TNF-α inhibitors: Data from clinical trials and national registries. *J Rheumatol Suppl.* 2014;91:56–64.

81. Holzschuh EL et al. Use of video directly observed therapy for treatment of latent tuberculosis infection—Johnson County, Kansas, 2015. *MMWR Morb Mortal Wkly Rep.* 2017;66(14):387–9.

82. Reichman LB, Felton CP, and Edsall JR. Drug dependence, a possible new risk factor for tuberculosis disease. *Arch Intern Med.* 1979;139(3):337–9.

83. Caylà JA, García de Olalla P, Galdós-Tangüis H, Vidal R, López-Colomés JL, Gatell JM, and Jansà JM. The influence of intravenous drug use and HIV infection in the transmission of tuberculosis. *AIDS.* 1996;10(1):95–100.

84. Batki SL, Gruber VA, Bradley JM, Bradley M, and Delucchi K. A controlled trial of methadone treatment combined with directly observed isoniazid for tuberculosis prevention in injection drug users. *Drug Alcohol Depend.* 2002;66(3):283–93.

85. Menzies D, Fanning A, Yuan L, and Fitzgerald M. Tuberculosis among health care workers. *N Engl J Med.* 1995;332(2):92–8.

86. Ticona E, Huaroto L, Kirwan DE, Chumpitaz M, Munayco CV, Maguiña M, Tovar MA, Evans CA, Escombe R, and Gilman RH. Impact of infection control measures to control an outbreak of multidrug-resistant tuberculosis in a human immunodeficiency Virus Ward, Peru. *Am J Trop Med Hyg.* 2016 Dec 7;95(6):1247–56.

87. Nasreen S, Shokoohi M, and Malvankar-Mehta MS. Prevalence of latent tuberculosis among health care workers in high burden countries: A systematic review and meta-analysis. *PLOS ONE.* 2016 Oct 6;11(10):e0164034

88. Corbett EL et al. Nursing and community rates of *Mycobacterium tuberculosis* infection among students in Harare, Zimbabwe. *Clin Infect Dis.* 2007;44(3):317–23.

89. Uden L, Barber E, Ford N, and Cooke GS. Risk of tuberculosis infection and disease for health care workers: An updated meta-analysis. *Open Forum Infect Dis.* 2017 Aug 29;4(3):ofx137.

90. Schepisi MS, Sotgiu G, Contini S, Puro V, Ippolito G, and Girardi E. Tuberculosis transmission from healthcare workers to patients and co-workers: A systematic literature review and meta-analysis. *PLOS ONE.* 2015 Apr 2;10(4):e0121639.

91. United Nations Department of Economic and Social Affairs Population Division. *International Migration Report 2017.* Geneva: United Nations, 2017. Available at: http://www.un.org/en/development/desa/population/migration/publications/migrationreport/docs/MigrationReport2017_Highlights.pdf (accessed March 24, 2018).

92. Tuberculosis in England. *2017 Report Public Health England.* Available at: https://www.gov.uk/government/publications/tuberculosis-in-england-annual-report.

93. Baussano I, Mercadante S, Pareek M, Lalvani A, and Bugiani M. High rates of *Mycobacterium tuberculosis* among socially marginalized immigrants in low-incidence area, 1991–2010, Italy. *Emerg Infect Dis.* 2013;19(9):1437–45.

94. Pareek M, Watson JP, Ormerod LP, Kon OM, Woltmann G, White PJ, Abubakar I, and Lalvani A. Screening of immigrants in the UK for imported latent tuberculosis: A multicentre cohort study and cost-effectiveness analysis. *Lancet Infect Dis.* 2011;11(6):435–44.

95. Walker TM et al. A cluster of multidrug-resistant *Mycobacterium tuberculosis* among patients arriving in Europe from the Horn of Africa: A molecular epidemiological study. *Lancet Infect Dis.* 2018 Jan 8. pii: S1473-3099(18)30004-5.

96. Abarca Tomás B, Pell C, Bueno Cavanillas A, Guillén Solvas J, Pool R, and Roura M. Tuberculosis in migrant populations. A systematic review of the qualitative literature. *PLOS ONE.* 2013;8(12):e82440.

97. Walker CL, Duffield K, Kaur H, Dedicoat M, and Gajraj R. Acceptability of latent tuberculosis testing of migrants in a college environment in England. *Public Health.* 2018;158:55–60.

98. Story A, Aldridge RW, Abubakar I, Stagg HR, Lipman M, Watson JM, and Hayward AC. Active case finding for pulmonary tuberculosis using mobile digital chest radiography: An observational study. *Int J Tuberc Lung Dis.* 2012;16(11):1461–7.

99. Aldridge RW et al. High prevalence of latent tuberculosis and bloodborne virus infection in a homeless population. *Thorax.* 2018 Jan 29. pii: thoraxjnl-2016-209579.

100. Dara M et al. Tuberculosis control in prisons: Current situation and research gaps. *Int J Infect Dis.* 2015;32:111–7.

101. European Centre for Disease Control. *Mathematical Modelling of Screening strategies for latent tuberculosis infection in countries with low tuberculosis incidence.* Stockholm, 2018. Available at: https://ecdc.europa.eu/sites/portal/files/documents/Technical-Report_LTBI_math_modelling.pdf (accessed March 25, 2018).

102. teWaterNaude JM et al. Tuberculosis and silica exposure in South African gold miners. *Occup Environ Med.* 2006;63:187–92.

103. Cowie RL. The epidemiology of tuberculosis in gold miners with silicosis. *Am J Respir Crit Care Med.* 1994; 150: 1460–2.

104. Paul R. Silicosis in Northern Rhodesian copper miners. *Arch Environ Health.* 1961;2:96–109.

105. Burke RM, Schwartz LP, and Snider DE Jr. The Ottawa County project: A report of a tuberculosis screening project in a small mining community. *Am J Public Health.* 1979 69(4):340–7.

106. Knight D, Ehrlich R, Fielding K, Jeffery H, Grant A, and Churchyard G. Trends in silicosis prevalence and the healthy worker effect among gold miners in South Africa: A prevalence study with follow up of employment status. *BMC Public Health.* 2015;15:1258.

107. Monaco A. Antituberculosis chemoprophylaxis in silicotics. *Bull Int Union Tuberc.* 1964;35:51–6.

108. Hong Kong Chest Service/Tuberculosis Research Centre, Madras/British Medical Research Council. A double-blind placebo-controlled clinical trial of three antituberculosis chemoprophylaxis regimens in patients with silicosis in Hong Kong. *Am Rev Respir Dis.* 1992;145(1):36–41.

109. International Diabetes Federation. *Diabetes Atlas.* 9th edition, 2019. Available at: http://diabetesatlas.org/en/resources/ (accessed February 25, 2018).

110. Workneh MH, Bjune GA, and Yimer SA. Prevalence and associated factors of tuberculosis and diabetes mellitus comorbidity: A systematic review. *PLOS ONE.* 2017 Apr 21;12(4):e0175925.

111. Al-Rifai RH, Pearson F, Critchley JA, and Abu-Raddad LJ. Association between diabetes mellitus and active tuberculosis: A systematic review and meta-analysis. *PLOS ONE.* 2017 Nov 21;12(11):e0187967.

112. Rayfield EJ, Ault MJ, Keusch GT, Brothers MJ, Nechemias C, and Smith H. Infection and diabetes: The case for glucose control. *Am J Med.* 1982 Mar;72(3):439–50.

113. Stalenhoef JE, Alisjahbana B, Nelwan EJ, van der Ven-Jongekrijg J, Ottenhoff TH, van der Meer JW, Nelwan RH, Netea MG, and van Crevel R. The role of interferon-gamma in the increased tuberculosis risk in type 2 diabetes mellitus. *Eur J Clin Microbiol Infect Dis.* 2008 Feb;27(2):97–103.

114. Bailey SL, Ayles H, Beyers N, Godfrey-Faussett P, Muyoyeta M, du Toit E, Yudkin JS, and Floyd S. The association of hyperglycaemia with prevalent tuberculosis: A population-based cross-sectional study. *BMC Infect Dis.* 2016;16(1):733.

115. Bailey SL, and Ayles H. Association between diabetes mellitus and active tuberculosis in Africa and the effect of HIV. *Trop Med Int Health.* 2017;22:261–8.

116. Lin HH, Wu CY, Wang CH, Fu H, Lönnroth K, Chang YC, and Huang YT. Association of obesity, diabetes, and risk of tuberculosis: Two population-based cohorts. *Clin Infect Dis.* 2018;66(5):699–705.

117. Lee MR, Huang YP, Kuo YT, Luo CH, Shih YJ, Shu CC, Wang JY, Ko JC, Yu CJ, and Lin HH. Diabetes mellitus and latent tuberculosis infection: A systemic review and meta-analysis. *Clin Infect Dis.* 2017 Mar 15;64(6):719–27.

118. Andrew OT, Schoenfeld PY, Hopewell PC, and Humphreys MH. Tuberculosis in patients with end-stage renal disease. *Am J Med.* 1980;68(1):59–65.

119. Belcon MC, Smith EK, Kahana LM, and Shimizu AG. Tuberculosis in dialysis patients. *Clin Nephrol.* 1982;17(1):14–8.

120. Hussein MM, Mooij JM, and Roujouleh H. Tuberculosis and chronic renal disease. *Semin Dial.* 2003;16(1):38–44.

121. Lundin AP, Adler AJ, Berlyne GM, and Friedman EA. Tuberculosis in patients undergoing maintenance hemodialysis. *Am J Med.* 1979;67(4):597–602.

122. Dobler CC, McDonald SP, and Marks GB. Risk of tuberculosis in dialysis patients: A nationwide cohort study. *PLOS ONE.* 2011;6(12):e29563.

123. Ostermann M, Palchaudhuri P, Riding A, Begum P, and Milburn HJ. Incidence of tuberculosis is high in chronic kidney disease patients in South East England and drug resistance common. *Ren Fail.* 2016;38(2):256–61.

124. Tamayo-Isla RA, de la Cruz MC, and Okpechi IG. Mycobacterial peritonitis in CAPD patients in Limpopo: A 6-year cumulative report from a single center in South Africa. *Perit Dial Int.* 2016;36(2):218–22.

125. Foster R, Ferguson TW, Rigatto C, Lerner B, Tangri N, and Komenda P. A retrospective review of the two-step tuberculin skin test in dialysis patients. *Can J Kidney Health Dis.* 2016;3:28.

126. British Thoracic Society Standards of Care Committee and Joint Tuberculosis Committee, Milburn H, Ashman N, Davies P, Doffman S, Drobniewski F, Khoo S, Ormerod P, Ostermann M,

and Snelson C. Guidelines for the prevention and management of *Mycobacterium tuberculosis* infection and disease in adult patients with chronic kidney disease. *Thorax.* 2010;65(6):557–70.

127. Naylor H, Robichaud J. Decreased tacrolimus levels after administration of rifampin to a patient with renal transplant. *Can J Hosp Pharm.* 2013;66(6):388–92.

128. Feld R, Bodey GP, and Gröschel D. Mycobacteriosis in patients with malignant disease. *Arch Intern Med.* 1976;136(1):67–70.

129. Simonsen DF, Farkas DK, Horsburgh CR, Thomsen RW, and Sørensen HT. Increased risk of active tuberculosis after cancer diagnosis. *J Infect.* 2017;74(6):590–8.

130. Edwards LB, Livesay VT, Acquaviva FA, and Palmer CE. Height, weight, tuberculous infection, and tuberculous disease. *Arch Environ Health.* 1971;22:106–12.

131. Palmer CE, Jablon S, and Edwards PQ. Tuberculosis morbidity of young men in relation to tuberculin sensitivity and body build. *Am Rev Tuberc.* 1957;76(4):517–39.

132. Lo ̈nnroth K, Williams BG, Cegielski P, and Dye C.A consistent log- linear relationship between tuberculosis incidence and body mass index. *Int J Epidemiol.* 2010;39:149–55.

133. Saag LA, LaValley MP, Hochberg NS, Cegielski JP, Pleskunas JA, Linas BP, and Horsburgh CR. Low body mass index and latent tuberculous infection: A systematic review and meta-analysis. *Int J Tuberc Lung Dis.* 2018;22(4):358–65.

134. Compher C. The impact of protein-calorie malnutrition on drugs. In: Boullata J, Armenti V (eds.). *Handbook of Drug- Nutrient Interactions.* Totowa, NJ, USA: Humana Press, 2005.

135. Cegielski JP, Arab L, and Cornoni-Huntley J. Nutritional risk factors for tuberculosis among adults in the United States, 1971–1992. *Am J Epidemiol.* 2012;176:409–22.

136. Allison ST. Pulmonary tuberculosis after subtotal gastrectomy. *N Engl J Med.* 1955;252(2):862–3.

137. WHO Korea 2016. Available at: https://extranet.who.int/sree/Reports?opReplet&name=%2FWHO_HQ_Reports%2FG2%2FPROD%2FEXT%2FTBCountryProfile&ISO2=KR&LANEN&outtypehtml.

138. Jung WJ et al. Treatment outcomes of patients treated for pulmonary tuberculosis after undergoing gastrectomy. *Tohoku J Exp Med.* 2016 Dec;240(4):281–6.

139. Jung WJ et al. Risk factors for tuberculosis after gastrectomy in gastric cancer. *World J Gastroenterol.* 2016 Feb 28;22(8):2585–91.

140. Bruce RM, and Wise L. Tuberculosis after jejunoileal bypass for obesity. *Ann Intern Med.* 1977;87:574–6.

141. Pickleman JR, Evans LS, Kane JM, and Freeark RJ. Tuberculosis after jejunoileal bypass for obesity. *JAMA.* 1975;234:744.

142. Alhajri K, Alzerwi N, Alsaleh K, Yousef HB, and Alzaben M. Disseminated (miliary) abdominal tuberculosis after laparoscopic gastric bypass surgery. *BMJ Case Rep.* 2011 May 12;2011. pii: bcr1220103591.

143. Webb GB. The effect of the inhalation of cigarette smoke on the lungs. *American Review of Tuberculosis.* March 1918;2:25–7.

144. Jayes L, Haslam PL, Gratziou CG, Powell P, Britton J, Vardavas C, Jimenez-Ruiz C, Leonardi-Bee J, and Tobacco Control Committee of the European Respiratory Society. SmokeHaz: Systematic reviews and meta-analyses of the effects of smoking on respiratory health. *Chest.* 2016;150(1):164–79.

145. Bishwakarma R, Kinney WH, Honda JR, Mya J, Strand MJ, Gangavelli A, Bai X, Ordway DJ, Iseman MD, and Chan ED. Epidemiologic link between tuberculosis and cigarette/biomass smoke exposure: Limitations despite the vast literature. *Respirology.* 2015;20(4):556–68.

146. van Zyl-Smit RN, Brunet L, Pai M, and Yew WW. The convergence of the global smoking, COPD, tuberculosis, HIV, and respiratory infection epidemics. *Infect Dis Clin North Am.* 2010;24:693–703.

147. Slama K, Chiang CY, Enarson DA, Hassmiller K, Fanning A, Gupta P, and Ray C. Tobacco and tuberculosis: A qualitative systematic review and meta-analysis. *Int J Tuberc Lung Dis.* 2007 Oct;11(10):1049–61.

148. Lin HH, Ezzati M, and Murray M. Tobacco smoke, indoor air pollution and tuberculosis: A systematic review and meta-analysis. *PLoS Med.* 2007 Jan;4(1):e20.

149. Bates MN, Khalakdina A, Pai M, Chang L, Lessa F, and Smith KR. Risk of tuberculosis from exposure to tobacco smoke: A systematic review and meta-analysis. *Arch Intern Med.* 2007 Feb 26;167(4):335–42.

150. Dogar OF, Pillai N, Safadr N, Shah SK, Zahid R, and Siddiqi K. Second-hand smoke and the risk of tuberculosis: A systematic review and a meta-analysis. *Epidemiol Infect.* 2015;143:3158–72.

151. Menzies D, Gardiner G, Farhat M, Greenaway C, and Pai M. Thinking in three dimensions: A web-based algorithm to aid the interpretation of tuberculin skin test results. *Int J Tuberc Lung Dis.* 2008 May;12(5):498–505

152. The Online TST/IGRA Interpretor. Available at: http://www.tstin3d.com/en/calc.html (accessed February 27, 2018).

153. Jordan TJ, Lewit EM, and Reichman LB. Isoniazid preventive therapy for tuberculosis. Decision analysis considering ethnicity and gender. *Am Rev Respir Dis.* 1991;144(6):1357–60.

154. Saukkonen JJ et al. An official ATS statement: Hepatotoxicity of antituberculosis therapy. *Am J Respir Crit Care Med.* 2006;174:935–52.

155. Fountain FF, Tolley E, Chrisman CR, and Self TH. Isoniazid hepatotoxicity associated with treatment of latent tuberculosis infection: A 7-year evaluation from a public health tuberculosis clinic. *Chest.* 2005 Jul;128(1):116–23.

156. Fountain FF, Tolley EA, Jacobs AR, and Self TH. Rifampin hepatotoxicity associated with treatment of latent tuberculosis infection. *Am J Med Sci.* 2009;337(5):317–20.

157. Stuurman AL, Vonk Noordegraaf-Schouten M, van Kessel F, Oordt-Speets AM, Sandgren A, and van der Werf MJ. Interventions for improving adherence to treatment for latent tuberculosis infection: A systematic review. *BMC Infect Dis.* 2016;16:257.

158. Liu Y, Birch S, Newbold KB, and Essue BM. Barriers to treatment adherence for individuals with latent tuberculosis infection: A systematic search and narrative synthesis of the literature. *Int J Health Plann Manage.* 2018;33(2):e416–433.

159. Interrante JD, Haddad MB, Kim L, and Gandhi NR. Exogenous reinfection as a cause of late recurrent tuberculosis in the United States. *Ann Am Thorac Soc.* 2015;12(11):1619–26.

160. Schiroli C et al. Exogenous reinfection of tuberculosis in a low-burden area. *Infection.* 2015 Dec;43(6):647–53.

161. Shen G, Xue Z, Shen X, Sun B, Gui X, Shen M, Mei J, and Gao Q. The study recurrent tuberculosis and exogenous reinfection, Shanghai, China. *Emerg Infect Dis.* 2006;12(11):1776–8.

162. Moore DA. What can we offer to 3 million MDRTB household contacts in 2016? *BMC Med.* 2016;14:64.

163. van der Werf MJ, Langendam MW, Sandgren A, and Manissero D. Lack of evidence to support policy development for management of contacts of multidrug-resistant tuberculosis patients: Two systematic reviews. *Int J Tuberc Lung Dis.* 2012;16(3):288–96.

164. van der Werf MJ, Sandgren A, and Manissero D. Management of contacts of multidrug-resistant tuberculosis patients in the European Union and European Economic Area. *Int J Tuberc Lung Dis.* 2012;16(3):426.

165. Attamna A, Chemtob D, Attamna S, Fraser A, Rorman E, Paul M, and Leibovici L. Risk of tuberculosis in close contacts of patients with multidrug resistant tuberculosis: A nationwide cohort. *Thorax*. 2009 Mar;64(3):271.

166. Bamrah S, Brostrom R, Dorina F, Setik L, Song R, Kawamura LM, Heetderks A, and Mase S. Treatment for LTBI in contacts of MDR-TB patients, Federated States of Micronesia, 2009–2012. *Int J Tuberc Lung Dis*. 2014 Aug;18(8):912–8.

167. Seddon JA, Hesseling AC, Finlayson H, Fielding K, Cox H, Hughes J, Godfrey-Faussett P, and Schaaf HS. Preventive therapy for child contacts of multidrug-resistant tuberculosis: A prospective cohort study. *Clin Infect Dis*. 2013;57(12):1676–84.

168. Schaaf HS, Gie RP, Kennedy M, Beyers N, Hesseling PB, and Donald PR. Evaluation of young children in contact with adult multidrug-resistant pulmonary tuberculosis: A 30-month follow-up. *Pediatrics*. 2002 May;109(5):765–71.

169. Marks SM, Mase SR, and Morris SB. Systematic review, meta-analysis, and cost-effectiveness of treatment of latent tuberculosis to reduce progression to multidrug-resistant tuberculosis. *Clin Infect Dis*. 2017 Jun 15;64(12):1670–7.

170. Moro RN, Borisov AS, Saukkonen J, Khan A, Sterling TR, Villarino ME, Scott NA, Shang N, Kerrigan A, and Goldberg SV. Factors associated with noncompletion of latent tuberculosis infection treatment: Experience from the PREVENT TB trial in the United States and Canada. *Clin Infect Dis*. 2016;62(11):1390–400.

171. Gupta A et al. Postpartum tuberculosis incidence and mortality among HIV-infected women and their infants in Pune, India, 2002–2005. *Clin Infect Dis*. 2007;45(2):241–9.

172. Malhamé I, Cormier M, Sugarman J, and Schwartzman K. Latent tuberculosis in pregnancy: A systematic review. *PLOS ONE*. 2016 May 5;11(5):e0154825.

173. Gómez-Reino JJ, Carmona L, Angel Descalzo M, and BIOBADASER Group. Risk of tuberculosis in patients treated with tumor necrosis factor antagonists due to incomplete prevention of reactivation of latent infection. *Arthritis Rheum*. 2007;57(5):756–61.

174. Tubach F et al. Risk of tuberculosis is higher with anti-tumor necrosis factor monoclonal antibody therapy than with soluble tumor necrosis factor receptor therapy: The three-year prospective French Research Axed on Tolerance of Biotherapies registry. *ArthritisRheum*. 2009;60(7):1884–94.

175. Mariette X, Vencovsky J, Lortholary O, Gomez-Reino J, de Longueville M, Ralston P, Weinblatt M, and van Vollenhoven R. The incidence of tuberculosis inpatients treated with certolizumab pegol across indications: Impact of baseline skin test results, more stringent screening criteria and geographic region. *RMD Open*. 2015;1(1):e000044.

176. Brassard P, Kezouh A, and Suissa S. Antirheumatic drugs and the risk of tuberculosis. *Clin Infect Dis*. 2006;43(6):717–22.

177. Wallis RS, Broder MS, Wong JY, Hanson ME, and Beenhouwer DO. Granulomatous infectious diseases associated with tumor necrosis factor antagonists. *Clin Infect Dis*. 2004;38(9):1261–5.

178. Kay J, Fleischmann R, Keystone E, Hsia EC, Hsu B, Mack M, Goldstein N, Braun J, and Kavanaugh A. Golimumab 3-year safety update: An analysis of pooled data from the long-term extensions of randomised, double-blind, placebo-controlled trials conducted in patients with rheumatoid arthritis, psoriatic arthritis or ankylosing spondylitis. *Ann Rheum Dis*. 2015;74(3):538–46.

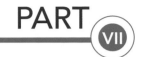

PART VII

OFFICIAL STATEMENTS: COMPARISON OF NATIONAL AND INTERNATIONAL RECOMMENDATIONS

Treatment Guidelines for Active Drug-Susceptible and Drug-Resistant Pulmonary Tuberculosis, and Latent Tuberculosis Infection

LYNN E. SOSA AND LLOYD N. FRIEDMAN

INTRODUCTION

This chapter is designed to compare and give guidance on options for treatment recommended by established national and international organizations. Generally, practitioners should follow the guidelines specified by the organization that represents the geographical location of the treatment facility. These recommendations are a guide and should not be substituted for the detailed information in the guidelines themselves and should not be substituted for the opinion of an expert consultant. Although many of these regimens can be applied to the treatment of extrapulmonary disease, it would be prudent to refer to the chapter on Extrapulmonary Tuberculosis for guidance, as well as, where indicated, the chapters on Pulmonary Tuberculosis, Tuberculosis and Human Immunodeficiency Virus Co-infection, Tuberculosis in Childhood and Pregnancy, and Drug Resistant Tuberculosis.

- ATS: American Thoracic Society
- CDC: Centers for Disease Control and Prevention
- CTS: Canadian Thoracic Society
- Curry: Curry International Tuberculosis Center
- ERS: European Respiratory Society
- IDSA: Infectious Disease Society of America
- IUATLD: International Union Against Tuberculosis and Lung Disease
- NICE: National Institute for Health and Care Excellence
- NTCA: National Tuberculosis Controllers Association
- WHO: World Health Organization

Drug Abbreviations: Am = amikacin; Bdq = bedaquiline; Cfz = clofazimine; Clv = clavulanic acid; Cs = cycloserine; Dlm = delaminid; E = ethambutol; Fq = fluoroquinolone (Lfx or Mfx); H = isoniazid; H^H = high-dose isoniazid; Ipm-Cln = imipenem-cilastatin; Km = kanamycin; Lfx = levofloxacin; Lzd = linezolid; Mfx = moxifloxacin; Mpm = meropenem; P = rifapentine; PAS = para-aminosalicylic acid; Pto/Eto = prothionamide/ethionamide; R = rifampin; S = streptomycin; Trd = terizidone; Z = pyrazinamide

GUIDELINES FOR READING THE TABLES

The first number reflects the number of months to administer the drugs.

Numbers within *parentheses* reflect number of times per week; if no parentheses are present, daily therapy is indicated.

Within each column, the *first row* represents the initiation phase, and the *second row* is the continuation phase. For example, 2HRZE represents 2 months of initial therapy with isoniazid, rifampin, pyrazinamide and ethambutol, and on the line following, 4HR represents 4 months of maintenance therapy with isoniazid and rifampin. Similarly, 2HRZE (3) represents 2 months of isoniazid, rifampin, pyrazinamide, and ethambutol given thrice weekly. Usually, the drug dosages for intermittent therapy are higher than for daily therapy.

DRUG-SENSITIVE TUBERCULOSIS

The usual therapy for drug-sensitive tuberculosis (TB) comprises four drugs for 2 months, dropping ethambutol once the organism is known to be sensitive to isoniazid, rifampin, and pyrazinamide; then continuing maintenance isoniazid and rifampin for 4 months. In the United States,[1] if the person has cavitary disease *and* is culture positive 2 months after starting treatment, maintenance therapy is extended to 7 months for

Table 20.1 Drug-sensitive tuberculosis treatment regimens[1–6]

	WHO	ATS/CDC/IDSA	ERS	NICE	CTS	IUATLD
Daily	2HRZE 4HR	2HRZE 4–7HR[a]	2HRZE 4HR	2HRZE 4HR	2HRZE 4–7HR[a]	2HRZE 4HR
Intermittent	2HRZE (3) 4HR (3)	2HRZE (3) 4HR (3) or 2HRZE (daily for 14 days then twice weekly) 4HR (2) or 2HRZE (daily) 4HR (2)		2HRZE (3) 4HR (3)	2HRZE (daily) 4–7HR (3)	

[a] ATS/CDC/IDSA and IUATLD guidelines state that the maintenance phase be extended to 7 months for cavitary disease that is culture positive at 2 months.[1,6] For CTS, extend maintenance phase to 7 months for cavitary disease, or for persistent smear or culture positivity at 2 months, or HIV coinfection.[5] As noted in the text, clinicians can use their clinical judgment to extend therapy.

a total of 9 months of therapy (see Table 20.1). Consideration also can be given to extending therapy for cavitary disease *or* a positive 2-month culture based on clinical expertise, such as extensive disease or the existence of medical comorbidities that might cause a delay in response. HIV-positive individuals who are not on antiretroviral therapy should have maintenance therapy extended to 7 months. Decisions on when to start antiretroviral therapy, as well as drug interactions, in persons with TB who are newly diagnosed with HIV may be found in the chapter on Tuberculosis and Human Immunodeficiency Virus Co-infection.

Individuals should receive therapy weekdays by directly observed therapy (DOT), be evaluated monthly by the clinician, and obtain a sputum for acid-fast bacilli (AFB) each month until 2 consecutive monthly sputum examinations are negative. Ethambutol should be discontinued once the organism is known to be pansensitive. HIV-positive persons and persons with cavitary disease should take a daily regimen. It is considered acceptable to give only five doses per week by DOT, even if the individual

does not take the weekend doses. If an individual is intolerant to one of the drugs and it must be discontinued, the individual should be treated as if resistant to that drug (e.g., if isoniazid is stopped because of hepatitis, then an isoniazid monoresistant regimen should be used).[1,9]

ISONIAZID MONORESISTANT TB

In most cases, isoniazid monoresistant TB can be cured with a 6-month regimen without using injectable drugs. (Table 20.2).[1,3–9]

MULTIDRUG-RESISTANT TB

Multidrug-resistant tuberculosis (MDR-TB) can be treated, according to the WHO, without injectable agents in a regimen that usually lasts for at least 18 months. The prioritization of medications is noted in Table 20.3.[7] It is essential that the person be taking at least four medications to which the organism is sensitive for the first 24 weeks, at which time bedaquiline is discontinued

Table 20.2 Isoniazid monoresistant TB treatment regimens[1,3–5,9]

	WHO	ATS/CDC/ERS/IDSA	NICE	CTS	IUATLD
Daily	6RZELfx[a]	6RZEFq[a,b] or For less extensive disease: 2RZEFq 4REFq	2RZE 7–10RE	6–9RZE±Fq or 2RZE 10RE	Is not addressed in current guidance; is addressed in older statement.
Intermittent				2RZE (daily) 4–7RZE (3) or 2RZE (daily) 10RE (3) or 2RZEFq (daily) 4–7REFq (3)	

[a] Recommend extending therapy to 9 months for cavitary disease, extensive disease or a positive sputum culture at 2 months, based on guidance for drug-sensitive TB.
[b] Assess resistance to other drugs in the regimen wherever possible.

Table 20.3 Drugs recommended by WHO for the injectable-free treatment of MDR-TB and rifampin-resistant TB (these groupings are intended to guide the design of long regimens)[7]

Group A (include all three if possible)	Levofloxacin Bedaquiline[a] Linezolid
Group B (add at least one if all of the Group A medications are not used	Clofazimine Cycloserine or terizidone
Group C (add to complete a regimen of at least four, preferably five, drugs when medicines from Groups A or B cannot be used)	Ethambutol Delamanid[a] Pyrazinamide (if sensitive) Imipenem-cilastatin[b] or meropenem[b] Amikacin or streptomycin (only if sensitive, and hearing tests available) Ethionamide or prothionamide Para-aminosalicylic acid

[a] Evidence on the safety and effectiveness of bedaquiline or delaminid beyond 6 months was insufficient for review. Evidence on concurrent use of bedaquiline and delamanid are insufficient for review.[7]

[b] Amoxicillin−clavulanic acid is administered with every dose of imipenem−cilastatin or meropenem since it is the only convenient way to give clavulanic acid, but it is not counted as a separate agent and should not be used as a separate agent.[7]

leaving three effective drugs for the remainder of treatment. Ideally, fluoroquinolone testing at a minimum should be performed before starting treatment. It is preferred that all three drugs from group A and at least one drug from group B be used. WHO suggests starting five drugs in case one drug has to be discontinued due to side effects.[7] The person should be culture negative (i.e., three consecutive negative monthly cultures) for at least 15 months from the time of the first negative culture of the series. If amikacin is started, it is recommended for at least 6 months. Streptomycin is an acceptable alternative. Kanamycin and capreomycin are not considered acceptable drugs due to high rates of failure. There is no definite cutoff, in terms of months treated, to define treatment failure; data show that the percentage of treatment failure if culture positive at 5, 6, 7, and 8 months is 10.3%, 16.4%, 24.7%, and 44.5%, respectively.[7] The ATS/CDC/ERS/IDSA guidelines[9] also recommend an all-oral regimen starting with five drugs (see Table 20.4).

MDR-TB TREATMENT REGIMENS

Table 20.4 shows multiple long daily regimens (12–21 months) and one short daily regimen (at least 9 months) for MDR-TB. The long regimens are standard. The short intensive WHO regimen includes additional drugs plus an injectable agent, although a recent WHO communication allows for substitution of bedaquiline for the injectable agent.[10] In persons with MDR-TB who were not previously treated with second-line drugs, do not have central nervous system or disseminated TB, and in whom resistance to fluoroquinolones and second-line injectable agents (or bedaquiline if substituted) was excluded or is considered highly unlikely, the short intensive MDR-TB regimen may be used instead of the long regimen; these individuals must not previously have received any TB treatment for 1 month or more. Amikacin may be substituted for kanamycin, although now it is recommended that bedaquiline be substituted for the injectable agent so that it is an all-oral regimen.[3–5,7–10]

RIFAMPIN MONORESISTANT TB

The WHO regimen for rifampin monoresistance is exactly the same as the MDR-TB regimen.[7] The new ATS/CDC/ERS/IDSA guidelines do not address rifampin monoresistance; the recommendations from the Curry International Tuberculosis Center do address it (Table 20.5).[11] One can be less aggressive with rifampin monoresistance in some developed countries because, where better resources are available, one can be more confident that rifampin is the only resistant drug. Before the inclusion of rifampin in TB regimens in 1980, isoniazid and ethambutol for 18 months was the standard regimen and was used with great success. Although there are no direct studies, it is felt that this regimen can be shortened to 12 months if a fluoroquinolone such as levofloxacin is added and pyrazinamide is used for the first 2 months. Although an injectable has been suggested to shorten the regimen, the goal is to avoid injectable agents wherever possible.

EXTENSIVELY DRUG-RESISTANT TUBERCULOSIS

Extensively drug-resistant tuberculosis (XDR-TB) is defined as resistance to isoniazid and rifampin, a fluoroquinolone, and one of the following three injectable agents: amikacin, kanamycin, or capreomycin.[9]

For pre-XDR and XDR-TB, one can use the same approach as the ATS/CDC/ERS/IDSA recommendations for MDR-TB treatment in terms of number of susceptible drugs, initially five if possible, but with a longer duration of treatment (15–24 months after culture conversion).[9] The WHO recommendations also can be adapted. Expert consultation is necessary.

NEW XDR-TB REGIMEN

Pretomanid was approved by the United States Food and Drug Administration as part of a three-drug regimen to treat highly resistant TB (predominantly XDR-TB but also MDR-TB that is

Table 20.4 MDR-TB treatment regimens[3–10]

WHO	ATS/CDC/ERS/IDSA	NICE	CTS	IUATLD
Long course (at least 18 months total): Start with at least four drugs (preferably five) to which the organism is sensitive: All three from Group A plus at least one, preferably two, from Group B plus drugs from Group C if at least four drugs cannot be chosen from Groups A and B. At 24 weeks, Bdq is discontinued and the remaining three to four drugs are used for 15 months after culture conversion.	Use at least five drugs to which the organism is sensitive, preferably drugs not used previously for the person. Strategy for building a regimen is as follows: Choose a later generation Fq (Lfx or Mfx), Bdq, Lzd, Cfz and Cs/Trd If a regimen of five drugs cannot be achieved, and the clinician and individual agree to an injectable drug, add Am or S after confirming the organism is sensitive If a regimen of five drugs still cannot be achieved or an all-oral regimen is preferred, add Dlm, E (only if susceptible and/or Z (only if susceptible) to create a five-drug regimen. Other drugs include Pto/Eto (usually use only if susceptible) or Imp-Cln or Mpm or PAS or H^H (if no high-level isoniazid resistance) Treat with the initial regimen for 5–7 months after culture conversion. Since Bdq is only approved for 24 weeks, this may require adding at 24 weeks an additional drug to which the organism is sensitive or, if the clinician approves, renewing Bdq. After the initial regimen is complete, reduce to four drugs and treat for a total duration of 15–21 months after culture conversion.	Use at least six drugs to which isolate is sensitive; consult with expert.	Start with at least four drugs to which the isolate is sensitive, including Fq and an injectable agent for at least 8 months, then continue with at least three drugs for a continuation phase of 12–16 months. Minimum total duration of 20 months.	4-6 AmMfxPtoH^{H}CfzEZ 5 MfxCfzEZ^a
Short course: 9 months (The length of initial therapy can be extended depending on sputum smear conversion) 4 MfxKmEtoCfzH^{H}ZE 5 MfxCfzZE WHO recently (December 2019) recommended substituting 6 months of Bdq for the injectable agent.[10] Lfx may be substituted for Mfx.				

^{a} Can substitute Gfx for Mfx, if available.[8]

Table 20.5 Rifampin monoresistant TB regimens[4–9,11]

WHO	USA: Curry	ERS	NICE	CTS	IUATLD
See MDR-TB	2HZEFq 10–16HEFq *or* 18HZE (if unable to take Fq) For both regimens above, can use an injectable for 2 months if extensive or cavitary disease	No specific rec found	See MDR-TB	2HZEFq 10–16HEFq (daily or thrice weekly) Can consider the use of an injectable agent for 2 months if extensive cavitary disease *or* 2HZS[a] 7HZS (daily or thrice weekly)[a] *or* 2HZEFq 16HE (daily or thrice weekly)	See MDR-TB

[a] Can substitute a different injectable. The latest literature suggests amikacin.[9]

nonresponsive or treatment intolerant). The regimen comprises bedaquiline, pretomanid, and linezolid for 6 months with an option to extend for a longer duration and is an all-oral regimen. Six months after completion of treatment, the regimen showed an efficacy of 90% which was defined as two consecutive negative cultures and no relapse in the subsequent 6 months. This is much better than the average historical control regimen efficacy of 14% for the treatment of XDR-TB.[12]

LATENT TUBERCULOSIS INFECTION

For many years, the standard for the treatment of presumably pansensitive latent tuberculosis infection (LTBI) was either 9 or 6 months of isoniazid. More recently, shorter regimens have been shown to be equivalent and are fast gaining popularity because of increased adherence, safety, and economy of resources (Table 20.6).[4–6,13,14]

Table 20.6 Latent TB infection regimens[4-6,13,14]

	WHO	NTCA/CDC	ERS	NICE	CTS	IUATLD
Daily	6H *or* 9H *or* 3HR *or* 36H (HIV+ in high TB transmission settings) 4R (alternative) *or* 1HP (alternative)	4R[a] (preferred for HIV−) *or* 3HR[b] (preferred for HIV+ and HIV−) *or* 6H (alternative for HIV+[b] and HIV−[a]) *or* 9H[b] (alternative for HIV+ and HIV−) *or* 2 HRZE[c]	No specific rec found	3HR *or* 6H	9H (standard regimen) *or* 6H *or* 3HR *or* 4R	9H *or* 36H (HIV+ in high TB burden areas) *or* 4R *or* 3HR *or* 1HP (HIV+ only)
Intermittent	3HP (1)	3HP (1)[a,d] (preferred for HIV+ and HIV−) *or* 6H (2)[e] *or* 9H (2)[e]			6–9H (2) *or* 3HR (2) *or* 3HP (1)	3HP (1)

[a] Strong recommendation.
[b] Conditional recommendation.
[c] HRZE may be initiated in a person in whom there is a substantial possibility of active TB disease. If cultures are ultimately negative, and it is determined the patient has LTBI, the person will have received 2 months of RZ as part of the HRZE regimen and treatment of LTBI is complete (it has been shown that 2RZ is an effective regimen, but because of the risk of fatal hepatotoxicity, it is not used).[14]
[d] 12 doses isoniazid and rifapentine once a week by DOT or self-administered therapy (SAT).[14]
[e] Should only be used in individuals who cannot take or adhere to other regimens [NCTA/CDC. Treatment of LTBI in the US: Practical Consideration—A Guide for Healthcare Providers; 2020, In Press]. Should always be used with DOT.[14]

Some of the nuances of treatment of LTBI are discussed in the bullets below:

- Nine months of isoniazid versus 6 months of isoniazid: 9 months is clearly a more effective regimen. The very study that is cited to justify the usefulness of a 6-month regimen is the same study that showed that it is less effective.[15] The study compared 12 months versus 6 months of isoniazid. Although nearly comparable for all participants who took a 12 versus a 6 month regimen, when analyzed only for those who were adherent, a 12-month regimen was 93% effective versus a 6-month regimen which was 69% effective. The 12-month regimen was clearly superior, but was subsequently shortened to 9 months when it was shown that most of the benefit of a 12-month regimen had already occurred by 9–10 months of therapy.[16]

- The WHO recommends 36 months of isoniazid preventive therapy for individuals who are HIV-positive who reside in high TB incidence countries[13] (see also the chapter on Tuberculosis and Human Immunodeficiency Virus Co-infection for information about this and other regimens, as well as drug interactions with antiretroviral therapy).

- WHO now recommends one month of isoniazid and rifapentine for HIV-positive and HIV-negative individuals with LTBI.[13] The IUATLD recommends this treatment only for HIV-positive individuals.[6]

- If a person with LTBI is a contact to a person with TB who is resistant to either isoniazid or rifampin, that drug should not be used.

- For a person with LTBI who was a known contact to someone with MDR-TB, a fluoroquinolone for 6–12 months with or without a second drug, based on source isolate sensitivities, can be used. Pyrazinamide generally should be avoided.[9]

CIRCUMSTANCES WHERE IT IS NOT CLEAR WHETHER THE PATIENT HAS ACTIVE OR INACTIVE TB

It often is found that an individual has a fibrotic lesion or density in an upper lobe and a positive test for LTBI. If it is not clear whether the radiographic abnormality represents active or inactive disease, and there is reasonable concern that it is active, a chest radiograph or chest CT can be used as a baseline evaluation, a sputum culture for acid fast bacilli should be obtained, and the person can be started on HRZE. If, after 2 months, the culture is negative and the chest radiograph or CT is unchanged, then the disease most likely is inactive; the person has received adequate treatment for LTBI and the drugs can be stopped. This is because rifampin and pyrazinamide for 2 months was proved to be an effective regimen to treat LTBI, but is no longer recommended, as noted earlier. If the culture is negative and the chest radiograph or CT improves, the person can be considered to have culture-negative TB and treatment with isoniazid and rifampin

can continue for another 2 months for a total of 4 months of therapy. If the culture is positive, the person is treated for the usual 6 months.[1] If it is very unlikely that the lesion is active, cultures can be obtained and, if negative, a standard LTBI regimen can be administered.

REFERENCES

1. Nahid P et al. ATS/CDC/IDSA clinical practice guidelines: Treatment of drug-susceptible tuberculosis. *Clin Infect Dis.* 2016;63:e147–95.

2. *Guidelines for Treatment of Drug-Susceptible Tuberculosis and Patient Care*, 2017 update. Geneva: World Health Organization; 2017. Licence: CC BY-NC-SA 3.0 IGO.

3. Migliori GB et al. European union standards for tuberculosis care. *Eur Respir J.* 2012;39:807–19, doi: 10.1183/09031936.00203811

4. National Institute for Health and Care Institute. Tuberculosis: NICE Guideline. http://nice.org.uk/guidance/ng33

5. Canadian Tuberculosis Standards: 7th edition, Available at: https://strauss.ca/OEMAC/wp-content/uploads/2013/11/Canadian_TB_Standards_7th-edition_English.pdf

6. Dlodlo RA et al. *Management of Tuberculosis: A Guide to Essential Practice.* Paris, France: International Union Against Tuberculosis and Lung Disease, 2019.

7. *WHO Consolidated Guidelines on Drug-Resistant Tuberculosis Treatment.* Geneva: World Health Organization, 20, 2019. Licence CC BY-NC-SA 3.0 IGO.

8. Piubello A et al. *Field Guide for the Management of Drug-Resistant Tuberculosis.* Paris, France: International Union Against Tuberculosis and Lung Disease, 2018.

9. Nahid P et al. Treatment of drug-resistant tuberculosis. An Official ATS/CDC/ERS/IDSA Clinical Practice Guideline. *Am J Respir Crit Care Med.* 2019;200(10):e93–142.

10. WHO. Rapid Communication: Key changes to the treatment of drug-resistant tuberculosis. December 2019. https://www.who.int/tb/publications/2019/WHO_RapidCommunicationMDR_TB2019.pdf?ua=1

11. Curry International Tuberculosis Center and California Department of Public Health. *Drug-resistant tuberculosis: A survival guide for clinicians*, 3rd ed., 2016.

12. Conradie F et al. Treatment of highly drug-resistant pulmonary tuberculosis. *NEJM.* 2020;382:893–902.

13. *WHO Consolidated Guidelines on Tuberculosis: tuberculosis preventive treatment.* Geneva: World Health Organization; 2020. Licence: CC BY-NC-SA 3.0 IGO.

14. Sterling TR et al. Guidelines for the treatment of latent tuberculosis infection: Recommendations from the National Tuberculosis Controllers Association and CDC, 2020. *MMWR Recomm Rep.* 2020;69:1–11.

15. IUATLD. Efficacy of various durations of isoniazid preventive therapy for tuberculosis: Five years of follow-up in the IUAT trial. *International Union Against Tuberculosis Committee on Prophylaxis. Bull World Health Org* 1982;60(4):555–64.

16. Comstock GW. How much isoniazid is needed for prevention of tuberculosis among immunocompetent adults? *Int J Tuberc Lung Dis.* 1999;3:847–50.

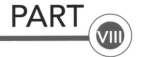

PART VIII

CONTROL

PART

CONTROL

21

Tuberculosis Epidemic Control
A Comprehensive Strategy to Drive Down Tuberculosis

SALMAAN KESHAVJEE, TOM NICHOLSON, AAMIR J. KHAN, LUCICA DITIU, PAUL E. FARMER, AND MERCEDES C. BECERRA

INTRODUCTION

Tuberculosis (TB) has been a curable disease since the 1950s. In the more than six decades since then, knowledge has been amassed about how to ameliorate its social causes, prevent its transmission, and treat both its clinical and quiescent forms.[1,2] In many high-income settings, this knowledge has been used with great success. Elsewhere, this is far from the case: more than 4,000 people die from this curable and preventable airborne disease each day, mostly in low-income and middle-income settings.[3] Distressed by the status quo, in 2012 more than 500 scientists, policy makers, and advocates from around the world signed the Zero TB Declaration, which called for "a new global attitude" in the fight against TB, and argued that, with the right set of interventions, the planet could move rapidly toward zero deaths from TB.[4]

Although TB incidence has declined over the past 25 years, it has done so at a glacial pace of approximately 1.5% annually.[5] At this rate, it will take another two centuries to eliminate the disease. This reality reflects the limited set of interventions recommended in the last three decades for, and implemented in, low-income and middle-income settings—a shadow of the comprehensive set of strategies that has brought the TB epidemic to heel in other places.[1,2] Rather than aggressively finding all cases of TB, preventing the disease in those at highest risk, and focusing on populations and places of highest transmission, most low-income and middle-income settings have focused narrowly on the diagnosis and treatment of those people sick with TB who manage to access care on their own. An over-reliance on standardized treatment and sputum smear microscopy—a low-sensitivity visual diagnostic test that cannot determine drug resistance—has sidelined not only individuals whose illness is characterized by a lower bacillary load, such as children and individuals with HIV, but also those with extrapulmonary forms or drug-resistant TB.[6] Early detection and treatment of both active disease and quiescent (the so-called latent) infection, along with efforts to control transmission in health care and congregate settings, have been recommended belatedly but have yet to be widely scaled up.[7] Much of the policy framing to date has been driven by concerns over cost, which has overridden both the scientific and moral imperatives to implement proven interventions that could inflect the global TB curve more rapidly.[6-8] Although standardization of treatment contributed to improved clinical outcomes for some people with TB, the absence of a comprehensive approach for fighting TB in high-burden settings has led to predictable and alarming results.[3,9,10]

More than 10 million people still fall sick from TB every year, including 1 million children.[3,11] More than 3 million patients with TB remain undetected and continue to transmit the disease in their families and communities. Appropriate treatment for drug-resistant TB remains the exception rather than the rule, allowing further transmission of these mutant strains. Most known contacts receive no post-exposure therapy even though it is a standard intervention in most high-income settings. Finally, and most damning of all, nearly 2 million people still die each year from TB—a preventable and curable disease.[3]

Ending the TB epidemic requires the urgent deployment of a comprehensive package of effective, tried-and-tested interventions in settings with high burdens of TB. This comprehensive approach must happen in tandem with the development of effective point-of-care diagnostics, highly effective and shorter treatment regimens, and vaccines. In this chapter, we review a set of proven epidemic-control strategies for combating the disease. Their wider and more systematic application, evidence suggests, will result in quantitatively greater and more rapid progress in tackling the global TB epidemic.[1,2,12-18] Separately, the effect of each strategy might be modest; in combination, however, global experience and mathematical modelling suggest that they will have a swift and dramatic effect on TB incidence and mortality.[1,2]

Key messages of this chapter

TB case reduction is stagnant, but it can be accelerated. This requires a comprehensive approach comprising three components:

Search Actively—Test Properly
 + Delays in diagnosis contribute to the spread of TB
 + Targeted active case-finding finds more people with TB earlier
 + Active case-finding requires proper testing and diagnostic tools
 + Active case-finding reduces TB transmission in communities
 + Active case-finding can reduce the global burden of TB

Treat Effectively—Support through Treatment
 + Effective TB treatment rapidly reduces infectiousness
 + Widespread testing for drug resistance can ensure effective treatment
 + Strengthening health systems can reduce treatment delays
 + Patients need to be supported throughout treatment

Prevent Exposure—Treat Exposure
 + Protecting people from exposure prevents future TB cases
 + Preventive therapy for high-risk groups reduces new TB cases
 + Shorter preventive therapy regimens can reduce the treatment burden
 + Preventive therapy can also reduce new cases of drug-resistant TB
 + Preventive therapy can have a population-level impact

A growing coalition is calling for the urgent, widespread implementation of these tried-and-tested approaches to stopping the disease.[4,19] This will mean applying evidence-based strategies to search for and diagnose everyone who is sick with TB, to treat them promptly and effectively with the best medicines that cause the least adverse events, and to prevent future TB cases by stopping TB transmission and treating TB infection. These strategies will need to be implemented all at once in an integrated fashion in order to have the maximum effect.[2] This approach is aligned with the Stop TB Partnership's Global Plan to End TB, the principles of the World Health Organization's end TB strategy, and the targets that emerged from the 2018 United Nations High-Level Meeting on TB.[20–22] Multiple local coalitions are working to operationalize this comprehensive approach in geographically defined zones. This network of coalitions is called the Zero TB Initiative.[23,24]

Where—and how rapidly—can TB rates actually drop toward elimination? Policy discussion about so-called TB elimination (defined as less than one TB case per million population per year) is often only in reference to countries where TB incidence is already below 10 per 100,000 population per year.[25] Notably, only about 12% of the world's population lives in those countries.[26] In contrast, more than 45% of the world's population lives in countries where TB case rates exceed 100 per 100,000 per year. Thus, one step in the required paradigm shift is the perspective that—regardless of the size of the current local TB burden—every community coalition can aspire to drive down TB rates toward

elimination. Indeed, as a first step toward closing this gap in global health equity, local coalitions can devise plans to reduce TB case rates to below 10 per 100,000 per year.

Similarly, a new perspective is needed about how rapidly case reductions can be achieved. As noted, at the global level, since 2000 the number of new TB cases has declined at just 1.5% per year.[5] In many settings, high TB case rates are essentially stagnant, with almost no change year after year. However, there are several locations where annual reductions in TB case rates have exceeded 15%. What these settings had in common was the simultaneous use of multiple strategies targeted in geographically defined zones: we refer to this as a *comprehensive approach* to driving down TB rates.

In this chapter, we will review examples of rapid TB declines (Part I) and review the three strands of activities that must be deployed simultaneously as a comprehensive approach: SEARCH—TREAT—PREVENT (Part II). Local coalitions can use these experiences and framework to inform how to tailor their own efforts to drive down TB rates one community at a time.

PART I: THE CASES

We identified illustrative examples in the literature where annual declines per year exceeded 5%. These are summarized in Table 21.1 and described in the following section.

Table 21.1 Examples of rapid declines in TB case rates in geographically defined zones

#	Where	When	TB cases per 100K	Years	Overall % decline	Annual % decline per year
1	Greenland[28]	1956	2,000	6	66	17
2	State of Alaska[29–35]	1955	300	5	67	20
3	(Western) Palm Beach County[36,37]	1997	80	5	66	21
4	New York City[38]	1992	50	5	55	15
5	Two neighborhoods in Smith County, Texas[39]	1996	40	10	>98	31
6	State of Tennessee[40,41]	2002	7	10	55	8

GREENLAND

Greenland is the world's largest island and part of the Kingdom of Denmark. In the early 1950s, a survey estimated that 2% of the population had TB—an incidence rate of approximately 2,000/100,000 population.[42] In 1955, the population of the island was approximately 22,000. By then, Greenland had begun programs to reduce its TB burden, including "better" case-finding, "effective" hospitalizations and chemotherapy, and BCG vaccination for newborns and young children.

In 1955, a dedicated TB ship began annual visits to all villages on the island, offering free examinations for all, which included chest radiography, sputum examinations, TST, and BCG vaccination. Each year, the ship visited 90% of the population, with nearly 100% coverage achieved after two years. In 1956, the program added an interventional study through which about half of all villages received isoniazid preventive therapy, excluding individuals already on treatment for active TB and those under the age of 15. This meant that isoniazid preventive therapy was used to treat nearly 20% of the entire population of Greenland (half of the adults in the country who did not have active TB).

The comprehensive approach was ongoing, and 5 years after the start of the intervention TB incidence had declined from 2,000/100,000 to 1,051/100,000: a decline of nearly half. Six years after the isoniazid intervention began, the TB rate had declined by 66%—a decline of 17% per year.

STATE OF ALASKA

In 1959, Alaska became a US state.[29,30,32,33,35,46] Prior to that, it was a US territory, having been purchased from Russia in 1867. In 1952, with a population of 190,000, the case rate for TB in Alaska was 379/100,000. BCG vaccination had been initiated in 1949 and was ongoing until 1956, when it was discontinued. In 1953, a United States Public Health Service commission was convened to provide recommendations on how to reduce rates of TB in Alaska. These recommendations included intensified case finding and outpatient treatment.

In 1955, an ambulatory chemotherapy program was introduced whereby patients received treatment for TB in their homes, rather than through lengthy hospital stays. In 1957, a randomized-controlled trial of isoniazid preventive therapy was initiated in the Bethel area; this trial randomized households to receive isoniazid or placebo in an effort to better understand the utility of community-wide preventive therapy for reducing TB in areas with a high disease burden. The only individuals who did not receive preventive therapy were those already on treatment for active TB, those with medical history suggesting epilepsy, and infants under 2 months of age. In the time that isoniazid was administered, the intervention group experienced a 68% reduction in rates of TB compared to the households that received placebo. Based on this success, isoniazid preventive therapy was expanded to the whole community in this area in 1963.

Five years after the interventions began, there had been a nearly 70% decline in TB case rates—from 299.1/100,000 to 98.2/100,000; an annual decline of 20%. By the early 1990s, Alaska's rate of TB was comparable to that of the rest of the United States: around 10 cases or less per 100,000 population.

WESTERN PALM BEACH COUNTY

Palm Beach County is in the southeastern US state of Florida.[36,37] The western portion of the county historically had higher rates of TB than the eastern portion: the average annual rate of TB cases in 1994–1997 was 81/100,000 in the western region, compared to 9.1 cases/100,000 population in the eastern region. In 1993, a team of investigators from the Palm Beach County Health Department, the Florida Department of Health, the CDC, Emory University, and Dartmouth Medical School gathered in order to develop a survey to assess the prevalence of both active and latent TB in western Palm Beach County.

A non-governmental organization, diverse and representative of the community, was formed in order to increase participation in the survey (which earlier assessments had indicated would be too low to gather meaningful measurements). This group initiated a community-based participatory intervention to reduce fears around stigma, confidentiality, and community reputation. They disseminated health messages about signs and symptoms of TB, availability of free treatment, rationale for the survey, and the importance of participation through a press conference; television and radio appearances; booths at community events; visits to local churches and clubs; and outreach to high-risk populations. The survey itself was conducted in a random selection of households in the region. Participants received TST and those with a positive result were referred to clinicians who performed chest radiography; participants then received treatment for active or latent TB as needed.

Concurrently, the county health department continued passive case-finding, and the intervention staff built a partnership with the health department and assisted in administering LTBI treatment to recently infected high-risk contacts of infectious TB patients. This approach resulted in a steep decline in TB rates in this region, which was faster than that observed in the eastern portion of the county. In 2002–2005, the average annual TB case rate was 25/100,000; an almost 70% reduction (a decline of nearly 20% per year) compared to 1994–1997; by 2006–2009, the rate was 19/100,000—a more than 75% reduction from the years prior to the intervention. Over this period, the average annual case rate in the eastern portion of the county decreased from 9.1/100,000 in 1994–1997 to 7.2/100,000 in 2006–2009—a roughly 20% decline.

NEW YORK CITY

In 1988, the number of TB cases in New York City had more than doubled compared to 10 years earlier; the number of TB patients tripled from 1978 to 1992.[50] New York City's population at that time was 7.3 million. From 1988 to 1994, funding for the New York City Department of Health increased 10-fold; the interventions deployed with these increased resources allowed for a more than 50% decline in TB case rates, from the 1992 peak of 51.3/100,000 to 23.3/100,000 in 1997.

Interventions introduced in this period included outreach workers traveling to patients' homes to support treatment; improvement of infection control to reduce nosocomial infection; downsizing of large shelters and provision of non-congregate housing for people living with HIV; improvement of TB care among incarcerated persons; and introduction of a four-drug regimen for treatment of TB disease. Laboratory testing methods were improved, drug susceptibility testing increased, a higher index of suspicion was used in diagnosis, and preventive therapy was expanded in high-risk groups.

With increased resources and improvements in case-finding, case notification rates continued to climb in 1988–1992. Subsequent to the peak case rate in 1992, TB rates declined by 15% per year over 5 years; by 2016, the rates had declined by more than 85% since the 1992 peak.

TWO NEIGHBORHOODS IN SMITH COUNTY, TEXAS

Texas is a large state in the United States.[39] In 1996, a team of researchers from the University of Texas, the Texas Department of Health, and the Smith County Health Office sought to assess whether targeting interventions to neighborhoods with high burdens of TB could help to reduce future cases of the disease in those geographic areas. The Texas Department of State Health Services shared with the researchers the addresses of all cases of TB that were reported in Smith County from 1985 to 1995, along with the addresses of all individuals with positive TST results from 1993 to 1995.

With the addresses provided by the government, the team used a geographic information system to map cases of TB and instances of positive TST within Smith County, Texas. The mapping showed two neighborhoods with an unusually high TB burden, an average case rate of 39.6/100,000 in a population of 3,153 enumerated residents—five times the average in the rest of the county. The coalition launched a community-wide screening intervention in these two neighborhoods, including: communication materials shared in churches and schools; public service announcements in local periodicals and TV/radio; door-to-door visits made by field workers to explain the project and offer free TSTs; free chest radiography and evaluation in mobile clinics for those participants with positive TSTs; treatment for those with active TB; and latent TB infection treatment for participants who had a positive TST result but who did not have active TB.

In the 10 years subsequent to the initial mapping, the team again mapped the cases of TB in Smith County. They found that, from 1996 to 2006, there had been no TB cases in the two neighborhoods targeted by the interventions; there was only one case in 2007. Rates of TB in the rest of the county and state had also declined, but much more slowly. In the two target neighborhoods, there was an annual decline in TB cases of 31%; in the county, the rate of TB declined at a rate of 5% per year, and in the state of Texas it declined at an annual rate of 4%.

STATE OF TENNESSEE

Tennessee is a state in the United States that had a population of 5.7 million in the year 2000.[52,53] At that time, Tennessee's TB case notification rate (6.7/100,000 in 2000) had been above the national annual rate for two decades. With state funding, the Tennessee Department of Health initiated a statewide TB screening program—at the time, the only program of its kind—integrated with other public health services.

The program began in 2002 and, by the end of 2006, had screened almost 170,000 individuals who presented at county health departments for other public health services, and at some community sites (such as jails, shelters, and other high-risk settings). It sought to distinguish high-risk individuals who could benefit from TST from low-risk individuals among whom usage of TST could be limited, and to prevent development of active TB by expanding treatment of latent TB infection.

In 2006, Tennessee's incidence of TB had approached and then dropped below the national rate. In 2010, Tennessee had three cases of TB/100,000 population, compared to the US rate of 3.6/100,000—an annual decline of 8% per year. (The state's TB case notification rate fell below the national rate for the first time in more than 20 years.) From 2000 to 2011, Tennessee experienced a 64% reduction in TB case notification, compared to the national reduction of 41%.

PART II: THE APPROACH

The preceding examples, among others, show the simultaneous use of multiple strategies in one location. We summarize them as a set of Search, Treat, and Prevent components of a comprehensive approach to more rapidly drive down TB rates in specific geographic areas.

SEARCH: SEARCH ACTIVELY, TEST PROPERLY

A person who is infected with TB bacteria can become sick with active TB disease. This can happen as quickly as a few weeks or months after infection, or as long as decades later. People with TB infection who become sick can transmit the infection to their families, communities, and places of work. Therefore, a crucial step in stopping the transmission of TB—and a fundamental tenet of tuberculosis epidemic control—is to actively search and treat people who are sick with TB or who have TB infection.

Of the more than 10 million people who became sick with TB in 2016, only 6.3 million were recorded and reported by national governments.[54] This has been consistent over the last decade—yearly, almost 4 million people sick with TB and MDR-TB are "missed" by health systems. These people may be sick with TB and are never diagnosed or are treated in the private sector and were not recorded by national or international registers. Those who are not diagnosed or treated continue to transmit TB infection in their families, communities, and places of work. The large proportion of missed people with TB is a major cause of the slow progress in stopping the global TB epidemic.

DELAYS IN DIAGNOSIS CONTRIBUTE TO THE SPREAD OF TB

In most of the world, people with TB are diagnosed with the disease only after they seek care for their symptoms at a health care facility. A person can have TB for a long period without noticeable symptoms or with symptoms that are not severe enough for them to seek care. By the time people are sick enough to seek care, they may have been infectious for a long time.

Diagnosing people only after they seek care directly contributes to the spread of TB. A study of TB patients and their contacts in the United States found that patients with undiagnosed TB were more likely to pass on the TB infection to their contacts; the longer the delay in diagnosis, the more likely they were to have transmitted the infection. More than half of patients in the study had a delay of at least 90 days between having their first symptom and starting TB treatment, and 40% of the contacts of those patients had been infected with TB.[55]

TARGETED ACTIVE CASE-FINDING FINDS MORE TB CASES EARLIER

Targeted active case-finding involves actively seeking out and screening people who are at higher risk of becoming sick with TB.[56] The strategy reduces transmission rates because it finds more people with TB and diagnoses them earlier, so that those who are infectious can be treated before they transmit TB to more people. Currently, targeted active case-finding activities for TB focus primarily on just a few of the key populations and groups with high exposure: contacts of people who have TB, including children; people living with HIV; and people who seek care at health facilities in areas where TB is prevalent.

Targeted active case-finding is effective in finding new TB cases among key populations and groups with high risk, and works better than mass screening of the entire population. Across many studies in low- and middle-income countries that examined the rates at which people sick with TB transmitted the infection to their contacts, an average of more than 3% of contacts had active TB disease and more than 50% of contacts had TB infection.[57] The risk was highest during the first year of exposure, for children under 5 years of age, and for people living with HIV.[58] A review of studies that used targeted active case-finding to screen people living with HIV for TB symptoms found that, on average, the strategy identified one additional case of TB for every 100 people who were screened.[59] Many studies carried out in a range of settings have examined the impact of screening people who visit general healthcare facilities for TB, which finds new TB cases in an average of 5%–10% of the people screened.[60,61,62,63] To optimize effectiveness, active case-finding efforts should be informed by local epidemiologic data.[1,64]

Table 21.2 summarizes the estimates of the percentage of new TB cases that will be found among people screened using different active case-finding activities.

Table 21.2 Expected yield of various active case-finding activities

Type of active case-finding activity	Expected % of new TB cases
Screening household contacts of TB patients in low-/middle-income countries	1–5
Screening people at general healthcare facilities in high TB-burden areas	5–10
Screening people treated for HIV in low-/middle-income countries with HIV prevalence >5%	1–25

ACTIVE CASE-FINDING REQUIRES PROPER TESTING AND DIAGNOSTIC TOOLS

Active case-finding activities are only as effective as the tests and diagnostic tools that are used. Countries with the highest TB burdens still rely heavily—and spend resources—on an older diagnostic test called sputum smear microscopy, in which a patient's sputum sample is examined under a microscope for the presence of TB mycobacteria.

Compared with newer and more sensitive diagnostic methods, sputum smear microscopy is very unreliable: it has an overall failure rate of around 50%, meaning that half of people tested are "smear negative" despite having TB; in children, it fails to detect TB approximately 90% of the time.[65] In people living with HIV, it fails to detect TB more than 70% of the time.[66] Sputum smear microscopy cannot detect TB that develops outside of the lungs (extrapulmonary TB), nor can it determine if the person has drug-resistant TB.[67]

Although they are generally less infectious than smear-positive patients, smear-negative patients can also transmit the disease to others. A study in the United States of more than 1,500 TB patients found that at least 17% had contracted TB from a smear-negative patient and around 27% had contracted it via a chain of transmission that began with a smear-negative patient.[68]

Relying only on smear microscopy for diagnosis causes many people who are sick with TB to remain undiagnosed and untreated while they continue to be infectious. More sensitive diagnostic tests are available that can detect a higher proportion of TB cases. These include combinations of the following diagnostic tools: radiography (chest X-ray); mycobacteriological culture; molecular diagnostic tests (such as the Xpert MTB/RIF test); and clinical algorithms.[69] Bacteriological culture of a patient's sputum sample is a very accurate diagnostic method (some types can also test for drug resistance) but the results can take 2–6 weeks, while new types of molecular diagnostic tests take only hours or days to identify people with drug-resistant TB.

Clinical algorithms for diagnosing TB can help to identify and promptly treat patients with forms of TB disease that are not confirmed by microbiological tests. Chest X-ray is a key tool in clinical algorithms because it is much more sensitive than sputum smear microscopy in detecting TB in the lungs. X-ray can also detect the most common forms of extrapulmonary TB. Children have trouble producing the sputum needed for TB diagnostic tests, including tests for drug resistance, so they should be treated for TB based upon clinical diagnosis.[70] Clinical algorithms are an essential tool in diagnosing TB in children and people living with HIV, most of whom have smear-negative pulmonary TB or extrapulmonary TB that is not easily detectable using currently available diagnostic tools.[71]

ACTIVE CASE-FINDING REDUCES TB TRANSMISSION IN COMMUNITIES

Using targeted active case-finding reduces the rates at which TB disease and TB infection are transmitted in communities. A study in Brazil examined the effect of screening household contacts of people with TB. After 5 years, the communities where active case-finding was carried out had 10% fewer reported TB cases, which

Table 21.3 Projecting impact of increased TB case finding[73]

If 25% more TB cases are diagnosed and treated, then after 10 years:

- 40%–44% fewer people will die from TB-related causes (mortality)
- 22%–27% fewer people will be get TB each year (incidence)
- 30%–33% fewer people will be sick with TB (prevalence)

was 15% lower than the number of cases reported in communities where household contacts were not screened.[13] Studies in Zambia and South Africa reported similar results after 4 years: communities where household contacts of TB patients were screened had 18% lower rates of TB among adults and 55% lower rates of TB infection among children compared with communities where active case-finding was not used.[72]

ACTIVE CASE-FINDING CAN REDUCE THE BURDEN OF TB

The benefits of active case-finding accumulate over time, because finding and treating people with infectious TB prevents them from transmitting the disease to others. Projecting forward, mathematical models based on data from the current TB epidemics in China, India, and South Africa predict that targeted active case-finding can have a substantial impact on TB mortality, incidence, and prevalence (Table 21.3).[73]

This goal of a 25% increase in the number of detected cases is feasible with active case-finding activities. One study analyzed 19-year-long active case-finding activities, which were associated with a 35% increase in reported TB cases.[74] Active case-finding activities are also highly cost-effective interventions because they help stop transmission. Active case-finding activities need to be linked directly to the delivery of prompt, effective treatment.

TREAT: TREAT EFFECTIVELY, SUPPORT THROUGH TREATMENT

Until they are treated effectively, people sick with TB disease remain infectious. Stopping the global TB epidemic will require treating people with the correct medications as quickly as possible after diagnosis.

For people with TB disease that is not drug resistant, treatment generally involves taking four different first-line drugs for a period of 6 months. That regimen will not cure drug-resistant TB disease, which requires treatment with a combination of five or more effective second-line drugs for as long as two years. The treatments for both types of TB disease are lengthy and the medicines used can cause side effects, so a key component of TB care delivery is to support each patient in completing the entire treatment regimen.

EFFECTIVE TB TREATMENT RAPIDLY REDUCES INFECTIOUSNESS

Diagnosis must be followed by prompt effective treatment, because people who are diagnosed with TB but are not treated immediately are more likely to transmit TB to others. Long delays between diagnosis and treatment further increase the risk of transmission. A study in China found that people who were treated 30 days or more after diagnosis had a significantly higher chance of transmitting TB and, after 90 days without treatment, were 2.3 times as likely to transmit it.[75]

Evidence gathered over the past 60 years has shown that effective TB treatment very quickly reduces the chance that a patient will infect others, even while the patient is still culture-positive or smear-positive. A pivotal study in India during the 1950s found that TB patients being treated effectively in their homes were no more likely to transmit TB to their family members than TB patients who were being treated in sanatoria and isolated from their families.[76]

Studies that expose guinea pigs to patients with TB have shown that effective treatment makes a TB patient non-infectious very rapidly, often within 24 hours. In an early study, TB patients who had started treatment were 98% less likely to transmit TB to the guinea pigs than patients who had not yet started treatment; more recent studies have reported that patients receiving no or inadequate treatment for drug-resistant TB were the source of virtually all transmission to guinea pigs. Patients being treated for drug-resistant TB were not infectious, even those who had started treatment within the past 2 weeks.[77]

WIDESPREAD TESTING FOR DRUG RESISTANCE CAN ENSURE EFFECTIVE TREATMENT

Some people develop drug-resistant TB (DR-TB) because they became sick with drug-susceptible TB in the past, but did not receive a complete and effective treatment regimen. However, people who are sick with DR-TB can also pass the DR-TB infection to other people, and are doing so at increasing rates. In fact, globally, most patients sick with DR-TB including multidrug-resistant TB (MDR-TB) have never previously been diagnosed with TB disease.

For example, in 2013, within the WHO European region, 14% of patients who had never been previously treated for TB had MDR-TB.[67] Although the proportion of MDR-TB among patients who have previously been treated for TB is higher—in the WHO European region it is almost 50%—there are fewer actual patients in the retreatment group.

Some TB programs do not test a patient with TB for drug resistance until a standard first-line drug regimen (taking 6 months) has been unsuccessful. Once a sample is collected for conventional testing of drug resistance, the results can take further weeks or months. Thus, patients may have infectious, untreated, drug-resistant disease for many months before being started on effective treatment. Treatment with inappropriate first-line drugs can cause patients with drug-resistant TB to develop more resistance to additional types of TB drugs (known as amplification of resistance); these patients also tend to have worse treatment outcomes and are more likely to relapse with TB after undergoing months of treatment.[79]

As with drug-susceptible TB, patients with drug-resistant TB quickly stop spreading the infection once they are treated with the correct regimen.[77] Widespread testing for drug-resistant TB using new rapid molecular testing can shorten the delay in treating patients with the correct regimen, substantially reducing the time they are infectious. Such programs have been implemented in countries with high rates of drug-resistant TB and have proven to be feasible.

For example, a TB hospital in Russia tested all patients with symptoms suggestive of TB for drug resistance using Xpert within 2 days of admission. Within 10 months, more than 150 patients with MDR-TB were identified and started appropriate treatment within 5 days of diagnosis.[80] The microscopic observation drug susceptibility (MODS) assay is a rapid test that can diagnose TB and test for drug resistance. In certain districts of Peru, the MODS assay was used to screen every patient who started treatment for TB. The result was a significant decrease in the time it took to diagnose patients with drug-susceptible TB (from 118 days to 33 days) and patients with MDR-TB (from 158 to 52 days).[81]

Standardized risk criteria can be used to guide decisions about treatment for drug-resistant TB in cases where tests for drug resistance are unavailable or the test results are pending. For example, if a child is clinically diagnosed with TB and lives in the same household as an adult with drug-resistant TB, then the child would be treated for drug-resistant TB. In the households of people with drug-resistant TB (source cases), when another person in a household also became sick with TB (secondary cases), the secondary case had the same pattern of drug resistance as the source case more than 50% of the time.[82]

STRENGTHENING HEALTH SYSTEMS CAN REDUCE TREATMENT DELAYS

Reducing the delay between diagnosis and treatment is critical for stopping transmission and ensuring that patients have the best chance for a good treatment outcome. Delays in initiating treatment for TB have been widely reported. For example, a study in South Africa reported that only 20% of patients with drug-resistant TB had started treatment within the 2 weeks after their diagnosis. MDR-TB patients faced an average delay of 17 days between diagnosis and treatment, despite having rapid nucleic acid test (Xpert MTB/RIF) results available within hours.[83] Gaps in the health delivery systems can exacerbate treatment delay at multiple points in the process, but protocols can be put in place to initiate effective treatment promptly. Such practices include collecting accurate contact information for patients at the first diagnostic visit and optimizing the processes of receiving, accessing, and communicating results to patients.

PATIENTS NEED TO BE SUPPORTED THROUGHOUT TREATMENT

Patients can face numerous obstacles that result in treatment delays and uncompleted treatments. Not only must they be able to access treatment after diagnosis, but they must be willing and able to start and maintain the lengthy treatment regimen. Patients may choose to decline or stop treatment for various reasons: they may not feel very sick from the disease; treatment may interfere with their ability to work; or the nearest health facility may entail travelling long distances. Having TB remains stigmatized in many communities, causing some patients to become isolated or depressed. Additionally, TB is driven by poverty and is itself a driver of poverty, so specific support strategies are required to make treatment feasible for people suffering from the disease (Table 21.4).

Integrated care can reduce the burden of time and effort that TB treatment can impose upon patients, making them more likely to complete treatment. Depending on the specific setting, TB care

Table 21.4 Examples of strategies for supporting patients through TB treatment[16,17,86]

- Following up actively with people who do not start treatment
- Providing incentives and enablers for patients to start treatment
- Monitoring patients during treatment
- Providing transportation assistance and/or food assistance as needed
- Providing social support through treatment supporters and patient support networks
- Providing cash transfers to patients and/or their families

might be integrated into other public healthcare services such as HIV care, diabetes care, or maternal–child health programs.[84] Partnerships with community advocates and other public sectors can bolster TB detection and treatment efforts, as can partnering with private hospitals and providers in areas where many patients seek care in the private sector.[85] Approaches that address economic and social barriers to treatment adherence and completion are also important for a comprehensive TB program to be successful.[86]

PREVENT: PREVENT EXPOSURE, TREAT EXPOSURE

An estimated one-quarter of the global population is infected with TB (1.7 billion people), but most of those people will not become sick with active TB disease.[87] People who are infected with TB but who are not sick make up a reservoir of potential future cases of TB, and it has been estimated that roughly 10% of them will eventually become sick with TB disease, 5% within the first 2 years after infection. A recent re-analysis of the published literature concludes that the vast majority of TB disease will occur within two years of TB infection.[88] Even if health systems were able to find and instantly treat every new case of TB, or if there were an effective new vaccine for preventing TB, the epidemic would still not be stopped. People who are already infected will continue to become future TB cases and continue to spread the disease. Shrinking that reservoir of people who are infected with TB is the only way to stop the epidemic.[89] This will require protecting people from exposure to TB mycobacteria and treating people who have been exposed to TB with preventive therapy.

PROTECTING PEOPLE FROM EXPOSURE PREVENTS FUTURE TB CASES

TB is an airborne disease that can be spread anywhere by any untreated patient with pulmonary TB, but transmission of TB is more likely in crowded, poorly ventilated settings and inside homes or healthcare facilities where people are sick with TB. In healthcare facilities, patients and staff can be protected from exposure by implementing simple practices such as isolating and providing paper masks for people with symptoms suggestive of TB[90] and improving ventilation by opening windows and doors.[91] Another strategy is screening people who live or work in settings with a higher exposure risk—such as mines, prisons, and factories—so that they can be treated and protect others from infection.

PREVENTIVE THERAPY FOR HIGH-RISK GROUPS REDUCES NEW TB CASES

People who are infected with TB bacteria have a 10% risk of becoming sick with TB disease at some point in their lives. Testing a person for TB infection can be done using the tuberculin skin test (TST) or the interferon gamma-release assay (IGRA) blood test. If a person tests positive for TB infection, then treatment with appropriate preventive therapy can significantly reduce the person's chance of developing active TB disease. Treatment with isoniazid given daily for at least 6 months is the most common regimen for preventive therapy, but there are also other therapies that are shorter, easier to deliver, and shown to be as effective (e.g., isoniazid and rifapentine given once weekly for 3 months).[78] Decades of clinical studies have shown that preventive therapy can keep people with TB infection from becoming sick with TB. In adults with TB infection who do not have HIV and have otherwise healthy immune systems, isoniazid preventive therapy can reduce the risk of developing active disease by 60%, and one person will be saved from TB if 35 infected people take isoniazid for 6 months.[51]

Although the average person infected with TB has a 10% lifetime risk of becoming sick with the disease at some point in their lives, some groups of people have an even higher risk of becoming sick with TB if they are infected with the TB bacteria, including: children, people living with HIV, and people who have other types of chronic illnesses.[49] However, preventive therapy can significantly reduce the chance that people in these high-risk groups will become sick with TB if they are infected.

Among children with TB infection under the age of 16 years, preventive treatment with isoniazid reduces the risk of becoming sick with TB by more than 60%.[78] Adults living with HIV who are also infected with TB have a 30% chance of developing active disease if they do not receive preventive therapy; treatment with 3–12 months of isoniazid therapy reduces that risk by between 32% and 62%.[48] People infected with both HIV and TB who are being treated for HIV with antiretroviral therapy have a 60% lower chance of developing active TB, so combining TB preventive therapy with antiretroviral therapy has an even more powerful effect.[47]

SHORTER PREVENTIVE THERAPY REGIMENS CAN REDUCE THE TREATMENT BURDEN

The length of treatment and the potential side effects can make it difficult for patients to complete preventive therapy regimens, and health systems can have difficulty administering and monitoring patients' treatments. However, preventive therapy regimens are available that are shorter but highly effective, and can ease the burden on both patients and health systems. These regimens include: 3–4 months of treatment with rifampin once daily; 3–4 months of treatment with rifampin plus isoniazid once daily; or 3 months of treatment with rifapentine plus isoniazid once weekly.[89]

PREVENTIVE THERAPY CAN ALSO REDUCE NEW CASES OF DRUG-RESISTANT TB

Clinical studies are still underway, and observational evidence suggests that appropriate preventive therapy can also protect persons exposed to drug-resistant TB from developing active TB disease.[45] A systematic review of 21 observational studies of MDR-TB preventive therapy found it to be 90% effective in preventing MDR-TB in close contacts and it was also cost-effective.[44]

PREVENTIVE THERAPY CAN HAVE A POPULATION-LEVEL IMPACT

In the 1950s, a groundbreaking study in the United States investigated using isoniazid preventive therapy to treat household contacts of people with TB. In households where contacts were treated, the number of new TB cases was 60% lower than in households where contacts were not treated; this reduced risk of developing TB was sustained for 20 years.[43] More recent studies in Brazil looked at the effect of active case-finding combined with preventive therapy for household contacts of TB patients. After 5 years, the number of new TB cases was 10% lower in those communities, compared with a 5% increase of new TB cases in communities where household contacts were not screened.[13] Another study screened patients enrolled in HIV clinics in Brazil and treated those who had TB infection with preventive therapy, which reduced the number of new TB cases among the clinics' patient populations by between 25% and 30%.[27]

CONCLUSIONS

Local coalitions seeking to drive down TB rates can design a comprehensive strategy that integrates these three strands of activities—SEARCH, TREAT, and PREVENT—and that is tailored to the local epidemic. These efforts require collaboration among many stakeholders committed to driving down TB rates in specific locations: the public sector at the municipal, regional, and national levels; the private sector; academia; and civil society groups. The Zero TB Initiative is a learning community that promotes shared learning and disseminates lessons from these coalitions.[23]

REFERENCES

1. Lönnroth K, Jaramillo E, Williams BG, Dye C, and Raviglione M. Drivers of tuberculosis epidemics: The role of risk factors and social determinants. *Social Sci Med*. 2009; 68:2240–6.
2. Dye C, Glaziou P, Floyd K, and Raviglione M. Prospects for tuberculosis elimination. *Annu Rev Public Health*. 2013; 34:271–86.
3. World Health Organization. Global Tuberculosis Report 2014. Geneva: WHO, 2014.
4. Zero TB Declaration. Treatment Action Group. Available at http://www.treatmentactiongroup.org/tb/advocacy/zero-declaration (accessed July 19, 2015).
5. WHO. *Global Tuberculosis Report 2015*. Geneva, Switzerland: World Health Organization, 2015.
6. Keshavjee S, Farmer PE. Tuberculosis, drug resistance and the history of modern medicine. *N Engl J Med*. 2012;367(10):931–6.

7. McMillan CW. *Discovering Tuberculosis: A Global History 1900 to the Present.* New Haven and London: Yale University Press, 2015.

8. Walsh JA, and Warren KS. Selective primary health care: An interim strategy for disease control in developing countries. *N Engl J Med.* 1979;301:967–74.

9. Obermeyer Z, Abbott-Klafter J, and Murray CJL. Has the DOTS strategy improved case finding or treatment success? An empirical assessment. *PLOS ONE.* 2008;3(3):e1721. doi:10.1371/journal.pone.0001721

10. De Cock KM, and Chaisson RE. Will DOTS do it? A reappraisal of tuberculosis control in countries with high rates of HIV infection. *Int J Tuberc Lung Dis.* 1999;3(6):457–65.

11. Jenkins HE, Tolman AW, Yuen CM, Parr JB, Keshavjee S, Pérez-Vélez CM, Pagano M, Becerra MC, and Cohen T. Incidence of multidrug-resistant tuberculosis disease in children: Systematic review and global estimates. *Lancet.* 2014;383(9928):1572–9.

12. Frieden TR, Fujiwara PI, Washko RM, and Hamburg MA. Tuberculosis in New York City—Turning the tide. *N Engl J Med.* 1995;333(4):229–33.

13. Cavalcante SC, Durovni B, Barnes GL, Souza FB, Silva RF, Barroso PF, Mohan CI, Miller A, Golub JE, and Chaisson RE. Community-randomized trial of enhanced DOTS for tuberculosis control in Rio de Janeiro, Brazil. *Int J Tuberc Lung Dis.* 2010;14(2):203–9.

14. Bamrah S et al. Treatment for LTBI in contacts of MDR-TB patients, Federated States of Micronesia, 2009–2012. *Int J Tuberc Lung Dis.* 2014;18(8):912–8.

15. Graham NM et al. Effect of isoniazid chemoprophylaxis on HIV-related mycobacterial disease. *Arch Intern Med.* 1996;156:889–94.

16. Keshavjee S et al. Treating multi-drug resistant tuberculosis in Tomsk, Russia: Developing programs that address the linkage between poverty and disease. *Ann New York Acad Sci.* 2008;1136:1–11.

17. Rocha C et al. The innovative socio-economic interventions against tuberculosis (ISIAT) project: An operational assessment. *Int J Tuberc Lung Dis.* 2011;15(5):S50–57.

18. Comstock GW. Isoniazid prophylaxis in an underdeveloped area. *Am Rev Respir Dis.* 1962;86:810–22.

19. Keshavjee S, Dowdy D, and Swaminathan S. Stopping the body count: A comprehensive approach to move towards zero tuberculosis deaths. *Lancet.* 2015;386:e46–7.

20. Available at: http://www.stoptb.org/global/plan/plan2/ (accessed May 31, 2019).

21. Available at: https://www.who.int/tb/strategy/end-tb/en/ (accessed May 21, 2019).

22. Resolution A/RES/73/3 adopted by the United Nations General Assembly on 10 October 2018 following approval by the high-level meeting of the General Assembly on the fight against tuberculosis on 26 September 2018. Available at: https://www.who.int/tb/unhlmonTBDeclaration.pdf

23. Available at: https://www.zerotbinitiative.org/ (accessed May 31, 2019).

24. *Proceedings: The emerging role of municipalities in the fight against tuberculosis.* Dubai, UAE: Harvard Medical School Center for Global Health Delivery—Dubai, 2015. Available at: https://www.zerotbinitiative.org/http://ghd-dubai.hms.harvard.edu/files/ghd_dubai/files/municipalities_v1n3april2015.pdf (accessed September 4, 2018).

25. WHO. *Towards Tuberculosis Elimination: An Action Framework for Low-Incidence Countries.* Geneva, Switzerland: World Health Organization, 2014.

26. World Health Organization. Global tuberculosis database. Available at: http://www.who.int/tb/data/en/ (accessed April 24, 2018).

27. Durovni B et al. Effect of improved tuberculosis screening and isoniazid preventive therapy on incidence of tuberculosis and death in patients with HIV in clinics in Rio de Janeiro, Brazil: A stepped wedge, cluster-randomised trial. *Lancet Infect Dis.* 2013;13:852–58.

28. Horwitz O, Payne PG, and Wilbek E. Epidemiological basis of tuberculosis eradication: 4. The isoniazid trial in Greenland. *Bull WHO.* 1966;35(4):509–26.

29. Chandler B. Alaska's ongoing journey with tuberculosis: A brief history of tuberculosis in Alaska and considerations for future control. *State of Alaska Epidemiol Bull: Recomm Rep.* 2017;19(1).

30. Fraser RI. Tuberculosis in Alaska in 1965. *Alaska Med.* 1965;7:12–5.

31. Comstock GW, Baum C, and Snider DE, Jr. Isoniazid prophylaxis among Alaskan Eskimos: A final report of the Bethel isoniazid studies. *Am Rev Respir Dis.* 1979;119(5):827–30.

32. Comstock GW, Ferebee SH, and Hammes LM. A controlled trial of community-wide isoniazid prophylaxis in Alaska. *Am Rev Respir Dis.* 1967;95(6):935–43.

33. Comstock GW, Philip RN. Decline of the tuberculosis epidemic in Alaska. *Public Health Rep.* 1961;76:19–24.

34. Hanson ML, Comstock GW, and Haley CE. Community isoniazid prophylaxis program in an underdeveloped area of Alaska. *Public Health Rep.* 1967;82(12):1045–56.

35. Porter ME, and Comstock GW. Ambulatory chemotherapy in Alaska. *Public Health Rep.* 1962;77:1021–32.

36. O'Donnell MR et al. Sustained reduction in tuberculosis incidence following a community-based participatory intervention. *Public Health Action.* 2012;2(1):23–6. doi:10.5588/pha.11.0023.

37. O'Donnell MR et al. Racial disparities in primary and reactivation tuberculosis in a rural community in the southeastern United States. *Int J Tuberc Lung Dis.* 2010;14(6):733–40.

38. Frieden TR et al. Tuberculosis in New York City—Turning the tide. *NEJM.* 1995;333(4):229–33.

39. Cegielski JP et al. Eliminating tuberculosis one neighborhood at a time. *Am J Public Health.* 2014;104(Suppl 2):S225–33.

40. Cain KP et al. Moving toward tuberculosis elimination: Implementation of a statewide targeted tuberculin testing in Tennessee. *Am J Respir Crit Care Med.* 2012;186(3):273–9.

41. American Lung Association. Trends in Tuberculosis Morbidity and Mortality. American Lung Association Research and Health Education, Epidemiology and Statistics Unit. 2013. Available at: http://www.lung.org/assets/documents/research/tb-trend-report.pdf

42. Horwitz O, Payne PG, and Wilbek E. Epidemiological basis of tuberculosis eradication: The isoniazid trial in Greenland. *Bull WHO.* 1966;35(4):509–26.

43. Comstock GW, Baum C, and Snider DE Jr. Isoniazid prophylaxis among Alaskan Eskimos: A final report of the Bethel isoniazid studies. *Am Rev Respir Dis.* 1979;119:827–30.

44. Marks SM, Mase SR, and Morris SB. Systematic review, meta-analysis, and cost-effectiveness of treatment of latent tuberculosis to reduce progression to multidrug–resistant tuberculosis. *Clin Infect Dis.* 2017 Jun 15;64(12):1670–7.

45. Seddon JA, Fred D, Amanullah F, Schaaf HS, Starke JR, Keshavjee S, Burzynski J, Furin JJ, Swaminathan S, and Becerra MC. *2015 Post-Exposure Management of Multidrug-Resistant Tuberculosis Contacts: Evidence-Based Recommendations. Policy Brief No. 1.* Dubai, United Arab Emirates: Harvard Medical School Center for Global Health Delivery-Dubai.

46. Hanson ML, Comstock GW, and Haley CE. Community isoniazid prophylaxis program in an underdeveloped area of Alaska. *Public Health Rep.* 1967:82(12):1045–56.

47. Golub JE et al. The impact of antiretroviral therapy and isoniazid preventive therapy on tuberculosis incidence in HIV-infected patients in Rio de Janeiro, Brazil. *AIDS.* 2007;21:1441–8.

48. Akolo C, Adetifa I, Shepperd S, and Volmink J. Treatment of latent tuberculosis infection in HIV infected persons. *Cochrane Database Syst Rev.* 2010;20:CD000171.

49. Getahun H, Matteelli A, Chaisson RE, and Raviglione M. Latent *Mycobacterium tuberculosis* infection. *N Engl J Med.* 2015;372:2127–35.

50. Frieden TR et al. Tuberculosis in New York City—turning the tide. *N Engl J Med.* 1995;333(4):229–33.

51. Smieja MJ, Marchetti CA, Cook DJ, and Smaill FM. Isoniazid for preventing tuberculosis in non-HIV infected persons. *Cochrane Database Syst Rev.* 2000;2:CD001363.

52. Cain KP et al. Moving toward tuberculosis elimination: Implementation of a statewide targeted tuberculin testing in Tennessee. *Am J Respir Crit Care Med.* 2012;186(3):273–9. doi: 10.1164/rccm.201111–2076OC.

53. American Lung Association. *Trends in Tuberculosis Morbidity and Mortality.* American Lung Association Research and Health Education, Epidemiology and Statistics Unit, 2013. Available at: http://www.lung.org/assets/documents/research/tb-trend-report.pdf

54. Global Tuberculosis Report 2017. Geneva: World Health Organization; 2017.

55. Golub JE et al. Delayed tuberculosis diagnosis and tuberculosis transmission. *Int J Tuberc Lung Dis.* 2006;10:24–30.

56. Yuen CM, Amanullah F, Dharmadhikari A, Nardell EA, Seddon JA, Vasilyeva I, Zhao Y, Keshavjee S, and Becerra MC. Turning off the tap: Stopping tuberculosis transmission through active case-finding and prompt effective treatment. *Lancet.* 2015;386:2334–43.

57. Morrison J, Pai M, and Hopewell PC. Tuberculosis and latent tuberculosis infection in close contacts of people with pulmonary tuberculosis in low-income and middle-income countries: A systematic review and meta-analysis. *Lancet Infect Dis.* 2008;8(6):359–68.

58. Fox GJ, Barry SE, Britton WJ, and Marks GB. Contact investigation for tuberculosis: A systematic review and meta-analysis. *Eur Respir J.* 2013;41:140–56.

59. Kranzer K, Houben RM, Glynn JR, Bekker LG, Wood R, and Lawn SD. Yield of HIV-associated tuberculosis during intensified case finding in resource-limited settings: A systematic review and meta-analysis. *Lancet Infect Dis.* 2010;10:93–102.

60. Khan AJ et al. Engaging the private sector to increase tuberculosis case detection: An impact evaluation study. *Lancet Infect Dis.* 2012;12(8):608–16.

61. Baily GV, Savic D, Gothi GD, Naidu VB, and Nair SS. Potential yield of pulmonary tuberculosis cases by direct microscopy of sputum in a district of South India. *Bull WHO.* 1967;37(6):875–92.

62. Aluoch JA et al. Study of case-finding for pulmonary tuberculosis in outpatients complaining of a chronic cough at a district hospital in Kenya. *Am Rev Resp Dis.* 1984;129(6):915–20.

63. Sanchez-Perez HJ, Hernan MA, Hernandez-Diaz S, Jansa JM, Halperin D, and Ascherio A. Detection of pulmonary tuberculosis in Chiapas, Mexico. *Ann Epidemiol.* 2002;12(3):166–72.

64. Theron G, Jenkins HE, Cobelens F, Abubakar I, Khan AJ, Cohen T, and Dowdy DW. Data for action: Collection and use of local data to end tuberculosis. *Lancet.* 2015;386(10010):2324–33.

65. Murray CJ, Styblo K, and Rouillon A. Tuberculosis in developing countries: Burden, intervention and cost. *Bull Int Union Tuberc Lung Dis.* 1990;65:6–24.

66. Lawn SD et al. Screening for HIV-associated tuberculosis and rifampicin resistance before antiretroviral therapy using the Xpert MTB/RIF assay: A prospective study. *PLoS Med.* 2011;8:e1001067.

67. WHO. Global Tuberculosis Report 2014. Geneva, Switzerland: World Health Organization, 2014.

68. Behr MA et al. Transmission of *Mycobacterium tuberculosis* from patients smear-negative for acid-fast bacilli. *Lancet.* 1999;353:444–49.

69. WHO. *Systematic Screening for Active Tuberculosis: Principles and Recommendations.* Geneva: World Health Organization, 2013.

70. WHO. *Guidance for National Tuberculosis Programmes on the Management of Tuberculosis in Children.* 2nd ed. Geneva, Switzerland: World Health Organization, 2014.

71. Getahun H et al. Development of a standardized screening rule for tuberculosis in people living with HIV in resource-constrained settings: Individual participant data meta-analysis of observational studies. *PLoS Med.* 2011;8:e1000391.

72. Ayles H et al. and the ZAMSTAR team. Effect of household and community interventions on the burden of tuberculosis in southern Africa: The ZAMSTAR community-randomised trial. *Lancet.* 2013;382:1183–94.

73. Azman AS, Golub JE, and Dowdy DW. How much is tuberculosis screening worth? Estimating the value of active case finding for tuberculosis in South Africa, China, and India. *BMC Med.* 2014;12:216.

74. Creswell J, Sahu S, Blok L, Bakker MI, Stevens R, and Ditiu L. A multi-site evaluation of innovative approaches to increase tuberculosis case notification: Summary results. *PLOS ONE.* 2014;9:e94465.

75. Lin X, Chongsuvivatwong V, Lin L, Geater A, and Lijuan R. Dose response relationship between treatment delay of smear-positive tuberculosis patients and intra-household transmission: A crosssectional study. *Trans R Soc Trop Med Hyg.* 2008;102(8):797–804.

76. Kamat SR et al. A controlled study of the influence of segregation of tuberculous patients for one year on the attack rate of tuberculosis in a 5-year period in close family contacts in South India. *Bull World Health Organ.* 1966;34:517–32.

77. Dharmadhikari AS et al. Rapid impact of effective treatment on transmission of multidrug-resistant tuberculosis. *Int J Tuberc Lung Dis.* 2014;18:1019–25.

78. WHO. *Latent Tuberculosis Infection: Updated and Consolidated Guidelines for Programmatic Management.* Geneva: World Health Organization, 2018.

79. Lew W, Pai M, Oxlade O, Martin D, and Menzies D. Initial drug resistance and tuberculosis treatment outcomes: Systematic review and meta-analysis. *Ann Intern Med.* 2008;149:123–34.

80. Barrera E, Livchits V, and Nardell E. F-A-S-T: A refocused, intensified, administrative tuberculosis transmission control strategy. *Int J Tuberc Lung Dis.* 2015;19:381–84.

81. Mendoza-Ticona A et al. Effect of universal MODS access on pulmonary tuberculosis treatment outcomes in new patients in Peru. *Public Health Action.* 2012;2:162–67.

82. Shah NS, Yuen CM, Heo M, Tolman AW, and Becerra MC. Yield of contact investigations in households of patients with drug-resistant tuberculosis: Systematic review and meta-analysis. *Clin Infect Dis.* 2014;58:381–91.

83. Naidoo P et al. A comparison of multidrug-resistant tuberculosis treatment commencement times in MDRTBPlus line probe assay and XpertR MTB/RIF-based algorithms in a routine operational setting in Cape Town. *PLOS ONE.* 2014;9:e103328.

84. Detjen A, Gnanashanmugam D, and Talens A. *A Framework for Integrating Childhood Tuberculosis into Community-Based Child Health Care. Washington, DC*: CORE Group, 2013.

85. Khan MS, Salve S, and Porter JD. Engaging for-profit providers in TB control: Lessons learnt from initiatives in south Asia. *Health Policy Plan.* 2015;30(10):1289–95.

86. Ortblad KF, Salomon JA, Barnighausen T, and Atun R. Stopping tuberculosis: A biosocial model for sustainable development. *Lancet.* 2015;386:2354–6.

87. Houben RMGJ, and Dodd PJ. The global burden of latent tuberculosis infection: A re-estimation using mathematical modelling. *PLoS Med.* 2016;13(10):e1002152.

88. Behr MA, Edelstein PH, and Ramakrishnan L. Revisiting the timetable of tuberculosis. *BMJ.* 2018;362:k2738.

89. Rangaka MX et al. Controlling the seedbeds of tuberculosis: Diagnosis and treatment of tuberculosis infection. *Lancet.* 2015;386:2344–53.

90. Dharmadhikari AS et al. Surgical face masks worn by patients with multidrug-resistant tuberculosis: Impact on infectivity of air on a hospital ward. *Am J Respir Crit Care Med.* 2012;185(10):1104–9.

91. Lygizos M et al. Natural ventilation reduces high TB transmission risk in traditional homes in rural KwaZulu-Natal, South Africa. *BMC Infect Dis.* 2013;13:300.

RELATED ASPECTS

22

Animal Tuberculosis

CATHERINE WILSON

INTRODUCTION

Mycobacterial infection can clinically affect a wide range of animal species including humans, and several mycobacterial species have the potential to cause zoonotic disease. *Mycobacterium bovis* infection is currently one of the most significant veterinary public health concerns worldwide and may account for a substantial loss of productivity of cattle. This can lead to a significant economic impact for farmers, impacting on the trade of livestock and associated products both within a country and internationally. Incidence of *M. bovis* in the human population of most higher middle income countries (HMICs) has decreased significantly since the nineteenth century due to the widespread introduction of milk pasteurization, but the disease remains endemic in the cattle and human population in many countries across the world. Disease control in cattle is challenging, particularly in areas where *M. bovis* has a significant reservoir in the wildlife population. Solutions to eradicate the disease completely are currently being sought in many countries across the world.

HISTORY

Columella was the first to document the incidence of tuberculosis in cattle in 40 AD. In the seventeenth and eighteenth centuries, the term "Persucht" was recorded in Germany, referring to the grape-like lesions documented on clinical examination, most likely to describe the disease currently known as bovine tuberculosis. At this point, the grape-like symptoms were considered to be a symptom of syphilis and their identification in cattle resulted in more rigorous control of disposal of the carcasses of affected animals. However, once the misconception that syphilis was the cause of this clinical sign was corrected, these control measures were discarded.

It was not until 1882 that Robert Koch first discovered the bacilli *Mycobacterium tuberculosis*, the main causative agent of tuberculosis in humans. Koch postulated at this time that the tuberculous disease also affecting cattle was not pathogenic to man. Theobald Smith, however, disproved this theory in 1898 by demonstrating that there was only a small difference between the mycobacteria that cause disease in humans and cattle.[1] Koch later accepted Smith's theory, under the assumption that the bovine form of tuberculosis was a less pathogenic form in humans than cows, and the reverse to be true upon transmission from humans to cattle.

The first route of transmission of *M. bovis* from cattle to humans was found to be by ingestion of unpasteurized cows' milk.[1] It was initially thought that eradication of zoonotic tuberculosis should be carried out by banning the sale of milk from tubercular cows, and eradicating tuberculosis in cattle.[2] In 1901 the British Government opted to establish a Royal Commission to perform further investigations in an effort to establish whether tuberculosis in animals and humans was the same and investigate the potential main transmission routes from cattle to humans.[1] This report was completed in 1911, and concluded that it is possible that *M. bovis* transmitted from cows can infect humans, and may cause clinical disease in both species. The main infection route to humans was found to be via ingestion of infected cows' milk, especially for children,[3] and meat ingestion was concluded to be a much lesser risk.

Following this conclusion, control measures were slowly implemented in the United Kingdom and in 1913 the Tuberculosis Order offered local authorities the power to remove infected animals from farmers' herds. In spite of the high prevalence of infected animals among herds, little was done to prevent the spread of disease and eradication was considered to be only an option for the wealthy cattle owners; the action of this Order was suspended during World War I. The general consensus appeared to be that although the disease was of great economic importance, its presence in the country was largely inevitable. However, over time, the Tuberculosis Order evolved, and in 1925 the government started to offer compensation to farmers for animals withdrawn from herds due to the presence of clinical signs of tuberculosis, a chronic cough, tuberculosis of the udder, weight loss, or tubercular milk. Under this Order, 15,000 cattle were slaughtered, an estimated 2500 of which were producing tubercular milk. In fact, the instigation of the Tuberculosis Order prompted the formation of veterinary services across all areas of the United Kingdom.

Initially there was a resistance to milk pasteurization across the United Kingdom due to both a public preference for raw milk, and the presence of powerful economic forces in the dairy industry that were reluctant to instigate the pasteurization procedure on a large scale. The practice first began in 1923, and by 1938, 98% of milk on sale in London was pasteurized. Over this same period the death rate due to abdominal tuberculosis fell dramatically to 9% for children under 5 years of age in London in comparison to children in more rural areas, where pasteurization of milk prior to ingestion was much less common, which fell to only 25% of the level recorded in 1923.[1]

In 1934, the Cattle Disease Committee reported that over 40% of cattle in the UK herds were infected with TB, and that 0.5% of cattle were suffering from tuberculous mastitis. Two thousand five hundred humans were reported to die annually due to zoonotic tuberculosis, 6% of the total mortality rate in the United Kingdom in the 1930s.[4] This prompted the Cattle Diseases Committee to assert that the only solution to this problem was total eradication of tuberculosis from cattle in the United Kingdom. In 1935, the Tuberculosis (Attested Herds) Scheme was launched by the government providing a reward for the owners of "clean" herds and subsidizing the cost of tuberculin tests in herds that have only a small percentage of reactors.

It was not until 1950 that a national compulsory tuberculosis eradication scheme was introduced by the government in the United Kingdom, and compensation for reacting cattle and movement restrictions of affected herds were effectively enforced. Initially, the scheme was introduced only in areas with the highest numbers of affected herds, and gradually was extended out to reach herds across the whole of the United Kingdom by 1960.[1] Following strict implementation of these policies, the incidence of infected cattle dramatically decreased, and in the late 1970s, the lowest prevalence of the disease yet was recorded in the United Kingdom. The number of cattle slaughtered annually decreased significantly over this period, and the percentage of tested herds

offering positive reactions dropped from 3.5% in 1961 to 0.49% in 1979. However, as has remained until this day, the incidence of disease remained higher in the South West of England compared to the remainder of Great Britain.[5]

The disease became notifiable to the State Veterinary Service in England, Wales, and Scotland under Sections 32 and 34 of the Animal Health Act 1981. The Act has since been variously amended by various instruments and the latest versions are available on the UK Government website (www.legislation.gov.uk).

It has never been possible to implement universal compulsory pasteurization of milk in England and Wales, despite advice from the Advisory Committee for the Microbiological Safety of Food, which independently reports to the Food Standards Agency. Currently, it is legally possible in England and Wales to sell milk from a cattle herd that is classed as Officially Tuberculosis Free (OTF) to the public.

Tuberculosis remains a major concern in animals in the United Kingdom. Between 1990 and 2004 there was an annual increase of 14% of new herd breakdowns of infections of tuberculosis, as detected by routine surveillance.

In 2004, 4.6 million cattle were tested in 44,720 herd tests across the United Kingdom. Overall in Great Britain at that time there were 93 million cattle herds, and a total of 9 million cattle and calves. These tests revealed 3339 new tuberculosis herd breakdowns, which was 7.5% of the total herds tested. Of these, 1702 breakdowns were confirmed, which equated to 3.6 confirmed herd breakdowns for every 100 nonrestricted cattle herds tested. Nearly 20,000 cattle were slaughtered as tuberculin test reactors in Great Britain in 2004. There were also 3000 cattle removed from herds that were "direct contacts," i.e., those with a negative or inconclusive tuberculin test, but presented too high a risk of infection with *M. bovis*. In 2003, although approximately 50% of the new infections were from herds including dairy cattle, the incidence of tuberculosis in dairy herds was comparable to beef and other herd types (Figure 22.1). Updated figures for the incidence and prevalence of tuberculosis among cattle herds in Great Britain are published quarterly by the Department for Environment, Food and Rural Affairs.[125]

The main aim of eradication of bovine tuberculosis from countries where the disease is endemic has proved to be challenging. This is mainly due to the reservoir of the disease in wildlife. One of the successful eradication stories took place in Australia in the 1970s following a long, 27-year period of abattoir surveillance and culling of affected wildlife reservoirs of water buffalo as part of the Brucellosis and Tuberculosis Eradication Campaign to reduce the reservoir of tuberculosis. Australia was declared free of bovine tuberculosis in 1997. In the United Kingdom and Republic of Ireland the badger (*Meles meles*) became a source of concern as a possible wildlife reservoir of the disease and potential source of infection for cattle in the mid-1970s.[1] In 1989, tuberculosis was made a notifiable disease of deer under the Tuberculosis (Deer) Order 1989 (as amended). Evidence does not suggest that other wild or feral animals (e.g. deer, fox and wild boar) pose a substantial national threat to cattle, although further work needs to be undertaken. Although there is no compulsory testing scheme for this species, postmortem inspection and notification of suspect lesions to the APHA is statutory for farmed, park, or wild deer.

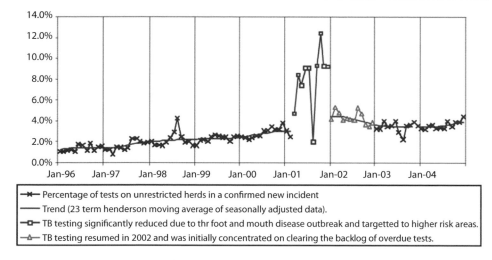

Figure 22.1 Confirmed new incidences of bovine TB in Great Britain, expressed as a percentage of unrestricted cattle herds tested during the period 1996–2004. The monthly number of TB breakdowns has been divided by the number of tuberculin herd tests carried out each month to account for the seasonality of cattle testing, most of which takes place between October and April. (From Anon Tuberculosis statistics DEFRA (2005). Available online http://www.defra.gov.uk/animalh/tb/stats/dec2004.htm.) (Permission: http://www.nationalarchives.gov.uk/legal/copyright/.)

Culling schemes of other animals which act as reservoirs of *M. bovis* for cattle and humans have taken place worldwide, for example, that of the brushtail possum in New Zealand, with limited effect on the provision of control of the disease.

To this day tuberculosis in animals remains a major veterinary public health concern across the world. This chapter aims to expand on these concerns.

ETIOLOGY

Mycobacteria of veterinary importance have been broken up into three groups.

1. *Obligate primary pathogens*: These mycobacteria require the presence of a mammalian host to continue their life cycle and include those of *M. tuberculosis* complex and *Mycobacterium lepraemurium*.
2. *Saphrophytes*: These mycobacteria are normally found existing on dead or decaying matter but have the potential to become facultative pathogens causing symptoms of either local or disseminated disease. They can be further categorized into fast- or slow-growing opportunistic non-tuberculous mycobacteria and include mycobacteria such as *M. avium*.
3. *Mycobacteria that are difficult to grow*: These bacteria are so challenging to grow that it is impossible to determine their natural environmental niche. This group of bacteria is responsible for feline leprosy and canine leproid granuloma syndrome.

Over the last few years, genomic sequencing has begun to play a role in clarifying these taxonomic divisions.[7,8] The lack of clarity in taxonomy has meant that specific mycobacteria are more easily classified according to their clinical presentation of disease, speed and ability to grow on culture media, and the mycobacteria's biochemical properties. The etiological agents of tuberculosis in animals and their classification still remain the subject of debate.[9]

M. bovis is the main etiological agent of bovine tuberculosis. It carries the highest risk of zoonotic transmission and the greatest economic impact to humans. This acid-fast, aerobic, Gram-positive, nonmotile, non-sporulating, rod-shaped, and slow-growing bacillus can survive for long periods of time in the environment (between 18 and 332 days) at temperatures ranging between 12°C and 24°C.

M. bovis has been classified as part of the *M. tuberculosis* complex. This complex includes genetically related bacilli including *M. tuberculosis*, *Mycobacterium microti*, first discovered in the vole population, *Mycobacterium caprae*, the main agent that causes tuberculous disease in goats, and *Mycobacterium pinnipedii*, which usually clinically affects marine dwelling mammals such as seals and sea lions. This complex has a 99.9% similarity at a nucleotide level and almost identical 16S rRNA sequences.[10] *M. tuberculosis*, the host-restricted mycobacteria that is the main mycobacterium to cause disease in humans, has evolved as a separate lineage of the MTB complex.[11] Non-tuberculous mycobacteria are all those mycobacteria that are not part of the complex and contain fewer identical nucleotide sequences. These mycobacteria still have pathogenic potential and include the *M. avium* complex, the species of which include *M. avium* and *M. avium paratuberculosis (MAP)*, the mycobacterium that is implicated in Crohn's disease in humans and is the causative agent of Johne's disease in cattle and sheep.

PATHOGENESIS AND TRANSMISSION OF TUBERCULOSIS

Mycobacteria can infect a very broad range of hosts. *M. bovis*, which is the main agent responsible for tuberculosis in domestic animals and wildlife, has the broadest host range of the Mycobacterium complex group. Alternatively, *M. tuberculosis* rarely affects species other than humans, although cases in dogs have been occasionally reported.

Cattle are the natural host of *M. bovis*. These mycobacteria are distributed worldwide and most terrestrial animals and some birds are susceptible to these bacteria. Some host species, for example cattle, humans, pigs and goats are "maintenance" hosts, in which infection can become established and cause clinical disease while other species such as dogs and cats can act as "spillover" hosts, in which infection does not transmit onwards to other members of the same species. The innate resistance of "spillover" hosts' immune systems is one of the reasons as to why these species do not go on to develop clinical disease when exposed to an infected individual of the same species. Other epidemiological factors, such as population density, husbandry, and habitat also affect the degree of interaction between the susceptible and the infected individuals and therefore the potential for clinical infection to occur.

M. bovis is a highly contagious, chronic debilitating disease of the maintenance hosts. Characteristically, tubercles, or nodular granulomas, may be seen on postmortem examination in the lymph nodes or affected tissue. The resulting caseation and calcification, excluding the skeletal muscles, contribute to the clinical symptoms of the disease. In all maintenance hosts, the disease can be contracted either via aerosol or ingestion, causing a non-pulmonary or pulmonary form of the disease and clinical symptoms of either form can take months or years to develop.

As expected, the clinical symptoms of the pulmonary form include a chronic cough due to granulomatous, caseous, necrotizing inflammation in the lungs and associated lymph nodes,[12] the commonest of which to be affected are the bronchial, mediastinal, retropharyngeal, and portal lymph nodes. Enlargement of other lymph nodes can also be detected and tubercles can also be discovered in the liver, spleen and body cavities. In advanced cases of the disease, enlarged lymph nodes have the potential to cause significant obstruction, for example, of the trachea, alimentary tract, or blood vessels. Enlargement of the peripheral lymph nodes can be viewed on external examination, and these nodes have the potential to rupture and their caseous contents to drain. Symptoms due to the involvement of the digestive tract may include intermittent diarrhea and bloating, due to the presence of enlarged mediastinal lymph nodes and retropharyngeal lymph node enlargement can lead to dysphagia. Clinical symptoms can therefore be attributed to the organs involved and may vary between cases. They may include weight loss, weakness, inappetence, fluctuating fever, an intermittent hacking cough, diarrhea, anorexia, and induration of the udder, depending on the manifestation of the disease. Tuberculous mastitis in cattle is a major public health concern, as the disease can spread easily from infected cattle to both calves and humans consuming the milk, and mastitis caused by *M. bovis* is clinically indistinguishable from other forms of mastitis.

An understanding of the immune response of the host will help to understand the pathogenesis of the disease.[13] During the initial infection a cell-mediated response, with activity of T cells and macrophages, predominates. As the infection progresses, the immune response converts to humoral and there is a change from the T helper 1 to T helper 2 immune response. A deviation of interleukin responses also occurs, which can be detected on investigation by cytokine analysis.

The most common route of transmission of *M. bovis* between animals is via the respiratory system and therefore humans handling potentially infected cattle should take appropriate precautions. Cutaneous or mucosal transmission routes are extremely rare, especially in industrialized countries, where the bacilli load is much smaller. Previously in the United Kingdom, cutaneous transmission was the source of localized skin, tendon, and lymph node lesions, and otitis and conjunctivitis commonly afflicted milking staff or farm workers in regular contact with infected cattle.[3] The incidence of tuberculosis caused by *M. bovis* in humans is associated with the efficiency of tuberculosis control strategies.

In the United Kingdom, ingestion of infected milk was the main transmission route of *M. bovis* from cattle to man before the advent of pasteurization.[1] In countries where milk pasteurization is common and widespread, transmission of *M. bovis* to humans from cattle is now a much-decreased risk. Where milk pasteurization is not present or well controlled, transmission of *M. bovis* from cattle to humans continues to occur.[14] The infective dose of tuberculosis has been thought to be 10–100 cfu by inhalation and much higher, in millions, to cause disease by ingestion.[15] One cow in a 100 cattle herd infected with *M. bovis* and shedding bacilli into the milk is sufficient to contaminate the entire bulk milk tank, with the potential to infect a human. *M. bovis* can remain present and viable in unpasteurized milk for a long period of time, but will only replicate within the udder. Currently in the United Kingdom, due to the instigation of tuberculosis control programmes and milk pasteurization, infection via ingestion of infected milk is rare in humans and currently only 0.5% of all infected cattle slaughtered appear to be shedding *M. bovis* bacilli into the milk at the time of death.

Transmission of *M. bovis* to humans from any other animals apart from cattle is thought to occur only sporadically. Normally only those humans with regular contact with other potentially infected maintenance hosts are likely to be infected, such as deer farm owners. Published information documenting transmission from deer to humans is very limited, and no reports have been published in the literature originating from the United Kingdom. One report has documented transmission to a human from an elk (*Cervus elaphus canadensis*) in Canada.[16] In the United Kingdom, there is a high prevalence of *M. bovis* in the wild deer population, and tuberculosis outbreaks have been confirmed in a small number of farmed deer herds,[17] therefore, the potential reservoir for transmission does exist.

EPIDEMIOLOGY

Natural infection with *M. bovis* has been described in many different species of wild and domestic animals across the world.[18] The host range of this bacteria is much broader than that of *M. tuberculosis* and the complex epidemiology of this pathogen has complicated its eradication.[19] To some degree, all terrestrial mammals are susceptible to infection and infection rate depends on exposure, innate resistance, immunological pathways, type of husbandry and ecology, and characteristic pathology of the disease.[20]

Cattle are the major maintenance host of *M. bovis*, and therefore are capable of maintaining the infection within their population. "Spillover" hosts can be defined as those in which the animal species may become infected, but are not particularly effective at transmitting the infection between other members of the same species. In the case of *M. bovis*, these spillover hosts include, among others, humans, cats, and dogs.

Within the cattle species, different breeds have been found to show differing susceptibilities to disease. *Bos taurus*, a European lineage of cattle, is more susceptible to disease than *Bos indicus*, or zebu cattle.[21] Zebu cattle appear to have an innate resistance to infection with mycobacteria. In the United Kingdom and Republic of Ireland, Holstein cattle have been shown to pass a significant degree of heritability of resistance to bovine tuberculosis infection on to their young.[22-24] The modern Friesian breed of cattle was developed in the 1940s by Dutch cattle breeders as a hardier and more "tuberculosis-resistant" dairy cow.[25] Greater genetic variation is expected between beef cattle in comparison to dairy cattle, as the latter are more homogenous in terms of breeding history. Normally dairy herds are more intensively managed than beef cattle due to the nature of their production systems, and this closer and more regular contact between cattle, as well as the longer life expectancy of a dairy cow in comparison to beef cattle, increases the probability of a higher prevalence of *M. bovis* within the dairy population. Geographically, *M. tuberculosis* infection has been found to be much less prevalent in areas where cattle farming is more extensive, for example, South America, Asia and Africa, although a higher incidence has been reported across the world in ranch cattle, potentially as the extensively reared cattle cluster around watering points at ranches to drink.

The main route of transmission of *M. bovis* among cattle and spillover hosts is via aerosolized droplets from infected individuals. The mycobacterial organisms can also be secreted in sputum, feces, urine, vaginal, and uterine discharges, as well as from any draining fluid from ruptured peripheral lymph nodes.[26] Ingestion of unpasteurized infected milk or milk products is also an excellent medium for transmission for both calves and humans. If no pasteurization has occurred, mycobacteria present in milk can remain infectious for extended periods of time. This may be up to 200 days in milk and 322 days in certain types of cheese. Environmental transmission of *M. bovis* can occur, as aerosolized particles may contaminate fomites at pasture or inside housing. The mycobacteria may, more rarely, be transmitted by contact with contaminated feces or urine from infected animals.[27] Movement of cattle across the country spreads the bacteria, as infected cattle spread the infection to naïve areas containing susceptible animals.

Eradication of *M. bovis* has occurred in some areas such as Australia, some states of the United States, Germany and some countries in South America, normally following strict test and slaughter policies, and eradication of the disease to an appropriate extent in wildlife reservoirs.

In the United Kingdom and Ireland, the Eurasian badger (*M. meles*) is an additional maintenance host for *M. bovis*. Krebs[5] declared this species to be a significant reservoir of infection for cattle, so impeding the eradication of the disease in cattle.[5,28] There is a split of opinion as to whether badgers present a significant reservoir of infection in endemically infected areas in the United Kingdom, and whether this infection is passed onto the environment from badgers to infect other species.[28]

In Africa, generally, a high prevalence of bovine tuberculosis has been reported in cattle, buffalo,[56] monkeys, and deer. *M. bovis* infection is widespread and endemic among cattle and humans in Ethiopia, and has been for many years. This country has the largest livestock population in Africa with a total of 56 million cattle, 29 million sheep, and 29 million goats. The exact current prevalence of bovine tuberculosis infection in cattle is unknown, but suspected to be anywhere between 7.9% and 49%[53] of the cattle population affected, and the prevalence in dairy herds ranges between 15.6% and 50%. Most of the prevalence surveys have been based on results from the intradermal skin test and postmortem inspection of cattle carcasses at abattoirs. Prevalence studies in various parts of Ethiopia have confirmed that exotic breeds are more likely to be affected than zebu cattle.[54]

The main route of transmission in Ethiopia between animals and man is the ingestion of unpasteurized milk, leading to the development of the extrapulmonary form of tuberculosis in humans. As well as the consequences due to human infection, the productivity of the cattle, including the milk yield, is decreased, and the economic impact of bovine tuberculosis infection in Ethiopia has been described.

In Ethiopia, there are four categories of livestock production systems, which are variously affected by bovine tuberculosis infection:

1. Integrated crop—livestock extensive production system
2. Pastoral livestock production system
3. Smallholder production system
4. Intensive production systems

Eighty-five percent of the country's livestock production occurs in system 1, where crop production is the primary target and animals are kept for draught power and seasonal milk and meat production in the semiarid and highland areas. Animal husbandry is traditional, with low hygiene standards. Those who implement the pastoralist production system derive the bulk of their food supply from animals in the lower altitude areas of the country. The cattle herds are either constantly or partially mobile. This system covers 12% of the total livestock production and 61% of the total land area of the country. The smallholder production system mainly occurs near towns, and is mainly practised in highland areas where dairy animals are reared for milk production and subsistence. Prevalence of bovine tuberculosis in these systems has not been adequately surveyed but has been thought to be low, mainly due to the extensive nature of the production systems. One survey found a 3.5% prevalence in Asela, Southeast Ethiopia. However, drinking raw milk is a common practice for cattle owners in these areas, so the risk of human infection with bovine tuberculosis remains.

There are a small number of intensive production systems, mainly located in urban and peri-urban areas, for which milk and milk product production is the main concern. The animals in these more intensive systems are normally housed and managed more intensively, so increasing the risk of spreading *M. bovis*. Overall targets for milk and meat production are mainly met by the introduction of exotic breeds to increase productivity. However, these exotic, non-native breeds have an increased susceptibility to bovine tuberculosis and this has created a conducive environment for the spread of infection and an increased risk to humans, particularly those drinking unpasteurized milk or milk products. Around dairy farms in the Debre Zeit areas, Holsteins were reported to have a prevalence of bovine tuberculosis infection of 55% whereas that in cross-bred cattle was found to be 23%. However, when kept under more intensive feed-lot conditions, tubercular zebu cattle can experience a depression in weight gain and up to a 60% morbidity rate[55] demonstrating that under more intensive environmental conditions, zebu cattle have an increased predisposition to clinical symptoms of disease, in comparison to their counterparts reared in less intensive environments.

TRANSMISSION OF INFECTION BY INGESTION

MILK

Prior to the advent of pasteurization, the main transmission route of *M. bovis* from cattle to humans, was via ingestion of infected milk. Bovine tuberculosis used to be an endemic disease of humans in the United Kingdom; however, currently, the total annual infection of humans with *M. bovis* is likely to be between 0.5% and 15% in all cases of tuberculosis confirmed in the United Kingdom, similar to the prevalence of *M. bovis* infection detected in humans in other industrialized countries. Sale of unpasteurized milk and dairy products is not illegal in England and Wales, as it is in Scotland, as long as it is clearly labelled as such and sold directly from the site where it was produced. It is possible for *M. bovis* infections to reactivate later on in life and currently the demographics of human *M. bovis* cases in the United Kingdom is most often the older generation who drank unpasteurized milk as children in the 1940s–1950s and doctors are seeing reactivation of the disease in this population at this late stage of their lives, following incomplete eradication of *M. bovis* post treatment.

CHEESE AND OTHER MILK PRODUCTS

It has been found that *M. bovis* can survive well in mature, unpasteurized cheeses as they are less likely than other bacteria to be affected by the potentially more extreme pH of the cheese.[29] Not much work has been carried out to look at the impact of the cheese-making process on *M. bovis* but it has been confirmed that the storage and ripening of certain cheeses does lead to the full inactivation of the bacterium if it was originally present in the raw milk. Currently, there are no validated laboratory techniques that would certify a non-heat-treated dairy product as *M. bovis* "free".

MEAT AND MEAT PRODUCTS

Every carcass slaughtered at a UK slaughterhouse is inspected postmortem. In reference to tuberculosis infection, particular attention is paid to any lesions in the lungs or lymph nodes, and therefore 59% of cattle with visible tuberculosis lesions but not displaying clinical signs are identified at this point.[30] This inspection process complements the National Tuberculosis Testing Scheme, and is especially important in areas of the country where annual tuberculosis testing does not take place.

Occupational exposure of humans is an additional risk factor for contracting *M. bovis* infection. Time spent within close contact of infected animals offers the opportunity for inhalation of aerosolized bacteria from the lungs of an infected cow. Infection through broken skin, although rare, is also a possibility. It may be possible for a carcass to appear entirely normal on gross postmortem and yet contain hematogenously disseminated bacilli that are able to cause infection post consumption. Cross contamination of lesions may also occur during postmortem processing potentially introducing bacilli into the food chain during unhygienic carcass dressing and contamination of muscle surfaces.[31] However, the risk of tuberculous infection from the ingestion of infected meat is minimal and far less efficient than inhalation. The higher doses of tuberculosis bacteria that may cause disease are only found in milk from infected cattle[32] and would be almost impossible to find in skeletal muscle tissue with a lower mycobacterial load and no visible tuberculosis lesions. In developing countries where there is potential for undercooking of meat, the risk of infection by ingestion of meat may be slightly higher, especially in areas where meat hygiene inspection occurs only sporadically.[33]

INFECTION OF OTHER ANIMAL SPECIES

Wild animals have been implicated in the transmission of *M. bovis* to livestock, and potentially play a role in zoonotic transmission of the disease to humans. In the United Kingdom and Ireland, the badger (*M. meles*) is the principal wild animal infected. In other parts of Europe, goats (*Capra hircus*),[40] species of deer, mostly the red deer (*C. elaphus*), fallow deer (*Damam dama*), roe deer (*Capreolus capreolus*), and wild boar[41] are affected. In North America and Canada, bison (*Bison bison*),[43] elk (*C. canadensis*)[44], and white-tailed deer (*Odocoileus virginianus*)[45] play an important role in the transmission of *M. bovis*. In Africa, many species that warrant local conservation are affected, which poses a threat to the survival of local populations.[46] The brush-tailed possum (*T. vulpecula*) and ferret (*Mustela furo*) in New Zealand,[35] the Cape buffalo (*Syncerus caffer*) in some parts of South Africa, the Kaufe Lechwe antelope (*Kobus leche kafuensis*), and the white-tailed deer (*O. virginianus*) in Michigan, USA[47,48] are all considered to be maintenance hosts of *M. bovis*.

In non-maintenance or spillover hosts, or dead-end hosts,[48] transmission of *M. bovis* is self-limiting as a maintenance host is required to be present within the ecosystem for this to occur. These spillover hosts may act as an incidental source of *M. bovis* for cattle.[48] Examples of true dead-end hosts may be horses and sheep. Pigs, goats, farmed wild boar, dogs, cats and camelids in the United Kingdom should be treated as potential amplifier hosts as they have the potential to act as a source of infection for other animals and man.[49]

BADGERS (*M. MELES*)

Badgers are an important reservoir and maintenance host for *M. bovis* in the United Kingdom and Republic of Ireland and there are areas where the disease is endemic in the badger population.[20] A greater number of male badgers are infected than female badgers, likely due to the males increased roaming behavior and tendency toward aggression allowing transmission of the disease via bite wounds. However, the majority of infections appear to be via the respiratory route, with open submandibular abscesses often being the first clinical sign noted. The communal social structure of the badger population, with social grooming and sleeping in groups, provides an excellent environment in which *M. bovis* can be spread. A large proportion of infected badgers will survive for more than 12 months after the initial infection, and mortality induced by *M. bovis* infection appears to have only a small part to play in badger population numbers.

Badgers with advanced *M. bovis* infection shed the bacilli in their urine and this is thought to be the primary infection source for cattle. In some populations where there are recently infected cattle herds, up to 50% infection rate of badgers has been recorded, and the risk of transmission increases as badger density increases. Behavioral studies to determine the degree of interaction between badgers and cattle on pasture has found this to be minimal, and the badgers preferred not to occupy fields occupied by cows and did not approach within 10–15 m of a cow.[34] The conclusion was that, rather than direct aerosol transmission between badgers and cattle, if disease spread between badgers and cattle does occur, it is likely through contact with or ingestion of badger urine or feces. The risk of infection to humans directly from badgers is thought to be very low, because close contact between humans and badgers is limited.[35] The risk to those humans working more directly with badgers, such as government officials involved in collecting road carcasses, wildlife center employees, veterinary surgeons, farmers, and residents of rural areas has been found, unsurprisingly, to be higher.

POSSUMS (*TRICHOSURUS VULPECULA*)

Brush-tailed possums are indigenous to Australia but have colonized New Zealand and provide a significant reservoir of *M. bovis* for infection of cattle and man in this country, but not in Australia. The first tuberculous lesion detected in a possum was noted in 1967 by a possum trapper. Subsequently, endemic populations of *M. bovis*-infected possums was found in all areas where tuberculosis from cattle was difficult to eradicate. Transmission between possums is either by aerosol or pseudo-vertical (via the joey) routes. Lesions in possums can be widely disseminated, and the disease is normally fatal after 2–3 months from the onset of clinical disease. Breakdown of infection in previously susceptible cattle herds can occur in the presence of only one infected possum. A cross-sectional survey of possums in New Zealand in 1994 showed a local prevalence of *M. bovis* infection of up to 20% in clustered areas, but the overall prevalence of infection of possums in New Zealand was 1.2%.[36]

DEER

Farmed and wild deer are susceptible to infection with *M. bovis*.[37] The disease was first reported in farmed deer in New Zealand and currently tuberculosis is considered to be the most important bacterial disease in farmed deer in New Zealand and the United Kingdom.[38] It has been suggested that farmed deer are more susceptible to the disease than wild deer. Griffin found that the immune response of red deer to infection varies,[39] and that there was a high heritability of resistance to *M. bovis* infection in red deer under experimental conditions. Susceptibility to disease varies depending on genotype, previous exposure to disease, nutritional status of the herd and level of sex hormones.[38] Pathogenesis of the disease varies with the site of infection. Wild deer or farmed

deer in contact with cattle that are susceptible to disease have the potential to act as a reservoir of infection for cattle. There is the possibility that captive, farmed deer can act as maintenance hosts of *M. bovis*, and a tuberculosis control programme has been sporadically introduced in the United Kingdom and New Zealand among farmed deer populations to help prevent this.[117,118]

SMALL RUMINANTS (SHEEP AND GOATS)

Goats are much more susceptible to infection with *M. bovis* than sheep. However, there is minimal epidemiological significance of goats acting as a reservoir of *M. bovis* disease.

PIGS

The disease incidence in pigs normally reflects that of the cattle population. The first historical report was made in 1969 by Myers and Steele that in 1921 in the United States 12% of pigs which were slaughtered under Federal Inspection Law were found to have tuberculous lesions. The origin of these pigs was traced and it was found that all of the infected pigs had been fed unpasteurized milk or dairy products, and were kept together with cattle. In fact, this is the most common route of infection in pigs. As with other species, the prevalence of disease in pigs is found to increase with age, and as most intensively farmed pigs are slaughtered for meat before the age of 6 months therefore *M. bovis* disease does not manifest as too severe a clinical problem in this species. Transmission between pigs has been found to be insignificant and lesions are normally localized. Pulmonary lesions are infrequent, therefore pigs represent an insignificant infection source for cattle.

GOATS

Goats are fairly susceptible to TB and most commonly develop either pulmonary infection or tuberculous mastitis. Bacilli have the potential to be shed in the milk of lactating goats.[15] Reports of clinical cases of tuberculosis have been reported in goats in Spain.[50] In Spain, goats are considered to be a maintenance host as are cattle. In Germany between 1999 and 2001, a goat-adapted strain, *M. bovis* subsp *caprae*, was responsible for a third of all zoonotic tuberculosis cases reported.[51]

CATS AND DOGS

The incidence of clinical tuberculosis caused by *M. bovis* in dogs and cats has decreased over the last 100 years, most likely due to the ingestion of milk or offal from tubercular cattle on farms, or from living in close proximity to humans infected with tuberculosis and inhaling sputum particles. Tuberculosis in cats has documented to be caused mainly by *M. bovis* and *M. microti*[9] with fewer cases of *M. avium* and non-tuberculous mycobacteria.[119] In dogs, *M. tuberculosis* was found to cause 75% of cases; the remainder was mostly *M. bovis* and a small proportion of *M. avium*.[52]

OTHER MYCOBACTERIA

Members of the *M. tuberculosis* complex include the following mycobacteria: *M. tuberculosis*, *Mycobacterium africanum*, *Mycobacterium canetti*, *M. bovis*, *M. microti*, *Mycobacterium orygis*, *M. caprae*, *M. pinnipedii*, and the recently recognized *Mycobacterium mungi*.[58] WHO reported that there were 9 million new cases and 1.5 million deaths due to these mycobacteria in 2014.

Non-tuberculous mycobacterial (NTM) infections are present worldwide and are found in many different environmental niches. They are harmless to most individuals and rarely cause human disease. Species of NTM associated with human disease include *M. avium*, *Mycobacterium intracellulare*, *Mycobacterium kansasii*, *Mycobacterium fortuitum*, *Mycobacterium chelonae*, *Mycobacterium szulgai*, *M. paratuberculosis*, and *Mycobacterium scrofulaceum*. The majority of NTM infections have been reported in countries in which tuberculosis is not endemic, as the chances of missing NTM infection are higher in countries where tuberculosis is already present. Currently, the individual mycobacteria causing mycobacterial infection are not routinely characterized worldwide. Therefore, some NTM cases in humans with positive Ziehl–Neelsen (ZN) stains will be misclassified as MTB.[59] This may result in a patient receiving routine treatment for *M. tuberculosis* for which the NTM strain may be resistant. Additionally, occasional mixed strain infections of NTM and MTB infections have been reported.[60,61]

A brief epidemiology of several other mycobacteria are described below:

- *M. tuberculosis*: This mycobacterium classically causes disease in humans and is the most common agent to cause tuberculosis. However, although animal infection is uncommon, it has been described among some species (birds, elephants, and other mammals) that have had prolonged and close contact with humans. Transmission of *M. tuberculosis* between animals and humans has not been reported.
- *M. microti*: The name of this serovar of tuberculosis translates directly as "vole," as it was the first mycobacterium discovered to cause disease in voles during investigations into the cause of cyclic population density changes in this species. Field voles, bank voles, wood mice, and shrews are all susceptible to infection with *M. microti*. *M. microti* has also been documented to cause disease in cats[62] and other larger animals[63] and very occasional reports of human infection are recorded, totalling 13 patients worldwide.[64–67]
- *Mycobacterium avium complex* (MAC): MAC, which includes *M. avium*, *M. intracellulare* and *Mycobacterium chimaera*, is the most important cause of NTM-related pulmonary disease in humans.[68,69] MAC are widely distributed in the environment and rarely cause human disease. Factors such as host susceptibility, pathogen virulence, and environmental risk factors likely play a role in the pathogenesis of the disease. Often patients with MAC also suffer from concurrent immunologic or genetic disorders that predispose to lung infections or bronchiectasis. However, MAC disease can be seen in some patients with no other lung or immune abnormalities.[70]
- *M. avium*: This serovar of tuberculosis causes disease in birds, pigs, cats, humans, and dogs[71] and is the most frequently isolated NTM mycobacteria in humans. The clinical signs produced are often indistinguishable from that of the *M. tuberculosis* complex and therefore it is often considered to be within the same group.
- *M. avium paratuberculosis* (MAP): This mycobacterial infection causes a chronic granulomatous infection of the gastrointestinal tract of domestic ruminants and wildlife worldwide, and is the NTM of greatest importance in the field of

veterinary medicine,[72] particularly for cattle and sheep. MAP is extremely resistant to destruction and can survive pasteurization, and for up to a year in the environment. Transmission of the disease may occur horizontally via the fecal–oral route, and vertically from infected dams to calves, and the incubation period varies between 2 and 7 years.[73] The most common route of introduction of infection into a previously MAP-free herd is via the introduction of previously infected cattle into the herd, or breaks in on-farm biosecurity.

Infection with *M. avium paratuberculosis* (MAP) is also known as Johne's disease and is found worldwide. Clinical symptoms of the condition can be attributed to the presence of chronic granulomatous inflammation within the gastrointestinal tract; with diarrhea and weight loss occuring in cattle in advanced stages of MAP infection. Most infected cattle will be in the subclinical stage of disease; less than 5% of the cattle display clinical signs of illness. Fecal culture and antibody detection are the most common diagnostic methods to determine prevalence,[74] although there is a decrease in sensitivity of tests for those animals with subclinical disease. In the United States, it was reported in 2009 that up to 68% of the dairy herds contained clinically infected cattle, with the prevalence lower in beef herds. It has been estimated that for every cow showing clinical signs of advanced Johne's disease, it is likely that 15–25 others in the herd are also infected. Once clinical signs occur there is no known cure for the disease and culling presents the most economic option.

In sheep, the disease is characterized by emaciation, but not chronic diarrhea as in cattle. In many infected flocks, ewe mortality can reach as high as 5%–10% annually due to Johne's disease.

Although *M. avium* subsp. *paratuberculosis* has not been confirmed as a zoonotic agent, there has been suspicion that this bacilli may play some role in the development of Crohn's disease in humans and one meta-analysis has demonstrated a positive association between the two.[75]

- *M. caprae*: This zoonotic mycobacteria was first characterized in 1999. The major route of human acquisition appears to be from livestock, mainly goats or cattle. No clear evidence of human to human transmission has been reported. *M. caprae* has only been found in 0.3% of all tuberculosis cases, and its range is almost entirely confined to Europe. The low incidence is thought to be due to the European-wide introduction of public health measures to prevent zoonotic TB transmission, including milk pasteurization and culling infected cattle. Incidence of *M. caprae* infection is highest in Spain, where this Mycobacteria represents 7.4% of all *M. tuberculosis* complex isolates from animals.[76]
- *M. leprae*: This bacterium is the etiological agent of leprosy in humans, and gives rise to a chronic granulomatous disease primarily affecting the skin and peripheral nerves. The bacterium can be grown in several species of experimental animals, including the armadillo, nonhuman primates, and rodents. Naturally occurring leprosy has been reported in wild nine-banded armadillos (*Dasypus troglodytes*) and three species of nonhuman primates (chimpanzees (*Pan troglodytes*), sooty mangabey monkeys (*Cercocebus atys*) and cynomolgus macaques (*Macaca fascicularis*)), therefore qualifying leprosy as a zoonosis.

- *M. lepraemurium*: This causes a leprosy-like disease affecting rats and mice, primarily affecting the viscera and skin and very rarely the peripheral nerves. Naturally acquired murine leprosy has been observed in rats, mice, cats and dogs, but not in humans or any other species. Therefore, it appears that murine leprosy is not a zoonosis.[77]

DIAGNOSTIC TESTS

In humans, the clinical signs observed due to infection by *M. tuberculosis* or *M. bovis* are indistinguishable radiographically, pathologically or by direct smear analysis. Prior to 1970, UK laboratories did not make an attempt to distinguish the strains,[4] a practice that currently continues in some European countries and, until recently, the United States.[78] This is not of grave concern clinically in humans as the treatment of most mycobacterial organisms remains the same. However, *M. bovis* does have an intrinsic resistance to the drug pyrazinamide, so the use of this drug is not recommended when cases of zoonotic tuberculosis infection are suspected.[3] Epidemiologically it would be extremely useful to be aware of the exact cause and the potential transmission route of the clinical disease. Therefore, accessible and cost-effective tests to distinguish these strains of bacilli would be extremely useful. Currently, in order to achieve an accurate diagnosis between strain cultures, biochemical tests and DNA analysis are necessary[9] are time-consuming and not cost-effective. Many reports have been made of misdiagnosis of tuberculosis in human patients.[79]

The accurate use of molecular markers to differentiate *M. bovis* and *M. tuberculosis* is also difficult. Organisms of the MTBC complex have been found to have a 99.9% similarity rate between nucleotide levels, and identical 16rRNA sequences.[11]

Due to the zoonotic potential of some mycobacterial infections affecting animals, care should be taken when handling the potentially affected tissue, and awareness to all involved should be made of the potential zoonotic risk of disease. *M. bovis* is classified as a Hazard Class 3 biological agent, according to the Control of Substances Hazardous to Health (COSHH) Regulations 1999. Tuberculosis is a notifiable disease in any animal, so if the disease is suspected and the legislation of the country in which the diagnosis is made stipulates, care should be taken that the correct procedures are followed to inform the relevant authorities. Aseptic practice and an aerosol mask when handling samples is normally adequate to reduce the risk of transmission via aerosol or ingestion, and attention should be drawn to wear gloves when handling the biopsy site or biopsy material. The body of any confirmed, euthanized case should be cremated, not buried, so that any infective bacilli present in the carcass can be destroyed.

DIAGNOSTIC TESTS OF CATTLE

SINGLE INTRADERMAL COMPARATIVE CERVICAL TUBERCULIN TEST

The intradermal skin test is the first-line test of routine surveillance to be carried out in the field in the United Kingdom. In areas of the United Kingdom where tuberculosis has been discovered in cattle, regular testing is carried out at a predetermined frequency until such a time as eradication from the herd has occurred, if possible.

The intradermal skin test involves subcutaneous injection in the skin of the mid-cervical region of cattle using an antigenic *M. bovis* purified protein derivative (PPD) mixture, "tuberculin," which is sourced from heat-killed bacteria.[80] Robert Koch was the first to purify this PPD solution in 1882[3] and bovine PPD remains to this day the most commonly used agent in the field to diagnose bovine tuberculosis. A delayed-type hypersensitivity inflammatory response occurs following injection, causing skin swelling at the inoculation site. Measurement of the diameter of this swelling 72 hours after inoculation correlates with previously determined values; the larger the diameter of the skin swelling, the greater the delayed-type hypersensitivity reaction and therefore the more likely that the cow has previously reacted immunogenically to this stimulus, therefore, the higher the likelihood that a cell-mediated response to *M. bovis* has already previously occurred.

M. bovis (PPD) antigenic compounds are shared by many other mycobacteria,[81] including members of the *M. avium intracellulare* complex.[82] Therefore, *M. avium* antigens are injected as a control agent, separately to either the mid-cervical region, at the same time as the *M. bovis* antigen injection, making the intradermal skin test comparative. These antigens are often found in the environment, and may confound the outcome of the *M. bovis* diagnostic tests.[83] Comparing the difference in the diameter of the skin reactions between the *M. bovis* and *M. avium* antigens determines the difference in size of the delayed-type hypersensitivity and therefore allows for the discrimination to be made whether the cow is infected with *M. bovis*, or solely sensitized to environmental mycobacteria.

Established standards differentiate the diameter of the skin reaction, so the cattle are classified with the largest diameter of *M. bovis* skin reaction as "reactors," medium sized as "inconclusive," or "negative" for those that match or have a smaller diameter than the control, *M. avium*.

The sensitivity of the intradermal skin test has been reported to be 80%.[84] Although some animals may present with physical signs of tuberculosis infection or postmortem changes, they may not respond to the intradermal skin test[85] due to the presence of advanced disease, very initial disease, i.e., prior to 6 weeks postinfection, testing of a cow within 6 weeks of calving, or the administration of a variable dose using a multidrug syringe. Therefore, currently in the United Kingdom, tissue samples are still submitted for culture at postmortem from cattle with a negative single intradermal comparative cervical tuberculin test (SICCT) that have shown physical clinical signs of disease or have suspicious postmortem findings.

Alternatively, specificity of the intradermal skin test can also be considered to be on the lower side, with false positives recorded with evidence of a delayed-type hypersensitivity reaction and no visible lesions discovered on postmortem examination.[85] However, as a public health measure, under Annex B of European Directive 64/432/EEC, all skin test reactors are considered to be affected by tuberculosis and are therefore slaughtered, regardless of the bacterial culture results.

An increased frequency of the SICCT test affects test performance. In the United Kingdom, tests are not validated if they are carried out more frequently than 30 days apart. The antigens injected during the test may modulate the cell-mediated immunity of the cow and depress the response to subsequent skin tests.[86] Therefore, should disease confirmation be required within this time period, an alternative test should be performed.

INTERFERON-GAMMA TEST

The interferon-gamma test was first documented and initially used in Australia during the Brucellosis and Tuberculosis Eradication Program.[87,88] This ELISA (enzyme-linked immunosorbent assay) detected cell-mediated resistance of interferon-gamma to tuberculosis using whole blood following incubation with PPD-b.[89] Individual sensitivity of this test is higher than the tuberculin skin test described previously, which is felt to be superior to detect an infected herd. With a higher sensitivity, the interferon-gamma test is thought to be better served to more accurately detect infected individuals within herds,[89] and if there is detection of the cytokine interferon-gamma, a preferentially positive result is indicated.[90] The SICCT and interferon-gamma tests detect infection at different stages of disease. The tuberculin skin test is more widely used as a first-line detection test in cattle in the United Kingdom, one other benefit of this test being that the results of the test are quick, more cost-effective to gather and do not require a well-equipped laboratory to generate results.

Unfortunately, a negative interferon-gamma reaction and absence of visible lesions on postmortem examination with a positive intradermal skin test does not confirm that the cow is free of infection.

POSTMORTEM EXAMINATION

All carcasses following slaughter in the United Kingdom are routinely grossly inspected for the presence of visible tuberculosis lesions. Routine postmortem examination detects approximately 9%–12% of newly diagnosed tuberculosis cases in the United Kingdom annually, with the remainder detected on antemortem testing. Between 1998 and 2006, 30%–53% of slaughterhouse cases reported as suspected tuberculosis to the Meat Hygiene Service have yielded a final diagnosis of M. bovis.

Following slaughter, all confirmed tuberculosis reactors are submitted for postmortem examination with the aim not just to validate the antemortem testing, but to assess the severity of disease and provide epidemiological information about the nature of the bacilli present. Genotyping tests are carried out on the tissues to determine the latest strain responsible for tuberculosis herd breakdown. In the United Kingdom, postmortem examination of cattle is carried out at The Veterinary Laboratories Agencies, which are government-run institutions serving the country. The isolation rate of tuberculosis bacilli from reactors with visible lesions is normally approximately 90%, although gross lesions on postmortem cannot be considered confirmatory of disease.[91] Postmortem testing determines the risk of infection to other animals within the same herd as well as to human contact, and following on from this to ascertain the number of follow-up tests likely required to restore the herd's tuberculosis-free status, as well as to what degree contact animals and humans need to be monitored for the development of the disease in the future.

Where cases of tuberculosis have been confirmed by antemortem diagnosis but no visible lesions are present or grow on postmortem examination, the Animal and Plant Health Agency (APHA) will carry out histological diagnosis to provide a presumptive answer within 2 weeks.

LABORATORY CULTURE

Definitive diagnosis of M. bovis can be made microbiologically from tissue from the lesion.[30] Samples suitable to submit for culture include sputum, pleural fluid, or prepared tissues, for example, a lung or lymph node biopsy. Selective laboratory culture using an acid-fast stain such as ZN can provide confirmation of this slow-growing bacteria after 6–8 weeks of incubation at 37°C. Should acid-fast organisms grow that do not show the typical growth pattern of M. bovis, a multiplex PCR (polymerase chain reaction) test is carried out to help in the differentiation of MAC or other organisms of the Mycobacterium genus. This primary technique has currently replaced bio-typing in the United Kingdom for tuberculosis identification.

Bacterial culture methods are not currently found to be highly sensitive, although they are very specific. Sensitivity is particularly lost when pooled samples of lymph nodes from a suspected cow with no visible lesions are submitted.[30] European Directive 64/432/EEC, Section 1, Annex B, describes techniques to identify M. bovis from clinical and biological specimens but does not provide specific directives to diagnose and confirm M. bovis infections in cattle, although methods used may conform to those specified in Chapter 2.3.3 (Bovine TB of the World Organisation for Animal Health [OIE] Manual of Standards for Diagnostic Tests and Vaccines).

GENETIC WORK

In the United Kingdom, the APHA routinely determines the genotype of tuberculosis isolates from cattle in order to provide more information about epidemiology of this disease across the country while monitoring for new tuberculosis herd breakdowns and their spread. Spoligotyping, a technique to analyze polymorphisms in various repeats of DNA sequences, was the principal technique used for molecular typing in the 1990s and earlier 2000s.[92,93] In 1998, Frothingham[94] provided a method to analyze the highly polymorphic DNA loci of M. bovis to analyze finer discrimination between strains, which is used in tandem with spoligotyping by the APHA. The main feature of this is the ability to differentiate the isolates of the most prevalent and widespread tuberculosis strain, SB0140, found in cattle and badgers in the United Kingdom.[95] The APHA has amassed spoligotyping data from over 31,000 M. bovis strains detected in the United Kingdom between 1997 and 2004 from cattle, badgers, deer, and other mammals (APHA, unpublished). Of these, 6500 isolates also have variable number tandem repeat (VNTR) data, and therefore comprise the largest collection of M. bovis genotype isolates within Europe. This epidemiologic resource has helped scientists to investigate the spread and incidence of M. bovis isolates across the United Kingdom over this period, and the evolution of the MTBC complex.[11] VNTR typing was used to good effect in the 13-year outbreak of bovine tuberculosis in Switzerland, which occurred after a 15-year period of time during which no bovine tuberculosis was diagnosed in the country. The VNTR data found that the 17 isolates tested from outbreaks across the country were identical, caused by the *M. bovis* spoligotype SB0120, indicating a single source of infection.[97] Comparison of one previously archived sample of bovine tuberculosis from infection in Switzerland 15 years earlier using MIRU-VNTR testing showed an identical VNTR profile, insinuating that the infectious agent had persisted in the dairy herd for nearly 15 years prior to reactivation.

Several candidate genes are being assessed for their use as genetic markers of *M. bovis*. Once these genes are discovered, the aim is to assess whether they have the potential to alter the disease phenotype of cattle. One marker gene includes the bovine natural resistance-associated macrophage protein gene (NRAMP1), which has been ubiquitously identified in mice models and humans. The survival of *M. bovis* BCG appears to be linked to the presence of a resistant allele of this gene.[98] Small comparative epidemiologic studies have been carried out to examine plausible genes within cattle populations, however these are normally scientifically underpowered to determine significant associations.

In the future, it is likely that a whole genome approach will be used to investigate the single-nucleotide polymorphism (SNP) numbers and determine the degree of disease-associated variation. A whole genome sequencing approach will determine the presence of particular disease-associated variants and in humans has the potential to identify the genotype present in cases of drug-resistant tuberculosis and mechanisms that influence the phenotype. This initial whole genome approach will identify the most polymorphic areas of the genome, and the chromosome that corresponds to the genetic information of the phenotype of interest. Potentially, findings show that a specific allelic combination occurs more commonly in the diseased population. The linkage disequilibrium, or occurrence in members of a population of linked genes in nonrandom proportions, of *M. bovis* infections in cattle appears to be much smaller than that of *M. tuberculosis* affecting humans, likely due to the occurrence of nonrandom mating in cattle and their smaller population size,[99,100] which acts to reduce the overall number of SNPs. There are currently 800,000 SNPs in current bovine genome SNP arrays, and this may be sufficient to effectively map the entirety of the bovine genome.

DIAGNOSTIC TESTS IN DOGS AND CATS

As previously mentioned, the potential for zoonotic transmission of mycobacterial infections from dogs and cats is a concern. Should a dog and cat infected with a zoonotic strain be detected but the threat to human health be found to be minimal, diagnostic tests in dogs and cats can be carried out with a slightly different focus to that of cattle and other herd animals where containment of the spread of this zoonotic disease within the herd is of extreme importance.

Diagnosis of infection with the *Mycobacterium tuberculosis* complex relies on a combination of histopathology, mycobacterial culture and molecular testing. Suggestive historical and clinical findings will prompt testing for the infection.

The dog or cat should be thoroughly evaluated to determine the location of infection and severity of the disease, extent of systemic involvement and local infection, in order to determine the likely prognosis for this specific animal. The most common findings on physical examination of cats infected with *M. bovis* and *M. microti* are single or multiple cutaneous nodular lesions. Multifocal peripheral lymphadenopathy may be present. The results of serum biochemistry and hematology are often non-specific. Biochemical and hematological tests, if performed, will normally identify nonspecific changes. The presence of ionized hypercalcemia is a poor prognostic indicator[101] as it suggests a higher burden of granulomatous disease.

Radiography can be used to assess if there is respiratory involvement. Changes may be variable and potentially not be specific or diagnostic for the disease. They may include tracheobronchial lymphadenopathy, interstitial to alveolar lung infiltration, lobar consolidation, and pleural effusion. Abdominal radiography or ultrasound may demonstrate hepatomegaly or splenomegaly, lymphadenopathy, mineralization of the mesenteric lymph nodes, or ascites. Assessment of bones by radiography may also reveal areas of bony lysis and sclerosis, osteoarthritis, discospondylitis, or periosteitis.

Specific tests that can be undertaken are similar to those available for other animals, and include the interferon-gamma test, which is available from the APHA in the United Kingdom.[103] Intradermal skin testing results are often unreliable in cats, as they do not tend to show a strong reaction.[104,105] False-negative results can occur in both cats and dogs.

To generate confirmation that mycobacteria are involved, fine-needle aspiration or biopsy samples of affected tissues should be obtained and stained with ZN stain or similar. On microscopy of stained tissue, the number of acid-fast organisms present within macrophages may vary and depend on the specific mycobacteria present, the location of the granuloma, and the nature and strength of the host immune response. A mixed population of often heavily vacuolated histiocytes and smaller numbers of degenerate or nondegenerate neutrophils and small lymphocytes may also be seen. Once the organisms have been viewed microscopically, it is important to perform a culture as the gold-standard method to determine the mycobacterial species involved and establish the potential zoonotic risk of the infection, the source of the infection, and options available for treatment. However, often tissues in which acid-fast staining organisms are seen may fail to grow mycobacteria in the laboratory, and culture is continued for as long as 8–12 weeks as the organisms grow very slowly, to maximize the opportunity for diagnosis.

Other diagnostic techniques available include molecular PCR, which is particularly useful when bacteriological culture results are not available,[106–109] mycobacterial interspersed repetitive unit-variable-number tandem repeat (MIRU-VNTR)[120] and spoligotyping. Using this technique, bacteria can be identified within tissue aspirates or buffy coat preparations separated from the blood.

HISTOPATHOLOGY

There are several presentations of tuberculous masses that may be viewed on biopsy or postmortem examination. Large, solid, tumor-like masses or multiple small disseminated masses throughout the body may lead to a similar diagnosis. Often the gross appearance of the mass is a grayish-white color, with haemorrhagic edges and a soft purulent center due the presence of caseous necrosis. Lesions in the lungs are often a grayish red color, and may be associated with serosanguinous pleural fluid. Renal lesions typically occur as infarcts within the cortex, and intestinal lesions include ulceration of Peyer's patches, with the presence of submucosal tubercles.

Histopathological reports for the disease will often report the presence of foamy macrophages and granulomatous inflammation, some necrotic areas, and a variable number of acid-fast bacilli within and outside macrophages.[107] Lymphocytes and fibroblasts may also be present, but multinucleate giant cells are often absent, or rarely seen.[105,101]

Calcification may be seen within larger tubercles, potentially surrounded by zones of histiocytic cells and a well-defined fibrous capsule.[105]

Feline leprosy may generate either lepromatous or tuberculous lesions, while a diagnosis of tuberculosis may generate only tuberculous lesions.[107]

TREATMENT

CATTLE

M. bovis infections detected in cattle are not suitable for treatment due to the zoonotic and infectious nature of the disease. The public health and risk of infection to other herd members is too great and the treatment period is too long and uneconomic to make treatment of cattle a viable option. The treatment period required to effectively cure a cow would be 4–12 months of daily dosing, with the potential for relapse of infection once treatment is ceased. An additional problem that is posed by the concept of treating cattle is the potential for drug residues to be left in milk, meat and other products consumed by humans. Given that human drug resistance to standard tuberculosis treatment is a serious concern, the use of large proportions of the same drugs in cattle may serve to exacerbate this problem, and increase the degree of multidrug-resistant infections among the human population.

Currently, however, drug-resistant isolates of *M. bovis* have rarely been reported. Due to the infrequency of treatment of the disease in cattle, the selective pressure for resistance is likely to be low and so apart from the innate resistance of this mycobacteria to pyrazinamide, it would be expected currently that most *M. bovis* infections be susceptible to routine mycobacterial treatment, if required.

COMPANION ANIMALS

Consideration can be given to treatment of companion animals under the guidance of the treating veterinary surgeon. The potential for dissemination of zoonotic bacteria is lower in these species than in production animals, as generally companion animals are housed in much smaller groups, and can be contained indoors, with less opportunity for dissemination of infection among numerous animals as would occur in a herd situation. However,

regardless of this, the zoonotic potential of the infection should be carefully considered, and public health authorities should be notified if a diagnosis of MTBC infection is made in a cat or dog.

Prior to the onset of treatment of a confirmed case of a mycobacterial infection in a dog or a cat, several factors should be taken into consideration with all of the human members of the household where the animal resides.

i. In cases where there is any human individual suffering any degree of immunocompromise within a household (e.g., the recipient of an organ transplant or an individual undergoing chemotherapy treatment) euthanasia of the dog or cat, rather than treatment, would be advised to limit the risk of harm to the human.

ii. The nature of the symptoms of disease displayed by the dog or cat. If the disease appears to be generalized, respiratory tract involvement is present, or there are cutaneous lesions that are continually draining fluid, the risk of zoonotic transmission is increased, and euthanasia rather than treatment should be considered.

iii. The owners of suitable candidates for treatment should understand that the treatment is long term and a challenge to maintain should the patient be noncompliant. The drugs used to treat tuberculosis have some degree of inherent toxicity and the financial cost of the ongoing drug treatment and monitoring can be very high. The owner should also be made aware that while some drug therapies may act to suppress the tuberculosis infection, eradication may not take place, and once treatment finishes the infection may recrudesce. Therefore, treatment for an indefinite period of time may be required.

However, having considered these points, treatment of cutaneous uncomplicated forms of tuberculosis in dogs and cats does often offer a good prognosis. Treatment protocols normally involve an initial and continuation phase of treatment with antibiotics. Currently, the initial recommendation would be treatment with three drugs for 2 months, followed by a continuation phase of two drugs for at least 4 months. The exact regime will depend on the type and severity of disease. Although antimicrobial susceptibility testing can be carried out on affected tissues, it has been found that the sensitivity results in vitro do not always match those in vivo. Surgical excision of affected tissues can be carried out to submit for analysis and further culture work, but again, the use of these tissue specimens for an accurate culture and sensitivity result may not always provide a successful result. There is a risk of wound dehiscence and local recurrence of infection should attempts be made to surgically remove large portions of infected tissue. However for the local cutaneous signs of disease surgical excision could be considered.

Culture and sensitivity can take up to 6 weeks or more to generate a result, and in the interim time, treatment with a fluoroquinolone antibiotic has been advised, although consideration should be offered to the reported side effects of treatment with this drug to cats. Currently, this route of treatment is only advised in cases of localized cutaneous infection and generally it is more sensible to institute the recommended double or triple therapy once a diagnosis has been made as this therapy offers the best chance of clinical resolution. Treatment with a single fluoroquinolone increases the opportunity for the bacteria to develop resistance to this single antibiotic. If triple or double therapy is initiated prior to culture results being known, it is strongly advised to continue the same treatment once the diagnosis of a mycobacterial infection has been made. Ideally, the exact mycobacteria should be known prior to treatment. In many cases, culture results of suspected *M. bovis* cases in cats are negative, but ZN positive stains may be seen on cytology or histopathology. In these cases where a very high suspicion of infection with tuberculosis exists, the owners should be counselled about the risks and complications of treatment prior to initiation.

In cats, treatment with three oral tablets daily may present a compliance issue and the owner may struggle with this regimen for a protracted period of time. Should this be the case, treatment should continue with two drugs alone, normally for a longer period of 6–9 months.[64] The most effective combination for treatment in cats is considered to be a combination of rifampicin, isoniazid, and ethambutol. There are some newer, less toxic drugs available that may be worth considering. The fluoroquinolones have the potential to treat infection, e.g., marbofloxacin and clarithromycin can be used effectively to treat tuberculosis in animals, especially in combination with rifampicin. Clinical experience denotes the most effective treatment regime to be an initial phase of treatment with rifampicin–fluoroquinolone combination and clarithromycin or azithromycin, followed by continuation of the treatment with rifampicin and a fluoroquinolone or an azithromycin or clarithromycin alternative. To ease administration, medication can be administered as a liquid in a single syringe, or all three tablets together in a gelatin capsule. Should resistance to drug therapy develop, a rifampicin, isoniazid, ethambutol combination may be considered. There is natural resistance to the treatment of *M. bovis* with pyrazinamide, as previously mentioned.

The prognosis following treatment of infection in dogs and cats depends on the mycobacteria involved and the extent and severity of infection. *M. microti* has often shown a favorable response to treatment. Many cases can obtain a long-term remission of infection, although response to treatment should be guarded.

CONTROL

GENERAL PRINCIPLES OF CONTROL

From a pathogenic and economic perspective, of all the mycobacteria that can infect animals, the most important to control is *M. bovis*. An important consideration is the route of disease transmission, which in the case of *M. bovis* can be either by aerosol or ingestion, and the linkages and interfaces by which effective transmission of the mycobacteria is achieved.

CONTROL OF THE DISEASE IN CATTLE

Cattle are considered the maintenance hosts of *M. bovis*, able to maintain the infection within their own population. On-farm control of *M. bovis* in cattle is extremely important. In order to eliminate the disease in an endemic area, regular herd surveillance

is essential, both for noninfected herds to monitor for new breakouts of infection, and currently infected herds to monitor the progression of disease within the herd. This can best be achieved by regular herd testing, which normally takes place using the SICCT or potentially interferon-gamma assay, and rigorous monitoring of carcasses during meat hygiene inspection.[110] Treatment of infected cattle is not economically feasible, and the positive animal is slaughtered with the aim to eliminate the disease and reduce the spread of infection.[84]

On-farm hygiene and biosecurity considerations are also extremely important to prevent the spread of infection. This will decrease any indirect spread via fomites if feed and water troughs are regularly disinfected and appropriate personal protective clothing is utilized when handling animals or infected carcasses. Ideally, infected carcasses should be cremated or, if this is not a possibility, buried at least 4 ft below the ground. The rodent population should be kept under control to reduce spread of infection.

Diagnostic tests including DNA fingerprinting techniques such as variable number of tandem repeat (VNTR) typing and spoligotyping help to determine the strain of *M. bovis* present within a herd and have epidemiological value to control disease by helping to trace the route of infection and ensuring that adequate control strategies are instigated.[15,92,111]

Currently, the UK Government is midway through implementing a 25-year plan for the eradication of bovine tuberculosis from this country which was first unveiled in 2013. The Department for the Environment, Food and Rural Affairs (DEFRA) has divided the country into three areas; "low-risk area," "edge area," and "high-risk area," to reflect differences in how the disease is spread and the number of infected cattle detected upon routine testing in each region. In the high-risk areas of the South West and Midlands, the focus of control is to contain the disease in cattle and wildlife and reverse the spread of the disease northwards. The final goal of this scheme is to move the status of low-risk areas to that of "OTF," thereby easing the economic burden of TB control in the United Kingdom and facilitating trade with other countries. The target is for most of England to achieve OTF status by 2025, and the whole country by 2038. This strategy leans heavily on the experience of New Zealand.

Attempts are made to control tuberculosis in the United Kingdom by testing every cattle herd at least every 1–4 years, funded by the UK taxpayer. The exact frequency is calculated according to the specific numbers of reactors in a certain geographical area recorded over the last 2, 4, or 6 years in compliance with the Directive 64/432/EEC. Increased surveillance can be instigated at a local level as necessary and any herd that represents a local or public health risk will be tested annually, in addition to herds where new breakouts of bovine tuberculosis are detected. Herds at a higher risk of TB infections include, for example, those which produce unpasteurized milk for sale or those that hire out bulls for mating, will be tested annually.

Should macroscopic tuberculosis lesions be detected at the slaughterhouse during carcass processing, a report will be made by the Meat Hygiene Service to the Local State Veterinary Service. Tracings will be carried out to determine the origin of the infected cattle and bacteriological and pathological samples will be submitted from in-contact herd members to the APHA.

As described earlier, the primary test used for screening for tuberculosis in herds in the United Kingdom is the SICCT. This uses inoculation with *M. avium* subsp. *avium* and *M. bovis* tuberculin to assess previous sensitization to these allergens. The test is carried out in accordance with the procedure described by the Commission Regulation 1226/2002 (Annex B to Directive 64/432/EEC). The interferon-gamma test is used as a second-line test to supplement the SICCT test, particularly in areas where there is protracted and extensive breakdown of tuberculosis control.[113]

Milk from reactor animals has been banned from sale under any circumstances following instigation of the EU Food Hygiene Regulation 853/2004 in England, Wales and Scotland. This regulation states, however, that sale of milk from nonreactor animals in the same herd is permitted as long as it has been correctly heat-treated. Herds from which raw milk is sold should be registered under Regulation 4 of DEFRA's Dairy Hygiene Inspectorate. Testing of the dairy premises for *M. bovis* are carried out free of charge with a frequency according to the appreciated risk within the local area and for the specific herd. The producer must pay for the microbiological testing of the milk for *M. bovis*, but not for more general bacterial contaminants.

Unpasteurized milk from herds that have been declared as OTF can be sold by dairy farmers directly from the holding where it is produced, as long as the milk is clearly labelled as raw, as defined by the Council Directive 64/432/EEC. The Animal and Plant Health Agency has advised that annual testing should be performed on all herds from which unpasteurized milk is sold for human consumption. This is more frequent than in OTF herds where milk is pasteurized before consumption or use in order to catch any tuberculosis-reactor cattle before the bacilli become well established in the udder and shed into the milk.

Should tuberculosis be suspected during meat inspection in any part of the carcass or offal, a more detailed postmortem examination is carried out than normal, following specific governmental requirements. Should generalized tuberculosis lesions be detected, the entire offal and carcass are condemned and do not enter the human food chain. If a single lesion is found on any organ or the associated lymph nodes, only the affected part of the animal is removed from the food chain, as any residual contamination of muscle should be deactivated during the cooking process. A tuberculin reactor cow can only be deemed fit for human consumption should it be entirely free of tuberculosis lesions following a thorough postmortem inspection. Reactors, if present, should be slaughtered at the end of the production line, in order to minimize cross contamination. During the early studies of investigation of the pathogenesis of tuberculosis in animals it was quickly realized by Francis[114] that surveillance and control at postmortem was an important requirement to minimize zoonotic transmission of disease. The very first link between infected meat and human tuberculosis infection had been postulated years before, in 1893, by Brehrend,[115] who called for effective meat inspection. This call was reinforced by Ostertag[116] who claimed that humans could contract tuberculosis from eating infected meat. Actually, the current evidence of this route of transmission from cattle to humans is weak or nonexistent[96] and the risk for consumption in industrialized countries is extremely low. The route of ingestion causing infection in animals has not been documented in many

countries over decades. In the United Kingdom, there has never been documented evidence of gastrointestinal transmission of *M. bovis* to humans due to consumption of infected meat, however, given the infectious and zoonotic nature of the disease, caution is warranted.

CONTROL OF DISEASE IN WILDLIFE MAINTENANCE HOSTS

Wildlife such as badgers or brush-tailed possums can also be considered to be maintenance hosts of *M. bovis*, as these species are able to maintain the infection within their own population, and control among these groups should be considered in order to eliminate the disease. Eradicating any possible contact between wildlife and cattle limits the spread of infection, although this is not always feasible. Culling or vaccinating of an adequate level of affected wildlife species are strategies that are currently employed in an effort to effect control of bovine tuberculosis in the UK.

In New Zealand, following recognition that possums infected with bovine tuberculosis were a significant source of persistent infection in cattle in the early 1970s, the Ministry of Agriculture and Fisheries began to carry out possum control operations in areas where there was a persistent tuberculosis problem in cattle. Possum control proved to be difficult to achieve and in 1991–1992 there remained 20 areas in New Zealand where *M. bovis* infection was present in the possum populations. Eighty-three percent of test reactor cattle and those under movement restriction were found to live in these regions. From a financial perspective, the budget for tuberculosis control in New Zealand in the 1992–1993 financial year was NZ$21.82 million, and a total of NZ$5.1 million was spent on possum control. These methods helped to decrease the spread of *M. bovis* in cattle in this country, but the disease in New Zealand still has not been eradicated.

Since the discovery that badgers are maintenance hosts for *M. bovis* in the 1970s, limitation of bovine tuberculosis in the badger population of the United Kingdom and Republic of Ireland has been an important consideration to aid control of the disease among cattle populations. The Kreb's report, published in 1997,[5] concluded that despite there being compelling evidence that badgers were involved in transmitting the infection to cattle, the effectiveness of badger culling could not be quantified using available data. A recommendation was made to establish the Randomised Badger Culling Trial (RBCT) in order to quantify the impact of culling badgers on incidence of TB in cattle and determine the effectiveness of strategies to reduce the risk of a TB cattle herd breakdown. This took place from 1998 to 2005 and was overseen by the Independent Scientific Group (ISG). During this period, nearly 8,900 badgers were culled across large areas where there was a high risk of bovine TB. The conclusions of this trial, published in June 2007, were that although badgers were a clear source of cattle TB, badger culling could make no meaningful contribution to cattle TB control in Britain. In addition, weaknesses in the cattle testing regimes mean that cattle themselves contributed significantly to the persistence of TB in all areas where the disease occurs, and in some parts of Britain cattle were likely to be the main source of infection. However, a different review of the basic data presented in this report made by the then Government Chief

Scientific Advisor Sir David King in 2007 at the government's request produced a different interpretation; that badger culling "would have a significant effect on reducing TB in cattle". It would appear that the reasons for the differences in the conclusions in the two reports occurred as the ISG's report took economic feasibility into account when making its calculations, while Sir David King's group of experts did not include practicalities or costs in their considerations. DEFRA published a (bovine) Tuberculosis Eradication Programme for England in 2011* and the pilot badger cull in South West England was announced in December 2011. Licences to cull badgers were granted to land owners by Natural England under the *Protection of Badgers Act 1992* and the *Wildlife and Countryside Act 1981* with provisions to cover culling for four years. This pilot cull was initiated in 2013, with an aim to eradicate 70% of the badger population in each 150 km² the culling areas over a six-week period. To minimize perturbation (movement of badgers disturbed by culling out of their own territories and consequently spreading disease), land owners were requested to identify natural barriers to badger movements, and establish the culling areas with these at their edge.† Badgers were culled using a controlled shooting method, as well as cage trapping and shooting. In 2015, the British Veterinary Association (BVA) concluded that it could not be demonstrated that controlled shooting could be carried out humanely and effectively. Although the Association remained supportive of the cull as a necessary part of a comprehensive strategy for controlling and eradicating bovine tuberculosis, they called on the government to revert only to the method of cage trapping and shooting method to deliver the badger cull by a safer and more humane and effective route. The long-term effect of badger culling on the prevalence of tuberculosis in the English cattle population remains to be seen. Some limited assessment was performed in 2016 and concluded that "reductions in TB incidence were associated with culling in the first two years in the intervention areas, when compared to areas with no culling." However, the authors did acknowledge that the interim data analysed originated only from two years" worth of data from only two of the culling sites; further analysis was necessary.[121]

In 2018, the Godfray Report identified that it would be desirable to move from a lethal to a non-lethal control strategy for badger control.[122] The government has since advised that the control strategy will move towards use of the BCG vaccine in badgers to vaccinate against tuberculosis, retaining the option of culling in areas where the bovine tuberculosis is rife and epidemiological evidence points to a significant disease reservoir in badgers. Over time it is thought that this will reduce the number of new cases and increase the herd immunity of badgers to the disease. A pilot study was undertaken between 2010 and 2014,[123] the results of which suggest that badger vaccination had no effect on the incidence of TB in cattle, although this study had limitations and bias and further studies need to be carried out. Badgers have a lifespan[124] of 3—5 years, so a cyclical plan of either culling or vaccination control methods every four years is predicted to be effective to reduce the disease in the badger population. Plans for a roll out of badger vaccination in the UK are to be carried out by DEFRA as part of its drive to eradicate bovine TB, with the aim to wind down the current badger cull programme by the mid- to late 2020s.

VACCINATION

A successful vaccine targeting *M. bovis* in cattle and other animals has not yet been developed, although efforts are underway. The bacillus Calmette—Gùerin (BCG) vaccine, a live-attenuated strain of *M. bovis*, is recommended to be administered to babies, children and adults under the age of 35 who are at risk of catching tuberculosis. The safety of this live vaccine for humans is well investigated and documented and the efficacy of live vaccines is always greater than killed. However, the use of the BCG vaccine is not permitted in the United States as field trials have repeatedly demonstrated that the protection offered does not appear to protect all members of a vaccinated population, and delayed-type hypersensitivity induced by the vaccine causes humans to react positively to the tuberculin skin test used to diagnose active tuberculosis infection, therefore reducing the value of this test, should it be required as part of a diagnostic investigation, although the interferon-gamma test for latent infection does not cross react with BCG or MAC.

Used alone, the BCG vaccine does not provide cost-effective or useful protection against infection of *M. bovis* in cattle. The current BCG vaccine does not have a high enough efficacy to provide full protection against tuberculosis, and is currently administered to cattle to provide a "Ring Vaccination" initiative in exposed herds where a breakout of TB infection has occurred. The same concern with this vaccine exists in cattle as in humans, as cattle that have received the BCG vaccine may offer a false-positive reaction to the tuberculin SICCT and therefore cattle infected with tuberculosis, and those which have been vaccinated, cannot be differentiated. The rational development of an effective vaccine for cattle involves the development of the optimal combination of *M. bovis* antigens that are required for protective immunity. Diagnostic tests based on antigens not incorporated into the vaccine would allow differentiation of the immune response generated by either vaccination or infection.

The BCG vaccination is licensed for intramuscular use in badgers in the United Kingdom, although an oral formulation, which would be easier and more cost-effective to administer, has also been trialed.[55] Wales is the only country currently implementing a BCG vaccination trial in this species, and the results of this trial are yet to be published.

CONTROL OF DISEASE SPREAD TO "SPILLOVER" HOSTS

In the domestic situation, cats and dogs can be considered the main spillover hosts of *M. bovis*, i.e., they are not very effective at transmitting the disease to other members of their own species or to other species, including humans. Consideration needs to be given to mechanisms to reduce transmission of mycobacteria from "maintenance" hosts to "spillover" hosts, as by definition no further transmission of disease will occur from a "spillover" host. An important consideration to limit the spread of disease is to limit the degree of contact of "spillover" hosts with any infected

---

* Defra, bTB Eradication Programme for England, July 2011.
† Defra, Update on measures to tackle bTB, 14 December 2011.

material from "maintenance" hosts. The main source of transmission of *M. bovis* infection is ingestion of infected milk or inhalation of aerosolized mycobacteria. In Scotland, selling of unpasteurized milk is illegal. This has not currently been achieved completely in England, as unpasteurized milk may currently be sold from certified "tuberculosis-free" herds. However, since the majority of herds across the United Kingdom began to sell pasteurized milk alone, the rate of human, cat, and dog infection has decreased.

Control of transmission via the aerosol route is an important consideration for farm workers, veterinary surgeons, or abattoir workers, who all have regular contact with cattle, and therefore the potential to inhale aerosolized droplets. This can be done most effectively by the use of personal protective clothing during animal and carcass handling and regular assessment of cattle as a source of infection.

CONTROL IN LOW INCOME COUNTRIES

There are many reasons to explain why it is difficult to implement standard control methods for tuberculosis in animals in HMICs in practice in low income countries. In low income countries, limiting steps to tuberculosis control may include a lack of knowledge about the disease prevalence and transmission, some degree of technical and financial limitation, lack of veterinary infrastructure, and cultural or geographical barriers to implementing a successful disease control strategy. In some areas of Ethiopia, some efforts to control bovine tuberculosis have been made on the Government State farms. At Mojo State Dairy Farm in Central Ethiopia in 1997, 55% of the positive reactor cattle were culled post-diagnosis, the farm was closed and healthy or negative cattle were transferred to other farms.[112] These steps have helped to decrease the prevalence of bovine tuberculosis in these herds. Control methods, however, are generally not well practiced on small-holder farms. In Ethiopia, the mobility of the pastoralist or semi-pastoralist herds makes any control practices hard to implement, even without consideration of the social and economic factors involved. Therefore currently, a test and slaughter policy is not yet established.

Alaku[55] has identified steps to be implemented as fundamental practice to initiate the control of bovine tuberculosis in Ethiopia. These steps can also be considered in other countries where there is currently no control programme for the disease.

1. Cattle over the age of 6 months should be permanently marked or identified using a systematic approach.
2. Hygiene and management practices should be implemented to increase biosecurity. Cattle should be kept further from human dwellings to decrease opportunities for transmission. Creation of legislation is necessary to register individual dairy farms, and notify vets of cattle purchases, sales, or transfers.
3. Regular testing and meat inspection practices are required to identify infected individuals. Ideally testing of infected herds should occur in a predetermined pattern to establish whether there are any changes in the rate of new infections, and biannual testing programs should be put in place for those herds that have gained disease-free status, to confirm that this disease-free status remains (Figure 22.2).

4. A system of insurance or initiation of a government policy to reimburse farmers for the loss of individual cattle will make it possible for a farmer to maintain their livelihood should an infected cow need to be removed from the herd. It is extremely rare to find such a system in low income countries, however, the current practice of condemnation in low income countries is not well studied or documented.

RISK TO HUMANS

The major risk to humans of mycobacterial infections from animals worldwide is the risk of infection with *M. bovis*. The most common transmission route of the mycobacteria from cattle to humans occurs due to ingestion of unpasteurized, infected milk. The important public health issue has ensured that *M. bovis* has been made a listed disease by the World Organization of Animal Health (OIE). In addition to the impact of illness on the human population, *M. bovis* has a significant economic impact on international trade of animals and animal products.[18]

As knowledge of the mycobacteria has increased over the last 100 years, control measures have been set in place in some countries to limit to the spread of the disease, and currently in the United Kingdom the risk to humans of infection with *M. bovis* from cattle is low.

Risk to humans is higher where no control mechanisms have been set in place or where there is a lack of public health education. In African countries such as Ethiopia, where the level of milk pasteurization is generally low, and certainly not generally regulated or controlled, infection of humans due to ingestion of infected milk remains high. In the United Kingdom, should a tuberculosis-reactor cow be detected on farm, the Government Local Authority and State Veterinary Service offer verbal and written advice to avoid consumption of milk from reactor animals; however, there is no legal obligation for the farmer to follow this recommendation.

Risk of human infection by exposure to *M. bovis* or other zoonotic mycobacteria is heightened by the presence of any concurrent cause of immunosuppression such as HIV/AIDS infection, malnutrition, and concurrent disease, thus increasing the likelihood of developing clinical signs of disease.

Another group of individuals at risk are those who work regularly in close contact with infected cattle, for example, farm workers, abattoir workers, and veterinary surgeons. *M. bovis* bacilli can be aerosolized and infected particles be easily inhaled by humans or other cattle in close contact, in addition to oral transmission by infected milk.

The Health Protection Agency and Animal and Plant Health Agency in the United Kingdom are the bodies that are able to provide information about the incidence of confirmed human cases of *M. bovis* infections, and so are able to annually quantify the risk to humans in the United Kingdom from *M. bovis* infection. Consideration will be made as to the demographics of the diseased individual; older members of the population with a limited travel history are thought to have been exposed to the bacteria while drinking unpasteurized milk years previously, while the younger generation are more likely to be infected during travel abroad.

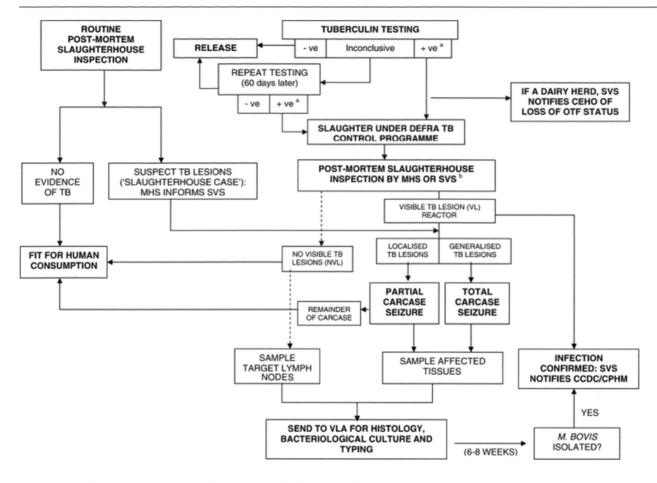

Figure 22.2 Schematic representation of the protocols for the testing of cattle and meat inspection for bovine tuberculosis in Great Britain, 2000. (Adapted from: Advisory Committee on the Microbiological Safety of Foods. Report on *Mycobacterium bovis*: A review of the possible health risks to consumers of meat from cattle with evidence of *Mycobacterium bovis* infection. Hayes: Food Standards Agency Publications; 2002). (Permission: http://www.nationalarchives.gov.uk/legal/copyright/.)

CONCLUSION

M. bovis infection remains an economically important disease across the world. Although efforts to eradicate the disease have been successful in several countries including Australia, France and the majority of the United States, across many countries of the world the disease remains endemic in the cattle population. Successful disease control requires a thorough understanding of the epidemiology and transmission of the disease within and between the human, domestic and wild animal population. Tailoring a range of control methods using a multipronged approach is the sole route by which complete eradication of bovine tuberculosis can and will be achieved.

REFERENCES

1. Pritchard DG. A century of bovine tuberculosis 1888–1988: Conquest and controversy. *J Comp Pathol*. 1988;99(4):357–99.
2. Collins CH. The bovine tubercle bacillus. *Br J Biomed Sci*. 2000;57:234–40.
3. Grange J, and Yates M. Zoonotic aspects of *Mycobacterium bovis* infection. *Vet Microbiol*. 1994;40(1–2):137–51.
4. Hardie RM, and Watson JM. *Mycobacterium bovis* in England and Wales: Past, present and future. *Epidemiol Infect*. 1992;109:23–33.
5. Krebs JR, Anderson RM, Clutton-Brock T, Morrison WI, Young D, and Donnelly C. Bovine Tuberculosis in Cattle and Badgers. 1997.
6. O'Connor REO. *Badgers and Bovine Tuberculosis in Ireland*. 1989.
7. Katoch VM. Newer diagnostic techniques for tuberculosis. *Indian J Med Res*. 2004;120:418–28.
8. Tortoli E. Impact of genotypic studies on mycobacterial taxonomy: The new mycobacteria of the 1990s. *Clin Microbiol Rev*. 2003;16:319–54.
9. Rastogi N, Legrand E, and Sola C. The mycobacteria: An introduction to nomenclature and pathogenesis. *Rev Sci Tech L'OIE [Internet]*. 2001;20(1):21–54. Available at: http://doc.oie.int:8080/dyn/portal/index.seam?page=alo&aloId=29767

10. Huard RC et al. Novel genetic polymorphisms that further delineate the phylogeny of the *Mycobacterium tuberculosis* complex. *J Bacteriol [Internet]*. 2006;188(12):4271–87. Available at: http://jb.asm.org/cgi/content/abstract/188/12/4271%5Cnd:%5Cjournals%5Chuard2006.pdf

11. Brosch R et al. A new evolutionary scenario for the *Mycobacterium tuberculosis* complex. *Proc Natl Acad Sci USA [Internet]*. 2002;99(6):3684–9. Available at: http://www.pubmedcentral.nih.gov/articlerender.fcgi?artid=122584&tool=pmcentrez&rendertype=abstract

12. Domingo M, Vidal E, and Marco A. Pathology of bovine tuberculosis. *Res Vet Sci*. 2014;97(S):S20–9.

13. Wang J et al. Expression pattern of interferon-inducible transcriptional genes in neutrophils during bovine tuberculosis infection. *DNA Cell Biol*. 2013;32(8):480–6.

14. Ashford D, Whitney E, and Raghunathan P. Epidemiology of selected mycobacteria that infect humans and other animals. *Rev Sci Tech Off Int Epiz*. 2001;20(1):325–37.

15. O'Reilly LM, and Daborn CJ. The epidemiology of *Mycobacterium bovis* infections in animals and man: A review. *Tuber Lung Dis*. 1995;76(Suppl. 1):1–46.

16. TB and deer farming: Return of the king's evil? *Lancet*. 1991;338(8777):1243–4.

17. Delahay RJ, De Leeuw ANS, Barlow AM, Clifton-Hadley RS, and Cheeseman CL. The status of *Mycobacterium bovis* infection in UK wild mammals: A review. *Veterinary J*. 2002;164:90–105.

18. Cousins DV, and Roberts JL. Australia's campaign to eradicate bovine tuberculosis: The battle for freedom and beyond. *Tuberculosis*. 2001;21(5):5–15.

19. Grange JM, and Collins CH. Bovine tubercle bacilli and disease in animals and man. *Epidemiol Infect*. 1987;99(2):221–34.

20. Morris RS, Pfeiffer DU, and Jackson R. The epidemiology of *Mycobacterium bovis* infections. *Vet Microbiol*. 1994;40(1–2):153–77.

21. Ameni G, and Erkihun A. Bovine tuberculosis on small-scale dairy farms in Adama Town, Central Ethiopia, and farmer awareness of the disease. *Rev Sci Tech*. 2007;26(3):711–9.

22. Brotherstone S et al. Evidence of genetic resistance of cattle to infection with *Mycobacterium bovis*. *J Dairy Sci [Internet]*. 2010;93(3):1234–42. Available at: http://www.sciencedirect.com/science/article/pii/S0022030210000901

23. Bermingham ML et al. Genome-wide association study identifies novel loci associated with resistance to bovine tuberculosis. *Heredity (Edinb)*. 2014;112(5):543–51.

24. Richardson IW, Bradley DG, Higgins IM, More SJ, Jennifer M, and Berry DP. Variance components for susceptibility to *Mycobacterium bovis* infection in dairy and beef cattle. *Genet Sel Evol*. 2014;46(1).

25. Theunissen B. Breeding without Mendelism: Theory and practice of dairy cattle breeding in the Netherlands 1900–1950. *J Hist Biol*. 2008;41:637–76.

26. Gilbert M, Mitchell A, Bourn D, Mawdsley J, Clifton-Hadley R, and Wint W. Cattle movements and bovine tuberculosis in Great Britain. *Nature*. 2005;435(7041):491–6.

27. Goodchild AV, and Clifton-Hadley RS. Cattle-to-cattle transmission of *Mycobacterium bovis*. *Tuberculosis (Edinb)*. 2001;81(1–2):23–41.

28. Gallagher J, and Clifton-Hadley RS. Tuberculosis in badgers: A review of the disease and its significance for other animals. *Res Vet Sci*. 2000;69:203–17.

29. Keogh BP. Reviews of the progress of dairy science: Section B. The survival of pathogens in cheese and milk powder. *J Dairy Res*. 1971;38:91–111.

30. Corner LA. Post mortem diagnosis of *Mycobacterium bovis* infection in cattle. *Vet Microbiol*. 1994;40(1–2):53–63.

31. Francis J. Route of infection in tuberculosis. *Aust Vet J*. 1972;48:663–669.

32. Zanini MS, Moreira EC, Lopes MT, Mota P, and Salas CE. Detection of *Mycobacterium bovis* in milk by polymerase chain reaction. *Zentralbl Veterinarmed B [Internet]*. 1998;45(8):473–9. Available at: http://www.ncbi.nlm.nih.gov/pubmed/9820115

33. Cosivi O et al. Zoonotic tuberculosis due to *Mycobacterium bovis* in developing countries. *Emerg Infect Dis*. 1998;4(1080–6040; 1):59–70.

34. Benham PFJ, and Broom DM. Interactions between cattle and badgers at pasture with reference to bovine tuberculosis transmission. *Br Vet J*. 1989;145(3):226–41.

35. Gallagher J, Monies R, Gavier-Widen M, and Rule B. Role of infected, non-diseased badgers in the pathogenesis of tuberculosis in the badger. *Vet Rec [Internet]*. 1998;142(26):710–4. Available at: http://www.ncbi.nlm.nih.gov/pubmed/9682428

36. Pfieffer D. The role of a wildlife reservoir in the epidemiology of Bovine Tuberculosis. 1994.

37. Cliftonhadley RS, and Wilesmith JW. Tuberculosis in deer—A review. *Vet Rec [Internet]*. 1991;129(1):5–12. Available at: http://www.ncbi.nlm.nih.gov/pubmed/1897111

38. De Lisle GW, and Havill PF. Mycobacteria isolated from deer in New Zealand. *N Z Vet J*. 1985;33(8):138–40.

39. Griffin JFT, and Mackintosh CG. Tuberculosis in deer: Perceptions, problems and progress. *Vet J*. 2000;160:202–19.

40. Rodríguez S et al. *Mycobacterium caprae* infection in livestock and wildlife, Spain. *Emerg Infect Dis*. 2011;17(3):532–5.

41. Vicente J et al. Wild boar and red deer display high prevalences of tuberculosis-like lesions in Spain. *Vet Res*. 2006;37(1):107–19.

42. Jackson R, Morris RS, Cooke MM, Coleman JD, De Lisle GW, and Yates GF. Naturally occurring tuberculosis caused by *Mycobacterium bovis* in brushtail possums (*Trichosurus vulpecula*): III. Routes of infection and excretion. *N Z Vet J*. 1995;43(7):322–7.

43. Himsworth CG et al. Comparison of test performance and evaluation of novel immunoassays for tuberculosis in a captive herd of wood bison naturally infected with *Mycobacterium bovis*. *J Wildl Dis [Internet]*. 2010;46(1):78–86. Available at: http://www.jwildlifedis.org/doi/10.7589/0090-3558-46.1.78

44. Thoen CO, Quinn WJ, Miller LD, Stackhouse LL, Newcomb BF, and Ferrell JM. *Mycobacterium bovis* infection in North American elk (*Cervus elaphus*). *J Vet Diagn Invest [Internet]*. 1992;4(4):423–7. Available at: http://www.ncbi.nlm.nih.gov/pubmed/1457545

45. Waters WR et al. Antigen recognition by serum antibodies in white-tailed deer (*Odocoileus virginianus*) experimentally infected with *Mycobacterium bovis*. *Clin Diagn Lab Immunol [Internet]*. 2004;11(5):849–55. Available at: http://www.ncbi.nlm.nih.gov/pmc/articles/PMC515268/pdf/0075-04.pdf

46. Renwick AR, White PCL, and Bengis RG. Bovine tuberculosis in Southern African wildlife: A multi-species host-pathogen system. *Epidemiol Infect*. 2007;135:529–40.

47. Barron MC, Pech RP, Whitford J, Yockney IJ, De Lisle GW, and Nugent G. Longevity of *Mycobacterium bovis* in brushtail possum (*Trichosurus vulpecula*) carcasses, and contact rates between possums and carcasses. *N Z Vet J*. 2011;59(5):209–17.

48. de Lisle GW, Mackintosh CG, and Bengis RG. *Mycobacterium bovis* in free-living and captive wildlife, including farmed deer. *Rev Sci Tech*. 2001;20(1):86–111.

49. Dinkla ET, Haagsma J, Kuyvenhoven J V, Veen J, and Nieuwenhuijs JH. Tuberculosis in imported alpacas—a zoonosis—Now what? (see comments). *Tijdschr Diergeneeskd*. 1991;116(9):454–60.

50. Gutierrez M, Samper S, Jimenez MS, Van Embden JDA, Marin JFG, Martin C. Identification by spoligotyping of a caprine genotype in *Mycobacterium bovis* strains causing human tuberculosis. *J Clin Microbiol*. 1997;35(12):3328–30.

51. Kubica T, Rüsch-Gerdes S, and Niemann S. *Mycobacterium bovis* subsp. *caprae* caused one-third of human *M. bovis*-associated tuberculosis cases reported in Germany between 1999 and 2001. *J Clin Microbiol*. 2003;41(7):3070–7.

52. Thorel MF, Huchzermeyer HF, and Michel AL. *Mycobacterium avium* and *Mycobacterium intracellulare* infection in mammals. *Rev Sci Tech L Off Int Des Epizoot*. 2001;20(1):204–18.

53. Regassa A et al. A cross-sectional study on bovine tuberculosis in Hawassa town and its surroundings, Southern Ethiopia. *Trop Anim Health Prod*. 2010;42(5):915–20.

54. Ameni G, Aseffa A, Engers H, Young D, Hewinson G, and Vordermeier M. Cattle husbandry in Ethiopia is a predominant factor affecting the pathology of bovine tuberculosis and gamma interferon responses to mycobacterial antigens. *Clin Vaccine Immunol*. 2006;13(9):1030–6.

55. Alaku B. A review on epidemiology of Bovine tuberculosis in Ethiopia. *Acad J Anim Dis*. 2017;6(3):57–66.

56. Grange JM, and Yates MD. The time-table of tuberculosis. *Respir Med*. 1995;89:313–4.

57. Raviglione MC, Snider DE, and Kochi A. Global epidemiology of tuberculosis. Morbidity and mortality of a worldwide epidemic. *JAMA*. 1995;273(3):220–6.

58. Alexander KA et al. Novel *Mycobacterium tuberculosis* complex pathogen, *M. mungi*. *Emerg Infect Dis*. 2010;16(8):1296–9.

59. Gopinath K, and Singh S. Non-tuberculous mycobacteria in TB-endemic countries: Are we neglecting the danger? *PLOS Negl Trop Dis*. 2010;4(4).

60. Wolinsky E. Mycobacterial diseases other than tuberculosis. *Clin Infect Dis*. 1992;15(1):1–12.

61. Aliyu G et al. Prevalence of non-tuberculous mycobacterial infections among tuberculosis suspects in Nigeria. *PLOS ONE*. 2013;8(5).

62. Gunn-Moore DA, Jenkins PA, and Lucke VM. Feline tuberculosis: A literature review and discussion of 19 cases caused by an unusual mycobacterial variant. *Vet Rec*. 1996;138(0042–4900; 3):53–8.

63. Oevermann A, Pfyffer GE, Zanolari P, Meylan M, and Robert N. Generalized tuberculosis in Llamas (*Lama glama*) due to *Mycobacterium microti*. *J Clin Microbiol*. 2004;42(4):1818–21.

64. Van Soolingen D et al. Use of various genetic markers in differentiation of *Mycobacterium bovis* strains from animals and humans and for studying epidemiology of bovine tuberculosis. *J Clin Microbiol*. 1994;32(10):2425–33.

65. Horstkotte MA et al. *Mycobacterium microti* llama-type infection presenting as pulmonary tuberculosis in a human immunodeficiency virus-positive patient. *J Clin Microbiol*. 2001;39(1):406–7.

66. Niemann S et al. Two cases of *Mycobacterium microti*-derived tuberculosis in HIV-negative immunocompetent patients. *Emerg Infect Dis*. 2000;6(5):539–42.

67. Foudraine NA, van Soolingen D, Noordhoek GT, Reiss P,. Pulmonary tuberculosis due to *Mycobacterium microti* in a human immunodeficiency virus-infected patient. *Clin Infect Dis*. 1998;27(6):1543–4.

68. Tortoli E. Microbiological features and clinical relevance of new species of the genus *Mycobacterium*. *Clin Microbiol Rev*. 2014;27(4):727–52.

69. Hoefsloot W et al. The geographic diversity of nontuberculous mycobacteria isolated from pulmonary samples: An NTM-NET collaborative study. *Eur Respir J*. 2013;42(6):1604–13.

70. Honda JR et al. Pathogenic nontuberculous mycobacteria resist and inactivate cathelicidin: Implication of a novel role for polar mycobacterial lipids. *PLOS ONE*. 2015;10(5).

71. Thorel MF, Huchzermeyer H, Weiss R, and Fontaine JJ. *Mycobacterium avium* infections in animals. Literature review. *Vet Res*. 1997;28(5):439–47.

72. Manning EJ, and Collins MT. *Mycobacterium avium* subsp. paratuberculosis: Pathogen, pathogenesis and diagnosis. *Rev Sci Tech [Internet]*. 2001;20(1):133–50. Available at: http://europepmc.org/abstract/med/11288509

73. Whittington RJ, Marshall DJ, Nicholls PJ, Marsh IB, and Reddacliff LA. Survival and dormancy of *Mycobacterium avium* subsp. *paratuberculosis* in the environment. *Appl Environ Microbiol*. 2004;70(5):2989–3004.

74. Lombard JE. Epidemiology and economics of paratuberculosis. *Vet Clin N Am Small Anim Pract*. 2011;27:525–35.

75. Waddell LA, Rajic A, Stärk KDC, and McEwen SA. The zoonotic potential of *Mycobacterium avium* ssp. *Paratuberculosis*: A systematic review and meta-analyses of the evidence. *Epidemiol Infect*. 2015;143:3135–57.

76. Rodriguez-Campos S et al. Limitations of spoligotyping and variable-number tandem-repeat typing for molecular tracing of *Mycobacterium bovis* in a high-diversity setting. *J Clin Microbiol*. 2011;49(9):3361–4.

77. Rojas-Espinosa O, and Lovik M. *Mycobacterium leprae* and *Mycobacterium lepraemurium* infections in domestic and wild animals. *Rev Sci Tech*. 2001;20(1):219–51.

78. LoBue PA, and Moser KS. Use of isoniazid for latent tuberculosis infection in a public health clinic. *Am J Respir Crit Care Med.* 2003;168(4):443–7.

79. Gutierrez M, Castilla J, Noguer I, Diaz P, Arias J, and Guerra L. Anti-tuberculosis drug consumption as an indicator of the epidemiological situation of tuberculosis in Spain. *Gac Sanit.* 1999;13(4):275–81.

80. Waddington K. To stamp out "So Terrible a Malady": Bovine tuberculosis and tuberculin testing in Britain, 1890–1939. *Med History.* 2004;48:29–48.

81. Andersen P, Munk ME, Pollock JM, and Doherty TM. Specific immune-based diagnosis of tuberculosis. *Lancet.* 2000;356:1099–104.

82. Biet F, Boschiroli ML, Thorel MF, and Guilloteau LA. Zoonotic aspects of *Mycobacterium bovis* and *Mycobacterium avium*-intracellulare complex (MAC). *Vet Res.* 2005;36:411–36.

83. Pollock JM, Welsh MD, and McNair J. Immune responses in bovine tuberculosis: Towards new strategies for the diagnosis and control of disease. *Vet Immunol Immunopathol.* 2005;108(1–2):37–43.

84. De La Rua-Domenech R. Human *Mycobacterium bovis* infection in the United Kingdom: Incidence, risks, control measures and review of the zoonotic aspects of bovine tuberculosis. *Tuberculosis.* 2006;86:77–109.

85. Doherty ML, and Cassidy JP. New perspectives on bovine tuberculosis. *Vet J.* 2002;163(2):109–10.

86. Coad M, Clifford D, Rhodes SG, Hewinson RG, Vordermeier HM, and Whelan AO. Repeat tuberculin skin testing leads to desensitisation in naturally infected tuberculous cattle which is associated with elevated interleukin-10 and decreased interleukin-1 beta responses. *Vet Res.* 2010;41(2):14.

87. Rothel JS, Jones SL, Corner LA, Cox JC, and Wood PR. A sandwich enzyme immunoassay for bovine interferon-gamma and its use for the detection of tuberculosis in cattle. *Aust Vet J.* 1990;67(4):134–7.

88. Waters WR, Maggioli MF, McGill JL, Lyashchenko KP, and Palmer MV. Relevance of bovine tuberculosis research to the understanding of human disease: Historical perspectives, approaches, and immunologic mechanisms. *Vet Immunol Immunopathol.* 2014;159(3–4):113–32.

89. Neill SD, and Pollock JM. Testing for bovine tuberculosis—More than skin deep. *Vet J.* 2000;160(1):3–5.

90. Wood PR et al. Field comparison of the interferon-gamma assay and the intradermal tuberculin test for the diagnosis of bovine tuberculosis. *AustVetJ.* 1991;68(0005–0423 (Print)):286–90.

91. Malama S, Muma JB, Godfroid J. A review of tuberculosis at the wildlife-livestock-human interface in Zambia. *Infect Dis Poverty.* 2013;2.

92. Kamerbeek J et al. Simultaneous detection and strain differentiation of *Mycobacterium tuberculosis* for diagnosis and epidemiology. *J Clin Microbiol.* 1997;35(4):907–14.

93. Durr PA, Clifton-Hadley RS, and Hewinson RG. Molecular epidemiology of bovine tuberculosis—II. Applications of genotyping. *Rev Sci Tech L'OIE [Internet].* 2000;19(3):689–701. Available at: http://doc.oie.int:8080/dyn/portal/index.seam?page=alo&aloId=29700

94. Frothingham R, and Meeker-O'Connell WA. Genetic diversity in the *Mycobacterium tuberculosis* complex based on variable numbers of tandem DNA repeats. *Microbiology.* 1998;144(5):1189–96.

95. Smith I. *Mycobacterium tuberculosis* pathogenesis and molecular determinants of virulence. *Clin Microbiol Rev [Internet].* 2003;16(3):463–96. Available at: http://cmr.asm.org/content/16/3/463.short

96. Kleeberg HH. Human tuberculosis of bovine origin in relation to public health. *Rev Sci Tech Off Int Epiz.* 1984;3(1):11–32.

97. Ghielmetti G et al. Epidemiological tracing of bovine tuberculosis in Switzerland, multilocus variable number of tandem repeat analysis of *Mycobacterium bovis* and *Mycobacterium caprae. PLOS ONE.* 2017;12(2).

98. Qureshi T, Templeton JW, and Adams LG. Intracellular survival of *Brucella abortus, Mycobacterium bovis* BCG, *Salmonella dublin,* and *Salmonella typhimurium* in macrophages from cattle genetically resistant to *Brucella abortus* 18. *Vet Immunol Immunopathol.* 1996;50(0165–2427):55–65.

99. Buchanan CC, Torstenson ES, Bush WS, and Ritchie MD. A comparison of cataloged variation between international HapMap consortium and 1000 genomes project data. *J Am Med Informatics Assoc.* 2012;19(2):289–94.

100. Kim ES, and Kirkpatrick BW. Linkage disequilibrium in the North American Holstein population. *Anim Genet.* 2009;40(3):279–88.

101. Ellis MD, Davies S, McCandlish IAP, Monies R, Jahans K, and Rua-Domenech R. *Mycobacterium bovis* infection in a dog. *Vet Rec [Internet].* 2006;159(2):46–8. Available at: http://www.bvapublications.com

102. Martinez ME, Gonzalez J, Sanchez-Cabezudo MJ, Pena JM, Vazquez JJ, Felsenfeld A. Evidence of absorptive hypercalciuria in tuberculosis patients. *Calcif Tissue Int [Internet].* 1993;53(6):384–7. Available at: 8293351

103. Rhodes SG, Gruffydd-Jones T, Gunn-Moore D, and Jahans K. Adaptation of IFN-gamma ELISA and ELISPOT tests for feline tuberculosis. *Vet Immunol Immunopathol.* 2008;124(3–4):379–84.

104. Hawthorne VM, Jarrett WFH, Lauder I, Martin WB, Roberts GBS. Tuberculosis in man, dog, and cat. *Br Med J.* 1957;2(5046):675–8.

105. Kaneene JB et al. Epidemiologic investigation of *Mycobacterium bovis* in a population of cats. *Am J Vet Res.* 2002;63(11):1507–11.

106. Aranaz A, Liébana E, Pickering X, Novoa C, Mateos A, and Domínguez L. Use of polymerase chain reaction in the diagnosis of tuberculosis in cats and dogs. *Vet Rec [Internet].* 1996;138(12):276–80. Available at: http://www.ncbi.nlm.nih.gov/pubmed/8711884

107. Kipar A, Schiller I, and Baumgärtner W. Immunopathological studies on feline cutaneous and (muco)cutaneous mycobacteriosis. *Vet Immunol Immunopathol.* 2003;91(3–4):169–82.

108. Malik R et al. Infections of the subcutis and skin of dogs caused by rapidly growing mycobacteria. *J Small Anim Pract [Internet]*. 2004;45(10):485–94. Available at: http://www.ncbi.nlm.nih.gov/pubmed/15517689

109. Brodin P et al. Bacterial artificial chromosome-based comparative genomic analysis identifies *Mycobacterium microti* as a natural ESAT-6 deletion mutant. *Infect Immun*. 2002;70(10):5568–78.

110. Smith RL, Tauer LW, Schukken YH, Lu Z, and Grohn YT. Minimization of bovine tuberculosis control costs in US dairy herds. *Prev Vet Med*. 2013;112(3–4):266–75.

111. Biffa D, Bogale A, Godfroid J, and Skjerve E. Factors associated with severity of bovine tuberculosis in Ethiopian cattle. *Trop Anim Health Prod*. 2012;44(5):991–8.

112. Grange J. The Global Burden of Tuberculosis. 1999.

113. Vordermeier M, Goodchild A, Clifton-Hadley R, and de la Rua R. The interferon-gamma field trial: Background, principles and progress. *Vet Rec [Internet]*. 2004;155(2):37–8. Available at: http://www.ncbi.nlm.nih.gov/pubmed/15285281

114. Francis J, Choi CL, and Frost AJ. The diagnosis of tuberculosis in cattle with special reference to bovine PPD tuberculin. *Aust Vet J*. 1973;49:246–51.

115. Behrend H. *Cattle Tuberculosis and Tuberculous Meat*. London: Calder-Turner, 1893.

116. Ostertag. The use of the flesh and the milk of tuberculous animals. *J Comp Pathol Ther*. 1899;XII:240.

117. Busch F, Bannerman F, Liggett S, Griffin F, Clarke J, Lyashchenko KP, Rhodes S. Control of bovine tuberculosis in a farmed red deer herd in England *Veterinary Record* 2017;180:68.

118. Buddle BM, de Lisle GW, Griffin JFT, Hutchings SA. Epidemiology, diagnostics, and management of tuberculosis in domestic cattle and deer in New Zealand in the face of a wildlife reservoir. *NZ Vet J* 2015;63(suppl. 1): 19–27.

119. Gunn-Moore D, McFarland S, Brewer J, Cranshaw T, Clifton-Hadley R, Kovalik M, Shaw D. Mycobacterial disease in cats in Great Britain: I. Culture results, geographical distribution and clinical presentation of 339 cases. *J Feline Med Surg*. 2011;13(12):934–44.

120. Sykes JE, Gunn-Moore DA. Mycobacterial infections. In: Sykes JE (ed.). *Canine and Feline Infectious Diseases*, Elsevier/Saunders, 2014, 418–36.

121. Brunton LA et al. Assessing the effects of the first 2 years of industry-led badger culling in England on the incidence of bovine tuberculosis in cattle 2013–2015. *Ecology and Evolution*, 4 August 2017.

122. Godfray C, Donnelly C, Hewinson G, Winter M, Wood J. *Bovine TB Strategy Review*, October 2018.

123. APHA. A descriptive analysis of the effect of the badger vaccination on the incidence of bovine tuberculosis in cattle within the Badger Vaccine Deployment Project area, using observational data. 2016.

124. Gov.UK. A strategy for achieving bovine tuberculosis free status for England. 2018 review—government response. 2020.

125. DEFRA: Quarterly publication of National Statistics on the incidence and prevalence of tuberculosis (TB) in cattle in Great Britain to end March 2020. [Internet]. [cited 2020 Jul 20]. Available from: https://assets.publishing.service.gov.uk/government/uploads/system/uploads/attachment_data/file/892569/bovinetb-statsnotice-Q1-quarterly-17jun20.pdf.

Index